TOPICAL TABLE OF CONTENTS

CLINICAL DISORDERS

Topic	Chapter	Page
Congenital Heart Disease		
Integrated clinical approach	12	90
Echocardiography	33	420
Fast CT	58	871
MRI	46, 47	672, 692
Valvular Heart Disease		
Integrated clinical approach	10	84
Basic physiology	5	50
Echocardiography	30	365
Fast CT	53	820
Intraoperative echocardiography	39	566
MRI	46, 47	672, 692
Transesophageal echocardiography	38	533
Ischemic Heart Disease		
Integrated clinical approach	9	81
Basic physiology	2	8
Contrast echocardiography	35	480
Coronary angiography	23	220
Digital angiography	24	251
Echocardiography	37	522
Fast CT	54	829
Infarct avid imaging	65	1012
Intravascular ultrasound	40	581
Metabolic imaging	66, 71	1020, 1113
MRI	48	719
PET	70, 71	1093, 1113
Stress echocardiography	36	503
Tc-99m perfusion imaging	62, 63, 64	963, 971, 996
Thallium-201 imaging	62, 63, 64	963, 971, 996
Ultrasonic tissue characterization	41	606

Topic	Chapter	Page
Cardiomyopathy		
Integrated clinical approach	11	87
Echocardiography	31	395
MRI	49	744
PET	72	1171
Pericardial Disease		
Integrated clinical approach	13	93
Echocardiography	32	404
Fast CT	57	863
MRI	49	744
Cardiac Masses		
Echocardiography	34	452
Fast CT	57	863
Indium-111 thrombus imaging	67	1034
MRI	49	744
Cardiovascular Trauma		
Integrated clinical approach	14	95
Diseases of the Great Vessels		
Integrated clinical approach	15	98
Aortography	21	199
Fast CT	56	852
MRI	47	692
Pulmonary angiography	22	208
Transesophageal echocardiography	38	533

MARCUS

Cardiac Imaging

A COMPANION TO BRAUNWALD's

HEART DISEASE

MARCUS
Cardiac
Imaging

SECOND EDITION

A COMPANION TO BRAUNWALD's

HEART DISEASE

VOLUME 1

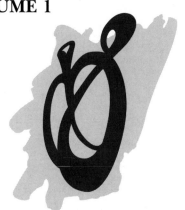

EDITOR IN CHIEF

DAVID J. SKORTON, M.D.
Professor of Medicine and Electrical and Computer
 Engineering
Co-Director, The University of Iowa Hospitals and Clinics
 Adolescent and Adult Congenital Heart Disease Clinic
Vice President for Research
The University of Iowa
Consulting Physician, Department of Veterans Affairs Medical
 Center
Iowa City, Iowa

ASSOCIATE EDITORS

HEINRICH R. SCHELBERT, M.D.
Professor of Pharmacology and Radiological Sciences
Vice Chair
Department of Molecular and Medical Pharmacology
UCLA School of Medicine
Principal Investigator, Laboratory of Structural Biology and
 Molecular Medicine
Medical Director, Nuclear Medicine Clinic
UCLA Medical Center
University of California at Los Angeles
Los Angeles, California

GERALD L. WOLF, Ph.D., M.D.
Professor of Radiology
Harvard Medical School
Director, Center for Imaging and Pharmaceutical Research
Massachusetts General Hospital
Boston, Massachusetts

BRUCE H. BRUNDAGE, M.D.
Professor of Medicine and Radiologic Sciences
UCLA School of Medicine
Chief, Division of Cardiology, Harbor-UCLA Medical Center
Scientific Director, Saint John's Cardiovascular Research
 Center
Torrance, California

CONSULTING EDITOR

EUGENE BRAUNWALD, M.D.
Hersey Professor of the Theory and Practice of Medicine
Harvard Medical School
Chairman, Department of Medicine
Brigham and Women's Hospital
Boston, Massachusetts

W.B. SAUNDERS COMPANY
A Division of Harcourt Brace & Company
PHILADELPHIA LONDON TORONTO
MONTREAL SYDNEY TOKYO

W.B. SAUNDERS COMPANY
A Division of Harcourt Brace & Company

The Curtis Center
Independence Square West
Philadelphia, Pennsylvania 19106

Library of Congress Cataloging-in-Publication Data

Marcus cardiac imaging: a companion to Braunwald's heart disease / David J.
Skorton . . . [et al.]. — 2nd ed.

p. cm.

Rev. ed. of: Cardiac imaging / edited by Melvin L. Marcus . . . [et al.]. 1991.

Companion to: Heart disease / edited by Eugene Braunwald. 4th ed. ©1992.
Includes bibliographical references and index.

ISBN 0–7216–4687–5 (set)

1. Heart—Imaging.   2. Heart—Diseases—Diagnosis.   I. Marcus, Melvin.
II. Braunwald, Eugene.   III. Heart Disease.   [DNLM: 1. Diagnostic
Imaging.   2. Heart Diseases—diagnosis.   3. Skorton, David J.
WG 141 M322 1996]

RC683.5.I42C37   1996   616.1′20754—dc20

DNLM/DLC   95–19482

Marcus Cardiac Imaging:
A Companion to Braunwald's Heart Disease, Second Edition

ISBN
Volume 1 0–7216–7127–6
Volume 2 0–7216–7128–4
Two-Volume Set 0–7216–4687–5

Printed in the United States of America.

Last digit is the print number: 9   8   7   6   5   4   3   2   1

Dedications

In memory of my parents,
Pauline and Sam Skorton.

D.J.S.

To my wife, Barbara, my daughter, Kristina, and my son, Mark,
for their continued patience, support, and encouragement.

H.R.S.

To David, Darin, Alvera, Cindy, and Delia,
who supported my heart, especially in difficult times.

G.L.W.

To my wife, Rita,
for her constant, unselfish support and love,
without which none of this would have been possible.

B.H.B.

Contributors

NICOLE AEBISCHER, MD
Chef de clinique, Department of Cardiology, Centre Hôpitalier Universitaire Vaudois (CHUV), Lausanne, Switzerland
Echocardiographic Assessment of Ventricular Systolic Function

BENICO BARZILAI, M.D.
Associate Professor of Medicine, Washington University School of Medicine; Associate Physician, Barnes Hospital, St. Louis, Missouri
Ultrasonic Characterization of Cardiovascular Tissue

MALCOLM R. BELL, M.B.B.S.
Associate Professor of Medicine, and Consultant in Cardiovascular Diseases and Internal Medicine, Mayo Clinic and Foundation, Rochester, Minnesota
Measurement of Myocardial Perfusion Using Electron-Beam (Ultrafast) Computed Tomography

GEORGE A. BELLER, M.D.
Ruth C. Heede Professor of Cardiology and Professor of Internal Medicine, University of Virginia School of Medicine; Chief, Cardiovascular Division, Department of Internal Medicine, University of Virginia Health Sciences Center, Charlottesville, Virginia
Myocardial Imaging for the Assessment of Myocardial Viability

KEVIN S. BERBAUM, PH.D.
Adjunct Professor, Department of Radiology, University of Iowa, Iowa City, Iowa
Perceptual Aspects of Cardiac Imaging

DANIEL G. BLANCHARD, M.D.
Assistant Professor of Medicine, University of California, San Diego, School of Medicine; Director, Noninvasive Cardiac Laboratories, UCSD Medical Center, San Diego, California
Cardiac and Extracardiac Masses: Echocardiographic Evaluation

PAUL A. BOTTOMLEY, PH.D.
Russell H. Morgan Professor of Radiology, The Johns Hopkins University School of Medicine, Baltimore, Maryland
Cardiac Magnetic Resonance Spectroscopy: Principles and Applications

GARY M. BROCKINGTON, M.D.
Assistant Professor of Medicine, Tufts University School of Medicine, Boston; Director of Cardiac Pacing, Faulkner Hospital, Jamaica Plain, Massachusetts
Echocardiography in Pericardial Diseases

BRUCE H. BRUNDAGE, M.D.
Professor of Medicine and Radiological Sciences, UCLA School of Medicine; Chief, Division of Cardiology, Harbor-UCLA Medical Center; Scientific Director, Saint John's Cardiovascular Research Center, Torrance, California
Goals of Cardiac Imaging; Valvular Heart Disease; Myocarditis and Cardiomyopathy; Pericardial Disease; Diseases of the Great Vessels

RICHARD C. BRUNKEN, M.D.
Staff Physician, Department of Nuclear Medicine, The Cleveland Clinic Foundation, Cleveland, Ohio
Evaluation of Myocardial Substrate Metabolism in Ischemic Heart Disease

DENIS B. BUXTON, PH.D.
Associate Professor of Molecular and Medical Pharmacology, UCLA School of Medicine, Los Angeles, California
Principles of Myocardial Metabolism

EDWARD G. CAPE, PH.D.
Assistant Professor, University of Pittsburgh, Schools of Medicine and Engineering; Director, Cardiac Dynamics Laboratory, Division of Cardiology, Children's Hospital of Pittsburgh, Pittsburgh, Pennsylvania
Principles and Instrumentation for Doppler

MELVIN D. CHEITLIN, M.D.
Professor of Medicine, University of California, San Francisco; Chief of Cardiology Service, San Francisco General Hospital, San Francisco, California
The Chest Radiograph in the Adult Patient

MICHAEL P. CHWIALKOWSKI, Ph.D.
Professor, Department of Electrical Engineering, University of Texas, Arlington, Arlington, Texas
Quantitative Magnetic Resonance Imaging of the Heart

C. DAVID COOKE, M.S.E.E.
Assistant Professor of Radiology, Emory University School of Medicine, Atlanta, Georgia
Radionuclide Imaging: Principles and Instrumentation

JOHN MICHAEL CRILEY, M.D.
Professor of Medicine and Radiological Sciences, UCLA School of Medicine; Faculty, Division of Cardiology, Harbor-UCLA Medical Center, Torrance, California
Principles of Valvar Function

BIBIANA CUJEC, M.D.
Associate Professor of Medicine, University of Saskatchewan; Director, Echocardiography Laboratory Staff Cardiologist, Royal University Hospital, Saskatoon, Saskatchewan, Canada
Echocardiography in Pericardial Diseases

S. JAMES CULLOM, Ph.D.
Assistant Professor of Radiology, Emory University School of Medicine; Department of Mechanical Engineering, Georgia Institute of Technology; Associate Director, Nuclear Medicine Physics, Emory University Hospital, Atlanta, Georgia
Radionuclide Imaging: Principles and Instrumentation

JOHANNES CZERNIN, M.D.
Assistant Professor of Pharmacology and Medicine, Department of Molecular and Medical Pharmacology, UCLA School of Medicine, Los Angeles, California
Metabolic Imaging With Single-Photon Emitting Tracers

SETH T. DAHLBERG, M.D.
Assistant Professor, Departments of Nuclear Medicine and Medicine, University of Massachusetts Medical Center, Worcester, Massachusetts
Single-Photon Emitting Tracers for Imaging Myocardial Perfusion and Cell Membrane Integrity

ANTHONY N. DeMARIA, M.D.
Professor of Medicine, University of California at San Diego School of Medicine; Chief, Division of Cardiology, University of California at San Diego, San Diego, California
Cardiac and Extracardiac Masses: Echocardiographic Evaluation

LINDA L. DEMER, M.D., Ph.D.
Associate Professor of Medicine and Cardiology, UCLA School of Medicine; Chief, Division of Cardiology, UCLA Medical Center, Los Angeles, California
Evaluation of Myocardial Blood Flow in Cardiac Disease

ALBERT DE ROOS, M.D.
Department of Diagnostic Radiology, University Hospital Leiden, Leiden, The Netherlands
Congenital Heart Disease Assessed With Magnetic Resonance Techniques

ROBERT R. EDELMAN, M.D.
Professor of Radiology, Harvard Medical School; Director of Magnetic Resonance, Beth Israel Hospital, Boston, Massachusetts
Magnetic Resonance Imaging Assessment of Ischemic Heart Disease

STEVEN R. FLEAGLE, B.S.E.E.
Technical Director, Cardiovascular Image Processing Laboratory, College of Medicine, The University of Iowa, Iowa City, Iowa
Quantitative Methods in Cardiac Imaging: An Introduction to Digital Image Processing

EDWARD D. FOLLAND, M.D.
Professor of Medicine, University of Massachusetts Medical School; Chief, Cardiology, and Director, Cardiac Catheterization Laboratory, Medical Center of Central Massachusetts, Worcester, Massachusetts
Echocardiographic Assessment of Ventricular Systolic Function

THOMAS L. FORCE, M.D.
Assistant Professor of Medicine, Harvard Medical School; Staff Cardiologist, Massachusetts General Hospital, Boston, Massachusetts
Echocardiographic Assessment of Ventricular Systolic Function

ELYSE FOSTER, M.D.
Associate Professor of Clinical Medicine and Anesthesia, and Associate Director, Adult Echocardiography Laboratory, University of California, San Francisco, California
Transesophageal Echocardiography

MICHAEL W. FRANK, M.D.
Instructor, Department of Surgery, Northwestern University Medical School, Chicago, Illinois
Principles of Myocardial Perfusion

E. A. FRANKEN, Jr., M.D.
Professor of Radiology, University of Iowa, Iowa City, Iowa
Perceptual Aspects of Cardiac Imaging

JAMES R. GALT, Ph.D.
Assistant Professor of Radiology, Emory University School of Medicine, Atlanta; Assistant Chief, Nuclear Medicine Service, Veterans Affairs Medical Center (Atlanta), Decatur, Georgia
Radionuclide Imaging: Principles and Instrumentation

ERNEST V. GARCIA, Ph.D.
Professor of Radiology, Emory University School of Medicine; Director, Emory Center for Positron Emission Tomography (P.E.T.), Emory University Hospital, Atlanta, Georgia
Radionuclide Imaging: Principles and Instrumentation

EDWARD A. GEISER, M.D.
Professor of Medicine, Director, Echocardiography, and Associate Director, General Clinical Research Center, University of Florida, College of Medicine, Gainesville, Florida
Echocardiography: Physics and Instrumentation

EDWARD M. GELTMAN, M.D.
Professor of Medicine, Washington University; Director, Heart Failure–Transplant Program; Medical Director, Cardiac Diagnostic Laboratory, Barnes Hospital, St. Louis, Missouri
Assessment of Myocardial Perfusion and Metabolism in the Cardiomyopathies

RAYMOND J. GIBBONS, M.D.
Professor of Medicine, Mayo Medical School; Consultant, Cardiovascular Diseases, Mayo Clinic, Rochester, Minnesota
Equilibrium Radionuclide Angiography

STANTON A. GLANTZ, Ph.D.
Professor of Medicine, University of California, San Francisco, San Francisco, California
Principles of Ventricular Function

ANTOINETTE S. GOMES, M.D.
Associate Professor of Radiology and Medicine, UCLA Medical Center, Los Angeles, California
Pulmonary Angiography

LEENA M. HAMBERG, Ph.D.
Instructor in Radiology, Harvard Medical School; Medical Physicist, Massachusetts General Hospital, Boston, Massachusetts
Principles of Nuclear Magnetic Resonance Relaxation

SCOTT M. HANDLEY, Ph.D.
Research Scientist, Washington University, St. Louis, Missouri
Ultrasonic Characterization of Cardiovascular Tissue

CHARLES B. HIGGINS, M.D.
Professor and Vice-Chairman, Radiology, School of Medicine, University of California, San Francisco, San Francisco, California
Contrast Agents for Cardiac Magnetic Resonance Imaging

JOHN W. HIRSHFELD, Jr., M.D.
Professor of Medicine, University of Pennsylvania; Director, Cardiac Catheterization Laboratory, University of Pennsylvania Medical Center, Philadelphia, Pennsylvania
Radiographic Contrast Agents

MARK R. HOLLAND, Ph.D.
Research Scientist, Washington University, St. Louis, Missouri
Ultrasonic Characterization of Cardiovascular Tissue

W. GREGORY HUNDLEY, M.D.
Cardiology Fellow, The University of Texas Southwestern Medical Center at Dallas, Parkland Hospital, Dallas, Texas
Quantitative Magnetic Resonance Imaging of the Heart

GEORGE J. HUNTER, M.D.
Assistant Professor of Radiology, Harvard Medical School; Assistant Radiologist, Massachusetts General Hospital, Boston, Massachusetts
Cardiomyopathies, Cardiac Masses, and Pericardial Disease: Value of Magnetic Resonance in Diagnosis and Management

TAREK S. HUSAYNI, M.D.
Director of Noninvasive Imaging, The Heart Institute for Children, Christ Hospital and Medical Center, Oak Lawn, Illinois
Ultrafast Computed Tomography Evaluation of Congenital Cardiovascular Disease in Children and Adults

GARY D. HUTCHINS, Ph.D.
Associate Professor of Radiology, Indiana University School of Medicine, Indianapolis, Indiana
Imaging the Cardiac Autonomic Nervous System

JEFFREY M. ISNER, M.D.
Professor of Medicine and Pathology, Tufts University School of Medicine; Chief, Cardiovascular Research, St. Elizabeth's Medical Center, Boston, Massachusetts
Intravascular Ultrasound

LYNNE L. JOHNSON, M.D.
Professor of Medicine, Brown University School of Medicine; Director of Nuclear Cardiology, Rhode Island Hospital, Providence, Rhode Island
Imaging Acute Myocardial Necrosis (Monoclonal Antibodies and Technetium-99m Pyrophosphate)

MARYL R. JOHNSON, M.D.
Associate Professor of Medicine, Rush Medical College; Associate Medical Director, Rush Heart Failure and Cardiac Transplant Program, Rush-Presbyterian-St. Luke's Medical Center, Chicago, Illinois
Principles and Practice of Coronary Angiography

ALAN S. KATZ, M.D.
Assistant Professor of Medicine, Brown University School of Medicine; Director, Echocardiography Laboratory, The Miriam Hospital, Providence, Rhode Island
Echocardiographic Assessment of Ventricular Systolic Function

SANJIV KAUL, M.D.
Professor of Medicine, University of Virginia; Director, Cardiac Imaging Center, University of Virginia Medical Center, Charlottesville, Virginia
Myocardial Perfusion and Other Applications of Contrast Echocardiography

RICHARD E. KERBER, M.D.
Professor of Medicine, Department of Internal Medicine, University of Iowa Hospital and Clinics, Iowa City, Iowa
Echocardiography in Coronary Artery Disease; Myocardial Ischemia and Infarction

ALLAN L. KLEIN, M.D.
Associate Professor of Medicine, Health Science Center, Ohio State University, Columbus; Staff Cardiologist, Director of Cardiovascular Imaging Research, and Associate Director, Echocardiography Laboratory, The Cleveland Clinic Foundation, Cleveland, Ohio
Doppler-Echocardiographic Evaluation of Diastolic Function

FRANCIS J. KLOCKE, M.D.
Professor of Medicine and Director, Feinberg Cardiovascular Research Institute, Northwestern University School of Medicine, Chicago, Illinois
Principles of Myocardial Perfusion

ARTHUR J. LABOVITZ, M.D.
Professor of Medicine and Director of Echocardiography, St. Louis University School of Medicine, St. Louis, Missouri
Cardiomyopathies

JEFFREY A. LEPPO, M.D.
Professor of Medicine and Nuclear Medicine, and Clinical Director, Nuclear Medicine, University of Massachusetts Medical Center, Worcester, Massachusetts
Single-Photon Emitting Tracers for Imaging Myocardial Perfusion and Cell Membrane Integrity

NADJA M. LESKO, M.D.
Director of Radiology, Northern Hospital of Surrey County, Mt. Airy, North Carolina
Imaging of the Valves and Great Vessels

KERRY M. LINK, M.D.
Department of Radiology, Bowman Gray School of Medicine, Winston-Salem, North Carolina
Imaging of the Valves and Great Vessels

JAMSHID MADDAHI, M.D.
Professor of Molecular and Medical Pharmacology (Nuclear Medicine) and Radiological Sciences, University of California at Los Angeles School of Medicine, Los Angeles, California
Myocardial Perfusion Imaging for the Detection and Evaluation of Coronary Artery Disease

G. B. JOHN MANCINI, M.D.
Eric W. Hamber Professor, University of British Columbia; Head, Department of Medicine, Vancouver Hospital and Health Sciences Centre, Vancouver, British Columbia, Canada
Digital Angiography

WARREN J. MANNING, M.D.
Assistant Professor of Medicine and Radiology, Harvard Medical School; Associate Director, Non-Invasive Cardiac Imaging, and Co-Director, Cardiac MR Center, Beth Israel Hospital, Boston, Massachusetts
Magnetic Resonance Imaging Assessment of Ischemic Heart Disease

CYNTHIA H. McCOLLOUGH, PH.D.
Assistant Professor of Radiologic Physics, Mayo Medical School; Consultant in Diagnostic Radiology, Mayo Clinic, Rochester, Minnesota
Ultrafast Computed Tomography: Principles and Instrumentation

PASCAL MERLET, M.D.
Head of Clinical Section, Service Hôpitalier Frédéric Joliot, Département de Recherche Médicale, Commissariat à l'Energie Atomique, Orsay, France
Positron Emission Tomography: Evaluation of Cardiac Receptors and Neuronal Function

JAMES G. MILLER, PH.D.
Professor of Physics, Research Professor of Medicine, and Director, Laboratory for Ultrasonics, Washington University, St. Louis, Missouri
Ultrasonic Characterization of Cardiovascular Tissue

TODD D. MILLER, M.D.
Associate Professor of Medicine, Mayo Medical School; Consultant, Cardiovascular Diseases, Mayo Clinic, Rochester, Minnesota
Equilibrium Radionuclide Angiography

R. JOE NOBLE, M.D.
Clinical Professor of Medicine, Indiana University School of Medicine; Consultant in Cardiology, St. Vincent Hospital and Health Care Facility, Indianapolis, Indiana
A Clinician's Perspective: The Place of Imaging in Cardiac Diagnosis

LYLE J. OLSON, M.D.
Assistant Professor of Medicine, Mayo Medical School; Consultant, Division of Cardiovascular Diseases and Internal Medicine, Mayo Clinic and Mayo Foundation, Rochester, Minnesota
Valvular Heart Disease

NATESA G. PANDIAN, M.D.
Associate Professor of Medicine and Radiology, Tufts University School of Medicine; Director of Cardiovascular Imaging and Hemodynamic Laboratory, New England Medical Center, Boston, Massachusetts
Echocardiography in Pericardial Diseases

ELÉONORE PAQUET, M.D.
Associate Professor of Medicine, University of Montreal, Montreal Heart Institute, Montreal, Canada
Cardiomyopathies, Cardiac Masses, and Pericardial Disease: Value of Magnetic Resonance in Diagnosis and Management

ALFRED F. PARISI, M.D.
Professor of Medicine, Brown University School of Medicine; Chief of Cardiology, The Miriam Hospital, Providence, Rhode Island
Echocardiographic Assessment of Ventricular Systolic Function

ALAN S. PEARLMAN, M.D.
Professor of Medicine, University of Washington School of Medicine; Director, Echocardiography Laboratory, University of Washington Medical Center, President, American Society of Echocardiography, Seattle, Washington
Assessment of Systolic Function With Doppler Echocardiography

JULIO E. PÉREZ, M.D.
Professor of Medicine, Cardiovascular Division, Washington University School of Medicine; Director of Echocardiography and Physician, Barnes Hospital, St. Louis, Missouri
Ultrasonic Characterization of Cardiovascular Tissue

RONALD M. PESHOCK, M.D.
Professor, Radiology and Internal Medicine, University of Texas Southwestern Medical Center at Dallas, Southwestern Medical School, Dallas, Texas
Quantitative Magnetic Resonance Imaging of the Heart

STEVEN PORT, M.D.
Clinical Professor of Medicine, University of Wisconsin Medical School, Madison, Wisconsin
First-Pass Radionuclide Angiography

SIDNEY A. REBERGEN, M.D.
Department of Diagnostic Radiology, University Hospital Leiden, Leiden, The Netherlands
Congenital Heart Disease Assessed With Magnetic Resonance Techniques

STUART RICH, M.D.
Professor of Medicine, and Chief, Section of Cardiology, University of Illinois at Chicago Medical Center, Chicago, Illinois
Evaluation of Coronary Artery Disease by Electron-Beam Computed Tomography

RICHARD A. ROBB, Ph.D.
Professor of Biophysics and of Computer Science, and Director, Biomedical Imaging Resource, Mayo Foundation and Clinic, Rochester, Minnesota
Ultrafast Computed Tomography: Principles and Instrumentation

JOHN A. RUMBERGER, Ph.D., M.D.
Associate Professor of Medicine, and Consultant in Cardiovascular Diseases and Internal Medicine, Mayo Clinic and Foundation, Rochester, Minnesota
Measurement of Myocardial Perfusion Using Electron-Beam (Ultrafast) Computed Tomography

THOMAS RYAN, M.D.
Associate Professor of Medicine, and Director of Echocardiography, Duke University School of Medicine, Durham, North Carolina
Stress Echocardiography

MAYTHEM SAEED, D.V.M., Ph.D.
Associate Professor of Radiology, University of California, San Francisco, School of Medicine, San Francisco, California
Contrast Agents for Cardiac Magnetic Resonance Imaging

COLLEEN SANDERS, M.D.
Associate Professor of Radiology, University of Alabama at Birmingham, Birmingham, Alabama
Role of Aortography in the Age of Imaging

DANY E. SAYAD, M.D.
Cardiology Fellow, University of Texas Southwestern Medical Center at Dallas, Parkland Memorial Hospital, Dallas, Texas
Quantitative Magnetic Resonance Imaging of the Heart

HEINRICH R. SCHELBERT, M.D., PH.D.
Professor of Pharmacology and Radiological Sciences, and Vice Chair, Department of Molecular and Medical Pharmacology, UCLA School of Medicine; Principal Investigator, Laboratory of Structural Biology and Molecular Medicine; Medical Director, Nuclear Medicine Clinic, UCLA Medical Center, University of California at Los Angeles, Los Angeles, California
Goals of Cardiac Imaging; Coronary Artery Disease; Metabolic Imaging With Single-Photon Emitting Tracers; Principles of Positron Emission Tomography; Evaluation of Myocardial Blood Flow in Cardiac Disease; Evaluation of Myocardial Substrate Metabolism in Ischemic Heart Disease; Appendix I: Radiation Dosimetry

NELSON B. SCHILLER, M.D.
Professor of Medicine, Radiology, Anesthesiology, and Director, Adult Echocardiography Laboratory, University of California, San Francisco, San Francisco, California
Transesophageal Echocardiography

HEIKO SCHÖDER, M.D., PH.D.
Postdoctoral Scholar, Department of Pharmacology, Division of Nuclear Medicine, UCLA School of Medicine, Los Angeles, California
Appendix I: Radiation Dosimetry

STEVEN L. SCHWARTZ, M.D.
Associate Professor of Medicine, Tufts University School of Medicine; Associate Director, Cardiovascular Imaging and Hemodynamic Laboratory, New England Medical Center, Boston, Massachusetts
Echocardiography in Pericardial Diseases

SATISH SHARMA, M.D.
Associate Professor of Medicine, Brown University School of Medicine; Chief of Cardiology, Veterans Administration Medical Center, Providence, Rhode Island
Echocardiographic Assessment of Ventricular Systolic Function

FLORENCE H. SHEEHAN, M.D.
Research Professor, Department of Medicine, Division of Cardiology, University of Washington, Seattle, Washington
Principles and Practice of Contrast Ventriculography; Applications of Contrast Ventriculography

DAVID J. SKORTON, M.D.
Professor of Medicine and Electrical and Computer Engineering, and Co-Director, The University of Iowa Hospitals and Clinics Adolescent and Adult Congenital Heart Disease Clinic, and Vice President for Research, The University of Iowa; Consulting Physician, Department of Veterans Affairs Medical Center, Iowa City, Iowa
Goals of Cardiac Imaging; Quantitative Methods in Cardiac Imaging: An Introduction to Digital Image Processing; Congenital Heart Disease; Cardiovascular Trauma; Ultrasonic Characterization of Cardiovascular Tissue

A. REBECCA SNIDER, M.D.
Pediatric Cardiologist, Baltimore, Maryland
Two-Dimensional and Doppler Echocardiography in the Evaluation of Congenital Heart Disease

HEINZ SOCHOR, M.D.
Professor of Cardiology, University of Vienna Medical School, Vienna, Austria
Metabolic Imaging With Single-Photon Emitting Tracers

STEVEN SOLOMON, PH.D.
Cardiovascular Research Institute, University of California, San Francisco, School of Medicine, San Francisco, California
Principles of Ventricular Function

KIRK T. SPENCER, M.D.
Assistant Professor of Medicine, University of Chicago, Chicago, Illinois
Echocardiography in Coronary Artery Disease: Myocardial Ischemia and Infarction

WILLIAM STANFORD, M.D.
Professor, Department of Radiology, College of Medicine, University of Iowa; Director, Cardiovascular Radiology, University of Iowa Hospitals and Clinics, Iowa City, Iowa
Evaluation of Cardiovascular Structure and Function With Electron-Beam Computed Tomography; The Great Vessels: Imaging by Electron-Beam Computed Tomography; Cardiac Masses and Pericardial Disease: Imaging by Electron-Beam Computed Tomography

WILLIAM J. STEWART, M.D.
Associate Professor of Medicine, Ohio State University; Director, Echocardiography Laboratory, and Co-Director, Cardiac Valve Management Center, Cleveland Clinic Foundation, Cleveland, Ohio
Intraoperative Echocardiography

JOHN R. STRATTON, M.D.
Professor of Medicine, Division of Cardiology, University of Washington; Staff Cardiologist, Seattle VA Medical Center, Seattle, Washington
Thrombosis Imaging With Indium-111–Labeled Platelets

ANDRÉ SYROTA, M.D., Ph.D.
Professor of Biophysics and Nuclear Medicine, Université Paris Sud; Head of Service Hôpitalier Frédéric Joliot, Département de Recherche Médicale, Commissariat à l'Energie Atomique, Orsay, France
Positron Emission Tomography: Evaluation of Cardiac Receptors and Neuronal Function

DAVID M. SZCZESNIAK, M.D.
Resident, Mayo Clinic, Rochester, Minnesota
Imaging of the Valves and Great Vessels

DIETER SZOLAR, M.D.
Research Fellow, University of California, San Francisco, School of Medicine, San Francisco, California
Contrast Agents for Cardiac Magnetic Resonance Imaging

A. JAMIL TAJIK, M.D.
Chair, Division of Cardiovascular Diseases and Internal Medicine, Mayo Clinic and Foundation; Thomas J. Watson, Jr., Professor in Honor of Dr. Robert L. Frye, Mayo Medical School, Rochester, Minnesota
Valvular Heart Disease

JAMES D. THOMAS, M.D.
Professor of Medicine and Biomedical Engineering, The Ohio State University, Columbus; Director of Cardiovascular Imaging, Department of Cardiology, Cleveland Clinic Foundation, Cleveland, Ohio
Doppler-Echocardiographic Evaluation of Diastolic Function

BRAD H. THOMPSON, M.D.
Assistant Professor, Department of Radiology, University of Iowa College of Medicine, Iowa City, Iowa
The Great Vessels: Imaging by Electron-Beam Computed Tomography; Cardiac Masses and Pericardial Disease: Imaging by Electron-Beam Computed Tomography

BYRON F. VANDENBERG, M.D.
Associate Professor of Medicine, Department of Internal Medicine, The University of Iowa College of Medicine, Iowa City, Iowa
Ultrasonic Characterization of Cardiovascular Tissue

ERNST E. van der WALL, M.D.
Department of Cardiology, University Hospital Leiden, Leiden, The Netherlands
Congenital Heart Disease Assessed With Magnetic Resonance Techniques

JOHN R. VOTAW, Ph.D.
Assistant Professor of Radiology, Emory University, Atlanta, Georgia
Radionuclide Imaging: Principles and Instrumentation

ROBERT G. WEISS, M.D.
Associate Professor of Medicine and Radiology, Cardiology Division, The Johns Hopkins University School of Medicine; Attending Physician, The Johns Hopkins Hospital, Baltimore, Maryland
Cardiac Magnetic Resonance Spectroscopy: Principles and Applications

ROBERT M. WEISS, M.D.
Assistant Professor, Department of Internal Medicine, University of Iowa College of Medicine; Staff Cardiologist, University of Iowa Hospitals and Clinics and Department of Veterans Affairs Medical Center, Iowa City, Iowa
Evaluation of Cardiovascular Structure and Function With Electron-Beam Computed Tomography

ROBERT W. WEISSKOFF, PH.D.
Assistant Professor, Radiology, Harvard Medical School, Boston; Director of NMR Physics Research, Massachusetts General Hospital NMR Center, Charlestown, Massachusetts
Principles and Instrumentation for Cardiac Magnetic Resonance Imaging

MICHAEL F. WENDLAND, PH.D.
Associate Professor, University of California, San Francisco, School of Medicine, San Francisco, California
Contrast Agents for Cardiac Magnetic Resonance Imaging

JAMES S. WHITING, PH.D.
Adjunct Associate Professor, Department of Radiological Sciences, University of California, Los Angeles; Director, Department of Medical Physics and Imaging, Cedars-Sinai Medical Center, Los Angeles, California
Principles and Instrumentation for Radiography

DuWAYNE L. WILLETT, M.D.
Instructor of Internal Medicine, Division of Cardiology, The University of Texas Southwestern Medical Center at Dallas; Attending Physician, Cardiology, Zale Lipsky University Hospital and Parkland Hospital, Dallas, Texas
Quantitative Magnetic Resonance Imaging of the Heart

GERALD L. WOLF, PH.D., M.D.
Professor of Radiology, Harvard Medical School; Director, Center for Imaging and Pharmaceutical Research, Massachusetts General Hospital, Boston, Massachusetts
Goals of Cardiac Imaging; Principles of Nuclear Magnetic Resonance Relaxation

CHRISTOPHER J. WOLFKIEL, PH.D.
Research Assistant Professor of Medicine, and Director, Ultrafast CT Laboratory, University of Illinois at Chicago Medical Center, Chicago, Illinois
Evaluation of Coronary Artery Disease by Electron-Beam Computed Tomography

AJIT P. YOGANATHAN, PH.D.
Professor of Chemical, Mechanical and Bioengineering, Georgia Institute of Technology, Atlanta, Georgia
Principles and Instrumentation for Doppler

ELIAS A. ZERHOUNI, M.D.
Professor of Radiology and Biomedical Engineering, The Johns Hopkins University School of Medicine; Director, Thoracic Imaging and MRI, The Johns Hopkins Hospital, Baltimore, Maryland
Integrated Cardiac Magnetic Resonance Examination

DOUGLAS P. ZIPES, M.D.
Professor of Cardiology, Indiana University School of Medicine, Indianapolis, Indiana
Imaging the Cardiac Autonomic Nervous System

Foreword

The dramatic reductions in cardiovascular mortality and morbidity during the past three decades represent one of the major triumphs of twentieth-century medicine. Striking advances in three major areas are responsible—diagnosis, therapy, and prevention. The first of these, cardiac diagnosis, has improved almost entirely as a consequence of the spectacular developments in cardiac imaging. In the five years since the publication of the first edition of this book, the technologies available for cardiac imaging have progressed exponentially, and the contributions made by cardiac imaging to every aspect of cardiac care have expanded with unexpected rapidity.

As we approach the end of the century, it is clear that the public expectations of the medical profession are increasing. Patients, their families, and those who pay for medical care require first and foremost an accurate clinical assessment—not merely a diagnosis. In the case of patients with cardiac disease, both anatomic and functional evaluations are required, and clinicians now have a broad array of cardiac imaging techniques available to them for accomplishing these tasks. While this book presents the cardiologist, cardiovascular radiologist, and cardiovascular surgeon with the information required to use and interpret the entire gamut of contemporary imaging techniques, it goes much further by providing the understanding required to employ these complex and sometimes costly techniques intelligently. In an era of cost-conscious medicine, it is essential to select the appropriate technique without paying for unnecessary or redundant information. An entire new section of this edition, "Integrated Clinical Approach to Diagnosis Using Imaging Methods," guides clinicians to the specific technique required for addressing specific clinical issues.

This second edition is much more than a revision and an updating of an exemplary text. A new editor, Dr. Bruce H. Brundage, has joined the editorial group, and his influence on the second edition is clearly felt. Approximately one half of the chapters are new to this edition or were written by new authors, and both volumes are replete with spectacular new illustrations, which constitute the cornerstone of any work on imaging. The editors and authors of this book are not only technical experts but also experienced and thoughtful clinicians, and this combined expertise is interwoven throughout the text.

A number of excellent review articles, manuals, and texts are now available to aid physicians in the clinical applications of cardiac imaging. Rarely are such works also helpful in selecting the appropriate imaging technique for solving specific problems. In my estimation, none accomplishes these twin tasks with greater clarity, precision, and judgment than does the second edition of *Marcus Cardiac Imaging*. I am proud of its continued companionship to the new (fifth) edition of *Heart Disease: A Textbook of Cardiovascular Medicine*.

Eugene Braunwald, M.D.
Boston, Massachusetts

Preface

Imaging techniques continue to be immensely important in the management of patients with known or suspected cardiovascular disease. The widespread use of imaging technology in clinical diagnosis and the rapid development of new knowledge and methods in the research laboratory and at the bedside have dictated the need for an updated edition of this book. Virtually all modalities of cardiac imaging have experienced growth and development since the first edition of *Cardiac Imaging*. Echocardiographers have further embraced transesophageal echocardiography as an important method of assessing cardiac structure and function in the clinic, emergency room, and operating suite. The revised chapter on transesophageal echocardiography by Schiller and Foster is a lucid and comprehensive "textbook within a textbook" that will be useful to new and experienced echocardiographers alike. Intravascular ultrasound techniques are acquiring an increasingly important role and are discussed in a new chapter by Isner. All the other chapters in the echocardiography section have been updated and revised. Chapters on fast computed tomography have also been updated. In this section, the chapter by Rumberger and Bell is an extremely useful review of applicable principles of perfusion imaging. Radionuclide methods have focused to a greater extent on the assessment of myocardial viability, and this important area is discussed in a new chapter by Beller. Further experience with newer, technetium-based single-photon emitting radionuclides has necessitated extensive updating in Part 7. A new chapter by Dahlberg and Leppo discusses single-photon emitting tracers for assessing perfusion and cell membrane integrity. Also, imaging of myocardial neuronal activity with single-photon emitting tracers has further developed; the new chapter by Hutchins and Zipes provides a detailed account of this topic. Positron emission tomography (PET) continues to mature; the chapters on PET have been revised carefully. They emphasize new accomplishments and their clinical applications as well as the potential role of absolute myocardial blood flow measurements. The entire magnetic resonance imaging (MRI) section of the second edition has been extensively rewritten, including basic principles of relaxation, imaging, spectroscopy, contrast agents, and quantitation. A new chapter by Zerhouni summarizes the enormous amount of information that can be obtained in a 1-hour integrated cardiac MRI examination. The expanded MR glossary will be valuable for all students of this technology.

Although one thrust of the book continues to be sophisticated, *high-tech* imaging methods, we have attempted to further emphasize general issues that span different techniques and simpler methods. A new chapter by Cheitlin on the chest roentgenogram emphasizes the usefulness of this simple yet effective imaging method. An entirely new section, *The Integrated Clinical Approach to Diagnosis Using Imaging Methods,* is intended to help guide the busy clinician through the often bewildering maze of seemingly redundant diagnostic imaging choices. Finally, a new appendix has been added, detailing useful information on radiation dosimetry. In all, the book has undergone a major revision: Of the 73 chapters in this edition, 21 are by new authors, 14 are new chapters, and 1 appendix is new.

The features of the book that were popular in the first edition have been retained. The introductory section (Part 1) again features clear descriptions of the aspects of cardiovascular physiology relevant to imaging studies of cardiac function, perfusion, and metabolism as well as discussion of digital image processing and perceptual considerations in imaging. Each imaging modality is described comprehensively, from physics and instrumentation through clinical applications. Abundant use is made of figures, with full-color illustrations appearing in each volume. Finally, the reference lists have been updated to supply the reader with the latest information for further learning.

Dr. Eugene Braunwald continues to be an important force in the conceptualization and implementation of this project. We again gratefully acknowledge his inspiration and support during the preparation of this second edition of our text.

We also thankfully acknowledge Carolyn Frisbie, Catherine Dowty, Leah Voigt, Eileen Rosenfeld, and Diane Dalton for their efforts in organizational aspects of the project as well as manuscript preparation. We again were fortunate to work with Richard Zorab and his colleagues Nellie McGrew, Leslie E. Hoeltzel, Gina Scala, Mike Carcel, and others at W.B. Saunders Company; these consummate professionals guided us through the project with good humor and patience.

The second edition of the text is named *Marcus Cardiac Imaging* in acknowledgment and honor of the late Dr. Melvin L. Marcus, founding editor of the book. Mel Marcus' dedication to excellence in the principles and practice of cardiac imaging was an inspiration in the preparation of this second edition.

The text continues to target cardiologists, cardiology fellows, radiologists, nuclear medicine physicians, radiology trainees, cardiac surgeons, internists, and others who employ cardiac imaging methods with the ultimate goal of improvement in patient care.

David J. Skorton, M.D.
Bruce H. Brundage, M.D.
Heinrich R. Schelbert, M.D.
Gerald L. Wolf, Ph.D., M.D.

Contents

Volume 1

PART 1

INTRODUCTION ____ 1

CHAPTER **1**

Goals of Cardiac Imaging ____ 1
David J. Skorton, M.D. ■ Bruce H. Brundage, M.D. ■ Heinrich R. Schelbert, M.D. ■ Gerald L. Wolf, Ph.D., M.D.

CHAPTER **2**

Principles of Myocardial Perfusion ____ 8
Francis J. Klocke, M.D. ■ Michael W. Frank, M.D.

CHAPTER **3**

Principles of Ventricular Function ____ 19
Steven Solomon, Ph.D. ■ Stanton A. Glantz, Ph.D.

CHAPTER **4**

Principles of Myocardial Metabolism ____ 34
Denis B. Buxton, Ph.D.

CHAPTER **5**

Principles of Valvar Function ____ 50
John Michael Criley, M.D.

CHAPTER **6**

Quantitative Methods in Cardiac Imaging: An Introduction to Digital Image Processing ____ 58
Steven R. Fleagle, B.S.E.E. ■ David J. Skorton, M.D.

CHAPTER **7**

Perceptual Aspects of Cardiac Imaging ____ 72
E. A. Franken, Jr., M.D. ■ Kevin S. Berbaum, Ph.D.

CHAPTER **8**

A Clinician's Perspective: The Place of Imaging in Cardiac Diagnosis ____ 78
R. Joe Noble, M.D.

PART 2

INTEGRATED CLINICAL APPROACH TO DIAGNOSIS USING IMAGING METHODS ____ 81

CHAPTER **9**

Coronary Artery Disease ____ 81
Heinrich R. Schelbert, M.D.

CHAPTER **10**

Valvular Heart Disease ____ 84
Bruce H. Brundage, M.D.

CHAPTER **11**

Myocarditis and Cardiomyopathy ____ 87
Bruce H. Brundage, M.D.

CHAPTER **12**

Congenital Heart Disease ____ 90
David J. Skorton, M.D.

CHAPTER **13**

Pericardial Disease ____ 93
Bruce H. Brundage, M.D.

CHAPTER **14**

Cardiovascular Trauma ____ 95
David J. Skorton, M.D.

CHAPTER **15**

Diseases of the Great Vessels ____ 98
Bruce H. Brundage, M.D.

PART 3

CONVENTIONAL RADIOGRAPHY AND ANGIOGRAPHY ____ 102

CHAPTER **16**

Principles and Instrumentation for Radiography ____ 102
James S. Whiting, Ph.D.

CHAPTER **17**

The Chest Radiograph in the Adult Patient ____ 126
Melvin D. Cheitlin, M.D.

CHAPTER **18**

Radiographic Contrast Agents ____ 144
John W. Hirshfeld, Jr., M.D.

CHAPTER **19**

Principles and Practice of Contrast Ventriculography ____ 164
Florence H. Sheehan, M.D.

CHAPTER **20**

Applications of Contrast Ventriculography ____ 187
Florence H. Sheehan, M.D.

CHAPTER **21**

Role of Aortography in the Age of Imaging _____ 199

  Colleen Sanders, M.D.

CHAPTER **22**

Pulmonary Angiography _____ 208

  Antoinette S. Gomes, M.D.

CHAPTER **23**

Principles and Practice of Coronary Angiography _____ 220

  Maryl R. Johnson, M.D.

CHAPTER **24**

Digital Angiography _____ 251

  G. B. John Mancini, M.D.

P A R T **4**

ECHOCARDIOGRAPHY _____ **273**

CHAPTER **25**

Echocardiography: Physics and Instrumentation _____ 273

  Edward A. Geiser, M.D.

CHAPTER **26**

Principles and Instrumentation for Doppler _____ 291

  Edward G. Cape, Ph.D. ■ Ajit P. Yoganathan, Ph.D.

CHAPTER **27**

Echocardiographic Assessment of Ventricular Systolic Function _____ 297

  Alan S. Katz, M.D. ■ Thomas L. Force, M.D. ■ Edward D. Folland, M.D.
  ■ Nicole Aebischer, M.D. ■ Satish Sharma, M.D. ■ Alfred F. Parisi, M.D.

CHAPTER **28**

Assessment of Systolic Function With Doppler Echocardiography _____ 324

  Alan S. Pearlman, M.D.

CHAPTER **29**

Doppler-Echocardiographic Evaluation of Diastolic Function _____ 336

  James D. Thomas, M.D. ■ Allan L. Klein, M.D.

CHAPTER **30**

Valvular Heart Disease _____ 365

  Lyle J. Olson, M.D. ■ A. Jamil Tajik, M.D.

CHAPTER **31**

Cardiomyopathies _____ 395

  Arthur J. Labovitz, M.D.

CHAPTER **32**

Echocardiography in Pericardial Diseases _____ 404

  Bibiana Cujec, M.D. ■ Gary M. Brockington, M.D. ■ Steven L. Schwartz,
  M.D. ■ Natesa G. Pandian, M.D.

CHAPTER **33**

Two-Dimensional and Doppler Echocardiography in the Evaluation of Congenital Heart Disease _____ 420

  A. Rebecca Snider, M.D.

CHAPTER **34**

Cardiac and Extracardiac Masses: Echocardiographic Evaluation _____ 452

  Daniel G. Blanchard, M.D. ■ Anthony N. DeMaria, M.D.

CHAPTER **35**

Myocardial Perfusion and Other Applications of Contrast Echocardiography _____ 480

  Sanjiv Kaul, M.D.

CHAPTER **36**

Stress Echocardiography _____ 503

  Thomas Ryan, M.D.

CHAPTER **37**

Echocardiography in Coronary Artery Disease: Myocardial Ischemia and Infarction _____ 522

  Kirk T. Spencer, M.D. ■ Richard E. Kerber, M.D.

CHAPTER **38**

Transesophageal Echocardiography _____ 533

  Nelson B. Schiller, M.D. ■ Elyse Foster, M.D.

CHAPTER **39**

Intraoperative Echocardiography _____ 566

  William J. Stewart, M.D.

CHAPTER **40**

Intravascular Ultrasound _____ 581

  Jeffrey M. Isner, M.D.

CHAPTER **41**

Ultrasonic Characterization of Cardiovascular Tissue _____ 606

  Julio E. Pérez, M.D. ■ Mark R. Holland, Ph.D. ■ Benico Barzilai, M.D. ■
  Scott M. Handley, Ph.D. ■ Byron F. Vandenberg, M.D. ■ James G. Miller,
  Ph.D. ■ David J. Skorton, M.D.

Color Plates 1 to 21 follow page 296.

Volume 2

P A R T **5**

MAGNETIC RESONANCE IMAGING _____ **629**

CHAPTER **42**

Principles of Nuclear Magnetic Resonance Relaxation _____ 629

Leena M. Hamberg, Ph.D. ■ *Gerald L. Wolf, Ph.D., M.D.*

CHAPTER **43**

Principles and Instrumentation for Cardiac Magnetic Resonance Imaging _____ 639

Robert W. Weisskoff, Ph.D.

CHAPTER **44**

Contrast Agents for Cardiac Magnetic Resonance Imaging _____ 652

Maythem Saeed, D.V.M., Ph.D. ■ *Michael F. Wendland, Ph.D.* ■ *Dieter Szolar, M.D.* ■ *Charles B. Higgins, M.D.*

CHAPTER **45**

Integrated Cardiac Magnetic Resonance Examination _____ 667

Elias A. Zerhouni, M.D.

CHAPTER **46**

Congenital Heart Disease Assessed With Magnetic Resonance Techniques _____ 672

Albert de Roos, M.D. ■ *Sidney A. Rebergen, M.D.* ■ *Ernst E. van der Wall, M.D.*

CHAPTER **47**

Imaging of the Valves and Great Vessels _____ 692

Kerry M. Link, M.D. ■ *David Szczesniak, M.D.* ■ *Nadja M. Lesko, M.D.*

CHAPTER **48**

Magnetic Resonance Imaging Assessment of Ischemic Heart Disease _____ 719

Warren J. Manning, M.D. ■ *Robert R. Edelman, M.D.*

CHAPTER **49**

Cardiomyopathies, Cardiac Masses, and Pericardial Disease: Value of Magnetic Resonance in Diagnosis and Management _____ 744

George J. Hunter, M.D. ■ *Eléonore Paquet, M.D.*

CHAPTER **50**

Quantitative Magnetic Resonance Imaging of the Heart _____ 759

Ronald M. Peshock, M.D. ■ *W. Gregory Hundley, M.D.* ■ *DuWayne L. Willett, M.D.* ■ *Dany E. Sayad, M.D.* ■ *Michael P. Chwialkowski, Ph.D.*

CHAPTER **51**

Cardiac Magnetic Resonance Spectroscopy: Principles and Applications _____ 784

Robert G. Weiss, M.D. ■ *Paul A. Bottomley, Ph.D.*

P A R T **6**

FAST COMPUTED TOMOGRAPHY _____ **793**

CHAPTER **52**

Ultrafast Computed Tomography: Principles and Instrumentation _____ 793

Cynthia H. McCollough, Ph.D. ■ *Richard A. Robb, Ph.D.*

CHAPTER **53**

Evaluation of Cardiovascular Structure and Function With Electron-Beam Computed Tomography _____ 820

Robert M. Weiss, M.D. ■ *William Stanford, M.D.*

CHAPTER **54**

Evaluation of Coronary Artery Disease by Electron-Beam Computed Tomography _____ 829

Stuart Rich, M.D. ■ *Christopher J. Wolfkiel, Ph.D.*

CHAPTER **55**

Measurement of Myocardial Perfusion Using Electron-Beam (Ultrafast) Computed Tomography _____ 835

John A. Rumberger, Ph.D., M.D. ■ *Malcolm R. Bell, M.B.B.S.*

CHAPTER **56**

The Great Vessels: Imaging by Electron-Beam Computed Tomography _____ 852

William Stanford, M.D. ■ *Brad H. Thompson, M.D.*

CHAPTER **57**

Cardiac Masses and Pericardial Disease: Imaging by Electron-Beam Computed Tomography _____ 863

William Stanford, M.D. ■ *Brad H. Thompson, M.D.*

CHAPTER **58**

Ultrafast Computed Tomography Evaluation of Congenital Cardiovascular Disease in Children and Adults _____ 871

Tarek S. Husayni, M.D.

P A R T **7**

RADIONUCLIDE IMAGING _____ **887**

CHAPTER **59**

Principles and Instrumentation _____ 887

Ernest V. Garcia, Ph.D. ■ *John R. Votaw, Ph.D.* ■ *S. James Cullom, Ph.D.* ■ *James R. Galt, Ph.D.* ■ *C. David Cooke, M.S.E.E.*

CHAPTER **60**

First-Pass Radionuclide Angiography _____ 923

Steven Port, M.D.

CHAPTER **61**

Equilibrium Radionuclide Angiography _____ 941

Raymond J. Gibbons, M.D. ■ *Todd D. Miller, M.D.*

CHAPTER **62**

Single-Photon Emitting Tracers for Imaging Myocardial Perfusion and Cell Membrane Integrity _____ 963

Seth T. Dahlberg, M.D. ■ *Jeffrey A. Leppo, M.D.*

CHAPTER **63**

Myocardial Perfusion Imaging for the Detection and Evaluation of Coronary Artery Disease _____ 971

Jamshid Maddahi, M.D.

CHAPTER **64**

Myocardial Imaging for the Assessment of Myocardial Viability _____ 996

George A. Beller, M.D.

CHAPTER **65**

Imaging Acute Myocardial Necrosis (Monoclonal Antibodies and Technetium-99m Pyrophosphate) _____ 1012

Lynne L. Johnson, M.D.

CHAPTER **66**

Metabolic Imaging With Single-Photon Emitting Tracers _____ 1020

Johannes Czernin, M.D. ■ *Heinz Sochor, M.D.* ■ *Heinrich R. Schelbert, M.D.*

CHAPTER **67**

Thrombosis Imaging With Indium-111–Labeled Platelets _____ 1034

John R. Stratton, M.D.

CHAPTER **68**

Imaging the Cardiac Autonomic Nervous System _____ 1052

Gary D. Hutchins, Ph.D. ■ *Douglas P. Zipes, M.D.*

PART **8**
POSITRON EMISSION TOMOGRAPHY _____ **1063**

CHAPTER **69**

Principles of Positron Emission Tomography _____ 1063

Heinrich R. Schelbert, M.D.

CHAPTER **70**

Evaluation of Myocardial Blood Flow in Cardiac Disease _____ 1093

Heinrich R. Schelbert, M.D. ■ *Linda L. Demer, M.D.*

CHAPTER **71**

Evaluation of Myocardial Substrate Metabolism in Ischemic Heart Disease _____ 1113

Richard C. Brunken, M.D. ■ *Heinrich R. Schelbert, M.D.*

CHAPTER **72**

Assessment of Myocardial Perfusion and Metabolism in the Cardiomyopathies _____ 1171

Edward M. Geltman, M.D.

CHAPTER **73**

Positron Emission Tomography: Evaluation of Cardiac Receptors and Neuronal Function _____ 1186

André Syrota, M.D., Ph.D. ■ *Pascal Merlet, M.D.*

APPENDIX **I**

Radiation Dosimetry _____ 1205

Heiko Schöder, M.D. ■ *Heinrich R. Schelbert, M.D.*

APPENDIX **II**

Glossary of NMR Terms _____ 1209

INDEX _____ i

Color Plates 22 to 35 follow page 892.

CHAPTER

1 Goals of Cardiac Imaging

David J. Skorton, M.D.
Bruce H. Brundage, M.D.
Heinrich R. Schelbert, M.D.
Gerald L. Wolf, Ph.D., M.D.

**CURRENT CAPABILITIES AND NEEDS IN
    DIAGNOSTIC CARDIAC IMAGING** _____ 1
Anatomy _____ 1
Chamber Function _____ 2
Valvular Function _____ 3

Myocardial Perfusion _____ 4
Myocardial Metabolism _____ 5
Tissue Characterization _____ 5
CONCLUSIONS _____ 6

Clinicians who care for patients with cardiovascular disease can intervene in powerful ways to favorably alter the course of most disorders. Optimal use of the potent therapeutic options available depends on highly specific diagnosis. Current diagnostic goals are not merely oriented toward placing a patient into a broad category of disease. Instead, the modern diagnostician aims for a comprehensive and specific evaluation of anatomy and physiology to guide optimal management of the patient.

The diagnostic process still begins with the history and physical examination, usually followed by obtaining the resting electrocardiogram and chest roentgenogram. Based on this initial information, tentative diagnostic hypotheses are formed. The clinician evaluates these initial hypotheses by employing an array of diagnostic tools, including biochemical analyses of blood and urine; electrocardiographic recordings at rest, with graded exercise, during daily activities, and within the heart chambers; and several sophisticated methods of imaging the heart and vasculature. With the exception of electrocardiographic and electrophysiologic testing, the most commonly used laboratory diagnostic procedures in current practice are the imaging techniques. Thus, cardiac imaging has become a dominant force in modern cardiovascular diagnosis.

This chapter prepares the reader by briefly reviewing the goals of cardiac imaging as part of the comprehensive approach to diagnostic evaluation. Through cardiac imaging methods, a clinician first attempts to visualize cardiac *anatomy* and to derive quantitative descriptors. Anatomic assessment includes determination of the size, shape, and structure of the cardiac chambers, valves, great vessels, and the coronary arteries. Next, chamber and valvular *function* are addressed, including evaluation of systolic and diastolic function and assessment of the severity of valvular stenosis or regurgitation.

The most widely used cardiac imaging methods offer information restricted chiefly to anatomy and function. In the last decade, however, rapid progress in the laboratory and at the bedside has placed three additional goals within the reach of clinical utility: assessment of myocardial *perfusion*, *metabolism*, and *tissue characteristics*.[1] Particularly in the present era of aggressive intervention to minimize the deleterious effects of acute myocardial ischemia and to reduce coronary arterial occlusion, the clinician desires accurate information concerning myocardial perfusion. Ideally, this information would include regional and transmural estimates of cardiac perfusion at rest, with pharmacologic vasodilation or exer-

cise stress, and during acute ischemia.[2] At a more basic level, investigators and clinicians seek insights into myocardial metabolism under normal and abnormal conditions.[3, 4] The metabolic information sought includes details of myocardial uptake of fuel substrates, certain aspects of intermediary metabolism, and myocardial bioenergetics, especially the kinetics of high-energy phosphate metabolism. Finally, the clinician seeks information regarding myocardial tissue composition,[5] including identification of abnormal deposition of collagen, iron, amyloid, or other substances, delineation of the nature of intracardiac masses, and identification of acutely and chronically ischemic myocardium.

Thus, the goals of cardiac imaging are broad. How do current, widely available techniques measure up to these goals, and what needs are still to be met in cardiac imaging? Answers to these questions are attempted briefly in this chapter, with citations to primary sources. The individual chapters that follow provide reviews of particular topics in much greater detail.

CURRENT CAPABILITIES AND NEEDS IN DIAGNOSTIC CARDIAC IMAGING

Anatomy

Chest roentgenography, echocardiography, radionuclide ventriculography, and selective left heart angiography are commonly used to assess the anatomy of the heart and great vessels. Properly performed and interpreted, chest roentgenography permits qualitative identification of enlargement of each cardiac chamber and gives important information on the physiologic state of the pulmonary vasculature, especially in chronic disorders. Echocardiography,[6] radionuclide imaging,[7] and angiography[8] permit quantitative assessment of left ventricular volume. Echocardiography[9] and angiography[10] also permit estimates of left ventricular mass. Because echocardiography provides clear delineation of wall thickness, it has been the method most widely used for estimation of left ventricular mass, especially in patients with left ventricular hypertrophy related to hypertensive and valvular heart disease.[11] Because contrast angiography depicts only the intracardiac blood pool, assessment of ventricular mass is less precise and usually requires assumptions concerning the distribution of wall thickness in the normal and abnormal heart. The shortcomings of standard transthoracic echocardiography include the difficulties of the examination in some patients and the need to approximate the shape of the left ventricle with the use of simple geometric models. Even methods that utilize "Simpson's rule" based on echocardiographic data suffer from an important theoretical limitation: The various echocardiographic images used to integrate mass or volume across the entire left (or right) ventricle are not truly mutually parallel; they are obtained at somewhat arbitrary orientations based in part on the patient's thoracic habitus and on the availability of acoustic "windows" at particular anatomic sites. The problems of acoustic access and the varying orientation of images produced by transthoracic echocardiography are alleviated with the use of transesophageal echocardiography (TEE).[12] Extremely clear depiction of anatomy is possible with TEE, and three-dimensional (3D) reconstructions have become available through the use of multiple TEE images.[13]

Assessment of right ventricular volume or mass is more difficult, since the complex shape of this chamber defies accurate representation by a simple geometric model. Echocardiography may be used to assess right ventricular volume,[14] although this approach is not widely applied in clinical practice.

Increased accuracy in determination of ventricular mass and volume requires high-resolution methods that can delineate endocardial and epicardial surfaces in multiple, mutually parallel sections, preferably within the same cardiac cycle, or within only a few cardiac cycles. This accurate and precise volumetric information for both ventricles appears to be available through the use of fast computed tomographic (CT) methods.[15–17] In this chapter, we use the term "fast CT" to indicate either of two approaches to rapid-acquisition CT: slip-ring or electron beam CT (the latter method was previously termed "ultrafast CT"). Although currently requiring many cardiac cycles for acquisition, standard spin-echo and "cine" techniques of magnetic resonance imaging (MRI) also permit very accurate anatomic assessment.[18–20] The recent commercial availability of echo-planar and other ultrafast MRI methods permits extremely rapid MRI image acquisition, facilitating dynamic cardiac imaging.[21, 22]

In addition to the determination of global left ventricular mass, the assessment of regional ventricular wall thickness in selected patients is important, as in the subject with suspected left ventricular aneurysm or localized scar from prior myocardial infarction. Echocardiography provides excellent information on regional wall thickness and systolic thickening[23] in patients in whom good-quality studies are obtained. Computed tomography and MRI appear to provide quantitative data that are extremely accurate and precise in this application.[24–25]

Clinicians often need to determine the size and shape of the thoracic aorta to evaluate the patient with suspected aneurysm, coarctation, dissection, or rupture. Both echocardiography and angiography permit excellent delineation of aortic root size and anatomic characteristics. Transthoracic echocardiography is less consistently useful than is aortography in the definition of proximal aortic dissection.[26] Angiography fulfills this goal but requires an invasive left heart catheterization. Again, the newer tomographic methods of transesophageal echocardiography,[27] fast CT,[28] and MRI[29] permit superb noninvasive assessment of the size and shape of the thoracic aorta, including identification of aneurysm, dissection, and rupture. Furthermore, MRI permits acquisition of images along arbitrarily oriented planes, potentially permitting the entire thoracic aorta to be viewed in a single image. Currently, aortography is generally considered the definitive diagnostic procedure; however, in many instances transesophageal echocardiography, CT, and MRI all are reasonable approaches to the diagnosis of aortic dissection. The specific choice in any particular center depends on local availability and expertise. The portability of echocardiography makes it the procedure of choice when the clinician desires to evaluate a patient with suspected aortic dissection at the bedside, in the critical care unit, or in the operating room.

Delineation of the detailed anatomy of the coronary arteries has remained the domain of selective coronary angiography. Early studies identified a large degree of interobserver and intraobserver variability in the assessment of percent coronary arterial narrowing,[30] the parameter most commonly derived from angiograms. This variability is probably still substantial in current practice. Furthermore, in patients with multivessel coronary disease, the physiologic significance of a particular coronary stenosis may not be defined by the standard arteriographic technique of visually estimating percent diameter stenosis.[31] Improved determination of the absolute size of the arterial lumen in normal and atherosclerotic regions, and of the physiologic significance of individual stenosis, is offered by quantitative, computer-based angiographic analyses.[32–34] These techniques are being applied to both digital and film-based cineangiographic data, chiefly in the research setting, with promising results. For example, assessment of subtle changes in arterial lumen morphology in serial studies of atherosclerosis progression or regression clearly requires quantitative analyses.[35, 36]

Noninvasive assessment of some portions of the coronary arterial tree and of coronary bypass grafts may be accomplished using fast CT,[37–39] MRI,[40] or echocardiography, particularly transesophageal approaches.[41] In particular, MRI and echocardiography permit the assessment of both luminal anatomy and blood flow. However, the methods do not currently challenge selective coronary angiography in assessing coronary anatomy throughout the vascular tree.

Recently, miniaturization of ultrasound transducers has permitted the development of catheter-mounted probes, allowing intravascular ultrasound examinations.[42, 43] These high-frequency devices yield images in which not only lumen but also arterial wall thickness and composition[43] may be evaluated. Some recent studies have shown abnormalities in wall (intimal) thickness in regions judged normal on angiography.[42] The ultimate value of these methods in the routine clinical management of individual patients remains to be determined.

An additional capability recently offered by modern cardiac imaging techniques is that of three-dimensional reconstruction of cardiac anatomy.[44] The clinician usually assesses the three-dimensional characteristics of the heart by mentally "reassembling" anatomic data from multiple echocardiographic or angiographic images. Three-dimensional computer-based reconstruction techniques seek to replace this process of mental reassembly with a computer-generated model of the heart capable of showing regional changes in chamber size, shape, and function. These advanced methods are now possible through the application of techniques involving digital processing of cardiac images. Promising results have been obtained by applying three-dimensional reconstruction approaches to data acquired from echocardiograms,[13, 45–47] CT scans,[48] MRI images,[49, 50] and tomographic radionuclide scans.[51] Further application of three-dimensional reconstruction and display technology should offer the clinician more precise assessment of cardiac anatomy from noninvasive imaging data. One clinical setting in which high-resolution tomographic imaging with three-dimensional reconstruction will probably be of increasing value is complex congenital heart disease. In particular, standard MRI is already making a contribution to the diagnosis of patients with congenital heart disease[52, 53]—especially after surgery—and three-dimensional reconstruction methods may add to the value of MRI in this setting. Imaging of the coronary arteries may also benefit from three-dimensional reconstructions of tomographic images.

Chamber Function

Ventricular systolic performance is an important determinant of prognosis in virtually all etiologies of heart disease. The choice of medical versus surgical therapy in coronary artery disease or in chronic valvular disease often depends, in part, on measurements of global left ventricular function, at rest and with exercise. Current approaches focus largely on systolic performance of the left ventricle. Ejection phase indices,[54] such as ejection fraction, give estimates of global ventricular performance based on data from echocardiograms, angiograms, radionuclide ventriculograms, CT scans, and MRI studies. Although clinically useful, ejection phase indices are highly dependent on afterload. Isovolumic phase indices,[54] such as dP/dt, are directly obtainable only with high-fidelity intraventricular pressure measurements and are affected to some extent by ventricular preload. Doppler echocardiography permits the accurate measurement of aortic outflow velocity patterns, which also offer insight into ventricular function and are particularly useful in serial studies.[55]

The evaluation of *regional* systolic ventricular performance (whether assessed with wall motion or with wall thickening) offers important insights into the extent of acute and chronic myocardial ischemic injury.[56] Coronary artery disease may be identified based on the visualization of transient regional ventricular contraction abnormalities during spontaneous chest discomfort or after exercise or pharmacologic stress.[57] Myocardium that is "stunned" or "hibernating" may exhibit persistent contraction abnormalities despite remaining viable. In this setting, stimulation of myocardium with infusion of catecholamines (e.g., dobutamine) may reveal improvement of wall contraction on echocardiography, yielding information on myocardial viability.[58]

Despite the widespread clinical use of global and regional systolic functional indices, important problems remain in their application. First is the aforementioned load dependence of most of these measures, which often makes comparisons of studies between patients, and even comparisons of serial studies in the same patient, difficult to interpret. The second problem is that measures of global ventricular function that depend on geometric assumptions in their calculation (e.g., angiographic and echocardiographic ejection fractions) may be inaccurate in patients whose ventricles do not conform to these ideal geometric figures. Echocardiographic, CT, and MRI methods based on Simpson's rule approximations reduce this dependence on geometric assumptions. This applies also to radionuclide ventriculography based solely on counts recovered from the left and right ventricular cavities, corresponding to cavitary blood volume. Thus, the approach does not rely on any geometric assumptions. Finally, regional left ventricular contraction patterns are heterogeneous in the normal heart,[59] and this heterogeneity must be considered during the interpretation of regional contraction patterns. A relatively new approach to assessing regional ventricular contraction is so-called magnetic resonance "tagging." In this approach, manipulation of the magnetic resonance pulse sequence selectively alters the magnetization of specific ventricular segments, causing them to display an intensity different from that of the surrounding myocardium. Thus, the motion of the specific tissue region can be followed throughout the heart cycle, permitting accurate, precise assessment of regional myocardial function.[60] This technique offers unusual insights into regional ventricular mechanics.

Because of these and other difficulties, research continues toward improvements in the assessment of left ventricular systolic function. Substantial recent work has been directed toward developing relatively load-independent indices of function. The left ventricular pressure-volume relationship has been used to generate end-systolic indices of ventricular function that appear to give information concerning inherent left ventricular contractility that is less load-dependent than that given by standard ejection phase indices.[54] Similarly, the increased geometric accuracy of left ventricular anatomic analysis by CT and MRI promises more accurate estimation of absolute left ventricular volumes as well as of ejection fraction. Finally, three-dimensional reconstruction techniques performed throughout the cardiac cycle may offer additional information in the assessment of left ventricular systolic function.

Assessment of right ventricular performance is even more complex, partly because of the unusual shape of the right ventricle, which precludes the use of simple geometric models for volumetric or ejection fraction analyses. Currently, first-pass radionuclide scintigraphy appears to be the most widely available accurate and reliable method of determining right ventricular ejection fraction.[61] Echocardiography offers information on right ventricular function,[62] and fast CT[15] and MRI[19, 20] appear to be accurate alternatives to radionuclide imaging for determining right ventricular function.

Although the largest body of work concerning left ventricular function has focused on systolic performance, the importance of diastolic function in cardiac symptoms and in therapeutic considerations has become increasingly clear. For example, pulmonary congestion and resultant dyspnea may occur as the result of elevated left ventricular diastolic pressure due to impaired left ventricular filling function, even in cases of normal or supernormal systolic performance. Often, the constellation of normal systolic and abnormal diastolic function is related to myocardial hypertrophy, as in hypertrophic cardiomyopathy or severe hypertensive heart disease.

Diastolic function has proved to be a difficult parameter to evaluate quantitatively in the clinical setting. Diastole comprises a complex series of events and does not constitute merely a passive phase of ventricular filling.[63] Isovolumic relaxation and early, rapid diastolic filling are related to active myocardial relaxation with transport of calcium into the sarcoplasmic reticulum. Following the active phases of isovolumic relaxation and rapid ventricular filling, a period of diastasis occurs, with a small volume of filling depending mainly on passive (elastic) properties of the left ventricular myocardium. Finally, in patients in sinus rhythm, atrial systole completes ventricular filling with the rapid addition of a variable bolus of blood, depending on atrial size and function as well as on left ventricular compliance. Because of these various diastolic phases, each with its own mechanism of ventricular filling, the interpretation of diastolic ventricular performance is complex. High-fidelity pressure measurement in the catheterization laboratory yields indices of isovolumic relaxation, such as $-dP/dt$. On the other hand, the measurement of left ventricular end-diastolic (or pulmonary artery wedge) pressure provides information on average or late diastolic filling. Finally, Doppler echocardiographic indices of diastolic function commonly provide information on early versus late relative filling.[64] The various mechanisms of ventricular filling responsible for the phases of diastolic function may make it difficult to compare functional parameters derived from different portions of diastole using different methods.

Some recent research in diastolic ventricular function has focused on measurement of intrinsic muscle properties with the use of finite element analysis methods and other techniques for assessing global and regional stress-strain characteristics of the myocardium. Finite element analysis techniques have been used with echocardiographic,[65] CT,[66] and angiographic[67] image data. The finite element method (a mathematical approach for assessing regional mechanical characteristics of complexly shaped objects) and other stress-strain analyses are computationally demanding and not available for routine clinical use. Thus, continuing attention is being directed to interpretation of global filling curves, such as those generated by echocardiographic, radionuclide, and CT techniques.

Like global systolic function, diastolic ventricular muscle function is load-dependent.[54] Furthermore, the regional pattern of left ventricular filling appears to be heterogeneous,[68] as is the pattern of regional systolic performance. Thus, the assessment of diastolic function is a complex process and remains a challenging task for imaging or hemodynamic-based techniques.

Valvular Function

The management of valvular heart disease accounts for an important portion of modern cardiovascular practice. The etiology of valvular disease is progressively changing, with less chronic rheumatic heart disease and a greater prevalence of degenerative and congenital disorders. Despite the change in etiology, however, the physiologic principles related to the assessment of valvular disorders remain similar to those that have been clarified over the past several decades. Clinical and physiologic assessment of stenotic valve lesions focuses on the estimation of transvalvular pressure drop (gradient) and of stenotic orifice area as well as evaluation of ventricular function. The evaluation of valvular regurgitation is oriented toward determination of the amount of regurgitation and its subsequent physiologic effects on atrial and ventricular function.

The laboratory evaluation of patients with stenotic valve lesions changed substantially with the development of accurate quantitative methods of Doppler echocardiography.[69] Pulsed, continuous-wave, and color Doppler echocardiography have had an important impact on the diagnostic process in patients with stenotic valve lesions.[70] Echocardiography can be used to accurately identify abnormal valvular morphology, to measure transvalvular gradient and valve area, and to identify other physiologic sequelae of the valve disorder, such as left ventricular hypertrophy related to aortic valve stenosis. Because the transvalvular gradient for any given stenotic orifice size is directly related to transvalvular flow, estimation of the blood volume passing through the orifice of interest is additional information required to fully assess the severity of valvular stenosis. Echocardiographic techniques have been developed to assess aortic valve orifice area based on the measurement of transvalvular flow and gradient. A variation of this approach, employing the so-called "continuity equation," has also been used for the diagnosis of the severity of aortic stenosis.[71] Mitral valve stenotic orifice area may be determined by direct imaging of the flow-limiting orifice in two-dimensional echocardiographic images of adequate quality as well as by estimation of valve area from mitral pressure half-time data.[72]

These echocardiographic methods of assessing stenotic valve areas and gradients are accurate enough to very reliably distinguish trivial from significant valvular stenosis. In intermediate degrees of stenosis, technical limitations of echocardiography may sometimes add enough variability to the measurements to make clinical decisions more difficult. For example, methods of assessing valve stenosis by echocardiography that depend on measurements of chamber or annular dimensions (to calculate flow volume) suffer from variability in these anatomic measurements introduced by the sometimes inadequate image quality of echocardiograms. This difficulty in measuring left ventricular outflow tract dimension, for example, probably explains some of the variability found in estimates of aortic valve areas by the continuity equation when compared with invasive hemodynamic data.[71] Although not performed in every patient with known or suspected valvular disease, TEE permits improved anatomic imaging of valves and great vessels. Further improvements in the technology of echocardiography are likely to continue to improve the precision and accuracy of assessment of stenotic valve severity. Overall, ultrasound continues to be the method of choice in the initial assessment of stenotic lesions. In expert hands, echocardiographic assessment permits decisions to be made regarding the need for valve surgery without additional invasive hemodynamic or angiographic studies.

The assessment of valvular regurgitation is more complex than that of valvular stenosis. The degree of regurgitation through a particular valve depends on several factors, including the size of the regurgitant orifice, cardiac function, the resistance of the downstream vascular bed, and the compliance of the chamber receiving the regurgitant flow. The most widely used laboratory technique for identification of valvular regurgitation is echocardiography. Both transthoracic echocardiography and TEE are useful in the assessment of valvular regurgitation. In addition to its use in the diagnosis of valvular regurgitation, TEE is useful intraoperatively to assess the results of valvular repair. Doppler techniques may be used to identify regurgitation and to offer a semiquantitative assessment of its severity.[73] The advent of color Doppler flow mapping techniques has added spatial information to the semiquantitative assessment of valvular regurgitation.[74] Doppler estimates compare favorably with angiographic parameters of valvular regurgitation.[73] Angiographic estimates, however, which are commonly used as an independent standard, are themselves subjective, imprecise,[75] and likely to depend on loading conditions and other factors. Thus, an important goal of recent research in assessing valvular regurgitation has been to develop more quantitative indices of regurgitation based on noninvasive measurements of regurgitant volume or fraction,[76] regurgitant orifice size, and other parameters. The precise geometric measurements necessary for calculation of biventricular stroke volumes, which are needed to estimate regurgitant volume and fraction, may be achieved through the use of echocardiographic, CT, or MRI techniques. Doppler ultrasound permits as-

sessment of regurgitation severity based on other attributes of regurgitant flow dynamics, such as a measure of flow convergence as the blood nears the orifice of the incompetent valve.[77] Improving the assessment of valvular regurgitation remains an important diagnostic goal for cardiac imaging.

Myocardial Perfusion

The present emphasis on interventional maneuvers (e.g., thrombolysis, angioplasty, atherectomy) in coronary artery disease has intensified the desire to obtain accurate and reproducible estimates of regional myocardial perfusion. The currently available imaging techniques do not permit determination of absolute regional perfusion. The assessment of epicardial coronary arterial anatomy with the use of angiographic techniques is a commonly employed indirect method of predicting abnormalities in regional coronary flow and flow reserve. Clinicians commonly interpret severe coronary artery stenosis (e.g., greater than 50 percent reduction in luminal diameter) as indicating a hydraulically significant obstruction likely to lead to perfusion deficits under conditions of stress. As alluded to previously, however, visual assessment of percent diameter stenosis is not always an accurate indication of the physiologic significance of individual coronary stenoses, particularly in the common setting of diffuse, multivessel coronary disease.[31]

Semiquantitative estimates of perfusion may be obtained through use of inert gas washout methods as well as coronary sinus thermodilution techniques.[78] Although both inert gas washout and selective cardiac vein sampling have been used to estimate regional ventricular perfusion, these methods are beset by a variety of difficulties that discourage their common clinical use.[78] Myocardial perfusion imaging with thallium-201 (^{201}Tl) or technetium-99m (^{99m}Tc) sestamibi is the only commonly available method used to depict the relative distribution of myocardial blood flow and, thus, to identify regional defects in myocardial perfusion. However, the approach does not offer information on absolute regional perfusion. Although this modality is widely employed, images of myocardial perfusion obtained with these agents may also suffer from photon attenuation and thus demonstrate false or artifactual perfusion abnormalities.

Several approaches, still investigational, have recently been introduced as means of estimating regional myocardial perfusion. These approaches may be divided into those that evaluate the kinetics of an indicator traversing the cardiac microvasculature and those that evaluate myocyte uptake of an indicator. Several different substances can be used as indicators for the study of regional perfusion via analysis of tracer transit through the coronary circulation. These indicators include iodinated contrast material studied with radiographic or CT imaging systems,[79, 80] ultrasonic contrast material studied with echocardiographic imaging techniques,[81, 82] and magnetic resonance contrast agents studied with MRI.[83, 84] Whether the imaging sensor is an x-ray image intensifier, a CT detector, an echocardiographic transducer, or an MRI coil, the resulting data frequently consist of indicator appearance and washout curves, which may be evaluated with the use of the mathematics of indicator-dilution theory.[85] Thus, to yield accurate estimates of perfusion, the indicator and subsequent imaging procedure must follow the assumptions of indicator-dilution theory. These assumptions are satisfied to varying degrees by the different imaging methods. For example, some early attempts at CT-based perfusion measurements were hampered by factors such as the prolonged duration of initial indicator appearance (the so-called input function) after intravenous infusion.[86] The perfusion estimate has been rendered more accurate by aortic root injection of a contrast agent, resulting in reasonably accurate calculation of absolute perfusion by CT.[87] Other improvements in the estimation of myocardial perfusion by CT continue to be reported.[80]

At present, the most mature approach to estimating absolute regional myocardial blood flow is the use of positron-emitting tracers of blood flow with dynamic positron emission tomography (PET). Partially extracted tracers such as nitrogen-13 (^{13}N)-ammonia and rubidium-82 (^{82}Rb) and freely diffusible tracers such as oxygen-15 (^{15}O)-water have been used to measure myocardial perfusion.[88] Although not very widely available, the PET methods offer estimates of regional perfusion in milliliters per minute per gram of myocardium in the clinical setting.

Magnetic resonance techniques may also supply data on myocardial perfusion through the use of contrast agents. These contrast substances shorten proton nuclear magnetic resonance relaxation time in areas of normal perfusion, and in the future, contrast-enhanced MRI techniques may become clinically useful as methods of assessing myocardial perfusion in a quantitative, noninvasive fashion.[84]

Myocardial Metabolism

One of the important unmet goals of cardiac diagnosis is the evaluation of the biochemistry of myocardium in patients with heart disease. Cardiac metabolism represents the link between perfusion and mechanical function and is of importance in virtually all cardiac disorders, including ischemic, valvular, myopathic, and congenital diseases. Until recently, virtually no information on myocardial metabolism was available clinically except for the calculation of lactate extraction via coronary sinus sampling methods.

Again, the recent emphasis on interventional techniques in acute myocardial ischemia has intensified the search for methods of noninvasive evaluation of salient aspects of myocardial metabolism. The reason for this intensified effort may be demonstrated by consideration of a clinical scenario. A patient presents for evaluation with severe chest discomfort and a history of known coronary heart disease. An abnormal electrocardiogram may be the result of prior ischemic injury; electrocardiographic conduction abnormalities may make even this determination difficult. Assessment of regional myocardial contraction may reveal regional wall motion disturbances. These wall motion abnormalities are nonspecific, however, and may be found in acute ischemia, acute and chronic myocardial infarction, and stunned or hibernating tissue. Abnormal levels of serum cardiac enzymes indicate injury but do not localize its site. Finally, even if measurements of myocardial perfusion were widely available, an area of decreased perfusion could represent acute injury, prior infarction in an area now replaced with scar, or a mixture of both. Only the assessment of regional myocardial metabolism or direct evaluation of tissue characteristics (discussed later) could differentiate chronic from acute injury in this setting. The addition of a measure of substrate uptake to the determination of perfusion has helped differentiate irreversibly damaged from potentially viable myocardium in acute and chronic ischemic settings.[59, 90] Hypoperfused but viable tissue exhibits a decrement in perfusion on PET scans performed with a tracer of perfusion but demonstrates normal or increased uptake of glucose (a so-called "mismatch"). On the other hand, irreversibly damaged tissue exhibits a concordant decrease in both perfusion and fuel substrate uptake.[90]

Various aspects of myocardial metabolism can be evaluated by different techniques. Both single-photon emission computed tomography (SPECT) and PET methods may be used to assess the uptake and turnover of myocardial fuel substrates, such as fatty acids and their analogues.[91] Other aspects of substrate or intermediary metabolism such as glucose utilization,[92] oxidative metabolism,[93] and adrenergic receptor characteristics[94] may also be studied with PET techniques. Magnetic resonance spectroscopy, especially that employing phosphorus-31 (^{31}P), offers important insights into myocardial bioenergetics, specifically the metabolism of high-energy phosphate compounds.[95–98] Proton and carbon spectroscopy also may offer data on aspects of intermediary metabolism and on other myocardial biochemical features of clinical interest.

These evolving technologies are likely to provide new insights into disease-specific abnormalities of myocardial substrate and energy metabolism. They offer the possibility of demonstrating, localizing, and measuring the metabolic consequences of structural abnormalities as well as the effects of treatment. Conversely, they offer the possibility of identifying metabolic abnormalities that ultimately result in structural changes; thus, they may permit early detection of disease. At the same time, they may offer new and important insights into the physiology of the human heart.

At present, none of the emerging methods of myocardial metabolic imaging is widely available, although PET systems are commercially obtainable and are in use in many academic medical centers in the United States for both research and direct clinical applications. Recent research in metabolic imaging has brought the clinician far closer to the goal of assessing the biochemistry of the myocardium in health and disease.

Tissue Characterization

Just as assessment of perfusion and metabolism represents the link between myocardial vascular and cellular function, research into "tissue characterization" may supply definitive data on the physical status or composition of the myocardium. The goal of tissue characterization is to identify abnormalities in myocardial architecture (as in hypertrophic cardiomyopathy) or material properties (as in ischemia), the deposition of abnormal substances (as in amyloidosis), and the replacement of myocardium with collagen (as in chronic infarction).

Currently, information on regional myocardial tissue characteristics is inferred by indirect means, such as the observation of abnormalities in regional wall motion or the lack of uptake of ^{201}Tl or ^{99m}Tc-sestamibi. Abnormalities in wall motion not related to acute myocardial ischemia may be attributed to previous injury and subsequent scar formation. Decreased wall thickness is also suggestive of fibrosis. A deficit in regional ^{201}Tl uptake that is not reversible after a period of rest or after administration of an additional dose of tracer (reinjection) is commonly assumed to represent scar. Unfortunately, both of these findings are nonspecific. For example, investigators have estimated that as many as 50 percent of regions demonstrating "fixed" defects of thallium uptake may, in fact, represent chronically ischemic but potentially viable tissue.[99] The only currently available method of directly identifying myocardial tissue abnormalities in vivo is endomyocardial biopsy. This technique is useful but is limited by the shallowness of the biopsy, by other sampling problems, and by the invasiveness of the method. Thus, the goal of tissue characterization research is to identify directly, but in a noninvasive fashion, abnormalities in the composition or physical state of myocardium.

The two methods that appear most promising for noninvasive tissue characterization are ultrasound and MRI. Ultrasound interacts differently with abnormal versus normal myocardium. For example, ultrasound is reflected more strongly by acutely ischemic and infarcted tissue than by normal tissue; it is strongly reflected by scar from infarction as well.[100, 101] Similarly, changes in the two-dimensional pattern or "texture" of tissue echoes imaged on standard two-dimensional echocardiograms may indicate the presence of infarction, or of specific cardiomyopathies such as amyloidosis or hypertrophic cardiomyopathy.[102] Ultrasound tissue characterization techniques have also been used successfully in intravascular studies to identify atheroma and calcification in vessel wall.[43] Based on these and other promising data, investigative efforts continue into methods of ultrasound tissue characterization.

Magnetic resonance methods offer a great wealth of information on cardiac anatomy, function, and, perhaps, perfusion as the result of high-resolution imaging techniques. In addition, as mentioned previously, spectroscopic methods may provide unique information on myocardial metabolism. In addition to these lines of information, magnetic resonance techniques may also be useful in tissue characterization through the study of proton relaxation times. Spin-lattice (T1) or spin-spin (T2) relaxation times are altered by a variety of changes in tissue structure, including ischemia and infarction.[103–107] Although the precise mechanisms of alteration of magnetic resonance relaxation in ischemic disease are not yet fully elucidated, the use of MRI techniques for tissue characterization appears promising.

CONCLUSIONS

Modern cardiac imaging techniques represent the predominant laboratory methods of diagnosis in the mid-1990s. The field of cardiac imaging currently resides at the threshold between structural-functional imaging and the assessment of myocardial perfusion, metabolism, and tissue characteristics. The extremely promising results of recent research into all these areas strongly suggest that all five goals of cardiac imaging will soon be realized to some extent for clinical use.

References

1. Skorton, D.J., and Collins, S.M.: New directions in cardiac imaging. Ann. Intern. Med. 102:795, 1985.
2. Marcus, M.L., Wilson, R.F., and White, C.W.: Methods of measurement of myocardial blood flow in patients: A critical review. Circulation 76:245, 1987.
3. Schelbert, H.R.: Blood flow and metabolism by PET. Cardiol. Clin. 12(2):303, 1994.
4. Syrota, A., and Jehenson, P.: Complementarity of magnetic resonance spectroscopy, positron emission tomography and single photon emission tomography for the in vivo investigation of human cardiac metabolism and neurotransmission. Eur. J. Nucl. Med. 18:897, 1991.
5. Vandenberg, B.F., and Skorton, D.J.: Ultrasound tissue characterization of the myocardium. In Chambers, J., and Monaghan, M.J. (eds.): Echocardiography: An International Review. New York, Oxford University Press, 1993, p. 83.
6. Schiller, N.B., Shah, P.M., Crawford, M., et al.: American Society of Echocardiography Committee on Standards, Subcommittee on Quantitation of Two-Dimensional Echocardiograms: Recommendations for quantitation of the left ventricle by two-dimensional echocardiography. J. Am. Soc. Echocardiogr. 2:358, 1989.
7. Stadius, M.L., Williams, D.L., Harp, G., et al.: Left ventricular volume determination using single-photon emission computed tomography. Am. J. Cardiol. 55:1185, 1985.
8. Wynne, J., Green, L.H., Mann, T., et al.: Estimation of left ventricular volumes in man from biplane cineangiograms filmed in oblique projections. Am. J. Cardiol. 41:726, 1978.
9. Devereux, R.B., and Reichek, N.: Echocardiographic determinants of LV mass in man: Anatomic validation of the method. Circulation 55:613, 1977.
10. Rackley, C.E., Dodge, H.T., Coble, Y.D., Jr., et al.: A method for determining left ventricular mass in man. Circulation 29:666, 1964.
11. Liebson, P.R., Devereux, R.B., and Horan, M.J.: Hypertension research: Echocardiography in the measurement of LV wall mass. Hypertension 9(Suppl. II):2, 1987.
12. Seward, J.B., Khandheria, B.K., Oh, J.K., et al.: Transesophageal echocardiography: Technique, anatomic correlations, implementation and clinical applications. Mayo Clin. Proc. 63:649, 1988.
13. Roelandt, J.R., ten Cate, F.J., Vletter, W.B., et al.: Ultrasonic dynamic three-dimensional visualization of the heart with a multiplane transesophageal imaging transducer. J. Am. Soc. Echocardiogr. 7(3 Pt. 1):217, 1994.
14. Aebischer, N.M., and Czegledy, F.: Determination of right ventricular volume by two-dimensional echocardiography with a crescentic model. J. Am. Soc. Echocardiogr. 2:110, 1989.
15. Reiter, S.J., Rumberger, J.A., Feiring, A.J., et al.: Precision of measurements of right and left ventricular volume by cine computed tomography. Circulation 74:890, 1986.
16. Feiring, A.J., Rumberger, J.A., Reiter, S.J., et al.: Determination of left ventricular mass in dogs with rapid-acquisition cardiac computed tomographic scanning. Circulation 72:1355, 1985.
17. Roig, E., Georgiou, D., Chomka, E.V., et al.: Reproducibility of left ventricular myocardial volume and mass measurements by ultrafast computed tomography. J. Am. Coll. Cardiol. 18:990, 1991.
18. Florentine, M.S., Grosskreutz, C.L., Chang, W., et al.: Measurement of left ventricular mass in vivo using gated nuclear magnetic resonance imaging. J. Am. Coll. Cardiol. 8:107, 1986.
19. Kondo, C., Caputo, G.R., Semelka, R., et al.: Right and left ventricular stroke volume measurements with velocity-encoded cine MR imaging: In vitro and in vivo validation. AJR 157:9, 1991.
20. Pattynama, P.M.T., Lamb, H.J., Van der Geest, R., et al.: Reproducibility of measurements of right ventricular volumes and myocardial mass with MR imaging. Magn. Reson. Imaging 13:53, 1995.
21. Hunter, G.J., Hamberg, L.M., Weisskoff, R.M., et al.: Measurement of stroke volume and cardiac output within a single breath hold with echo-planar MR imaging. J. Magn. Reson. Imaging 4:51, 1994.
22. Pearlman, J.D., and Edelman, R.R.: Ultrafast magnetic resonance imaging: Segmented turboflash, echo-planar, and real-time nuclear magnetic resonance. Radiol. Clin. North Am. 32:593, 1994.
23. Lieberman, A.N., Weiss, J.L., Jugdutt, B.J., et al.: Two-dimensional echocardiog-

raphy and infarct size: Relationship of regional wall motion and thickening to the extent of myocardial infarction in the dog. Circulation 63:739, 1981.
24. Stanford, W., Galvin, J.R., Weiss, R.M., et al.: Ultrafast computed tomography in cardiac imaging: A review. Semin. Ultrasound CT MR 12:45, 1991.
25. Peshock, R.M., Rokey, R., Malloy, C.M., et al.: Assessment of myocardial systolic wall thickening using nuclear magnetic resonance imaging. J. Am. Coll. Cardiol. 14:653, 1989.
26. Khandheria, B.K., Tajik, A.J., Taylor, C.L., et al.: Aortic dissection: Review of value and limitations of two-dimensional echocardiography in a six-year experience. J. Am. Soc. Echocardiogr. 2:17, 1989.
27. Smith, M.D., Cassidy, J.M., Souther, S., et al.: Transesophageal echocardiography in the diagnosis of traumatic rupture of the aorta. N. Engl. J. Med. 332:356, 1995.
28. Thompson, B.H., and Stanford W.: Utility of ultrafast computed tomography in the detection of thoracic aortic aneurysms and dissections. Semin. Ultrasound CT MR 14:117, 1993.
29. Link, K.M., and Lesko, N.M.: The role of MR imaging in the evaluation of acquired disease of the thoracic aorta. AJR 158:1115, 1992.
30. Zir, L.M., Miller, S.W., Dinsmore, R.E., et al.: Interobserver variability in coronary angiography. Circulation 53:627, 1976.
31. White, C.W., Wright, C.B., Doty, D.B., et al.: Does the visual interpretation of the coronary arteriogram predict the physiological significance of a coronary stenosis? N. Engl. J. Med. 310:819, 1984.
32. Fleagle, S.R., Johnson, M.R., Wilbricht, C.J., et al.: Automated analysis of coronary arterial morphology in cineangiograms: Geometric and physiologic validation in humans. IEEE Trans. Med. Imag. 8:387, 1989.
33. Reiber, J.H.C.: Morphologic and densitometric quantitation of coronary stenoses: An overview of existing quantitation techniques. In Reiber, J.H.C., and Serruys, P.W. (eds.): New Developments in Quantitative Coronary Arteriography. Dordrecht, Kluwer Academic, 1988, p. 34.
34. Brown, B.G., Bolson, E., Frimer, M., et al.: Quantitative coronary arteriography: Estimation of dimensions, hemodynamic resistance, and atheroma mass of coronary artery lesions using the arteriogram and digital computation. Circulation 55:329, 1977.
35. Hong, M.K., Mintz, G.S., Popma, J.J., et al.: Limitations of angiography for analyzing coronary atherosclerosis progression or regression. Ann. Intern. Med. 121:348, 1994.
36. Brown, G., Albers, J.J., Fisher, L.D., et al.: Regression of coronary artery disease as a result of intensive lipid-lowering therapy in men with high levels of apolipoprotein B. N. Engl. J. Med. 323:1289, 1990.
37. Napel, S., Rutt, B.K., and Pflugfelder, P.: Three-dimensional images of the coronary arteries from ultrafast computed tomography: Method and comparison with two-dimensional arteriography. Am. J. Card. Imaging 3:237, 1989.
38. Stanford, W., Brundage, B.H., MacMillan, R., et al.: Sensitivity and specificity of assessing coronary bypass graft patency with ultrafast computed tomography: Results of a multicenter study. J. Am. Coll. Cardiol. 12:1, 1988.
39. Stanford, W., Galvin, J.R., Thompson, B.H., et al.: Nonangiographic assessment of coronary artery bypass graft patency. Int. J. Card. Imaging 9:77, 1993.
40. Manning, W.J., Li, W., and Edelman, R.R.: A preliminary report comparing magnetic resonance coronary angiography with conventional angiography. N. Engl. J. Med. 328:828, 1993.
41. Iliceto, S., Marangelli, V., Memmola, C., et al.: Transesophageal Doppler echocardiography evaluation of coronary blood flow velocity in baseline conditions and during dipyridamole-induced coronary vasodilation. Circulation 83:61, 1991.
42. St. Goar, F.G., Pinto, F.J., Alderman, E.L., et al.: Intracoronary ultrasound in cardiac transplant recipients: In vivo evidence of "angiographically silent" intimal thickening. Circulation 85:979, 1992.
43. Linker, D.T., Kleven, A., Grønningsæther, ÅA., et al.: Tissue characterization with intra-arterial ultrasound: Special promise and problems. Int. J. Card. Imaging 6:255, 1991.
44. Collins, S.M., Chandran, K.B., and Skorton, D.J.: Three-dimensional cardiac imaging. Echocardiography 5:311, 1988.
45. Moritz, W.E., Pearlman, A.S., McCabe, D.H., et al.: An ultrasonic technique for imaging the ventricle in three dimensions and calculating its volume. IEEE Trans. Biomed. Eng. 30:482, 1983.
46. Gopal, A.S., Keller, A.M., Rigling, R., et al.: Left ventricular volume and endocardial surface area by three-dimensional echocardiography: Comparison with two-dimensional echocardiography and nuclear magnetic resonance imaging in normal subjects. J. Am. Coll. Cardiol. 22:258, 1993.
47. Schneider, A.T., Hsu, T.L., Schwartz, S.L., et al.: Single, biplane, multiplane, and three-dimensional transesophageal echocardiography. Cardiol. Clin. 11:361, 1993.
48. Collins, S.M., Yashodhar, P., Rumberger, J.A., et al.: Three-dimensional reconstruction of the contracting canine heart using cine computed tomography. 1985 Computers in Cardiology. Long Beach, CA, IEEE Computer Society, 1985, p. 67.
49. Laschinger, J.C., Vannier, M.W., Gronemeyer, S., et al.: Noninvasive three-dimensional reconstruction of the heart and great vessels by ECG-gated magnetic resonance imaging: A new diagnostic modality. Ann. Thorac. Surg. 45:505, 1988.
50. Kuwahara, M., and Eiho, S.: 3D heart image reconstructed from MRI data. Comput. Med. Imaging Graph. 15:241, 1991.
51. Miller, T.R., Starren, J.B., and Grothe, R.A., Jr.: Three-dimensional display of positron emission tomography of the heart. J. Nucl. Med. 29:530, 1988.
52. White, R.D.: Magnetic resonance imaging of congenital heart disease. In Pohost, G.M. (ed.): Cardiovascular Applications of Magnetic Resonance. Mt. Kisco, NY, Futura Publishing Company, 1993, p. 59.
53. Link, K.M., and Lesko, N.M.: Magnetic resonance imaging in the evaluation of congenital heart disease. Magn. Reson. Q. 7:173, 1991.

54. Braunwald, E.: Assessment of cardiac function. *In* Braunwald, E. (ed.): Heart Disease: A Textbook of Cardiovascular Medicine. 4th ed. Philadelphia, W.B. Saunders, 1992, p. 419.

55. Berk, M.R., Evans, J., Knapp, C., et al.: Influence of alterations in loading produced by lower body negative pressure on aortic blood flow acceleration. J. Am. Coll. Cardiol. 15:1069, 1990.

56. Collins, S.M., Kerber, R.E., and Skorton, D.J.: Quantitative analysis of left ventricular regional function by imaging methods. *In* Miller, D.D. (ed.): Clinical Cardiac Imaging. New York, McGraw-Hill, 1988, p. 223.

57. Ryan, T., Segar, D.S., Sawada, S.G., et al.: Detection of coronary artery disease using upright bicycle exercise echocardiography. J. Am. Soc. Echocardiogr. 6:186, 1993.

58. LaCanna, G., Alfieri, O., Giubbini, R., et al.: Echocardiography during infusion of dobutamine for identification of reversible dysfunction in patients with chronic coronary artery disease. J. Am. Coll. Cardiol. 23:617, 1994.

59. Feiring, A.J., Rumberger, J.A., Reiter, S.J., et al.: Sectional and segmental variability of left ventricular function: Experimental and clinical studies using ultrafast computed tomography. J. Am. Coll. Cardiol. 12:415, 1988.

60. Young, A.A., Imai, H., Chang, C.N., et al.: Two-dimensional left ventricular deformation during systole using magnetic resonance imaging with spatial modulation of magnetization. Circulation 89:740, 1994.

61. Rezai, K., Weiss, R., Stanford, W., et al.: Relative accuracy of three scintigraphic methods for determination of right ventricular ejection fraction: A correlative study with ultrafast CT. J. Nucl. Med. 32:429, 1991.

62. Tomita, M., Masuda, H., Sumi, T., et al.: Estimation of right ventricular volume by modified echocardiographic subtraction method. Am. Heart J. 123:1011, 1992.

63. Gilbert, J.C., and Glantz, S.A.: Determinants of left ventricular filling and of the diastolic pressure-volume relation. Circ. Res. 64:827, 1989.

64. St. Goar, F.G., Masuyama, T., Alderman, E.L., et al.: Left ventricular diastolic dysfunction in end-stage dilated cardiomyopathy: Simultaneous Doppler echocardiography and hemodynamic evaluation. J. Am. Soc. Echocardiogr. 4:349, 1991.

65. McPherson, D.D., Skorton, D.J., Kodiyalam, S., et al.: Finite element analysis of myocardial diastolic function using three-dimensional echocardiographic reconstructions: Application of a new method for study of acute ischemia in dogs. Circ. Res. 60:674, 1987.

66. Pao, Y.C., and Ritman, E.L.: Estimation of passive and active muscle properties of working heart. *In* Proceedings of the International Conference on Finite Elements in Biomechanics. Tucson, AZ, 1980. Vol. 2. 1980, p. 657.

67. Ray, G., Chandran, K.B., Nikravesh, P.E., et al.: Estimation of local elastic modulus of the normal and infarcted left ventricle from angiographic data. *In* Saha, S. (ed.): Proceedings of the 4th New England Bioengineering Conference. Elmsford, NY, Pergamon Press, 1976, p. 173.

68. Rumberger, J.A., Weiss, R.M., Feiring, A.J., et al.: Patterns of regional diastolic function in the normal human left ventricle: An ultrafast computed tomography study. J. Am. Coll. Cardiol. 14:119, 1989.

69. Hatle, L., and Angelsen, B. (eds.): Doppler Ultrasound in Cardiology: Physical Principles and Clinical Applications. 3rd ed. Philadelphia, Lea & Febiger, 1994.

70. van den Brink, R.B., Verheul, H.A., Hoedemaker, G., et al.: The value of Doppler echocardiography in the management of patients with valvular heart disease: Analysis of one year of clinical practice. J. Am. Soc. Echocardiogr. 4:109, 1991.

71. Otto, C.M., and Pearlman, A.S.: Doppler echocardiography in adults with symptomatic aortic stenosis: Diagnostic utility and cost-effectiveness. Arch. Intern. Med. 148:2553, 1988.

72. Hatle, L., Angelsen, B., and Tromsdal, A.: Noninvasive assessment of atrioventricular pressure half-time by Doppler ultrasound. Circulation 60:1096, 1979.

73. Enriquez-Sarano, M., Bailey, K.R., Seward, J.B., et al.: Quantitative Doppler assessment of valvular regurgitation. Circulation 87:841, 1993.

74. Chen, C., Koschyk, D., Brockhoff, C., et al.: Noninvasive estimation of regurgitant flow rate and volume in patients with mitral regurgitation by Doppler color mapping of accelerating flow field. J. Am. Coll. Cardiol. 21:374, 1993.

75. Croft, C.H., Lipscomb, K., Matthis, K., et al.: Limitations of qualitative grading in aortic or mitral regurgitation. Am. J. Cardiol. 53:1593, 1984.

76. Reiter, S.J., Rumberger, J.A., Stanford, W., et al.: Quantitative determination of aortic regurgitant volumes in dogs by ultrafast computed tomography. Circulation 76:728, 1987.

77. Bargiggia, G.S., Tronconi, L., Sahn, D.J., et al.: A new method for quantification of mitral regurgitation based on color flow Doppler imaging of flow convergence proximal to regurgitant orifice. Circulation 84:1481, 1991.

78. Marcus, M.L.: Methods of measuring coronary blood flow. *In* Marcus, M.L. (ed.): The Coronary Circulation in Health and Disease. New York, McGraw-Hill, 1983, p. 25.

79. Hodgson, J.McB., LeGrand, V., Bates, E.R., et al.: Validation in dogs of a rapid digital angiographic technique to measure relative coronary blood flow during routine cardiac catheterization. Am. J. Cardiol. 5:188, 1985.

80. Wolfkiel, C.J., and Brundage, B.H.: Measurement of myocardial blood flow by UFCT: Towards clinical applicability. Int. J. Card. Imaging 7:89, 1991.

81. Feinstein, S.B., Lang, R.M., Dick, C.D., et al.: Contrast echocardiography during coronary arteriography in humans: Perfusion and anatomic studies. J. Am. Coll. Cardiol. 11:59, 1988.

82. Kaul, S., Kelly, P., Oliner, J.D., et al.: Assessment of regional myocardial blood flow with myocardial contrast two-dimensional echocardiography. J. Am. Coll. Cardiol. 13:468, 1989.

83. Saeed, M., Wendland, M.F., Masui, T., et al.: Dual mechanisms for change in myocardial signal intensity by means of a single MR contrast medium: Dependence on concentration and pulse sequence. Radiology 186:175, 1993.

84. Edelman, R.R., and Li, W.: Contrast-enhanced echo-planar MR imaging of myocardial perfusion: Preliminary study in humans. Radiology 190:771, 1994.

85. Zierler, K.L.: Theoretical basis of indicator-dilution methods for measuring flow and volume. Circ. Res. 10:393, 1962.

86. Rumberger, J.A., Feiring, A.J., Lipton, M.J., et al.: Use of ultrafast CT to quantitate regional myocardial perfusion: A preliminary report. J. Am. Coll. Cardiol. 9:59, 1987.

87. Weiss, R.M., Otoadese, E.A., Noel, M.P., et al.: Quantitation of absolute regional myocardial perfusion using cine computed tomography. J. Am. Coll. Cardiol. 23:1186, 1994.

88. Kuhle, W., Porenta, G., Huang, S.C., et al.: Quantification of regional myocardial blood flow using ^{13}N-ammonia and reoriented dynamic positron emission tomographic imaging. Circulation 86:1004, 1992.

89. Brunken, R., Schwaiger, M., Grover-McKay, M., et al.: Positron emission tomography detects tissue metabolic activity in myocardial segments with persistent thallium perfusion defects. J. Am. Coll. Cardiol. 10:557, 1987.

90. Tillisch, J., Brunken, R., Marshall, R., et al.: Reversibility of cardiac wall-motion abnormalities predicted by positron tomography. N. Engl. J. Med. 314:884, 1986.

91. Schelbert, H.R., Henze, E., Sochor, H., et al.: Effects of substrate availability on myocardial C-11 palmitate kinetics by positron emission tomography in normal subjects and patients with ventricular dysfunction. Am. Heart J. 111:1055, 1986.

92. Choi, Y., Brunken, R., Hawkins, R., et al.: Factors affecting myocardial 2-[F-18]fluoro-2-deoxy-D-glucose uptake in positron emission tomography studies of normal humans. Eur. J. Nucl. Med. 20:308, 1993.

93. Armbrecht, J.J., Buxton, D.B., Brunken, R.C., et al.: Regional myocardial oxygen consumption determined noninvasively in humans with [1-^{11}C] acetate and dynamic positron tomography. Circulation 80:863, 1989.

94. Merlet, P., Delforge, J., Syrota, A., et al.: Positron emission tomography with ^{11}C CGP-12177 to assess β-adrenergic receptor concentration in idiopathic dilated cardiomyopathy. Circulation 87:1169, 1993.

95. de Roos, A., Doornbos, J., Rebergen, S., et al.: Cardiovascular applications of magnetic resonance imaging and phosphorus-31 spectroscopy. Eur. J. Radiol. 14:97, 1992.

96. Bottomley, P.A., Hardy, C.J., and Roemer, P.B.: Phosphate metabolite imaging and concentration measurements in human heart by nuclear magnetic resonance. Magn. Reson. Med. 14:425, 1990.

97. Scholz, T.D., Grover-McKay, M., Fleagle, S.R., et al.: Quantitation of the extent of acute myocardial infarction by phosphorus-31 nuclear magnetic resonance spectroscopy. J. Am. Coll. Cardiol. 18:1380, 1991.

98. Bottomley, P.A.: MR spectroscopy of the human heart: The status and the challenges. Radiology 191:593, 1994.

99. Liu, P., Kiess, M.C., Okada, R.D., et al.: The persistent defect on exercise thallium imaging and its fate after myocardial revascularization: Does it represent scar or ischemia? Am. Heart J. 110:996, 1985.

100. Skorton, D.J., Melton, H.E., Jr., Pandian, N.G., et al.: Detection of acute myocardial infarction in closed-chest dogs by analysis of regional two-dimensional echocardiographic gray-level distributions. Circ. Res. 52:36, 1983.

101. Pérez, J.E., and Miller, J.G.: Ultrasonic backscatter tissue characterization in cardiac diagnosis. Clin. Cardiol. 14(Suppl. V):V-4, 1991.

102. Chandrasekaran, K., Aylward, P.E., Fleagle, S.R., et al.: Feasibility of identifying amyloid and hypertrophic cardiomyopathy with the use of computerized quantitative texture analysis of clinical echocardiographic data. J. Am. Coll. Cardiol. 13:832, 1989.

103. Johnston, D.L.: Myocardial tissue characterization with magnetic resonance imaging techniques. Am. J. Card. Imaging 8:140, 1994.

104. de Roos, A., van der Wall, E.E., Bruschke, A.V.G., et al.: Magnetic resonance imaging in the diagnosis and evaluation of myocardial infarction. Magn. Reson. Q. 7:191, 1991.

105. Saeed, M., Wendland, M.R., Yu, K.K., et al.: Identification of myocardial reperfusion with echo planar magnetic resonance imaging: Discrimination between occlusive and reperfused infarctions. Circulation 90:1492, 1994.

106. Wisenberg, G., Prato, F.S., Carroll, S.E., et al.: Serial nuclear magnetic resonance imaging of acute myocardial infarction with and without reperfusion. Am. Heart J. 115:510, 1988.

107. Reeves, R.C., Evanochko, W.T., Canby, R.C., et al.: Demonstration of increased myocardial lipid with postischemic dysfunction ("myocardial stunning") by proton nuclear magnetic resonance spectroscopy. J. Am. Coll. Cardiol. 13:739, 1989.

2 Principles of Myocardial Perfusion

Francis J. Klocke, M.D.
Michael W. Frank, M.D.

NORMAL CORONARY PHYSIOLOGY _____ 8
Determinants of Myocardial Oxygen Demand _____ 8
Clinical Indices of Myocardial Oxygen Demand _____ 8
Determinants of Coronary Blood Flow _____ 9
  Driving Pressure _____ 9
  Resistance (Impedance) _____ 9
    Basal Viscous Resistance (R_1) _____ 9
    Autoregulatory Resistance (R_2) _____ 9
    Compressive Resistance (R_3) _____ 10
Control of Autoregulatory Resistance _____ 10
Calculations of Coronary Resistance _____ 11
Steady-State Relationships Between Coronary Artery Pressure and Coronary Blood Flow _____ 11
Coronary Flow Reserve _____ 11
CORONARY ARTERY DISEASE _____ 11
Effects of Individual Stenotic Lesions _____ 11
Relation Between Flow and Stenosis Resistance _____ 12

Relation Between Degree of Stenosis and Stenosis Resistance: Importance of Small Changes in Caliber of Severe Stenoses _____ 12
Dynamic Changes in Stenosis Resistance _____ 12
Arterial Remodeling and Arteriographic Estimates of Stenosis Severity _____ 14
Coronary Flow Reserve in Coronary Artery Disease _____ 14
Use of Relative Rather than Absolute Flow Reserve in Perfusion Imaging _____ 14
Coronary Collateral Circulation _____ 15
CONSIDERATIONS IN CHOOSING AN IMAGING TECHNIQUE FOR CORONARY FLOW MEASUREMENT _____ 17
Technical Issues _____ 17
Analytical Issues _____ 17
Normal Spatial Variation of Myocardial Perfusion _____ 17
Validation Studies _____ 17

NORMAL CORONARY PHYSIOLOGY

Determinants of Myocardial Oxygen Demand

Any consideration of myocardial perfusion needs to emphasize the pivotal relationship between myocardial oxygen requirements and coronary blood flow[1] (Fig. 2–1). Because the heart has a limited and short-lived capacity for anaerobic metabolism, its steady-state metabolic needs can be considered solely in terms of oxidative metabolism. Oxygen extraction within the coronary circulation is high under basal conditions; that is, the oxygen saturation of coronary sinus blood is typically only 20 to 30 percent (corresponding to a Po_2 of approximately 20 mm Hg). Changes in myocardial oxygen demand therefore mandate quantitatively similar changes in coronary flow.

Although the determinants of myocardial oxygen demand are complex, approximately 80 percent of oxygen requirements are accounted for by the following three factors.[2]

Afterload

Afterload is defined as the stress, that is, the force per unit area, developed by myocardial fibers as they shorten. It is directly proportional to ventricular systolic pressure and radius of curvature and inversely proportional to myocardial wall thickness. As discussed later, systolic arterial pressure is often used clinically as an index of wall stress. Wall tension, that is, the force per unit length developed as myocardial fibers shorten, is a less frequent surrogate. In keeping with the lower systolic pressure in the right ventricle, right ventricular oxygen demand is normally a small fraction of that in the left ventricle.

Heart Rate

Effects of heart rate relate primarily to the number of contractions per minute. Increases in rate also have a small positive inotropic effect.

Contractility

Myocardial contractility is a major determinant of the heart's oxygen demand and can vary substantially with changes in inotropic state caused by hemodynamic or metabolic events or pharmacologic interventions. Quantitative assessments of contractility in humans remain problematic; among the numerous hemodynamic indices that have been proposed, peak ventricular dP/dt is probably used most commonly.

Experimental studies indicate that oxygen demand per gram of tissue is normally greater in the inner layers of the heart (subendocardium) than in the outer (subepicardium).[3, 4] The greater oxygen demand is accommodated by a greater flow per gram[5] and slightly larger oxygen extraction[6] in the subendocardium.

Clinical Indices of Myocardial Oxygen Demand

Clinically, attention most frequently focuses on the left ventricle. Because of the ease with which it can be measured, the "double product" of systemic arterial systolic pressure and heart rate is commonly used as an index of total left ventricular oxygen consumption. Although the double-product index does not deal directly with changes in contractile state, ventricular volume, or wall thickness, it has proven value in estimating increases in left ventricular oxygen demand during exercise testing.

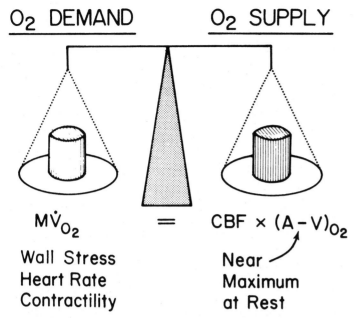

O₂ DEMAND — O₂ SUPPLY

$$M\dot{V}O_2 = CBF \times (A-V)O_2$$

Wall Stress
Heart Rate
Contractility

Near
Maximum
at Rest

FIGURE 2-1. Schematic representation of the normal balance between myocardial oxygen demand and supply. $M\dot{V}O_2$ = myocardial oxygen consumption; CBF = coronary blood flow; $(A-V)O_2$ = coronary arteriovenous oxygen difference. (From Klocke, F. J., and Ellis, A. K.: Physiology of the coronary circulation. *In* Parmley, W. W., and Chatterjee, K. [eds.]: Cardiology. Philadelphia, J.B. Lippincott, 1990, p. 101, with permission.)

Determinants of Coronary Blood Flow

Driving Pressure

Driving pressure across the coronary bed has traditionally been taken as the difference between aortic and right atrial pressures or, because right atrial pressure is normally only a few millimeters of mercury, as aortic pressure alone. Some investigators believe that left ventricular diastolic pressure is a preferable index of the "backpressure" opposing coronary inflow, particularly in situations in which ventricular diastolic pressure is elevated. Studies in recent years have demonstrated that the minimum aortic pressure required for forward flow in the coronary bed is at least 2–5 mm Hg greater than right atrial or left ventricular diastolic pressure, even when the bed is maximally dilated.[7-9] Backpressure determined in this fashion is now commonly referred to as "zero-flow" pressure and is abbreviated as $P_{f=0}$ or P_{ZF}. With vasomotor tone operative, $P_{f=0}$ is substantially higher (e.g., 20 mm Hg) than during vasodilation and plays a dynamic, rather than static, role in coronary flow regulation.

The question of the appropriate value of "backpressure" bears importantly on calculations of coronary vascular resistance. Since $P_{f=0}$ cannot ordinarily be determined in clinical situations, values calculated with the use of right atrial or ventricular diastolic pressure are better viewed as indices, rather than as absolute values, of coronary resistance.

Resistance (Impedance)

Although impedance to coronary flow is usually considered only in terms of resistance, it also includes the effects of inertia and capacitance. Capacitive effects reflect fluctuations of intravascular volume during a cardiac cycle. Differences in the phasic patterns of coronary inflow and outflow are well known; that is, the preponderance of coronary inflow occurs during diastole, whereas coronary outflow is primarily systolic. Although these capacitive effects cancel out over the entire cardiac cycle, they affect instantaneous patterns of flow during the cycle and can alter normal flow patterns in situations such as aortic insufficiency.

There remains no question, however, that coronary vascular resistance is the single most important determinant of coronary flow. Coronary resistance can be modeled as the sum of three functional components (Fig. 2–2).

Basal Viscous Resistance (R_1)

Basal viscous resistance refers to the minimum possible resistance of the entire coronary bed. It corresponds to the resistance during diastole with the coronary vessels fully dilated and depends most importantly on the vascular cross-sectional area of the coronary bed. In situations such as ventricular hypertrophy, vascular cross-sectional area per unit weight of myocardium is reduced; that is, the degree of vascular proliferation is less than that of myocardial tissue. Basal viscous resistance also varies with viscosity. In addition, it is normally somewhat less in the inner (subendocardial) portion of the myocardial wall than in the outer; that is, there is an inherent transmural gradient of capillary density favoring the subendocardium.[10, 11]

Autoregulatory Resistance (R_2)

Autoregulatory resistance refers to the caliber of arterial and arteriolar vessels and the number of open capillaries. Although the caliber of conduit as well as resistance vessels can change in response to a variety of stimuli, approximately 75 percent of autoregulatory resistance arises from vessels less than 200 μm in diameter, that is, from arterioles.[12] Because resistance is inversely propor-

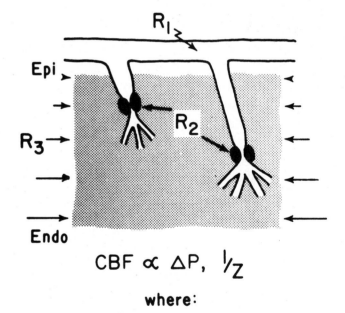

$$CBF \propto \Delta P, \frac{1}{Z}$$

where:

$$\Delta P = P_{Ao} - \text{"back pressure"}$$

Z = Impedance:

– Resistance ($R_{1,2,3}$)

– Capacitance

– Inertia

FIGURE 2-2. Schematic diagram of the coronary arterial circulation in the normal heart, illustrating the three functional components of coronary resistance. Epi = subepicardium; Endo = subendocardium; $R_{1,2,3}$ = viscous, autoregulatory, and compressive components of coronary resistance; ΔP = coronary driving pressure; P_{Ao} = aortic pressure; Z = coronary input impedance. (Adapted from Klocke, F. J., and Ellis, A. K.: Physiology of the coronary circulation. *In* Parmley, W. W., and Chatterjee, K. [eds.]: Cardiology. Philadelphia, J.B. Lippincott, 1990, p. 102, with permission.)

tional to the fourth power of vessel radius (Poiseuille's law), small changes in arteriolar dimension can affect autoregulatory resistance profoundly.

Changes in autoregulatory resistance represent the primary mechanism by which coronary flow adjusts to changing metabolic demand and is maintained constant in the face of changes in coronary artery pressure at a constant level of demand. Under basal conditions autoregulatory resistance is quite high; that is, there is normally sufficient vasodilator reserve to allow coronary flow to increase by a factor of 4 to 6 at normal levels of coronary arterial pressure.[13] The ability of autoregulatory resistance to decrease in response to increased myocardial oxygen demand or decreased coronary artery pressure has pivotal importance during stressful interventions and disease states. It also plays an important role in myocardial reactive hyperemia, that is, the increase in blood flow that follows a period of brief coronary occlusion[14] (Fig. 2–3). Changes in autoregulatory resistance are adjusted on a local basis; that is, hyperemia following a coronary occlusion occurs only in the distribution of the occluded artery.

Autoregulatory resistance plays an important role in the vulnerability of the subendocardium to myocardial ischemia.[15] Because myocardial oxygen demand is higher in the inner portions of the ventricular wall than in the outer portions, subendocardial flow needs to exceed subepicardial flow by approximately 20 percent. As noted below, subendocardial flow is limited by compressive resistance during systole. Therefore, diastolic flow in the subendocardium must exceed flow in the subepicardium by more than 20 percent if demand and flow are to remain in balance. (Although capillary density and oxygen extraction are higher in the subendocardium, these differences are insufficient in and of themselves to achieve the necessary increment in diastolic oxygen delivery.) Accordingly, autoregulatory vessels are relatively dilated under basal conditions, and coronary vasodilator reserve is normally less in the subendocardium than elsewhere.

Compressive Resistance (R_3)

Compressive resistance refers to the actions of local forces within the ventricular wall on the coronary blood vessels. The effects of compressive resistance are significant throughout the cardiac cycle but are especially large during systole; that is, coronary inflow is reduced to a small fraction of that occurring during diastole. The systolic effects of compressive resistance vary across the myocardial wall, in concert with the pressure difference between the ventricular cavity and the pericardial space. Because of the "throttling" effect of contraction on intramyocardial blood vessels, flow to the inner layers of myocardium is minimal during systole. Accordingly, the subendocardium is more vulnerable to ischemia than the subepicardium in situations in which inflow is limited, for example, coronary artery disease. Importantly, flow to the inner layers of myocardium can also be limited during diastole, when ventricular diastolic pressure is increased.[16]

Control of Autoregulatory Resistance

As noted previously, autoregulatory resistance is closely coupled to local metabolic activity and can be influenced by a variety of factors. In any given situation, several factors are likely to be acting in concert. These factors can be considered as follows.

Metabolic Factors

Adenosine, PO_2, PCO_2, pH, lactic acid, potassium, and phosphate each have been proposed, at various times, as the primary metabolic regulator of coronary resistance.[17] Over the years Berne and co-workers have amassed a large body of evidence favoring adenosine, which has proved to be a maximum coronary vasodilating agent in pharmacologic testing.[18] However, vasodilatory responses in vivo are little affected after administration of the enzyme adenosine deaminase, which converts adenosine to inosine, a vasoactively inert nucleoside. PO_2 and PCO_2 appear to play a significant but not exclusive role in response to changing metabolic demand.[19]

Neurohumoral Factors

Coronary arterial and arteriolar vessels are subject to neurohumoral influences through direct autonomic innervation as well as in response to agents reaching them through the coronary circulation.[17] Neural effects can be reflex as well as direct and are often difficult to separate from effects induced metabolically as the result of hemodynamic changes in myocardial oxygen demand.

Adrenergic innervation of coronary vessels involves both constrictor and dilator mechanisms. α-Adrenergic vasoconstriction is clearly important clinically as well as experimentally. Experimentally, α-adrenergic vasoconstriction has been shown to limit metabolically induced vasodilation during interventions that substantially increase myocardial metabolic demand, for example, treadmill exercise.[20] Clinically, it appears involved in at least some circumstances in which coronary vascular resistance fails to decrease (or even increases) in response to hemodynamic changes indicating an increased myocardial oxygen demand.[21, 22]

Myogenic Factors

Myogenic behavior refers to intrinsic responses of resistance vessels to changes in transmural pressure; that is, distention of a vessel by an increase in intraluminal pressure stimulates contraction of vascular smooth muscle, whereas a decrease in transmural pressure results in vasodilation. Myogenic behavior has now been convincingly demonstrated in coronary vessels and appears to be most prominent in smaller arterioles (80 to 100 μm in diameter).[23] It appears to play a particular role in maintaining flow constant during changes in coronary artery pressure.

Endothelial Factors

In the early 1980s it became apparent that the luminal size of epicardial (i.e., conduit) coronary arteries is influenced statically

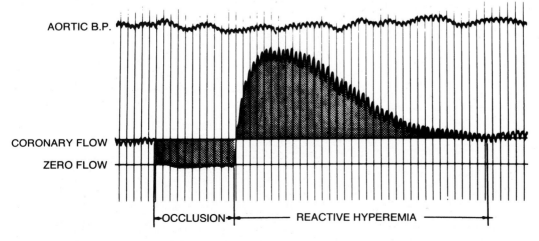

FIGURE 2–3. Coronary reactive hyperemia. Mean coronary artery pressure and flow are shown before, during, and after a brief period of coronary artery occlusion. Coronary flow rises severalfold above its preocclusion value during the postocclusion period. When the duration of occlusion is 20 seconds or more, the peak flow during the hyperemic period is thought to reflect maximal coronary vasodilation, that is, maximal coronary flow reserve. (Reprinted by permission from Olsson, R. A.: Myocardial reactive hyperemia. Circ. Res. 37:263–270, 1975.) (Copyright 1975, American Heart Association.)

AORTIC B.P.

CORONARY FLOW

ZERO FLOW

OCCLUSION ← → REACTIVE HYPEREMIA

and dynamically by vasoactive substances produced within the endothelium of the arterial wall. During the past few years it has also become clear that endothelium-derived factors influence the behavior of coronary resistance vessels.

The vasoactive factor referred to as "endothelium-derived relaxing factor" (EDRF) was identified by Furchgott and Zawadski in 1980[24] and is now known to be nitric oxide (or a closely related substance). It is synthesized continuously by coronary vascular endothelium and influences the degree of relaxation of adjacent vascular smooth muscle. In normal physiologic circumstances, the rate of EDRF production—and therefore the caliber of the coronary vascular lumen—is directly related to coronary blood flow. Changes in EDRF production accompanying changes in flow may be mediated mechanically, that is, by changes in shear stress at the endothelial surface. Also, EDRF plays a pivotal role in the effects of several clinically relevant agents, for example, acetylcholine, bradykinin, and substance P. When one of these substances is injected into a coronary artery, EDRF production normally increases, leading to vascular smooth muscle relaxation and vasodilation.

Prostacyclin is another important compound produced by coronary vascular endothelium.[25] This agent, which relaxes vascular smooth muscle and inhibits platelet aggregation, is produced through the cyclooxygenase enzyme complex, which also catalyzes the production of thromboxane A_2, a powerful vasoconstricting agent produced by blood platelets. It has been postulated that balance between endothelial production of prostacyclin and platelet production of thromboxane A_2 may play an important role in local hemostasis and vascular integrity. Coronary vascular endothelium interacts importantly with leukocytes, as well as with platelets. Leukotrienes, which originate from the same precursor as for prostaglandins and thromboxanes (arachidonic acid), are synthesized through the lipoxygenase, rather than the cyclooxygenase, enzyme system and demonstrate important vasoconstrictor activity. Endothelins are additional and uniquely powerful vasoconstricting peptides produced by endothelium. They, too, are under active study clinically as well as experimentally.[26]

Calculations of Coronary Resistance

At least 10 different approaches have been proposed for calculating coronary vascular resistance from measurements of pressure and flow.[27] Technical issues relate to the appropriate value of coronary backpressure; the use of mean versus instantaneous flow, or full-thickness versus subendocardial or subepicardial flow; and the effects of nonresistive components of impedance. Conceptual issues often arise when one is attempting to assess changes in vascular smooth muscle tone in a setting in which other components of resistance, for example, compressive resistance, may also vary. Because of these issues, modest changes in any calculated value of coronary resistance must be interpreted cautiously.

Steady-State Relationships Between Coronary Artery Pressure and Coronary Blood Flow

Figure 2–4 demonstrates steady-state relationships between coronary blood flow and mean coronary artery pressure at varying levels of myocardial oxygen demand.

Coronary Flow Reserve

Coronary flow reserve is defined as the ratio of flow during maximum vasodilation to flow under resting conditions, that is, immediately before vasodilation. As noted earlier, the coronary circulation normally has sufficient vasodilator reserve to allow flow in the left ventricle to increase by a factor of 4 to 6 at normal levels of coronary arterial pressure. The first accurate measurements of coronary reserve in humans were made by Marcus and colleagues in the early 1980s using, initially, an epicardial Doppler velocity probe in the operating room[13] and, subsequently, an intravascular Doppler probe in the cardiac catheterization laboratory.[28] In retrospect, earlier measurements in humans, reporting lower levels of reserve, were compromised by the use of less than maximum

vasomotor stimuli or measurement techniques that became inadequate at high levels of flow.

Factors Affecting Measured Values

Several factors can alter the value of coronary reserve in normal individuals as well as in patients.[29–31] Because flow varies directly with pressure during maximum vasodilation, the absolute value of flow reserve varies when vasodilation is accompanied by a change in arterial pressure. The flow-pressure relation during maximum vasodilation is also affected by the magnitude of compressive resistance, that is, heart rate and ventricular diastolic pressure, and by blood viscosity, that is, with anemia or polycythemia. Flow reserve may vary transmurally, in concert with transmural differences in the summated effects of the individual components of resistance. Finally, an increase in the "resting" level of flow causes a decrease in the calculated value of flow reserve independent of any other effects. These factors need to be considered when one interprets values of flow reserve, particularly when measurements are repeated in individuals or measurements between groups are compared.

Vasodilating Agents

The pharmacologic agents used to produce maximum coronary vasodilation clinically include intravenous dipyridamole, intravenous adenosine, intracoronary adenosine, and intracoronary papaverine. Dipyridamole acts by inhibiting cellular uptake and metabolism of endogenously produced adenosine. Maximal dilation is not achieved in a small percentage (10 to 25 percent) of patients, even when the standard dose (0.56 mg/kg over 4 minutes) is exceeded.[31] Because flow to abdominal viscera also increases, interfering effects of radioactivity in the liver and spleen on myocardial radionuclide scans can be greater than those during exercise tests. Possible side effects include nausea, emesis, dizziness, headache, perspiration, mild hypotension, tachycardia, and chest discomfort. Chest pain is occasionally severe (probably reflecting subendocardial ischemia due to a coronary "steal") and is accompanied by ST depression, ventricular dysfunction, or both. Although these effects can usually be reversed with intravenous aminophylline, dipyridamole is not recommended in unstable angina or acute ischemic states.

Intravenous adenosine has been used by several laboratories in recent years. Side effects similar to those of dipyridamole are viewed by some investigators as more common and troublesome. Impairment of sinus and/or atrioventricular nodal function is an additional concern. Adenosine effects usually abate within 1 to 2 minutes after the drug has been discontinued. Intracoronary adenosine is especially useful in invasive studies; systemic effects are noticeably less common when the smaller local dose is administered. Because intracoronary papaverine occasionally produces ventricular tachycardia, it is used less frequently.

Other pharmacologic agents, for example, nitroglycerin and nitroprusside, have not been shown to achieve maximum coronary vasodilation in the normal coronary vascular bed. The same is true of several interventions used reasonably frequently. Pacing-induced tachycardia provides only a modest stimulus for vasodilation (Fig. 2–4). The vasodilatory stimulus is normally also submaximal for interventions such as pacing plus handgrip, the cold pressor test, and the administration of radiographic contrast agent or catecholamines. The level of vasodilation occurring during treadmill or bicycle exercise can be substantially greater than that during these interventions, but it depends on the level of exercise and increment in myocardial oxygen demand achieved.

An additional important issue is that several flow measurement techniques become problematic when coronary flow increases more than two- to threefold. This point is discussed further subsequently.

CORONARY ARTERY DISEASE

Effects of Individual Stenotic Lesions

Important insights into the static and dynamic factors governing the functional effects of a coronary stenosis have developed during

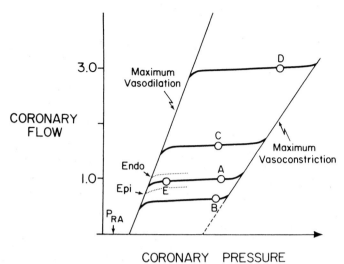

FIGURE 2–4. Steady-state relationships between coronary flow and coronary arterial pressure at varying levels of myocardial oxygen demand. The coronary bed can be considered to operate between the extremes of maximum vasodilation (*left, above*) and maximum vasoconstriction (*right, below*). Because the backpressure to coronary flow exceeds coronary venous pressure, the minimum coronary arterial pressure required for forward flow exceeds right atrial pressure by at least a few millimeters of mercury. The level of flow required to maintain an appropriate balance between myocardial oxygen demand and supply is determined by the level of myocardial metabolic activity. The heavy lines depict the average relationship between mean full-cycle flow and pressure for the entire myocardial wall at four levels of oxygen demand. The range of pressure over which flow remains relatively constant at any level of demand, that is, the "autoregulatory" range, lies between the bounds of maximum vasodilation and vasoconstriction. Point A may be considered to represent the normal basal condition, which is assigned a relative flow level of 1.0. Point B falls on a line corresponding to a lower metabolic demand and may represent the heart's operating point during the bradycardia of sleep. The reduced level of flow reflects autoregulatory vasoconstriction. Point C depicts a moderate increase in oxygen demand that may accompany pacing-induced tachycardia. There is relatively little change in arterial pressure, and the increase in flow primarily involves autoregulatory vasodilation. Point D represents a moderate level of muscular exercise. The increased myocardial metabolic demand causes coronary flow to increase to three times its resting value. The increased flow reflects a moderate increase in arterial pressure and a major decrease in autoregulatory resistance. Note that maximum vasodilation, which would correspond to at least a fivefold increment in flow at a normal level of coronary pressure, has not been reached. Point E represents an area of left ventricle perfused through a severely stenotic coronary artery. A pressure gradient across the stenotic lesion causes coronary pressure to be substantially less than simultaneous aortic pressure, which is at the level represented by point A. Flow in the area supplied by the stenotic artery is maintained at a normal (or nearly normal) level by vasodilation; that is, autoregulatory reserve is used to a greater degree than usual under resting conditions to maintain the normal supply-demand relationship. Transmural differences in flow (corresponding to transmural differences in demand) are shown by the dotted lines above and below the line depicting average values for the entire myocardium. Should poststenotic pressure fall further, or should metabolic demand increase, maximum vasodilation will occur earlier in the subendocardium. (From Klocke, F. J., and Ellis, A. K.: Physiology of the coronary circulation. *In* Parmley, W. W., and Chatterjee, K. [eds.]: Cardiology. Philadelphia, J.B. Lippincott, 1990, p. 105, with permission.)

1fpthe past 2 decades.[32–34] In considering these factors, it is helpful to view the stenotic lesion independently of the distal coronary bed and to focus on factors determining the pressure gradient across the stenosis—in the same fashion as is done for valvar aortic stenosis.

Figure 2–5 schematically illustrates factors governing energy losses and, therefore, pressure drop across a stenosis. The transstenotic gradient varies with flow and is potentially influenced by viscous losses, separation losses, and turbulence. Five points are noteworthy. First, separation losses are proportional to flow raised to the second power and become increasingly prominent as flow increases. Second, separation losses are also accentuated, in a nonlinear fashion, by increasing severity of stenosis. Third, for any given level of flow, the most important determinant of stenosis severity is the minimal cross-sectional area within the stenosis, which appears as a second-order term in the expression of both viscous and separation losses. Fourth, in evaluating an intervention that may change the resistance of a clinically important stenosis, emphasis ideally should be placed on the minimal cross-sectional area within the stenosis, expressed in absolute terms. Fifth, because the effects of stenosis length are manifested through viscous rather than separation losses, stenosis length usually plays a less important role than minimal cross-sectional area does in clinically important stenoses.

Relation Between Flow and Stenosis Resistance

As just discussed, when the transstenotic pressure gradient is plotted against flow, the relationship is curvilinear. As shown in Figure 2–6, stenosis resistance can be expressed as the tangent to this relationship at any given level of flow. As flow increases, stenosis resistance also increases, as reflected by the steeper slope of the tangent at the point of increased flow. Thus, the functional severity of even a rigid stenosis increases with effort, and the symptomatic implications of any stenotic lesion depend in part on the degree of activity a patient is likely to achieve. Flow-related increases in stenosis resistance contribute to effort-related angina.

Because the magnitude of pressure drop across a stenosis varies with flow, important changes in functional stenosis severity also occur during each cardiac cycle. Phasic measurements of pressure gradient and velocity are now possible in some clinical circumstances and should be included in experimental studies of stenosis behavior whenever possible.

Relation Between Degree of Stenosis and Stenosis Resistance: Importance of Small Changes in Caliber of Severe Stenoses

Figure 2–7 further explores the relation between transstenotic pressure gradient and flow. Pressure gradient is plotted against coronary flow, with relations shown for concentric stenoses 30, 50, 70, 80, and 90 percent in diameter. The tangents to the relations reflect stenosis resistance at a given level of flow. In the inset, individual values of stenosis resistance are plotted against degree of stenosis. Stenosis resistance increases relatively slowly in diameter narrowing below 70 percent, but then it almost doubles between 70 and 80 percent and doubles again between 80 and 90 percent. Even with technically excellent arteriograms, distinctions in degree of narrowing in this upper range of narrowing are difficult. It is not surprising, therefore, that patients with apparently similar lesions on arteriography can vary greatly in their clinical presentation and that small changes in degree of stenosis can have important clinical effects in individual cases.

Dynamic Changes in Stenosis Resistance

It is recognized that portions of the atherosclerotic arterial wall remain susceptible to constrictor or dilator effects of vascular smooth muscle. One early and convincing example of vasodilation was provided by Brown and co-workers in the early 1980s.[35] Using quantitative arteriographic measurements of the cross-sectional area of the lumen of human coronary stenoses, these researchers demonstrated that luminal area increases systematically in response to intracoronary or sublingual nitroglycerin and that stenosis vasodilation plays an important role in the clinically beneficial effects of nitroglycerin. Also, it is now clear that dynamic reductions in the caliber of a stenotic lumen sometimes play an important role in

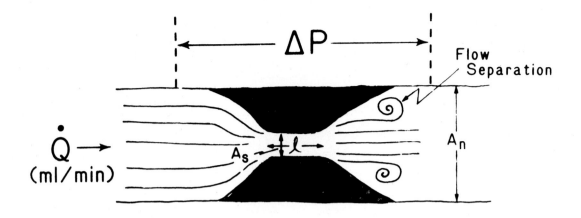

$$\Delta P = \underbrace{f_1\left(\frac{1}{A_s^2}, \ell, \dot{Q}\right)}_{\text{VISCOUS}} + \underbrace{f_2\left(\frac{1}{A_s^2}, \frac{1}{A_n^2}, \dot{Q}^2\right)}_{\text{SEPARATION}}$$

FIGURE 2–5. Factors governing energy losses across a stenosis. Illustrated is a stenosed artery with a flow $\dot{Q}$, expressed as volume of flow per unit of time, that is, milliliters per minute. Minimal cross-sectional area within the stenosis is designated as A_s, and stenosis length as l. The cross-sectional area of the normal portion of the artery is A_N. The fine lines indicate streamline laminar flow patterns before, within, and beyond the stenosis. Downstream of the stenosis, flow profiles show separation from the vessel wall, with resultant vortex formation. The total pressure reduction across the stenosis (ΔP) is influenced by three factors: viscous losses, separation losses, and turbulence. Although the magnitudes of both viscous and separation losses are flow-dependent, separation losses are proportional to $\dot{Q}^2$ rather than $\dot{Q}^1$. The role of turbulence remains poorly defined. (Reprinted with permission from Klocke, F. J.: Clinical and experimental evaluation of the functional severity of coronary stenoses. Newsletter of the Council on Clinical Cardiology, American Heart Association 7:1–9, 1982. Copyright 1982, American Heart Association.)

clinical syndromes. Vasoconstricting neurohumoral and endothelial-related factors include α-adrenergic agonists, serotonin, thromboxane A_2, histamine, endothelin, and platelet-related factors. A small thrombus can also narrow a stenotic lumen crucially; as a thrombus is being formed, platelet activation serves as an amplifying factor for the release of vasoconstrictor substances, and a vicious cycle of increasing luminal compromise can be readily visualized.

Endothelial involvement in the atherosclerotic process has important adverse effects on normal vasodilator mechanisms. As noted previously, EDRF and prostacyclin are normally produced continuously by coronary vascular endothelium. Epicardial arterial caliber increases when EDRF production is augmented by an increase in coronary flow or intracoronary acetylcholine injection. These mechanisms can be blunted in atherosclerotic vessels, to a degree that can reverse the response of luminal size to a variety of interventions. One example of this circumstance is "paradoxical vasoconstriction" of stenotic epicardial arteries as a response to intracoronary acetylcholine;[36] the usual EDRF-related vasodilator

FIGURE 2–6. Relation between the pressure drop across concentric stenoses (ΔP), which narrow luminal diameter by 50, 70, and 90 percent, and flow through the stenosis ($\dot{Q}$). The residual luminal cross-sectional areas, calculated on the basis of a normal internal diameter of 3.0 mm and cross-sectional area of 7.1 mm², are 1.8, 0.6, and 0.1 mm². The letters S and D on the 50 percent stenosis line illustrate a situation in which diastolic flow is, as usual, three times greater than systolic flow and is accompanied by a greater pressure gradient. Systolic (S) and diastolic (D) pressure gradients on the 90 percent stenosis line are much larger, and diastolic flow cannot increase by the usual amount because of the rapid increase in stenosis resistance with flow. In the in vivo state, changes in pressure drop and flow during each cardiac cycle are modified further by instantaneous changes in downstream impedance related to ventricular contraction and intravascular capacitance. An increase in resistance related to increased flow for the 70 percent stenosis is also illustrated. The tangent to the lower level of flow reflects stenosis resistance under resting conditions (R_{BASAL}). The tangent to the higher level of flow ($R_{\uparrow DEMAND}$) has a steeper slope, reflecting the flow-related increase in stenosis resistance that occurs without any change in stenosis geometry. (Reprinted with permission from Klocke, F. J.: Clinical and experimental evaluation of the functional severity of coronary stenoses. Newsletter of the Council on Clinical Cardiology, American Heart Association 7:1–9, 1982. Copyright 1982, American Heart Association.)

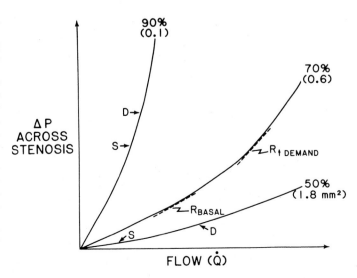

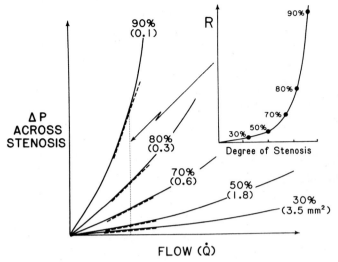

FIGURE 2–7. Relation between the pressure drops (ΔP) across stenoses narrowing internal arterial diameter by 30, 50, 70, 80, and 90 percent and flow (Q̇). Numbers in parentheses below each percent diameter stenosis represent residual luminal cross-sectional area, again calculated on the basis of a normal internal diameter of 3.0 mm and cross-sectional area of 7.1 mm². The vertical dotted line depicts the level of flow required for basal metabolic needs. Stenosis resistances for this level of flow are shown as the dashed tangent lines to the individual ΔP-Q̇ relations. In the inset on the right, stenosis resistance (Rₛ) is plotted as a function of degree of stenosis. (Adapted from Stiel, G. M., et al.: Circulation 80:1603–1609, 1989. Reprinted with permission from Klocke, F. J.: Clinical and experimental evaluation of the functional severity of coronary stenoses. Newsletter of the Council on Clinical Cardiology, American Heart Association 7:1–9, 1982. Copyright 1982, American Heart Association.)

response is replaced by a direct constrictor action on smooth muscle. Other examples, including net vasoconstrictor responses to pacing, exercise, cold pressor testing, and mental stress, involve coronary resistance as well as conduit vessels and presumably reflect the failure of endothelial-related dilator mechanisms to override concomitant stimuli to vasoconstriction.[37] Currently, there is also interest in the effects of estrogen on normal and atherosclerotic vessels; for example, the administration of estrogen to ovariectomized atherosclerotic cynomolgus monkeys has been reported to reverse a paradoxical vasoconstrictor response to acetylcholine.[38]

Arterial Remodeling and Arteriographic Estimates of Stenosis Severity

Many of us have traditionally thought of coronary stenoses only in terms of atherosclerotic proliferation, implicitly assuming a fixed external arterial diameter and a one-to-one correlation between amount of atherosclerotic material and reduction in lumen size. It is clear now, however, that atherosclerosis involves a complex remodeling of the entire arterial wall.[39–42] The atherosclerotic process proceeds in an outward as well as inward direction and involves an increase in external arterial diameter as well as a reduction in luminal diameter. As illustrated in Figure 2–8, arterial enlargement and local differences in degrees of enlargement and proliferation importantly affect luminal diameter and arteriographic measurements of percentage of narrowing.

Coronary Flow Reserve in Coronary Artery Disease

Figure 2–9 illustrates how coronary vasodilator reserve compensates for the effects of epicardial coronary stenoses under resting conditions. Coronary flow is plotted against coronary arterial pressure, with flow under resting conditions designated as 1.0 and the normal coronary pressure-flow point shown with a large circle. The horizontal distances between the normal operating point and the

various degrees of stenosis (smaller circles) reflect the pressure gradients across the stenoses. Progressive arteriolar dilation allows flow to be maintained until stenosis diameter is narrowed by approximately 90 percent. Because a portion of vasodilator reserve is used to maintain flow at the normal level, less reserve remains when flow needs to increase above the resting value.

Figure 2–10 illustrates why measurements of coronary flow reserve seem so attractive for determining the functional severity of stenotic lesions. Flows at rest and during maximal vasodilation are connected by the thin dashed lines, which are curvilinear because of the effects of flow separation mentioned earlier. The amount of flow that can be achieved during maximal vasodilation varies inversely with degree of stenosis. Initially, it would appear that stenoses in the clinically difficult range between 50 and 90 percent should be readily separated by a measurement of flow reserve. However, as discussed previously, the numeric value of flow reserve in any one patient varies with changes in arterial pressure and with other hemodynamic variables, such as heart rate and ventricular preload. Additional confounding factors in coronary disease are myocardial scarring and ventricular hypertrophy, both of which reduce flow reserve independently of other factors.

Figure 2–11 is adapted from a study by the University of Iowa investigators that nicely defined the reciprocal relation between flow reserve and degree of stenosis in humans.[43] In studying coronary patients, these investigators prudently chose to include only those with a discrete single stenosis and no evidence of myocardial hypertrophy, left ventricular dysfunction, previous myocardial infarction, or angiographically apparent collateral circulation. Although the overall relationship between flow reserve and percent stenosis was clear, confidence limits for individual measurements were quite wide, for example, varying from 1.2 to 4.2 in cases of stenosis 70 percent in diameter. Some of this variation may have been related to the invariable diffuseness of coronary atherosclerosis and differences in the distal coronary bed, that is, to functional differences not reflected in the measurement of a single stenosis diameter. In a group of apparently normal patients studied concurrently, however, flow reserve varied from approximately 3.8 to about 8.2. Thus, although group differences in flow reserve have been invaluable in defining coronary pathophysiology, the use of individual measurements to make patient care decisions requires seasoned clinical judgment.

Use of Relative Rather than Absolute Flow Reserve in Perfusion Imaging

When one attempts to identify a regional deficit in perfusion in a coronary patient, an approach based on comparing different regions within the left ventricle can avoid some of the pitfalls of numeric measurements of flow reserve. When perfusion imaging is combined with a stress test or pharmacologic vasodilation, one is really assessing whether flow reserve is reduced on a regional basis; that is, the focus is on the presence or absence of a regional difference rather than on absolute values. The minimal difference that can be appreciated varies with the imaging technique employed and the physical characteristics of the patient. Although there are few data that directly assess this minimal difference, a difference of at least 30 percent is probably needed for most techniques under resting conditions. Because the myocardial extraction of commonly used tracers varies inversely with flow, the magnitude of difference required during vasodilation is often greater than that at rest.

Interpretive issues that arise when one is utilizing estimates of relative flow reserve are depicted in Figure 2–12. It schematically illustrates three situations that would produce similar defects on perfusion images but have significantly different clinical implications. Consider first a patient with a stenosis of approximately 90 percent who develops angina at a workload of 3 metabolic equivalents (METs) during a treadmill exercise test. Extrapolating from the studies of Kitamura and colleagues, a flow of 1.6 times that of

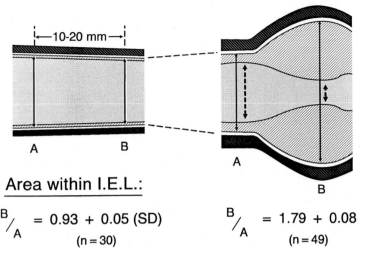

Area within I.E.L.:

$$\frac{B}{A} = 0.93 + 0.05 \text{ (SD)}$$
$$(n = 30)$$

$$\frac{B}{A} = 1.79 + 0.08$$
$$(n = 49)$$

FIGURE 2–8. This figure was prepared using data from a study by Stiel and colleagues[41] of human coronary arteries fixed at a normal arterial pressure. The proximal portion of a normal artery is shown on the left, and a stenotic atherosclerotic coronary artery on the right. The intima is shown by the diagonally striped area adjacent to the vessel lumen; the thin white line on the abluminal side of the intima is the internal elastic membrane (I.E.L.). As shown at point A, the atherosclerotic process in the diseased artery encroaches on luminal area, but the degree of encroachment is attenuated by an increase in overall arterial diameter. Point B further illustrates that atherosclerotic enlargement is accentuated at points of clinically recognizable stenosis. The local increase in degree of enlargement can be expressed in terms of the ratio of the areas contained within the internal elastic membrane at points B and A *(solid arrows)*. In Stiel's series of patients, this ratio averaged 1.79 in diseased arteries, as opposed to 0.93 in nondiseased normally tapering arteries. It is important to note that the percent luminal narrowing that would be calculated on routine arteriography depends on the relative luminal diameters at points B and A in the atherosclerotic artery *(dashed arrows)*. Each diameter is the result of a process involving both atherosclerotic proliferation and local arterial enlargement. The degrees of proliferation and enlargement differ substantially at the two points. Thus, factors underlying local differences in degree of proliferation and enlargement have an important effect on measurements of percent stenosis. (Redrawn from Klocke, F. J.: Cognition in the era of technology: "Seeing the shades of gray." J. Am. Coll. Cardiol. 16:763–769, 1990, with permission from the American College of Cardiology.)

control is required for this level of work and is achieved in the nonstenotic portion of the ventricle.[44] However, flow reserve in the stenotic area is limited to 1.1 (a 30 percent reduction), and angina develops. Consider next a patient with a stenosis of approximately 75 percent who becomes ischemic at a workload of 10 METs. The

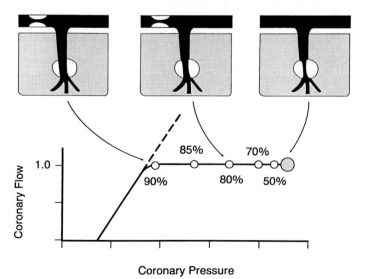

FIGURE 2–9. Use of coronary vasodilator reserve to compensate for effects of coronary stenoses under basal conditions. Progressive arteriolar vasodilation *(top diagrams)* allows coronary flow to be maintained until stenosis diameter *(open circles on lower graph)* is narrowed by approximately 90 percent. (Redrawn from Klocke, F. J.: Cognition in the era of technology: "Seeing the shades of gray." J. Am. Coll. Cardiol. 16:763–769, 1990, with permission from the American College of Cardiology.)

required flow is 3.4 times that of control, but the stenotic area can reach only 2.4 times control (again a 30 percent reduction). Although the relative perfusion deficits are similar, the therapeutic implications of angina developing at 3 and 10 METs differ appreciably. Last, consider an asymptomatic patient with a stenosis of approximately 60 percent who has been given dipyridamole. Assuming maximum vasodilation in the nonstenotic area (and no decrease in aortic pressure), a fivefold flow increment may be expected. The stenotic area can increase only to 3.5 times the resting value; that is, again there is a 30 percent regional "deficit." This deficit is not accompanied by any appreciable increase in local myocardial oxygen demand and is not associated with ischemia. Although it may be diagnostically useful in identifying an asymptomatic stenotic lesion, it would ordinarily have little therapeutic impact.

Although this last example suggests that pharmacologic stress imaging may be more sensitive than exercise testing for diagnostic screening, this is probably not the case. Because the myocardial extraction of radionuclide imaging agents varies inversely with flow, myocardial tracer content typically increases with flow only to a level approximately 2.5 times the resting level.[45] Thus, the third example in Figure 2–12 may not be appreciated with currently used imaging agents; that is, tracer content may be similar in the stenotic and nonstenotic areas.

As also noted previously, coronary reserve is normally less in the subendocardium than in outer layers of the ventricular wall. Thus, perfusion imaging techniques that have sufficient resolution and other features to allow subendocardial flow to be assessed selectively would be advantageous.

Coronary Collateral Circulation

Although coronary collateral vessels have been studied extensively in animals, the extrapolation of findings to humans is compli-

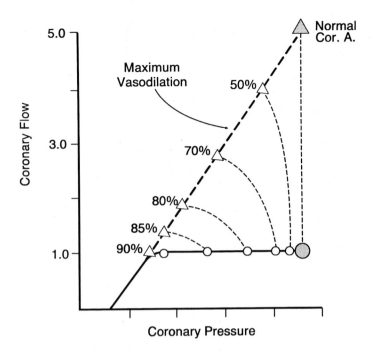

FIGURE 2-10. Use of coronary flow reserve to evaluate the functional significance of stenotic lesions. Coronary flow rates at rest and during vasodilation are connected by curvilinear dashed lines; the lines are curvilinear because of the effects of flow separation (see Fig. 2–5). Cor. A. = coronary artery. (Redrawn from Klocke, F. J.: Cognition in the era of technology: "Seeing the shades of gray." J. Am. Coll. Cardiol. 16:763–769, 1990, with permission from the American College of Cardiology.)

cated by variations in the collateral circulation among different species and by limitations of animal models of human coronary artery disease.[46] There is agreement that collaterals develop only when a stenotic lesion is severe enough to produce a substantial transstenotic pressure drop. Although vessels with diameters as small as 100 μm can be visualized angiographically, angiographic quantification of the functional capacity of collaterals remains problematic. The spatial extent of collateralization is now also being assessed with contrast echocardiography (using intracoronary injection of contrast agent).[47]

The collateral circulation typically becomes flow-limiting during exercise or other periods of increased myocardial oxygen demand.[48] In patients with occluded native coronary arteries, myocardial segments served by the occluded vessels were reported as early as 1978[49] to have better contractile function when collaterals are present than when they are absent. It is accepted that pre-existent collateral vessels decrease the rate and extent of myocardial necrosis at the time of native artery occlusion. Flow per unit weight in collateral-dependent myocardium can be reduced compared with

that of adjacent normally perfused myocardium under resting conditions in patients with well-developed collaterals.[50] One reason for the reduced flow may be the lower arterial pressure in the collateralized segment. In patients with total or near-total occlusive lesions, arterial pressure distal to the lesion is often only 25 to 50 percent of aortic pressure. A low arterial perfusion pressure places the collateral-dependent myocardium at or near the lower breakpoint of the autoregulatory pressure-flow relation (see Figs. 2–4 and 2–9). Therefore, it is not surprising that coronary reserve is limited and that regional ischemia and dysfunction frequently occur during modest increases in myocardial oxygen demand.

One important feature of studies of collateral vessels in experimental animals is their response to a variety of vasoactive agents. Collateral vessels in canine and porcine hearts have been reported to constrict in response to indomethacin, aspirin, ergonovine, vasopressin, serotonin, and thromboxane A_2 and to dilate in response to nitroglycerin, arachidonic acid, acetylcholine, bradykinin, atrial natriuretic peptide, and calcitonin gene–related peptide.[51–58] Prostaglandins[51] and EDRF (nitric oxide)[59] appear to have tonic vasodilat-

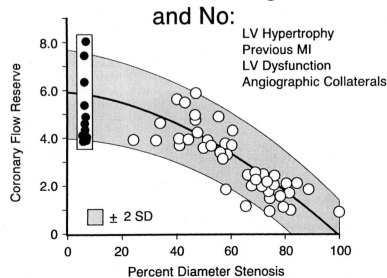

FIGURE 2-11. Data of Wilson and associates[43] defining the reciprocal relation between coronary flow reserve (measured with a Doppler velocity catheter) and degree of stenosis (measured arteriographically) in humans. Values in normal patients are shown with solid circles, and values in coronary patients with open circles. See text for discussion. (Redrawn and reprinted with permission from Wilson, R. F., Marcus, M. L., and White, C. W.: Prediction of the physiologic significance of coronary arterial lesions by quantitative lesion geometry in patients with limited coronary artery disease. Circulation 75:723–732, 1987. Copyright 1987, American Heart Association.)

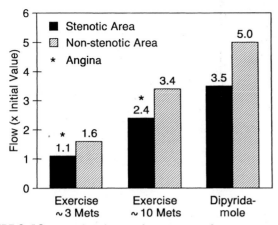

FIGURE 2-12. Examples of regional 30 percent reductions in vasodilated flow that have different clinical implications. *Left,* Exercise with angina at a low workload. *Center,* Exercise with angina at a high workload. *Right,* Dipyridamole infusion. (Redrawn from Klocke, F. J.: Cognition in the era of technology: "Seeing the shades of gray." J. Am. Coll. Cardiol. 16:763–769, 1990, with permission from the American College of Cardiology.)

ing activity. Whereas not all these findings may apply to humans, the effects of vasoactive factors are an important consideration in human collateral vessels as well as in those of experimental animals. The possibility of therapeutically augmenting myocardial angiogenesis in collateral-dependent areas of myocardium is under active investigation.[60-62]

CONSIDERATIONS IN CHOOSING AN IMAGING TECHNIQUE FOR CORONARY FLOW MEASUREMENT

Technical Issues

Technical issues, such as radiation scatter, spatial and temporal resolution, partial volume effects, and attenuation correction, are enormously important in all imaging approaches and need to be considered carefully in each application of each technology. Subsequent chapters address these complex issues as they apply to individual technologies.

Analytical Issues

Analytical issues vary with both flow measurement technique and imaging agent. Arbitrary flow measurement "indices" derived from plots of indicator signal versus time require careful justification. Calculations of flow for tracers manifesting extravascular exchange require more complex (i.e., distributed) models than is the case for intravascular indicators. Although this point is not always appreciated, radiographic contrast agents fall into the "exchangeable" category of imaging agent; as with most other diffusible tracers, their degree of exchange is flow-dependent.[63] As noted previously, the inverse relationship between flow and myocardial extraction of commonly used tracers is an important limiting factor at the high flows potentially achieved with pharmacologic vasodilating agents. Calculations of flow now frequently include factors intended to correct for decreasing extraction of tracer as flow increases; the validity of these corrections needs to be established experimentally in each case.

Another analytical issue relates to intramyocardial blood volume, which increases noticeably during coronary vasodilation. The increment in intravascular volume causes an increase in indicator signal independently of flow and must be taken into consideration. Some intravascular indicators present further problems; for example, the intensity of an echocardiographic signal originating from a micro-

bubble varies with the fourth power of bubble radius. In so-called "first-pass" approaches, indicators that remain present in the left ventricular cavity during the time their signals are being measured in the myocardium cause formidable complexities, for example, x-ray beam hardening and scatter, echocardiographic acoustic shadowing, and count spillover of gamma- or positron-emitting tracers. Additional problems, which cannot be dealt with quantitatively, arise in first-pass approaches employing indicators having rapid transit times and small volumes of distribution.[64]

Normal Spatial Variation of Myocardial Perfusion

It is often not appreciated that measurements of myocardial blood flow involve tradeoffs between spatial resolution of the imaging technique and normal spatial variation in myocardial perfusion.[64-68] Bassingthwaighte and colleagues demonstrated that flows in small segments of a normally perfused left ventricle vary considerably, that is, from one third of mean flow to more than twice mean flow.[67] The degree of flow dispersion (SD/mean) is inversely related to the size of segments examined and falls to approximately 15 percent when 1-g segments are examined.[68] This spatial variation in flow occurs within transmural layers and is not explained by variations in flow between the subendocardium and the subepicardium. Because vasodilated levels of flow in small segments are not matched to resting levels, spatial variation of flow reserve exceeds the spatial variation of resting flow.[69]

The detection of a difference in flow between two areas of the ventricle can be significantly confounded by these inherent spatial variations in flow. Canty[64] pointed out that regions of interest that include several grams of myocardium are needed to detect perfusion differences that are less than 20 percent of mean flows. As illustrated in Figure 2–13, such regions would represent a few positron emission tomography (PET) voxels and several hundred voxels of a high-resolution technique, such as electron beam computed tomography (CT) or magnetic resonance imaging (MRI).

Validation Studies

Useful "validation" studies comparing flow measurements using positron emission tomography to measurements employing radioactive microspheres (the accepted flow measurement standard in experimental animals) have been reported in recent years.[70-74] An initial report correlating microsphere flows with an index of mean

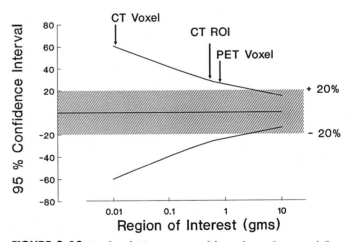

FIGURE 2–13. Predicted 95 percent confidence limits for normal flow variation about the mean as a function of size of region of interest. Observed variability in perfusion increases as image resolution improves and voxel size becomes smaller. To detect perfusion differences exceeding 20 percent of mean values *(dashed horizontal lines)*, several grams of tissue must be examined. (From Canty, J. M., Jr.: Methods of assessing coronary blood flow and flow reserve. Am. J. Cardiac Imaging 7:222–232, 1993, with permission.)

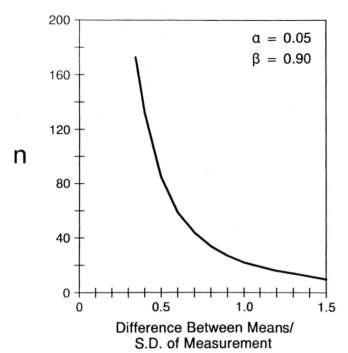

FIGURE 2–14. Size of patient groups needed to provide a 90 percent probability of identifying a group difference in a parameter such as coronary flow at $P = .05$. The abscissa represents the quotient of the actual difference in group means and the standard deviation of the measurement technique used to quantify the parameter being evaluated. For example, if one was designing a study to identify a 20 percent difference in resting coronary flow in two patient groups and the standard deviation of the flow measurement technique was 25 percent, each group should include 34 patients. As measurement variability increases, the likelihood of an "underpowered" study increases precipitously. (Data from Table 7–2 in reference 77.)

transit time obtained with magnetic resonance imaging has also been published.[75] Measurements using flow models that include corrections for decreasing extraction of tracer as flow increases and that correlate with microsphere flows at vasodilated as well as resting levels of flow are now being used to assess group differences in flow reserve noninvasively.[76]

Although microsphere and imaging measurements of myocardial flow can be made to correlate well over a wide range of flow rates, confidence limits for individual imaging measurements remain quite wide and need to be considered carefully in clinical studies. Since 95 percent confidence limits are often 50 percent of resting flow, the identification of modest reductions in resting flow in individual patients, or between patient groups, can require rather large patient groups[77] (Fig. 2–14).

References

1. Klocke, F. J., and Ellis, A. K.: Physiology of the coronary circulation. In Parmley, W. W., and Chatterjee, K. (eds.): Cardiology. Vol. 1. Philadelphia, J.B. Lippincott, 1990, pp. 101–114.
2. Parmley, W. W., and Tyberg, J. V.: Determination of myocardial oxygen demand. Prog. Cardiol. 5:19, 1976.
3. Mirsky, I.: Left ventricular stresses in the intact human heart. Biophys. J. 9:189, 1969.
4. Yoran, C., Covell, J. W., and Ross, J., Jr.: Structural basis for the ascending limb of left ventricular function. Circ. Res. 32:297, 1973.
5. Hoffman, J. I. E., and Buckberg, G. D.: Transmural variations in myocardial perfusion. Prog. Cardiol. 5:37, 1976.
6. Monroe, R. G., Gamble, W. J., LaFarge, C. G., et al.: Transmural coronary venous oxygen saturations in normal and isolated hearts. Am. J. Physiol. 228:318, 1975.
7. Klocke, F. J., Mates, R. E., Canty, J. M., Jr., et al.: Coronary pressure-flow relationships: Controversial issues and probable implications. Circ. Res. 56:310, 1985.
8. Farhi, E. R., Klocke, F. J., Mates, R. E., et al.: Tone-dependent waterfall behavior during venous pressure elevation in isolated canine hearts. Circ. Res. 68:392, 1991.
9. Satoh, S., Klocke, F. J., and Canty, J. M., Jr.: Tone-dependent coronary arterial-

10. venous pressure differences at the cessation of venous outflow during long diastoles. Circulation 88:1238, 1993.
10. Wüsten, B., Buss, D. D., Deist, H., et al.: Dilatory capacity of the coronary circulation and its correlation to the arterial vasculature in the canine left ventricle. Basic Res. Cardiol. 72:636, 1977.
11. Archie, J. P., Jr.: Minimum left ventricular coronary vascular resistance in dogs. J. Surg. Res. 25:21, 1978.
12. Chilian, W. M., Eastham, C. L., and Marcus, M. L.: Microvascular distribution of coronary vascular resistance in beating left ventricle. Am. J. Physiol. 251:H779, 1986.
13. Marcus, M., Wright, C., Doty, D., et al.: Measurements of coronary velocity and reactive hyperemia in the coronary circulation of humans. Circ. Res. 49:877, 1981.
14. Olsson, R. A.: Myocardial reactive hyperemia. Circ. Res. 37:263, 1975.
15. Rouleau, J., Boerboom, L. E., Surjadhana, A., et al.: The role of autoregulation and tissue diastolic pressures in the transmural distribution of left ventricular blood flow in anesthetized dogs. Circ. Res. 45:804, 1979.
16. Aversano, T., Klocke, F. J., Mates, R. E., et al.: Preload-induced alterations in capacitance-free diastolic pressure-flow relationships. Am. J. Physiol. 246:H410, 1984.
17. Feigl, E. O.: Coronary physiology. Physiol. Rev. 63:1, 1983.
18. Berne, R. M., and Rubio, R.: Coronary circulation. In Berne, R. M. (ed.): Handbook of Physiology. Section II. The Cardiovascular System. Bethesda, MD, American Physiological Society, 1979, p. 873.
19. Broten, T. P., and Feigl, E. O.: Role of myocardial oxygen and carbon dioxide in coronary autoregulation. Am. J. Physiol. 262:H1231, 1992.
20. Murray, P. A., and Vatner, S. F.: Alpha-adrenoreceptor attenuation of the coronary vascular response to severe exercise in the conscious dog. Circ. Res. 45:654, 1979.
21. Mudge, G. H., Jr., Grossman, W., Mills, R. M., Jr., et al.: Reflex increase in coronary vascular resistance in patients with ischemic heart disease. N. Engl. J. Med. 295:1333, 1976.
22. Friedman, P. L., Brown, E. J., Jr., Gunther, S., et al.: Coronary vasoconstrictor effect of indomethacin in patients with coronary-artery disease. N. Engl. J. Med. 305:1171, 1981.
23. Kuo, L., Davis, M. J., and Chilian, W. M.: Myogenic activity in isolated subepicardial and subendocardial coronary arterioles. Am. J. Physiol. 255:H1558, 1988.
24. Furchgott, R. F., and Zawadski, J. V.: The obligatory role of endothelial cells in the relaxation of arterial smooth muscle by acetylcholine. Nature 288:373, 1980.
25. Cannon, P. J.: The role of the endothelium in coronary vasomotion: New insights. Prim. Cardiol. 15:15, 1989.
26. Rubanyi, G. M., and Parker Botelho, L. H.: Endothelins. FASEB J. 5:2713, 1991.
27. Marcus, M. L.: The Coronary Circulation in Health and Disease. New York, McGraw-Hill, 1983, pp. 107–109.
28. Wilson, R. F., Laughlin, D. E., Ackell, P. H., et al.: Transluminal, subselective measurement of coronary artery blood flow velocity and vasodilator reserve in man. Circulation 72:82, 1985.
29. Hoffman, J. I. E.: Maximal coronary flow and the concept of coronary vascular reserve. Circulation 70:153, 1984.
30. Klocke, F. J.: Measurements of coronary flow reserve: Defining pathophysiology versus making decisions about patient care. Circulation 76:1183, 1987.
31. Marcus, M. L., and Harrison, D. G.: Physiologic basis for myocardial perfusion imaging. In Marcus, M. L., Schelbert, H. R., Skorton, D. J., et al. (eds.): Cardiac Imaging: A Companion to Braunwald's Heart Disease. Philadelphia, W.B. Saunders, 1991.
32. Gould, K. L.: Dynamic coronary stenosis. Am. J. Cardiol. 45:286, 1980.
33. Mates, R. E., Gupta, R. L., Bell, A. C., et al.: Fluid dynamics of coronary artery stenosis. Circ. Res. 42:152, 1978.
34. Klocke, F. J.: Clinical and experimental evaluation of the functional severity of coronary stenoses. Newslett. Council Clin. Cardiol., American Heart Association 7:1, 1982.
35. Brown, B. G., Balson, E., Peterson, R. B., et al.: The mechanisms of nitroglycerin action: Stenosis vasodilation as a major component of the drug response. Circulation 64:1089, 1981.
36. Ludmer, P. L., Selwyn, A. P., Shook, T. L., et al.: Paradoxical vasoconstriction induced by acetylcholine in atherosclerotic coronary arteries. N. Engl. J. Med. 315:1046, 1986.
37. Selwyn, A. P., Yeung, A. C., Ryan, T. J., Jr., et al.: Pathophysiology of ischemia in patients with coronary artery disease. Prog. Cardiovasc. Dis. 35:27, 1992.
38. Williams, J. K., Adams, M. R., Herrington, D. M., et al.: Effects of short-term estrogen treatment on vascular responses of coronary arteries. J. Am. Coll. Cardiol. 20:452, 1992.
39. Glagov, S., Weisenberg, E., Zarins, C. K., et al.: Compensatory enlargement of human atherosclerotic coronary arteries. N. Engl. J. Med. 316:1371, 1987.
40. Zarins, C. K., Weisenburg, E., Kolettis, G., et al.: Differential enlargement of artery segments in response to enlarging atherosclerotic plaques. J. Vasc. Surg. 7:386, 1988.
41. Stiel, G. M., Stiel, L. S. G., Schofer, J., et al.: Impact of compensatory enlargement of atherosclerotic coronary arteries on angiographic assessment of coronary artery disease. Circulation 80:1603, 1989.
42. Klocke, F. J.: Cognition in the era of technology: "Seeing the shades of gray." J. Am. Coll. Cardiol. 16:763, 1990.
43. Wilson, R. F., Marcus, M. L., and White, C. W.: Prediction of the physiologic significance of coronary arterial lesions by quantitative lesion geometry in patients with limited coronary artery disease. Circulation 75:723, 1987.
44. Kitamura, K., Jorgensen, C. R., Gobel, F. L., et al.: Hemodynamic correlates of myocardial oxygen consumption during upright exercise. J. Appl. Physiol. 32:516, 1972.

45. Glover, D. K., and Okada, R. D.: Myocardial kinetics of Tc-MIBI in canine myocardium after dipyridamole. Circulation 81:628, 1990.
46. Gregg, D. E., and Patterson, R. E.: Functional importance of the coronary collaterals. N. Engl. J. Med. 303:1404, 1980.
47. Sabia, P. J., Powers, E. R., Jayaweera, A. R., et al.: Functional significance of collateral blood flow in patients with recent acute myocardial infarction: A study using myocardial contrast echocardiography. Circulation 85:2080, 1992.
48. Bache, R. J., and Schwartz, J. S.: Myocardial blood flow during exercise after gradual coronary occlusion in the dog. Am. J. Physiol. 245:H131, 1983.
49. Schwarz, F., Flameng, W., Ensslen, R., et al.: Effects of collaterals on left ventricular function at rest and during stress. Am. Heart J. 95:570, 1978.
50. Arani, D. T., Greene, D. G., Bunnell, I. L., et al.: Reductions in coronary flow under resting conditions in collateral-dependent myocardium of patients with complete occlusion of the left anterior descending coronary artery. J. Am. Coll. Cardiol. 3:668, 1984.
51. Altman, J., Dulas, D., and Bache, R. J.: Effect of cyclooxygenase blockade on blood flow through well-developed coronary collateral vessels. Circ. Res. 70:1091, 1992.
52. Altman, J. D., Dulas, D., Pavek, T., et al.: Effect of aspirin on coronary collateral blood flow. Circulation 87:583, 1993.
53. Bache, R. J., Foreman, B., and Hautamaa, P. V.: Response of canine coronary collateral vessels to ergonovine and alpha-adrenergic stimulation. Am. J. Physiol. 261:H1019, 1991.
54. Foreman, B. W., Dai, X. Z., and Bache, R. J.: Vasoconstriction of canine coronary collateral vessels with vasopressin limits blood flow to collateral-dependent myocardium during exercise. Circ. Res. 69:657, 1991.
55. Wright, L., Homans, D. C., Laxson, D. D., et al.: Effect of serotonin and thromboxane A_2 on blood flow through moderately well developed coronary collateral vessels. J. Am. Coll. Cardiol. 19:687, 1992.
56. Altman, J., Dulas, D., Pavek, T., et al.: Endothelial function in well-developed canine coronary collateral vessels. Am. J. Physiol. 264:H567, 1993.
57. Foreman, B., Dai, X. Z., Homans, D. C., et al.: Effect of atrial natriuretic peptide on coronary collateral blood flow. Circ. Res. 65:1671, 1989.
58. Quebbeman, B. B., Dulas, D., Altman, J., et al.: Effect of calcitonin gene–related peptide on well-developed coronary collateral vasculature. J. Cardiovasc. Pharmacol. 21:774, 1993.
59. Frank, M. W., Harris, K. R., Ahlin, K. A., et al.: Endothelial-derived relaxing factor (nitric oxide) has a tonic vasodilating action on coronary collateral vessels. J. Am. Coll. Cardiol. Feb. 95, Special Issue, p. 261A.
60. Takeshita, S., Zheng, L. P., Brogi, E., et al.: Therapeutic angiogenesis: A single intraarterial bolus of vascular endothelial growth factor augments revascularization in a rabbit ischemic hind limb model. J. Clin. Invest. 93:662, 1994.
61. Unger, E. F., Banai, S., Shou, M., et al.: Basic fibroblast growth factor enhances myocardial collateral flow in a canine model. Am. J. Physiol. 266:H1588–H1595, 1994.
62. Banai, S., Jaklitsch, M. T., Shou, M., et al.: Angiogenic-induced enhancement of collateral blood flow to ischemic myocardium by vascular endothelial growth factor in dogs. Circulation 89:2183, 1994.
63. Canty, J. M., Jr., Judd, R., Brody, A. S., et al.: First-pass entry of nonionic contrast agent into the myocardial extravascular space: Effects on radiographic estimates of transit time and blood volume. Circulation 84:2071, 1991.
64. Canty, J. M., Jr.: Methods of assessing coronary blood flow and flow reserve. Am. J. Cardiac Imaging 7:222, 1993.
65. Falsetti, H. L., Carroll, R. J., and Marcus, M. L.: Temporal heterogeneity of myocardial blood flow in anesthetized dogs. Circulation 52:848, 1975.
66. Schänzenbacher, P., and Klocke, F. J.: Inert gas measurements of myocardial perfusion in the presence of heterogeneous flow documented by microspheres. Circulation 61:590, 1980.
67. King, R. B., Bassingthwaighte, J. B., Hales, J. R. S., et al.: Stability of heterogeneity of myocardial blood flow in normal awake baboons. Circ. Res. 57:285, 1985.
68. Bassingthwaighte, J. B., King, R. B., and Roger, S. A.: Fractal nature of regional myocardial blood flow heterogeneity. Circ. Res. 65:578, 1989.
69. Austin, R. E., Aldea, G. S., Coggins, D. L., et al.: Profound spatial heterogeneity of coronary reserve: Discordance between patterns of resting and maximal myocardial blood flow. Circ. Res. 67:319, 1990.
70. Herrero, P., Markham, J., Shelton, M. E., et al.: Noninvasive quantification of regional myocardial perfusion with rubidium-82 and positron emission tomography: Exploration of a mathematical model. Circulation 82:1377, 1990.
71. Kuhle, W. G., Porenta, G., Huang, S. C., et al.: Quantification of regional myocardial blood flow using ^{13}N-ammonia and reoriented dynamic positron emission tomographic imaging. Circulation 86:1004, 1992.
72. Bergmann, S. R.: Quantification of myocardial perfusion with positron emission tomography. In Bergmann, S.R., and Sobel, B. E. (eds.): Positron Emission Tomography of the Heart. Mt. Kisco, NY, Futura Publishing, 1992.
73. Muzik, O., Beanlands, R. S. B., Hutchins, G. D., et al.: Validation of nitrogen-13 ammonia tracer kinetic model for quantification of myocardial blood flow using PET. J. Nucl. Med. 34:83, 1993.
74. Bol, A., Melin, J. A., Vanoverschelde, J. L., et al.: Direct comparison of [^{13}N]ammonia and [^{15}O]water estimates of perfusion with quantification of regional myocardial blood flow by microspheres. Circulation 87:512, 1993.
75. Wilke, N., Simm, C., Zhang, J., et al.: Contrast-enhanced first-pass myocardial perfusion imaging: Correlation between myocardial blood flow in dogs at rest and during hyperemia. Magn. Reson. Med. 29:485, 1993.
76. Czernin, J., Muller, P., Chan, S., et al.: Influence of age and hemodynamics on myocardial blood flow and flow reserve. Circulation 88:62, 1993.
77. Machin, D., and Campbell, M. J.: Comparing two means. In Machin, D., and Campbell, M. J. (eds.): Statistical Tables for the Design of Clinical Trials. Chap. 7. Oxford, Blackwell Scientific Publications, 1987, pp. 79–88.

CHAPTER

3 Principles of Ventricular Function

Steven Solomon, Ph.D.
Stanton A. Glantz, Ph.D.

CARDIAC MUSCLE ____ 20
Sarcomere Structure and Function ____ 20
  Anatomy ____ 20
  Active Length-Tension Relationship ____ 20
  Passive Length-Tension Relationship ____ 20
Excitation-Contraction Coupling ____ 20
  Role of Calcium ____ 20
  Calcium Cycle ____ 22
Calcium, Contraction, and Inotropic Agents ____ 22
  Effect of Changing the Action Potential ____ 23
  Effect of Changing Ion Concentration ____ 23
  Time and Frequency Effects on Contraction ____ 23
  Cardiovascular Drugs and Inotropic Agents ____ 23
  Effects of Disease ____ 23
VENTRICULAR MECHANICS ____ 24

Stress-Strain and Pressure-Volume Relations ____ 24
Cardiac Cycle ____ 24
DETERMINANTS OF VENTRICULAR FUNCTION ____ 25
Determinants of Diastolic Function ____ 25
  Passive Components of Filling ____ 25
  Active Components of Filling ____ 26
    Relaxation ____ 26
  Passive Diastolic Pressure-Volume Relation ____ 26
  Factors Affecting the Atrioventricular Pressure Gradient ____ 27
    Effect of Changing Left Atrial Pressure ____ 27
    Effect of Changing Afterload ____ 27
    Diastolic Suction ____ 27
  Ventricular Interaction and the Pericardium ____ 27

Effects of Cardiovascular Drugs on Diastolic Function _____ 28
Determinants of Systolic Function _____ 29
  Contractility _____ 29
  Frank-Starling Mechanism _____ 29
  Afterload _____ 30
  Heart Rate _____ 30
Systolic Ventricular Interaction _____ 30
Effects of Cardiovascular Drugs on Systolic Function _____ 30
Coronary Blood Flow and Ischemia _____ 30
Cardiac Hypertrophy _____ 31
Myocardial Energetics _____ 31
SUMMARY _____ 32

The heart is a pump that delivers oxygenated blood and nutrients to all of the body's organs, including the heart itself, and then returns the deoxygenated blood to the lungs. Blood is also pumped to the kidneys and liver to remove metabolic waste products. This pump consists of four cardiac chambers, which accept blood into the heart, then eject the blood to the lungs and body. To appreciate how the heart functions, one must examine the properties that are intrinsic to the cardiac muscle fibers, the dynamic properties of the cardiac chambers, and their relationship with the heart's external environment.

CARDIAC MUSCLE

The function of the heart is controlled by several properties intrinsic to the cardiac muscle (myocardium) itself. In skeletal muscle, each cell acts as a discrete subunit, and the force in the muscle as a whole is regulated by the number of cells that contract. Because the heart contracts all the time, this arrangement would not be an efficient method for the heart to regulate the force it generates. Instead, all the muscle cells contract during each beat, and each cell varies the force it develops. As a result, the same factors that affect the performance of isolated cardiac muscle influence the performance of the whole heart. These factors include the resting fiber length (preload), the load after the muscle starts to shorten (afterload), the contractile or inotropic state of the muscle, and the frequency of electrical stimulation (heart rate).

Sarcomere Structure and Function

Anatomy

The myocardium is composed of a branching network of nucleated muscle fibers 10 to 20 μm wide and 50 to 100 μm long (Fig. 3–1). Each of these fibers contains bundles of myofilaments arranged in repeating subunits called sarcomeres. The sarcomeres are composed of myosin (thick filaments) and actin (thin filaments). The thick filaments overlap the thin filaments and in cross section appear as a hexagonal array. When calcium is released into the sarcomeres, cross-bridges form from the myosin to sites on the actin, causing the sarcomere to shorten and develop force. Globular heads from the myosin form cross-bridges by attaching to the actin. In an action similar to that of a ratchet, the thin filaments are pulled toward the center of the sarcomere, resulting in tension development and shortening. When the calcium is removed from the sarcomere, the myosin and actin dissociate and the sarcomere relaxes.

Active Length-Tension Relationship

The amount of force developed depends on the length of the sarcomere before it is stimulated. In cardiac muscle, as the sarcomere rest length increases from 1.7 to 2.0 μm, the developed force increases (Fig. 3–2, _bottom_). According to the so-called sliding-filament model for muscle contraction and relaxation,[1] the active length-tension relation depends on the degree of overlap of the thick and thin filaments see (Fig. 3–2, _top_). At lengths below 2.0 μm, the 1.0-μm actin filaments overlap the other thin filaments, which interfere with cross-bridge formation. As the sarcomere is stretched (1.7 to 2.0 μm), the amount of double overlap decreases,

allowing more cross-bridges to attach, increasing the developed tension. Beyond this length (2.0 to 2.2 μm), the amount of force developed plateaus because of an absence of cross-bridge sites on the central 0.2-μm region of the thick filament. The sarcomere active length-tension relationship is manifested in the whole heart as the Frank-Starling mechanism, where developed pressure (force) and stroke volume (shortening) increase as end-diastolic volume (initial sarcomere length) of the heart increases.

Passive Length-Tension Relationship

The resting tension in the myocardium is low at physiologic muscle lengths. As isolated cardiac muscle is passively stretched, small increases in tension are observed[2, 3] (see Fig. 3–2, _bottom_). This situation contrasts with that of skeletal muscle, whose tension does not rise appreciably as the resting muscle length is increased. At lengths above 2.0 μm, tension increases rapidly, and the sarcomere becomes very stiff as it is stretched to 2.3 to 2.4 μm. At these tensions, sarcomeres resist any further stretch, which would irreversibly damage them. The connective tissue content of the cardiac muscle gives it the ability to develop this high resting tension. The sarcomere passive length-tension relationship contributes to the diastolic pressure-volume relationship of the whole heart.

Excitation-Contraction Coupling

Role of Calcium

The electrical impulses that drive the heart originate in a group of pacemaker cells in the sinoatrial node at the top of the heart. The sinoatrial node begins a depolarizing wave that spreads across the atria to and through the specialized conduction system to the left and right ventricles, causing them to contract. Calcium is the link that couples electrical excitation of muscle to mechanical contraction. Muscle contraction results from the interaction of actin and myosin, adenosine triphosphate (ATP), and calcium ions. Figure 3–3 shows the movement of calcium during a single cardiac cycle. The sarcoplasmic reticulum is a network of small tubules that surrounds the sarcomeres and stores calcium ions, which are released into the sarcomere when the cell is depolarized. ATP-dependent calcium pumps then remove the calcium from the sarcomere back to the sarcoplasmic reticulum, and the cell relaxes. The contraction reaction is modulated by the regulatory proteins troponin and tropomyosin, located on the actin filament. When calcium binds to troponin, the tropomyosin shifts, uncovering the active sites and allowing the myosin filaments to bind with the actin filaments, which produces tension development and shortening.

ATP is the source of energy for the muscle's contractile machinery. The ATPase activity of myosin hydrolyzes ATP, transferring the energy from ATP to the actin-myosin system, which results in muscle contraction. ATP is hydrolyzed during the detachment of the myosin cross-bridge from the actin active site, allowing the myosin cross-bridge to attach to another actin active site. ATP is also required to provide the energy needed for the ion pumps that remove calcium from the sarcomere to relax the muscle.

The force developed in the heart muscle depends on the concentration of calcium in proximity to the myosin ATPase sites, because the system is not saturated with calcium. The relationship between the concentration of calcium and the percentage of maximum tension resembles a sigmoid curve. This relationship is similar to

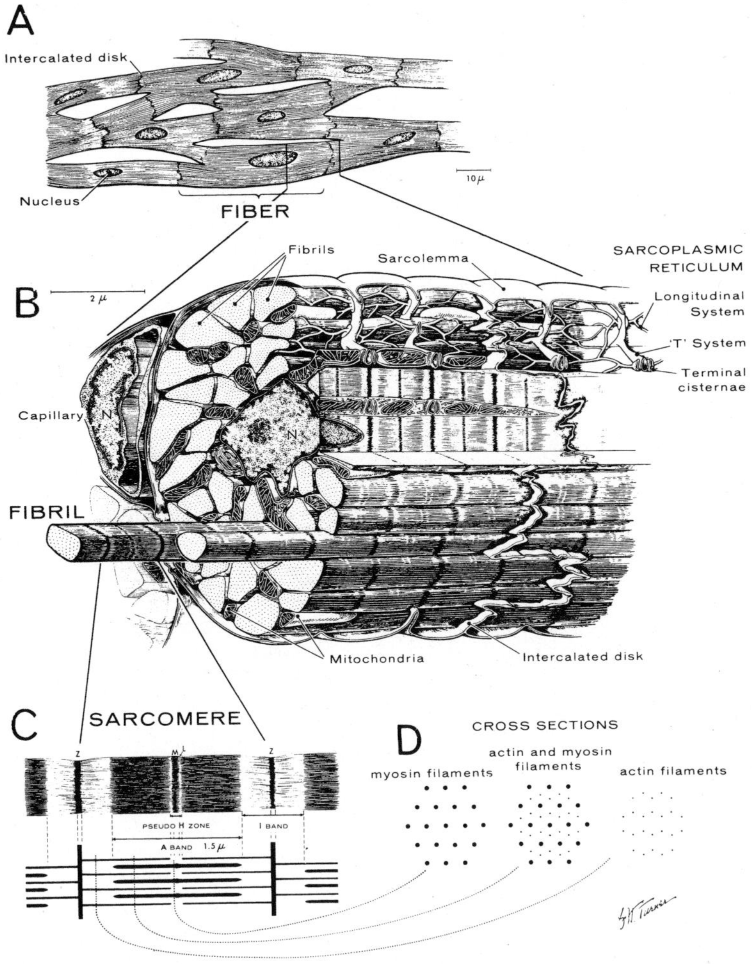

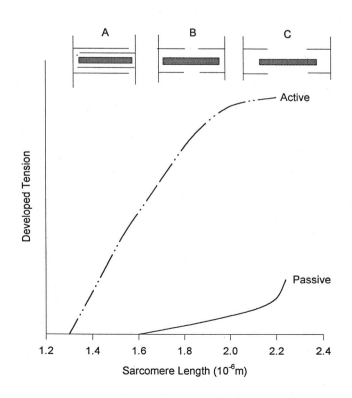

FIGURE 3–1. Schematic drawing of myocardial muscle. *A,* The structure of the myofibril bundle, transverse and longitudinal tubules, and sarcolemma. *B,* An individual sarcomere from a fibril, showing the light and dark regions that constitute the actin and myosin filaments, respectively. *C,* Three cross sections through different regions of the sarcomere. The first cross section, through the middle of the sarcomere, shows the hexagonal arrangement of myosin only. The second cross section, through the overlapping region of actin and myosin filaments, illustrates the location of actin with respect to myosin. The third cross section shows actin filaments only. (From Braunwald, E., Ross, J., Jr., and Sonnenblick, E.H.: Mechanisms of Contraction of the Normal and Failing Heart. 2nd ed. Boston, Little, Brown, 1976, p. 3, with permission.)

FIGURE 3–2. *Top,* The sarcomere of a myofilament at different lengths, showing the relative amount of overlap between actin thin filaments and myosin thick filaments. *A,* At short lengths (1.5 to 2.0 μm), there is double overlap of the thin filaments with thick filaments. *B,* At 2.0 μm, the thin filaments no longer overlap. *C,* At greater lengths, the number of possible cross-bridge attachments decreases. *Bottom,* The active and passive sarcomere length-tension relationship is shown. With small increments of sarcomere length, the passive tension curve develops little force until lengths exceeding 2.0 μm. The active length-tension curve increases until 2.0 μm, at which point the amount of developed tension plateaus.

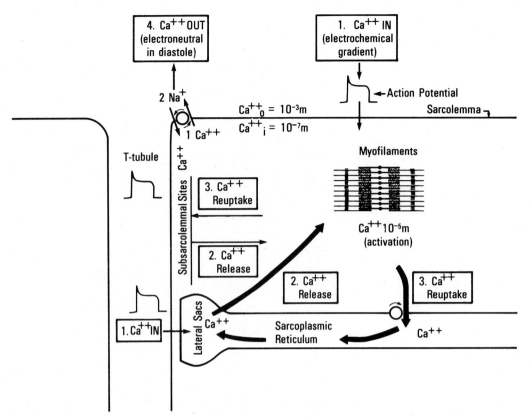

FIGURE 3–3. Schematic of the movement of calcium during the cardiac cycle. *1,* Calcium moves across the sarcolemma after being stimulated by an action potential. *2,* The inward movement of calcium triggers the release of a much larger concentration of calcium from the sarcoplasmic reticulum, with additional releases from subsarcolemmal calcium sites. *3,* Calcium is taken up by the sarcoplasmic reticulum in an ATP-dependent process and in an ATP-independent process at the subsarcolemmal calcium sites. *4,* Calcium inside the cell is exchanged for extracellular sodium (in a 1:2 ratio) across the sarcolemma. (From Best, C.H., and Taylor, N.B.: Cardiovascular system. *In* West, J.B. [ed.]: Physiologic Basis of Medical Practice. Baltimore, Williams & Wilkins, 1985, p. 191, with permission.)

the one between the concentration of calcium and ATPase activity in the presence of the troponin-tropomyosin complex. Comparing the sigmoidal calcium concentration–maximum tension relation with the calcium sensitivity of myosin ATPase alone shows that the regulatory proteins troponin and tropomyosin are required and that they confer calcium sensitivity on the ATPase.

The intracellular levels of calcium regulate the contraction and relaxation of cardiac muscle. Modulation of calcium during the cardiac cycle occurs at several sites within the cell. Many cardiovascular drugs and disease states can alter the cellular mechanisms that control the movement of calcium within the cell, resulting in altered excitation-contraction coupling events and the subsequent mechanical behavior of the myocardium and cardiac pump. Therefore, it is important to understand the normal movement of calcium within the cell and the effect of cardiovascular drugs and disease states on the regulation of various calcium-mediated processes.

Calcium Cycle

When the cell is depolarized, sodium enters the sarcolemma, followed by an influx of calcium. Near the end of the action potential, the calcium inflow stops, and potassium ions flow out, which repolarizes the cell. Although the amount of calcium entering the cell is much less than that needed to activate contraction, this calcium stimulates the release of calcium from the sarcoplasmic reticulum. The sarcoplasmic reticulum contains much more calcium than is necessary for a single contraction, and only part of it is released into the sarcomere during each cardiac cycle. This calcium-mediated calcium release produces contraction, and the remaining calcium in the sarcoplasmic reticulum acts as a contractile reserve. The end of contraction is due to the reuptake of calcium by the sarcoplasmic reticulum, an active ATP-dependent process.

During diastole, the filling phase of the cardiac cycle, an ion-exchange mechanism in the sarcolemma removes calcium from the cell.[4] The sarcoplasmic reticulum functions to keep the intracellular calcium concentration low. This low intracellular calcium concentration produces a high concentration of calcium outside the cell,

which creates a gradient for the inward movement of calcium. The ion pump in the sarcolemma exchanges two sodium ions for one calcium ion. Therefore, the rate of calcium movement into and out of the cell depends on the sodium gradient created by the sodium-potassium pump. This gradient influences the ability of the cell to contract as well as the cell's contractile reserve.

Calcium, Contraction, and Inotropic Agents

Because the activation of cardiac muscle by calcium is well below the maximum, there is a large reserve for modulation of the inotropic (contractile) state of the myocardium. The importance of this reserve is that it allows the heart to respond to the changing demands of the body. A positive inotropic response increases the developed peak force in a contraction without changing initial sarcomere length. Conversely, a negative inotropic response decreases the developed peak force in a contraction without changing initial sarcomere length. When the demand for cardiac output increases (as occurs when one is exercising), the amount of calcium released to the heart can be increased to increase muscle force development and shortening and, therefore, cardiac output to meet the new demands. The relationship between calcium and inotropic state can be described by events that influence the movement of and sensitivity to calcium. Four pathways can alter the inotropic state: (1) that which modulates the availability of free calcium for activation of the sarcomeres, (2) that which modulates the ability of the sarcomeres to respond to a given amount of bound calcium, (3) that which modulates the affinity of the sarcomeres for free calcium, and (4) that which changes the availability or use of the ATP required for contraction and relaxation. The increase in peak force due to a positive inotrope also increases the rate of force development and the rate of fall of force. Several mechanisms affect the inotropic state of the sarcomeres, including the action potential, ion concentration, time- and frequency-dependent changes, effects of cardiovascular drugs, and disease.

Effect of Changing the Action Potential

When the duration of the plateau of an action potential or the degree of depolarization is increased, a positive inotropic response occurs on the subsequent contraction. A current applied during a single action potential in an isolated papillary muscle augments the duration of the action potential.[5] This prolonged action potential has a very small effect on the degree of contraction of that beat. The following beat shows a positive inotropic effect, resulting from the increased duration of depolarization in the preceding beat. This result shows that the extra calcium is buffered in a store with no effect on the immediate beat but is released on the subsequent beat and produces an inotropic response. Any events that increase the excitability of the cell (lower threshold potential), decrease the recovery time required by the cell before it can be restimulated (shorter refractory period), or increase the conducting properties of the cells increase the ability of the cells in the heart to depolarize and increase the magnitude of the resulting contraction. Changes in the opposite direction depress the inotropic state.

Effect of Changing Ion Concentration

Any cardiovascular or hormonal agents that affect the sodium-calcium exchange or the sodium-potassium pump will modulate the ability of the heart muscle to contract. The ions that influence the contractile state of the myocardium are calcium, sodium, and potassium. To investigate the ionic flows across the membrane of isolated cardiac muscle for a given voltage step of depolarization, the voltage across the membrane is held constant (voltage clamping). Then the current flow across the membrane can be determined and the calcium current (the amount of calcium ion flow) can be measured. Increasing the level of depolarization by increasing the voltage across the membrane in amplitude and duration produces an increase in intracellular stores of calcium. This increase in the intracellular stores results in an increase in tension development and contraction force. Decreasing the external sodium concentration decreases the sodium gradient across the sarcolemma, decreasing the concentration of intracellular calcium by decreasing the rate of sodium-calcium exchange. A reduction in the external concentration of potassium produces a decrease in the intracellular concentration of potassium, increasing the intracellular sodium and decreasing the sodium gradient. This decrease in the sodium gradient results in an increase in intracellular calcium and a positive inotropic effect.

Time and Frequency Effects on Contraction

The frequency of stimulation of the myocardium directly affects the heart's inotropic response. An increase in the frequency of stimulation produces an initial decrease in the force of contraction, which, over time, increases to a higher level of peak-force development. This change in the force-frequency relation is called the "force treppe" and reflects a positive inotropic response to increased stimulation frequency. The increased rate initially produces a decrease in calcium release, because reuptake is not complete, resulting in a reduced peak tension. A delay in the removal of calcium by the sodium-calcium exchange pump may also occur, which contributes to the decrease in developed tension. As the intracellular calcium stores increase, the amount of available calcium and the rate of uptake in the sarcoplasmic reticulum increase, increasing the amount of free calcium released per beat and, thus, peak-developed tension. The reverse effect occurs with a decrease in the frequency of contraction, resulting in an initial increase in the force of contraction and eventually a settling into a steady state lower than baseline. The force-frequency response allows the heart to increase its output, even with the decrease in the duration of systole that occurs as heart rate increases by increasing its performance. This important mechanism is utilized during exercise when the duration of the cardiac cycle and its components—ventricular filling and ejection—are shortened. This increase in the force of contraction allows the heart to meet the increasing demands of the body by increasing cardiac output in the presence of a reduced ejection time. As the interval of recovery is increased, the calcium stores can fully recover and return the force of contraction to normal.

Cardiovascular Drugs and Inotropic Agents

Several types of cardiovascular drugs and inotropic agents modify the diastolic and systolic performance of the myocardium. The ability to modulate the mechanisms that regulate myocardial function leads to therapies that are applied when the myocardium is dysfunctional. These drugs alter the concentration of calcium in the cell and the sensitivity of the myofilaments to calcium, resulting in positive or negative changes in inotropic state. Understanding the mechanisms that underlie the activity of the drugs and their effects on calcium regulation is important in the treatment of systolic and diastolic dysfunction.

Digitalis is a positive inotrope that increases ventricular function and cardiac output. It increases the trans-sarcolemmal sodium gradient by inhibiting the sodium-potassium pump, leading to an increase in the sodium-calcium exchange rate. This increased exchange rate produces an increase in intracellular calcium concentration, while a decrease in the sodium gradient that is normally higher outside the cell results in increased force of contraction. Calcium-channel blockers increase the atrioventricular pressure gradient by increasing the rate of relaxation and, subsequently, the rate and volume of early ventricular filling, resulting in an increased diastolic performance.[6, 7] Calcium-channel blockers decrease the concentration of calcium in the cell by blocking entry via the sarcolemma, which provides an increased concentration of intracellular calcium to be removed by the sarcoplasmic reticulum. The blockade of calcium channels results in a decrease in the heart rate, prolonging diastole and increasing the rate of ventricular relaxation by allowing the sarcoplasmic reticulum a longer time for calcium reuptake, resulting in increased ventricular filling.

Pharmacologic studies have shown that cyclic adenosine monophosphate (cAMP) levels are depressed in the failing myocardium and may contribute to the inability of the cells to handle calcium, resulting in systolic contractile and diastolic relaxation abnormalities. Like calcium, cAMP regulates excitation-contraction coupling in the heart. It functions by activating protein kinases, which phosphorylate proteins at several subcellular sites, including the sarcolemma, the sarcoplasmic reticulum, and the troponin-tropomyosin complex. Phosphorylation of the calcium channels not only increases the rate of calcium entry, resulting in an increase in the force of contraction, but also augments the uptake of calcium by the sarcoplasmic reticulum and increases the rate of relaxation. Therefore, the use of agents that increase cAMP diminishes the systolic and diastolic dysfunction resulting from hypertrophic cardiomyopathy.[8]

β-Adrenergic blockers slow the heart rate and improve the balance between myocardial oxygen supply and demand. They act by decreasing the cAMP levels, decreasing the amount of calcium flux into the cell. β-Adrenergic blockers produce a negative inotropic response, whereas β-adrenergic agonists not only increase cAMP levels, increasing calcium entry and force production, but also increase the reuptake of calcium by the sarcoplasmic reticulum, resulting in faster (better) ventricular relaxation. β-Adrenergic blockers promote increased filling by increasing filling time but, most important, they allow the myocardium to reinstate a normal intracellular calcium concentration, which results in decreased diastolic tone (reduced formation of actomyosin complexes throughout diastole) and diastolic pressures.[9] Catecholamines, such as epinephrine and norepinephrine, increase cAMP levels by increasing the inward flow of calcium into the cell, resulting in a positive inotropic effect. Catecholamines also increase the calcium sensitivity of the ATPase in the sarcoplasmic reticular calcium pump, which increases calcium flux and, therefore, the contractile state of the heart.

Effects of Disease

Several disease states have been related to changes in calcium handling that result in myocardial dysfunction. In Syrian hamsters with dilated cardiomyopathy, systolic dysfunction is due to decreased availability of calcium in the sarcoplasmic reticulum.[10, 11] A decrease in the calcium stores reduces the calcium available for contraction and the amount of calcium accessible for contractile reserve. Ischemia is associated with increases in diastolic and systolic calcium uncoupled from force production. This ion-mechanical uncoupling shows that decreased responsiveness of the sarcomeres to calcium leads to contractile dysfunction and abnormalities in diastolic relaxation.[12, 13]

VENTRICULAR MECHANICS

The intact heart is a pump that meets the functional demands of the body. The pressure and volume within the cardiac chambers result from forces acting both on and within the myocardium. The cardiac cycle begins with the electrical depolarization of a region of specialized atrial tissue (sinoatrial node) and is followed by the contraction of the right and left atria, which is slightly offset in time. After a delay in another region of specialized tissue at the junction of the atria and the ventricle, the atrioventricular node, the ventricles contract. They are also slightly offset in time from each other. These electrical events stimulate mechanical contraction by the atria and ventricles to produce pressure changes within the chambers and the flow of blood into and out of the chambers. The relationship between chamber pressure and volume depends on the equilibrium between the ventricular chamber pressure and the stresses in the myocardium, which, in turn, depends on the size and thickness of the ventricular chamber and the elasticity of the myocardium.

Stress-Strain and Pressure-Volume Relations

The pressure-volume relation of the ventricle is determined by the intrinsic properties of the myocardial wall and the geometry of the chamber.[14] This relationship reflects the balance between two forces: the force within the ventricle, pushing out against the walls (pressure), and the force in the wall, holding the tissues together (stress). As the ventricle fills, it stretches the muscle that makes up the wall. When cardiac muscle is stretched, it becomes stiffer because of its intrinsic elastic properties, so it requires greater force to produce additional increases in length. When the ventricle fills, the relationship between pressure and volume reflects the equilibrium between these forces.

Within the myocardium, the local forces and deformations are normalized as stress and strain. Stress (σ) is defined as the force per unit area in a material. Thus, all things being equal, for a given stress in a material, the total force increases as the material gets thicker. Deformation is often normalized as Lagrangian strain (ϵ), defined as the measured fractional extension above an equilibrium length (x_0), the length of muscle when not subject to any forces, divided by that equilibrium length: $\epsilon = (x - x_0)/x_0$. Strain is important because it ties local deformation of the equilibrium length of the muscle to equilibrium volume of the chamber (V_0), the volume at zero transmural pressure. Muscle stress and strain can be related by an exponential equation that describes the elastic properties of the myocardium, $\sigma = \alpha(e^{\beta\epsilon} - 1)$,[15] where α and β are elastic constants.

While the precise relationship between stress in the wall and pressure in the chamber depends on the exact geometry of the cavity and distribution of wall thickness,[16, 17] to a first approximation the Laplace relation, $\sigma = (Pr)/(2h)$, where stress (σ) equals pressure (P) times radius (r) divided by twice the wall thickness (h), describes the relationship between wall stress and cavity pressure. The Laplace law shows that the wall stress increases with increased pressure and chamber radius and decreases in inverse proportion to wall thickness. Chamber radius, in turn, depends on chamber volume (i.e., $V = k\pi r^3$, where the constant (k) depends on the shape of the ventricular cavity).[18] Combining the Laplace law with

an exponential relation between stress and strain describing the elastic properties of the myocardium[19] shows that the pressure-volume relation can be described with three things: the elastic properties of the myocardium, the wall thickness, and the left ventricular equilibrium volume. This work showed that the material properties of the myocardium are coupled through shell geometry to the pressure and volume of the ventricular chamber, which determines diastolic elastic function. There is a similar relationship between cavity pressure, wall force, and deformation during systole, except that the relationship between stress and strain in activated muscle is different from that observed in relaxed muscle.[20]

Cardiac Cycle

A pressure-volume relation is one way of describing the activity of the ventricular chamber during the cardiac cycle (Fig. 3–4), including passive diastolic filling and active contraction. The diastolic pressure-volume curve determines the end-diastolic volume that is achievable with a given filling pressure. The end-systolic pressure-volume relation describes the contractile performance of the ventricular chamber. During a typical cardiac cycle, the closing of the aortic valve marks the beginning of isovolumic relaxation (point 1), which ends at point 2, where diastolic filling begins. During isovolumic relaxation, the cells are repolarizing, the reuptake of calcium by the sarcoplasmic reticulum is proceeding, and the stress and strain of the myocardium are at a minimum. The ventricle begins to fill along its diastolic pressure-volume curve (point 2→3). The ventricular volume increases, increasing chamber wall strain and stress, which results in increased pressure. The amount of filling determines the performance of the ventricle by stretching the myocardial wall and, thus, the sarcomeres. As the active length-tension relation illustrated, the greater the stretch of the sarcomeres prior to stimulation, the greater the developed force. At the beginning of systole, a wave of electrical activity depolarizes the cells in the myocardial walls, generating the calcium-stimulated release, resulting in the synchronous contraction of the sarcomeres and, subsequently, the myocardial chambers. At

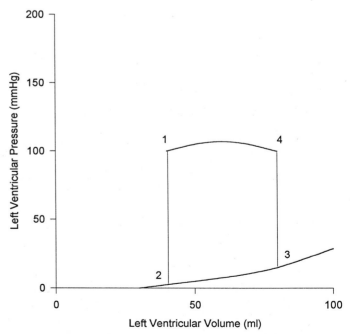

FIGURE 3–4. Left ventricular pressure-volume loop and the diastolic pressure-volume curve. Point 1 shows the end-systolic pressure and volume at the end of ventricular ejection. The ventricle isovolumically relaxes (point 2), until the ventricle begins to fill (points 2 to 3). The end of filling is the end-diastolic pressure-volume point (point 3), when the ventricle begins to contract isovolumically, until the beginning of ejection at point 4. The change in volume during systole (points 4 to 1) is the stroke volume.

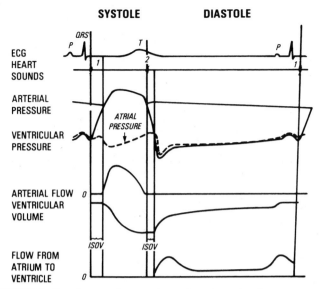

FIGURE 3–5. Schematic drawing shows the relationship between various pressures, volume, and flows. The numbers associated with pressure-volume loop correspond to the numbers in that in Figure 3–4. ECG = electrocardiogram. (From Best, C.H., and Taylor, N.B.: Cardiovascular system. *In* West, J.B. [ed.]: Physiologic Basis of Medical Practice. Baltimore, Williams & Wilkins, 1985, p. 208, with permission.)

point 3, the ventricle begins to contract isovolumically, until the ventricular pressure exceeds the aortic pressure (point 4). Point 4 shows the onset of ventricular ejection, which proceeds until ventricular pressure drops below aortic pressure (point 1). This systolic contraction causes the left ventricle to expel part of its total blood volume.

Figure 3–5 presents another view of the cardiac cycle in terms of the time-dependent events that characterize ventricular function. Left ventricular pressure falls rapidly during relaxation, and at the moment of crossover with the left atrial pressure (PCO) the mitral valve opens and flow starts. The initial slow increase in mitral flow is due to motion of the closed leaflets toward the ventricle; no forward flow or ventricular volume change has occurred, and there is only a change in the shape of the ventricular chamber. After the onset of mitral flow, left ventricular pressure continues to fall, but at a decreased rate, because deactivation has slowed and filling relengthens the sarcomeres, increasing wall stress. Minimum left ventricular pressure is reached at a value determined by the interaction of the active relaxation of force and passive stretch. Therefore, it depends on the rate of relaxation and end-systolic volume, which determine where on its passive pressure-volume curve filling starts. Minimum left ventricular pressure, a function of the rate of relaxation and end-systolic volume, and left atrial pressure are the components of the atrioventricular pressure gradient that determine early diastolic filling.

When the ventricular end-systolic volume is less than the equilibrium volume, the myocardial wall stores elastic energy during systole, just as a compressed spring stores energy. As the myocardium relaxes, this energy is released, reducing the ventricular pressure and increasing the atrioventricular pressure gradient. This increase in the pressure gradient facilitates the filling of the ventricle, which maintains end-diastolic volume and systolic function. Changing the contractile state of the myocardium or the rate of relaxation of the ventricular chamber affects the end-diastolic and end-systolic volume of the ventricle and alters stroke volume and cardiac output. Left atrial pressure falls at the onset of filling, because the left atrium empties faster than it fills via the pulmonary veins. In fact, pulmonary venous flow is quite large in early diastole, so the atrium acts as both a reservoir and a conduit during early ventricular filling.[21] Flow reaches zero as the mitral valve closes.[22]

Following closure of the atrioventricular valve, the ventricle begins to shorten and develop pressure against the blood inside the chamber. This is a period of isovolumic contraction because the chamber volume remains constant. Once the ventricular pressure exceeds the aortic pressure, the aortic valve opens and ejection into the aorta begins. Following peak systolic pressure before the aortic valve closes, the ventricle begins to relax. As the ventricular pressure falls below the aortic pressure, the valve closes and the period of isovolumic relaxation begins again.

DETERMINANTS OF VENTRICULAR FUNCTION

Determinants of Diastolic Function

The pressure difference between the left atrium and the left ventricle, the atrioventricular pressure gradient, provides the motive force for filling. This force is produced by the time-independent passive mechanical properties of the ventricle and the atrium and by the active ventricular properties (Table 3–1). Myocardial elastic forces, a function of the amount of early filling, chamber geometry, and elastic recoil of the chamber due to elastic energy stored in the myocardium from the previous systole, all contribute to the ventricular component of the gradient and, subsequently, to the transmitral flow pattern. The rate of change of the atrioventricular pressure gradient also influences the early filling pattern. The factors that are important at different times during the diastolic period are shown in Figure 3–6.

Passive Components of Filling

The study of ventricular filling and the factors that determine the pattern of filling are important in understanding the diastolic function of the heart. The motive force for left ventricular filling is the atrioventricular pressure gradient,[22] which depends on the active and passive properties of the atrium and ventricle and determines the ventricular filling pattern. These factors include preload, afterload, contractility, and heart rate. Diastolic suction, which is the effect of elastic recoil of the ventricular wall on ventricular filling, is also an important aspect of filling and needs to be addressed in any discussion of left ventricular filling dynamics.[23, 24]

Left atrial pressure at the time of mitral valve opening and the rate of relaxation are important determinants of the early transmitral velocity pattern.[25, 26] Many studies have investigated the effect of varying these parameters to determine how they influence the atrioventricular pressure gradient. The small early atrioventricular pressure difference provides the motive force for the rapid acceleration of mitral flow to its peak (E-point, or peak rapid filling rate, PRFR) (see Fig. 3–5). Flow then rapidly decelerates, and

TABLE 3–1. DETERMINANTS OF SYSTOLIC AND DIASTOLIC VENTRICULAR PROPERTIES

	Systolic Determinants	Diastolic Determinants
Relaxation		X
Elastic recoil		X
Left atrial compliance		X
Venous return		X
Mitral impedance		X
Ventricular stiffness	X	X
Inotropic state	X	X
Afterload	X	
Chamber mass	X	X
Ventricular interaction	X	X
Heart rate	X	X
Chamber geometry	X	X
Coronary vascular tone	X	X

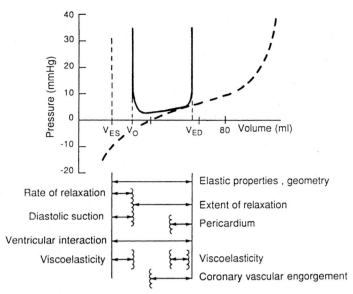

FIGURE 3–6. Factors that affect the diastolic pressure at various times during diastole. Myocardial elasticity, chamber geometry, and ventricular interaction are important throughout diastole. Active relaxation and diastolic suction (the effect of elastic recoil from the previous systole) are important early in diastole, because they influence the atrioventricular pressure gradient and the rate of early ventricular filling. In late diastole, ventricular interaction and the pericardium become increasingly important. Viscoelastic and coronary vascular engorgement have a small effect during late diastole. The dashed line shows the passive diastolic pressure-volume relation due to purely elastic properties of the myocardium. The solid line is a pressure-volume relation during a typical cardiac cycle. V_0 = the equilibrium volume of the chamber with zero transmural pressure; V_{ed} = end-diastolic volume; V_{es} = end-systolic volume. (From Gilbert, J.C., and Glantz, S.A.: Determinants of left ventricular filling and of the diastolic pressure-volume relation. Circ. Res. 64[5]:827–852, 1989, with permission. Copyright 1989, American Heart Association.)

although the pressure gradient soon becomes zero, often reversing slightly, forward mitral flow continues because of inertia.[27] The atrial contraction then reaccelerates mitral flow to a second peak (A-point), from which flow decelerates and pressure falls as the atrium empties and relaxes. Volume infusion and inotropic agents have been used to study the effect of altering left atrial pressure on the transmitral velocity pattern.[25, 28] This work showed that mitral flow that was reduced because of a decrease in the rate of left ventricular relaxation could be overcome by increasing left atrial pressure. This finding suggests that left atrial pressure plays a larger role in the determination of mitral flow than the rate of relaxation. Changing afterload by altering the resistance of the aorta has been used as a tool to change the rate of relaxation. An increase in afterload, decreasing the rate of relaxation, produces a decreased atrioventricular pressure gradient. The decrease in the atrioventricular pressure gradient results in a reduced volume flow into the ventricle, although the peak rate of filling is increased, because the atrium sees a stiffer ventricular chamber owing to an increase in ventricular load.

End-systolic volume clamping, that is, occluding the mitral orifice during late systole to prevent filling, has been used to separate the passive effects of filling from the active process of relaxation.[23, 29] End-systolic volume clamping showed that the elastic properties of the heart augment the transmitral flow pattern by contributing to the atrioventricular pressure gradient.[30] Each of these factors will be discussed because of the effect they have on altering the atrioventricular pressure gradient.

Active Components of Filling

Relaxation

Relaxation refers to the process by which the myocardium returns to its initial length and tension following a contraction.[31] The

onset of left ventricular filling occurs before the end of relaxation from the previous systole. The ventricular diastolic pressure-volume relation is influenced by the extent and rate of myocardial relaxation from the previous systole. The rate of relaxation affects the atrioventricular pressure gradient, which is the motive force behind early ventricular filling. The efficient and complete reuptake of calcium from the sarcomeres by the sarcolemma and sarcoplasmic reticulum produces a fast rate of relaxation to a low minimum ventricular pressure, which facilitates high left ventricular filling rates. The rate and extent of relaxation are influenced by changes in load, heart rate, and neurohumoral effects. An impaired (slowed) rate of relaxation manifests as a decreased rate of left ventricular pressure fall. This decreased rate of relaxation reduces mitral flow early in diastole, because it decreases the atrioventricular pressure gradient, resulting in less early ventricular filling.

The time course of left ventricular isovolumic relaxation can be described with an exponential decline to a zero asymptote.[32] This characterization was further refined by adding a nonzero asymptote to the exponential.[24] The relaxation rate is calculated from the time constant of an assumed exponential isovolumic pressure fall is described by:

$$P = (P_0 + P_\infty)e^{-t/\tau} - P_\infty$$

where P_0 = pressure at time zero, P_∞ = asymptote of an exponential pressure decay at $t = \infty$, τ = time constant, t = time following dP/dt_{min}.

To separate the effects of relaxation from the effects of deformation and to determine the role relaxation plays as an active component of diastolic function, it is necessary to prevent the ventricle from filling. By occluding the mitral orifice mechanically at end-systole with a volume clamp,[24] filling was prevented, allowing relaxation to proceed to completion without stretching any elastic elements. The rate of ventricular relaxation is slowed after incremental increases in stretch owing to mitral inflow into the ventricular chamber. The duration of relaxation is also increased when compared with nonfilling beats. These results show that the rate of ventricular relaxation depends on ventricular volume.[33] Inotropic state and heart rate influence the rate of relaxation. Increasing the inotropic state increases the rate of relaxation when compared with low inotropic states. Similarly, an increase in the heart rate produces an increase in contractility, which results in a decrease in the duration of contraction and leads to an earlier onset of relaxation. Thus, the rate of relaxation is determined by the passive ventricular properties of the ventricular chamber. The rate of relaxation depends on absolute volume, its interaction with internal restoring forces (elastic ventricular properties), and stretch due to filling. These factors determine the performance of the ventricular chamber, and inotropic state and heart rate influence the roles these factors play.

Passive Diastolic Pressure-Volume Relation

The diastolic pressure-volume curve for the normal canine left ventricle is typically curvilinear, being essentially linear at low ventricular end-diastolic volumes and becoming steeper at the upper limit of normal end-diastolic pressures (approximately 10 mm Hg) and above.[19] It approximates a logarithmic relation, and as the chamber becomes progressively filled during each diastole, instantaneous ventricular chamber stiffness increases (larger dP/dt). This response is consistent with the muscle's exponential stress-strain relation, which shows that the muscle gets stiffer (larger $d\sigma/d\epsilon$) as it is stretched. The geometric relationship between increases in chamber volume and strain in the wall accounts for the relatively linear ventricular pressure-volume curve at low volumes, despite the fact that the myocardial stress-strain curve is exponential. Chamber radius, and so circumference and wall strain, increase as $V^{1/3}$, which increases more slowly at low volumes than at higher ones.[19] At low volumes, when the ventricular pressure increase is small, the chamber is very distensible, but at larger volumes, the ventricle becomes stiffer, so small volume increases produce large pressure increases.

The left ventricle normally operates on the flat part of the curve, but during an acute volume load, the left ventricle operates on a stiffer portion of the passive diastolic pressure-volume relation. A stiff ventricle, such as occurs in left ventricular hypertrophy, exhibits a larger increase in pressure for a given increase in volume when compared with a normal ventricle. The increase in stiffness in the hypertrophied heart is due to the increase in the size of the myocytes becoming less distensible (greater h in the Laplace relationship), an increase in the number of sarcomeres in parallel, and the accumulation of myocardial collagen matrix, increasing the elastic stiffness of the myocardium itself. Thus, an increase in stiffness can result from an increase in filling pressure (with the heart functioning on a steeper portion of the diastolic pressure-volume curve) or can be due to an intrinsically stiffer chamber that has a steeper pressure-volume curve at a given end-diastolic pressure.

Factors Affecting the Atrioventricular Pressure Gradient

Effect of Changing Left Atrial Pressure

Left atrial pressure is a primary determinant of the atrioventricular pressure gradient, which is the motive force behind mitral flow. When left atrial pressure is increased, such as by volume infusion, the increase in left atrial pressure at mitral valve opening is greater than the increase in minimum left ventricular pressure. This increase in the gradient produces an increase in the peak rate of filling, despite a slowed relaxation because of an increase in filling volume.[25] The increase in filling rate demonstrates that the increased transmitral pressure difference overcame the effects of a decrease in the rate of relaxation. A decrease in left atrial pressure, induced by nitroglycerin, reflects systemic venodilation and was found to decrease both the peak rate of filling and the time constant of relaxation.[28] Similar results accompany the altering of left atrial pressure with lower-body negative pressure[34] or balloon inflation in the inferior vena cava. The relation between peak filling velocity and left atrial pressure before mitral valve opening is approximately linear over the entire physiologic range of left atrial pressure, when left ventricular pressure is held constant.[26] This linear relationship between peak filling velocity and left atrial pressure before mitral valve opening suggests that left atrial pressure strongly influences ventricular diastolic function.

Effect of Changing Afterload

The effect of loading on rate of left ventricular relaxation, left atrial pressure, and minimum left ventricular pressure reflects the important effect of these determinants on the atrioventricular pressure gradient and, subsequently, on the mitral flow pattern. In isolated cardiac muscle, changing afterload significantly affects the rate of relaxation.[35] Both the extent and the velocity of shortening decrease as the afterload is increased, and, conversely, muscle performance increases as the afterload is decreased. In an intact heart, when afterload is pharmacologically increased, a weak but statistically significant correlation is found between the peak rate of flow and the time constant of relaxation, generating large increases in peak left ventricular pressure and left ventricular end-diastolic pressure.[25] The increase in afterload causes an increase in end-diastolic volume and pressure, forcing the heart to function on a steeper portion of the passive diastolic pressure-volume curve (producing a stiffer ventricular chamber). The Frank-Starling mechanism is called on to maintain cardiac output, resulting in a decrease in the functional reserve capacity of the ventricular chamber.

Diastolic Suction

The equilibrium volume (V_0) is defined as the volume of the ventricle at zero transmural pressure. The normally contracting ventricle can reach end-systolic volumes both above and below the equilibrium volume, depending on the loading conditions and inotropic state. When the end-systolic volume is below V_0, stored energy in the muscle produces a negative ventricular pressure in early diastole. This stored energy provides an internal restoring force that facilitates filling by contributing to the atrioventricular pressure gradient. This suction is a passive component of filling because there are no contractile forces involved. The finding of a negative pressure gradient from the base to the apex of the ventricle is further evidence of elastic recoil.[27] This is also compatible with a model of diastolic function that treats the apex as recoiling during early diastole and contributing to filling by actively drawing blood into the ventricular chamber.[36] The remainder of filling results from an atrial contraction, during which a positive atrioventricular pressure gradient (left atrial pressure is greater than left ventricular pressure) exists.

Higher inotropic states lead to smaller end-systolic volumes and increase the likelihood that the ventricle will contract to below V_0. Diastolic suction (elastic ventricular recoil) at small end-systolic volumes due to an increased inotropic state or a reduced afterload produces a decreased left atrial pressure at the onset of mitral flow. During exercise, diastolic suction plays a larger role when a large stroke volume is subjected to a decreased diastolic period.[37] During increased contractility, diastolic suction is also increased, independent of end-systolic volume.[23, 38] These findings suggest that diastolic suction plays an increasingly important role in maintaining diastolic function during times of increasing demands on the heart.

Ventricular Interaction and the Pericardium

The ventricular chambers share a common septum, and the right ventricular output becomes the left ventricular input. Ventricular interaction describes the influence of one chamber on the performance of the other chamber because of these mechanical connections. The chamber interaction shifts the diastolic pressure-volume relation in response to changing ventricular loading conditions. Several studies have shown that there are both direct and series components of mechanical interaction between the ventricles during the cardiac cycle.[18, 39–41]

The interventricular septum is a composite of shared fibers connecting the left and right ventricular free walls to each other. Direct interventricular interaction involves septal shifting that changes the chamber geometry and, consequently, affects ventricular filling by decreasing the distensibility of the opposite ventricle. This interaction depends on the elastic properties of the septum and the transseptal pressure gradient. The transseptal pressure gradient depends on the chamber volumes and the loading conditions on the individual ventricles and affects the ventricular pressure-volume relation. The ventricular pressure-volume relation is shifted up by an increase in the contralateral ventricular pressure.[42]

The series component arises from the series arrangement of the chambers, in which the output of one chamber determines the input of the other.[18, 39] This interaction maintains the balance between the outputs of the right and left ventricles, because the Frank-Starling mechanism adjusts the output of the left ventricle to match that of the right ventricle on a beat-to-beat basis. A change in right ventricular output is transmitted across the pulmonary circulation and appears in the left ventricular filling one beat after the initial change.[43] Thus, series interaction is also an important determinant of left ventricular end-diastolic volume.

The pericardium is a bag that surrounds the heart's four chambers and increases the magnitude of direct mechanical interaction, because the four chambers of the heart compete for space within the relatively stiff pericardium.[44] The left and right ventricular diastolic pressures are coupled by the intact pericardium. The effect of the pericardium depends on the chamber volumes. As the volumes in the chambers are increased, ventricular pressures increase, and the interaction between the left and the right ventricles increases. This increase in chamber interaction is due to the pericardium moving onto a steep part of its pressure-volume curve, which produces a tighter coupling between the right and the left chambers.[45]

The determination of pericardial pressure has been controversial.

The use of a flat balloon placed into the pericardial space to measure contact pressure between the ventricular epicardium and pericardium has shown that pericardial pressure is positive and contributes to interventricular pressure throughout the normal range of diastolic pressures. The change in pericardial pressure is closely approximated by the change in the right ventricular end-diastolic pressure and is, therefore, similar to right atrial pressure.[46] This result suggests that right ventricular transmural pressure is negligible. Other studies have shown that the right ventricular pericardial pressure is always positive; therefore, right ventricular diastolic pressure does not equal pericardial pressure.[40, 47] To reconcile these two findings it was shown that the pericardium operates differently at different volumes.[48] At low volumes, pericardial pressure is near zero, while at higher volumes the pericardial pressure is a substantial fraction of the left ventricular end-diastolic pressure. Right ventricular end-diastolic pressures are greater than the pericardial pressures at low volumes. At higher volumes, when the pericardium had a restraining effect on filling, both pericardial and right ventricular end-diastolic pressures increased in a similar fashion. The pericardial pressure is near zero until right ventricular diastolic pressure is greater than 4 mm Hg; then pericardial pressure correlates with right ventricular end-diastolic pressure. Normal left ventricular end-diastolic pressure (8 to 10 mm Hg) coincides with the onset point of pericardial constraint, where there is a linear relationship between the pericardial pressure and increases in left ventricular end-diastolic pressure.[48] This response shows that the left ventricle usually operates near the unstressed volume of the pericardium, where the pericardial pressure is small. At high left ventricular filling pressures (greater than about 10 mm Hg) pericardial stiffness increases left ventricular diastolic pressures. Thus, at low chamber pressures, the pericardial pressure is close to zero and does not play a role in chamber filling. At higher chamber volumes, the pericardium significantly constrains chamber filling. This increase in constraint enhances diastolic ventricular interdependence at the upper limit of the normal range of left ventricular pressure.

To determine the relative roles of the direct and series ventricular interaction in the in situ heart, Slinker and Glantz[18] used the time delay between a change in right ventricular output and left ventricular input to separate these components. They found that direct interaction is about 50 percent as important as series interaction in determining left ventricular end-diastolic size with an intact pericardium. After removing the pericardium, the importance of direct interaction falls to about 20 percent of series interaction because of a reduction in pericardial constraint. Without the presence of the stiffer pericardial sac encasing the four chambers, a change in volume in the more compliant chambers does not have a large effect on the contralateral chamber. Wall thickness also affects the relative roles of ventricular interaction by reducing the role of direct interaction and the pericardium with increased wall thickness. An increase in ventricular pressure in a chamber with a thicker interventricular septum does not interact as much with the contralateral ventricle because the thicker septum is stiffer.[47] In contrast with normal hearts, removal of the pericardium had no significant effect on direct ventricular interaction, suggesting that the mechanical properties of the chamber are more reliant on the myocardium in the hypertrophied hearts.

Effects of Cardiovascular Drugs on Diastolic Function

The primary goal in treating filling abnormalities is to reduce the effects of diastolic dysfunction, such as pulmonary congestion, and to reduce the factors responsible for the dysfunction. Pulmonary congestion is the result of increased arterial pressures producing increased atrial and ventricular chamber pressures to maintain cardiac output. These increased chamber pressures are then transmitted back into the lungs, increasing pulmonary capillary pressure, resulting in fluid buildup in the lungs. Diuretics reduce pulmonary congestion by increasing the excretion of salt and water by the kidneys. Diuretics decrease left ventricular filling pressures, reducing left atrial pressure, and shift the operating range of the left ventricle to a flatter portion of the end-diastolic pressure-volume curve. This response decreases the stress and strain placed on the chamber for the heart to operate, decreasing the heart's oxygen requirements and increasing the reserve capacity of the heart to respond to changing demands.

Venous dilators, such as nitroprusside, produce their effect by relaxing venous smooth muscle and acting as a potent arteriolar dilator. Nitroprusside reduces right ventricular filling and volume by decreasing venous return. Nitroprusside also decreases afterload. This decrease in venous return and afterload increases cardiac output while shifting blood from the heart to the periphery. This redistribution of blood volume accounts for a downward shift in the diastolic pressure-volume relation, decreasing the end-diastolic pressure by 50 percent.[49] The end-diastolic volume decreases less than 10 percent, maintaining or even increasing stroke volume, resulting in an increase in cardiac output by as much as 50 percent in patients with heart failure. Because the diastolic pressure-volume curve shifts downward, stroke volume is maintained despite a large decrease in end-diastolic pressure (Fig. 3–7). This downward shift in response to nitroprusside has been abolished in dogs following pericardial excision, because the heart is no longer restricted by the stiff pericardium.[50] This shift reflects the important role of the pericardium and ventricular interaction in modulating this effect. If the vasodilator caused the ventricle to simply move down a single diastolic pressure-volume relation, maintaining stroke volume would have been impossible, because the end-diastolic volume corresponding to the reduced end-diastolic pressure would be too low to maintain stroke volume and cardiac output. The stroke volume was maintained because the entire pressure-volume curve shifted downward owing to ventricular interaction. Therefore, direct end-diastolic ventricular interaction is an important factor in the heart, maintaining stroke volume in the presence of falling end-diastolic pressure.

To improve cardiac output in an impaired ventricle, the loading conditions on the heart must be reduced. Angiotensin-converting enzyme (ACE) inhibitors, besides decreasing systemic vascular re-

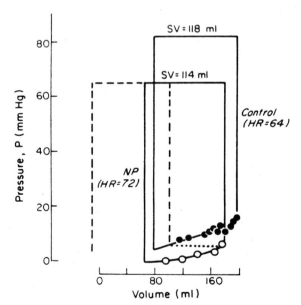

FIGURE 3–7. Diastolic pressure-volume curve from a patient. This plot shows the shift in the pressure-volume curve in response to a vasodilator to maintain stroke volume. The stroke volume was maintained by shifting the pressure-volume curve downward. If the vasodilator caused the ventricle to move down the original diastolic pressure-volume curve, the end-systolic volume would have become negative (*dashed line*), which is incompatible with life. Therefore, by shifting downward, the left ventricle could function on a lower end-diastolic pressure and maintain stroke volume. SV = stroke volume; NP = nitroprusside; HR = heart rate. (From Alderman, E.L., and Glantz, S.A.: Acute hemodynamic interventions shift the diastolic pressure-volume curve in man. Circulation 54[4]:662–671, 1976, with permission.)

sistance and increasing systemic venous capacitance, improve diastolic filling by blocking the production of angiotensin II, which directly impairs ventricular relaxation. Angiotensin II is a potent vasoconstrictor that is degraded into angiotensin III, which stimulates the release of aldosterone, producing an increase in preload by increasing sodium and water resorption. ACE inhibitors act by inhibiting the conversion of angiotensin I to angiotensin II, producing a drop in afterload. Because the formation of angiotensin II is prevented, it cannot be degraded to angiotensin III. Thus, the stimulation and release of aldosterone do not occur, and there is no increase in sodium and water resorption, resulting in a decrease in preload. These effects produce an increase in cardiac output secondary to an improvement in ventricular relaxation and a decrease in end-diastolic pressure and afterload. Conversely, angiotensin, a powerful vasoconstrictor, increases right ventricular pressure and shifts the diastolic pressure-volume curve upward.[51]

In patients with hypertension, calcium antagonists and β-adrenergic blockers have been shown to speed relaxation and improve diastolic filling. Calcium-channel blockers produce an increase in the peak filling rate and decrease the time to peak filling. These drugs also slow the heart rate and improve the balance between myocardial oxygen supply and demand. Because the diastolic time is increased, the sarcoplasmic reticulum has more time to sequester the cytosolic calcium, increasing the extent of ventricular relaxation and lowering filling pressures. β-Adrenergic blockers also function by decreasing the heart rate and increasing filling time. A more important effect of this class of drugs is the increase in oxygen efficiency. Both calcium-channel blockers and β-adrenergic blockers improve diastolic function by producing a regression of hypertrophy, correcting abnormal calcium transport, reducing region asynchrony, normalizing relaxation, and balancing myocardial oxygen demand and supply. The positive or negative effect of calcium antagonists and β-adrenergic blockers on diastolic function depends on the source of the hypertrophy, but they potentially play an important role in improving cardiac function in hypertrophic cardiomyopathy, hypertension, and coronary artery disease.

Determinants of Systolic Function

Contractility

As discussed earlier, cardiac muscle has two ways of modulating the amount of force and shortening when it contracts: changes in muscle length, which affect thin- and thick-filament overlap and, therefore, available cross-bridge sites, and changes in the amount of calcium available, which triggers cross-bridge formation. Changes in end-diastolic volume change the strain on the myocardium and, thus, modulate systolic function via the Frank-Starling mechanism. A variety of neurohumoral and pharmacologic agents alter calcium availability and change the inotropic state of the heart. Agents that increase available calcium and increase developed pressure and ejection are called positive inotropic agents.

Frank-Starling Mechanism

As already discussed, in an isolated muscle, developed force increases as the rest length increases. This provides the physiologic basis for the Frank-Starling relationship in the intact heart, where an increase in the end-diastolic volume of the ventricle results in an increase in ventricular stroke volume or stroke work. The Frank-Starling mechanism operates on a beat-to-beat basis to adjust ventricular performance to changes in venous return and balance the stroke volumes of the right and left ventricles. There is a linear relationship between stroke work and end-diastolic volume,[52] with the curve shifting upward (more stroke work for a given end-diastolic volume) when drugs are administered to increase inotropic state.[53, 54] This specific manifestation of the Frank-Starling mechanism has been called preload recruitable stroke work (PRSW). The Frank-Starling mechanism also plays an important compensatory role during a variety of disease states.

The end-systolic pressure-volume relationship is another mani-

festation of the Frank-Starling relationship. When the volume in the ventricle is varied, the peak pressure of the isometric contractions falls along a straight line at a given inotropic state.[55] In addition, the end-systolic pressure-volume point of an ejecting pressure-volume loop falls along this isovolumic pressure-volume relation. The end-systolic pressure represented on a pressure-volume diagram shows that there is a linear relationship between the end-systolic pressure and volume of ejecting and nonejecting beats for a given contractile state (Fig. 3–8). This relationship is called the end-systolic pressure-volume relation. The line intersects with the volume axis at V_d, the dead volume, the minimum volume to which the ventricular chamber can contract. The slope of the end-systolic pressure-volume relation equals the end-systolic elastance, E_{es}, or maximum elastance, E_{max} (elastance is the reciprocal of stiffness, so E_{max} is the active systolic analogue of passive diastolic stiffness). The introduction of a positive inotrope does not affect V_d but increases the slope of the relation and rotates the isovolumic pressure-volume relation up and to the left, whereas a negative inotrope rotates the isovolumic pressure-volume relation down and to the right.

The slope of the end-systolic pressure-volume relation (E_{max}) has been used as an index of contractility to reflect changes in inotropic state of the heart, independent of preload and afterload conditions. Preload independence can be tested by fixing arterial pressure while varying end-diastolic volume to see whether the end-systolic corner of the loops falls along the same end-systolic pressure-volume relation. Afterload independence can be determined by varying the aortic resistance. Unfortunately, the end-systolic pressure-volume relation has been found to be curvilinear[56, 57] and afterload dependent.[58] These changes in linearity and influence by arterial impedance on the end-systolic pressure-volume relation are limitations of an ideal index of myocardial contractility, which should be independent of loading conditions. These findings sug-

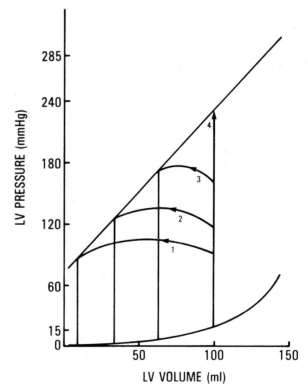

FIGURE 3–8. Schematic shows left ventricular pressure-volume relation at increasing end-diastolic volumes. Peak pressure increases during isovolumic contractions (beats 2 and 3) with same end-diastolic volumes. Stroke volume decreases (beats 2 and 3) for the same end-diastolic volumes at higher left ventricular pressures. (From Best, C.H., and Taylor, N.B.: Cardiovascular system. *In* West, J.B. [ed.]: Physiologic Basis of Medical Practice. Baltimore, Williams & Wilkins, 1985, p. 213, with permission.)

gest that the inotropic state of the myocardium should be created by examining relative changes in slope and linearity of the end-systolic pressure-volume relation. At present, preload recruitable stroke work appears to be the most reliable index of systolic performance, because it exhibits a linear relation, despite wide variations in afterload and inotropic state.[54] The preload recruitable stroke work is linear and reliable, because stroke work is determined by integrating the entire cardiac cycle. In contrast, the end-systolic pressure-volume relation is based on a single point in the cardiac cycle.

Afterload

A change in the afterload, the load after the muscle starts to shorten, on the ventricular chamber affects the performance of the myocardium. A sudden increase in aortic pressure at a given end-diastolic volume reflects the effects of a pure change in afterload. An increase in afterload results in a decrease in stroke volume and a decrease in the velocity of ejection in the beat immediately following the increase in afterload. There is an inverse relationship between afterload and the extent of shortening and the velocity of ejection for a given end-diastolic volume. This inverse relationship is due to the increase in chamber volume reducing the degree of shortening and the increase in time required to develop sufficient force to overcome the load on the chamber. Following the beat immediately after the afterload perturbation, compensatory use of the Frank-Starling mechanism restores the stroke volume of a healthy heart to normal.

Heart Rate

The main effect of increases in heart rate on cardiac function is to increase cardiac output because cardiac output = heart rate × stroke volume. Heart rate also modulates systolic performance by its effect on the inotropic state of the heart. By increasing the heart rate, an increase in contractility occurs because of the force-frequency relation. In an isolated heart preparation, the positive inotropic effect of an increased heart rate, as quantified by the slope of the end-systolic pressure-volume relation, is not enhanced beyond 120 beats per minute, until reaching values above 200 beats per minute, where it continues to increase modestly.[59] This positive inotropic response is the result of an increase in calcium availability because of a gradual buildup of calcium entering the cell with each beat.

Indexes of diastolic filling are also influenced by heart rate. Heart rate is directly related to peak filling rate and inversely related to time to peak filling. The early and late diastolic filling waves constitute most of the filling during diastole. The late filling wave (atrial contraction) occurs after a time following the early filling wave. Therefore, the effects of any changes in heart rate on filling are buffered by the interval between early and late filling. However, at rates above 95 beats per minute, the peak filling rate and time to peak filling rate become sensitive to changes in the duration of the cardiac cycle. At high heart rates, the active and passive ventricular properties of filling overlap with atrial systole.[60] Small changes in cardiac cycle length at high heart rates dramatically affect the rate of peak filling and, subsequently, the volume of transmitral flow. This effect of heart rate on filling effectively limits the maximum rate that the heart can use to augment cardiac output.

Systolic Ventricular Interaction

Systolic ventricular interaction also determines systolic performance in response to changes in loading conditions. Because the two ventricles share a common interventricular septum and muscle fibers in their free walls, they interact directly. A change in the right ventricular diastolic pressure affects left ventricular diastolic pressure. Therefore, a change in right ventricular loading alters left ventricular filling and, subsequently, systolic performance. Systolic direct ventricular interaction due to septal displacement increases cardiac output under normal physiologic conditions.[61] An acute increase in right ventricular afterload results in an increase in peak systolic pressure and reduces the rate of relaxation in the left ventricle of the same beat. This change in right ventricular loading conditions and the resultant decrease in left ventricular relaxation show that direct interventricular interaction is involved in modulating the systolic performance.

Effects of Cardiovascular Drugs on Systolic Function

Digoxin (digitalis) produces an increase in the contractile state of the myocardium and increases the velocity of ejection. It increases the slope of the end-systolic pressure-volume relation, resulting in an increase in stroke volume. These inotropic effects are produced by inhibiting the exchange of sodium and potassium, which increases intracellular sodium. The increase in intracellular sodium increases the amount of calcium exchange that enters the cell, increases calcium binding to the myofilaments, and increases the force of contraction. In addition, digoxin produces an increase in vagal tone that slows the atrioventricular conduction rate, increasing filling time and cardiac output. It also affects the kidneys by inhibiting the sodium-potassium ATPase pump, resulting in diuresis and decreased loading pressures.

Receptors that respond to catecholamines are called adrenergic. The inotropic state of the heart is modulated by the level of adrenergic tone. A decrease in blood pressure detected by the arterial baroreceptors results in a reflex-positive inotropic response to raise blood pressure. During conditions of increased sympathetic tone, stimulation of the vagus nerve results in a negative inotropic effect on the atria. Drugs can also alter inotropic state. There are at least two major types of adrenergic receptors, α and β, and several subtypes. α-Receptors are innervated by the sympathetic vasoconstrictor nerves and respond to circulating norepinephrine, which has little β-stimulating activity. β-Receptors cause vasodilation. Dobutamine is a synthetic sympathomimetic amine that stimulates β_1-, β_2-, and α_1-receptors by increasing the contractile state of the myocardium and decreasing the load on the ventricular chamber. β_1-Receptors have inotropic activity, β_2-receptors produce a vasodilatory response, and α_1-receptors cause a vasoconstriction response, counteracting the vasodilatory activity. Dobutamine has a greater affinity for β_1-receptors, resulting in an increased force of contraction with mild vasodilatory effects.

Dopamine is a dose-dependent catecholamine that can act as a diuretic, improve contractility, or increase afterload, depending on the dose. The response to this catecholamine, which stimulates α_1-receptors, β-receptors, and dopaminergic receptors, differs, depending on the dose. At low doses, it produces dopaminergic responses in the kidney and increases renal blood flow, producing an increase in the rate of fluid excretion, decreasing systemic pressure by reducing volume. For midlevel doses, β-receptors are stimulated, resulting in an increased heart rate and positive inotropic effects, which improves contractile state and cardiac output. At high doses the α-receptors are stimulated and produce vasoconstriction. These and other drug therapies, such as diuretics, can be used to improve the performance of a failing or dysfunctional heart.

Coronary Blood Flow and Ischemia

The coronary circulation is the series of vessels located within the myocardium that are responsible for delivering blood to the myocardium. The major determinants of coronary blood flow include aortic pressure, myocardial extravascular compression, myocardial metabolism, and neural control. During diastole, blood flow is supplied to the coronaries, while during systole, flow is impeded because the myocardium compresses the coronary circulation. Coronary arterial pressure does not affect left ventricular peak systolic pressure when coronary pressure is within the normal physiologic range. Below this range, the peak contractile performance of the ventricle decreases.[62] This fall in ventricular performance is reflected as a decrease in the slope of the end-systolic pressure-volume relation and may be related to the limit of coronary autoregulatory reserve.[63] Therefore, coronary artery pressure below the critical pressure becomes a major determinant of ventricular contractility.

Regional ischemia due to a local blockage of blood flow to an area of the myocardium produces changes in ventricular wall properties, vascular properties, and blood volume. A decrease in regional coronary blood flow leads to regional mechanical dysfunction, which, when it is large enough, impairs chamber function. During ischemia, systolic function is reduced in the myocardium. A decrease in systolic performance leads to an increase in end-diastolic volume, which increases diastolic pressure and produces higher ventricular stresses and increased strain in the myocardium. These changes force the heart to function on a steeper portion of the diastolic pressure-volume curve. The ischemia also impairs ventricular relaxation, leading to a shorter and lower velocity filling pattern, which results in a decrease in filling. Calcium accumulates in the cytosol because the ability of the sarcoplasmic reticulum to sequester calcium is diminished.

The heart can maintain overall systolic performance with reduced regional systolic function.[64] Regions of the heart outside the ischemic area are stretched to a greater extent than normal because of the increased diastolic pressure produced by a stiffer myocardium. Increased diastolic stretch results in an increase in developed systolic force because of the Frank-Starling mechanism, which is called on from the increase in end-diastolic chamber length to compensate for the initial decrease in systolic performance in the ischemic region. When systolic function is reduced in an area near the ischemic region of the myocardium, those areas far from the ischemic region show an increase in systolic performance.[65, 66] Thus, reduced systolic performance in an ischemic region is accompanied by a compensatory lengthening in the myofilaments of the normal regions to reduce the overall global effects of regional ischemia.

Ischemia can be divided into supply-induced and demand-induced ischemia.[67] Supply-induced ischemia is caused by a decrease in myocardial perfusion, which decreases systolic work, resulting in a rightward shift in the diastolic pressure-volume curve.[68, 69] This type of flow-limited ischemia produces an acidotic myocardium, reducing contractile function and increasing end-diastolic volume. Supply-induced ischemia due to coronary occlusion decreases the supply of oxygen by decreasing the blood flow to the myocardium, resulting in a decrease in the rate of ventricular relaxation.

Pacing-induced ischemia is a form of demand ischemia. The work done by the heart is increased, increasing oxygen demand, and coronary flow cannot meet the increased demand. This form of ischemia was found to shift the pressure-volume relation upward[67, 70] and rightward,[71] suggesting that the response of the diastolic pressure-volume relation is not determined solely by the type of ischemia present. During pacing-induced ischemia, the diastolic pressure-volume relation shifted upward in the filling beat without any effect on the curve in a nonfilling beat.[70] These findings suggest that this upward shift in the pressure-volume relation is due to a stretch-induced increase in the release of calcium into the myofilaments. This stretch activation during rapid filling increases the effective chamber stiffness by increasing the active stiffness of some of the myocardium during diastole, resulting in an upward shift in the ventricular diastolic pressure-volume curve.

Other studies have found that demand-and-supply ischemia produces shifts in various directions.[72–74] With these contradictory results, it would appear that trying to determine the size and direction of the shift of the diastolic pressure-volume curve from the type of ischemia produces unclear results. Left ventricular end-systolic elastance, an index of contractility, most accurately reflects both the direction and the size of the shift of the end-systolic pressure-volume relation during pacing-induced ischemia.[75] A heart that demonstrates good contractile function before the ischemic event will increase its effective chamber stiffness, producing an upward shift in the diastolic pressure-volume curve, whereas a heart with limited contractile function before ischemia will dilate and produce a rightward shift in the diastolic pressure-volume relation.

Cardiac Hypertrophy

Hypertrophy is the process whereby the adult heart grows through an increase in the size of cardiac cells. Hypertrophy occurs as a compensatory response to maintain stroke volume in the presence of an increase in chamber stress or strain and is produced by several types of disease states. Hypertrophy can be divided into two basic types, pressure overload and volume overload.

Hypertension is the most common cause of pressure-overload hypertrophy of the left ventricle. Hypertension increases the aortic pressure experienced by the ventricular chamber during systole, requiring the left ventricular systolic pressure to increase to maintain stroke volume. Aortic stenosis, a narrowing of the aortic valve area, also produces pressure-overload hypertrophy. The heart responds to the increased resistance to outflow by developing concentric hypertrophy. Concentric hypertrophy is an increase in the wall thickness of the left ventricular wall that does not affect the size of the ventricular chamber. Hypertrophy occurs as a means of normalizing the increase in stress on the ventricular chamber, and the extent of the response is governed by the Laplace law.[76] During pressure-overload hypertrophy, the stroke volume is maintained, but the end-systolic pressure-volume relation is shifted up and to the left in a manner similar to that seen in a heart with increased inotropic state because of the increase in wall thickness and, thus, total wall force and chamber pressure development. This increase in force development also increases oxygen consumption. The increase in oxygen consumption is coupled with studies that show that there is a reduction in capillary density[77] and coronary reserve.[78] Because of the growth in the myocardial walls, the ability of the coronaries to dilate is limited. Thus, during an increase in demand, the epicardial vessels cannot enlarge sufficiently in the hypertrophic myocardium, further reducing the capacity to deliver oxygen, resulting in ischemic myocardium.

Volume-overload hypertrophy can occur as the result of a variety of disease states, including congestive heart failure, mitral regurgitation, aortic regurgitation, and systemic arteriovenous fistula. All these diseases increase the volume load and, thus, the passive strain on the ventricular chamber.[76] During congestive heart failure, volume-overload hypertrophy is produced by a decrease in the ability of the myocardium to contract. The ventricular chamber responds to a volume load by increasing its size eccentrically. Eccentric hypertrophy produces an enlarged ventricular chamber without significant change in wall thickness. Under conditions in which the contractility of the chamber is not reduced, the eccentric hypertrophy produces a significant increase in stroke volume. In the case of valvular regurgitation, the increase in stroke volume maintains the amount of blood ejected from the heart by dilating sufficiently to overcome the amount of regurgitant flow during systole or diastole. During heart failure, the myocardium is in a reduced contractile state, and the increase in chamber volume maintains stroke volume in the presence of a diminished ejection fraction. Volume-overload hypertrophy requires the Frank-Starling mechanism to maintain stroke volume, shifting the end-diastolic pressure-volume relation to the right and onto a steeper (stiffer) portion of the passive diastolic pressure-volume curve, resulting in a reduced functional reserve.

Myocardial Energetics

ATP is converted to mechanical energy, which is used to produce contractile force in the myocardium. When the myocardium shortens against a load, external work is produced. Force generated without shortening produces internal work (elastic potential energy). The production of ATP is essentially aerobic, and a steady supply of oxygen is required. When the supply of oxygen is interrupted, the ability of the myocardium to contract is diminished. Oxygen consumption increases with increases in pressure and volume load in the heart.[79] Myocardial function depends on oxygen supply through the coronary circulation. Therefore, oxygen con-

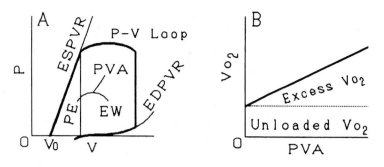

FIGURE 3–9. *A,* The end-systolic (ESPVR) and end-diastolic (EDPVR) pressure-volume relations described in terms of ventricular energetics. Total mechanical energy generation of the ventricle is quantified as the pressure-volume area (PVA), consisting of external mechanical work (EW) performed during systole and elastic potential energy (PE) stored in the myocardium at end-systole. *B,* This plot shows the relationship between pressure-volume area (PVA) and oxygen consumption (Vo₂). This relationship has two components: unloaded Vo₂, energy used for basal metabolism and excitation-contraction coupling, and excess Vo₂, the effective energy used for generating total mechanical energy. (From Suga, H., et al.: Circ. Res. 63:61–71, 1988, with permission.)

sumption (Vo_2) can be used as a measure of total energy used by the heart.

Ventricular energetics is based on the total mechanical energy generation of the ventricle.[55] Total mechanical energy is quantified as the pressure-volume area that is bound by the end-systolic pressure-volume relation and the passive diastolic pressure-volume relation. This area consists of an area for external work, the pressure-volume loop, and the area for mechanical or elastic potential energy (Fig. 3–9A). The pressure-volume area consists of external mechanical work performed during systole and elastic potential energy stored in the myocardium at end-systole. Pressure-volume area allows myocardial contractile efficiency, the fraction of the total energy contraction that appears as mechanical work (efficiency = (cardiac work/min)/Vo_2), to be determined directly and can be quantified by a specific area in the pressure-volume relation. This measure of total mechanical energy extends the pressure-volume relation to include cardiac energetics and mechanoenergetic coupling under a variety of loading and contractile conditions.

The relationship between pressure-volume area and oxygen consumption (Vo_2) is divided into unloaded Vo_2 and excess Vo_2 (Fig. 3–9B). The unloaded Vo_2 consists of basal metabolism and excitation-contraction coupling. Basal metabolism includes energy used for the maintenance of intracellular ionic environment and cellular structures and energy loss in futile cycles; in particular, 5 to 20 percent of basal metabolism is used in the sodium-potassium pump. The Vo_2 for excitation-contraction coupling corresponds to the activation heat or force-independent component of the active heart in excess of basal metabolic heat. The excess Vo_2 is the effective energy used for generating the total mechanical energy. The excess Vo_2 indicates reciprocally the efficiency of the energy conversion, from total Vo_2 to total mechanical energy, as measured by the pressure-volume area. The efficiency computed by comparing excess Vo_2 with pressure-volume area is called contractile efficiency and is approximately 44 percent.

The major determinants of oxygen consumption in the intact contracting heart include heart rate, developed chamber pressure, chamber wall shortening, and inotropic state. There is a linear relationship between an increase in heart rate and Vo_2. A doubling of the heart rate results in a doubling of the Vo_2. There is also a linear relation between the peak systolic pressure and Vo_2. Wall shortening due to ejection contributes about 15 percent to the total oxygen consumption of an isovolumically contracting ventricular chamber. An increase in the positive inotropic state increases the Vo_2. Since the basal metabolic Vo_2 does not change, the increase reflects an increase in excitation-contraction coupling. It is important to note that Vo_2 is linearly related to pressure-volume area and that it is independent of load and contractility. The relation of Vo_2 to pressure-volume area presents these basic concepts of the heart under normal cardiac conditions. Understanding the coupling between mechanics and energetics is essential to understanding the pathophysiology of various cardiomyopathies.

SUMMARY

The heart functions to meet the changing demands of the body by pumping oxygenated blood and nutrients to the organs and then collecting the deoxygenated blood and metabolic waste products to be removed by the lungs, kidneys, and liver. This process is facilitated by properties intrinsic to the myocardium, the mechanics of the cardiac chambers, and the pericardium. All these factors interact to determine how the heart functions to maintain cardiac output.

The structure of the sarcomere regulates the extent of stretch of the cardiac chambers and maintains stroke volume at high pressures and reduced contractility. Calcium is a primary component for modulating the contractile state of the myocardium. The amount of calcium released is regulated by the action potential and inotropic agents. These factors affect the way the individual sarcomeres function as part of the cardiac chamber.

The material properties of the heart are coupled through shell geometry to the pressure and volume of the ventricular chamber, which can be described with the use of a stress-strain relationship. The determinants of the atrioventricular pressure gradient, including left atrial pressure, relaxation, chamber compliance, elastic recoil, and afterload, influence the mitral filling pattern. Because the ventricular chambers share a common septum, the function of each chamber influences the performance of the contralateral chamber. These chambers are enclosed by the pericardium, which is stiffer than the cardiac chambers and, thus, plays a role in cardiac function. All these properties of the heart, from those intrinsic to the sarcomeres, to the ventricular mechanics, to those that influence the heart externally, are interrelated and function together to maintain myocardial performance and meet the demands of the body.

References

1. Huxley, A.F.: Muscular contraction. J. Physiol. 243:1, 1974.
2. Spotnitz, H.M., Sonnenblick E.H., and Spiro, D.: Relation of ultrastructure to function in the intact heart: Sarcomere structure relative to pressure-volume curves of the intact left ventricles of dogs and cats. Circ. Res. 18:49, 1966.
3. Spiro, D., and Sonnenblick, E.H.: Comparison of contractile process in heart and skeletal muscle. Circ. Res. 15(Suppl. 2):14, 1964.
4. Marban, E., Kitakaze, M., Chacko, V.P., et al.: Ca²⁺ transients in perfused hearts revealed by gated ¹⁹F NMR spectroscopy. Circ. Res. 63:673, 1988.
5. Antoni, H., Jacob, R., and Kaufmann, R.: Mechanical response of the frog and mammalian myocardium to changes in the action potential duration by constant current pulses. Pflugers Archiv. Eur. J. Physiol. (Berlin) 306:33, 1969.
6. Hanrath, P., Mathey, D.G., Kremer, P., et al.: Effect of verapamil on left ventricular isovolumic relaxation time and regional left ventricular filling in hypertrophic cardiomyopathy. Am. J. Cardiol. 45:1258, 1980.
7. Alvares, R.F., Shaver, J.A., Gamble, W.H., et al.: Isovolumic relaxation period in hypertrophic cardiomyopathy. J. Am. Coll. Cardiol. 3:71, 1984.
8. Gwathmey, J.K., Warren, S.E., Briggs, G.M., et al.: Diastolic dysfunction in hypertrophic cardiomyopathy: Effect on active force generation during systole. J. Clin. Invest. 87:1023, 1991.
9. Bristow, M.R., Hershberger, R.E., Port, J.D., et al.: Beta-adrenergic pathways in nonfailing and failing human ventricular myocardium. Circulation 82(Suppl. 2):I12, 1990.
10. Wikman-Coffelt, J., Stefenelli, T., Wu, S.T., et al.: [Ca²⁺]i transients in the cardiomyopathic hamster heart. Circ. Res. 68:45, 1991.
11. Bentivegna, L.A., Ablin, L.W., Kihara, Y., et al.: Altered calcium handling in left ventricular pressure-overload hypertrophy as detected with aequorin in the isolated, perfused ferret heart. Circ. Res. 69:1538, 1991.
12. Kihara, Y., Grossman, W., and Morgan, J.P.: Direct measurement of changes in intracellular calcium transients during hypoxia, ischemia, and reperfusion of the intact mammalian heart. Circ. Res. 65:1029, 1989.
13. Levine, M.J., Harada, K., Meuse, A.J., et al.: Excitation-contraction uncoupling during ischemia in the blood perfused dog heart. Biochem. Biophys. Res. Commun. 179:502, 1991.

14. Gilbert, J.C., and Glantz, S.A.: Determinants of left ventricular filling and of the diastolic pressure-volume relation. Circ. Res. 64:827, 1989.

15. Glantz, S.A.: Ventricular pressure-volume curve indices change with end-diastolic pressure. Circ. Res. 39:772, 1976.

16. Bovendeerd, P.H., Huyghe, J.M., Arts, T., et al.: Influence of endocardial-epicardial crossover of muscle fibers on left ventricular wall mechanics. J. Biomech. 27:941, 1994.

17. Nielsen, P.M., Le Grice, I.J., Smaill, B.H., et al.: Mathematical model of geometry and fibrous structure of the heart. Am. J. Physiol. 260(4 Part 2):H1365, 1991.

18. Slinker, B.K., and Glantz, S.A.: End-systolic and end-diastolic ventricular interaction. Am. J. Physiol. 251(5 Part 2):H1062, 1986.

19. Glantz, S.A., and Kernoff, R.S.: Muscle stiffness determined from canine left ventricular pressure-volume curves. Circ. Res. 37:787, 1975.

20. Suga, H., and Sagawa, K.: Instantaneous pressure-volume relationship and their ratio in the excised, supported canine left ventricle. Circ. Res. 35:117, 1974.

21. Keren, G., Meisner, J.S., Sherez, J., et al.: Interrelationship of mid-diastolic mitral valve motion, pulmonary venous flow, and transmitral flow. Circulation 74:36, 1986.

22. Yellin, E.L., Peskin, C., Yoran, C., et al.: Mechanisms of mitral valve motion during diastole. Am. J. Physiol. 241:H389, 1981.

23. Hori, M., Yellin, E.L., and Sonnenblick, E.H.: Left ventricular diastolic suction as a mechanism of ventricular filling. Jpn. Circ. J. 46:124, 1982.

24. Yellin, E.L., Hori, M., Yoran C., et al.: Left ventricular relaxation in the filling and nonfilling intact canine heart. Am. J. Physiol. 250(4 Part 2):H620, 1986.

25. Ishida, Y., Meisner, J.S., Tsujioka, K., et al.: Left ventricular filling dynamics: Influence of left ventricular relaxation and left atrial pressure [published erratum appears in Circulation 74(3):462, 1986]. Circulation 74:187, 1986.

26. Choong, C.Y., Abascal, V.M., Thomas, J.D., et al.: Combined influence of ventricular loading relaxation on the transmitral flow velocity profile in dogs measured by Doppler echocardiography. Circulation 78:672, 1988.

27. Courtois, M., Kovacs, S.J, Jr., and Ludbrook P.A.: Transmitral pressure-flow velocity relation: Importance of regional pressure gradients in the left ventricle during diastole. Circulation 78:661, 1988.

28. Choong, C.Y., Herrmann, H.C., Weyman, A.E., et al.: Preload dependence of Doppler-derived indexes of left ventricular diastolic function in humans. J. Am. Coll. Cardiol. 10:800, 1987.

29. Meisner, J.S., Nikolic, S., Tamura, T., et al.: Development and use of a remote-controlled mitral valve. Ann. Biomed. Eng. 14:339, 1986.

30. Nikolic, S., Yellin, E.L., Tamura, K., et al.: Passive properties of canine left ventricle: Diastolic stiffness and restoring forces [published erratum appears in Circ. Res. 62(6): preceding 1059, 1988]. Cir. Res. 62:1210, 1988.

31. Ariel, Y., Gaasch, W.H., Bogen, D.K., et al.: Load-dependent relaxation with late systolic volume steps: Servo-pump studies in the intact canine heart. Circulation 75:1287, 1987.

32. Weiss, J.L., Frederiksen, J.W., and Weisfeldt, M.L.: Hemodynamic determinants of the time-course of fall in canine left ventricular pressure. J. Clin. Invest. 58:751, 1976.

33. Nikolic, S., Yellin, E.L., Tamura, K., et al.: Effect of early diastolic loading on myocardial relaxation in the intact canine left ventricle. Circ. Res. 66:1217, 1990.

34. Takahashi, T., Katsuragawa, S., Abe, C., et al.: Quantitative analysis of global and regional cardiac performance in normal subjects and patients with coronary artery disease by rest/exercise radionuclide blood-pool study. Jpn. Circ. J. 50:935, 1986.

35. Brutsaert, D.L., Rademakers, F.E., and Sys, S.U.: Triple control of relaxation: Implications in cardiac disease. Circulation 69:190, 1984.

36. Robinson, T.F., Factor, S.M., and Sonnenblick, E.H.: The heart as a suction pump. Sci. Am. 254:84, 1986.

37. Cheng, C.P., Igarashi, Y., and Little, W.C.: Mechanism of augmented rate of left ventricular filling during exercise. Circ. Res. 70:9, 1992.

38. Udelson, J.E., Bacharach, S.L., Cannon, R.O, III, et al.: Minimum left ventricular pressure during beta-adrenergic stimulation in human subjects: Evidence for elastic recoil and diastolic "suction" in the normal heart. Circulation 82:1174, 1990.

39. Elzinga, G., Grondelle, R. van., Westerhof, N., et al.: Ventricular interference. Am. J. Physiol. 226:941, 1974.

40. Santamore, W.P., Lynch, P.R., Meier, G., et al.: Myocardial interaction between the ventricles. J. Appl. Physiol. 41:362, 1976.

41. Janicki, J.S., and Weber, K.T.: The pericardium and ventricular interaction, distensibility, and function. Am. J. Physiol. 238:H494, 1980.

42. Maruyama, Y., Ashikawa, K., Isoyama, S., et al.: Mechanical interactions between four heart chambers with and without the pericardium in canine hearts. Circ. Res. 50:86, 1982.

43. Appleyard, R.F., and Glantz, S.A.: Pulmonary model to predict the effects of series ventricular interaction. Circ. Res. 67:1225, 1990.

44. Glantz, S.A., Misbach, G.A., Moores, W.Y., et al.: The pericardium substantially affects the left ventricular diastolic pressure-volume relationship in the dog. Circ. Res. 42:433, 1978.

45. Holt, J.P.: The normal pericardium. Am. J. Cardiol. 26:455, 1970.

46. Tyberg, J.V., Taichman, G.C., Smith, E.R., et al.: The relationship between pericardial pressure and right atrial pressure: An intraoperative study. Circulation 73:428, 1986.

47. Slinker, B.K., Chagas, A.C., and Glantz, S.A.: Chronic pressure-overload hypertrophy decreases direct ventricular interaction. Am. J. Physiol. 253(2 Part 2):H347, 1987.

48. Applegate, R.J., Johnston, W.E., Vinten-Johansen, J., et al.: Restraining effect of intact pericardium during acute volume loading. Am. J. Physiol. 262(6, Part 2):H1725, 1992.

49. Tyberg, J.V., Keon, W.J., Sonnenblick, E.H., et al.: Mechanics of ventricular diastole. Cardiovasc. Res. 4:423, 1970.

50. Spotnitz, H.M., and Kaiser, G.A.: The effect of the pericardium on pressure-volume relations in the canine left ventricle. J. Surg. Res. 11:375, 1971.

51. Alderman, E.L., and Glantz, S.A.: Acute hemodynamic interventions shift the diastolic pressure-volume curve in man. Circulation 54:662, 1976.

52. Misbach, G.A., and Glantz, S.A.: Changes in the diastolic pressure-diameter relation after ventricular function curves. Am. J. Physiol. 237:H644, 1979.

53. Glower, D.D., Spratt, J.A., Snow, N.D., et al.: Linearity of the Frank-Starling relationship in the intact heart: The concept of preload recruitable stroke work. Circulation 71:994, 1985.

54. Feneley, M.P., Skelton, T.N., Kisslo, K.B., et al.: Comparison of preload recruitable stroke work, end-systolic pressure-volume and dP/dtmax–end-diastolic volume relations as indexes of left ventricular contractile performance in patients undergoing routine cardiac catheterization. J. Am. Coll. Cardiol. 19:1522, 1992.

55. Sagawa, K.: The ventricular pressure-volume diagram revisited. Circ. Res. 43:677, 1978.

56. Burkhoff, D., Sugiura, S., Yue, D.T., et al.: Contractility-dependent curvilinearity of end-systolic pressure-volume relations. Am. J. Physiol. 252(6, Part 2):H1218, 1987.

57. Kass, D.A., Beyar, R., Lankford, E., et al.: Influence of contractile state on curvilinearity of in situ end-systolic pressure-volume relations. Circulation 79:167, 1989.

58. Baan, J., and Van der Velde, E.T.: Sensitivity of left ventricular end-systolic pressure-volume relation to type of loading intervention in dogs. Circ. Res. 62:1247, 1988.

59. Maughan, W.L., Sunagawa, K., Burkhoff, D., et al.: Effect of heart rate on the canine end-systolic pressure-volume relationship. Circulation 72:654, 1985.

60. Bonow, R.O.: Left ventricular diastolic function in hypertrophic cardiomyopathy. Herz 16:13, 1991.

61. Slinker, B.K., Goto, Y., and LeWinter, M.M.: Systolic direct ventricular interaction affects left ventricular contraction and relaxation in the intact dog circulation. Circ. Res. 65:307, 1989.

62. Sunagawa, K., Maughan, W.L., Friesinger, G., et al.: Effects of coronary arterial pressure on left ventricular end-systolic pressure-volume relation of isolated canine heart. Circ. Res. 50:727, 1982.

63. Downey, J.M.: Myocardial contractile force as a function of coronary blood flow. Am. J. Physiol. 230:1, 1976.

64. Sasayama, S., and Suga, H.: Symposium on mechanics of contraction and relaxation of the ischemic myocardium: Opening remarks. Jpn. Circ. J. 51:60, 1987.

65. Theroux, P., Ross, J., Jr., Franklin, D., et al.: Regional myocardial function and dimensions early and late after myocardial infarction in the unanesthetized dog. Circ. Res. 40:158, 1977.

66. Janz, R.F., and Waldron, R.J.: Predicted effect of chronic apical aneurysms on the passive stiffness of the human left ventricle. Circ. Res. 42:255, 1978.

67. Serizawa, T., Carabello, B.A., and Grossman W.: Effect of pacing-induced ischemia on left ventricular diastolic pressure-volume relations in dogs with coronary stenoses. Circ. Res. 46:430, 1980.

68. Paulus, W.J., Serizawa, T., and Grossman, W.: Altered left ventricular diastolic properties during pacing-induced ischemia in dogs with coronary stenoses: Potentiation by caffeine. Circ. Res. 50:218, 1982.

69. Bronzwaer, J.G., de Bruyne, B., Ascoop, C.A., et al.: Comparative effects of pacing-induced and balloon coronary occlusion ischemia on left ventricular diastolic function in man. Circulation 84:211, 1991.

70. Shintani, H., and Glantz, S.A.: Influence of filling on left ventricular diastolic pressure-volume curve during pacing ischemia in dogs. Am. J. Physiol. 266(4, Part 2):H1373, 1994.

71. Applegate, R.J., Walsh, R.A., and O'Rourke, R.A.: Comparative effects of pacing-induced and flow-limited ischemia on left ventricular function [see comments]. Circulation 81:1380, 1990.

72. Bertrand, M.E., Lablanche, J.M., Traisnel, G., et al.: Coronary arterial angiographic findings during transient myocardial ischemia. Can. J. Cardiol. (Suppl. A):205A, 1986.

73. Wijns, W., Serruys, P.W., Slager, C.J., et al.: Effect of coronary occlusion during percutaneous transluminal angioplasty in humans on left ventricular chamber stiffness and regional diastolic pressure-radius relations. J. Am. Coll. Cardiol. 7:455, 1986.

74. Kass, D.A., Midei, M., Brinker, J., et al.: Influence of coronary occlusion during PTCA on end-systolic and end-diastolic pressure-volume relations in humans. Circulation 81:447, 1990.

75. Takano, H., and Glantz, S.A.: Left ventricular contractility predicts how end-diastolic pressure-volume relation shifts during pacing-induced ischemia in dogs. Circulation 91:2423, 1995.

76. Nguyen, T.N., Chagas, A.C., and Glantz, S.A.: Left ventricular adaptation to gradual renovascular hypertension in dogs. Am. J. Physiol. 265(1, Part 2):H22, 1993.

77. Michel, J.B., Salzmann, J.L., Ossondo Nlom, M., et al.: Morphometric analysis of collagen network and plasma perfused capillary bed in the myocardium of rats during evolution of cardiac hypertrophy. Basic Res. Cardiol. 81:142, 1986.

78. Tomanek, R.J., Palmer, P.J., Peiffer, G.L., et al.: Morphometry of canine coronary arteries, arterioles, and capillaries during hypertension and left ventricular hypertrophy. Circ. Res. 58:38, 1986.

79. Sarnoff, S.J., Case, G.H., Welch, D.W., Jr., et al.: Performance characteristics and oxygen debt in a nonfailing metabolically supported, isolated heart preparation Am. J. Physiol. 192:141, 1958.

80. Braunwald, E., Ross, J., Jr., and Sonnenblick, E.H.: Mechanisms of Contraction of the Normal and Failing Heart. 2nd ed. Boston, Little, Brown, 1976.

81. Best, C.H., and Taylor, N.B.: Cardiovascular system. In West, J.B. (ed.): Physiologic Basis of Medical Practice. Baltimore, Williams & Wilkins, 1985.

82. Suga, H.: Ventricular energetics. Physiol. Rev. 70:247, 1990.

4 Principles of Myocardial Metabolism

Denis B. Buxton, Ph.D.

GENERAL CONSIDERATIONS _____ 34
ENERGY PRODUCTION IN
    MYOCARDIUM _____ 34
CARBOHYDRATE METABOLISM _____ 34
Glucose Uptake and Phosphorylation _____ 34
Glycogen Metabolism _____ 35
Glycolysis _____ 37
Pyruvate Metabolism _____ 38
Pyruvate Dehydrogenase _____ 38
Lactate Metabolism _____ 38
Malate-Aspartate Shuttle _____ 38
LIPID METABOLISM _____ 39
Fatty Acid Metabolism _____ 39
    Uptake and Activation _____ 39
    Transport of Acyl-CoA into
        Mitochondria _____ 40
    β-Oxidation _____ 41
Ketone Metabolism _____ 41
TRICARBOXYLIC ACID CYCLE ACTIVITY _____ 41
Electron Transport and ATP Synthesis _____ 42
Creatine Phosphate Shuttle _____ 43
Respiratory Control in Myocardium _____ 43
MYOCARDIAL SUBSTRATE
    INTERACTIONS _____ 43

Fasting _____ 43
Diabetes and Insulin _____ 43
Increased Work and Exercise _____ 44
Catecholamines _____ 44
Ischemia _____ 44
Reperfusion _____ 44
COMPARTMENTATION OF ENERGY
    UTILIZATION _____ 45
PROTEIN TURNOVER _____ 45
Protein Synthesis _____ 45
    Amino Acid Transport and Aminoacyl-tRNA
        Synthesis _____ 45
    Peptide-Chain Initiation _____ 45
PEPTIDE ELONGATION AND
    TERMINATION _____ 46
Protein Degradation _____ 46
REGULATION OF PROTEIN TURNOVER _____ 47
Insulin and Diabetes _____ 47
Starvation _____ 47
Hypertrophy _____ 47
Ischemia _____ 47
SUMMARY _____ 47

The myocardium displays eclectic substrate tastes, modifying its fuel selection in response to a wide range of influences, including nutritional status, hormonal signals, cardiac innervation, myocardial demand, and pathophysiologic status. The rate of energy production is closely linked to myocardial workload, allowing the heart to maintain its stores of high-energy phosphates, ATP, and phosphocreatine at relatively constant levels during changes in workload or substrate use. The aims of this chapter are to summarize the major myocardial energy-producing metabolic pathways and to discuss the regulation of these pathways under different physiologic and pathophysiologic conditions. Regulation of the protein synthetic and degradative pathways under varying metabolic conditions will also be addressed. For additional information on cardiac muscle metabolism, several comprehensive reviews are available.[1–3]

GENERAL CONSIDERATIONS

Regulation of biochemical pathways has traditionally been considered in terms of rate-limiting steps controlling the flux through the pathway. The elegant studies of Kacsar and Burns[4] have demonstrated that this concept is an oversimplification and that limitation of flux through a pathway cannot be attributed solely to a single step. However, for the purposes of this general overview of myocardial metabolism, the less rigorous approach of considering rate-limiting steps will be used, because the researchers doing most of the experimental work on myocardial metabolism have adopted this approach.

ENERGY PRODUCTION IN MYOCARDIUM

Under normoxic conditions, the vast majority of myocardial energy production takes place via the complete oxidation of fuels to CO_2 and H_2O. The pathways of oxidative myocardial energy production can be divided into three sections (Fig. 4–1). In the first section, the many fuels that can contribute to myocardial energy production are broken down into acetyl CoA and other intermediates in the tricarboxylic acid (TCA) cycle. In the second section, oxidation of acetyl CoA via the TCA cycle, yielding CO_2 and H_2O, is coupled to reduction of NAD^+ and FAD to NADH and $FADH_2$. Finally, NADH and $FADH_2$ are reoxidized by transfer of electrons to molecular oxygen via the electron-transport chain. Movement of electrons through the electron-transport chain is coupled to the vectorial pumping of protons out of the mitochondrion to form a proton gradient, and ATP synthesis is in turn coupled to return of protons down the gradient via ATPase.

The pathways for production of acetyl CoA from the various myocardial substrates will now be considered.

CARBOHYDRATE METABOLISM

Glucose Uptake and Phosphorylation

Entry of glucose into myocardial cells, a process that is acutely regulated by insulin and other stimuli, occurs via carrier-mediated, facilitated diffusion, requiring no energy or counter-ion. Facilitated transport of glucose is mediated by a family of glucose-transport

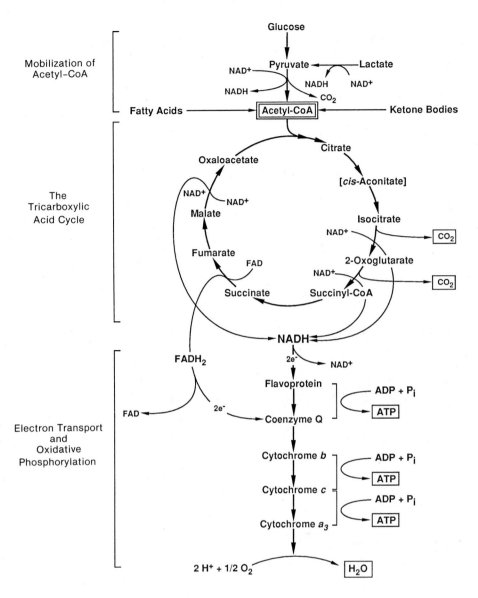

FIGURE 4–1. Catabolic breakdown of substrates. In the first stage, fuels are broken down to acetyl CoA by the individual catabolic pathways. In the second stage, acetyl CoA is oxidized to CO_2 by the TCA, producing reducing equivalents (reduced coenzymes). In the third stage, electrons flow from the reduced coenzymes to molecular oxygen via the electron-transport chain, leading to ATP synthesis via oxidative phosphorylation. (Modified from Lehninger, A.L.: Biochemistry. New York, Worth, 1975, p. 465, with permission.)

molecules, which are expressed in a tissue-dependent manner; six members of the family have been described so far.[5] The transporters contain 12 transmembrane helices, which are believed to form an aqueous pore.[5] In myocardium, two members of the transporter family are found, GLUT 1 and GLUT 4, and it has been proposed that GLUT 1 is responsible for basal glucose transport, whereas GLUT 4 is involved in up-regulation of glucose transport by insulin and other stimuli.[6] Insulin stimulation of glucose transport activity in myocardium occurs via increased maximum transport velocity (Vmax) rather than changes in the apparent affinity (K_M) of the carrier for glucose.[7] This is believed to be achieved at least in part by the reversible, stoichiometric, energy-dependent translocation of GLUT 4 transporters from an intracellular pool to the sarcolemmic surface.[6, 8] Glucose transport is accelerated by anoxia, increased cardiac work in the absence of insulin, and epinephrine and is inhibited by oxidation of fatty acids, ketone bodies, and pyruvate.[9] Transport of glucose is not limiting in the presence of adequate glucose levels with high insulin levels or at high workload, or in hypoxia, but it does limit glucose metabolism in the absence of insulin and at low workloads in normoxia.

Once inside the cell, glucose is phosphorylated by the ATP-dependent hexokinase reaction. When glucose transport is activated, phosphorylation of glucose becomes rate limiting. Hexokinase is present as three isozymes in muscle and is also found in both soluble and particulate forms.[1] Both forms are inhibited noncompetitively by glucose-6-phosphate, which appears to be the

major regulatory factor in vivo.[10] ADP and AMP also inhibit competitively with $Mg\text{-}ATP^{2-}$. Rates of glucose phosphorylation in vivo were found to correlate well with those predicted from the kinetic properties of the enzyme and intracellular concentrations of substrates and effectors.[10]

Glucose-6-phosphate can now enter one of three alternative pathways in myocardium (Fig. 4–2): storage as glycogen, glycolytic breakdown to pyruvate, or the pentose phosphate pathway. The pentose phosphate pathway yields ribose and NADPH primarily for biosynthetic purposes and is of little importance quantitatively in glucose oxidation.[11]

Glycogen Metabolism

Glycogen is synthesized and degraded by two separate pathways. Synthesis of glycogen proceeds via isomerization of glucose-6-phosphate to glucose-1-phosphate, followed by the uridine triphosphate (UTP)-dependent formation of uridine diphosphate glucose (UDPG) by UDPG pyrophosphorylase. UDPG is then transferred to the glycogen chain. The transfer of the α-glucosyl residue to the 4-glucosyl position of the chain is catalyzed by glycogen synthetase, which requires a primer of at least four glucose residues, formed by an additional enzyme and carrier protein, on which to work.[12] Another enzyme, 1,4-α-glucan branching enzyme, inserts branch points in the growing chain by transferring six or seven glucosyl residues from the end of the chain to form an α(1→6) linkage with

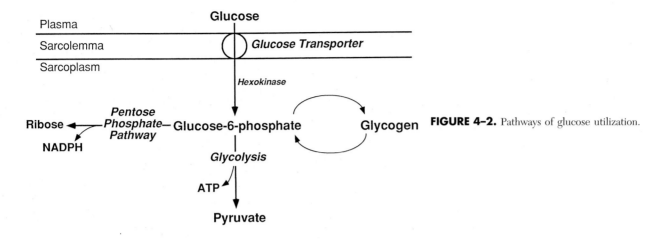

FIGURE 4–2. Pathways of glucose utilization.

the 6-hydroxyl of a glucosyl residue. The branched structure of glycogen allows more rapid mobilization of glucosyl residues, because degradation of glycogen can occur simultaneously on the multiple branches.

Degradation of glycogen requires glycogen phosphorylase, which cleaves the terminal $\alpha(1\rightarrow4)$ glycosidic linkage at the nonreducing end of the glycogen chain by phosphorylytic introduction of phosphoric acid. The products are glucose-1-phosphate and a glycogen chain with one less glucose unit. This is followed by isomerization of glucose-1-phosphate to glucose-6-phosphate by phosphoglucomutase. Because glycogen phosphorylase cannot cleave $\alpha(1\rightarrow6)$ glycosidic linkages, a debranching enzyme, a hydrolytic amylo-1,6-glucosidase, removes branch points, allowing glycogen phosphorylase to continue progressive cleavage of the glycogen chain.

Regulation of glycogen metabolism has been studied in depth for skeletal muscle, and it is generally assumed that cardiac muscle follows a similar pattern.[2] In skeletal muscle, glycogen phosphorylase and synthetase are regulated in a coordinated fashion, thus limiting futile cycling and providing a large amplification of the stimulus by means of the enzymatic cascade systems (Fig. 4–3). Glycogen phosphorylase exists in phosphorylated and dephosphorylated forms, with the phosphorylated enzyme termed *a* and the dephosphorylated enzyme *b*. Phosphorylation of the *b* form is catalyzed by phosphorylase kinase, and dephosphorylation of *a* by

the same protein phosphatase involved in activation of glycogen synthetase. Glycogen phosphorylase *a* is active in the absence of AMP at high concentrations of the substrates glycogen and Pi, requiring AMP only at low substrate concentrations. In contrast, phosphorylase *b* requires AMP for activity; the activation by AMP is antagonized by ATP and glucose-6-phosphate.

The enzyme responsible for covalent activation of phosphorylase, phosphorylase kinase, is also regulated in turn by phosphorylation-dephosphorylation. Activation by phosphorylation is catalyzed by cyclic AMP (cAMP)–dependent protein kinase, while protein phosphatase again carries out the dephosphorylation reaction. Activity of phosphorylase kinase is Ca^{2+} dependent, which allows glycogen breakdown to be coordinated to contractility on a beat-to-beat basis by the transient increase in cytosolic calcium concentration.

Glycogen synthetase also exists in dephosphorylated and phosphorylated forms, termed *a* and *b*, respectively. Cyclic AMP-dependent protein kinase and protein phosphatase catalyze interconversion of the two forms of glycogen synthetase. Glycogen synthetase *a* is active in the absence of glucose-6-phosphate and is only weakly inhibited by ATP, ADP, and Pi. Glucose-6-phosphate lowers the K_M for UDPG but has no effect on Vmax. In contrast, glycogen synthetase *b* requires a glucose-6-phosphate–mediated increase in Vmax for full activation, having only low activity in the absence of the effector. ATP, ADP, and Pi strongly inhibit glycogen synthetase

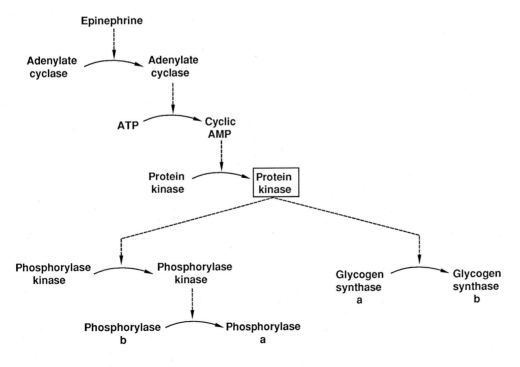

FIGURE 4–3. Regulation of glycogen phosphorylase and synthetase by covalent modification.

b competitively with glucose-6-phosphate. Under normal in vivo conditions, the *a* form is active, whereas the *b* form is inactive.

In myocardium, the importance of inactivation of glycogen synthetase during activation of phosphorylase is less clear than in skeletal muscle, because the synthetase appears to be 80 to 90 percent in the *b* form under basal conditions, and most studies show no further inactivation of glycogen synthetase in response to catecholamines, under conditions when glycogen phosphorylase was activated.[13, 14]

Glycolysis

The reactions involved in the breakdown of glucose to pyruvate by glycolysis are shown in Figure 4–4. The pathway can be divided into two halves. In the first half, the pathway goes from glucose to the triose phosphates dihydroxyacetone phosphate and glyceraldehyde-3-phosphate. ATP is utilized in two priming steps, while in the second half, from the triose phosphates to pyruvate, two ATP molecules are produced from each of the two triose phosphates, providing a net gain of two ATP molecules per glucose molecule.

In addition, two molecules of NADH are produced for production of ATP via the electron-transport chain after transfer of the reducing equivalents to the mitochondria via the malate-aspartate shuttle.

Regulation of glycolysis under most conditions is believed to reside at the level of 6-phosphofructo-1-kinase (PFK-1), an enzyme whose activity can be regulated in vivo by a large number of allosteric effectors.[15] The precise physiologic roles of the various effectors of PFK-1 are still not fully understood. PFK-1 is inhibited by ATP, phosphocreatine, and citrate and is activated by ADP, AMP, Pi, and its product fructose 1,6-bisphosphate (F1,6-P). Allosteric control of PFK-1 is sensitive to pH, showing decreased allosteric sensitivity as the pH is increased from 6.8 to 7.3.[16]

Increased citrate levels are believed to be important in inhibiting PFK-1 when fatty-acid oxidation rates are high[16] but cannot explain increased glycolysis observed in hearts perfused with insulin and glucose, when citrate levels also rise.[17] The relatively recent discovery of fructose-2,6-bisphosphate (F2,6-P) as a potent stimulator of PFK-1[18, 19] and demonstration that F2,6-P is required for in vitro activity of PFK-1 purified from perfused rat hearts[20] add an additional potential control mechanism. F2,6-P is synthesized from fructose-6-phosphate by 6-phosphofructo-2-kinase (PFK-2) and is

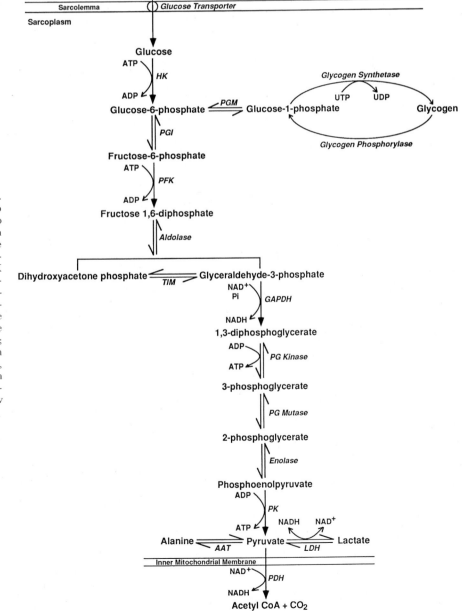

FIGURE 4–4. Glucose metabolism in myocardium. Under aerobic conditions, most glucose taken up will be broken down to pyruvate and ultimately to CO_2 and water via the tricarboxylic acid cycle. In hypoxia and ischemia, release of lactate and alanine is increased. HK = hexokinase; PGM = phosphoglucomutase; PGI = phosphoglucoisomerase; PFK = 6-phosphofructo-1-kinase; TIM = triosephosphate isomerase; GAPDH = glyceraldehyde 3-phosphate dehydrogenase; PG Kinase = phosphoglycerate kinase; PG Mutase = phosphoglycerate mutase; PK = pyruvate kinase; AAT = alanine aminotransferase; LDH = lactate dehydrogenase; PDH = pyruvate dehydrogenase. (Modified from Taegtmeyer, H.: Myocardial metabolism. *In:* Phelps, M., Mazziotta, J., and Schelbert, H. [eds.]: Positron Emission Tomography and Autoradiography: Principles and Applications for the Brain and Heart. New York, Raven Press, 1986, p. 149, with permission.)

broken down by fructose-2,6-bisphosphatase. Further experiments in perfused rat hearts demonstrated that changes in glycolytic rate induced by insulin or increased work correlated well with changes in the substrate, fructose-6-phosphate and the activator F2,6-P, but not with other effectors.[21, 22] An additional level of control of PFK-1 may consist of covalent modification; epinephrine activation appears to activate PFK-1 via covalent modification, possibly phosphorylation, in addition to changes in effector concentrations.[20, 23] There is also evidence for covalent activation of myocardial PFK-2 in response to insulin[24] and epinephrine,[20] and phosphorylation of PFK-2 by calcium-calmodulin protein kinase has been proposed as a potential cause of the decrease in K_m of PFK-2 in response to increased workload.[22]

When PFK-1 is activated, glyceraldehyde-3-phosphate dehydrogenase may become rate limiting for glycolysis under certain conditions, including ischemia[25] and very high workloads.[26] Regulation of glyceraldehyde-3-phosphate dehydrogenase occurs via product inhibition by NADH and 1,3-diphosphoglycerate. It is probable that glycolysis is limited by the rate of disposal of cytosolic NADH, which must be reoxidized either by the malate-aspartate shuttle or by lactate dehydrogenase (LDH).[26]

Pyruvate Metabolism

Pyruvate generated in the cytosol by glycolysis can undergo a number of different fates. Lactate dehydrogenase (LDH), a near-equilibrium cytosolic enzyme, converts pyruvate to lactate, regenerating NAD^+ from NADH simultaneously. This pathway is less important in normoxia but is increased in hypoxia, when the NAD^+ formed in this manner is important for maintenance of glycolysis. Similarly, formation of alanine by alanine aminotransferase, using glutamate as the amino-group donor, occurs primarily in the cytosol by means of a near-equilibrium reaction and is accelerated by hypoxia. Oxidation of pyruvate by pyruvate dehydrogenase and carboxylation to oxaloacetate by pyruvate carboxylase take place in the mitochondrial matrix and thus require transport of pyruvate across the inner mitochondrial membrane, which is achieved by the monocarboxylate carrier.[27] Pyruvate carboxylation to oxaloacetate represents a method by which the levels of TCA cycle intermediates can be increased, a process termed anaplerosis.

Pyruvate Dehydrogenase

Under normoxic conditions, the main route for pyruvate disposition is oxidation to acetyl CoA by pyruvate dehydrogenase (PDH). PDH consists of a high-molecular-weight complex containing multiple copies of three polypeptides catalyzing a series of reactions: pyruvate carboxylase, dihydrolipoyl acetyltransferase, and dihydrolipoyl dehydrogenase.[28] The pyruvate decarboxylase reaction is es-

sentially irreversible under physiologic conditions, and thus the enzyme represents a vital committed step in breakdown of carbohydrate and, hence, in myocardial fuel selection. Therefore, it is not surprising that the PDH complex is tightly regulated. Two interrelated regulatory mechanisms operate to control the activity of PDH, allosteric regulation and covalent modification by a phosphorylation-dephosphorylation cycle[28, 29] (Fig. 4–5).

Allosteric control is mediated by feedback inhibition by the reaction products NADH and acetyl CoA, competitively with NAD^+ and CoA, respectively. Phosphorylation of the pyruvate decarboxylase subunit of PDH is mediated by an intrinsic kinase activity tightly bound to the pyruvate dehydrogenase complex. PDH kinase activity is stimulated by high ratios of [ATP]/[ADP], [CoA]/[CoA], and [NADH]/[NAD$^+$] and is inhibited by pyruvate, Ca^{2+}, and Mg^{2+}. The products of the PDH reaction, acetyl CoA and NADH, thus regulate activity of the complex both directly allosterically and indirectly via kinase-mediated covalent inhibition. Removal of the phosphate is accomplished by a phosphatase, PDH phosphatase, which is not tightly bound to the PDH complex. The phosphatase is stimulated by Ca^{2+} and Mg^{2+}.

In diabetes and starvation, myocardial PDH is almost entirely in the inactive form, and reactivation of the enzyme by pyruvate or dichloroacetate, inhibitors of the kinase reaction, is inhibited.[2]

Lactate Metabolism

Exogenous lactate is readily taken up and metabolized by myocardium,[30] and evidence exists for a stereospecific transporter.[31] Lactate is then converted to pyruvate by LDH, and the pyruvate enters the TCA cycle as acetyl CoA produced by the PDH reaction. Under normoxic conditions, lactate utilization in dogs was proportional to the arterial lactate concentration, up to about 4.5 mM lactate, when approximately 90 percent of myocardial oxygen consumption (MVO_2) was supplied by lactate.[32] In hypoxia, lactate use is limited by high cytosolic NADH levels, pushing the LDH equilibrium toward lactate. Decreased pyruvate utilization by PDH also increases net lactate formation through the glycolytic pathway. Experiments in humans, using dual carbon-labeled substrates, have demonstrated that even during net chemical extraction of lactate, release of lactate from myocardium occurs.[33] In patients with coronary artery disease, lactate derived from exogenous glucose constitutes about 25 percent of lactate release at rest in the absence of clinical evidence for ischemia.[33]

Malate-Aspartate Shuttle

The inner mitochondrial membrane is impermeable to NAD^+ and NADH, which means that NADH formed in the cytosol by glycolysis must be transported into the mitochondrion by means of

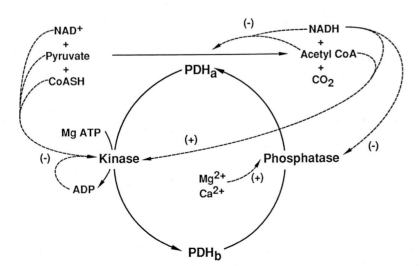

FIGURE 4–5. Regulation of PDH by allosteric and covalent mechanisms. In addition to direct-feedback product inhibition of the active pyruvate dehydrogenase PDH_a, substrates, products and metal ions modulate the reversible covalent inactivation to the phosphorylated PDH_b by allosteric effects on the kinase-phosphatase system.

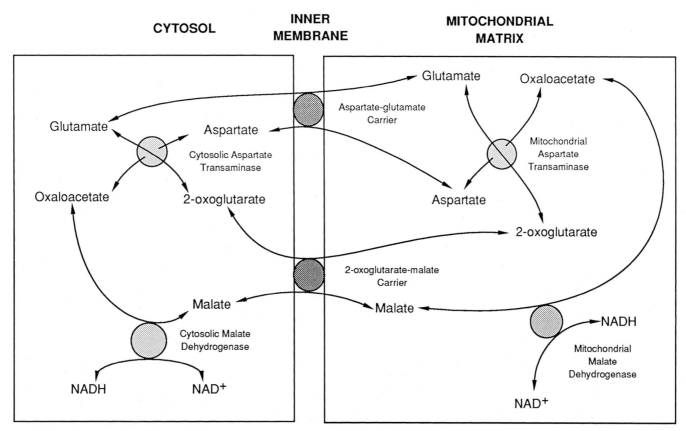

FIGURE 4–6. The malate-aspartate shuttle. The shuttle allows the reversible transfer of reducing equivalents, produced in the cytosol during breakdown of glucose to pyruvate, to the mitochondrial electron-transport chain. Three molecules of ATP are produced from ADP for each cytosolic NADH transferred to the mitochondrion. (Modified from Lehninger, A.L.: Biochemistry. New York, Worth, 1975, p. 535, with permission.)

an indirect mechanism. In cardiac muscle, this is achieved by the malate-aspartate shuttle (Fig. 4–6), in which oxaloacetate, generated by transamination of aspartate, is reduced to malate in the cytosol, regenerating NAD$^+$. Cytosolic malate undergoes electroneutral exchange with mitochondrial 2-oxoglutarate, and in the mitochondrion it is reoxidized to oxaloacetate by malate dehydrogenase. Transamination of oxaloacetate forms aspartate, which exchanges with glutamate across the mitochondrial membrane to complete the shuttle. Aspartate efflux in exchange for glutamate entry is accompanied by uptake of a proton, and thus the exchange is driven by the mitochondrial membrane potential.[2] It should be noted that when glucose is used as the myocardial fuel, flux through the malate dehydrogenase reaction is approximately double that through the other reactions of the TCA cycle because malate is also being delivered to the enzyme from the cytosol, bringing in the reducing equivalents from glycolysis.[2]

LIPID METABOLISM

Fatty Acid Metabolism

Uptake and Activation

It has long been recognized that under most conditions, fatty acids constitute the preferred fuel for myocardial energy supply.[34] Despite this fact, the metabolism of fatty acids, the main pathways of which are shown in Figure 4–7, is less well understood than carbohydrate metabolism. The heart is able to use both nonesterified fatty acids, which are bound largely to albumin in the circulation, and circulating triglycerides, which can be broken down by lipoprotein lipase found at the extracellular surface in myocardium

and other extrahepatic cells.[2] The relative importance of these two sources of fatty acid has not been well characterized. The uptake of fatty acid into cells is also poorly understood; uptake is generally believed to be by means of a simple diffusion process,[35] although some researchers have argued for the existence of a specific carrier in addition to diffusion processes.[36] Recent studies have demonstrated a membrane protein in myocyte membranes, with high binding affinity for long-chain fatty acids; a specific antibody against this protein was able to reduce both binding and uptake of long-chain fatty acid by myocytes. Generally, fatty acid uptake is governed by the circulating nonesterified fatty acid levels and the rate of intracellular fatty acid use.[2]

On entering the cell, fatty acids are bound to a soluble protein, termed fatty acid–binding protein.[37, 38] The physiologic significance of fatty acid–binding protein remains unclear at present.[38] However, the tissue concentration of fatty acid–binding protein has been shown to be regulated at the transcriptional level and probably also at the level of mRNA stability.[39] Metabolic situations leading to increased fatty acid oxidation generally result in increased levels of fatty acid–binding protein.[39, 40] These and similar findings have led to the hypothesis that fatty acid–binding protein may somehow be involved in directing fatty acids toward oxidation.

Subsequent metabolism of fatty acids requires activation by formation of a coenzyme A thioester. Acyl-CoA synthesis requires hydrolysis of ATP to give AMP and PPi. The location of the acyl-CoA synthetases responsible for this reaction is dependent on the chain length of the fatty acid; short-chain acyl-CoA synthetases, acting on fatty acids of C_8 or shorter, are present in the mitochondrion.[41] Thus, short-chain fatty acids can be oxidized by heart mitochondria in the absence of external carnitine or coenzyme A. In contrast, the long-chain fatty acids, which in general are of much greater physiologic importance, are activated to their CoA

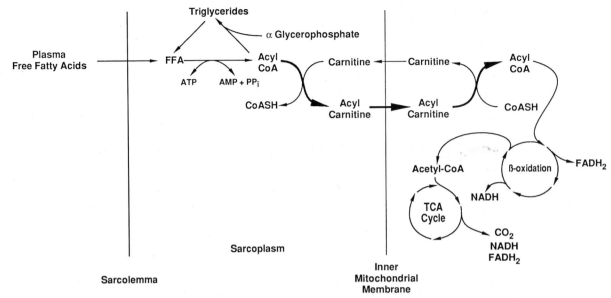

FIGURE 4–7. Metabolism of long-chain fatty acid in myocardium. After entry into the cell, the fatty acid must first be activated to form an acyl-CoA derivative. The acyl-CoA can then be transported into the mitochondrion via a carnitine-dependent shuttle, to undergo β-oxidation to acetyl CoA for entry into the TCA cycle, or esterified in the cytosol to form triglyceride.

derivatives via extramitochondrial acyl-CoA synthetases, of which the majority of the activity is bound to the mitochondrial outer membrane.[42]

After activation, long-chain acyl-CoA either can be esterified to form triglyceride, a process taking place in the cytosol, or can be oxidized to acetyl CoA, a process that takes place intramitochondrially. The regulation of partitioning between these two pathways is also not clear; increased net esterification of fatty acids into triglyceride occurs in ischemia, when fatty acid oxidation is inhibited, and also in starvation and diabetes, when fatty acid levels are elevated in the plasma. Thus, triglyceride synthesis rates may reflect in part the relative rates of fatty acid uptake from the plasma and disposition via mitochondrial oxidation.

Transport of Acyl-CoA into Mitochondria

Because activation of long-chain fatty acids takes place extramitochondrially, while β-oxidation occurs in the mitochondrial matrix, the long-chain acyl-CoA moieties must be transported into the mitochondrion before being oxidized (Fig. 4–8). Transport of long-chain acyl-CoA across the inner mitochondrial membrane occurs via a carnitine-dependent system involving two carnitine palmitoyltransferase enzymes, one present on each side of the inner mitochondrial membrane, and carnitine translocase, which catalyzes the stoichiometric exchange of carnitine and acylcarnitine across the inner mitochondrial membrane.[43] The outer carnitine palmitoyltransferase, CPT I, which catalyzes the freely reversible formation

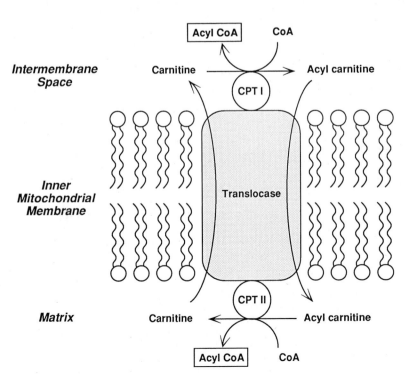

FIGURE 4–8. The carnitine shuttle. Acyl-CoA crosses the inner mitochondrial membrane via a carnitine-dependent shuttle system. The acyl group is first transferred to carnitine by the action of carnitine palmitoyltransferase I (CPT I) on the cytosolic face of the inner mitochondrial membrane. Acyl-carnitine then exchanges via a translocase with free carnitine across the inner mitochondrial membrane, and the acyl group is transferred back to form intramitochondrial acyl-CoA by a second transferase, CPT II, situated on the matrix side. (Modified from Stryer, L.: Biochemistry. New York, W.H. Freeman, 1988, p. 474, with permission.)

of acylcarnitine and CoA from acyl-CoA and carnitine, is located on the inner surface of the outer mitochondrial membrane.[44] Following translocation of the acylcarnitine across the inner mitochondrial membrane, acyl-CoA is re-formed by the inner carnitine palmitoyltransferase, CPT II. Transport of fatty acids into the mitochondrion appears to be an important regulatory step; myocardial CPT I is inhibited by malonyl CoA[45] and is more sensitive than liver CPT I to the effector.[46] Recent experiments have also demonstrated acute regulation of malonyl CoA levels by hormones.[47] Dichloroacetate, which activates PDH and inhibits palmitate oxidation, increased malonyl CoA levels in perfused heart, probably via increased provision of acetyl CoA for the enzyme synthesizing malonyl CoA, acetyl CoA carboxylase.

β-Oxidation

Oxidation of intramitochondrial acyl CoA requires the repetitive sequential action of four enzymes: acyl-CoA dehydrogenase, enoyl-CoA hydratase, 3-hydroxyacyl-CoA dehydrogenase, and 3-oxoacyl-CoA thiolase (Fig. 4–9). Each passage through the enzyme sequence results in the liberation of acetyl CoA, with concomitant shortening of the acyl-CoA by two carbons. Additional mitochondrial enzymes are responsible for the conversion of intermediates formed during oxidation of unsaturated fatty acids to normal β-oxidation intermediates.[43] Under normal conditions, intermediates of β-oxidation are present at only low concentrations in mitochon-

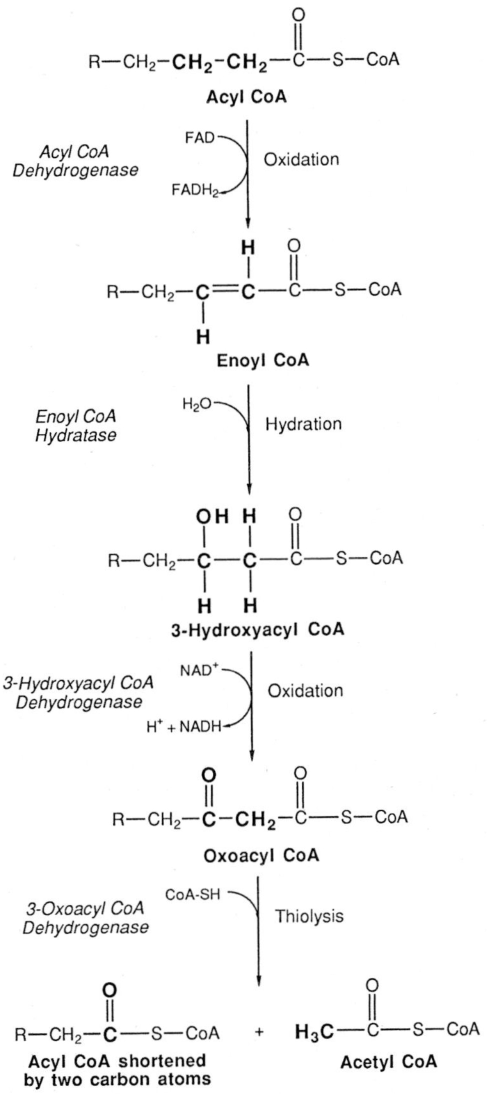

FIGURE 4–9. β-Oxidation of fatty acids.

dria. The intermediates also display anomalous turnover kinetics, leading to the suggestion that the β-oxidation enzymes are arranged in a loose complex that breaks apart during isolation of the enzymes, thus channeling the intermediates from enzyme to enzyme.[49] Thus, the free intermediates would represent leakage from the complex. Acetyl CoA formed by β-oxidation appears to enter the general mitochondrial acetyl CoA pool.[50]

Because ketogenesis is absent in myocardium, β-oxidation is tightly coupled to disposition of acetyl CoA via the TCA cycle, and it has been proposed that accumulation of acetyl CoA may regulate β-oxidation,[51] possibly by inhibiting the 3-oxoacyl-CoA thiolase.[52] Approximately 85 percent of myocardial CoA is found in the mitochondria, whereas carnitine is predominantly cytosolic, with only 9 percent being associated with the mitochondria.[53] This arrangement is believed to assist in directing fatty acid primarily toward oxidation in myocardium.

Ketone Metabolism

Myocardium represents the tissue with the highest rate of ketone body utilization, reflecting the continuous high-energy requirements of cardiac muscle.[54] Uptake of ketones at the plasma membrane is believed to occur by means of diffusion of the undissociated acids,[54] while at the mitochondrial membrane, in addition to diffusion, entry of the ionized ionic forms can also occur via the monocarboxylate carrier used by pyruvate.[55] Inside the mitochondrion, 3-hydroxybutyrate is converted to acetoacetate by 3-hydroxybutyrate dehydrogenase, an enzyme tightly bound to the inner mitochondrial membrane. The reaction, which also generates NADH from NAD^+, is reversible. Acetoacetate is then activated to acetoacetyl CoA in an unusual reaction catalyzed by 3-oxoacid-CoA transferase (Fig. 4–10), in which succinyl CoA acts as CoA donor with formation of succinate. Thus, in effect acetoacetyl CoA synthesis bypasses the succinate dehydrogenase reaction of the TCA cycle and, hence, the substrate level phosphorylation of GDP to GTP.[56] Acetoacetyl CoA is then cleaved by acetoacetyl CoA thiolase, with the net reaction being formation of two molecules of acetyl CoA from acetoacetyl CoA and CoA.[54] There is no evidence for regulation of ketone body metabolism at any particular step.[56] Utilization of ketone bodies in heart is linearly related to the plasma concentration at low concentrations, reaching a plateau at higher plasma concentrations.[57, 58]

Studies in isolated hearts have demonstrated an inability of ketone bodies to act as sole myocardial substrates at high workloads because of a relative inhibition of the TCA cycle at the 2-oxoglutarate dehydrogenase step. It has been proposed that this inhibition reflects sequestration of CoA in the form of acetyl CoA and acetoacetyl CoA and is overcome by glucose or other anaplerotic substrates.[56, 59]

TRICARBOXYLIC ACID CYCLE ACTIVITY

The TCA cycle represents the means by which acetyl CoA derived from the breakdown of glucose, fatty acid, ketone bodies, lactate, and pyruvate, in addition to other cycle intermediates derived from the metabolism of amino acids, is catabolized to CO_2 and H_2O, with the production of reduced coenzymes (NADH and $FADH_2$) and GTP. The reduced coenzymes can then donate electrons to the electron-transport chain, leading to synthesis of ATP and the reduction of molecular oxygen. Because the TCA cycle is responsible for approximately two thirds of the energy production from the major myocardial fuels under normoxic conditions, it is clear that flux through the TCA cycle must be closely coupled to myocardial energy demand. Determination of the mechanisms of regulation of the TCA cycle is complicated by the cyclical nature of the process, which makes interpretation of data more difficult than in a linear system.[60] The current state of knowledge on the regulatory mechanisms linking TCA cycle flux to myocardial

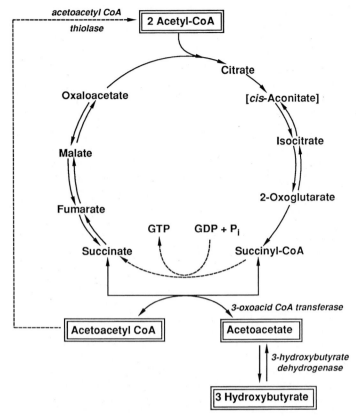

FIGURE 4–10. Mechanism of entry of ketone bodies into the TCA. Acetoacetyl CoA is synthesized using succinyl CoA as a CoA donor, thus bypassing the GTP-yielding substrate-level phosphorylation step catalyzed by succinyl CoA synthetase. Cleavage of acetoacetyl CoA yields two acetyl CoA units. (Modified from Taegtmeyer, H.: Myocardial metabolism. *In* Phelps, M., Mazziota, J., and Schelbert, H. [eds.]: Positron Emission Tomography and Autoradiography: Principles and Applications for the Brain and Heart. New York, Raven Press, 1986, p. 149, with permission.)

citrate synthesis as a regulatory step in the myocardial regulation of TCA cycle flux is still unclear.[61]

NAD-linked isocitrate dehydrogenase is strongly inhibited by NADH and is stimulated by ADP, and it appears to be the site most sensitive to changes in the [NADH]/[NADH⁺] ratio.[60] Results obtained in isolated heart mitochondria have demonstrated increased flux through isocitrate dehydrogenase in uncoupled mitochondria treated with oligomycin, which have a high [ATP]/[ADP] ratio but a low [NADH]/[NAD⁺] ratio, suggesting that the redox state of the mitochondrial nicotinamide adenine nucleotides may be of greater importance than the phosphorylation state of the adenine nucleotides in regulating NAD⁺-linked isocitrate dehydrogenase.[64]

The 2-oxoglutarate dehydrogenase reaction commits 2-oxoglutarate to oxidation, in contrast with the alternative fates of efflux from the mitochondrion as part of the malate-aspartate shuttle, or transamination.[65] 2-Oxoglutarate dehydrogenase is also inhibited by increases in the [NADH]/[NAD⁺] ratio and, in addition, is strongly inhibited by the product succinyl-CoA. The [succinyl CoA]/[CoA] ratio is increased in high mitochondrial energy states by the action of succinate thiokinase and nucleoside diphosphate kinase, tending to decrease flux through 2-oxoglutarate dehydrogenase.[66] The inhibitory effects of succinyl CoA are dependent on the relative concentrations of the substrate, 2-oxoglutarate, and the inhibitor succinyl CoA.

An additional level of control of TCA cycle flux may result from the Ca²⁺ sensitivity of the NAD-linked isocitrate dehydrogenase and 2-oxoglutarate dehydrogenase reactions, and also the PDH reaction feeding in acetyl CoA from glycolysis.[67] This mechanism may be of particular importance in catecholamine stimulation and is discussed in more detail in the section on the role of catecholamines in myocardial substrate interactions.

Thus, it is apparent that there are multiple mechanisms by which TCA cycle flux can be linked to the energy state of the mitochondrion, reflected by the [ATP]/[ADP] ratio and, probably of primary importance, the [NADH]/[NAD⁺] ratio, thus providing the tight coupling necessary between energy utilization and the provision of reducing equivalents via the TCA cycle for energy production via the electron-transport chain.

Electron Transport and ATP Synthesis

The reducing equivalents produced in oxidative reactions in the TCA cycle and elsewhere are transferred by the reduced coenzymes NADH and FADH₂ to the electron-transport chain contained in the inner mitochondrial membrane. Each of the reduced coenzymes donates a pair of electrons to the respiratory chain, in the process regenerating the oxidized forms of the coenzymes, which can then participate again as electron acceptors in oxidative reactions. The electrons then flow through the respiratory chain, which consists of three enzyme complexes linked by two mobile electron carriers, to the ultimate electron acceptor, molecular oxygen. In the process, the movement of electrons is coupled to the vectorial transport of protons through the enzyme complexes across the inner mitochondrial membrane from the matrix to the extramitochondrial space. Since the membrane is impermeable to protons, this leads to the formation of a proton gradient across the inner mitochondrial membrane. The return of protons down this proton gradient into the mitochondrial matrix occurs via ATP synthase, which spans the inner mitochondrial membrane; the flow of protons is tightly linked to the synthesis of ATP from ADP and orthophosphate.

The entry point into the respiratory chain differs for the two coenzymes; NADH, which has a high reduction potential, feeds electrons into the respiratory chain via NADH dehydrogenase. This leads to the synthesis of three molecules of ATP per electron pair, one in each of the proton-pumping enzyme complexes of the respiratory chain. For FADH₂, the reduction potential is lower, and so the electrons are passed to the protein pump, cytochrome

energy demand has been reviewed extensively.[2, 60, 61] The main points are summarized below.

The main role of the TCA cycle is the efficient oxidation of the acetyl group of acetyl CoA to CO₂ and H₂O, with the concomitant production of reducing equivalents for energy production. A secondary function of the TCA cycle is as a regulatory mechanism coordinating fatty acid metabolism and glycolysis.[2] Thus, increased β-oxidation and, hence, increased flux of acetyl CoA from fatty acid into the TCA cycle elevate citrate levels, leading to inhibition of PFK-1 and glycolysis.[2]

The main candidates for regulation of TCA cycle activity, based on identification of disequilibrium enzymes,[60] are citrate synthetase and the TCA cycle dehydrogenases, NAD-linked isocitrate dehydrogenase and 2-oxoglutarate dehydrogenase, which are linked directly to reduction of coenzymes. Citrate synthetase was assumed to be a rate-limiting enzyme because of its position in committing acetyl CoA to oxidation.[62] Whereas citrate synthetase is inhibited by NADH, ATP, and succinyl CoA in vitro, thus providing possible feedback regulation of the enzyme, the significance of these factors in vivo has been questioned.[2, 61] The possible functional and structural linkage of citrate synthetase and malate dehydrogenase[63] has been proposed as a means by which citrate synthetase is linked to the mitochondrial redox state.[61] Because the equilibrium of citrate synthetase favors citrate synthesis, whereas the equilibrium of malate dehydrogenase favors malate formation, the two enzymes will compete for oxaloacetate. Consideration of the two reactions as a unit demonstrates that, purely on the basis of thermodynamic equilibria, NADH will inhibit flux through citrate synthetase, whereas NAD⁺ will promote it.[61] However, the importance of

reductase, via the mobile electron carrier ubiquinol. Thus, the ATP yield from $FADH_2$ is two molecules of ATP per electron pair.

Since the inner mitochondrial membrane is also impermeable to adenine nucleotides, ATP, which is synthesized on the matrix side of the membrane, leaves the mitochondrion via a specific transport system, ATP-ADP translocase, which exchanges intramitochondrial ATP for extramitochondrial ADP. Exchange is driven by the positive membrane potential, as ATP has one more negative charge than ADP, and thus the membrane potential is decreased by one negative charge per ATP-ADP exchange.

Creatine Phosphate Shuttle

Excitable tissues, including cardiac and skeletal muscle and neural tissue, use a shuttle system involving creatine phosphate for the intracellular distribution of high-energy phosphate.[68] The free-energy change during ATP hydrolysis is dependent on the concentrations of the reactants:

$$\Delta G = \Delta G_0 + RT \log [ADP][Pi]/[ATP]$$

where ΔG_0 is the standard free energy change, R the gas constant, and T the absolute temperature. To achieve the high thermodynamic efficiency necessary in excitable tissues, the ADP concentration must be low, which limits the rate of ADP diffusion. In the absence of a shuttle system, there would be a gradient of free energy change for ATP hydrolysis; the energy yield from ATP hydrolysis would decrease with increasing distance from the mitochondria,[69] leading to insufficient free-energy change to drive cellular processes such as ion transport.[68]

To circumvent this problem, excitable tissues contain creatine kinases located at the sites of energy production (the mitochondria) and utilization (the myofibrils, sarcolemma, sarcoplasmic reticulum). Creatine kinase catalyzes the reversible transfer of a phosphoryl group from creatine phosphate to ADP and can thus act to buffer ATP levels. Because the standard free energy of hydrolysis for creatine phosphate is higher than that for ATP, creatine phosphate and creatine are closer to equilibrium, and a low creatine concentration is not necessary to maintain the free-energy change at adequate levels for cellular processes. The creatine phosphate shuttle thus allows high efficiency of energy transformation in combination with high-energy flux.[68]

Respiratory Control in Myocardium

Under normal conditions, the healthy myocardium has the ability to match energy production closely to the rate of myocardial energy utilization, but the regulatory mechanisms involved in this coordination are, as yet, incompletely understood. A number of models have been put forward to explain the control of myocardial respiration. These include (1) limitation of respiration by the availability of ADP and Pi,[70, 71] (2) regulation of the translocation of ATP and ADP by kinetic control by the substrates and electrophoretic control by the membrane potential,[72] and (3) the near-equilibrium hypothesis, in which a near equilibrium exists between the extramitochondrial adenylate system and the respiratory chain reactions across the first two energy-conserving sites. According to this hypothesis, MVo_2 is determined by the redox state of the mitochondrial free [NADH]/[NAD] couple.[73] This topic has been discussed in several reviews.[60, 74, 75] Thus, the mechanism or mechanisms of respiratory control remain a controversial area.

MYOCARDIAL SUBSTRATE INTERACTIONS

The selection of fuels by myocardium is governed by a number of factors.[2, 56] The utilization of a substrate is first dependent on its plasma concentration. While plasma glucose levels remain relatively constant, the concentrations of fatty acids, ketone bodies, and lactate in blood can vary widely with changes in nutritional status and with exercise. Increases in plasma concentrations of any of these substrates tend to lead to increased myocardial utilization of that substrate.[2] The presence and nature of alternative substrates also have a profound effect on utilization of a particular substrate. It has been pointed out[56] that the ease of access of a substrate to the TCA plays an important role in substrate selection. Thus, ketone bodies[57, 62] and lactate,[30] which have few control steps in their metabolic pathways, tend to be used preferentially in proportion to their plasma concentrations, while glucose and fatty acid oxidation pathways have more potential for regulation and thus are more affected by alternative substrates. Plasma levels of hormones can control both the provision of substrates in the circulation and myocardial uptake and oxidation of substrates.

The importance of fatty acids as the primary substrate for myocardium under normal conditions, and the "glucose-sparing" effects of lipid substrates in myocardium, have long been recognized.[34] Fatty acids and ketone bodies inhibit glucose utilization at multiple sites. Most important of these is inhibition of PFK-1. Metabolism of fatty acids and ketone bodies increases mitochondrial citrate levels as the result of increased mitochondrial acetyl CoA production and, hence, substrate effects on citrate synthetase.[76] Transport of citrate to the cytosol resulting in inhibition of PFK-1 occurs by citrate-malate exchange or efflux of 2-oxoglutarate and synthesis of citrate by cytosolic isocitrate dehydrogenase.[2] Inhibition of PFK-1 causes accumulation of glucose-6-phosphate, with resultant inhibition of hexokinase.[76] Transport of glucose into myocardium is inhibited by oxidation of fatty acids and ketone bodies, although the mechanism is unclear at present.[9] Last, oxidation of fatty acids or ketones inhibits PDH activity by increases in mitochondrial [acetyl CoA]/[CoA] and [NADH]/[NAD$^+$], with resultant allosteric inhibition of PDH in addition to covalent inactivation by stimulation of PDH kinase.[2, 17]

The regulation of fatty acid metabolism by alternative substrates has also been demonstrated, although the mechanisms are less well understood. Carbohydrate feeding of animals, with resultant increases in plasma glucose and insulin, decreases myocardial fatty acid uptake, in part by decreasing plasma fatty acid levels.[77] However, additional regulation at the level of the myocardium has been demonstrated both in vivo and in vitro. In vivo, inhibition of fatty acid oxidation has been demonstrated with glucose/insulin[78] and lactate,[30] and also by ketone bodies.[79] Similar results have been obtained in vitro.[80, 81] Interestingly, lactate, pyruvate, and glucose inhibited oxidation of long-chain but not medium-chain fatty acids in perfused hearts,[80, 81] consistent with an effect at the level of the transport of long-chain fatty acids into the mitochondrion. In contrast, ketones inhibited both oleate and octanoate oxidation, suggesting an intramitochondrial site of action.[81]

Fasting

Fasting leads to elevated plasma concentrations of free fatty acids and low levels of circulating insulin. Myocardial triglyceride and glycogen stores are increased, reflecting increased esterification of free fatty acid to triglyceride and inhibition of glycolysis in response to increased β-oxidation.[2] Perfused hearts from starved rats demonstrate decreased glucose transport, glycolysis, and PDH activity.[2, 76] Accumulation of citrate is observed in vivo and in vitro and is believed to be responsible for the inhibition of PFK-1, with consequent accumulation of glucose-6-phosphate and inhibition of hexokinase.[2, 76] PDH inhibition probably reflects increases in [acetyl CoA]/[CoA] and [NADH]/[NAD] in response to increased β-oxidation of fatty acids.

Diabetes and Insulin

Myocardial metabolism in diabetes demonstrates marked similarity to the situation in fasting. Rats made diabetic by administration of alloxan are characterized by high plasma levels of free fatty acids, elevated blood glucose concentrations, ketonemia, and undetectable levels of circulating insulin.[2] As observed in fasting, increased β-oxidation of fatty acids leads to accumulation of citrate, with concomitant inhibition of PFK-1 and glycolysis.[76] Despite the presence of high plasma levels of glucose, transport of glucose into myocardium is limited because of the absence of insulin. Treatment with insulin in vivo (but not in vitro) restores glucose transport, although the sensitivity of the glucose transport system to insulin is decreased.[2, 76] The percentage of active PDH is decreased by phosphorylation of the enzyme in diabetes, mediated at least in part by increases in [acetyl CoA]/[CoA] and [NADH]/[NAD]. There is some evidence for additional, as yet incompletely defined, inhibition of the reactivation of the enzyme by multisite phosphorylation.[82]

Increased Work and Exercise

Increased myocardial work leads to an increased rate of ATP utilization, with a consequent increase in TCA flux and oxygen consumption. Experiments in vitro have shown that consumption of free fatty acids is increased preferentially over glucose metabolism at higher workloads.[1, 2] Glucose was found to be unable to support maximal rates of cardiac work as the sole substrate, because of the inability to dispose of cytosolic NADH, with consequent inhibition of glyceraldehyde-3-phosphate dehydrogenase.[26]

In exercise in vivo, changes in plasma substrate concentrations are an additional factor. Exercise leads to increases in arterial plasma lactate concentrations from the low levels of about 1 mM found at rest to 5 or 12 mM with moderate or heavy exercise, respectively.[32] Exercise has been shown to lead to an increase in lactate oxidation,[83, 84] consistent with the increased plasma availability of lactate. In addition, myocardial glucose uptake and oxidation were also increased with exercise.[84]

Catecholamines

Stimulation of myocardium with catecholamines affects cardiac metabolism in a number of ways. Myocardial oxygen consumption (MVo_2) is increased, providing additional energy to fuel the chronotropic and inotropic actions of catecholamines on the heart. Experimental evidence suggests that the catecholamine-mediated stimulation of cardiac respiration may have both α- and β-adrenergic mechanisms. α-Adrenergic stimulation has been shown to activate Ca^{2+} influx into mitochondria via the Ca^{2+} uniporter,[85] while β-adrenergic stimulation increases cytoplasmic [Ca^{2+}], leading to enhanced mitochondrial Ca^{2+} uptake.[86] Increased mitochondrial [Ca^{2+}] is then believed to activate key Ca^{2+}-dependent intramitochondrial dehydrogenases, NAD-linked isocitrate dehydrogenase, 2-oxoglutarate dehydrogenase, and PDH phosphatase. Stimulation of PDH phosphatase by Ca^{2+} leads to dephosphorylation (and, hence, activation) of PDH, while Ca^{2+} lowers the K_m of the two TCA cycle dehydrogenases for their respective substrates, stimulating TCA cycle fluxes.[67]

Glucose metabolism is stimulated at several steps by catecholamines. α-Adrenergic activation stimulates glucose uptake[87] and activates PFK-1.[23] β-Adrenergic stimulation also stimulates glucose uptake[87] and activates glycogen phosphorylase, stimulating glycogen breakdown.[88] Activation of glycogen phosphorylase occurs via the cAMP-dependent phosphorylation cascade (see Fig. 4–3).

Ischemia

The alterations in substrate metabolism occurring in ischemia have been discussed in detail in extensive review articles.[3, 89] The main points are summarized below, concentrating on ischemia (reduction in blood flow), rather than anoxia (removal of oxygen from perfusate), in view of its greater relevance to clinical heart disease.

Reduction of blood flow resulting in decreased delivery of oxygen to myocardium leads to a reduction in TCA cycle flux approximately in proportion to flow,[90] reflecting the very limited capacity of myocardium to increase oxygen extraction. Tricarboxylic acid cycle flux is limited by elevated mitochondrial [NADH]/[NAD$^+$] in consequence of the oxygen limitation of respiratory chain, with resultant inhibition of the key dehydrogenase steps in the TCA cycle. PDH flux is also limited by elevated [NADH]; the relative contributions of allosteric and covalent control to the inhibition of flux are unclear.[91, 92] Ischemia is accompanied by a rapid decline in contractile function, thus decreasing myocardial energy demand.

In ischemia, glucose metabolism accounts for an increased percentage of the residual oxygen consumption, with concomitantly decreased fatty acid oxidation.[90] Metabolism of glucose is accelerated in oxygen deficiency at a number of steps. Utilization of both exogenous and endogenous glucose supplies is increased in ischemia. Transport of glucose is increased,[93] probably reflecting GLUT translocation to the plasma membrane; activation of glycogen phosphorylase leads to increased glycogen breakdown. PFK-1 activity is increased because of decreased inhibition by the decreased tissue ATP levels and stimulation by elevation of AMP and Pi.[94] Increased flux through PFK-1 decreases glucose-6-phosphate levels, relieving inhibition of hexokinase, which is also stimulated by elevated Pi levels.[94, 95] Overall, glycolytic flux is increased in ischemia, but the degree of stimulation is dependent on the extent of residual flow, and in very severe ischemia glycolysis falls below control heart levels.[96] Because PDH flux is limited, pyruvate is converted to lactate, with concomitant regeneration of NAD from NADH. Increased alanine production is also observed[97]; the probable source of the alanine is disposal of TCA cycle metabolites, rather than glycolysis.[97] As flow decreases, washout of tissue lactate, produced by glycolysis, and H$^+$, produced by breakdown of ATP, is inhibited. Accumulation of lactate prevents regeneration of NAD$^+$ via the LDH reaction, and the resulting increase in cytosolic NADH, produced by triose phosphate dehydrogenation, in conjunction with lactate itself, inhibits glyceraldehyde-3-phosphate dehydrogenase.[98] Thus, the accumulation of metabolites in ischemia prevents glycolysis from reaching the maximum levels observed in anoxia with normal flows. Whereas anaerobic glycolysis may account for more than 50 percent of the glycolytic flux in ischemic myocardium, because of the low yield of ATP from anaerobic glycolysis (2 moles of ATP per mole of glucose), compared with aerobic glycolysis (36 moles of ATP per mole of glucose) aerobic metabolism still contributes more than 90 percent of ATP production in ischemia in canine myocardium with 7 percent residual flow from collaterals.[89] The possibility exists, however, that compartmentation of ATP production may exist.

Unlike glucose metabolism, no anaerobic alternative exists for energy-producing metabolism of fatty acids. Increases in mitochondrial [NADH]/[NAD$^+$] rapidly inhibit β-oxidation. Production of β-hydroxy fatty acid by ischemic heart suggests that the NAD$^+$-dependent β-hydroxyacyl-CoA dehydrogenase may be the most sensitive locus.[99] Fatty acid uptake is decreased,[100] fatty acid activation is decreased by product inhibition, and transport of long-chain acyl-CoA into mitochondria is decreased.[101] Free fatty acids, acylcarnitine, and acyl-CoA accumulate in ischemia: the possible deleterious effects of accumulation of intermediates of fatty acid metabolism on cardiac function in ischemia have been reviewed elsewhere.[3]

Studies in humans in vivo have demonstrated similar metabolic patterns in ischemia. Increased glucose metabolism relative to blood flow has been demonstrated in ischemic myocardial segments, compared with normal myocardial segments in patients with abnormal wall motion.[102, 103] Pacing-induced stress increases glucose extraction and lactate production in patients with coronary artery disease[33, 104] and decreases oxidation of long-chain fatty acid.[105] Thus clinical studies have demonstrated a switch to glucose from fatty acid metabolism as well as increased anaerobic glucose utilization.

Reperfusion

The prolonged functional abnormalities following brief periods of regional myocardial ischemia, often referred to as stunned myocardium, are well established.[106] Reperfused myocardium also demonstrates profound metabolic disturbances. Myocardial ATP levels remain depressed following reperfusion,[107] but decreased ATP levels are not thought to be the cause of the contractile dysfunction. Glycogen levels also show prolonged depletion in reperfused myocardium.[108] Experiments using ^{13}C-glucose and magnetic resonance imaging in hearts made globally ischemic have shown that glycogen levels continued to fall in the early postreperfusion period, probably reflecting increased activity of glycogen phosphorylase as the result of elevated levels of inorganic phosphate.[109]

The changes in substrate metabolism observed in reperfusion have proved rather variable, probably reflecting differences in the experimental models used. In general, uptake and oxidation of fatty acids have been found to be decreased immediately following reperfusion,[110–112] with the return of fatty acid oxidation paralleling the return of function.[110, 112] However, oxidation of fatty acids remains the main source of energy in the reperfused myocardium.[111, 113] In dogs, glucose uptake has been found to be decreased immediately after reperfusion compared with normal myocardium.[110, 114, 115] Twenty-four hours after reperfusion, glucose metabolism is enhanced in the reperfused tissue compared with the remote tissue.[110, 114, 115] Measurements of glucose metabolic rates demonstrated that increased glucose metabolism in reperfused tissue compared with remote tissue was found only when the glucose metabolic rate was low in the remote tissue.[114] Thus, glucose metabolism in the reperfused tissue appears to be resistant to the normal suppression by factors such as increased plasma fatty acids. Increased anaerobic glucose utilization contributes to the enhanced glucose utilization seen 24 hours after reperfusion.[108] In patients with coronary artery disease, increased glucose metabolism was demonstrated after exercise-induced angina, in the presence of normal flow.[116]

The MVO_2 is generally lower in the reperfused territory, compared with that in control myocardium.[111, 115, 117–119] However, contraction and MVO_2 in reperfused myocardium can be enhanced by stimuli such as catecholamines or postextrasystolic potentiation, demonstrating that the tissue retains contractile reserve.[119, 120] A number of studies have demonstrated that MVO_2 is increased relative to cardiac work in reperfused myocardium.[121–123] Because ^{31}P magnetic resonance imaging spectroscopy measurements have shown the P:O ratio, the ratio of net ATP synthesis to MVO_2, to be normal in postischemic myocardium, uncoupling of the mitochondria can be ruled out.[124] Thus, the inefficiency appears to lie at a step or steps subsequent to ATP production, such as decreased myofilament responsiveness.[125]

COMPARTMENTATION OF ENERGY UTILIZATION

Studies in a number of laboratories have suggested that ATP derived directly from glycolysis via substrate-level phosphorylations at the phosphoglycerate kinase and pyruvate kinase steps may be used preferentially in the maintenance of membrane integrity in ischemia, whereas energy derived from oxidative metabolism is used for support of contractile function. Inhibition of glycolysis has been shown to lead to increased enzyme leakage,[126, 127] shortening of the action potential,[128] accelerated onset of contracture,[129] and increased extracellular K^+ accumulation[130, 131] with little effect on contractility, whereas inhibition of oxidative metabolism has a much greater effect on contractility than on membrane function.[130, 131] Preferential inhibition of ATP-sensitive K^+ channels in isolated guinea pig cardiomyocytes by glycolysis has also been demonstrated.[132] On the basis of these and other experimental results, it has been proposed that the glycolytic enzymes are positioned close to the sarcolemmal membrane, allowing ready utilization of glycolytically generated ATP at the ATP-sensitive K^+ channels and for other energy-dependent membrane processes. Conversely, the close proximity of the mitochondria to the myofibrils would allow ready utilization of ATP derived from oxidative metabolism for contractility.

PROTEIN TURNOVER

Myocardial protein turnover reflects a balance between the rates of protein synthesis and degradation, a balance that can be disturbed by a number of physiologic variations.[133] Myocardium shows an overall fractional protein synthesis rate of 8 to 9 percent per day in rabbits and rats,[134, 135] whereas individual proteins display markedly heterogeneous turnover rates.[136] The pathways of protein synthesis and degradation, and the factors controlling the balance between these two pathways, will be discussed later.

Protein Synthesis

The pathway for protein synthesis can conveniently be divided into three sections: amino acid transport and aminoacyl-tRNA synthesis, peptide-chain initiation, and elongation and termination of peptide chains.

Amino Acid Transport and Aminoacyl-tRNA Synthesis

Transport of amino acids into cells takes place via a number of transport systems with overlapping substrate specificities.[137] Availability of amino acids does not appear to limit cardiac protein synthetic rate when amino acids are available at physiologic concentrations.[133] Synthesis of aminoacyl-tRNA derivatives takes place by means of the enzymatic action of aminoacyl-tRNA synthetases specific for each amino acid and its corresponding tRNA. Interestingly, many of the tRNA synthetases are found as a loose complex in the cell.[138] Measurement of the specific activity of the aminoacyl-tRNA pools with the use of radiolabeled amino acids has demonstrated that it is generally greater than that of the intracellular amino acid pool but less than that of the extracellular pool, suggesting that extracellular amino acids are used for synthesis of aminoacyl-tRNA before mixing with the bulk intracellular amino acid pool.[133]

Peptide-Chain Initiation

Initiation of protein synthesis in mammalian cells has been reviewed[139] and is summarized in Figure 4–11. Initiation of protein synthesis utilizes a specific initiator transfer RNA (tRNA), methionyl-tRNA$_f$, which donates methionine exclusively into the N-terminal position of newly synthesized peptides; a separate methionine-accepting tRNA is used for incorporation of methionine into internal positions. Met-tRNA$_f$ binds to eukaryotic initiation factor 2 (eIF-2) in a GTP-dependent reaction to form a ternary complex. The ternary complex binds to a 43S ribosomal complex consisting of the 40S ribosomal subunit and eIF-3 and eIF-4C, forming a 43S preinitiation complex. The 43S preinitiation complex then binds to the 5′ end of messenger RNA (mRNA) and migrates to the initiation codon, AUG. eIF-4A, eIF-4B and eIF-4F are required, as well as ATP hydrolysis. Eukaryotic initiation factor 5 then promotes dissociation of the other initiation factors bound to the 40S subunit, as well as hydrolysis of the GTP that entered as part of the ternary complex. Finally the 60S ribosomal subunit joins to form an 80S initiation complex on the mRNA.

Regulation of protein synthesis initiation has been studied in most detail in the reticulocyte lysate, where protein synthesis is dependent on the continued presence of haemin. Inhibition of protein synthesis in the absence of haemin involves decreased 43S preinitiation complex formation, which is accompanied by an increase in the phosphorylation of one of the subunits of eIF-2 by a cAMP-independent protein kinase. However, the mechanism by which eIF-2 phosphorylation inhibits 43S complex formation is still not fully understood.[139] Decreased formation of 43S preinitiation complexes has also been demonstrated in skeletal muscle from starved or diabetic rats,[140, 141] suggesting that a similar regulatory mechanism may be operative in muscle tissue.

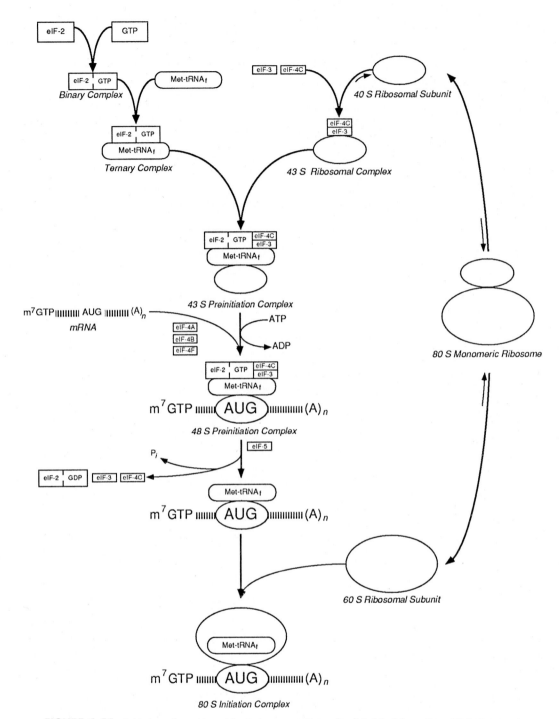

FIGURE 4-11. Initiation of protein synthesis in mammalian cells. (Modified from Pain, V.M.: Initiation of protein synthesis in mammalian cells. Biochem. J. 235:625–637, 1986.)

PEPTIDE ELONGATION AND TERMINATION

Elongation of peptides requires two elongation factors, EF-1 and EF-2.[142] EF-1 forms a ternary complex with GTP and charged aminoacyl-tRNA,[143] which binds to the acceptor site of the ribosomes, with hydrolysis of GTP. Peptide-bond formation, catalyzed by a peptidyltransferase activity located on the 60S ribosomal subunit, is then followed by translocation of the peptidyl-tRNA from the acceptor (A) site to the donor (P) site and translocation of the ribosome one codon along the mRNA. This reaction probably requires EF-2–mediated GTP hydrolysis.[144]

Termination occurs when a termination codon is reached by the A site, and requires binding of GTP and a specific release factor

RF.[145] In the presence of a termination codon in the A site and binding of RF and GTP, peptidyltransferase catalyzes the hydrolysis of the peptidyl-tRNA ester, releasing the completed polypeptide chain from the tRNA. Release of RF, the terminal tRNA, and the ribosomal subunits from the mRNA requires GTP hydrolysis; the released ribosomal subunits then enter the ribosomal subunit pool and are available for another round of protein synthesis, starting with the initiation process. A detailed account of the elongation and termination processes is available in a recent review.[142]

Protein Degradation

Protein degradation occurs via two pathways, lysosomal and non-lysosomal.[146] It has been proposed that lysosomal protein degradation has two components: first, macroautophagy, which is responsible for acceleration of protein degradation under various stimuli, and, second, microautophagy or basal autophagy, which is the sequestration of proteins through smaller vacuoles with high surface-to-volume ratios via invaginative or single-walled vesicular mechanisms and is responsible for basal levels of protein degradation. In muscle, macroautophagic protein degradation appears limited to nonmyofibrillar proteins, whereas myofibrillar protein degradation probably involves nonlysosomal calcium-activated disassembly of myofibrils into separate contractile proteins,[147] at least for the initial steps in myofibrillar degradation. The macroautophagic pathway appears to be the component of total protein breakdown suppressed by insulin and amino acids in perfused hearts and by food intake in vivo.[146]

REGULATION OF PROTEIN TURNOVER

Net protein turnover is determined by the relative rates of protein synthesis and degradation, which can be modified by a large number of physiologic stimuli.

Insulin and Diabetes

Perfusion of isolated hearts in the absence of insulin leads to dissociation of polyribosomal complexes and increased levels of ribosomal subunits, indicating decreased polypeptide initiation.[133] A negative nitrogen balance is also observed in such hearts, as protein degradation rates are double protein synthesis rates.[133, 134] Addition of insulin decreased protein degradation rates and increased protein synthesis rates, restoring a positive nitrogen balance.[133, 134] Addition of insulin to the perfusate increased latency of lysosomal enzymes, possibly indicating stabilization of the lysosomes.[148]

Diabetes was not found to lead to decreases in polyribosomal content and increases in levels of ribosomal subunits, indicating that initiation of protein synthesis remained rapid, relative to peptide elongation.[149] It has been proposed that increased plasma levels of fatty acids in diabetes maintain peptide-chain initiation because addition of fatty acids to perfused hearts mimicked the effect of insulin in maintaining peptide initiation and, thus, in preserving polyribosomal profiles.[149, 150] A reduced level of protein synthesis in diabetic rat hearts in vivo was found to reflect both a decreased number of ribosomes and decreased efficiency of protein synthesis per ribosome.[139] Tissue levels of EF-2 were decreased in diabetic rat hearts but recovered in parallel with protein synthesis rates after insulin treatment, suggesting a role for EF-2 in the impairment of diabetic protein synthesis efficiency.[151] The effect of diabetes on protein degradation has not been investigated in detail, but preliminary results indicate that protein degradation may be increased in diabetes.[133]

Starvation

Starvation leads to a decrease in myocardial mass and protein content, indicating a negative myocardial nitrogen balance.[134, 152] Prolonged starvation inhibits protein synthesis.[134, 135, 152] While the RNA content of cardiac muscle was decreased, the major effect of starvation was to decrease the efficiency of protein synthesis (the rate of protein synthesis was relative to RNA content).[134] Polyribosomal profiles were maintained without breakdown to ribosomal subunits, again indicating maintenance of peptide initiation, relative to elongation.[150] Elevated serum levels of fatty acids during fasting may again contribute to the relative maintenance of peptide initiation, in contrast with skeletal muscle, in which inhibition of protein synthesis initiation is observed during fasting.[149, 150] Starvation has been shown to have differential effects on the synthesis rates for different myocardial proteins; a disproportionate reduction of actin

synthesis relative to myosin heavy-chain and total-protein synthesis has been demonstrated,[135, 152] which is readily reversible on refeeding.[152] The decrease in actin synthesis could be explained, at least in part, by a disproportionately large decrease in actin mRNA.[152] It was also of interest that a similar disproportionate decrease in actin synthesis did not occur in skeletal muscle.[152]

The effects of starvation on protein degradation are less clear-cut, probably reflecting the greater methodologic difficulties involved in the estimation of protein degradation rates.[133] Whereas in vivo studies have found increased fractional rates of protein degradation in starvation,[134, 135] in vitro studies have found decreased degradation rates in cardiac tissue from fasted animals.[134, 153, 154] These results are thus likely to reflect the involvement of systemic factors in the regulation of protein degradation in vivo during starvation.

Hypertrophy

Cardiac hypertrophy is characterized by increases in flux through both the protein-synthetic and the protein-degradative pathways. Aortic banding leads to a rapid increase in cardiac muscle protein content.[155] Studies from several laboratories have demonstrated protein-synthetic rates in hypertrophy ranging from 165 to 400 percent of initial rates, and in each case the increase in the protein-synthetic rate was greater than the increase in myocardial growth, indicating that protein-degradative rates must also be increased.[155] Similarly, in left-ventricular hypertrophy induced in rabbits with thyroxine treatment, the rate of protein synthesis was increased in excess of the rate of total protein accumulation, again indicating an increase in left-ventricular protein-degradative rates.[156] An increased protein-synthetic rate was observed prior to significant changes in left-ventricular RNA content, suggesting that an increase in the efficiency of protein synthesis per ribosome is responsible, at least in part, for the increase in protein-synthetic rate.[156]

It has also been demonstrated that imposition of acute pressure overload in isolated perfused hearts leads to increased rates of myocardial protein synthesis, with some evidence suggesting that peptide-chain initiation was increased.[133] Protein degradation was not increased by acute pressure overload.[133]

Ischemia

The effects of oxygen deprivation on the rates of protein synthesis and degradation have been studied both in vitro and in vivo. In vitro, inhibition of both protein synthesis and degradation was observed in perfused rat hearts made ischemic by reduction of coronary flow.[133] Anoxia, induced by perfusion with buffer equilibrated with N_2-CO_2 instead of O_2-CO_2, caused a more profound inhibition of protein synthesis but a lesser inhibition of protein degradation, compared with that of ischemia. Energy deprivation was more severe in the anoxic hearts than in the ischemic hearts, as indicated by a greater decline in myocardial creatine phosphate levels.[133]

Exposure of rats to mild hypoxia in vivo (10 percent O_2 atmosphere) for 6 hours led to a modest decrease (20 percent) in the myocardial protein-synthesis rate, which was attributable to decreased efficiency of protein synthesis.[157] After 24 hours of mild hypoxia, protein-synthesis rates were found to be normal, however.[158] Short-term exposure to severe hypoxia (in a 5 percent O_2 atmosphere) for as little as 1 hour caused approximately a 50 percent inhibition of myocardial protein synthesis, decreased efficiency again being the cause.[158]

SUMMARY

This chapter has focused on the major metabolic pathways in myocardium and on their regulation under various physiologic and pathophysiologic conditions. Current understanding of the regulation of these pathways is by no means complete, particularly with respect to regulatory mechanisms in vivo. It is to be hoped that cardiac imaging will play an increasing role in furthering the understanding of these complex pathways in health and sickness.

References

1. Neely, J.R., and Morgan H.E.: Relationship between carbohydrate and lipid metabolism and the energy balance of heart muscle. Annu. Rev. Physiol. 36:414, 1974.
2. Randle, P.J., and Tubbs, P.K.: Carbohydrate and fatty acid metabolism. In Berne, R.M., Sperelakis, N., and Geiger, S.R. (eds.): Handbook of Physiology, Section 2: The Cardiovascular System. Bethesda, MD, The American Physiological Society, 1979.
3. Liedtke, A.J.: Alterations of carbohydrate and lipid metabolism in the acutely ischemic heart. Prog. Cardiovasc. Dis. 23:321, 1981.
4. Kacser, H.: The control of enzyme systems in vivo: Elasticity analysis of the steady state. Biochem. Soc. Trans. 11:35, 1983.
5. Mueckler, M.: Facilitative glucose transporters. Eur. J. Biochem. 219:713, 1994.
6. Kraegen, E.W., Sowden, J.A., Halstead, M.B., et al.: Glucose transporters and in vivo glucose uptake in skeletal and cardiac muscle: Fasting, insulin stimulation and immunoisolation studies of GLUT 1 and GLUT 4. Biochem. J. 295:287, 1993.
7. Cheung, J.Y., Conover, C., Regen, D.M., et al.: Effects of insulin on kinetics of sugar transport in heart muscle. Am. J. Physiol. 234:E70, 1978.
8. Simpson, I.A., and Cushman, S.W.: Hormonal regulation of mammalian glucose transport. Annu. Rev. Biochem. 55:1959, 1986.
9. Randle, P.J., Newsholme, E.A., and Garland, P.B.: Regulation of glucose uptake by muscle. 8. Effects of fatty acids, ketone bodies and pyruvate and of alloxan diabetes and starvation, on the uptake and metabolic fate of glucose in rat heart and diaphragm muscle. Biochem. J. 93:652, 1964.
10. England, P.J., and Randle, P.J.: Effectors of rat heart hexokinases and the control of rates of glucose phosphorylation in the perfused rat heart. Biochem. J. 105:907, 1967.
11. Green, M.H., and Landau, B.R.: Contribution of the pentose cycle to glucose metabolism in muscle. Arch. Biochem. Biophys. 111:569, 1965.
12. Krisman, C.R., and Barengo, R.: A precursor of glycogen biosynthesis: Alpha-1,4-glucan-protein. Eur. J. Biochem. 52:117, 1975.
13. Grably, S., and Rossi, A.: Changes in cardiac glycogen synthase and phosphorylase activities following stimulation of beta-adrenergic receptors in rats. Basic Res. Cardiol. 80:175, 1985.
14. McCullough, T.E., and Walsh, D.A.: Phosphorylation of glycogen synthase in the perfused rat heart. J. Biol. Chem. 254:7336, 1979.
15. Uyeda, K.: Phosphofructokinase. Adv. Enzymol. 48:193, 1979.
16. Mansour, T.E.: Phosphofructokinase. Curr. Top. Cell. Regul. 5:1, 1972.
17. Opie, L.H., Mansford, K.R.L., and Owen, P.: Effects of increased heart work on glycolysis and adenine nucleotides in the perfused heart of normal and diabetic rats. Biochem. J. 124:475, 1971.
18. Hers, H.G., and van Schaftigen, E.: Fructose 2,6-bisphosphate 2 years after its discovery. Biochem. J. 206:1, 1982.
19. Uyeda, K., Furuya, E., Richards, C.S., et al.: Fructose 2,6-P_2: Chemistry and biological function. Mol. Cell Biochem. 48:97, 1982.
20. Narabayashi, H., Lawson, J.W.R., and Uyeda, K.: Regulation of phosphofructokinase in perfused rat heart. J. Biol. Chem. 260:9750, 1985.
21. Lawson, J.W.R., and Uyeda, K.: Effects of insulin and work on fructose 2,6-bisphosphate content and phosphofructokinase activity in perfused rat hearts. J. Biol. Chem. 262:3165, 1987.
22. Depre, C., Rider, M.H., Veitch, K., et al.: Role of fructose 2,6-bisphosphate in the control of heart glycolysis. J. Biol. Chem. 268:13274, 1993.
23. Clark, M.G., and Patten, G.S.: Adrenaline activation of phosphofructokinase in rat heart mediated by α-receptor mechanism independent of cyclic AMP. Nature (Lond.), 292:461, 1981.
24. Rider, M.H., and Hue, L.: Activation of rat heart phosphofructokinase-2 by insulin in vivo. FEBS Lett. 176:484, 1984.
25. Rovetto, M.J., Lamerton, W.F., and Neely, J.R.: Mechanism of glycolytic inhibition in ischemic rat hearts. Circ. Res. 37:742, 1975.
26. Kobayashi, K., and Neely, J.R.: Control of maximum rates of glycolysis in rat cardiac muscle. Circ. Res. 44:166, 1979.
27. Mowbray, J.: A mitochondrial monocarboxylate transporter in rat liver and its possible function in cell control. Biochem. J. 148:41, 1975.
28. Reed, L.J.: Regulation of mammalian pyruvate dehydrogenase complex by a phosphorylation-dephosphorylation cycle. Curr. Top. Cell. Regul. 18:95, 1981.
29. Behal, R.H., Buxton, D.B., Robertson, J.G., et al.: Regulation of the pyruvate dehydrogenase multienzyme complex. Annu. Rev. Nutr. 13:497, 1993.
30. Drake, A.J., Papadoyannis, D.E., Butcher R.G., et al.: Inhibition of glycolysis in the denervated dog heart. Circ. Res. 47:338, 1980.
31. Mann G.E., Zlokovic B.V., and Yudilevich D.L.: Evidence for a lactate transport system in the sarcolemmal membrane of the perfused rabbit heart: Kinetics of unidirectional flux, carrier specificity and effects of glucagon. Biochim. Biophys. Acta 819:241, 1985.
32. Drake-Holland, A.J.: Substrate utilization. In Drake, A.J., and Noble, M.I. (eds.): Cardiac Metabolism. New York, John Wiley & Sons, 1983.
33. Wisneski, J.A., Gertz, E.W., Neese, R.A., et al.: Dual carbon-labeled isotope experiments using D-[6-^{14}C] glucose and L-[1,2,3-^{13}C3] lactate: A new approach for investigating human myocardial metabolism during ischemia. J. Am. Coll. Cardiol. 5:1138, 1985.
34. Bing, R.J.: The metabolism of the heart. In Harvey Lecture Series. New York, Academic Press, 1954/1955.
35. DeGrella, R.F., and Light, R.J.: Uptake and metabolism of fatty acids by dispersed adult rat heart myocytes. J. Biol. Chem. 255:9731, 1980.
36. Stremmel W.: Fatty acid uptake by isolated rat heart myocytes represents a carrier-mediated transport process. J. Clin. Invest. 81:844, 1988.
37. Glatz, J.F.C., Janssen, A.M., Baerwaldt, C.C.F., et al.: Purification and characterization of fatty acid-binding proteins from rat heart and liver. Biochim. Biophys. Acta 837:57, 1985.
38. Sweetser, D.A., Heuckforth, R.O., and Gordon, J.I.: The metabolic function of fatty-acid-binding proteins: Abundant proteins in search of a function. Annu. Rev. Nutr. 7:337, 1987.
39. Carey, J.O., Neufer, P.D., Farrar, R.P., et al.: Transcriptional regulation of muscle fatty acid-binding protein. Biochem. J. 298:613, 1994.
40. Van Breda, E., Keizer, H.A., Vork, M.M., et al.: Modulation of fatty acid–binding protein content of rat heart and skeletal muscle by endurance training and testosterone treatment. Pflugers Arch. 421:274, 1992.
41. Groot, P.G.E., Scholte, H.R., and Hulsmann, W.C.: Fatty acid activation: Specificity, localization and function. Adv. Lipid Res. 14:75, 1976.
42. De Jong, J.W., and Hülsmann, W.C.: A comparative study of palmitoyl-CoA synthetase activity in rat heart, liver and gut mitochondrial and microsomal preparations. Biochim. Biophys. Acta 197:127, 1970.
43. Bremer, J., and Osmundsen, H.: Fatty acid oxidation and its regulation. In Numa, S. (ed.): Fatty Acid Metabolism and Its Regulation. Amsterdam, Elsevier, 1984.
44. Murthy, M.S.R., and Pande, S.V.: Malonyl-CoA binding site and the overt carnitine palmitoyl transferase activity reside on opposite sides of the outer mitochondrial membrane. Proc. Natl. Acad. Sci. USA 84:378, 1987.
45. McGarry, J.D., Mills, S.E., Long, C.S., et al.: Observations on the affinity for carnitine, and malonyl CoA sensitivity of carnitine palmitoyl-transferase I in animal and human tissue. Biochem. J 214:21, 1983.
46. Saggerson, E.D., and Carpenter, C.A.: Carnitine palmitoyltransferase and carnitine octanoyltransferase activities in liver, kidney cortex, adipocyte, lactating mammary gland, skeletal muscle and heart: Relative activities, latency and effects of malonyl CoA. FEBS Lett. 129:229, 1981.
47. Awan, M.M., and Saggerson, E.D.: Malonyl-CoA metabolism in cardiac myocytes and its relevance to the control of fatty acid oxidation. Biochem. J. 295:61, 1993.
48. Saddik, M., Gamble, J., Witters, L.A., et al.: Acetyl-CoA carboxylase regulation of fatty acid oxidation in the heart. J. Biol. Chem. 268:25836, 1993.
49. Stanley, K.K., and Tubbs, P.K.: The role of intermediates in fatty acid oxidation. Biochem. J. 150:77, 1975.
50. Lopes-Cardozo, M., Klazinga, W., and van den Bergh, S.G.: Evidence for a homogeneous pool of acetyl CoA in rat liver mitochondria. Eur. J. Biochem. 83:635, 1978.
51. Oram, J.F., Bennetch, S.L., and Neely, J.R.: Regulation of fatty acid utilization in isolated perfused rat hearts. J. Biol. Chem. 248:5299, 1973.
52. Wang, H.-Y., Baxter, C.F., and Schulz, H.: Regulation of fatty acid β-oxidation in rat heart mitochondria. Arch. Biochem. Biophys. 289:274, 1991.
53. Oram, J.F., Wenger, J.J., and Neely, J.R.: Regulation of long chain fatty acid activation in heart muscle. J. Biol. Chem. 250:73, 1975.
54. Robinson, A.M., and Williamson, D.H.: Physiological roles of ketone bodies as substrates and signals in mammalian tissues. Physiol. Rev. 60:143, 1980.
55. Land, J.M., Mowbray, J., and Clark, J.B.: Control of pyruvate and β-hydroxybutyrate utilization in rat brain mitochondria and its relevance to phenylketonuria and maple syrup urine disease. J Neurochem 26:823, 1976.
56. Taegtmeyer, H.: Myocardial metabolism. In Phelps, M, Mazziotta, J., Schelbert, H. (eds.): Positron Emission Tomography and Autoradiography: Principles and Applications for the Brain and Heart. New York, Raven Press, 1986.
57. Wick, A.N., and Drury, D.R.: The effect of concentration on the rate of utilization of β-hydroxybutyric acid by the rabbit. J. Biol. Chem. 138:129, 1941.
58. Rudoph W., Maas D., Richter J., et al.: Über die Bedeutung von Acetoacetat und β-Hydroxybutyrat im Stoffwechsel des menschlichen Herzen. Klin. Wochenschr. 43:445, 1965.
59. Russell, R.R., and Taegtmeyer, H.: Pyruvate carboxylation prevents the decline in contractile function of rat hearts oxidizing acetoacetate. Am. J. Physiol. 261:H1756, 1991.
60. Williamson J.R.: Mitochondrial function in the heart. Annu. Rev. Physiol. 41:485, 1979.
61. Taegtmeyer H.: Six blind men explore an elephant: Aspects of fuel metabolism and the control of tricarboxylic acid cycle activity in heart muscle. Basic Res. Cardiol. 79:322, 1984.
62. Randle P.J., England P.J., and Denton R.M.: Control of the tricarboxylate cycle and its interactions with glycolysis during acetate utilization in the rat heart. Biochem. J. 117:677, 1970.
63. Srere, P.A., Halper, L.A., and Finkelstein, M.B.: Interaction of citrate synthase and malate dehydrogenase. In Srere, P.A., and Estabrook, R.W. (eds): Microenvironments and Metabolic Compartmentation. New York, Academic Press, 1978.
64. Hansford, R.G., and Johnson, R.N.: Steady state concentrations of coenzyme A-SH, coenzyme A thioester, citrate and isocitrate during tricarboxylate cycle oxidation in rabbit heart mitochondria. J. Biol. Chem. 250:8361, 1975.
65. Hansford, R.G.: Control of mitochondrial substrate oxidation. Curr. Top. Cell Regul. 10:217, 1980.
66. LaNoue, K.F., Walajtys, E.I., and Williamson, J.R.: Regulation of glutamate metabolism and interactions with the citric acid cycle in rat heart mitochondria. J. Biol. Chem. 248:7171, 1973.

67. Denton, R.M., and McCormack, J.G.: On the role of the calcium transport cycle in heart and other mammalian mitochondria. FEBS Lett. 119:1, 1980.

68. Kammermeier, H.: Why do cells need phosphocreatine and a phosphocreatine shuttle? J. Mol. Cell. Cardiol. 19:115, 1987.

69. Mainwood, G.W., and Rakusan, K.: A model for intracellular ion transport. Can. J. Physiol. Pharmacol. 60:98, 1982.

70. Chance, B., and Williams, G.R.: Respiratory enzymes in oxidative phosphophorylation. 1. Kinetics of oxygen utilization. J. Biol. Chem. 217:383, 1955.

71. Jacobus, W.E., Moreadith, R.W., and Vandegaer, K.M.: Mitochondrial respiratory control. J. Biol. Chem. 257:2397, 1982.

72. Klingenberg, M.: The ADP-ATP translocation in mitochondria: A membrane potential-controlled transport. J. Membr. Biol. 56:97, 1980.

73. Nishiki, K., Erecinska, M., and Wilson, D.: Energy relationships between cytosolic metabolism and mitochondrial respiration in rat heart. Am. J. Physiol. 234:C73, 1978.

74. Erecinska, M., and Wilson, D.F.: Regulation of cellular energy metabolism. J. Membr. Biol. 70:1, 1982.

75. Hansford, R.G.: Relation between mitochondrial Ca^{2+} transport and control of energy metabolism. Rev. Physiol. Biochem. Pharmacol. 102:1, 1985.

76. Newsholme, E.A., and Randle, P.J.: Regulation of glucose uptake by muscle. 7. Effects of fatty acids, ketone bodies and pyruvate, and of alloxan diabetes, starvation, hypophysectomy and adrenalectomy, on the concentrations of hexose phosphates, nucleotides and inorganic phosphate in perfused heart. Biochem. J. 93:641, 1964.

77. Goodale, W.T., Olson, R.E., and Hackel, D.B.: The effects of fasting and diabetes mellitus on myocardial metabolism in man. Am. J. Med. 27:212, 1959.

78. Schelbert, H.R., Henze, E., Schön, H.R., et al.: C-11 palmitate for the noninvasive evaluation of regional myocardial fatty acid metabolism with positron computed tomography. III. In vivo demonstration of the effects of substrate availability on myocardial metabolism. Am. Heart. J. 105:492, 1983.

79. Bassenge, E., Wendt, V.E., Schollmeyer, P., et al.: Effects of ketone bodies on cardiac metabolism. Am. J. Physiol. 208:162, 1965.

80. Bielefeld, D.R., Vary, T.C., and Neely, J.R.: Inhibition of carnitine palmitoyl-CoA transferase activity and fatty acid oxidation by lactate and oxfenicine in cardiac muscle. J. Mol. Cell. Cardiol. 17:619, 1985.

81. Forsey, R.G.P., Reid, K., and Brosnan, J.T.: Competition between fatty acids and carbohydrates or ketone bodies as metabolic fuels for the isolated perfused heart. Can. J. Physiol. Pharmacol. 65:401, 1987.

82. Sale, G.J., and Randle, P.J.: Occupancy of sites of phosphorylation in inactive rat heart pyruvate dehydrogenase phosphate in vivo. Biochem. J. 193:935, 1981.

83. Keul, J., Doll, E., Steim, H., et al.: Über den Stoffwechsel des menschlichen Herzens. III. Der oxidative Stoffwechsel des menschlichen Herzens unter verschiedenen Arbeitsbedingungen II. Pflügers Arch. 282:43, 1965.

84. Gertz, E.W., Wisneski, J.A., Stanley W.C., et al.: Myocardial substrate utilization during exercise in humans: Dual carbon-labeled carbohydrate isotope experiments. J. Clin. Invest. 82:2017, 1988.

85. Kessar, P., and Crompton, M.: The α-adrenergic-mediated activation of Ca^{2+} influx into cardiac mitochondria. Biochem. J. 200:379, 1981.

86. McCormack, J.G., and Denton, R.M.: The activation of pyruvate dehydrogenase in the perfused rat heart by adrenaline and other inotropic agents. Biochem. J. 194:639, 1981.

87. Clark, M.G., and Patten, G.S.: Adrenergic regulation of glucose metabolism in rat heart. J. Biol. Chem. 259:15204, 1984.

88. Williamson, J.R.: Metabolic effects of epinephrine in the isolated perfused rat heart. J. Biol. Chem. 239:2721, 1964.

89. Opie, L.H.: Effects of regional ischemia on metabolism of glucose and fatty acids. Circ. Res. 38:I52, 1976.

90. Opie, L.H., Owen, P., and Riemersma, R.A.: Relative rates of oxidation of glucose and free fatty acids by ischemic and non-ischemic myocardium after coronary artery ligation in the dog. Eur. J. Clin. Invest. 3:419, 1973.

91. Kobayashi, K., and Neely, J.R.: Effects of ischemia and reperfusion on pyruvate dehydrogenase in isolated rat hearts. J. Mol. Cell. Cardiol. 15:359, 1983.

92. Patel, T.B., and Olson, M.S.: Regulation of pyruvate dehydrogenase complex in ischemic rat heart. Am. J. Physiol. 246:H858, 1984.

93. Morgan, H.E., Randle, P.J., and Regen, D.M.: Regulation of glucose uptake by muscle. III. Effects of insulin, anoxia, salicylate and 2,4-dinitrophenol on membrane transport and intracellular phosphorylation of glucose in the isolated rat heart. Biochem. J. 73:573, 1959.

94. Morgan, H.E., Henderson, M.J., Regen D.M., et al.: Regulation of glucose uptake in muscle. I. The effects of insulin and anoxia on glucose transport and phosphorylation in the isolated perfused heart of the normal rat. J. Biol. Chem. 236:253, 1961.

95. Williamson, J.R.: Glycolytic control mechanisms. II. Kinetics of intermediate changes during the aerobic-anoxic transition in perfused rat heart. J. Biol. Chem. 214:5026, 1966.

96. Neely, J.R., Whitmer, J.T., and Rovetto, M.J.: Effect of coronary blood flow on glycolytic flux and intracellular flux in ischemic rat hearts. Circ. Res. 37:733, 1975.

97. Peuhkurinen, K.J., Takala, T.E.S., Nuutinen, E.M., et al.: Tricarboxylic acid cycle metabolites during ischemia in isolated perfused rat heart. Am. J. Physiol. 244:H281, 1983.

98. Mochizuki, S., and Neely, J.R.: Control of glyceraldehyde-3-phosphate dehydrogenase in cardiac muscle. J. Mol. Cell. Cardiol. 11:221, 1979.

99. Moore, K.H., Radloff, J.F., Hull F.E., et al.: Incomplete fatty acid oxidation by ischemic heart: β-Hydroxy fatty acid production. Am. J. Physiol. 239:H257, 1980.

100. van der Vusse, G.J., Roemen, T.H., Prinzen, F.W., et al.: Uptake and tissue content of fatty acids in dog myocardium under normoxic and ischemic conditions. Circ. Res. 50:538, 1982.

101. Wood, J.M., Hanley, H.G., Entman, M.L., et al.: Biochemical and morphological correlates of acute experimental ischemia in the dog. IV. Energy mechanisms during very early ischemia. Circ. Res. 44:52, 1979.

102. Marshall, R.C., Tillisch, J.H., Phelps, M.E., et al.: Identification and differentiation of resting myocardial ischemia and infarction in man with positron computed tomography ^{18}F-labeled fluorodeoxyglucose and N-13 ammonia. Circulation 67:766, 1983.

103. Tillisch, J., Brunken, R., Marshall, R., et al.: Reversibility of cardiac wall motion abnormalities predicted by positron tomography. N. Engl. J. Med. 314:884, 1986.

104. Most, A.S., Gorlin, R., and Soeldner, J.S.: Glucose extraction by the human myocardium during pacing stress. Circulation 45:92, 1972.

105. Grover-McKay, M., Schelbert, H.R., Schwaiger, M., et al.: Identification of impaired metabolic reserve by atrial pacing in patients with significant coronary artery stenosis. Circulation 74:281, 1986.

106. Braunwald, E., and Kloner, R.A.: The stunned myocardium: Prolonged, postischemic ventricular dysfunction. Circulation 66:1146, 1982.

107. DeBoer, L.W.V., Ingwall, J.S., Kloner, J.S., et al.: Prolonged derangements of canine myocardial purine metabolism after a brief coronary artery occlusion not associated with anatomic evidence of necrosis. Proc Natl Acad Sci USA 77:5471, 1980.

108. Schwaiger, M., Neese, R.A., Araujo, L., et al.: Sustained nonoxidative glucose utilization and depletion of glycogen in reperfused canine myocardium. J. Am. Coll. Cardiol. 13:745, 1989.

109. Kalil-Filho, R., Gerstenblith, G., Hansford, R.G., et al.: Regulation of myocardial glycogenolysis during post-ischemic reperfusion. J. Mol. Cell. Cardiol. 23:1467, 1991.

110. Schwaiger, M., Schelbert, H.R., Ellison D., et al.: Sustained regional abnormalities in cardiac metabolism after transient ischemia in the chronic dog model. J. Am. Coll. Cardiol. 6:336, 1985.

111. Myears, D.W., Sobel, B.E., and Bergmann, S.R.: Substrate use in ischemic and reperfused canine myocardium: Quantitative considerations. Am. J. Physiol. 253:H107, 1987.

112. Heyndrickx, G.R., Wijns, W., Vogelaers, D., et al.: Recovery of regional contractile function and oxidative metabolism in stunned myocardium induced by 1 hr circumflex coronary artery in chronically instrumented dogs. Circ. Res. 72:901, 1993.

113. Lopaschuk, G.D., Spafford, M.A., Davies, N.J., et al.: Glucose and palmitate oxidation in isolated working rat hearts reperfused after a period of transient global ischemia. Circ. Res. 66:546, 1990.

114. Buxton, D.B., and Schelbert, H.R.: Measurement of regional glucose metabolic rates in reperfused myocardium. Am. J. Physiol. 262:H2058, 1991.

115. Buxton, D.B., Vaghaiwalla Mody, F., Krivokapich, J., et al.: Quantitative assessment of prolonged metabolic abnormalities in reperfused canine myocardium. Circulation 85:1842, 1992.

116. Camici, P., Araujo, L.I., Spinks, T., et al.: Increased uptake of ^{18}F-fluorodeoxyglucose in postischemic myocardium of patients with exercise-induced angina. Circulation 74:81, 1986.

117. Buxton, D.B., Schwaiger, M., Vaghaiwalla Mody F., et al.: Regional abnormality of oxygen consumption in reperfusion assessed with $[1-^{11}C]$ acetate and positron emission tomography. Am. J. Card. Imaging 3:276, 1989.

118. Liedtke, A.J., DeMaison, L., Eggleston, A.M., et al.: Changes in substrate metabolism and effects of excess fatty acids in reperfused myocardium. Circ. Res. 62:535, 1988.

119. Hashimoto, T., Buxton, D.B., Krivokapich J., et al.: Responses of blood flow, oxygen consumption, and contractile function to inotropic stimulation in stunned canine myocardium. Am. Heart J. 127:1250, 1994.

120. Becker, L.C., Levine, J.H., Di Paula, A.F., et al.: Reversal of dysfunction in postischemic stunned myocardium by epinephrine and postextrasystolic potentiation. J. Am. Coll. Cardiol. 7:508, 1986.

121. Stahl, L.D., Weiss, H.R., and Becker, L.C.: Myocardial oxygen consumption, oxygen supply/demand heterogeneity, and microvascular patency in regionally stunned myocardium. Circulation 77:865, 1988.

122. Laxson, D.D., Homans, D.C., Dai, X.-Z., et al.: Oxygen consumption and coronary reactivity in post-ischemic myocardium. Circ. Res. 64:9, 1989.

123. Vinten-Johansen, J., Gayheart, P.A., Johnston, W.E., et al.: Regional function, blood flow, and oxygen utilization relations in repetitively occluded-reperfused canine myocardium. Am. J. Physiol. 261:H538, 1991.

124. Sako, E.Y., Kingsley-Hickman, P.B., From, A.H.L., et al.: ATP synthesis kinetics and mitochondrial function in the postischemic myocardium as studied by ^{31}P NMR. J. Biol. Chem. 263:10600, 1988.

125. Carrozza, J.P., Bentivegna, L.A., Williams, C.P., et al.: Decreased myofilament responsiveness in myocardial stunning follows transient calcium overload during ischemia and reperfusion. Circ. Res. 71:1334, 1992.

126. Bricknell, O.L., and Opie, L.H.: Effects of substrates on tissue metabolic changes in the isolated rat heart during underperfusion and on release of lactate dehydrogenase and arrhythmias during reperfusion. Circ. Res. 43:102, 1978.

127. Higgins, T.J.C., and Bailey, P.J.: The effects of cyanide and iodoacetate intoxication on enzyme release from the perfused rat heart. Biochim. Biophys. Acta 762:47, 1983.

128. McDonald, T.F., Hayahi, H., Ponnambalam, C., et al.: Cardiac Function Under Ischemia and Hypoxia. Nagoya, Japan, University of Nagoya Press, 1986.

129. Bricknell, O.L., Davies, P.S., and Opie, L.H.: A relationship between adenosine triphosphate, glycolysis and ischemic contracture in the isolated rat heart. J. Mol. Cell. Cardiol. 13:941, 1981.

130. Hasin, Y., and Barry, W.H.: Myocardial metabolic inhibition and membrane potential, contraction, and potassium uptake. Am. J. Physiol. 247:H322, 1984.

131. Weiss, J., and Hiltbrand, B.: Functional compartmentation of glycolytic vs. oxidative metabolism in isolated rabbit heart. J. Clin. Invest. 75:436, 1985.
132. Weiss, J.N., and Lamp, S.T.: Glycolysis preferentially inhibits ATP-sensitive K+ channels in isolated guinea pig myocytes. Science 238:67, 1987.
133. Morgan, H.E., Rannels, D.E., and McKee E.E.: Protein metabolism of the heart. *In* Berne RM, Sperelakis, N., and Geiger, S.R. (eds.): Handbook of Physiology: The Cardiovascular System I. Bethesda, MD, The American Physiological Society, 1979.
134. Preedy, V.R., Smith, D.M., Kearney, N.F., et al.: Rates of protein turnover in vivo and in vitro in ventricular muscle of hearts from fed and starved rats. Biochem. J. 222:395, 1984.
135. Samarel, A.M., Parmacek, M.S., Magid, N.M., et al.: Protein synthesis and degradation during starvation-induced cardiac atrophy in rabbits. Circ. Res. 60:933, 1987.
136. Zak, R., Martin, A.F., Prior G., et al.: Comparison of turnover of several myofibrillar proteins and critical evaluation of double isotope method. J. Biol. Chem. 252:3430, 1977.
137. Collarini, E.J., and Oxender, D.L.: Mechanisms of transport of amino acids across membranes. Annu. Rev. Nutr. 7:75, 1987.
138. Schimmel, P.R., and Söll, D.: Aminoacyl t-RNA synthetases: General features and recognition of transfer RNA. Annu. Rev. Biochem. 48:601, 1979.
139. Pain, V.M.: Initiation of protein synthesis in mammalian cells. Biochem. J. 235:625, 1986.
140. Harmon, C.S., Proud, C.G., and Pain, V.M.: Effects of starvation, diabetes and acute insulin treatment on the regulation of polypeptide initiation in rat skeletal muscle. Biochem. J. 223:687, 1984.
141. Kelly, F.J., and Jefferson, L.S.: Control of peptide chain initiation in rat skeletal muscle: Development of methods for preparation of native ribosomal subunits and analysis of the effects of insulin on formation of 40S initiation complexes. J. Biol. Chem. 260:6677, 1985.
142. Moldave, K.: Eukaryotic protein synthesis. Annu. Rev. Biochem. 54:1109, 1985.
143. Slobin, L.I.: Eukaryotic elongation factor Ts is an integral component of rabbit reticulocyte elongation factor-1. Eur. J. Biochem. 96:287, 1979.
144. Henriksen, O., Robinson, E.A., and Maxwell, E.S.: Interaction of guanine nucleotides with elongation factor-2. 1. Equilibrium dialysis studies. J. Biol. Chem. 250:720, 1975.
145. Tate, W.P., and Caskey, C.T.: The mechanism of peptide chain termination. Mol. Cell. Biochem. 5:115, 1974.
146. Mortimer, G.E., and Pösö, A.R.: Intracellular protein catabolism and its control during nutrient deprivation and supply. Annu. Rev. Nutr. 7:539, 1987.
147. Zeman, R.J., Kameyama, T., Matsumoto, K., et al.: Regulation of protein degradation in muscle by calcium. J. Biol. Chem. 260:13619, 1985.
148. Rannels, D.E., Kao, R., and Morgan, H.E.: Effect of insulin on protein turnover in heart muscle. J. Biol. Chem. 250:1694, 1975.
149. Rannels, D.E., Jefferson, L.S., Hjalmarson, A.C., et al.: Maintenance of protein synthesis in hearts of diabetic animals. Biochem. Biophys. Res. Commun. 40:1110, 1970.
150. Rannels, D.E., Hjalmarson, A.C., and Morgan, H.E.: Effects of non-carbohydrate substrates on protein synthesis in muscle. Am. J. Physiol. 226:528, 1974.
151. Vary, T.C., Nairn, A., and Lynch, C.J.: Role of elongation factor 2 in regulating peptide-chain elongation in the heart. Am. J. Physiol. 266.:E628, 1994.
152. Clark, A.F., and Wildenthal, K.: Disproportionate reduction of actin synthesis in hearts of starved rats. J. Biol. Chem. 261:13168, 1986.
153. Crie, J.S., Sanford, C.F., and Wildenthal, K.: Influence of starvation and refeeding on cardiac protein degradation in rats. J. Nutr. 108:22, 1980.
154. Curfman, G.D., O'Hara, D.S., Hopkins, B.E., et al.: Suppression of myocardial protein degradation in the rat during fasting: Effects of insulin, glucose and leucine. Circ. Res. 46:581, 1980.
155. Waterlow, J.C., Garlick, P.J., and Millward, D.J.: Protein turnover in the whole body and in whole tissues. *In* Protein Turnover in Mammalian Tissues and in the Whole Body. Amsterdam, North Holland, 1978.
156. Parmacek, M.S., Magid, N.M., Lesch, M., et al.: Cardiac protein synthesis and degradation during thyroxine-induced left-ventricular hypertrophy. Am. J. Physiol. 251:C727, 1986.
157. Preedy, V.R., Smith, D.M., and Sugden, P.H.: The effects of 6 hours of hypoxia on protein synthesis in rat tissues in vivo and in vitro. Biochem. J. 228:179, 1985.
158. Preedy, V.R., and Sugden, P.H.: The effects of fasting or hypoxia on rates of protein synthesis in vivo in subcellular fractions of the rat heart and gastrocnemius muscle. Biochem. J. 257:519, 1989.
159. Lehninger, A.L.: Biochemistry. New York, Worth, 1975.
160. Stryer, L.: Biochemistry. New York, W.H. Freeman, 1988.

CHAPTER

5 Principles of Valvar Function

John Michael Criley, M.D.

LEFT HEART VALVAR ANATOMY _____ **50**
Aortic Valve _____ **50**
Mitral Valve _____ **51**
NORMAL VALVE FUNCTION _____ **53**
Functional Anatomy (Integration of Pressure and Flow) _____ **54**

Atrial Pressure Waves _____ **55**
Transvalvar Flow Rate _____ **56**
DYSFUNCTION OF NORMAL CARDIAC VALVES _____ **56**
SURROGATE VALVAR FUNCTION _____ **57**
CONCLUDING REMARKS _____ **57**

Cardiac valves are remarkable in their structure, function, adaptability, and durability. Normal valves remain superior to any prosthetic device, despite the many breakthroughs in engineering designs and materials that have occurred. This chapter reviews normal valvar structure and function by integrating the anatomy and physiology of cardiac valves. An appreciation of this functional anatomy should serve to obviate common pitfalls based on faulty interpretation of cardiac images and intracardiac pressures. The primary focus is on the functional anatomy of cardiac valves of the left heart because these valves perform in a more critical environment and their dysfunction produces a greater impact than do analogous events in the right heart. It should be recognized that the right heart valves respond to analogous pressure and flow events, albeit slightly later and at considerably lower pressures than their counterparts in the left heart. Next, dysfunction of structurally normal valves is reviewed with an emphasis on the settings in which it occurs. The structure and function of pathologically altered valves is discussed only briefly because of extensive coverage elsewhere in this volume. Last, the recruitment of noncardiac valves as surrogates for cardiac valves is briefly discussed.

LEFT HEART VALVAR ANATOMY

The mitral and aortic valves constitute an integrated unit that provides inflow into and outflow from the left ventricle.[1, 2] Because the aortic valve has a central location in the heart, its position can be predicted by the intersection of imaginary cross-hairs centered over the cardiac silhouette in virtually any radiographic projection (Fig. 5–1). In an analogy to a world globe, the aorta is equivalent to the axis that remains central as the world spins around it. The mitral valve shares a common attachment with the aortic valve; its position can be predicted by its left caudal-dorsal spatial relation to the aorta.

Aortic Valve

The normal aortic valve is a tricuspid structure. Each of the symmetric cusps is semilunar in shape and suspended by attachments to a hemicircular limb of the tricornute annulus fibrosus (Figs. 5–2 and 5–3). During systole, the aortic orifice resembles an

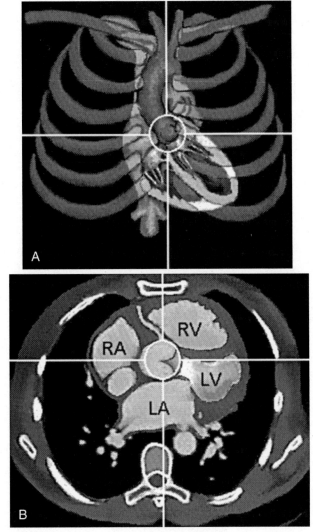

FIGURE 5–1. Location of the aortic valve. *A,* Frontal view. *B,* Tomographic cross section. The aortic valve is located in the center of the heart in both projections *(circle).* LA = left atrium; LV = left ventricle; RA = right atrium; RV = right ventricle.

outward-bulging equilateral triangle and the leaflets almost obliterate the sinuses of Valsalva. When closed, the cusps mutually support one another, and the sinuses are fully expanded. The leaflets and their respective sinuses are usually identified by their relation to the expected location of the coronary artery orifices: right, left, and noncoronary (or posterior). Other terminology is based on the cusps' location within the body (anterior, left posterior, and posterior).

The anatomical position of aortic root and valve at the "hub" of the heart in cross-sectional images places the aortic root in a position adjacent to every cardiac chamber (see Fig. 5–1B), with a relatively thin tissue barrier between this high-pressure structure and its surrounding low-pressure chambers. The aortic root is separated from the left ventricle to the left and caudally by thin aortic valve leaflets. The right ventricular outflow tract lies anteriorly (ventrally), the right atrium is to the right, and the left atrium is behind (dorsal). Aneurysmal dilations of the aortic sinuses or proximal aortic root project into these low-pressure chambers and, as a result, do not distort the external cardiac silhouette.

Mitral Valve

The mitral valve has a quadricuspid structure (see Fig. 5–3) consisting of an anterior leaflet, a middle scallop, and two commis-

sural scallops, anterolateral and posteromedial, aligned with their respective papillary muscles.[3] The latter three scallops constitute the posterior or mural leaflet; they are contiguous with the left atrial wall and are attached to the C-shaped mitral annulus (see Fig. 5–2).

The anterior mitral leaflet (also called the anteromedial, aortic, or septal leaflet) is contiguous with the left and noncoronary sinuses of the aortic valve. The integrated unit formed by the mitral and aortic valves includes a merger of the mitral and aortic annuli (see Fig. 5–2). The open portion of the incomplete mitral annulus is affixed to the tricornute aortic valve annulus. (Although the fibromuscular support structures of the mitral and aortic valves are not annular, or ring-like, they nevertheless have traditionally been termed rings or annuli.)

The anterior and posterior leaflets of the mitral valve are distinct not only in their structure but also in their function. The *anterior mitral leaflet* occupies about one quarter to one third of the circumference of the valve, and it serves a dual function. During diastole (see Fig. 5–3A) it forms the anterior wall of the inflow orifice, and during systole (see Fig. 5–3B) it becomes the posterior wall of the outflow orifice of the left ventricle. This transition requires a diastolic excursion of the anterior leaflet across the aortic vestibule toward the ventricular septum with concavity toward the atrium, followed by a complete reversal during systole as the leaflet swings toward the atrium and forms the posteromedial concave boundary of the cylindrical outflow tract. The anterior leaflet's long axis, which extends from its proximal attachment to the aortic annulus to its chordal attachments to the papillary muscles, undergoes considerably less bending than the posterior leaflet does during closure. As a result, it forms more of a wall than a floor when seen from inside the atrium during systole (see Fig. 5–3B).

The three scallops that make up the *posterior leaflet* occupy two thirds to three quarters of the mitral valve circumference.[3, 4] During systole, the leaflet inflates into a "croissant" shape (see Fig. 5–3B), engulfing and supporting the anterior leaflet with a broad appositional interface. When it is closed and viewed from an atrial aspect, the surface of the inflated posterior leaflet is at a shelf-like right angle to the atrial wall as it forms the atrial floor. The appositional surface with the anterior leaflet is at right angles to the atrial floor, and its concavity meets the convex atrial aspect of the latter. During diastole, the leaflet pivots on the annulus to a position parallel to the atrial wall and the direction of ventricular inflow (see Fig. 5–3A).

Understanding of the three-dimensional anatomy of the mitral valve is necessary for avoiding common pitfalls based on misinter-

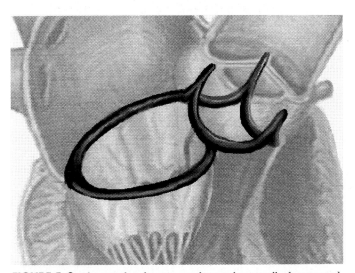

FIGURE 5–2. The mitral and aortic annuli are schematically diagrammed. The juxtaposition of the fibromuscular annuli of the mitral *(left)* and aortic *(right)* valves in the ostium of the left ventricle is demonstrated in a right posterior oblique (RPO) view.

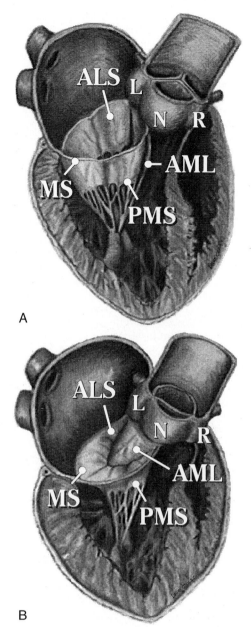

FIGURE 5–3. The mitral-aortic unit. *A*, Diastole. *B*, Systole. A right posterior oblique (RPO) view of the interior of the heart demonstrates the mitral and aortic valves in the ostium of the left ventricle. The posterior leaflet of the mitral valve consists of three cusps or scallops: middle scallop (MS), anterolateral scallop (ALS), and posteromedial scallop (PMS). The anterior mitral leaflet (AML) is contiguous with the left coronary (L) and noncoronary (N) sinuses of the aortic valve, forming the anterior wall of the inflow tract in *A* and the posterior wall of the outflow tract in *B*. R = right coronary sinus.

pretation of its angiographic or echocardiographic images. Levine and colleagues[5, 6] have stressed the need to appreciate the "saddle" shape (see Fig. 5–3B) of the mitral closure plane to avoid the mistaken diagnosis of "anterior leaflet prolapse" when the leaflet seemingly crosses the annular plane in apical echocardiographic views.

Another source of potential confusion is the "subaortic cone" (Fig. 5–4), which is often seen in left ventriculographic images of patients with left ventricular hypertrophy associated with aortic stenosis or hypertrophic cardiomyopathy.[7] This conical figuration is best seen in lateral and left anterior oblique projections and has its base at the aortic annulus and points located inferiorly and apically to that structure, giving the ventricular silhouette an hourglass

shape. The closed aortic valve confirms the diastolic timing of the image. The small and incompliant left ventricular cavity crowds the mitral valve, so as the anterior leaflet swings anteromedially in early diastole, its leading edge strikes the interventricular septum. This convergence of the anterior leaflet and septum forms the tip of the cone (see Fig. 5–4B). During angiography, the opacified blood pools in the vestibule below the aortic valve so that the submitral body and apex of the ventricle are separated by this narrow waist, giving an illusory appearance of "subaortic stenosis."

An accurate three-dimensional construct of the mitral valve can also dispel another area of potential confusion in the definition of

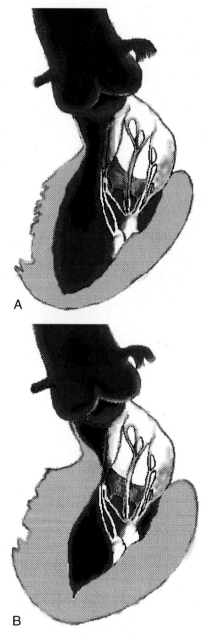

FIGURE 5–4. The left ventriculographic "cone." *A*, Normal left ventricle in diastole. *B*, Hypertrophic left ventricle in diastole. In the left anterior oblique (LAO) projection, unopacified blood (white) entering the opaque (black) left ventricle through the open mitral valve creates an hourglass figuration that may be misinterpreted as "outflow tract narrowing" if the diastolic timing of the ventriculographic image is not established by noting that the aortic valve is closed. In the hypertrophic left ventricle (*B*), the thick septum and widely open anterior leaflet meet, giving the impression that there is "tight stenosis" between the aortic vestibule above and the body of the ventricle below.

the boundaries of the left ventricular inflow tract. Because the mitral valve sleeve is invaginated within the cavity of the left ventricle (Fig. 5–5), left atrial pressures are recorded when a catheter lies within the sleeve. This atrial pressure zone is within the left ventricular silhouette in right anterior oblique and lateral projections and extends anteriorly (apically) to the aorta. When a catheter first emerges from the mitral valve and encounters pressure in the inflow tract of the left ventricle, it is midway into the left ventricular silhouette.

Angiographic depictions of the mitral valve can also lead to considerable confusion because the annular attachment of the an-terolateral scallop of the posterior leaflet projects anterior to the aortic valve in the right anterior oblique projection (Fig. 5–6; see also Fig. 5–5). If there is billowing or prolapse of this portion of the posterior leaflet (see Fig. 5–6), it bulges anterior to the aorta and is frequently thought to represent "anterior leaflet prolapse."

NORMAL VALVE FUNCTION

The efficiency of the heart as a pump is heavily dependent on the integrity of the cardiac valves. Cardiac valves ensure unimpeded

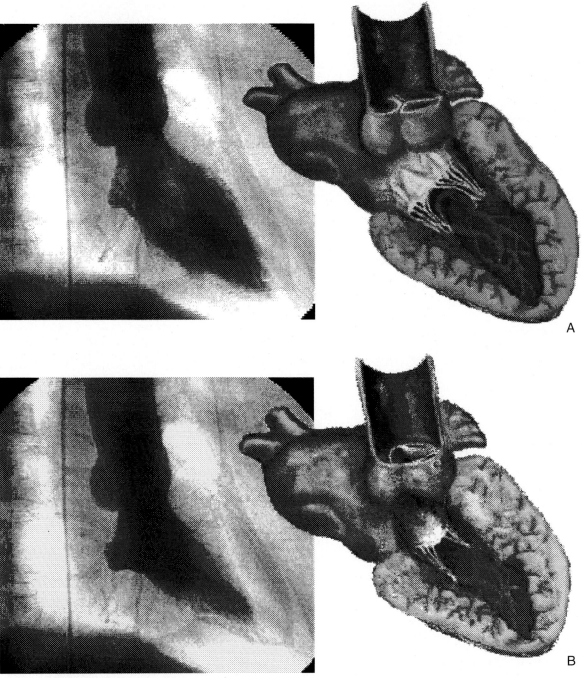

A

B

FIGURE 5–5. Normal left ventriculographic silhouette, right anterior oblique (RAO) projection. *A,* Diastole. *B,* Systole. Anatomical depictions of the left heart demonstrate the deep invagination of the mitral valve within the left ventricle in both diastole and systole. The chordae hold the leading edges of the mitral sleeve deep within the ventricle during systole, and flattening of the sleeve provides a concave posterior wall to the outflow tract below the aortic valve. These excursions of the anterior leaflet are not seen in an RAO radiographic projection but are well seen in orthogonal views (see Figs. 5–3 and 5–4), in which the anterior leaflet is a boundary-forming structure.

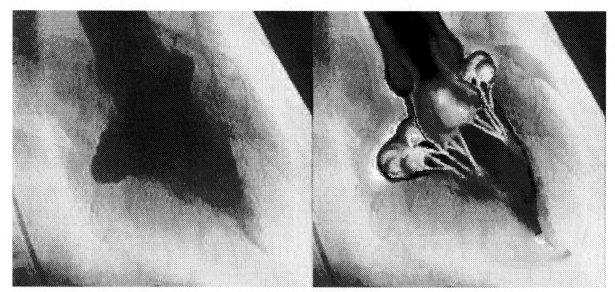

FIGURE 5–6. Systolic left ventriculographic silhouette in mitral prolapse, right anterior oblique (RAO) projection. Compared with Figure 5–5, the silhouette has projections both anterior and inferoposterior to the aortic valve. The anatomical depiction *(right)* demonstrates that the billowing posterior leaflet engulfs the concave anterior leaflet, forming both of the projections. The concavity of the anterior leaflet beneath the open aortic valve is also shown in the anatomical drawing, but this leaflet does not form a boundary in the ventriculogram.

anterograde flow when they are open and prevent retrograde flow when they are closed. Valvar dysfunction occurs when the valves fail to perform these functions as a result of intrinsic changes in the valve structure or extrinsic factors that impair performance.

Functional Anatomy (Integration of Pressure and Flow)

Valvar function is integrated in terms of pressure and flow relationships. In Figure 5–7, pressures in the chambers are denoted by the density of the shading in the individual drawings, the darkest shading representing pressures higher than 80 mm Hg. The figure is described in detail in the following paragraphs (the numerals in parentheses refer to numerals on the figure).

(1) *Rapid (passive) filling* follows opening of the mitral valve. The valve opens as the ventricular pressure achieves its nadir and the left atrial pressure is momentarily higher. Approximately 75 percent of the diastolic inflow volume *(large white arrow)*, which will contribute to the ventricular stroke volume, enters the ventricle passively at this time. The initiation of mitral valve opening actually begins while the left ventricular pressure is greatly in excess of atrial pressure, because active deformation of the isovolumically relaxing ventricle exerts a pull on apposed leaflets and anterograde flow begins within the valve sleeve. This initiation of intravalvar anterograde flow from atrium to valve causes a decline in atrial pressure, the *y descent,* which precedes and continues through valve opening and ends at the time of diastatic pressure equilibration.

The peak of the atrial *v wave* and the initiation of the *y descent* precede the left ventricular–left atrial pressure crossover because of the preopening increase in left atrial compliance that results from displacement of atrial volume into the valve sleeve, which invaginates into the ventricular inflow region (see Fig. 5–5) before the valve opens. Failure to appreciate this preopening decline in atrial pressure leads to overestimation of the mitral valve gradient if the determinations are made with the use of pulmonary capillary wedge pressures (as surrogate left atrial pressures) that are time-adjusted so that the *v wave* peak coincides with the left ventricular pressure crossover.

This initial *intravalvar* flow is depicted on the bimodal mitral flow profile (see Fig. 5–7) as a slow-rising deflection that occurs before the ventriculoatrial pressure crossover. After pressure crossover, the flow accelerates, and a small pressure gradient is depicted during peak inflow.

The ventricular pressure exhibits a *rapid filling wave,* beginning at the nadir and rising asymptotically toward a plateau as the rate of inflow declines.

(2) *Diastasis* occurs when the pressures in the atrium and ventricle equilibrate and inflow is reduced as the valve leaflets float toward apposition. Eddy currents on the ventricular surface of the valve leaflets and the declining inflow contribute to this partial closure. This mid-diastolic decline in left ventricular inflow is seen between the two peaks of the mitral valve flow signal (see Fig. 5–7).

(3) *Atrial systole* forcibly adds about 20 percent of the diastolic inflow volume shown on the mitral valve flow signal and is accompanied by a small pressure gradient between the atrium and ventricle. The *a wave* in the atrium results from atrial systolic contraction, and the impact of this inflow bolus causes a comparable or greater presystolic rise in left ventricular pressure. This ventricular *a wave* often exceeds that in the atrium because of elastic recoil, especially in hypertrophic ventricles. Active transport is followed by a wake and a reversal of the pressure gradient, which together initiate mitral valve closure.

Contraction of the mitral annulus[8–10] begins with atrial systole. The circumference progressively decreases throughout atrial and ventricular systole, until at peak systole it is about 75 percent of its relaxed dimension. Approximately two thirds of this annular constriction occurs during atrial systole, and the remainder occurs during the first half of ventricular systole. Muscle tissue within the valve leaflets also contracts during atrial systole, and this fiber shortening may contribute to atriogenic mitral valve closure. If atrial systole is dissociated from ventricular systole by atrioventricular block, the mitral valve may close completely as a consequence of these events associated with atrial contraction.[11]

(4) *Mitral valve closure,* which was initiated by the wake trailing the atrial systolic flow bolus *(tapered arrow),* is completed by contraction of the papillary muscles, the systolic rise in ventricular pressure, and the exceeding of pressure in the atrium by that in the left ventricle. The atrial *c wave* results from tensing of the mitral valve leaflets in response to their inflation by the ventricle. It is the pressure analog of mitral valve closure and the first heart sound. The black arrows in the drawing denote the abrupt

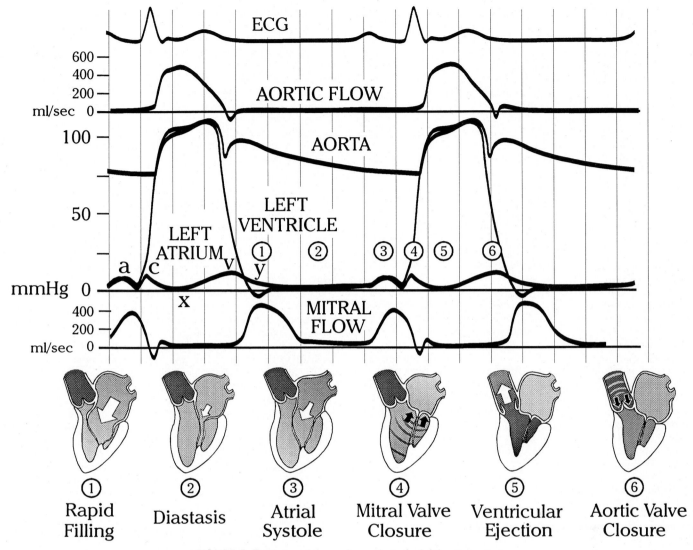

FIGURE 5–7. Phases of the cardiac cycle in the left heart. See text.

deceleration of the surge of blood propelled toward the left atrium as it impacts on the apposed and tensing mitral leaflets; this results in a "shock wave" that transmits the first heart sound toward the ventricular apex.

(5) *Ventricular ejection (white arrow)* ensues after the intracavitary pressure exceeds the aortic diastolic pressure, opening the aortic valve and propelling a column of blood anterograde into the aorta. A small pressure difference (impulse gradient) between the left ventricle and the aorta[11] is present during the period of most rapid outflow, shown on the aortic flow signal (see Fig. 5–7).

The initial systolic decline in atrial pressure, called the *x descent,* is followed by the *v wave,* which results from progressive filling of the atrium. Because the atria have no outlet and therefore serve as reservoirs during systole, the *v wave* increases in magnitude until the ventricle begins to relax in protodiastole, allowing blood to enter the mitral valve sleeve before mitral valve inflow into the ventricle.

As the ventricular outflow rate begins to decline in midsystole, a retrograde aortic pressure wave from the reflecting sites in the periphery, the *tidal wave,* reaches the aortic root, adding to the late systolic pressure magnitude and causing a reversal of the gradient between the left ventricle and the aorta. The momentum of the column of ejected blood permits anterograde flow to continue despite this reversal in gradient.[12] This momentum is lost after ventricular systolic contraction ceases and pressure in the left ventricle begins to decline.

(6) *Aortic valve closure* occurs as pressure in the left ventricle falls precipitously below aortic pressure, resulting in momentary flow reversal in the aortic root, as depicted in the aortic flow signal (see Fig. 5–7). The black arrows above the aortic valve cusps in the drawing represent the abrupt impact of the retrograde surge of blood on the tensed aortic valve leaflets. The shock wave that causes the aortic valve closure sound advances in an anterograde fashion. The brief "hangout" period[13, 14] between the abrupt protodiastolic pressure decline in the left ventricle and the dicrotic notch represents aortic valve closure in the aortic pressure pulse. The duration of this hangout is related to the compliance of the vascular bed; it is longer in the right heart, especially during inspiration, because of the compliance of the pulmonary vascular bed. Consequently, the pulmonic valve closes later than the aortic valve during inspiration,[13] because forward momentum in the pulmonary artery persists longer after the protodiastolic decline in right ventricular pressure.

Atrial Pressure Waves

Some additional comments about atrial waveforms are in order at this point. The atrial pressure may reflect the ventricle's rapid filling wave; if present, this atrial wave is termed the *h wave.*[15] It is a positive deflection in the atrium that results from the rebound of an exaggerated ventricular rapid filling wave on the upstream atrium, and it is often seen in the jugular and atrial pulse in cases of acute valvar regurgitation (Fig. 5–8) or constrictive pericarditis.

Early investigators[15] divided the *x descent* into *x* (presystolic) and *x'* (systolic) components, but this archaic terminology is rarely used today. Three mechanical events contribute to the systolic *x descent*: atrial relaxation, the descent of the cardiac base, and the systolic reduction of the cardiac volume contained within the pericardial sac. As blood is ejected from the ventricles, the intrapericardial pressure becomes subatmospheric because the girdle-like restraint of the pericardial sac on the cardiac chambers is relieved by their volume loss. Because the atria are relaxed, this negative pressure is exerted on the atrial walls and contributes to the *x descent* and to atrial filling.

The atrial *v wave* is a reflection of the left atrial volume, the rate of inflow during systole, and the left atrial compliance. Both atria progressively increase in volume during ventricular systole from venous inflow, and if atrioventricular valvar regurgitation is present, the rate and volume of filling are increased. The magnitude of the *v wave* is positively related to the volume of systolic filling and negatively related to the compliance of the chamber. A highly compliant chamber can accept a massive volume of mitral regurgitation without producing a large *v wave*, whereas a normally compliant atrium may produce a large *v wave* with a normal volume of venous inflow if its diastolic emptying is impaired by atrioventricular valvar stenosis or reduced compliance of the downstream ventricle.

The *y descent* reflects the relief of atrial pressure that accompanies isovolumic relaxation of the ventricle, mitral valve opening, and atrial outflow during the rapid filling period of the ventricle. The first derivative (negative dP/dt) of this decline is increased if the magnitude of the *v wave* or the rate of outflow is increased, as in mitral regurgitation (see Fig. 5–8). Conversely, the slope of the *y descent* is reduced by impaired atrial outflow, which is the case in mitral stenosis and hypertrophic cardiomyopathy.

Transvalvar Flow Rate

Valvar flow rates may be estimated by dividing the cardiac output by the period of time during which the valve is open[16]:

$$\text{Mitral Valve Flow in mL/sec} = \frac{\text{Cardiac Output in mL/min}}{\text{Diastolic Filling Time in sec/min}}$$

$$\text{Aortic Valve Flow in mL/sec} = \frac{\text{Cardiac Output in mL/min}}{\text{Systolic Ejection Time in sec/min}}$$

These formulas acknowledge the fact that the cardiac output can traverse the mitral valve (or tricuspid valve) only when it is open in diastole, and the aortic valve (or pulmonic valve) only in systole. The mean flow rate across the mitral valve may increase to more than 500 mL per second during exercise, when the cardiac output

increases and the available diastolic time decreases. These formulas do not take into account the effect of valvar regurgitation, which increases the flow rate across the valve by the addition of the regurgitant volume to the net forward flow. Severe mitral or aortic regurgitation can result in a threefold or fourfold increase in anterograde flow across the regurgitant valve.

An unrestricted valve can accommodate these flows without significant hemodynamic impact, but a stenotic valve requires a higher driving pressure as the flow rate increases. For example, tachycardia is poorly tolerated in mitral stenosis because the left atrial–left ventricular pressure gradient must quadruple in order to double the flow rate.

DYSFUNCTION OF NORMAL CARDIAC VALVES

Abnormal valve function can result from functional as well as structural alterations. Functional abnormalities of valve function can occur if anatomically normal valves are subjected to elevated pressures or to distorted chamber anatomy caused by either underfilling or overfilling of the affected ventricle.

The integrity of the mitral valve depends on the intricate coordination of its component parts and the geometry of its surrounding structures.[17] The mitral apparatus consists of leaflets, annulus, chordae, papillary muscles, and the ventricular walls supporting the papillary muscles. Ischemic dysfunction of the papillary muscles can lead to dramatic "Jekyll and Hyde" conversion of a normal mitral valve into a grossly incompetent valve,[18] and the resultant sudden volume overload on an ischemic ventricle can be life threatening (see Fig. 5–8).

The mitral apparatus can be "crowded" in a ventricle with concentric or asymmetric ingrowth hypertrophy and a resultant small chamber volume. The valve in this setting may be functionally stenotic or functionally incompetent, or both. If this type of ventriculovalvar disproportion leads to mitral incompetence, perturbations that increase the ventricular volume may improve valve competence. On the other hand, a greatly bloated ventricle, as in dilated cardiomyopathy[19] or severe aortic regurgitation, usually causes mitral regurgitation that improves with reductions in ventricular size. Diastolic mitral incompetence is also commonly seen with greatly dilated ventricles.

Pressure overload conditions affecting the left ventricle, such as aortic stenosis and systemic hypertension, can also cause mitral regurgitation, and the combined pressure and volume overload of renal failure can cause both mitral and aortic regurgitation.

Ventricular arrhythmias disrupt the sequence of contraction in the ventricles and often cause functional mitral and tricuspid regurgitation. Angiographic and echocardiographic observations during cardiopulmonary resuscitation demonstrate incompetence of the tricuspid valve and anterograde flow through the mitral valve during chest compression and incompetence of the aortic valve during relaxation between compressions.[20, 21]

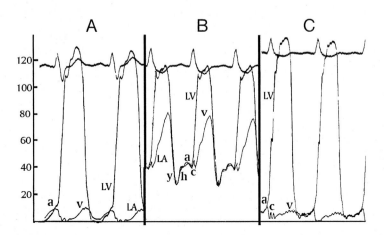

FIGURE 5–8. Left heart pressures in acute, intermittent mitral regurgitation ("Jekyll-Hyde syndrome"). *A,* Left ventricular (LV) and left atrial (LA) pressures are normal. *B,* Several minutes later, the patient complained of chest discomfort and went into acute pulmonary edema. The systolic pressure in the ventricle decreased, the *v wave* magnitude increased tenfold, and the left ventricular diastolic pressure rose from 8 to 40 mm Hg. An *h wave*, reflecting the ventricle's rapid filling wave, is seen before the *a wave*. *C,* After administration of isosorbide dinitrate, the patient's symptoms abated and the pressures returned to normal.

SURROGATE VALVAR FUNCTION

Venous valves can serve as surrogate or backup cardiac valves in the setting of pulsatile rapid increases in right atrial pressure,[20, 22] as may occur during cardiopulmonary resuscitation, coughing, and severe tricuspid regurgitation. These valves are prominent in the jugular and axillary veins and have been demonstrated to close competently when precipitous pressure fluctuations are imposed on the thorax or right atrium. They prevent these pressures from impacting on the capillary beds.

CONCLUDING REMARKS

Hemodynamic investigations and cardiovascular imaging modalities that have been developed in the last half of the 20th century have greatly enhanced the understanding of the functional anatomy of the cardiac chambers and valves. There has been a progressive improvement in the clarity of the images and, at the same time, a steady evolution toward noninvasive technology. The use of invasive diagnostic studies, even those that are seemingly indispensable at the current time, is certain to yield to procedures with lower risk and even greater diagnostic accuracy in the future.

However, the full potential of the technologies detailed here will be achieved only if those responsible for their interpretation have a thorough understanding of the integrated anatomical and hemodynamic alterations that result from cardiac disease. Structure and function are inextricably linked and equally important. It was the purpose of this chapter to provide a framework for appreciation of this linkage.

Acknowledgment

The author gratefully acknowledges the preparation of the illustrations in this chapter by David Criley.

References

1. Walmsley, R., and Watson, H.: The outflow tract of the left ventricle. Br. Heart J. 28:435, 1966.
2. McAlpine, W.A.: Heart and Coronary Arteries. New York, Springer-Verlag, 1975.
3. Ranganathan, N., Lam, J.H.C., Wigle, E.D., et al.: Morphology of the human mitral valve: II. The valve leaflets. Circulation 41:459, 1970.
4. du Plessis, L.A., and Marchand, P.: The anatomy of the mitral valve and its associated structures. Thorax 19:221, 1964.
5. Levine, R.A., Triuzli, M.O., Harrigan, P., et al.: The relationship of mitral annular shape to the diagnosis of mitral valve prolapse. Circulation 75:756, 1987.
6. Levine, R.A.: Mitral valve prolapse: Clinical impact of new diagnostic criteria and insights from three-dimensional echocardiography. J. Cardiol. 24(Suppl. 38):3, 1994.
7. Criley, J.M., Lewis, K.B., White, R.I., Jr., et al.: Pressure gradients without obstruction: A new concept of "hypertrophic subaortic stenosis." Circulation 32:881, 1965.
8. Tsakiris, A.G., von Bernuth, G., Rastelli, G.C., et al.: Size and motion of the mitral valve annulus in anesthetized intact dogs. J. Appl. Physiol. 30:611, 1971.
9. Ormiston, J.A., Shah, P.M., Tei, C., et al.: Size and motion of the mitral annulus in man: I. A two-dimensional echocardiographic method and findings in normal subjects. Circulation 64:113, 1981.
10. Ormiston, J.A., Shah, P.M., Tei, C., et al.: Size and motion of the mitral annulus in man: II. Abnormalities in mitral valve prolapse. Circulation 65:713, 1982.
11. Zaky, A., Steinmetz, E., and Feigenbaum, H.: Role of atrium in closure of mitral valve in man. Am. J. Physiol. 217:1652, 1969.
12. Murgo, J.P., Altobelli, S.A., Dorethy, J.F., et al.: Normal Ventricular Ejection Dynamics in Man during Rest and Exercise. Dallas, TX, American Heart Association Monograph 46:92, 1975.
13. Shaver, J.A., Nadolny, R.A., O'Toole, J.D., et al.: Pressure correlates of the second heart sound: An intracardiac sound study. Circulation 49:316, 1974.
14. Curtiss, E.I., Matthews, R.G., and Shaver, J.A.: Mechanism of normal splitting of the second heart sound. Circulation 51:157, 1975.
15. Lewis, T.: The Mechanism and Registration of the Heart Beat. London, Shaw & Sons, 1925.
16. Gorlin, R., and Gorlin, G.: Hydraulic formula for calculation of area of stenotic mitral valve, other cardiac valves and central circulatory shunts. Am. Heart J. 41:1, 1951.
17. Perloff, J.P., and Roberts, W.C.: The mitral apparatus: Functional anatomy of mitral regurgitation. Circulation 46:227, 1972.
18. Brody, W., and Criley, J.M.: Intermittent severe mitral regurgitation: Hemodynamic studies in a patient with recurrent left-sided heart failure. N. Engl. J. Med. 283:673, 1970.
19. Boltwood, C.M., Tei, C., Wong M., et al.: Quantitative echocardiography of the mitral complex in dilated cardiomyopathy: The mechanism of functional mitral regurgitation. Circulation 68:498, 1983.
20. Niemann, J.T., Rosborough, J.P., Hausknecht, M., et al.: Pressure synchronized cineangiography during experimental cardiopulmonary resuscitation. Circulation 64:985, 1981.
21. Werner, J.A., Greene, H.L., Janko, C.L., et al.: Visualization of cardiac valve motion in man during external chest compression using two-dimensional echocardiography: Implications regarding the mechanisms of flow. Circulation 63:1417, 1981.
22. Fisher, J., Vaghaiwalla, F., Tsitlik, J., et al.: Determinants and clinical significance of jugular venous valve competence. Circulation 65:188, 1982.

6 Quantitative Methods in Cardiac Imaging: An Introduction to Digital Image Processing

Steven R. Fleagle, B.S.E.E.
David J. Skorton, M.D.

ASSESSMENT OF ANATOMY AND
    FUNCTION _____ 58
General Considerations _____ 58
3-D Reconstruction of the Heart _____ 59
DIGITAL IMAGE PROCESSING: A PRIMER _____ 60

Digital Images and Their Characteristics _____ 60
Image Enhancement _____ 63
Segmentation _____ 69
Future Directions of Quantitative Image
    Processing _____ 70

Modern cardiac imaging encompasses an extremely broad variety of methods in which several energy forms are used to create diagnostically useful pictures of the cardiovascular system. At least two similarities are shared by all methods. First, modern modalities are based to a large and increasing degree on digital computer processing technology for creation, display, storage, and analysis of image data.[1, 2] Second, increasing use is being made of image quantitation in the clinical practice of cardiac imaging. For example, the subjective, visual assessment of coronary arterial narrowing caused by atherosclerosis may now be complemented by computer-based quantitative coronary arteriographic techniques that permit reproducible, precise delineation of minimal coronary lumen area and other important parameters of stenosis severity.[3, 4] The quantitative approaches have been found to be particularly important in assessing subtle changes in coronary atherosclerosis on serial studies.[5] Similarly, computer-based quantitation of the results of myocardial perfusion scintigraphy, including planar and single-photon emission computed tomograms, has been demonstrated.[6, 7] Many other examples may be considered as evidence of the trend toward image quantitation and its growing importance in cardiac diagnosis, prognostication, and treatment planning.

The orientation toward quantitation in imaging is a result of at least two evolutionary factors. First, the clinician caring for the patient with heart disease is becoming increasingly sophisticated in the assessment of cardiovascular physiology. For example, investigators and clinicians are demanding quantitative capabilities in the assessment of ventricular function and myocardial perfusion. Second, the increasing capabilities and decreasing costs of digital computing systems have permitted sophisticated computational devices to be integrated into modern imaging systems. From relatively simple measures, such as determinations of left ventricular ejection fraction, to more complex assessment of regional myocardial glucose uptake by positron emission tomography (PET) scanning, most modern imaging systems contain sufficient computing power for many forms of quantitative analysis. In addition, off-line computer systems can be used to supplement the capability of the main imaging system (e.g., in radionuclide scanning) or as an added capability offered by the original equipment vendor or other manufacturers (e.g., of echocardiography and coronary angiography equipment). These two factors—the need for quantitation and the capability for quantitation—are combining to make cardiovascular imaging an increasingly quantitative science.

This chapter presents some of the principles common to quantitation of cardiac images based on digital image processing methods. It begins with a brief review of an example of the evolution of quantitation in imaging: assessment of left ventricular anatomy throughout the heart cycle. This example demonstrates the progression from qualitative estimates of ventricular size and shape to a precise, dynamic three-dimensional representation of ventricular morphology. These advances in the assessment of ventricular anatomy and function are based in part on progress in the science of digital image processing, and the major portion of this chapter consists of a brief primer on that subject. Because the orientation of this book is toward the clinician, detailed and mathematically rigorous descriptions of image processing techniques are not within its scope. However, we hope to introduce the reader to enough of the basic concepts of image processing that new ideas and their implementation in clinical practice may be viewed in their proper perspective. This chapter presents general principles of digital processing; detailed descriptions of specific quantitative analyses are presented in the chapters dealing with particular imaging techniques.

QUANTITATION IN CARDIAC IMAGING: ASSESSMENT OF ANATOMY AND FUNCTION

General Considerations

Cardiac anatomy and function are assessed by ascertaining the size and shape of the cardiac chambers throughout the heart cycle. Although quantitative analysis of all four cardiac chambers is of physiologic and diagnostic importance, the majority of investigative and clinical work has pertained to evaluation of the size, shape, and function of the left ventricle because of its predominant role in many cardiac disorders. Early methods of assessing left ventricular anatomy and function were based on the assumption of an idealized geometric model, commonly a prolate ellipsoid,[8] to represent the shape of this chamber. Area-length angiographic methods and some echocardiographic and radionuclide techniques depend on this assumed prolate ellipsoid geometry to assess left ventricular volume, mass, and ejection fraction. However, the normal shape of the left ventricle does not precisely match that of a prolate ellipsoid. The match is even worse in disease, especially in ischemic disorders, in which wide local variations in shape occur. In these cases, methods of quantitation not based on the assumption of a limited geometric model are more generally applicable.

Since the advent of tomographic or "slice-like" imaging methods, various approaches have been used employing an approximation technique based on Simpson's rule to delineate left ventricular volume and mass throughout the heart cycle. In the current context, the term "Simpson's rule" is used to refer to the summation of the volumes of several tomographic slices through a part of the heart, such as the left ventricle, to obtain a total volume for the left ventricular cavity and total myocardial mass. The ideal approximation requires many mutually parallel slices through the left ventricle; the volume encompassed by the endocardium and epicardium in each slice, multiplied by the distance between slices, yields an estimate of left ventricular cavity and muscle volume; multiplication of the myocardial volume by the specific gravity of muscle (usually taken to be 1.05) yields left ventricular mass. Simpson's rule–based approximations of left ventricular volume or mass from echocardiographic,[9] computed tomographic (CT),[10] or magnetic resonance image (MRI)[11] data have supplied accurate and precise delineations of these variables.

Three important requirements form the basis for approximations of left ventricular volume and mass using Simpson's rule. First, endocardial and epicardial contours must be accurately identified in each tomographic slice. Second, the location of the imaging plane and of the patient during all slice acquisitions must be known precisely. Third, for techniques in which the slices are not all obtained within a single cardiac cycle (including echocardiography, CT, and MRI), stability of the cardiac cycle length and hemodynamics is required, because the calculated volume and mass will be "average" values across the several cardiac cycles required for image data acquisition. Similarly, nonideal electrocardiographic gating (triggering of the image acquisition process based on the electrocardiogram) may contribute to variability.

Three-Dimensional Reconstruction of the Heart

Complete evaluation of cardiac anatomy and function requires appreciation of not only cardiac size but cardiac shape throughout the heart cycle. The shape of the heart is complex and, as mentioned, does not precisely fit any simple geometric model. This is particularly true for the right ventricle and the atria. In the evaluation of cardiac shape, clinicians often use information from several individual images to conceptualize the three-dimensional shape of the portion of the heart under study. Because this conceptualization may be difficult even for the experienced observer, particularly in disorders of complex morphology, such as congenital heart disease, there has been growing interest in three-dimensional modeling of the cardiovascular system.[12] Reconstruction techniques originally developed for industrial and engineering applications, especially computer-aided design and manufacturing,[13] permit visualization of an object without the need for a physical model.

Three-dimensional image processing methods applied to biomedical images have already shown utility in planning of maxillofacial surgery[14] and in imaging of the spine and other bony structures.[15] Cardiovascular applications of three-dimensional reconstruction techniques are relatively recent but appear capable of providing accurate calculations of chamber volume[16] and mass as well as analysis of regional stress-strain characteristics of the heart. For example, three-dimensional reconstruction of the left ventricle, combined with high-fidelity intracavitary pressure measurements, may be used to evaluate regional stress-strain characteristics of the normal left ventricle and alteration of these characteristics in the setting of acute ischemia.[17] The great potential of sophisticated three-dimensional reconstruction techniques is just beginning to be appreciated in cardiovascular imaging.

Several basic steps must be followed for three-dimensional cardiac reconstruction from multiple tomographic images (Table 6–1).[18–20] Individual images must be acquired, along with information

TABLE 6–1. STEPS IN THREE-DIMENSIONAL CARDIAC RECONSTRUCTION AND ANALYSIS FROM MULTIPLE TOMOGRAPHIC IMAGES

Acquisition of several tomographic images encompassing the entire structure of interest
Registration of spatial position and orientation of each image
Identification and digitization of important image contours (e.g., endocardium)
Reconstruction of individual digitized image contours into a three-dimensional data structure
Display of three-dimensional reconstruction
Extraction of quantitative data

about the position and orientation of each image relative to other images or to a common reference system. This process of acquiring information on the relative orientation and position of various images is referred to as "spatial registration." The important structural contours in each image then must be identified, and their locations must be entered into the computer system. After the contours in each image have been spatially registered, they may be reconstructed into a three-dimensional data structure. Data "missing" between actual image slices must be interpolated, usually by use of polynomial curves or other similar procedures.

Display of the three-dimensional reconstructions has followed two basic approaches: wire-frame displays and shaded-surface displays. Wire-frame displays depict the important image contours along with lines interpolated between individual image slices (Fig. 6–1A). Calculations of volume, mass, and ejection fraction and stress-strain analysis may be expedited by the use of wire-frame structures. For structures of relatively simple shape, such as the left ventricle, wire-frame displays allow the form to be represented with an amount of data small enough to be easily manipulated. On the other hand, the multiplicity of lines in a wire-frame model of

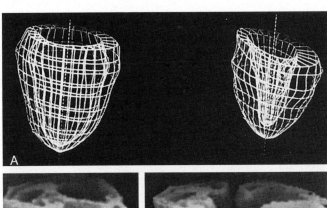

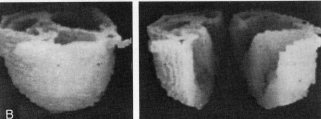

FIGURE 6–1. Three-dimensional reconstructions of the heart based on noninvasive imaging methods. *A*, Wire-frame display of reconstruction of the left ventricle from ultrafast computed tomographic (CT) images. At the left is an end-diastolic reconstruction, and at the right is an end-systolic reconstruction. *B*, Shaded-surface display of reconstruction produced from CT data. At the left is a reconstruction of the entire heart, and at the right the three-dimensional data structure has been "sectioned" mathematically, revealing details of internal anatomy. (*A*, From Collins, S.M., Chandran, K.B., and Skorton, D.J.: Three-dimensional cardiac imaging. Echocardiography 5:311, 1988, with permission; *B*, from Herman, G.T., and Liu, H.K.: Display of three-dimensional information in computed tomography. J. Comput. Assist. Tomogr. 1:155, 1977, with permission.)

a complex structure makes the display visually less appealing than a solid, shaded-surface display.

The shaded-surface reconstruction produces a display that appears to be a solid object, with shading effects calculated by the computer program (see Fig. 6–1B).[21] Qualitative visual evaluation of these structures is easier than that of wire-frame displays because the shaded-surface displays more closely resemble actual anatomical structures. However, these displays involve manipulation and storage of substantially more data than the wire-frame displays.

After the three-dimensional reconstruction information is available for a complete heart cycle (or for selected portions of the cycle), these images may be combined sequentially to produce cine loop animated displays of cardiac motion that closely resemble the actual cardiac appearance.

Three-dimensional reconstruction techniques have been applied to echocardiographic,[17, 19, 22–25] angiographic,[26, 27] CT,[21, 28, 29] radionuclide,[30] and MRI image data.[31, 32] Static cardiac geometry (e.g., left ventricular mass), left ventricular function, and complex stress-strain characteristics of the heart have all been assessed by use of three-dimensional reconstruction techniques. The continuing improvements in digital display and reconstruction technology and the increasing emphasis on digital picture archiving and communications systems (PACS) in departments of radiology will probably lead to increased use of cardiac three-dimensional reconstructions.

Newer imaging methods, coupled with the trend toward quantitation in cardiac imaging, are improving the assessment of left ventricular function. Part of the improved capability of modern imaging modalities must be credited to advances in the physics and engineering of energy sources and sensors used to produce images, demonstrated so dramatically in the development of PET scanning, fast CT, and MRI. Much of the progress must also be credited to the ingenious use of digital computational techniques—methods that permit rapid image reconstruction, flexible display, and unique data analysis. The following section provides an overview of the science that is so integral to modern imaging—digital image processing.

DIGITAL IMAGE PROCESSING: A PRIMER

Digital image processing is a type of computerized data processing in which an image is stored in a numerical format that can easily be manipulated and analyzed by a computer. With the use of the computational abilities of modern computers, quantitative analyses that were formerly almost impossible are now routine.

Computers have been used to analyze digital images for many years. Much of the early work in digital image processing was done at the Jet Propulsion Laboratory,[33] with the goal of maximizing the information extractable from images transmitted from exploration spacecraft. Since this work was begun in the early 1960s, many advances in the science of digital image processing have occurred, primarily owing to the decreased cost and increased availability of the imaging equipment needed by researchers. Medical image processing has benefited tremendously from nonbiological applications of image processing and, as one of the major applications, has also served to advance the general science of digital image processing.

Digital image processing has many important advantages over other techniques such as optical or analog image processing. These advantages include ease of implementation of new algorithms, relative immunity to noise generated during the application, and an abundance of available techniques. In contrast, the nondigital techniques are sometimes faster (most optical and analog operations are performed at video frame rates) and are occasionally more desirable in special, dedicated applications.[34]

Digital Images and Their Characteristics

Because computers work with numerical data, images must be represented in numerical form to permit computer manipulation and analysis. The process of transforming an image into numerical form is called digitization or analog-to-digital conversion. Many methods can be used to digitize images, largely because of the many diverse sources of images. For instance, the method of choice for digitization of echocardiographic images stored on videotape is not applicable to images stored on radiographic films. Images from videotape are available as an analog video signal (a time-varying voltage) when the tape is played; the voltage of the video signal at a particular point in time corresponds directly to the brightness of a portion of the image at that time. The film, however, contains a static, two-dimensional distribution (pattern) of film densities. In each case, the signal (voltage or density) at a particular portion of the image represents the feature of interest (e.g., backscattered ultrasound amplitude or x-ray exposure).

It is common for an image to be converted from its natural state of energy into a voltage by use of an appropriate transducer. A videocamera is an example of a transducer that converts energy in the form of light into a voltage signal that varies in proportion to the amount of light received. The videocamera accomplishes this in much the same way as a person reads text from a printed page: it scans across the image, line by line, and converts the brightness at each point in the line into a voltage. The most common method of scanning is from upper left to lower right, traversing in almost horizontal rows from top to bottom. The scanning process is rapid, usually being completed in less than 30 msec. The resulting voltage signal, in turn, must be converted into a signal that can be processed by a computer.

Conversion of the voltage signals that represent an image into digital form involves two steps: *sampling* (dividing the image into small areas) and *quantizing* (converting the intensity of each small area into a number). In the case of the video signal that results from scanning with the videocamera, the image is divided into small areas by measurement of the voltage at frequent time intervals as the scanning proceeds. Each interval is related to a particular region of the image. This process of digitization results in a digital image composed of an ordered array of *pixels* (picture elements). With each pixel is associated a gray level, which describes the intensity of that region, and a unique location. Figure 6–2 shows some of the steps taken during digitization of an image. In cases in which the location is described by three dimensions, the elements of the array are termed *voxels* (volume elements). For example, if the pixel dimensions in a CT image are 2×2 mm and the image "slice" thickness is 3 mm, each voxel represents a rectangular volume element of $2 \times 2 \times 3$ mm.

The term *resolution* is often used in relation to the characteristics of digital images. Spatial resolution, which is most commonly used, refers to how much structural detail can be represented in the image. The higher the spatial resolution, the finer the detail, or the closer together two objects can be and still be resolved as separate objects. Temporal resolution is determined by the number of images per unit time and defines how well a series of images can represent changes that occur over time. Imaging techniques with higher temporal resolution are able to represent events that occur more rapidly. Contrast resolution describes how well an image can differentiate among various intensity attributes, such as displaying differing tissues as separate shades (levels) of gray.

The number of pixels into which an image is divided (the matrix size), the size of each pixel (the spatial resolution), and the number and range of intensity levels each pixel can represent have important effects on the characteristics of digital images. The matrix size and spatial resolution are interrelated and sometimes confused. The matrix size is simply the number of pixels used to represent an image. If the region to be digitized, or the "field of view," is held constant, the matrix size and spatial resolution are directly related, as shown in Figure 6–3. Adding more pixels by making the matrix larger requires each pixel to be smaller in order to maintain the same field of view; as each pixel becomes smaller, the spatial resolution increases. Conversely, if the matrix size is decreased, each pixel must be larger in order to maintain the field of view, and the spatial resolution decreases. If the field of view is increased,

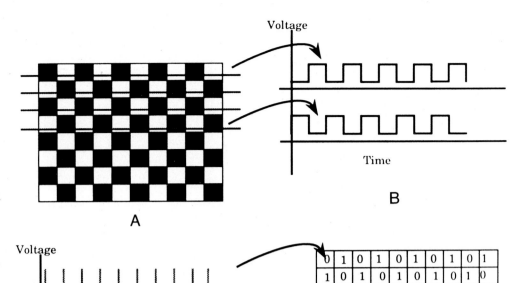

FIGURE 6–2. The concept of image digitization as implemented with a video camera. *A,* An "image" representing a checkerboard pattern. The horizontal lines drawn through the first four rows of the image indicate scan lines for a video camera. *B,* The resulting voltage signals from two of the scan lines. *C,* The voltage signals are sampled at points in time indicated by the vertical lines. *D,* The value of the voltage at each of these times is quantized (in this case as 0 or 1) and stored as a rectangular grid of numbers.

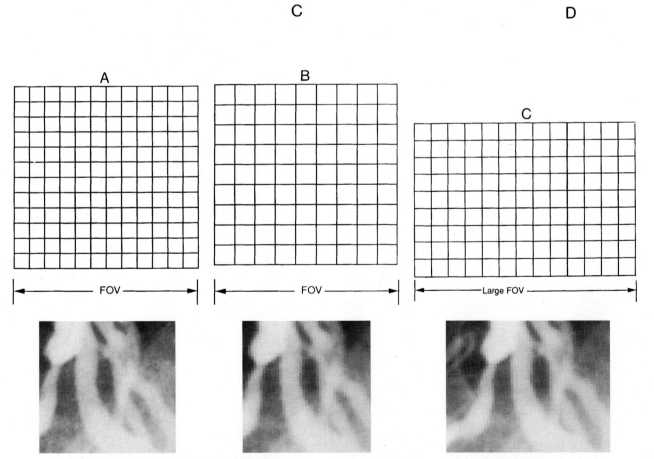

FIGURE 6–3. Relation between matrix size and spatial resolution. Each panel shows a schematic image matrix *(above)* and an example image *(below).* If the images in *A* are considered to have the standard spatial resolution and matrix size, then those in *B* have a lower spatial resolution because they have the same field of view (FOV) but a smaller matrix size. The images in panel *C,* on the other hand, have the same matrix size but a lower spatial resolution than *A* because the field of view has increased. Note that *B* and *C* have the same spatial resolution even though they have different matrix sizes and different fields of view.

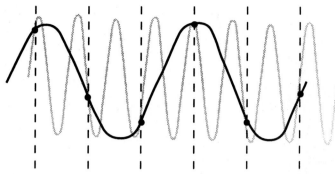

FIGURE 6–4. Effect of undersampling during the process of digitization. A time-varying voltage signal is represented as a sinusoidal wave pattern (*gray line*). The vertical, dashed lines indicate times at which the voltage values are sampled in the digitization process. The intersections of the vertical lines and the original sinusoid, indicated here by dots, are the voltage values measured at these times. The darker line through the dots indicates a signal that could be fit through the sampled points. This sampled signal differs from the original sinusoidal signal because the original signal was sampled at too low a frequency (not enough samples per unit time). The distortion of the original signal because of undersampling is often referred to as aliasing.

however, the matrix size can increase while spatial resolution stays the same (see Fig. 6–3). Thus, matrix sizes between different imaging devices must be carefully compared to ascertain the relation between matrix size and actual spatial resolution.

The lower the spatial resolution of a digital image, the poorer the approximation to the original data. Sufficient spatial resolution is determined by use of the Nyquist sampling theorem,[35, 36] which states that to preserve all information found in the original image, the image must be sampled spatially at a minimum of twice the highest *spatial frequency* found in the original image. Spatial frequency is defined as the number of gray level fluctuations over a given region of the image; high spatial frequencies are found at points in the image at which there are rapid gray level transitions, such as object borders. The "sharper" the border, the higher the spatial frequency. An image that contains high spatial frequencies needs high spatial resolution to represent it. *Undersampling* (i.e., use of a sampling rate that is less than twice the highest spatial

frequency) results not only in loss of some information but also in the introduction of image artifacts known as aliasing errors.[37] Aliasing errors occur when a signal is undersampled and information is lost. As shown in Figure 6–4, the sampled points seem to form a signal of lower frequency than that of the original data. In images, these artifacts of lower frequency may appear in the form of moiré patterns. An example of such a pattern is shown in Figure 6–5. Any aliasing errors introduced by undersampling are permanent, so care should be taken to avoid undersampling the image data. It can be difficult to determine the proper sampling frequency unless some information is available about the range of spatial frequencies to be expected in the data being digitized.

Errors introduced by representing pixels with too few gray levels are called *quantization* errors. Some quantization error usually occurs with digitization because the pixel can rarely assume as many values as the original, analog data. To use a familiar analogy, the column of mercury in a common thermometer can assume an infinite variety of lengths and thus is able to represent an infinite variety of temperatures, but a digital thermometer can indicate the temperature only in discrete units. In the case of image data, if a signal actually has a value of 104.63 and the nearest allowable pixel

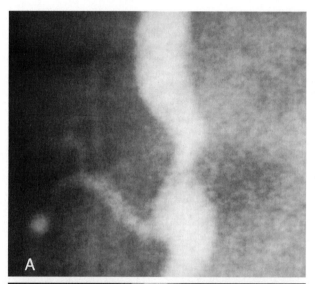

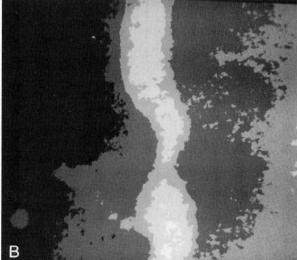

FIGURE 6–6. Effect of variable gray scale quantization on digital image appearance. *A*, Magnified image of a coronary arteriogram digitized with the use of a large number of gray levels. *B*, The same image data, digitized with the use of a smaller number of gray levels. The image quantized with fewer gray levels shows so-called false contours; artifactual edges have been produced because of inadequate gray level sampling.

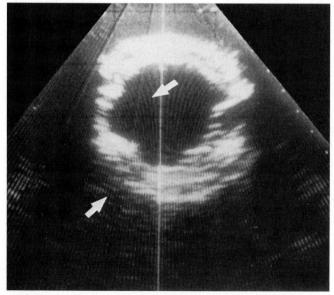

FIGURE 6–5. Illustration of a moiré pattern. The lines identified by the arrows are another undersampling artifact sometimes noted in digital images. (From Collins, S.M., and Skorton, D.J. [eds.]: Cardiac Imaging and Image Processing. New York, McGraw-Hill, 1986, p. 128, with permission.)

values are 104 and 105, the pixel is assigned a value of 105 and the difference of 0.37 is the quantization error. The effects of quantization errors can be just as dramatic as those of undersampling. The most common error is the appearance of false contours as edges in an area of an image that should exhibit a smoothly varying gray level. This effect can be seen in Figure 6–6.

The number of gray levels represented in a digital system is usually expressed as a power of two. This is a result of the binary representation of numbers by computers. The gray scale data are stored in binary digits or "bits" (0s or 1s). Each bit available in a binary number doubles the number of values (gray levels) that may be represented. Thus, an 8-bit system can represent four times more gray levels ($2^8 = 256$) than a 6-bit system ($2^6 = 64$). The number of bits available depends on the image storage or display device. Devices that store and display 6- or 8-bit images are most common, although newer technology is making 10- and 12-bit devices (1024 and 4096 gray levels, respectively) increasingly popular.

Because spatial resolution and pixel quantization can introduce errors, it seems logical to always sample at the highest possible rate and represent pixels with the largest possible number of gray levels. However, increasing the spatial resolution or the number of allowable gray levels increases digital data storage requirements and potentially increases the time required to analyze the image. In many cases, either of these improvements in image quality may require a much larger investment in both image acquisition time and equipment expense.

After manipulation by the computer, the digital image must be converted back into a form easily viewed by the human eye. This reverse process is termed digital-to-analog conversion or digital image display. Displays may be temporary (as on video monitors) or permanent (as on film recorders). Just as there are important considerations regarding image digitization, there are many factors that influence the proper display of digital images.[38] It is frequently not possible to display all the information available in the digital image. If the range of data (either spatially or in gray levels) exceeds the range of the available display, some transformation must be done. This may mean compressing the image data or omitting some information from the display. For example, with echocardiographic data, only a fraction of the broad dynamic range of the acoustic information available can be accommodated by common video displays. Most commercial echocardiographic systems therefore allow the user to adjust the compression of the data before display. Some common forms of data compression are shown in Figure 6–7. One should always keep in mind that the computer may be processing more information than is presented on the display.

Image Enhancement

One major application of digital image processing is the enhancement of images. Enhancement operations may be performed to improve the appearance of the image or to make quantitation easier or more accurate. Examples of such enhancement are accentuation of an important feature (e.g., the endocardial border) or removal of some undesirable feature of the image (e.g., noise).

Point Operations

Among the most common forms of image enhancement are gray level modification techniques. These operations are also called point operations because the operators (calculations) have no spatial dependencies. In other words, the output (processed) pixel gray level value depends only on the input (original) image pixel value at the same image location or "point." Point operators are, in general, easy to implement, and most modern image processing systems support point operations as part of their basic operation at or near video rates (i.e., the calculations can be performed at the rate of 30 frames per second).

Point operators are most efficiently implemented, in either hardware or software, through the use of a *lookup table*. A lookup table is simply a list of gray levels used to map the input pixel values to the output pixel values. The length of the list is equal to the number of possible input gray levels. At each location or address on the list, the desired output or processed gray level for an input pixel with that particular value is placed. To determine the output

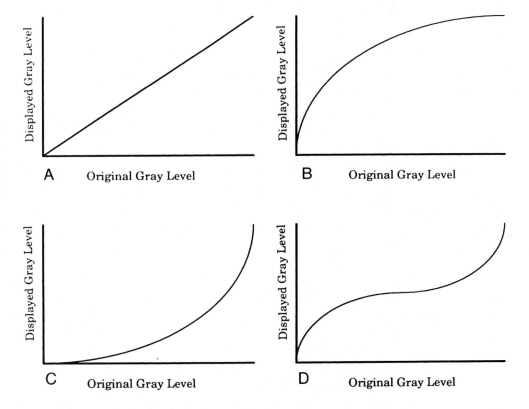

FIGURE 6–7. Four functions commonly used for gray scale compression in digital imaging. Each graph shows the displayed gray level plotted against the original gray level; notice that the original gray level range is wider than the displayed gray level range, necessitating compression. *A*, The data are compressed in a linear fashion. *B*, The function compresses higher gray levels more than middle gray levels. *C*, The function compresses lower gray levels more than higher ones. *D*, Middle-level gray levels are compressed the most.

for a particular input, the input value is used to "look up" the corresponding output value on the list. In Figure 6–8, for example, the third element of the list has a value of 18; therefore, whenever an input pixel has a value of 3, the output pixel will be assigned a value of 18. The advantage of using lookup tables is that there are usually many fewer elements in the lookup table than there are pixels in the image. For the same example, it may have been difficult to compute an output value of 18 for the input value of 3, but once this value has been calculated, it need not be done again, even if there are many pixels in the input image with a value of 3.

The ranges of input and output values in the lookup table are not necessarily the same. An important example is the pseudocolor display found in some medical imaging systems.[39, 40] In this sort of display, the input values are image intensities, but the output values are color hues or intensities instead of gray levels. The pseudocolor lookup table thus converts a gray scale image to a color image. The human eye is much more sensitive to variations in color than it is to small changes in gray scale.[41] By assigning colors to values that change quickly in the gray level range of interest, the pseudocolor display can amplify small differences in gray scale on the original image.

Lookup tables can be used to implement many different point operations (Fig. 6–9). One operation, histogram equalization, deserves special attention because of its important properties. Histogram equalization attempts to produce an image with a uniform gray level distribution or histogram. The *gray level histogram* is simply a plot of the number of occurrences of each particular gray level in an image; this is also the *probability density function* for gray levels in the image. In an image with a uniform histogram, all gray levels occur with the same frequency, which has the effect of spreading out the gray scale and increasing image contrast. If the image does not occupy the complete range of available gray levels, histogram equalization can be a powerful image enhancement technique (Fig. 6–10).

In contrast to the histogram equalization techniques, which depend only on the image gray level values, the "window" and "level" operations allow the user to isolate part of the image gray scale and expand this part to fill the full range of display gray levels available. These common point operations are found in almost all MRI and CT scanners and are implemented as interactive processes. The *window* is the range of input gray level values that is mapped to the entire range of the output display. The center gray level of the window is the *level*. Increasing the window size or "width" decreases contrast but displays a wider range of gray levels from the input image. Window and level displays are most commonly used when the available range of gray scales is high and exceeds the display capability of a standard monitor. The window can then be adjusted so that only a desired portion of the entire range of gray levels is displayed. A CT image is shown at different window and level settings in Figure 6–11.

Geometric Operations

Rotation, magnification, and translation of images are all examples of geometric transformations. Geometric transformations can all be considered special cases of polynomial or "rubber sheet" warping.[42] The basic idea is to map the input image into the output image in a manner described by the warping function. In this context, "warping" refers to changing some geometric characteristic of the image. Correction of an angiographic image for pincushion distortion is an example of corrective warping. Problems arise in polynomial warping because the locations of pixels in a digital image must have discrete integral coordinates. A pixel in the input image may be mapped to a location that lies between integral locations in the output image, two pixels may map to the same location, or the output image may have "holes" because no pixels were mapped there.

Two methods exist for mapping the input image pixels to the output image pixels. The first method starts by calculating the output location for a particular input pixel. If the output location falls between integral positions in the output image, the value assigned to the pixel is divided among the nearest neighboring output pixels. The value resulting from the input pixel need not be equally divided among the surrounding output pixels. Instead, the closer output locations can receive a proportionally larger share. This method is usually termed the "forward mapping" method.[42]

In the second method, known as the "reverse mapping"

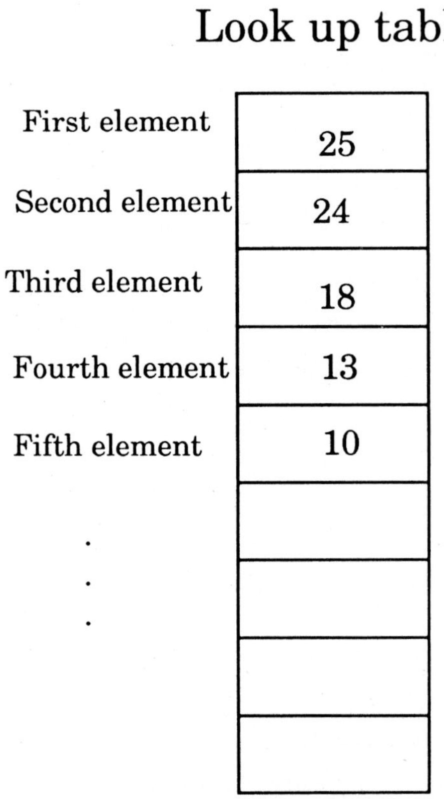

Look up table

First element	25
Second element	24
Third element	18
Fourth element	13
Fifth element	10
.	
.	
.	

FIGURE 6–8. The structure of a lookup table. The value of each input pixel is used as an address to "look up" a value in the table. This value is then used as the output value for the pixel.

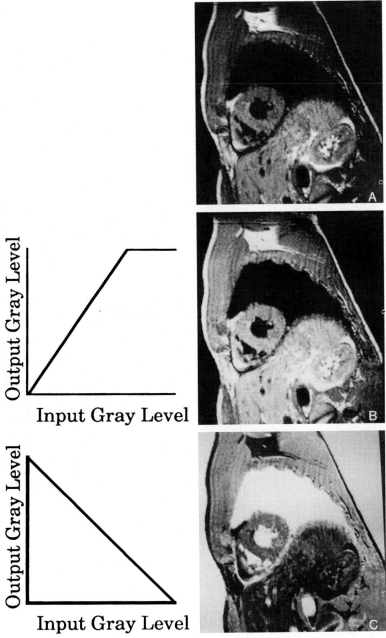

FIGURE 6–9. Effects of two lookup tables on magnetic resonance images. *A*, The original image. *B*, Graphical representation of the lookup table and resulting image for white stretching. *C*, Graphical representation of the lookup table and resulting image for gray level inversion.

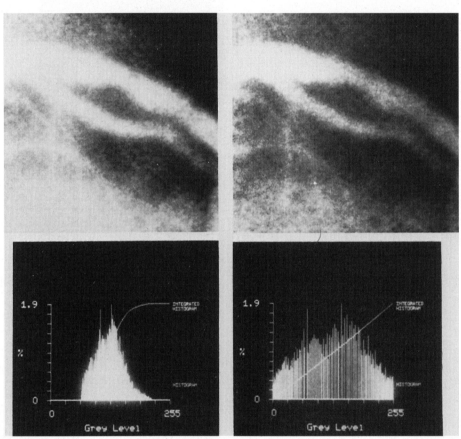

FIGURE 6–10. Effect of histogram equalization. Two images of a coronary arteriogram are shown at the top, each with its corresponding gray level histogram (display of the frequency of occurrence of all gray levels in the image) at the bottom. The image on the left is the original digitized image. The image on the right shows the alteration of image quality after histogram equalization, a process that spreads the gray levels in the image over the entire available display range. Notice the improved contrast in the image. (From Collins, S.M., and Skorton, D.J. [eds.]: Cardiac Imaging and Image Processing. New York, McGraw-Hill, 1986, p. 128, with permission.)

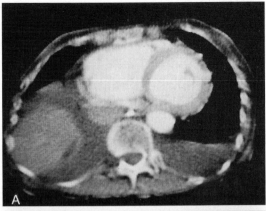

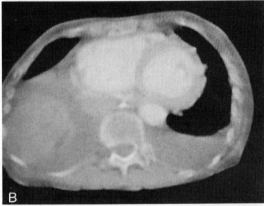

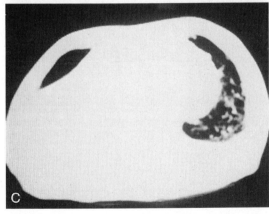

FIGURE 6–11. Window width and level adjustments can be used to examine objects with different intensities in the same digital image. *A,* Computed tomographic cardiac image with a fairly wide window and a medium level. *B,* The same image with a narrower window but the same level. *C,* Use of a narrow window and a low level permits visualization of the pulmonary vasculature.

method,[42] calculations are made in the opposite direction. Starting at an integral output location, the location of the input pixel is calculated. If this location falls between pixels in the input image, the output pixel value is interpolated from those of the four nearest neighbors in the input image. This method ensures that each pixel in the output image is assigned a value. However, sometimes a calculated input pixel location falls entirely outside the input image, and thus no data is available to map into the output image. The usual procedure when this occurs is to set the resulting output image value to zero.

In both methods, pixel values must be interpolated because of the discrete nature of the image matrix. The two most popular interpolation schemes are *nearest-neighbor* interpolation and *bilinear* interpolation. The nearest-neighbor method is a simple technique in which the pixel is interpolated by using the value of the closest pixel in the image matrix. This method, although fast and simple, can produce images that appear "blocky." The more complicated method of bilinear interpolation fits a mathematical surface (a hyperbolic paraboloid) to the four pixels surrounding the nonintegral location. Once the coefficients describing this surface are known, any point between those four neighbors may be found. Bilinear interpolation produces images that have no abrupt intensity transitions and thus do not appear blocky. It is, however, a computationally intensive task because a surface must be fit to each set of four neighboring pixels.

Geometric operations in general can be computationally intensive. Some may be implemented in software, but more complex operations usually require dedicated hardware.

Filtering Operations

Some of the most powerful image enhancement techniques can be grouped together in the general category of filtering operations. Filtering operations are image enhancement techniques that either accentuate or de-emphasize some feature of the image. Because image filtering received a large amount of attention in the early history of digital image processing research, there is a large body of literature on the subject.[43] This chapter introduces a few of the basic concepts, illustrated with some examples, and refers the interested reader to more in-depth reviews.[44–47]

For our purposes, filtering can be thought of as having two major functions: to remove noise from the image and to enhance edges. Most filtering operations can be described in two ways, in the spatial domain and in the frequency domain. As will be shown, there is a direct mathematical relation between these two domains that allows filters to be transformed from one domain to the other. Because of this relation, filtering operators can be expressed in either the spatial or the frequency domain, but most filters are more easily expressed in one domain or the other.

Spatial domain filters are described by an operation that is performed on a group of pixels called the "neighborhood." For example, a simple filter that removes noise from images is an averaging operator. This operator replaces each pixel value with the average value of that pixel and its neighbors. The more neighbors that are included, the more averaging, or smoothing, is performed. If the image noise is random, it is reduced by averaging; the image data, which are not random, are not removed by averaging. Spatial operations of this type are usually easy to apply and are often implemented through *mask operators*, which define a neighborhood size and a weighting function for each pixel in the neighborhood. The pixel in the center of the mask is replaced by the sum of all the pixel values, each multiplied by the respective weight of the mask. Mask operators can produce widely varying results, depending on their size and the particular weighting scheme employed. Figure 6–12 shows examples of some common mask operators and their effects on an image.

Before describing the frequency domain operators, it is appropriate to describe exactly what is meant by the frequency domain. The direct relation between the spatial domain and the frequency domain is known as the *Fourier transform*. The basis for the Fourier transform is that all images may be represented by a unique set of sinusoidal functions that vary in both frequency and phase (Fig. 6–13). The Fourier transform changes the representation of an image from spatial locations of gray scales to frequency amplitudes and phases. The Fourier transform is invertible (reversible), no information is lost, and if the process is reversed, the original data may be recovered. The motivation for using the frequency domain is that some operations are much easier to define in terms of frequencies and phases. High frequencies in images correspond to areas of rapidly changing gray levels (such as edges). Images with many edges contain more high frequencies than images without a large complement of edges.

Frequency domain filters usually fall into one of three classes: high-pass, low-pass, or bandpass. High-pass filters allow only relatively high frequencies to pass through and attenuate the low frequencies; low-pass filters allow only relatively low frequencies to

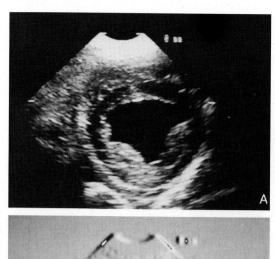

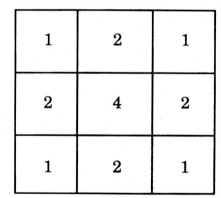

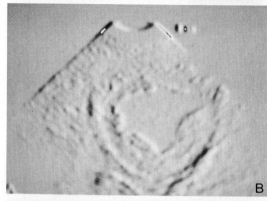

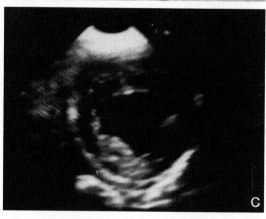

FIGURE 6–12. Effect of image filtering by the application of a mask. *A,* The original short-axis, two-dimensional echocardiographic image. *B,* An edge enhancement mask and the resulting image after the mask is applied. *C,* A smoothing mask and resulting image.

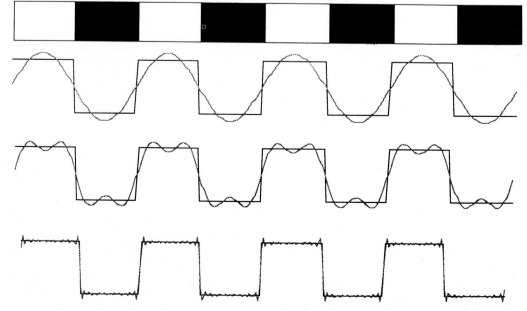

FIGURE 6–13. Illustration of the concept of Fourier transformation. The upper panel shows a digital "image" consisting of alternating black and white pixels. The second panel shows the representation of this image as alternating high and low values. Superimposed on this representation *(square waves)* is a single sine wave that may be used to approximate roughly this pattern of image intensities. The bottom two panels show increasingly accurate representation of the square-wave pattern by the addition of multiple sinusoids of varying phase and amplitude.

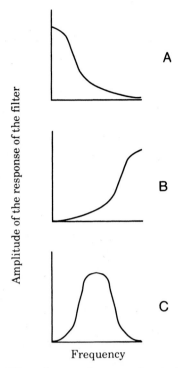

FIGURE 6–14. Effect of various frequency domain filters. Each graph shows how much each of the frequency components in the image is attenuated by the filter. *A,* Low-pass filter. Lower frequencies are allowed to pass at relatively high amplitude, but higher frequencies are reduced to a great extent. *B,* High-pass filter. Higher frequencies are permitted to pass at a high amplitude, but lower-frequency components of the signal are removed. *C,* Bandpass filter. Both the lowest and the highest frequencies are filtered, and middle-level frequencies are allowed to pass.

pass through; and bandpass filters allow a specific bandwidth (range) of frequencies to pass through (Fig. 6–14). Frequency domain filters are most easily applied after the image has been transformed into the frequency domain. The filtering may then be accomplished by multiplying each of the frequency components by the filter functions and then transforming the image back into the spatial domain.

The choice between a spatial and a frequency domain filter is usually based on a combination of representation, implementation, and efficiency. Some filters (e.g., an averaging filter) are easily represented in the spatial domain, whereas others (e.g., a high-pass filter) are more easily represented in the frequency domain.

Segmentation

Medical image processing problems often require isolation of a particular object or region of interest within an image. This process, known as segmentation, is sometimes the goal in itself, but more often it is a preprocessing step before further measurements of the object region can be made.[48, 49] For example, the left ventricular cavity area in an echocardiographic image must be separated or segmented from the remainder of the image before the area can be measured. Segmentation procedures can be divided into five categories: thresholding techniques, region-growing techniques, region-partitioning techniques, split-and-merge techniques, and border detection.

The simplest method of segmenting an image is through the use of *gray level thresholds*.[50] In this method, all pixels with values falling above a particular gray level (the threshold) are said to belong to one region; those whose values fall below the threshold belong to the other region. The difficulty in this method is finding the proper threshold. For images that have bimodal histograms, the "valley" or local minimum of the histogram can be used as

the threshold value[50] (Fig. 6–15). Alternatively, the distributions expected from the image can be fit to the histograms to determine the proper threshold.[51] Simple thresholding techniques are not useful in all cases. For example, using a gray level threshold to identify an object placed on a slowly varying background (which could be caused by camera shading) will fail because the threshold remains constant but the background and object intensities do not. A possible solution in this case is to perform the analysis adaptively on a regional basis, using a separate threshold for each region to compensate for the slowly varying background. A related technique is to use a multidimensional threshold. In this method, thresholds are picked for several image features. With color images, a separate threshold could be chosen for each color.

For many kinds of segmentation, thresholding techniques prove inadequate. A second type of segmentation technique is known as *region growing*. Region-growing techniques start with a "seed" location. The seed is a pixel or group of pixels known to be within the region, as indicated by an observer or perhaps determined automatically. From this seed, the region is "grown" by adding neighboring pixels that fit some criterion (e.g., their gray level is similar). The procedure stops when no neighboring pixels can be added to the region. An advanced form of this method starts with many seed locations and grows as many regions as needed until each pixel in the image belongs to a region.[52]

Region-partitioning techniques approach the segmentation problem in a related manner. These techniques start with the entire image as a region. The region is then divided or partitioned into smaller subregions, and the characteristics of the subregions are calculated and examined. If these characteristics meet a homogeneity requirement, the region is not partitioned further. If the homogeneity requirement is not met, the subregions are further partitioned until all subregions meet the requirement. When no regions can be partitioned further, the procedure stops.

By combining region-growing and region-partitioning techniques, a class of powerful *split-and-merge* techniques can be defined. Split-and-merge techniques first split the entire image into subregions. For each subregion, the neighboring subregions are examined to see if they are similar. Similar neighboring subregions are merged to form larger regions, and dissimilar subregions are split to form smaller subregions. When no more subregions can be split or merged, the procedure stops.

A completely different approach to segmentation is to identify not the regions but instead the boundaries between the regions. *Border detection* has been extensively studied in many applications of medical imaging,[4, 53, 54] with varying degrees of success. Traditionally, border detection consists of two steps. First, all pixels in the image or region of interest are evaluated for their potential to be

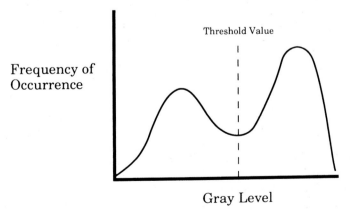

FIGURE 6–15. Concept of simple gray level thresholding. The gray level histogram displays the frequency of occurrence of all gray levels in an image. In the example shown, the histogram is bimodal; that is, two distinct populations of gray levels are present. The image may be divided into segments of high and low gray level by choosing a threshold level at the local minimum ("valley") of the histogram (*vertical line*).

points on the boundary. Second, the list of these candidate points is reduced by using the information contained in the first step. For example, the spatial gradient (change in gray level) across each point in the image could be determined and then those points with a gradient greater than some threshold value selected to be border points. There are many ways to implement both steps in border detection. A particularly interesting approach to the second procedure (that of selecting the boundaries) involves the use of graph-searching techniques to implement a minimum-cost search.[4] The problem is restated so that a "cost" is assigned to each pixel: the higher the probability that the particular pixel is a part of the border, the lower the assigned cost. Paths through the image may be found by connecting locations. Each path has an overall cost that is defined as the sum of the costs of all the locations along the path; the goal is to find the minimum-cost path. An exhaustive search of all paths through the image would always find this optimum path, but the large number of possible paths available precludes such a search in all but the simplest cases. Fortunately, intelligent heuristic search algorithms or dynamic programming techniques may be used to produce globally optimal borders with a reasonable amount of computation.

Future Directions of Quantitative Image Processing

The disciplines of image processing, computer graphics, signal processing, and artificial intelligence have all existed for more than 20 years, and each has made contributions to quantitation in medical imaging. The traditional distinctions among these disciplines have become blurred as techniques have been combined to solve specific problems. One illustration of this phenomenon is the dual representation of information as either the image data or a higher-level description. An example of such duality is the information contained in the geometry of the left ventricle, which can be represented as either a set of echocardiographic images or a three-dimensional mathematical model such as a prolate ellipsoid. Techniques from the various disciplines can be used to provide methods for transforming the image data into a description and vice versa. Specifically, computer graphic techniques transform the description into the image data, image and signal processing techniques enhance or modify the data, and pattern recognition, image processing, or artificial intelligence techniques transform image data and objects into descriptions.

In addition, image processing techniques can modify image data so that descriptions can be generated more easily. An example of the combination of these disciplines may be found in automated quantitative coronary angiography. A typical processing sequence involves some sort of preprocessing, for example with a smoothing filter (an image processing technique) followed by an edge operator (another image processing technique). A graph-searching technique (from the artificial intelligence discipline) is then applied to generate the borders of the coronary artery. These borders form the quantitative description of the part of the image data in which the researcher or clinician is interested. If multiple views of the coronary artery are obtained, the descriptions can be used to generate a three-dimensional model (from computer graphics) so that complex lesions may be more easily visualized. As awareness of these various disciplines and their interrelations increases, combinations of techniques will be used more commonly to solve specific problems.

Not only are separate techniques being combined to solve intricate problems in cardiac imaging, but the disciplines themselves are evolving to provide better individual tools to help solve these problems. An example is the development of three-dimensional analysis techniques. Much of three-dimensional analysis is a natural extension of two-dimensional image analysis. The three-dimensional techniques have, however, been limited by the computational abilities and display methods currently available. An example of an extension from two- to three-dimensional image processing is surface detection, which is related to the two-dimensional edge detection problem.[55] Because most cardiac analysis problems are inherently three-dimensional (or four-dimensional, if time is included),

many of the two-dimensional quantitative techniques will ultimately be replaced by higher-dimensional extensions.

In the short term at least, display of multidimensional data will still require the use of a traditional two-dimensional monitor. The reduction of multidimensional data for display will continue to be a computationally difficult problem. If the data can be represented as mathematical surfaces, shaded surface display techniques may be used. The advantage of these techniques is that numerous hardware accelerators are available that can display large data sets in real time, allowing the user to interact with the data. The drawback is that most medical data are not naturally represented by surfaces, so a segmentation step is required to produce the surfaces. This step is usually difficult because of the enormous amount of data present and the fact that most segmentation techniques require some manual correction to produce acceptable results. An entirely different approach is to visualize the data by volume rendering. In these techniques, all of the volume elements, or voxels, are displayed directly. These techniques do not require a segmentation step because they visualize the entire multidimensional volume directly. The limitation of this technique is the huge amount of data required to represent even the smallest data set. The sheer amount of data makes it difficult to implement usable volume visualization with hardware acceleration. Nonetheless, multidimensional presentation of data, with its potential to provide more usable information, continues to offer exciting opportunities.

The capabilities of modern digital computers are being increasingly applied to cardiovascular image data for the purposes of image enhancement, extraction of features of interest, derivation of quantitative data more objectively than is possible with visual interpretation, and extraction of information not easily extractable by simple visual means. The recent advances in fast CT scanning, color Doppler flow imaging, and ultrafast MRI have been possible because of the application of digital computer techniques for rapid image reconstruction and analysis. The need for quantitation and the ubiquitous presence of computers in modern imaging departments will undoubtedly increase the prevalence of computer image processing techniques, and of image quantitation in general, in modern cardiac imaging practice.

Acknowledgment

The authors acknowledge Carolyn Frisbie for expert preparation of the manuscript.

References

1. Buda, A.J., and Delp, E.J. (eds.): Digital Cardiac Imaging. Boston, Martinus Nijhoff, 1985.
2. Collins, S.M., and Skorton, D.J. (eds.): Cardiac Imaging and Image Processing. New York, McGraw-Hill, 1986.
3. Brown, B.G., Bolson, E., Frimer, M., et al.: Quantitative coronary arteriography: Estimation of dimensions, hemodynamic resistance, and atheroma mass of coronary artery lesions using the arteriogram and digital computation. Circulation 55:329, 1977.
4. Fleagle, S.R., Johnson, M.R., Wilbricht, C.J., et al.: Automated analysis of coronary arterial morphology in cineangiograms: Geometric and physiologic validation in humans. IEEE Trans. Biomed. Eng. 8:387, 1989.
5. Brown, G., Albers, J.J., Fisher, L.D., et al.: Regression of coronary artery disease as a result of intensive lipid-lowering therapy in men with high levels of apolipoprotein B. N. Engl. J. Med. 323:1289, 1990.
6. Garcia, E.V., DePuey, E.G., and DePasquale, E.E.: Quantitative planar and tomographic thallium-201 myocardial perfusion imaging. Cardiovasc. Intervent. Radiol. 10:374, 1987.
7. Van Train, K.F., Garcia, E.V., Cooke, C.D., et al.: Quantitative analysis of SPECT myocardial perfusion. *In* DePuey, E.G., Berman, D.S., Garcia, E.V. (eds.): Cardiac SPECT Imaging. New York, Raven Press, 1994.
8. Braunwald, E.: Assessment of cardiac function. *In* Braunwald, E. (ed.): Heart Disease. 4th ed. Philadelphia, W.B. Saunders, 1992, p. 419.
9. Schiller, N.B., Shah, P.M., Crawford, M., et al.: American Society of Echocardiography Committee on Standards, Subcommittee on Quantitation of Two-Dimensional Echocardiograms: Recommendations for quantitation of the left ventricle by two-dimensional echocardiography. J. Am. Soc. Echocardiogr. 2:358, 1989.
10. Feiring, A.J., Rumberger, J.A., Reiter, S.J., et al.: Determination of left ventricular mass in dogs with rapid-acquisition cardiac computed tomographic scanning. Circulation 72:1355, 1985.
11. Florentine, M.S., Grosskreutz, C.L., Chang, W., et al.: Measurement of left ventricular mass in vivo using gated nuclear magnetic resonance imaging. J. Am. Coll. Cardiol. 8:107, 1986.

12. Parker, D.L., and Muhlestein, B.: Vessel lumen imaging with digital subtraction angiography. *In* Zaret, B.L., Kaufman, L., Berson, A.S., et al. (eds.): Frontiers in Cardiovascular Imaging. New York, Raven Press, 1993, p. 179.

13. Ranky, P.G.: Computer Integrated Manufacturing. Englewood Cliffs, N.J., Prentice-Hall, 1986.

14. Hemmy, D.C., David, D.J., and Herman, G.T.: Three-dimensional reconstruction of craniofacial deformity using computed tomography. Neurosurgery 13:534, 1983.

15. Tessier, P., and Hemmy, D.: Three-dimensional imaging in medicine: A critique by surgeons. Scand. J. Plast. Reconstr. Surg. 20:3, 1986.

16. Aakhus, S., Mæhle, J., Bjoernstad, K.: A new method for echocardiographic computerized three-dimensional reconstruction of left ventricular endocardial surface: In vitro accuracy and clinical repeatability of volumes. J. Am. Soc. Echocardiogr. 7:571, 1994.

17. McPherson, D.D., Skorton, D.J., Kodiyalam, S., et al.: Finite element analysis of myocardial diastolic function using three-dimensional echocardiographic reconstructions: Application of a new method for study of acute ischemia in dogs. Circ. Res. 60:674, 1987.

18. Collins, S.M., Chandran, K.B., and Skorton, D.J.: Three-dimensional cardiac imaging. Echocardiography 5:311, 1988.

19. Geiser, E.A., Lupkiewicz, S.M., Christie, L.G., et al.: A framework for three-dimensional time-varying reconstruction of the human left ventricle: Sources of error and estimation of their magnitude. Comput. Biomed. Res. 13:225, 1980.

20. Roelandt, J.R.T.C., di Mario, C., Pandian, N.G., et al.: Three-dimensional reconstruction of intracoronary ultrasound images: Rationale, approaches, problems, and directions. Circulation 90:1044, 1994.

21. Herman, G.T., and Liu, H.K.: Display of three-dimensional information in computed tomography. J. Comput. Assist. Tomogr. 1:155, 1977.

22. Ariet, M., Geiser, E.A., Lupkiewicz, S.M., et al.: Evaluation of three-dimensional reconstruction to compute left ventricular volume and mass. Am. J. Cardiol. 54:415, 1984.

23. Linker, D.T., Moritz, W.E., and Pearlman, A.S.: A new three-dimensional echocardiographic method of right ventricular volume measurements: In vitro validation. J. Am. Coll. Cardiol. 8:101, 1986.

24. Moritz, W.E., Pearlman, A.S., McCabe, D.H., et al.: An ultrasonic technique for imaging the ventricle in three dimensions and calculating its volume. IEEE Trans. Biomed. Eng. 30:482, 1983.

25. Gopal, A.S., Keller, A.M., Rigling, R., et al.: Left ventricular volume and endocardial surface area by three-dimensional echocardiography: Comparison with two-dimensional echocardiography and nuclear magnetic resonance imaging in normal subjects. J. Am. Coll. Cardiol. 22:258, 1993.

26. Ray, G., Chandran, K.B., Nikravesh, P.E., et al.: Estimation of the local elastic modulus of the normal and infarcted left ventricle from angiographic data. *In* Saha, S. (ed.): Proceedings of the Fourth New England Bioengineering Conference. New York, Pergamon Press, 1976, p. 173.

27. Sasayama, S., Nonogi, H., Fujita, M., et al.: Three-dimensional analysis of regional myocardial function in response to nitroglycerin in patients with coronary artery disease. J. Am. Coll. Cardiol. 3:1187, 1984.

28. Collins, S.M., Yashodhar, P., Rumberger, J.A., et al.: Three-dimensional reconstruction of the contracting canine heart using cine computed tomography. *In* Ripley, K.L. (Proceedings ed.): 1985 Computers in Cardiology. Long Beach, CA, IEEE Computer Society, 1985, p. 67.

29. Ritman, E.L., Kinsey, J.H., Robb, R.A., et al.: Three-dimensional imaging of heart, lungs, and circulation. Science 210:273, 1980.

30. Miller, T.R., Starren, J.B., and Grothe, R.A., Jr.: Three-dimensional display of positron emission tomography of the heart. J. Nucl. Med. 29:530, 1988.

31. Kuwahara, M., Eiho, S.: 3D heart image reconstructed from MRI data. Comput. Med. Imaging Graph. 15:241, 1991.

32. Laschinger, J.C., Vannier, M.W., Gronemeyer, S., et al.: Noninvasive three-dimensional reconstruction of the heart and great vessels by ECG-gated magnetic resonance imaging: A new diagnostic modality. Ann. Thorac. Surg. 45:505, 1988.

33. Castleman, K.R.: Digital Image Processing. Englewood Cliffs, N.J., Prentice-Hall, 1979, p. 383.

34. Stark, H. (ed.): Applications of Optical Fourier Transforms. New York, Academic Press, 1982.

35. Rosenfeld, A., and Kak, A.: Digital Picture Processing. New York, Academic Press, 1976, p. 65.

36. Jain, A.K.: Fundamentals of Digital Image Processing. Englewood Cliffs, N.J., Prentice-Hall, 1989, p. 80.

37. Rosenfeld, A., and Kak, A.: Digital Picture Processing. New York, Academic Press, 1976, p. 75.

38. Castleman, K.R.: Digital Image Processing. Englewood Cliffs, N.J., Prentice-Hall, 1979, p. 39.

39. Collins, S.M., and Skorton, D.J. (eds.): Cardiac Imaging and Image Processing. New York, McGraw-Hill, 1986, p. 128.

40. Sonka, M., Hlavac, V., and Boyle, R.: Image Processing, Analysis and Machine Vision. London, Chapman & Hall, 1993, p. 60.

41. Gonzalez, R.C., and Wintz, P.: Digital Image Processing. Reading, Mass., Addison-Wesley, 1987, p. 13.

42. Castleman, K.R.: Digital Image Processing. Englewood Cliffs, N.J., Prentice-Hall, 1979, p. 110.

43. Pratt, W.K.: Digital Image Processing. New York, John Wiley & Sons, 1978, p. 279.

44. Castleman, K.R.: Digital Image Processing. Englewood Cliffs, N.J., Prentice-Hall, 1979, p. 190.

45. Jain, A.K.: Fundamentals of Digital Image Processing. Englewood Cliffs, N.J., Prentice-Hall, 1989, p. 267.

46. Pratt, W.K.: Digital Image Processing. New York, John Wiley & Sons, 1978, p. 291.

47. Rosenfeld, A., and Kak, A.: Digital Picture Processing. New York, Academic Press, 1976, p. 79.

48. Rosenfeld, A., and Kak, A.: Digital Picture Processing. Academic Press, New York, 1976, p. 256.

49. Sklansky, J.: Image segmentation and feature extraction. IEEE Trans. Syst. Man Cybern. SMC-8:237, 1978.

50. Ballard, D.H., and Brown, C.M.: Computer vision. Englewood Cliffs, N.J., Prentice-Hall, 1982, p. 152.

51. Chow, C.K., and Kaneko, T.: Automatic boundary detection of the left ventricle from cineangiograms. Comput. Biomed. Res. 5:388, 1972.

52. Zucker, S.: Region growing: Childhood and adolescence. Comput. Graph. Image Process. 5:382, 1976.

53. Ashkar, G.P., and Modestino, J.W.: The contour extraction problem with biomedical application. Comput. Graph. Image Process. 7:331, 1978.

54. Lester, J.M., Williams, H.A., Weintraub, B.A., et al.: Two graph searching techniques for boundary finding in white blood cell images. Comput. Biol. Med. 8:293, 1978.

55. Monga, O., and Deriche, R.: 3D edge detection using recursive filtering: Application to scanner images. *In* Proceedings, IEEE Computer Society Conference on Computer Vision and Pattern Recognition, in San Diego, CA. Washington, DC, IEEE Computer Society Press, 1989, p. 28.

7 Perceptual Aspects of Cardiac Imaging

E. A. Franken, Jr., M.D.

Kevin S. Berbaum, Ph.D.

MOTION AND PERCEPTION _____ 73
IMAGE SEARCH _____ 73
SOME COMMON PERCEPTUAL ERRORS AND
    STRATEGIES FOR AVOIDING THEM _____ 74

JUDGMENT CALLS AND THEIR
    EVALUATION _____ 75
PERCEPTION AND EVALUATION OF HEART
    DISEASE _____ 76

Evaluation of images encompasses three aspects: image quality, perception and recognition, and interpretation of findings. The body of knowledge concerning factors of importance for production of a quality image is substantial. Similarly, there is a considerable literature on interpretation of recognized findings, as evidenced by the multitude of publications on descriptive aspects of images. The perceptual process, wherein the information implicit in the image is transferred explicitly to the level of consciousness and decision-making, is less well studied. Understanding of the perceptual process requires study of human brain activity with its acknowledged imperfections. Errors of image perception and related decision-making are the subject of this chapter.

Because the discipline of clinical practice is an imperfect science, error is universal. Interpretations among competent practitioners differ in up to one third of clinically ambiguous situations.[1, 2] Both interobserver error (disagreement of conclusions made by different physicians) and intraobserver error (disagreement among multiple observations by the same person) can occur. For example, what previously seemed an ejection murmur may, on repeated physical examination, be found unequivocally to be mitral regurgitation. Errors are produced by three general mechanisms: biologic variability of the patient, fallibility of the observer, and variation in clinical judgment. In this chapter, we attempt to raise awareness of perceptual error in cardiac imaging, to familiarize the reader with common sources of error, to illustrate methods of evaluation and to discuss some strategies for minimization of error.

Prevalence of error in diagnostic imaging is in the same general range as that found elsewhere in clinical medicine. Although our understanding of the nature of such errors has improved considerably, their rate of occurrence in diagnostic imaging has not changed substantially in the last 50 years. The inherent tendency of the radiologist (and presumably of other physicians) is to underread a positive case (false-negative interpretation); this type of error accounts for about 80 percent of all mistakes.[1, 2] Although the highest rate of disagreement is found between individual observers (especially those with different backgrounds), a competent physician observer may disagree with his or her own interpretations in up to one fifth of cases.[1, 2]

Sources of imaging error are multiple. Obviously, more mistakes are made with a poor image than if pathologic anatomy is well demonstrated. Environmental factors can be of considerable importance. For instance, minimization of indirect light sources around an image produces substantial improvement in contrast resolution,[3] although it is the unusual physician who maximizes viewing conditions. Similarly, fine detail is best detected at short viewing distances (sometimes with a magnifying glass), and minimal contrast differences may best be noticed from several meters away (or with a minifying lens), but physicians seldom use multiple viewing distances.

Image factors involved in perception are fairly well understood and can be measured. High spatial resolution is needed for fine structures (e.g., Kerley's B lines). Contrast sensitivity allows recognition of minimal differences in density (e.g., mitral insufficiency on a left ventriculogram). Analysis of motion can be critical in recognition of abnormality.

It seems logical that knowledge and experience would be important in the minimization of clinical errors in imaging, but in fact lack of knowledge accounts for fewer than 5 percent of imaging mistakes in clinical practice.[1] Mindset (e.g., clinical prejudice) and physiologic state (e.g., boredom, distraction) are often factors.[2, 4] Because the human perceptual system is imperfect, error occurs as a result of inherent limitations in human perception and cognition. Any limitations in an individual's visual acuity create additional problems.[5]

A significant cause of error in imaging is the faulty judgment call. In the imperfect world of clinical medicine, the journey from black to white goes through several shades of gray, and individual judgment varies as to the points of separation. By *judgment call* we mean that, although an image feature may always be observed (repeatedly fixated), different observers (or the same observer at different times) may require different levels of apparent abnormality to report a finding as positive. Such judgment calls may be quite deliberate, as when the observer spends a great deal of time and worry on whether to raise a question of cardiac calcification after noting an ambiguous shadow on the chest radiograph. Conversely, based on one's training, knowledge, and experience (or on characteristics of the image), such a decision may be automatic, never rising to the level of conscious deliberation. For example, the pulmonary artery segment of the normal adolescent female is known to be prominent on the chest radiograph. If a seasoned observer is viewing the radiograph of such a person, the possibility that the patient has valvar pulmonic stenosis may never be logically deliberated—previous experience causes the observer to automatically discard this observation in the appropriate situation.

Distraction (e.g., internal noise) may cause error by preventing potential observations. For example, mitral valve calcification is much more likely to be detected with routine fluoroscopy of the heart than on a cineangiocardiogram of the pulmonary arterial tree. In the latter circumstance, the observer's perceptual attention is directed to opacified vessels rather than to other cardiac structures.

The perceptual processes of the observer can be considered as a system of hardware and software.[6] The hardware consists of those aspects of registration of the visual stimulus and processing of that representation that are common to all human observers—that is, they are hardwired and unaffected by learning. The software comprises those aspects of the observer's perception of the stimulus that are based on changes in the perceptual system that accompany learning. Hardware factors include visual acuity, edge gradients of abnormalities, retinal illusions such as Mach bands, and the "limited channel" that carries retinal information to the brain. The hardware aspect of the system has been extensively studied and can be reasonably well quantified. The software processing of images is more obscure and complex[7]; study of the software is known as the science of psychophysics.

Most studies involving the interaction of the physician observer and the diagnostic image have used radiologists as the experimental subjects. Our own investigations involving orthopedic physicians[8] and family practitioners indicate that the same mechanisms apply, although they may be weighed differently when the experienced clinician evaluates images.

There are two general theories regarding perception of images: top-down (concept- and context-driven processing) and bottom-up (data-driven processing).[9] Bottom-up theory suggests that the image data that impact the senses are sufficient to form a coherent percept. Top-down theory suggests that perception begins with a concept, an expectation, or a hypothesis that serves to generate specific tests on the sensory data. (Neither theory alone is sufficient to explain all of perception: a data-driven process is often needed to fetch the concept from memory and initiate a concept-driven process.) Experience with radiologists indicates that top-down theory better explains image perception in that group; that is, there is rapid processing of the entire image, which results in a global percept. This processing is followed by entry of new data into the percept as the observer uses foveal vision to fill in specific details.

The influence of context on perception also helps explain the role of experience. Radiologists are no better than lay persons at discovering simple objects in a camouflaged environment,[10] but given a medical image, which the physician is trained to recognize, vast differences between the radiologist and the layperson are demonstrated. An example to illustrate this phenomenon is the typical chest radiograph in tetralogy of Fallot, in which overall heart size is usually normal. The experienced observer immediately recognizes the unusual cardiac contour on a top-down basis (according to a learned set of features), and, after confirming the observation by gathering further information from the radiograph, gives a confident diagnosis. Unless the observer is trained to recognize a boot-shaped heart (coeur en sabot) as indicative of abnormality, the diagnosis is not made.

For an observer to identify a radiographic abnormality, it must be recognizable and separable from normal structures. To use the terminology of signal detection theory, the signal (abnormality) must be distinguishable from noise (background), or, put another way, there must be a favorable signal-to-noise ratio. For example, gross cardiomegaly is easily recognized on an otherwise normal chest radiograph because the heart is surrounded by aerated lung. In a neonate with failure of primary lung inflation, however, heart size cannot be evaluated because heart and lungs are of the same radiographic density. In the latter situation, the signal is indistinguishable from the noise. Another example is radiographic recognition of increased pulmonary vascularity in patients with left-to-right shunts. Unless pulmonary flow is greater than twice normal, the signal is not sufficient to be differentiated from the noise of normal pulmonary vascularity.

MOTION AND PERCEPTION

Motion can be a powerfully informative diagnostic cue because motion perception influences the perception of structure (form). For example, a number of researchers[11-17] have demonstrated that apparent motion can readily be seen when random-dot cinematograms are used as stimuli (Fig. 7-1). Each half of the cinematogram pair consists of a matrix of black and white squares or dots. The

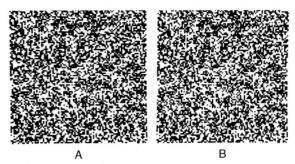

FIGURE 7-1. A pair of random-dot cinematograms of the type introduced by Julesz, which, when viewed alone, permit no global form to be seen. If *A* and *B* are spatially superimposed and temporally alternated, a form is seen in the center (in this case a small square) because elements in the region of the square have been displaced horizontally in *A* relative to *B*. This effect demonstrates that the perception of a structure may depend on prior perception of its motion.

sequence of black and white squares is random. If either half is viewed alone, the observer sees only a random pattern of dots but no global form. A central region depicting a square or some other form is identical in the two halves but displaced horizontally in one half relative to the other. Because global form cues become available only when the information from the two cinematograms is integrated, the perception of motion must logically precede the perception of form. The practical implication of this research is that elements of structure may be perceived based on motion even if the static images alternated to generate the motion do not themselves contain the information. In images with diagnostic low-contrast information, structures that are not apparent in the static views may become readily apparent in a cinematographic presentation.

A number of authors[18-21] have suggested that dynamic visual information is of greatest importance to survival of organisms and is therefore the most important determinant of perception. The most informative type of visual motion is believed to be relative motion (motion of an element relative to another element) rather than absolute motion (motion of an element relative to the observer). The results of a number of experiments argue that perception of relative motion is antecedent to that of object quality. It is therefore not surprising that relative motion in diagnostic images (e.g., motion of the heart wall) is informative.

Another way in which the motion of image elements may contribute to diagnosis derives from the influence of visual motion on visual search and attention. Selection of the location for each succeeding visual fixation depends on data acquired in the peripheral visual field. Initial analysis of peripherally imaged objects depends partly on their motion. The peripheral mechanisms may act as an early warning system of attention for control of eye movement, signaling the locations of unusual, unexpected, or informative events.[22] Temporal modulation in diagnostic images demonstrates changes or differences between images that may be particularly informative and directs attention towards these aspects.

In dynamic environments in which many stimulus elements are in motion, visual search may depend on specific characteristics of target motion that are known in advance.[23] If the stimulus elements move in various directions, prior knowledge of the target's direction of motion reduces search time. Because direction of motion is available at relatively early stages of visual processing, attention and eye movements can be voluntarily attuned to this information. Thus, even particular types of motion may be influential in guiding visual search.

IMAGE SEARCH

Visual search is one of the most common of human activities; it is employed, for example, when one searches for an entry in a phone book, attempts to locate a friend in a crowd, or looks for a book in a library. Evidence[24-27] suggests that when human beings search the visual field for some target item (e.g., a word, an object, a form), two types of cognitive activities are involved: an identification of the part of the visual field centered on the fovea, and a decision as to where in the peripheral visual field to next move the eyes. These two activities taken together are often referred to as *focal attention*. Identification seems to require the allotment of analysis mechanisms to a limited area of the visual field. Attentional mechanisms cannot work on the whole visual field simultaneously. Because of this spatial limitation on identification, any task that necessitates an analysis of a large part of the visual field will require successive fixations. A visual search is serial in nature, with steps in the search corresponding to eye movements. The decision as to where to next move the eyes is of great importance for the effectiveness of visual search.

In order to explain visual search, a stage of analysis has been postulated that is intermediate between the mechanisms responsible for stimulus registration and the sequential analysis of parts of the visual field that is referred to as focal attention. This is a preattentive stage of analysis in which the visual field is segmented into meaningful parts. This preattentive figural synthesis notion proposes that guidance of eye movement and focal attention depend on more complex aspects of the stimulus than those available in a receptor-level description. Other elements, such as perceptual tasks given to the observer, modify subsequent search.

Search patterns of physicians looking at radiographic images are similar to those observed in picture search experiments. For example, there is a strong tendency to fixate on edges and to exclude broad, uniform areas.[28-30] There appears to be preattentive segmentation that provides the perceptual system with information needed to carry out the search. In one report, tachistoscopic presentation of radiographs at an interval sufficiently brief to preclude eye movements (i.e., 0.2 second) still allowed 70 percent true-positive results (i.e., correct determination of abnormality in the presence of disease).[31] Visual search may therefore be described as beginning with a global response that establishes context and organizes subsequent fixations.

Another finding common to both picture and radiograph search experiments is that eye movement pattern is influenced by the search task. Kundel and Wright[28] showed that there is a difference between the eye movement pattern exhibited by subjects searching for lung nodules and that of subjects with a more general search task. In chest radiography, there is a definite evolution of the pattern of fixation from that of an untrained observer to that of a mature radiologist.[32] Such learned behavior is not that of a step-by-step organized search but a circumferential pattern that requires fewer fixations to sample the radiograph with the fovea.

Visual search and eye movement pattern are not synonymous. Attention can be directed sequentially at different organ systems without eye movements. Eye movements are ordinarily superimposed on the attentional pattern but do not follow it exactly.[28] Search may be quantitated by time. In one experiment, it was shown that experienced readers conclude their visual search while they are still making a significant number of true-positive observations and while the rate of true-positive observations is higher than that of false-positives (i.e., determinations of abnormality in the absence of disease).[33] Less experienced readers, who observed the radiographs for half again as long, found only 70 percent of the lesions found by more experienced observers. With neophyte observers, later observations are more likely to be false-positive interpretations.

Visual search experiments in which eye movements were recorded during inspection of radiographs have been used to determine particular sources of diagnostic error.[34, 35] *Scanning or sampling errors* occur when locations containing lesions are not covered by foveal fixation. *Recognition error* occurs when the viewer spends no more time attending to an unreported target than is spent attending to a normal anatomical structure. *Decision-making error* occurs when more time is spent attending to an unreported target than to a normal anatomical structure (three to four fixations in a cluster). In this case, the elements of the abnormality have been segmented, allowing increased interrogation with eye movements and fixation. However, the observer's criterion for apparent abnormality has not been met, so the lesion is not reported. Although different studies show different fractions of misses attributed to sampling, recognition, and decision-making, the results do indicate that most errors are related to recognition and decision-making rather than to sampling.[31, 34, 36]

Another area of research relevant to visual search of images is the effect of knowledge of clinical history on detection of lesions. Numerous studies involving radiologists indicate a powerful positive effect. Experiments with orthopedic surgeons[8] and family practitioners suggest that nonradiologists exhibit an even greater dependence on localizing clues to direct visual search. A true increase in perceptual ability, as well as improved decision-making, can be demonstrated when clinical information is made available.[8]

SOME COMMON PERCEPTUAL ERRORS AND STRATEGIES FOR AVOIDING THEM

Some situations are particularly apt to induce perceptual error. If there are two or more separate abnormalities on the radiograph (e.g., cardiomegaly and bronchogenic carcinoma), recognition of both abnormalities is considerably less likely than recognition of only one of them. This error, known as satisfaction of search, was thought to occur because the observer ceases the search after discovery of one abnormality. Our experiments indicate that termination of search is more strongly related to the task given,[37, 38] and that the satisfaction of search effect can be abolished by provision of an appropriate clinical history.[39] Undetermined perceptual mechanisms in the brain may subtract certain aspects of an image before the percept reaches the level of consciousness. Common foreign bodies such as safety pins are often overlooked for this reason, particularly if the perceptual task is related to a different end. Observers frequently fail to recognize visible abnormalities of the shoulder and abdomen on chest radiographs of patients with heart disease. The use of a checklist as the final step in evaluation of a radiograph has been suggested.

Certain strategies minimize perceptual effort in evaluation of images. Appropriate image quality and optimal viewing conditions are obvious aids. Because the light emanating from television monitors is much less than that from standard view boxes, it is of particular importance to reduce ambient light when viewing monitor displays.[40] Experience is of utmost importance. The differential diagnosis and imaging characteristics of the various types of atrial septal defects may be easily learned, but a neophyte in cardiology usually would not recognize a subtle puff of contrast material entering the right atrium after pulmonary arteriography until he or she has had experience with many similar studies. The minimum length of time required to gain the experience necessary for a good "eye" for cardiac studies has, to our knowledge, not been determined. Experience with plain film radiography[41] suggests that a year or less may be sufficient.

Having a directed perceptual task is of enormous benefit to a radiologist.[42, 43] This translates clinically into knowing the clinical history of the patient, so that the search of the radiograph may be directed toward abnormality. This access to clinical information may raise the number of false-positive observations slightly, but it is accompanied by a much greater increase in true-positive findings. This effect may be even more powerful for nonradiology physicians.[8]

Contrary to logical expectation, increased time for viewing of chest radiographs does not improve perception.[33, 38] Most observations are made after a short period of viewing. Although more positive diagnoses occur with prolonged viewing, many of these late diagnoses are false-positive interpretations. In some circumstances, prolonged viewing of images actually decreases observer accuracy because the rate of false-positive observations rises faster than that of true-positives.

Use of comparison radiographs facilitates interpretation by radiologists. Comparison radiographs facilitate discovery of abnormality as well as staging of any lesions detected. Length of previous training also changes the way in which observers use comparison films.[44]

Effects of motion are considerable in clinical interpretation of images such as those produced by cineangiography, but the mechanisms and nature of these effects are not well determined. For instance, "stacking" axial computed tomographic (CT) images and viewing them in rapid sequence is of considerable value in detection of chest and abdominal lesions.[45] Additional experimental work is necessary to evaluate the beneficial (or detrimental) effects of motion on perception in cardiovascular diagnosis.

Interpretation of images by more than one observer increases accuracy of diagnosis. Probabilities of true-positive and false-positive results are summated for the observers,[41] so the numbers of both increase. This approach is of value in studies in which sensitivity is of greatest importance. There are a variety of mechanisms for determining consensus diagnosis when multiple observers are involved. Such evaluations are necessary for formal investigations but are seldom needed in clinical practice.

JUDGMENT CALLS AND THEIR EVALUATION

A traditional method for evaluation of a diagnostic system involves analysis of a two-by-two decision matrix in which truth is crossed with the judgment of positive (abnormal) or negative (normal). With this characterization, difficulties arise in comparison of two diagnostic systems. For example, one system may not only yield more true-positive results but also more false-positive results. The fundamental problem with the decision matrix description of diagnostic systems is that it assumes a fixed threshold of abnormality on which a positive or negative judgment is based. Human decision-makers, however, can change the criterion of abnormality depending on costs of various kinds of errors. In other words, increases or decreases in the true-positive rate can be traded for increases or decreases in the false-positive rate. To overcome this problem, a family of decision matrices is needed to describe the performance of a diagnostic system. This is exactly what receiver operating characteristic (ROC) analysis involves.

With ROC analysis, the probability of a true-positive result is plotted as a function of the probability of a false-positive result. Each diagnostic system is forced to adopt several different criteria of abnormality. Each criterion leads to a decision matrix, thus becoming an ROC point relating the probabilities of true-positive and false-positive responses. The ROC curve can then be extrapolated from the points to describe the potential behavior of the system: every potential true-positive rate is related to its corresponding false-positive rate. This allows true-positive rates of different systems to be compared at a constant false-positive rate.

Figure 7–2 illustrates these points. Figure 7–2A presents three ROC points for one hypothetical diagnostic system (black) and three ROC points for another diagnostic system (white). In practice, each system tends to operate at a single point; however, that point may be anywhere on the curve for that system. If black operates at the highest point shown in Figure 7–2A and white operates at the lowest, there is no adequate way to tell whether the points for black and white lie on the same curve or matrix. To establish the underlying curve, both systems are forced to operate at several interior levels. The chief benefit of this kind of analysis is that a difference in true-positive rates between systems can be attributed either to simple changes in willingness to call a case normal or abnormal (the so-called response bias; see Fig. 7–2B) or to an actual difference in the systems' abilities to discriminate normal from abnormal (their relative accuracies; see Fig. 7–2A). Note that in both cases, the true-positive rates for black points are

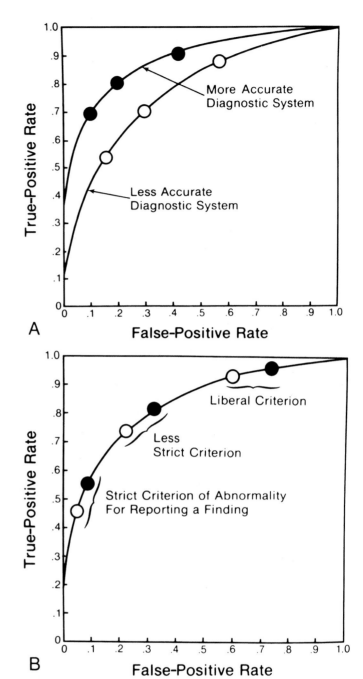

FIGURE 7–2. Receiver operating characteristic (ROC) points and curves for two hypothetical diagnostic systems (black and white) where black has either (A) greater accuracy or (B) simply a less stringent decision criterion of abnormality. Without relating true-positive rates to corresponding false-positive rates and forcing each system to operate at several criterion levels of apparent abnormality by which cases are called normal or abnormal, there is no way to determine whether one system is more accurate than the other.

always higher than those for the corresponding white points. In Figure 7–2B, however, differences in true-positive rates are completely compensated by differences in false-positive rates. In the one case, the ROC points for two diagnostic systems lie along the same fitted curve, with the placement of points being higher along the curve for one system (see Fig. 7–2B). In the other case, the ROC points for the two diagnostic systems lie along different curves (see Fig. 7–2A). Rigorous curve-fitting methods for derivation of separate parameters of ROC curves that describe detection accuracy and response bias have been developed,[46–48] and statistics may be used to analyze these parameters in order to generalize to various case and observer populations.[48, 49]

PERCEPTION AND EVALUATION OF HEART DISEASE

Disagreement and error in detection of heart disease have been known for years. In the early days of roentgenology, many elaborate attempts were made to quantitate heart size on the chest radiograph, with subsequent derivation of both simple and complex measurement techniques to differentiate the normal from the abnormal heart. It is now recognized that the chest radiograph cannot be used to recognize all patients with abnormal hearts; in other words, the sensitivity of the x-ray for this task is considerably less than 100 percent. Studies[50] indicate that the predictive value for individual evaluation of the chest radiograph for cardiomegaly (versus normal-sized heart) is about 70 percent, with wide observer variability. Computer-aided quantitative analysis offers no dramatic increase in accuracy.[51] With the supine radiograph, there is even greater overlap between normal and abnormal determinations.[52] Attempts to extend such judgments into determination of enlargement of specific chambers are much less successful, with sensitivity values of 30 to 40 percent, depending on the chamber being evaluated.

Recognition of increased vascularity in left-to-right shunts on chest radiographs is limited to those situations in which pulmonary flow is greater than twice normal. Unless the increased flow is of this magnitude, the "signal" of engorged vascular structures cannot be recognized within the "noise" of the normal pulmonary vessels, and interobserver agreement is poor.[53] In contrast, trained observers are quite accurate in diagnosis of congestive heart failure on plain films of the chest,[54] with correlation greater than 0.8 with measured pulmonary capillary wedge pressure. Accuracy can further be increased by use of consensus results from several observers and by assessing the degree of pulmonary blood flow redistribution and other specific signs of pulmonary venous hypertension.

Plain film diagnosis of the various types of congenital heart disease was attempted (with variable success) even before development of palliative and curative surgery for patients with such conditions. The subject has been a popular one for books and many descriptive reports. However, diagnostic sensitivity is suboptimal. There are marked differences in capabilities of physicians in this area, ranging from very poor to fair recognition of type and nature of disease.[55]

Although nuclear medicine studies are relied on for many clinical judgments in cardiology, observer performance studies in such cases are few. In one investigation[5] that assessed interpretation of myocardial images with ^{99m}Tc-labeled phosphates, there was so much inconsistency among observers that the authors suggested that "uncorrected visual defects could play an important role in the reading of nuclear medicine images." Even though cardiovascular nuclear medicine procedures have become much more technically sophisticated, there remains considerable overlap of normal and abnormal findings in lesion detection.[56]

With the notable exception of coronary arteriography, there have been few investigations of the reliability and reproducibility of diagnosis in angiocardiography. Motion effects are of obvious importance in evaluation of cinematographic studies, but formal perceptual investigations of these effects have been minimal. Cinecardiography is best for situations in which minimal changes in contrast are necessary for diagnosis or those in which motion of structures is important. An example is the puff of contrast material entering the left atrium from the left ventricle that is seen with minimal mitral insufficiency. Magnetic resonance imaging (MRI) now has a potential role here. Serial standard films from a film changer are of greatest benefit in situations in which spatial resolution must be optimal, such as determinations of the thickness of the pulmonary valve. Overall agreement between determinations

based on cine film versus cut film is 84 percent,[57] indicating that the experience of the observer and the nature of the abnormality are of considerably greater importance than the mechanism of image recording.

Interpretations of individual structures within the heart have about the same variability as do studies elsewhere in the body. Assessment of ventricular volumes by angiocardiography is inexact in comparison with analysis of autopsy material.[58] Reliability of angiographic diagnoses of ventricular aneurysm is good. Variability in "softer" diagnoses is considerable, with one observer's definite wall dyskinesia being another's normal heart.[59]

Observer performance studies in coronary artery examination are more numerous than in other aspects of cardiac imaging. A significant problem in such investigations is determination of a "gold standard"—that is, how to know truth in assessments of the degree of coronary artery narrowing. Interpretations of pathologic material, even with injection of resin into the arteries of a specimen, produce quantitative variations of up to 45 percent.[60] Except for severe stenosis, evaluations of angiograms by consensus panels angiograms are not reliable indicators of truth.[61] And measured degrees of arterial narrowing do not correlate well with actual perfusion through vessels.[62]

Most investigations of assessments of coronary artery narrowing show wide interpretive variation.[63, 64] This variability can be minimized with evaluation by multiple trained observers,[65] an effect that probably represents regression to the mean. The reader's experience may be of minimal importance.[66] Factors of particular importance in error generation include disease of distal segments, poor opacification, inadequate technical quality, and more severe disease. The left circumflex and distal left anterior descending arteries are the most common sites of disagreement.

For imaging studies, both intraobserver and interobserver variability are so high that the recording method is of minimal importance. For instance, one study[63] compared 16-mm cinecardiography with 70-mm serial images—two systems with substantial differences in resolution and image contrast. Accuracy of the two techniques was similar, but there were large interobserver differences in estimates of degree of arterial narrowing.

Because of recognized difficulties with the use of human observers for obtaining reproducible and reliable measurements of arterial stenosis, a variety of machine-based techniques have been advocated.[67–69] Published results indicate that measurements of structures by machines show much greater consistency than those made by human observers. What they do not address is validity: whether the electronic devices can give consistent results regarding arterial stenosis that accurately reflect dynamics of flow in the coronary arteries. Digital cardiac imaging may have the potential to quantify percentage narrowing, wall motion, and ejection fraction more accurately than angiocardiography.[70]

In contrast to the considerable rate of disagreement regarding arterial stenosis, observer assessment of extent of collateral circulation shows little variability. And subjective estimates of ejection fraction are as accurately reproducible as sophisticated quantitative methods.[71] Patency of coronary bypass grafts is more accurately and consistently assessed by coronary angiography than by alternative imaging methods.[72]

Information is now accumulating on the accuracy of cardiac diagnosis based on the newer imaging modalities. The use of ultrafast CT has been evaluated for determinations of several parameters: ventricular volume, left ventricular mass, ejection fraction, and patency of coronary artery grafts. In these aspects, the accuracy of results with ultrafast CT is comparable to or better than that achieved in other clinical studies.[73] Detection and quantification of heart calcification with this technique is of substantial value because interobserver variation has a negligible impact on the quantitative results.[74]

MRI has now emerged as a valuable tool in cardiac imaging. Interexamination variability seems to be of greater importance than observer variation in discovery and quantification of many cardiac parameters with MRI.[75] Similarly, there are reports of high reproducibility of classification of aortic regurgitation[76] and of automated border detection with MRI.[77] A cautious approach to these techniques is advisable, however; with time, they may well show the same variation as older methods.

In summary, errors of a perceptual and judgmental nature occur in evaluation of cardiac images in the same fashion (and probably at the same rate) as in other imaging categories. Awareness of error allows a realistic approach to image interpretation and avoidance of some of the common pitfalls. Avoidance methods include familiarity with the clinical histories of individual patients, use of previous examinations for comparison, readings by multiple observers, maximization of physical circumstances for interpretation sessions, and, if appropriate, use of motion to improve perception.

References

1. Smith, M.C.: Error and Variation in Diagnostic Radiology. Springfield, Ill., Charles C. Thomas, 1967.
2. Spodick, D.H.: On experts and expertise: The effect of variability in observer performance. Am. J. Cardiol. 36:592, 1975.
3. Baxter, B., Ravindra, H., and Normann, R.A.: Changes in lesion detectability caused by light adaptation in retinal photoreceptors. Invest. Radiol. 17:394, 1982.
4. Kundel, H.L., and Hendee, W.R.: The perception of radiologic image information. Invest. Radiol. 20:874, 1985.
5. Cuaron, A., Acero, A.P., Cardenas, M., et al.: Interobserver variability in the interpretation of myocardial images with Tc-99m–labeled diphosphonate and pyrophosphate. J. Nucl. Med. 21:1, 1980.
6. Jaffe, C.C.: Medical imaging, vision, and visual psychophysics. Med. Radiogr. Photo. 60:1, 1984.
7. Kundel, H.L.: Images, image quality and observer performance. Radiology 132:265, 1979.
8. Berbaum, K.S., Franken, E.A., Jr., and El-Khoury, G.Y.: Impact of clinical history on radiographic detection of fractures: A comparison of radiologists and orthopedists. AJR 153:1221, 1989.
9. Kundel, H.L., and Nodine, C.F.: A visual concept shapes image perception. Radiology 146:363, 1983.
10. Rackow, P.L., Spitzer, V.M., and Hendee, W.R.: Detection of low-contrast signals: A comparison of observers with and without radiology training. Invest. Radiol. 22:311, 1987.
11. Anstis, S.M.: Phi movement as a subtraction process. Vision Res. 10:1411, 1970.
12. Bell, H.H., and Lappin, J.S.: Sufficient conditions for discrimination of motion. Percept. Psychophys. 14:45, 1973.
13. Braddick, O.: The masking of apparent motion in random-dot patterns. Vision Res. 113:355, 1973.
14. Braddick, O.: A short-range process in apparent motion. Vision Res. 14:519, 1974.
15. Jules, B.: Foundations of Cyclopean Perception. Chicago, The University of Chicago Press, 1971.
16. Lappin, J.S., and Bell, H.H.: The detection of coherence in moving random-dot patterns. Vision Res. 16:161, 1976.
17. Lenel, J.C., and Berbaum, K.S.: Measurements of displacement and type of background in apparent motion with random-dot cinematograms. Am. J. Psychol. 97:563, 1984.
18. Boynton, R.M., and Boss, D.E.: The effect of background luminance and contrast upon visual search performance. Illuminating Eng. 66:173, 1971.
19. Boynton, R.M., Elworth, C., and Palmer, R.M.: Laboratory studies pertaining to visual air reconnaissance. Technical Report 55-304, Part 3. Dayton, OH, Wright Air Development Center, 1958.
20. Gibson, J.J.: The Perception of the Visual World. Boston, Houghton Mifflin, 1950.
21. Johannson, G.: Spatial temporal differentiation and integration in visual motor perception. Psychol. Rev. 35:379, 1976.
22. Breitmeyer, B.G., and Ganz, L.: Implications of sustained and transient channels for theories of visual pattern masking, saccadic suppression, and information processing. Psychol. Rev. 83:1, 1976.
23. Berbaum, K.S., Chung, C.S., and Loke, W.H.: Improved localization of moving targets with prior knowledge of direction of target motion. Am. J. Psychol. 99:509, 1986.
24. Beck, J.: Similarity grouping and peripheral discriminability under uncertainty. Am. J. Psychol. 85:1, 1972.
25. Haber, R.N., and Hershenson, M.: The Psychology of Visual Perception. 2nd ed. Chicago: Holt, Rinehart & Winston, 1980.
26. Neisser, U.: Decision-time without reaction-time: Experiments in visual scanning. Am. J. Psychol. 76:376, 1963.
27. Neisser, U.: Cognitive Psychology. New York: Appleton-Century-Crofts, 1967.
28. Kundel, H.L., and Wright, D.J.: The influence of prior knowledge on visual search strategies during the viewing of chest radiographs. Radiology 93:315, 1969.
29. Lewellyn-Thomas, E., and Landsdowne, E.L.: Visual search patterns of radiologists in training. Radiology 81:288, 1963.
30. Lewellyn-Thomas, E.: Search behavior. Radiol. Clin. North Am. 7:403, 1969.
31. Kundel, H.L., and Nodine, C.F.: Interpreting chest radiographs without visual search. Radiology 116:527, 1975.
32. Kundel, H.L., and LaFollette, P.S., Jr.: Visual search patterns and experience with radiological images. Radiology 103:523, 1972.
33. Christiansen, E.E., Murry, R.C., Holland, K., et al.: The effect of search time on perception. Radiology 138:361, 1981.
34. Kundel, H.L., Nodine, C.F., and Carmody, D.: Visual scanning, pattern recognition, and decision making in pulmonary nodule detection. Invest. Radiol. 13:175, 1978.
35. Nodine, C.F., and Kundel, H.L.: Using eye movements to study visual search and to improve tumor detection. Radiographics 7:1241, 1987.
36. Hu, C.E., Kundel, H.L., Nodine, C.F., et al.: Searching for bone fractures: A comparison with pulmonary nodule search. Acad. Radiol. 1:25, 1994.
37. Berbaum, K.S., Franken, E.A., Jr., Dorfman, D.D., et al.: Satisfaction of search in diagnostic radiology. Invest. Radiol. 25:133, 1990.
38. Berbaum, K.S., Franken, E.A., Jr., Rooholamini, S., et al.: Time-course of satisfaction of search. Invest. Radiol. 26:640, 1991.
39. Berbaum, K.S., Franken, E.A., Jr., Anderson, K.L., et al.: The influence of clinical history on visual search with single and multiple abnormalities. Invest. Radiol. 28:191, 1993.
40. Kundel, H.L.: Visual perception and image display terminals. Radiol. Clin. North Am. 24:69, 1986.
41. Hessel, S.J., Herman, P.G., and Swensson, R.G.: Improving performance by multiple interpretations of chest radiographs: Effectiveness and cost. Radiology 127:589, 1978.
42. Berbaum, K.S., Franken, E.A., Jr., Dorfman, D.D., et al.: Tentative diagnoses facilitate the detection of diverse lesions in chest radiographs. Invest. Radiol. 21:532, 1986.
43. Berbaum, K.S., Franken, E.A., Jr., Dorfman, D., et al.: Influence of clinical history upon detection of nodules and other lesions. Radiology 23:48, 1988.
44. Berbaum, K.S., Franken, E.A., Jr., and Smith, W.L.: The effect of comparison films upon resident interpretation of pediatric chest radiographs. Invest. Radiol. 20:124, 1985.
45. Berbaum, K.S., Franken, E.A., Jr., Honda, H., et al.: Evaluation of a PACS workstation for assessment of body CT studies. J. Comput. Assist. Tomogr. 14:853, 1991.
46. Dorfmann, D.D., and Alf, E.: Maximum likelihood estimation of parameters of signal-detection theory and determination of confidence intervals: Rating method data. J. Math. Psychol. 6:487, 1969.
47. Metz, C.E., Wang, P., and Kronman, H.B.: A new approach for testing the significance of differences between ROC curves measured from correlated data. In Deconick, F. (ed.): Information Processing in Medical Imaging. Rotterdam, Martinus Nijhoff, 1984, p. 432.
48. Dorfman, D.D., Berbaum, K.S., and Metz, C.E.: Receiver operating characteristic rating analysis: Generalization to the population of readers and patients with the jackknife method. Invest. Radiol. 27:723, 1992.
49. Hanley, J.A.: Alternative approaches to receiver operating characteristic analysis. Radiology 168:568, 1988.
50. Murphy, M.L., Blue, L.R., Thenabadu, N., et al.: The reliability of the routine chest roentgenogram for determination of heart size based on specific ventricular chamber evaluation at postmortem. Invest. Radiol. 20:21, 1985.
51. Nakamori, N., Doi, K., MacMahon, H., et al.: Effect of heart-size parameters computed from digital chest radiographs on detection of cardiomegaly. Invest. Radiol. 26:546, 1991.
52. van der Jagt, E.J., and Smits, H.J.: Cardiac size in the supine chest film. Eur. J. Radiol. 14:173, 1992.
53. Manninen, H., Remes, J., Partanen, K., et al.: Evaluation of heart size and pulmonary vasculature. Acta Radiol. 32:226, 1991.
54. Baumstark, A., Swensson, R.G., Hessel, S.J., et al.: Evaluating the radiographic assessment of pulmonary venous hypertension in chronic heart disease. AJR 141:877, 1984.
55. Steinbach, W.R., and Richter, K.: Multiple classification and receiver operating characteristic (ROC) analysis. Med. Decis. Making 7:234, 1987.
56. Gilland, D.R., Tsui, B.M., Metz, C.E., et al.: An evaluation of maximum likelihood-expectation maximization reconstruction for SPECT by ROC analysis. J. Nucl. Med. 33:451, 1992.
57. Bjork, L.: Cineangiocardiography of full-size angiocardiography? Radiology 86:663, 1966.
58. Ringertz, H.G., Rodgers, B., Lipton, M.J., et al.: Assessment of human right ventricular cast volume by CT and angiocardiography. Invest. Radiol. 20:29, 1985.
59. Zir, L.M., Miller, S.W., Dinsmore, R.E., et al.: Interobserver variability in coronary angiography. Circulation 53:527, 1976.
60. Robbins, S.L., Rodrigues, F.L., Wragg, A.L., et al.: Problems in the quantitation of coronary arteriosclerosis. Am. J. Cardiol. 18:153, 1966.
61. Galbraith, J.E., Murphy, M.L., and de Soyza, N.: Coronary angiogram interpretation. JAMA 240:2053, 1978.
62. Harrison, D.G., White, C.W., Hiratzka, L.F., et al: The value of lesion cross-sectional area determined by quantitative coronary angiography in assessing the physiologic significance of proximal left anterior descending coronary arterial stenoses. Circulation 69:1111, 1984.
63. Bjork, L., Spindola-Franco,H., Van Houten, F.X., et al: Comparison of observer performance with 16-mm cinefluorography and 70-mm camera fluorography in coronary arteriography. Am. J. Cardiol. 36:474, 1975.
64. Fisher, L.D., Judkins, M.P., Lesperance, J., et al: Reproducibility of coronary arteriographic reading in the coronary artery surgery study (CASS). Cathet. Cardiovasc. Diagn. 8:565, 1982.
65. Kussmaul, W.G., III, Popp, R.L., and Norcini, J.: Accuracy and reproducibility of visual coronary stenosis estimates using information from multiple observers. Clin. Cardiol. 15:154, 1992.
66. Fleming, R.M., Kirkeeide, R.L., and Smalling, R.W.: Patterns in visual interpretation of coronary arteriograms as detected by quantitative coronary arteriography. J. Am. Coll. Cardiol. 18:945, 1991.
67. LeFree, M.T., Simon, S.B., Mancini, G.B.J., et al.: A comparison of 35-mm cine

film and digital radiographic image recording: Implications for quantitative coronary arteriography: Film vs. digital coronary quantification. Invest. Radiol. 23:176, 1988.

68. Simons, M.A., Bastian, B.V., Bray, B.E., et al. Comparison of observer and videodensitometric measurements of simulated coronary artery stenoses. Invest. Radiol. 22:562, 1987.

69. Vas, R., Eigler, N., Miyazono, C., et al.: Digital quantification eliminates intraobserver and interobserver variability in the evaluation of coronary artery stenosis. Am. J. Cardiol. 56:718, 1985.

70. Dyet, J.F., Hartley, W., Cowen, A.R., et al.: Digital cardiac imaging: The death knell of cineangiography? Br. J. Radiol. 65:818, 1992.

71. Mueller, X., Stauffer, J.C., Jaussi, A., et al.: Subjective visual echocardiographic estimate of left ventricular ejection fraction as an alternative to conventional echocardiographic methods: Comparison with contrast angiography. Clin. Cardiol. 14:898, 1991.

72. Stanford, W., Galvin, J.R., Skorton, D.J., et al.: The evaluation of coronary bypass graft patency: Direct and indirect techniques other than coronary arteriography. AJR 156:15, 1991.

73. Marcus, M.L., Rumberger, J.A., Start, C.A., et al.: Cardiac applications of ultrafast computed tomography. Am. J. Card. Imaging 2:116, 1988.

74. Kaufmann, R.B., Sheedy, P.F., II, Breen, J.F, et al.: Detection of heart calcification with electron beam CT: Interobserver and intraobserver reliability for scoring quantification. Radiology 190:347, 1994.

75. Pattynama, P.M.T., Lamb, H.J., van der Velde, E.A., et al.: Left ventricular measurements with cine and spin-echo MR imaging: A study of reproducibility with variance component analysis. Radiology 187:261, 1993.

76. Dulce, M.C., Mostbeck, G.H., O'Sullivan, M., et al.: Severity of aortic regurgitation: Interstudy reproducibility of measurements with velocity-encoded cine MR imaging. Radiology 185:235, 1992.

77. Fleagle, S.R., Thedens, D.R., Stanford, W., et al.: Multicenter trial of automated border detection in cardiac MR imaging. J. Magn. Reson. Imaging 3:409, 1993.

CHAPTER

8 A Clinician's Perspective: The Place of Imaging in Cardiac Diagnosis

R. Joe Noble, M.D.

Authored in an editorial fashion by a clinician with no particular expertise or personal investment in any specific imaging technique, these remarks are intended to adumbrate a scheme for the use of, and to deal with the abuse of, cardiac imaging techniques in the diagnosis and management of patients with potential cardiovascular disease. Three prejudices on the part of the author should be acknowledged: first, his conviction that cardiovascular training programs over the past decade or so may have emphasized *tests*, both their performance and interpretation, at the expense of clinical decision-making based on history taking, physical examination, and clinical management. Second (perhaps as a consequence of the first) is the notion that testing is overdone in modern-day cardiology practice. Ordering tests would seem to compensate for a lack of clinical confidence.

These prejudices should not be misinterpreted as disparagements of the cardiac imaging currently available. On the contrary, an enormous amount of useful—even essential—information is provided by cardiac imaging techniques, much of it noninvasive. A standard echocardiogram can characterize much of the anatomic and functional state of the patient's heart and, with the addition of Doppler imaging, provide flow information as well. This information is provided at relatively low cost, at no risk, and in any conceivable clinical setting, including the outpatient office and the hospital. Portable cardiac imaging equipment is available to the intensive care unit; even mobile echocardiographic studies reach physicians and patients in many rural areas. The information provided by an echocardiogram is so useful that, rightly or wrongly, some cardiologists have substituted a standard echocardiogram for a standard chest radiograph in the evaluation of many cardiac patients. Similarly, characterization of myocardial perfusion with nuclear imaging techniques has proved indispensable to the functional assessment of many patients with ischemic heart disease.

The third prejudice is that the individual chapters in this book are penned by editors and authors who are rightfully acknowledged experts in their area of imaging, and who know the proper clinical utilization of the tests they describe. The *general comments* provided in this brief chapter must in no way supersede the *specific*

lessons taught in the chapters that follow. Other piquant prejudices will become evident with further reading.

Founded on experience with most of these techniques over the past many years, certain "rules" of utilization of imaging seem appropriate.

RULE NO. 1

Perhaps the most important, Rule No. 1 is that there are no rules. There are no blanket guidelines for ordering batteries of imaging tests for groups of patients with like illnesses. The individual physician must make a distinctive decision based on the specific patient with a unique illness and set of circumstances. Indeed, that is what physicians are paid to do. Parenthetically, the reader may query how a managed care organization could possibly dictate the proper selection of imaging techniques for the groups of patients under its management, but that is another question.

As an example, consider three elderly patients of identical age with identical classic symptoms of angina. The first patient looks his advanced age; he is sedentary and inactive; he has loud, long, high-pitched carotid bruits bilaterally and claudication whenever he does attempt to walk. No test of any sort is required to establish the diagnosis of coronary disease or to select medical therapy. The second patient, of identical age, has no concomitant illnesses and is moderately active. No imaging test is required for *diagnosis*, but, because of his advanced age, his physician would like to avoid intervention if possible. Prognostic information would be provided by an analysis of the *extent* of myocardial ischemia, best offered by a nuclear perfusion stress test. The third, equally elderly patient plays golf daily and would even like to continue with doubles tennis, but for the angina that persists in spite of aggressive medical treatment. Imaging tests short of visualization of the coronary anatomy would be superfluous to a decision on how best to intervene in a patient who has failed to respond to medical therapy, so the patient might best proceed directly to coronary cineangiography.

RULE NO. 2

The second guideline, probably of importance equal to the first, is that the cardiac images are not the final dictum on patient management. They are tests and tests only. Few are pathognomonic of a specific disease process. To rephrase, clinical decisions about specific patients are based not on tests but on the opinion of the expert clinician, derived from a painstaking history, a targeted physical examination, and an electrocardiogram. Then, the images or tests selected are those specifically designed to support or reject the clinical decision, never to dictate it. Testing is performed to answer specific clinical questions.

Indeed, when the information provided by the clinical image is at odds with the clinician's opinion, more often than not the good clinician is best advised to follow his or her clinical instincts rather than depend exclusively on the test. Thus, when the thallium-201 perfusion test report reads "normal" in a patient suspected of having severe coronary artery disease, the "normal" probably infers equal, though depressed, perfusion of all zones of myocardium fed by equally stenotic coronary arteries (multivessel disease). Retrospectively, this particular test should never have been ordered as a diagnostic test, since the clinician would have already decided on the need for coronary cineangiography; however, the test can be requested in order to provide functional information.

It is too easy to order a battery of tests on a reflex. Never is a select series of images or tests routinely indicated for any specific group of patients or disease processes. Instead, clinicians must ask what is it they need to know in order to make a good clinical decision. For instance, in a patient with suspected angina and a normal baseline electrocardiogram is the goal simply to establish the diagnosis of coronary disease? If so, stress electrocardiography will generally provide the answer. Is the extent of myocardial ischemia the question? A thallium-201 or sestamibi single-photon emission computed tomogram (SPECT) would best offer this information. Is it important to know the state of left ventricular function? An echocardiogram would provide this information, and stress echocardiography would also provide an approximation of perfusion and left ventricular dysfunction with ischemia. In addition, an assessment of resting ventricular function would be provided by a gated technetium-99m sestamibi perfusion scan or by a radionuclide ventriculogram; repeat studies following exercise provide direct or indirect information, respectively, about perfusion abnormalities.

RULE NO. 3

Despite these eristic comments, cardiac imaging can be decisive and helpful. So many cardiac imaging techniques have appeared and matured over the past 20 years that it is the rare clinician who can master all facets of these multiple techniques. Rule No. 3 states that good clinicians must be knowledgeable about those imaging techniques available to them.

Knowledge of an imaging technique implies more than familiarity with the procedure and results. The clinician ordering the test must know precisely what information can be provided by the image in a specific patient.

The clinician may pose the question, "Is the akinetic portion of the ventricle viable?" or, to rephrase, "May I reasonably expect a reversal of the myocardial dysfunction with either surgical or percutaneous revascularization?" The answer will not be provided by anatomic studies, that is, echocardiography, or coronary cineangiography and ventriculography. Positron emission tomography (PET) scanning, by demonstrating preserved metabolic activity, can detect viability; but this technique is relatively expensive and infrequently available to clinicians. Instead, thallium-201 scintigraphic distribution imaging after reinjection will accurately predict reversal of myocardial dysfunction with reperfusion. Transthoracic

or even transesophageal echocardiography with dobutamine infusion may play a role in this same determination.

For some specific disease processes, important correlates in diagnosis and prognosis have been derived with the use of some techniques but not others. Exercise radionuclide ventriculography (RNV) has been studied intensively, and specific guidelines have been developed for optimally timing operative intervention in patients with aortic regurgitation before irreversible left ventricular dilatation and dysfunction ensue. Consequently, radionuclide ventriculography is more helpful than a full cardiac catheterization in determining the date of surgery. Although other imaging techniques may provide useful information, the clinical correlates have not, as yet, been worked out to the degree that they have been with radionuclide ventriculography.

As another example that correlates imaging with prognosis, consider the preoperative risk assessment of the cardiac patient for noncardiac surgery. Generally, a history, a physical examination, and an electrocardiogram suffice to determine high or low risk. In patients with stable and mild angina, stress electrocardiography provides additional helpful information, and here the effort capacity of the patient is a better indicator of risk than any electrocardiographic change or, for that matter, thallium distribution on a scintigram. For patients who cannot exercise because of concomitant peripheral vascular or orthopedic disease, thallium-201 scintigraphy, pharmacologic (dobutamine or dipyridamole) echocardiography, and even ambulatory ischemia electrocardiographic monitoring are roughly equivalent in establishing perioperative risk. For patients who appear to be at high risk, and particularly those with angina despite intensive medical therapy, coronary angiography is required, without the additional preliminary testing.

Clinicians must know the potential shortcomings of the techniques that they request. Breast attenuation may preclude accurate measurement of apical perfusion with a thallium-201 scintigram, but this may be less of a problem with the technetium-99m sestamibi radioisotope. Interventricular septal hypoperfusion and septal wall motion abnormalities may inaccurately predict ischemia by thallium scintigraphy and echocardiography, respectively, in patients with left bundle branch block on the electrocardiogram; pharmacologic thallium-201 testing with dipyridamole or adenosine may improve on this diagnostic accuracy. Conversely, most clinicians believe that they can better judge the functional tolerance and prognosis of their patients with exercise rather than pharmacologic nuclear perfusion testing. An abnormal radionuclide ventriculogram seems to be less specific in the diagnosis of ischemia in women.

The safety of the pharmacologic agent infused is another consideration. The ordering physician must know that adenosine can provoke bronchospasm, and therefore it cannot be used in patients with asthma. Dipyridamole potentiates the action of adenosine, prolonging its activity, so adenosine is similarly contraindicated in patients receiving dipyridamole. By the same token, dipyridamole can induce or potentiate bronchospasm, and theophylline counteracts its behavior.

In other words, there is a great deal to be known about the specific sensitivity, specificity, diagnostic accuracy, and safety of each and all of the imaging techniques available.

RULE NO. 4

Rule No. 4 is probably one of those prejudices predicted in the introductory paragraphs. It is based on the axiom, "A picture is worth a thousand words." It may sound like "self-referral," but it is actually good medicine.

This clinician would opine that, according to Rule No. 4, when selecting specific imaging techniques, physicians should edge toward the techniques that they understand better, personally visualize, and hopefully interpret. The clinically responsible physician's personal visualization of an image supersedes the reading of another's report.

No doubt the numerical ejection fraction calculated by radionuclide ventriculography is quantitatively more accurate than that provided by cross-sectional echocardiography. However, for the physician who is responsible for managing a specific patient and who also understands echocardiography, actually visualizing that patient's ventricle on the monitor—noting the extent, degree, and distribution of hypokinesia and wall thickening and valve motion—is infinitely more meaningful than reading a number on a report. The view provides him or her with a qualitative aspect that should and does color clinical opinion and thus medical care.

Since more cardiologists are trained in echocardiography than in nuclear cardiology, it follows that more cardiologists will find useful information about the patient's ventricular size and function on an echocardiogram than on a radionuclide ventriculogram. For the cardiologists trained in nuclear cardiology, however, the reverse bias would pertain, in that viewing the multiple gated image acquisition analysis (MUGA) monitor would seem preferable. If the responsible physician is trained in neither, then this rule would not apply.

RULE NO. 5

Responsible physicians must investigate and learn the specificity, sensitivity, and diagnostic accuracy of the *laboratories* that they employ to perform the various cardiac imaging techniques. How accomplished are the technicians, how advanced the technology, and how talented the interpreter? Reading from a scientific manuscript that imaging technique A picked up 3 percent more of diagnosis X than technique B is of little solace if, in a given community, laboratory A employs poorly trained technicians to use an outdated instrument to record a poor-quality image interpreted by one not properly trained to do so.

The selection process between stress echocardiography and stress nuclear scintigraphy comes to mind when one applies this dictum. Indeed, the capability of the respective laboratories may be the only differentiating factor in the selection between two equally efficacious imaging techniques in the diagnosis of coronary disease.

Properly utilized, cardiac imaging has improved and will unequivocally continue to improve on our ability to manage patients with cardiovascular disease. A tremendous amount of information has been learned, and this information cannot remain the province of the imagers alone. Clinicians must share in this knowledge explosion if they hope to best represent their patients when ordering tests.

Recall that cardiac imaging is not static. Cardiac magnetic resonance imaging (MRI) is in its infancy; rapid advances in utilization of this technique are expected. Daily we learn more about the applicability of the available techniques, and there seems to be no doubt that in the near future, the currently available and new imaging techniques will provide additional information concerning myocardial metabolism and molecular biology. Positron emission tomography, single-photon emission computed tomography, and magnetic resonance imaging all provide some of this information even now. Abnormal tissue—that is, myocardial scar, myocardial infiltration with amyloid, and an abnormal myocardial architecture such as the septal abnormalities in hypertrophic cardiomyopathy—will be better characterized with the use of existing ultrasound and nuclear magnetic resonance technology as well as new techniques.

Imagers and clinicians, sharing technical and clinical experience such as that described in the text that follows, will continue to provide the most accurate, cost-effective testing necessary for optimal patient care.

CHAPTER

9 Coronary Artery Disease

Heinrich R. Schelbert, M.D.

DETECTION OF CORONARY ARTERY
   DISEASE ____ 81
Myocardial Blood Flow Imaging ____ 81
Dobutamine Stress Echocardiography ____ 81
Other Imaging Approaches ____ 82
CONSEQUENCES OF CORONARY ARTERY
   DISEASE ____ 82

Acute Myocardial Infarction ____ 82
Chronic Coronary Artery Disease ____ 83
   Radionuclide Approaches ____ 83
   Two-Dimensional Echocardiography ____ 83
SUMMARY AND CONCLUSIONS ____ 83

History taking and physical examination in the patient suspected of having coronary artery disease remain central to the diagnostic process. Coronary angiography, on the other hand, has retained its final role in determining the absence or presence of coronary artery disease. Whether a patient proceeds directly to angiography depends largely on the pretest probability of coronary artery disease as a function of age, gender, coronary risk factors, electrocardiographic findings, and symptomatology. Patients at both ends of the spectrum of pretest probability are unlikely to gain significantly from cardiac imaging approaches other than coronary angiography. For example, regardless of its outcome, an imaging procedure will have little, if any, effect on the post-test probability in a patient with a very high pretest or, conversely, with a very low pretest probability. Imaging approaches discriminate best between the absence and the presence of coronary artery disease in patients with intermediate pretest probabilities.[1] Yet, findings with imaging approaches often serve as measures of the extent and severity of coronary artery disease, contain prognostic information, permit an assessment of the consequences of coronary lesions on regional and global left ventricular blood flow and contractile function, and, thus, may decisively affect the therapeutic approach. This chapter seeks to discuss how best to utilize various imaging modalities ranging from ultrasound to radionuclide approaches, fast x-ray computed tomography (CT), and magnetic resonance imaging (MRI) for the detection of coronary artery disease, for characterizing its extent and severity, and for assessing the consequences of coronary lesions on regional myocardial blood flow and contractile function.

DETECTION OF CORONARY ARTERY DISEASE

As mentioned previously, history taking and physical examination remain essential steps in the diagnostic process. Most patients continue to undergo electrocardiographic stress testing, yet, because of its limited sensitivity and specificity this test is frequently

Dr. Schelbert is affiliated with the Laboratory of Structural Biology and Molecular Medicine, operated for the U.S. Department of Energy by the University of California under Contract #DE-AC03-76-SF00012. This work was supported in part by the Director of the Office of Energy Research, Office of Health and Environmental Research, Washington D.C., by Research Grants #HL 29845 and #HL 33177, National Institutes of Health, Bethesda, MD, and by an Investigative Group Award by the Greater Los Angeles Affiliate of the American Heart Association, Los Angeles, CA.

combined with an imaging test. Foremost among such imaging tests is myocardial blood flow imaging with thallium-201 (^{201}Tl)–labeled or, more recently, technetium-99m (^{99m}Tc)–labeled tracers of blood flow, such as ^{99m}Tc-sestamibi or ^{99m}Tc-tetrofosmin. Alternatively, an assessment of regional contractile function may be obtained with two-dimensional echocardiography before, during, and after exercise or during pharmacologic stress, for example, with intravenous dobutamine.

Myocardial Blood Flow Imaging

Both types of radiotracers, that is, ^{201}Tl- and ^{99m}Tc-labeled compounds offer comparably high diagnostic accuracies.[2] Separation of a stress-induced flow defect from a permanent one resulting from scar tissue formation requires delayed or redistribution imaging or reinjection of ^{201}Tl, while ^{99m}Tc compounds necessitate two separate tracer injections and imaging sessions, one at rest and another one during stress. More recent approaches employ both, ^{201}Tl for imaging resting myocardial blood flow and ^{99m}Tc-labeled compounds for imaging stress myocardial blood flow in the same patient.[3] In patients unable to exercise, pharmacologic stress testing with intravenous dipyridamole or adenosine is readily available without any loss in diagnostic accuracy.[2] Low-dose dobutamine may be equally effective for the detection of coronary artery disease with myocardial perfusion imaging; the approach may prove useful when vasodilators are contraindicated.

As an extension of radionuclide techniques, blood flow imaging with positron emission tomography (PET) offers a higher sensitivity and, especially, specificity, as it overcomes technical limitations such as scatter and attenuation of photons associated with the conventional planar or with single-photon emission computed tomography (SPECT) imaging. When both SPECT and PET imaging are available, PET appears of particular value in patients with only a modest pretest probability, in patients with probably mild coronary artery disease, and in patients prone to having image artifacts on SPECT, such as obese patients and women.

Dobutamine Stress Echocardiography

The use of incremental doses of intravenous dobutamine produces a β-receptor–mediated increase in regional contractile function and thus in myocardial oxygen demand. Such an increase may be impaired in the presence of coronary artery disease. Attenuated responses in systolic wall motion, or wall thickening, or both, or even deterioration of regional contractile function yields diagnostic accuracies that equal those achieved with radionuclide techniques.[4, 5] At the same time, patients may not always tolerate the maximal dobutamine doses needed to attain the highest accuracy. Thus, both ultrasound and radionuclide techniques may be complementary in some patients. In other patients, when transthoracic echocardiography yields diagnostically inadequate images, again radionuclide myocardial blood flow imaging may serve as an alternative, although other laboratories advocate the use of transesophageal stress echocardiography.[4, 6, 7]

Despite these complementary roles, both approaches to the detection of disease are largely competitive because they offer comparable diagnostic accuracies. Unless echocardiographic images are analyzed quantitatively, their evaluation for stress-induced changes may depend to some extent on the observer and his or her skills. While this also applies to radionuclide approaches, large databases of normal perfusion exist, so estimates of the extent and severity of flow defects and, thus, of the extent of coronary artery disease are relatively operator independent. Also, acquisition of diagnostically adequate images may not always be possible with echocardiography. On the other hand, echocardiography offers greater flexibility, that is, measurements can be made repeatedly and in real time. Thus, it appears that the use of one technique over the other at a given institution depends largely on the skills and diagnostic acumen of the personnel performing such studies. Relative to stress echocardiography as a comparative newcomer, a vast body of knowledge exists for myocardial blood flow imaging, especially with ^{201}Tl, which to some extent can be extrapolated to imaging with ^{99m}Tc-labeled compounds. Criteria exist that carry considerable prognostic information, especially for ^{201}Tl imaging. For example, increased lung uptake, multiple stress-induced flow defects, or a postexercise enlargement of the left ventricular cavity on thallium imaging identifies the high-risk patient who requires aggressive management, compared with the patient in whom perfusion imaging predicts a generally favorable prognosis and whose treatment may be, for the most part, medical.[2]

Other Imaging Approaches

While a number of imaging techniques, such as radionuclide ventriculography, have been largely abandoned for diagnosing the presence of coronary artery disease, other promising techniques are emerging. These include gated MRI and fast CT during physical and pharmacologic stress, using regional contractile function or tissue blood flow, or both, as delineated with contrast agents. Fast CT demonstrates coronary calcification and, thus, disease of the coronary artery wall. Although calcifications per se do not indicate hemodynamically significant coronary artery disease, their presence may be established with a "quantitative calcium score." Conversely, some investigators propose that the absence of calcifications rules out the presence of coronary artery disease.[8] Moreover, it now appears possible that MRI and echocardiography can visualize significant coronary stenoses located mostly in the proximal segments of the large epicardial vessels. Early results suggest that it may indeed become possible to measure coronary flow velocities entirely noninvasively with transesophageal echocardiography or with MRI. If such measurement is accomplished, this technique would offer noninvasive indices of the severity of coronary stenoses.[9, 10]

Last, traditional as well as most evolving technologies identify coronary artery disease via a regional luminal narrowing or its resulting regional abnormalities in blood flow or function. Yet, coronary disease may begin or, as in the case of transplant vasculopathy, manifest itself in the form of diffuse intimal thickening. Therefore, vascular abnormalities may, in fact, be detectable only with intravascular ultrasound, while all or most other imaging approaches, including coronary angiography, may remain within normal limits.

CONSEQUENCES OF CORONARY ARTERY DISEASE

Subtotal or complete occlusion of a coronary artery that develops over a period of years or occurs suddenly may result in a severe reduction in coronary blood flow at rest that is accompanied by an impairment or a cessation of regional contractile function. If resting coronary flow declines progressively over a prolonged period, the myocardium affected may down-regulate its function and "hibernate." Yet, if flow becomes compromised too severely, myocardium may sustain an irreversible injury and be replaced with scar tissue. In contrast, a sudden coronary occlusion may result in an acute myocardial infarction. Besides standard clinical findings, imaging techniques can be essential for characterizing the severity of the ischemic insult, for establishing the need for additional interventions, or for devising the course of therapy.

Acute Myocardial Infarction

Given the vast array of clinical and laboratory tests, the diagnosis of acute myocardial infarction usually poses little, if any, difficulties or challenges. Yet, difficulties may arise when the amount of infarcted myocardium is small or when the patient presents to the clinician late during the postinfarction period. In such instances, the presence of regional wall motion abnormalities on radionuclide angiography or on echocardiography or of a blood flow defect on radionuclide imaging may offer confirmatory evidence. These techniques may also be used for defining the location, if unidentifiable by electrocardiographic criteria, and, more importantly, the extent or amount of "infarcted myocardium." The latter seems to be accomplished most accurately with SPECT myocardial perfusion imaging. Yet, it must be remembered that neither of these approaches is specific for an acute event. In such a case, the use of radiolabeled antimyosin specific antibodies or of ^{99m}Tc-pyrophosphate discriminates an acute event from a chronic one. If coronary thrombolysis has been instituted, the questions facing the clinician include the following: (1) Has coronary blood flow been restored and myocardium been salvaged? (2) Does a residual stenosis persist that requires revascularization? and (3) If thrombolysis has not been instituted, did enough myocardium survive the ischemic insult so that interventional revascularization may restore contractile function?

Myocardial perfusion imaging with either ^{201}Tl or ^{99m}Tc compounds represents the most direct approach to assessing the restoration of blood flow at rest. Similarly, administration of ^{99m}Tc-labeled compounds, such as sestamibi, prior to the institution of any therapy in acute infarct patients "freezes" images of the myocardium at risk, which can be imaged several hours later. Comparison with images obtained several days or weeks later offers an assessment of how much myocardium has been salvaged.[11] Assessment of wall motion at rest with echocardiography early after thrombolysis may be of limited value, as reperfused myocardium may still be "stunned." On the other hand, responses in regional wall motion or wall thickening to low-dose dobutamine as seen on echocardiography may, in fact, be highly accurate in identifying stunned, and thus salvageable, myocardium.[12, 13]

Short of direct coronary angiography, both radionuclide techniques and echocardiography may identify the persistence of the residual stenosis. Moderate-level exercise or dobutamine may result in a new or larger perfusion defect, an attenuated response, or even deterioration of regional wall motion.

Similarly, both approaches appear suited to the identification of viable myocardium in the infarct zone. Resolution or improvement of a ^{201}Tl defect from the immediate postinjection period to the delayed images indicates the presence of viable myocardium as well as its extent, although the absence of redistribution does not necessarily establish the presence of only scar tissue. In this case, metabolic imaging with PET and ^{18}F-deoxyglucose or ^{11}C-acetate may establish the presence of viable myocardium and its amount and, thus, serve as a guide for patient management.[14] Echocardiography at rest may be useful in demonstrating residual wall thickening or wall motion as signs of viability.[12] The more severe the wall motion impairment, the less likely the presence of viable myocardium. Yet, echocardiography during dobutamine stress rather than at rest is more accurate in identifying viable myocardium. An added advantage of echocardiography, which applies also to planar radionuclide imaging, is that it can be performed at the bedside and, thus, in the safe environment of the coronary care unit.

The latter reason limits the use of MRI and fast CT in the acute infarct patient. As an evolving technique, ultrasound with echogenic bubbles used as a contrast agent may be of future utility in assessing the degree of residual blood flow and the degree to which blood flow has been restored. While currently limited to retrograde left ventricular or aortic root injections, the intravenous use of sonicated albumin microbubbles may, in fact, become feasible.[15]

Both echocardiography and equilibrium blood pool imaging are suitable for following regional and global left ventricular function in postinfarction patients. Such follow-up, especially in patients with relatively large infarctions, seems critical for identifying ventricular remodeling as well as for institution of adequate pharmacologic management. The fact that radionuclide angiocardiography does not depend on assumptions regarding the left ventricular geometry favors its use over echocardiography as being the more accurate approach to global left ventricular function, although echocardiography is more useful in assessing regional function. Competing with both approaches are MRI and fast CT. Both offer accurate measures of chamber sizes, regional and global systolic wall motion, and wall thickening and myocardial mass.

Chronic Coronary Artery Disease

The potential reversibility of sustained regional impairments of contractile function has been well established. Such reversible impairment may result from "stunning," "hibernation," or "repetitive stunning." The clinical challenge is to distinguish such reversibility from the nonreversibility of myocardial necrosis and scar tissue formation. Identification of such potentially irreversible impairment of contractile function, defined also as myocardial viability, is especially critical in patients with poor left ventricular function and congestive heart failure. The therapeutic choices range from pharmacologic management to revascularization and cardiac transplantation. These choices underscore the importance of the search for viability, since donor hearts are limited and the cost of cardiac transplantation is high and because revascularization in such patients is associated with a high perioperative morbidity and mortality. Identification of adequate amounts of viable myocardium affects the risk-to-benefit ratio of revascularization and heralds a potential improvement in global left ventricular function, congestive heart failure symptoms, and long-term survival.

Radionuclide Approaches

Traditionally, ^{201}Tl redistribution imaging has been used to search for viable myocardium. Yet, it has become clear that the conventional approach overestimates the amount of necrosis or scar tissue. The addition of tracer reinjection has markedly improved the performance of the ^{201}Tl approach.[16] The PET metabolic imaging approach has been explored and tested rather extensively, especially in patients with poor left ventricular function.[17] The value of identifying the presence and amount of metabolically active yet dysfunctional and hypoperfused myocardium as a predictor of a postrevascularization improvement in global left ventricular function has been well established. The method also identifies high-risk patients and patients who are likely to benefit most from revascularization in terms of improved survival and quality of life.[18] While the ^{201}Tl approach and its modifications generally perform well, metabolism imaging with PET appears to be superior in patients with very poor left ventricular function. This is not because of conceptual limitations of the ^{201}Tl technique but rather because of the higher spatial and contrast resolution of PET and, thus, diagnostically superior images. Among the various radionuclide approaches, adequate information on the long-term outcome of global left ventricular function, clinical symptoms, and long-term survival exists primarily for the PET technique; it is still largely missing for the more traditional ^{201}Tl approach.

Two-Dimensional Echocardiography

This imaging modality is gaining some acceptance as an alternative approach for the assessment of myocardial viability. Thus far, segment-to-segment comparisons between dobutamine echocardiography, ^{201}Tl imaging, PET blood flow metabolism patterns support the utility of dobutamine echocardiography as a possible alternative or true competitor to radionuclide imaging techniques. Missing are long-term outcomes of follow-up studies after revascularization in patients studied with dobutamine stress echocardiography. Currently available data suggest a high specificity but moderate sensitivity for dobutamine echocardiography in the detection of viable myocardium.[19–21]

Considering the evolution of dobutamine echocardiography, it appears that the approach will compete with the traditional, well-established and validated radionuclide ^{201}Tl approach and with the metabolic PET approach. On the other hand, it seems that the radionuclide techniques remain superior in affording estimates of the amount of viable myocardium. This information, in turn, is useful for predicting the gain in global left ventricular function and improvement in clinical symptomatology following revascularization. Yet, as is the case with detection of coronary artery disease, it is anticipated that the locally available skills, experience, and instrumentation will largely determine which test serves to identify the presence of myocardial viability at a given institution. Only if studies are technically inadequate or the results equivocal will echocardiography and radionuclide techniques be complementary.

Additional approaches for the assessment of myocardial viability are available, although they are less well established and are in a state of evolution. While the role of radionuclide imaging with ^{99m}Tc-sestamibi as well as that of radioiodinated fatty acids remains to be defined, the use of ^{18}F-deoxyglucose with conventional SPECT imaging approaches appears promising and encouraging.[22] There are also potential roles for gated MRI and fast CT. Wall thickness and the degree of impairment of wall motion and thickening offer some information on viability, which may be further supplemented with responses to dobutamine stimulation. Similarly, magnetic resonance spectroscopy or ultrasonic tissue characterization may offer additional information on the status of myocardial tissue and its metabolism and, thus, on myocardial viability.

SUMMARY AND CONCLUSIONS

History taking and physical examination remain critical in the diagnostic process of identifying the presence of coronary artery disease and in assessing its effects on global and regional contractile function. Also, coronary angiography continues to be the final arbiter in documenting the presence of coronary artery disease. Various other imaging techniques contribute significantly to the diagnostic process in the choice of the most appropriate and efficacious treatment. Foremost, at present, are radionuclide techniques, including SPECT and PET, and rest and stress echocardiography. Both general approaches are largely competitive. At times, when results are equivocal or when technically limited, both approaches may be complementary. Thus, it appears that local experience, skills, test availability, and diagnostic acumen as well as cost considerations largely determine which modality will be employed in a specific patient with a particular condition.

Acknowledgment

The author appreciates Eileen Rosenfeld's assistance in preparing this manuscript.

References

1. Turner, D., Battle, W., Deshmukh, H., et al.: The predictive value of myocardial perfusion scintigraphy after stress in patients without previous myocardial infarction. J. Nucl. Med. 19:249, 1978.
2. Maddahi, J., Rodrigues, E., Berman, D., et al.: State-of-the-art myocardial perfusion imaging. Cardiol. Clin. 12:199, 1994.
3. Berman, D., Kiat, H., Friedman, J., et al.: Separate acquisition rest thallium-201/ stress technetium-99m sestamibi dual-isotope myocardial perfusion single-photon emission computed tomography: A clinical validation study. J. Am. Coll. Cardiol. 22:1455, 1993.
4. Mairesse, G., Marwick, T., Vanoverschelde, J.-L. J., et al.: How accurate is dobutamine stress electrocardiography for detection of coronary artery disease? J. Am. Coll. Cardiol. 24:920, 1994.
5. Segar, D., Brown, S., Sawada, S., et al.: Dobutamine stress echocardiography: Correlation with coronary lesion severity as determined by quantitative angiography. J. Am. Coll. Cardiol. 19:1197, 1992.
6. Marwick, T., D'Hondt, A., Baudhuin, T., et al.: Optimal use of dobutamine stress for the detection and evaluation of coronary artery disease: Combination with echocardiography or scintigraphy, or both? J. Am. Coll. Cardiol. 22:159, 1993.
7. Frohwein, S., Klein, J., Lane, A., et al.: Transesophageal dobutamine stress echocardiography in the evaluation of coronary artery disease. J. Am. Coll. Cardiol. 24:823, 1995.
8. Wong, N., Vo, A., Abrahamson, D., et al.: Detection of coronary artery calcium by ultrafast computed tomography and its relation to clinical evidence of coronary artery disease. Am. J. Cardiol. 73:223, 1994.
9. Manning, W., Li, W., and Edelman, R.: A preliminary report comparing magnetic resonance coronary angiography with conventional angiography. N. Engl. J. Med. 328:828, 1993.
10. Tardif, J., Vannan, M., Taylor, K., et al.: Delineation of extended lengths of coronary arteries by multiplane transesophageal echocardiography. J. Am. Coll. Cardiol. 24:909, 1994.
11. Gibbons, R.: Perfusion imaging with ^{99m}Tc-sestamibi for the assessment of myocardial area at risk and the efficacy of acute treatment in myocardial infarction. Circulation 84:I37, 1991.
12. Watada, H., Ito, H., Oh, H., et al.: Dobutamine stress echocardiography predicts reversible dysfunction and quantitates the extent of irreversibly damaged myocardium after reperfusion of anterior myocardial infarction. J. Am. Coll. Cardiol. 24:624, 1994.
13. Salustri, A., Elhendy, A., Garyfallydis, P., et al.: Prediction of improvement of ventricular function after first acute myocardial infarction using low-dose dobutamine stress echocardiography. Am. J. Cardiol. 74:853, 1994.
14. Czernin, J., Porenta, G., Brunken, R., et al.: Regional blood flow, oxidative metabolism, and glucose utilization in patients with recent myocardial infarction. Circulation 88:884, 1993.
15. Skyba, D., Jayaweera, A., Goodman, N., et al.: Quantification of myocardial perfusion with myocardial contrast echocardiography during left atrial injection of contrast: Implications for venous injection. Circulation 90:1513, 1994.
16. Dilsizian, V., Rocco, T., Freedman, N., et al.: Enhanced detection of ischemic but viable myocardium by the reinjection of thallium after stress-redistribution imaging. N. Engl. J. Med. 323:141, 1990.
17. Schelbert, H.: Merits and limitations of radionuclide approaches to viability and future developments. J. Nucl. Cardiol. 1:S86, 1994.
18. Di Carli, M., Davidson, M., Little, R., et al.: Value of metabolic imaging with positron emission tomography for evaluating prognosis in patients with coronary artery disease and left ventricular dysfunction. Am. J. Cardiol. 73:527, 1994.
19. Cigarroa, C., deFilippi, R., Brickner, E., et al.: Dobutamine stress echocardiography identifies hibernating myocardium and predicts recovery of left ventricular function after coronary revascularization. Circulation 88:430, 1993.
20. Afridi, I., Kleiman, N., Raizner, A., et al.: Dobutamine echocardiography in myocardial hibernation: Optimal dose and accuracy in predicting recovery of ventricular function after coronary angioplasty. Circulation 91:663, 1995.
21. Mariani, M., Palagi, C., Donatelli, F., et al.: Identification of hibernating myocardium: A comparison between dobutamine echocardiography and study of perfusion and metabolism in patients with severe left ventricular dysfunction. Am. J. Card. Imaging 9:1, 1995.
22. Burt, R., Perkins, O., Oppenheim, B., et al.: Direct comparison of fluorine-18–FDG SPECT, fluorine-18–FDG PET and rest thallium-201 SPECT for detection of myocardial viability. J. Nucl. Med. 36:176, 1995.

CHAPTER

10 Valvular Heart Disease

Bruce H. Brundage, M.D.

AORTIC VALVE DISEASE _____ 84
Aortic Valve Stenosis _____ 84
Aortic Valve Regurgitation _____ 85
MITRAL VALVE DISEASE _____ 85
Mitral Valve Stenosis _____ 85
Mitral Valve Regurgitation _____ 85

TRICUSPID VALVE DISEASE _____ 86
Tricuspid Valve Stenosis _____ 86
Tricuspid Valve Regurgitation _____ 86
PULMONARY VALVE DISEASE _____ 86
PROSTHETIC VALVES _____ 86
SUMMARY _____ 86

History taking, physical examination, and electrocardiography are very useful in the assessment of valvular heart disease, but the evaluation is incomplete without cardiac imaging. Indeed, in most cases the imaging information is critical in planning the appropriate management of the disease. Multiple methods for imaging the heart are available to the clinician: chest roentgenography, cardiac catheterization with angiography, Doppler echocardiography, radioisotope imaging, magnetic resonance imaging (MRI), fast computed tomography (CT), and positron emission tomography (PET). Fast CT largely represents experience with electron-beam CT but, on occasion, can represent spiral CT capabilities as well. This chapter puts the use of cardiac imaging in the evaluation of valvular heart disease into perspective by indicating which imaging techniques are essential for each type of valvular abnormality; which are competing when two or more modalities provide similar information and there is controversy as to which one or ones are the best; and which are complementary (nice to have) but are not essential. Also highlighted are unresolved issues in which further development of imaging modalities is required to improve the management of valvular heart disease.

AORTIC VALVE DISEASE

Aortic Valve Stenosis

Stenosis of the aortic valve is usually not a difficult diagnosis to make because of the rather obvious findings on physical examination. However, once the diagnosis is suspected, imaging techniques play a very important role in determining severity and planning treatment. The initial evaluation certainly includes a posteroanterior and lateral chest roentgenogram. Evidence of congestive heart failure indicates a need for urgent evaluation and therapy. Heavy valve calcification, usually only seen on the lateral film, suggests that the stenosis is hemodynamically significant.[1]

Echocardiography of the aortic valve with Doppler assessment of the valve gradient has become essential in the evaluation of aortic valve stenosis.[2] The reliability of the gradient measurement is good enough that no further evaluation is usually necessary if the gradient is clinically insignificant. Large gradients warranting valve replacement are also reliably determined, and the main reason for cardiac catheterization is to perform coronary angiography. If there is no indication for coronary angiography, many clinicians believe that cardiac catheterization is unnecessary in patients with isolated aortic valve stenosis.[3]

With the development of high spatial and temporal resolution tomographic techniques, MRI and fast CT now provide very precise measurements of left ventricular mass, so these imaging methods may find an increasing role in monitoring the effects of aortic valve stenosis on the ventricle before and after valve replacement.[4, 5] These two imaging methods also provide very accurate three-dimensional measurements of the aortic root size, which is of some interest to the cardiovascular surgeon. However, echocardiographic measurements are usually of sufficient accuracy to make those by more expensive techniques unnecessary.

Imaging is a very important part of the evaluation of the patient with aortic stenosis. In the majority of cases, the chest roentgenogram, Doppler echocardiography, and coronary angiography provide all that is essential in managing the patient and for making all clinical decisions. Current state of the art and science leaves few unanswered questions.

Aortic Valve Regurgitation

For decades, the chest roentgenogram has been a useful imaging method for evaluating patients with aortic regurgitation. Assessment of left ventricular size is reasonably good with this technique, and left ventricular volume is an important predictor of prognosis.[6] The chest roentgenogram is still a useful and inexpensive method for following patients with aortic valve regurgitation.

Without question, Doppler echocardiography has become the primary method for evaluating patients with aortic valve regurgitation. Color flow Doppler techniques provide a reasonably good assessment of the severity of the regurgitation.[7, 8] Echocardiographic imaging of the aortic valve and root often can define the etiology of the regurgitation, such as identifying vegetations. Also, echocardiographic imaging can define the degree of ventricular enlargement and hypertrophy as well as determine the state of ventricular function, an important predictor of outcome.[9]

Radioisotope left ventricular angiography has been recommended as a method for following the state of left ventricular function in patients with aortic valve regurgitation.[10] Accurate measurement of left ventricular ejection fraction at rest and during exercise is possible with this imaging technique. Some clinical investigators have suggested that early detection of left ventricular dysfunction may be possible and is useful in determining when surgical intervention is necessary.[11]

Prior to aortic valve replacement, many patients undergo cardiac catheterization, although little additional information is obtained beyond that provided by coronary angiography. Patients with isolated aortic valve regurgitation probably do not need cardiac catheterization if coronary angiography is not indicated.

A chest roentgenogram and Doppler echocardiography are required in most patients with aortic valve regurgitation. Exercise nuclear angiography may be helpful in planning the timing of surgical valve replacement, although some investigators have indicated that the left ventricular volume measurements at rest are as good in guiding the timing of surgery.[12]

In some cases of aortic valve regurgitation, quantitation is problematic. Fast CT and MRI can provide accurate measurements of regurgitant fraction and left ventricular volume and mass.[4, 5, 13, 14] Occasionally, in some patients these tomographic imaging methods may be clinically useful in assessing the severity of the regurgitation.

In spite of major advances in the evaluation of aortic valve regurgitation by echocardiography, Doppler, and radioisotope methods, the timing of surgery can still be problematic in the asymptomatic or minimally symptomatic patient. Serial imaging is very helpful, but the search for a reliable sign of early but reversible left ventricular dysfunction goes on. Possibly, MRI or fast CT may provide more precise and accurate measurements of left ventricular stress-strain relationships. Even if such measurement is possible, however, there is no guarantee that such information will produce better clinical decisions. Perhaps improved understanding of myocardial metabolism will be provided by PET or magnetic resonance spectroscopy (MRS) and elucidate markers of early myocyte metabolic dysfunction.[15] Clearly, more insights are needed to assist the clinician in deciding when to operate on some patients with aortic valve regurgitation; future developments in imaging may provide some of the answers.

MITRAL VALVE DISEASE

Mitral Valve Stenosis

History taking and physical examination provide a large amount of information about the patient with mitral valve stenosis. The chest roentgenogram is a valuable adjunct. Beyond identifying left atrial enlargement, signs of pulmonary venous hypertension, chronic pulmonary edema, and pulmonary arterial hypertension nearly always indicate the need for surgical intervention. Doppler echocardiography provides critical information about the mitral valve gradient, the presence of left atrial thrombus, and the anatomy of the mitral valve apparatus, all necessary in the planning of surgery or balloon valvuloplasty.[16] Traditionally, cardiac catheterization has been performed before any planned intervention. However, many have challenged the need for catheterization in uncomplicated mitral valve stenosis.[17] In many cases, cardiac catheterization adds no additional information beyond that provided by the history, physical examination, electrocardiogram, chest roentgenogram, and Doppler echocardiogram study.

Fast CT and MRI can often provide excellent images of the mitral valve apparatus, define cardiac chamber size, measure myocardial mass, and detect the presence of left atrial thrombus. However, in most cases the echocardiographic images are of sufficient resolution that all necessary clinical decisions can be made. Occasionally, these more expensive and labor-intensive techniques are needed to clarify some particular issue, such as the presence of a left atrial appendage thrombus.[18] However, transesophageal echocardiography can also be used for this particular purpose.[19]

High resolution three-dimensional images of the mitral apparatus may help to better indicate which treatment choice is best: valve replacement, surgical valvuloplasty, or balloon valvuloplasty. Fast CT, MRI, and computer-processed echocardiographic images all have the potential for providing better definition of the mitral valve, chordae tendineae, and papillary muscles.

Mitral Valve Regurgitation

The chest roentgenogram is of some assistance in the evaluation of chronic mitral regurgitation but is of less help in acute mitral regurgitation. The greater the size of the left ventricle, the greater the regurgitant volume as long as ventricular contractility is reasonably well preserved. The relative low cost and ready availability of the chest film are additional features that preserve its place in the evaluation of the patient with mitral regurgitation.

Doppler echocardiography has achieved a central role in the evaluation of this lesion, as it has with other valvular abnormalities.[16] Assessment of left ventricular ejection fraction and end-systolic and end-diastolic volumes is key to planning the patient's management. Color flow Doppler imaging is useful in estimating the amount of regurgitation, and echocardiographic images of the valve structure may provide insights into the etiology, such as myxomatous changes with chordal rupture. Increasingly, Doppler echocardiography is replacing cardiac catheterization in the evaluation of mitral regurgitation. Catheterization is reserved for coronary arteriography, when indicated, and in the assessment of multivalvular disease.

As with aortic regurgitation, nuclear angiography has been of some value in serially assessing ventricular function in patients with mitral regurgitation, helping the clinician to decide when to recommend surgical treatment.[20]

The new tomographic imaging techniques, MRI and fast CT, can provide very accurate measurements of the regurgitant volume in patients with an isolated mitral leak. Accurate determinations of left ventricular mass and volume are also possible with these techniques, but there are no clinical studies that demonstrate that this information improves the management of patients. Clinicians are still greatly concerned about when to operate on asymptomatic or minimally symptomatic patients, fearing that waiting until symptoms occur in some cases may result in irreversible left ventricular dysfunction. Assessments with MRI and fast CT do not appear to have resolved this dilemma.

In recent years, surgeons have increasingly employed primary mitral valve repair instead of valve replacement in the treatment of mitral regurgitation. The success of the surgery is dependent largely on mitral valve anatomy. Improved imaging of the valve with echocardiography, transthoracically and transesophageally, has helped the surgeon in preoperative planning and intraoperative management. Three-dimensional imaging of the valve with echocardiography, MRI, and fast CT may provide the surgeon with additional insights in the future.

TRICUSPID VALVE DISEASE

Tricuspid Valve Stenosis

The decreasing incidence of rheumatic fever has made tricuspid valve stenosis very uncommon in the Western world. Other causes, such as carcinoid syndrome, are rare. When tricuspid valve stenosis is suspected, Doppler echocardiography provides the best initial evaluation.[21] Cardiac catheterization may be helpful in deciding when the obstruction is severe enough to warrant surgical treatment. There is little experience with the use of the newer imaging techniques, MRI and fast CT.

Tricuspid Valve Regurgitation

After the physical examination, the best method of evaluating tricuspid regurgitation is Doppler echocardiography. Other imaging modalities, including cardiac angiography, provide little additional information. Magnetic resonance imaging and fast CT can provide excellent images of the tricuspid pathology, such as Ebstein's anomaly, but echocardiographic images are sufficient in the majority of cases.[22] Surgical treatment is usually deferred until there are significant symptoms because a good surgical result is sometimes difficult to achieve. If the surgeon could be assured that valvuloplasty is feasible, surgical intervention might occur sooner in some patients. Better image resolution of the valve anatomy, particularly the leaflet body, would be helpful in this decision-making.

PULMONARY VALVE DISEASE

Most pulmonary valve disease is congenital in origin. The chest roentgenogram is helpful in confirming the pathologic nature of a pulmonic ejection systolic murmur. However, Doppler echocardiography provides the best noninvasive evaluation.[23] Valve anatomy and gradient can usually be deduced. In isolated pulmonic valve stenosis, cardiac catheterization provides little additional information. Whether MRI and fast CT will be of use remains unproven.

PROSTHETIC VALVES

The development of two-dimensional echocardiography and Doppler imaging has assisted the clinician greatly in the evaluation of prosthetic heart valves.[24] Transesophageal echocardiography has further improved assessment.[25] Cardiac angiography is often employed and still makes important contributions to the evaluation in some patients. Cineradiography can be very useful in the evaluation of metal-plastic valve prostheses. The technique can be performed quickly, without the use of contrast medium, and is particularly useful in emergency situations.[26] However, in a few cases these imaging techniques fall short, and on occasion MRI and fast CT have provided unique and clinically significant information, usually detecting a previously unrecognized myocardial abscess.[27] Patients with metallic valves and those with suspected valve dehiscence should not undergo MRI. There is still an occasional case in which all imaging modalities fail to provide the complete assessment of a prosthetic heart valve; therefore, further improvements in image resolution, largely through the reduction of artifacts, are needed.

SUMMARY

Imaging plays a critical role in the diagnosis and staging of valvular heart disease. Doppler echocardiography has become the cornerstone of the imaging evaluation. More and more, cardiac catheterization is being reserved only for patients who require coronary angiography. New developments in MRI, fast CT, and PET may further improve the assessment of patients with valvular disease by providing better information about valve anatomy and the state of myocardial contractility to assist the clinician in determining the appropriate time for surgical intervention.

References

1. Glancy, D. L., Freed, T. A., O'Brien, K. P., et al.: Calcium in the aortic valve: Roentgenologic and hemodynamic correlations in 148 patients. Ann. Intern. Med. 71:245, 1969.
2. Currie, P. J., Seward, J. B., Reeder, G. S., et al.: Continuous-wave Doppler echocardiographic assessment of severity of calcific aortic stenosis: A simultaneous Doppler-catheter correlative study in 100 adult patients. Circulation 71:1162, 1985.
3. Miller, F. A.: Aortic stenosis: Most cases no longer require invasive hemodynamic study. J. Am. Coll. Cardiol. 13:551, 1989.
4. Maddahi, J., Crues, J., Berman, D. S., et al.: Noninvasive quantification of left ventricular myocardial mass by gated proton nuclear magnetic resonance imaging. J. Am. Coll. Cardiol. 10:682, 1987.
5. Roig, E., Georgio, D., Chomka, E. V., et al.: Reproducibility of left ventricular myocardial volume and mass measurements by ultrafast computed tomography. J. Am. Coll. Cardiol. 18:990, 1991.
6. Spagnuolo, M., Kloth, H., Taranta, A., et al.: Natural history of rheumatic aortic regurgitation: Criteria predictive of death, congestive heart failure, and angina in young patients. Circulation 44:368, 1971.
7. Slater, J., Gindea, A. J., Freedberg, R. S., et al.: Comparison of cardiac catheterization and Doppler echocardiography in the decision to operate in aortic and mitral valve disease. J. Am. Coll. Cardiol. 17:1026, 1991.
8. Simpson, I. A., and Sahn, D. J.: Quantification of valvular regurgitation by Doppler echocardiography. Circulation 84(Suppl. I):I-188, 1991.
9. Henry, W. L., Bonow, R. O., Borer, J. S., et al.: Observations on the optimum time for operative intervention for aortic regurgitation: I. Evaluation of the results of aortic valve replacement in symptomatic patients. Circulation 61:471, 1980.
10. Boucher, C. A., Bingham, J. B., Osbakken, M. D., et al.: Early changes in left ventricular size and function after correction of left ventricular volume overload. Am. J. Cardiol. 47:991, 1981.
11. Borer, J. S., Bacharach, S. L., Green, M. V., et al.: Exercise-induced left ventricular dysfunction in symptomatic and asymptomatic patients with aortic regurgitation: Assessment with radionuclide cineangiography. Am. J. Cardiol. 42:351, 1978.
12. Bonow, R. O., Picone, A. L., McIntosh, C. L., et al.: Survival and functional results after valve replacement for aortic regurgitation from 1976 to 1983: Impact of preoperative left ventricular function. Circulation 72:1244, 1985.
13. Sechtem, U., Pflugfelder, P. W., Cassidy, M. M., et al.: Mitral or aortic regurgitation: Quantification of regurgitant volumes with cine MR imaging. Radiology 167:425, 1988.
14. Reiter, S. J., Rumberger, J. A., Stanford, W., et al.: Quantitative determination of aortic regurgitant volumes in dogs by ultrafast computed tomography. Circulation 76:728, 1987.
15. Cranney, G. B., Lotan, C. S., and Pohost, G. M.: Nuclear magnetic resonance imaging for assessment and follow-up of patients with valve disease. Circulation 84(Suppl. I):I-216, 1991.

16. Popp, R. L.: Echocardiography (Part I). N. Engl. J. Med. 323:101, 1990.
17. Leitch, J. W., Mitchell, A. S., Harris, P. J., et al.: The effect of cardiac catheterization upon management of advanced aortic and mitral valve disease. Eur. Heart J. 12:602, 1991.
18. Helgason, C. M., Chomka, E., Louie, E., et al.: The potential role for ultrafast cardiac computed tomography in patients with stroke. Stroke 20:465, 1989.
19. Edwards, L. C., III, and Louie, E. K.: Transthoracic and transesophageal echocardiography for the evaluation of cardiac tumors, thrombi, and valvular vegetations. Am. J. Card. Imaging 8:45, 1994.
20. Phillips, H. R., Levine, F. H., Cartes, J. E., et al.: Mitral valve replacement for isolated mitral regurgitation: Analysis of clinical course and late postoperative left ventricular ejection fraction. Am. J. Cardiol. 48:647, 1981.
21. Perez, J. E., Ludbrook, P. A., and Ahumada, G. G.: Usefulness of Doppler echocardiography in detecting tricuspid valve stenosis. Am. J. Cardiol. 55:601, 1985.
22. Miyatake, K., Okamoto, M., Kinoshita, N., et al.: Evaluation of tricuspid regurgitation by pulsed Doppler and two-dimensional echocardiography. Circulation 66:777, 1982.
23. Lima, C. O., Sahn, D. J., Valdes-Cruz, L. M., et al.: Noninvasive prediction of transvalvular pressure gradient in patients with pulmonary stenosis by quantitative two-dimensional echocardiography Doppler studies. Circulation 67:866, 1983.
24. Zabalgoitia, M.: Echocardiographic assessment of prosthetic heart valves. Curr. Probl. Cardiol. 17:271–325, 1992.
25. Deutsch, H. J., Bachmann, R., Sechtem, U., et al.: Regurgitant flow in cardiac valve prostheses: Diagnostic value of gradient echo nuclear magnetic resonance imaging in reference to transesophageal two-dimensional color Doppler echocardiography. J. Am. Coll. Cardiol. 19:1500, 1992.
26. Vogel, W., Stoll, H. P., Bay, W., et al.: Cineradiography for determination of normal and abnormal function in mechanical heart valves. Am. J. Cardiol. 71:225, 1993.
27. Bleiweis, M. S., Milliken, J. C., Baumgartner, F. J., et al.: Application of the ultrafast CT for diagnosis of perivalvular abcesses: Surgical implications. Chest 106:629, 1994.

CHAPTER

11 Myocarditis and Cardiomyopathy

Bruce H. Brundage, M.D.

MYOCARDITIS _____ 87
DILATED CARDIOMYOPATHY _____ 87
HYPERTROPHIC CARDIOMYOPATHY _____ 88
RESTRICTIVE CARDIOMYOPATHY _____ 88
SUMMARY _____ 88

Possibly the least well understood of all the forms of cardiac disease are the primary cardiomyopathies. Little is known about the pathogenesis of these diseases, whether congenital, infectious, or metabolic in etiology. Thus, for these diseases, the clinician takes a largely empirical approach to diagnosis and treatment. In both, however, imaging does play an important role. The primary focus of imaging is the left ventricle, although visualization of the atria, right ventricle, and pericardium can also be important. This chapter, as do the others in this section, defines the imaging techniques essential to the diagnosis and management of primary myocardial disease. Competing technologies are contrasted, and complementary but not nonessential imaging modalities are highlighted. Also discussed are areas in which knowledge is deficient and imaging technology may be helpful in the future.

MYOCARDITIS

The chest roentgenogram is often the first clue to the diagnosis of myocarditis, as the early symptoms are often nonspecific. Dilation of all four cardiac chambers is common, so the cardiac silhouette is usually enlarged. When pericarditis with pericardial effusion is also present, the enlargement may be massive. Doppler echocardiography is very useful in confirming the diagnosis by demonstrating global contractile dysfunction of both ventricles.[1] Any accompanying pericardial effusion is easily detected. Echocardiography is also good for detecting the presence of left atrial or ventricular thrombus. The lack of focal wall motion abnormalities and the demonstration of normal valve architecture are helpful in establishing the diagnosis of primary myocardial disease. Cardiac catheterization is often performed to obtain a myocardial biopsy, although the value of the biopsy has been questioned.[2, 3] The only other added value of cardiac catheterization is coronary angiography to exclude ischemic cardiomyopathy.

With the value of myocardial biopsy in question, some challenge the need for cardiac catheterization in patients with suspected myocarditis. As is discussed in a following section, there are other noninvasive methods that may exclude coronary artery disease as a cause of myocarditis. Therefore, a chest roentgenogram and Doppler echocardiographic study may be the only imaging techniques that are absolutely essential.

Occasionally, myocardial scanning with the radioisotope gallium-67 indicates inflammation.[4] However, this test yields negative results in the majority of patients and, thus, has not been widely used. Recently, several investigators have reported that indium-111–labeled antimyosin antibody may be useful in the detection of myocarditis, but clinical experience with this method is still limited.[5, 6] Magnetic resonance imaging (MRI) and fast computed tomography (CT) may occasionally be employed to define the presence of intracardiac thrombus when the echocardiogram is unclear.

In the future magnetic resonance spectroscopy (MRS) and positron emission tomography (PET) may provide metabolic insights regarding the pathogenesis of myocarditis, but at present their value is unknown. Sometimes, MRI can detect differences in the myocardial signal of transplanted hearts experiencing rejection. In the future, perhaps, MRI may be able to detect signal differences in inflamed myocardium.[7] Research efforts also continue to explore ultrasound's potential to detect signal differences between normal and pathologic myocardium.[8]

DILATED CARDIOMYOPATHY

Idiopathic dilated cardiomyopathy is almost certainly the final common pathway for a diverse group of primary myocardial diseases. Currently, the role of imaging has been largely to define the degree of cardiac dysfunction and to detect complicating problems, such as intracardiac thrombus.[9] The chest roentgenogram is useful for following the dilated cardiomyopathy patient to detect signs of worsening heart failure. Doppler echocardiography can detail the severity of ventricular dysfunction and detect the development of left atrial or ventricular thrombus.[10, 11] Coronary angiography is often performed to exclude the presence of advanced coronary artery disease because ischemic cardiomyopathy can present without a history of chest pain and appear clinically exactly the same as idiopathic dilated cardiomyopathy.[12, 13] When accurate measurements of left ventricular ejection fraction are required, as in clinical trials testing new drugs to treat heart failure and to prolong life, radioisotope methods are best.[14] However, in most clinical circumstances, the estimate of ejection fraction provided by echocardiography is sufficient.

The high spatial and temporal resolution of MRI and fast CT, coupled with their inherent three-dimensional depiction, can provide complete assessment of enlarged cardiac chambers as well as quantitative measurements of myocardial mass.[15, 16] Precise elucidation of volume, mass, wall stress, and function may prove helpful in the evaluation of medical therapy.[17] On occasion, when echocardiographic findings have been uncertain regarding the presence of an intracardiac thrombus, either MRI or fast CT has been used to clarify the situation.[18]

Nearly all the noninvasive imaging techniques have been tested to determine whether they can differentiate between ischemic cardiomyopathy and dilated cardiomyopathy. Echocardiography can distinguish between focal and global wall motion abnormalities, but, unfortunately, some patients with dilated cardiomyopathy may also have focal wall motion abnormalities.[19, 20] Myocardial scintigraphy with thallium-201 has also been evaluated as a means of differentiating between the two entities, but focal perfusion abnormalities characteristic of ischemic heart disease can also occur in dilated cardiomyopathy patients.[21–23] In some cases, PET assessment of myocardial metabolism may be helpful, but it does not always distinguish between the two.[24] Fluoroscopic detection of coronary calcium, a marker of coronary atherosclerosis, has been reported to successfully differentiate between ischemic cardiomyopathy and dilated cardiomyopathy, but corroborating studies have not been done.[25] Clearly, further studies on the differentiation of the two entities are warranted. Ultrasound tissue characterization, MRS, MRI, PET, and fast CT all have the potential to provide new approaches to this problem.[26–28]

HYPERTROPHIC CARDIOMYOPATHY

Rarely has an uncommon disease such as hypertrophic cardiomyopathy evoked so much clinical interest. Imaging has always played a central role in the evaluation of the disease. Early studies using left ventricular angiography suggested that the pathogenesis was the result of dynamic subvalvular obstruction. More recently, the development of echocardiography has greatly advanced the understanding of the pathophysiology. Doppler echocardiography plays a central role in the evaluation of the disease by defining the extent and distribution of the hypertrophy, elucidating the dynamic relationship between the mitral valve and the septum, quantifying the amount of mitral regurgitation, determining the role of diastolic dysfunction, and demonstrating the nature and degree of obstruction. In most cases, Doppler echocardiographic evaluation is the only form of imaging needed.[29–33]

Traditionally, cardiac catheterization was employed in most cases of symptomatic hypertrophic cardiomyopathy. Today, it is usually reserved for special circumstances, such as defining coronary anatomy and detecting myocardial bridges.

Both MRI and fast CT have also been used to evaluate patients with hypertrophic cardiomyopathy. With these modalities, the clinician can obtain detailed descriptions of the distribution of hypertrophy that differentiate between the septal, apical, and concentric forms of hypertrophy.[34, 35] In most cases, however, the depiction provided by two-dimensional echocardiography is satisfactory.

In spite of all the imaging information available, there remain many unanswered questions regarding this disease. Who benefits from surgical treatment? Who is at greatest risk for experiencing sudden death? Is permanent pacing of the ventricle an effective treatment?

Findings on PET have suggested that the metabolism in the hypertrophic septum is different from that in other areas of the left ventricle.[36] In the future, PET may provide even further metabolic insights.[37, 38] Tissue characterization with ultrasound, MRS, and fast CT may also improve our understanding of the pathogenesis of hypertrophic cardiomyopathy.[39–41] Dynamic high-resolution three-dimensional representations of the ventricular architecture throughout the cardiac cycle provided by fast CT or MRI may assist in the selection of the best form of therapy in the future. For a disease that has been so extensively studied with imaging techniques, it is remarkable how little is understood about its pathogenesis.

RESTRICTIVE CARDIOMYOPATHY

Restrictive cardiomyopathy is the least common form of primary myocardial disease and, not surprisingly, the most difficult to diagnose. Doppler echocardiography can suggest the diagnosis when ventricular systolic function is reasonably well preserved, when there is no significant ventricular hypertrophy, and when ventricular filling is found to be impaired.[42] Often, cardiac catheterization is required to differentiate, on a hemodynamic basis, between restrictive cardiomyopathy and constrictive pericarditis. In some cases, however, hemodynamic differentiation is impossible and imaging techniques, such as right atrial and coronary angiography, are employed in an attempt to determine whether the pericardium is abnormally thickened. More recently, MRI and fast CT have been used in difficult cases to define pericardial thickness.[43, 44] Consequently, in some cases several imaging techniques are necessary to establish the diagnosis of restrictive cardiomyopathy. In others, Doppler echocardiography may be all that is needed.[45, 46]

When restrictive cardiomyopathy is due to myocardial infiltration, such as in amyloidosis, cardiac imaging may suggest the diagnosis. The echocardiogram may detect an unusual "sparkle" in the myocardium, or technetium-99m pyrophosphate myocardial scintigraphy may "light up" the myocardium. Also, both MRI and fast CT have been used to diagnose arrhythmogenic right ventricular dysplasia by detecting fatty infiltration of the right ventricular myocardium. In many cases, however, there are no telltale images to clue the clinician. Hopefully, future developments in ultrasound and MRI tissue characterization will improve the ability to detect the myocardial changes associated with restrictive cardiomyopathies, infiltrative and otherwise. Also, metabolic imaging with PET and MRS may provide new insights.

SUMMARY

Imaging provides the clinician with much valuable information regarding the diverse group of diseases known as the cardiomyopathies. These diseases are uncommon to rare, so there is still much to be learned about their etiology, pathogenesis, and treatment. Imaging technologies offer real promise in contributing toward a better understanding of these diseases.

References

1. Pinamonti, B., Alberti, E., Cigalotto, A., et al.: Echocardiographic findings in myocarditis. Am. J. Cardiol. 62:285, 1988.
2. Maisch, B., Bauer, E., Hufnagel, G., et al.: The use of endomyocardial biopsy in heart failure. Eur. Heart J. 9(Suppl. H):59, 1988.
3. Chow, L. H., Radio, S. J., Sears, T. D., et al.: Insensitivity of right ventricular endomyocardial biopsy and the diagnosis of myocarditis. J. Am. Coll. Cardiol. 14:915, 1989.
4. O'Connell, J. B., Henkin, R. E., Robinson, J. A., et al.: Gallium-67 imaging in patients with dilated cardiomyopathy and biopsy-proven myocarditis. Circulation 70:58, 1984.
5. Dec, G. W., Palacios, I., Yasuda, T., et al.: Antimyosin antibody cardiac imaging: Its role in the diagnosis of myocarditis. J. Am. Coll. Cardiol. 16:97, 1990.
6. Lambert, K., Isaac, D., and Hendel, R.: Myocarditis masquerading as ischemic

heart disease: The diagnostic utility of antimyosin imaging. Cardiology 82:415, 1993.

7. Gagliardi, M. G., Bevilacqua, M., Di Renzi, P., et al.: Usefulness of magnetic resonance imaging for diagnosis of acute myocarditis in infants and children, and comparison with endomyocardial biopsy. Am. J. Cardiol. 68:1089, 1991.

8. Ferdeghini, E. M., Pinamonti, B., Picano, E., et al.: Quantitative texture analysis in echocardiography: Application to the diagnosis of myocarditis. J. Clin. Ultrasound 19:263, 1991.

9. Falk, R. H., Foster, E., and Coats, M. H.: Ventricular thrombi and thromboembolism in dilated cardiomyopathy: A prospective follow-up study. Am. Heart J. 123:136–142, 1992.

10. Acquatella, H., Rodriguez-Salas, L. A., and Gomez-Mancebo, J. R.: Doppler echocardiography in dilated and restrictive cardiomyopathies. Cardiol. Clin. 8:349, 1990.

11. Vigna, C., Russo, A., De Rito, V., et al.: Frequency of left atrial thrombi by transesophageal echocardiography in idiopathic and in ischemic dilated cardiomyopathy. Am. J. Cardiol. 70:1500, 1992.

12. Figulla, H. R., Kellermann, A. B., Stille-Siegener, M., et al.: Significance of coronary angiography, left heart catheterization, and endomyocardial biopsy for the diagnosis of idiopathic dilated cardiomyopathy. Am. Heart J. 124:1251, 1992.

13. Hare, J. M., Walford, G. D., Hruban, R. H., et al.: Ischemic cardiomyopathy: Endomyocardial biopsy and ventriculographic evaluation of patients with congestive heart failure, dilated cardiomyopathy and coronary artery disease. J. Am. Coll. Cardiol. 20:1318, 1992.

14. Goldman, M. R., and Boucher, C. A.: Value of radionuclide imaging techniques in assessing cardiomyopathy. Am. J. Cardiol. 46:1232, 1980.

15. Semelka, R. C., Tomei, E., Wagner, S., et al.: Interstudy reproducibility of dimensional and functional measurements between cine magnetic resonance studies in the morphologically abnormal left ventricle. Am. Heart J. 119:1367, 1990.

16. Gaudio, C., Tanzilli, G., Mazzarotto, P., et al.: Comparison of left ventricular ejection fraction by magnetic resonance imaging and radionuclide ventriculography in idiopathic dilated cardiomyopathy. Am. J. Cardiol. 67:411, 1991.

17. Doherty, N. E., III, Seelos, K. C., Suzuki, J. I., et al.: Application of cine nuclear magnetic resonance imaging for sequential evaluation of response to angiotensin-converting enzyme inhibitor therapy in dilated cardiomyopathy. J. Am. Coll. Cardiol. 19:1294, 1992.

18. Minor, R. L., Jr., Oren, R. M., Stanford, W., et al.: Biventricular thrombi and pulmonary emboli complicating idiopathic dilated cardiomyopathy: Diagnosis with cardiac ultrafast CT. Am. Heart J. 122:1477, 1991.

19. Sunnerhagen, K. S., Bhargava, V., and Shabetai, R.: Regional left ventricular wall motion abnormalities in idiopathic dilated cardiomyopathy. Am. J. Cardiol. 65:364, 1990.

20. Diaz, R. A., Nihoyannopoulos, P., Athanassopoulos, G., et al.: Usefulness of echocardiography to differentiate dilated cardiomyopathy from coronary-induced congestive heart failure. Am. J. Cardiol. 68:1224, 1991.

21. Glamann, D. B., Lange, R. A., Corbett, J. R., et al.: Utility of various radionuclide techniques for distinguishing ischemic from nonischemic dilated cardiomyopathy. Arch. Intern. Med. 152:769, 1992.

22. Juillière, Y., Marie, P. Y., Danchin, N., et al.: Radionuclide assessment of regional differences in left ventricular wall motion and myocardial perfusion in idiopathic dilated cardiomyopathy. Eur. Heart J. 14:1163, 1993.

23. Doi, Y. L., Chikamori, T., Takata, J., et al.: Prognostic value of thallium-201 perfusion defects in idiopathic dilated cardiomyopathy. Am. J. Cardiol. 67:188, 1991.

24. Mody, F. V., Brunken, R. C., Stevenson, L. P., et al.: Differentiating cardiomyopathy of coronary artery disease from nonischemic dilated cardiomyopathy utilizing positron emission tomography. J. Am. Coll. Cardiol. 17:373, 1991.

25. Johnson, A. D., Laiken, S. L., and Shabetai, R.: Noninvasive diagnosis of ischemic cardiomyopathy by fluoroscopic detection of coronary artery calcification. Am. Heart J. 96:521, 1978.

26. Goto, S., Aerbajinai, W., Ogawa, S., et al.: Progression of systolic dysfunction correlated with the ultrasonographically assessed myocardial tissue damage in patients with dilated cardiomyopathy. Cardiology 80:399, 1992.

27. Neubauer, S., Krahe, T., Schindler, R., et al.: ^{31}P magnetic resonance spectroscopy in dilated cardiomyopathy and coronary artery disease: Altered cardiac high-energy phosphate metabolism in heart failure. Circulation 86:1810, 1992.

28. Merlet, P., Delforge, J., Syrota, A., et al.: Positron emission tomography with ^{11}C CGP-12177 to assess β-adrenergic receptor concentration in idiopathic dilated cardiomyopathy. Circulation 87:1169, 1993.

29. Sasso, Z., Rakowski, H., Wigle, E. D., et al.: Echocardiographic and Doppler studies in hypertrophic cardiomyopathy. Cardiol. Clin. 8:217, 1990.

30. Klues, H. G., Roberts, W. C., and Maron, B. J.: Morphological determinants of echocardiographic patterns of mitral valve systolic anterior motion in obstructive hypertrophic cardiomyopathy. Circulation 87:1570, 1993.

31. Panza, J. A., Pertrone, R. K., Fananapazir, L., et al.: Utility of continuous-wave Doppler echocardiography in the noninvasive assessment of left ventricular outflow tract pressure gradient in patients with hypertrophic cardiomyopathy. J. Am. Coll. Cardiol. 19:91, 1992.

32. Schwammenthal, E., Block, M., Schwartzkopff, B., et al.: Prediction of the site and severity of obstruction in hypertrophic cardiomyopathy by color flow mapping and continuous-wave Doppler echocardiography. J. Am. Coll. Cardiol. 20:964, 1992.

33. Grigg, L. E., Wigle, E. D., Williams, W. G., et al.: Transesophageal Doppler echocardiography in obstructive hypertrophic cardiomyopathy: Clarification of pathophysiology and importance in intraoperative decision-making. J. Am. Coll. Cardiol. 20:42, 1992.

34. Park, J. H., Kim, Y. M., Chung, J. W., et al.: MR imaging of hypertrophic cardiomyopathy. Radiology 185:441, 1992.

35. Chomka, E. V., Wolfkiel, C. J., Rich, S., et al.: Ultrafast computed tomography: A new method for the evaluation of hypertrophic cardiomyopathy. Am. J. Noninvas. Cardiol. 1:140, 1987.

36. Grover-McKay, M., Schwaiger, M., Krivokapich, J., et al.: Regional myocardial blood flow and metabolism at rest in mildly symptomatic patients with hypertrophic cardiomyopathy. J. Am. Coll. Cardiol. 13:317, 1989.

37. Kurata, C., Tawarahara, K., Taguchi, T., et al.: Myocardial emission computed tomography with iodine-123–labeled beta-methyl-branched fatty acid in patients with hypertrophic cardiomyopathy. J. Nucl. Med. 33:6, 1992.

38. Nienaber, C. A., Gambhir, S. S., Mody, F., et al.: Regional myocardial blood flow and glucose utilization in symptomatic patients with hypertrophic cardiomyopathy. Circulation 87:1580, 1993.

39. Lattanzi, F., Spirito, P., Picano, E., et al.: Quantitative assessment of ultrasonic reflectivity in hypertrophic cardiomyopathy. J. Am. Coll. Cardiol. 17:1085, 1991.

40. Sakuma, H., Takeda, K., Tagami, T., et al.: ^{31}P MR spectroscopy in hypertrophic cardiomyopathy: Comparison with Tl-201 myocardial perfusion imaging. Am. Heart J. 125(5 Part I):1323, 1993.

41. Saito, H., Naito, H., Takamiya, M., et al.: Late enhancement of the left ventricular wall in hypertrophic cardiomyopathy by ultrafast computed tomography: A comparison with regional myocardial thickening. Br. J. Radiol. 64:993, 1991.

42. Pinamonti, B., Di Lenarda, A., Sinagra, G., et al.: Restrictive left ventricular filling pattern in dilated cardiomyopathy assessed by Doppler echocardiography: Clinical, echocardiographic and hemodynamic correlations and prognostic implications. J. Am. Coll. Cardiol. 22:808, 1993.

43. Masui, T., Finck, S., and Higgins, C. B.: Constrictive pericarditis and restrictive cardiomyopathy: Evaluation with MR imaging. Radiology 182:369, 1992.

44. Oren, R. M., Grover-McKay, M., Stanford, W., et al.: Accurate preoperative diagnosis of pericardial constriction using cine computed tomography. J. Am. Coll. Cardiol. 22:832, 1993.

45. Klein, A. L., Cohen, G. I., Pietrolungo, J. F., et al.: Differentiation of constrictive pericarditis from restrictive cardiomyopathy by Doppler transesophageal echocardiographic measurements of respiratory variations in pulmonary venous flow. J. Am. Coll. Cardiol. 22:193, 1993.

46. Mancuso, L., D'Agostino, A., Pitrolo, F., et al.: Constrictive pericarditis versus restrictive cardiomyopathy: The role of Doppler echocardiography in differential diagnosis. Int. J. Cardiol. 31:319, 1991.

CHAPTER

12 Congenital Heart Disease

David J. Skorton, M.D.

GOALS OF IMAGING IN CONGENITAL HEART DISEASE _____ 90
SPECIAL DIAGNOSTIC CONSIDERATIONS _____ 90
ESSENTIAL DIAGNOSTIC APPROACHES TO CONGENITAL HEART DISEASE _____ 90
SPECIFIC EXAMPLES _____ 91
Acyanotic Diseases _____ 91
Valvular Disease _____ 91

Shunt Lesions _____ 91
Coarctation of the Aorta _____ 91
Cyanotic Diseases _____ 92
Tetralogy of Fallot _____ 92
Ebstein's Anomaly _____ 92
Eisenmenger's Physiology _____ 92
Postoperative Patients _____ 92
UNANSWERED QUESTIONS _____ 92
CONCLUSIONS _____ 92

Congenital heart defects, among the most common birth defects, constitute an increasingly important area of cardiovascular care. The field of congenital heart disease has long been the province of pediatric cardiologists and cardiovascular surgeons. However, the great success of medical and, particularly, surgical interventions in this patient population is permitting the newborn with congenital heart disease to live through healthy infancy, childhood, and adolescence to a productive adult life.[1] The place of imaging methods in the diagnosis of congenital heart disease is a very prominent one; several imaging techniques shed light on congenitally abnormal cardiac anatomy and physiology. Choosing wisely among these various diagnostic alternatives can be difficult in this sometimes complex patient population.

GOALS OF IMAGING IN CONGENITAL HEART DISEASE

In the patient with congenital heart disease, imaging methods are used to make the diagnosis, to guide medical, catheter-based, or surgical therapy, and to evaluate surgical procedures in the operating room and postoperatively. The patient with congenital heart disease can be studied in utero (with fetal echocardiography), in the newborn nursery, and during infancy, childhood, adolescence, and adulthood. Thus, in this patient population, reproducibility reliable enough to allow serial examinations is an important goal.

The initial objective of imaging in congenital heart disease is precise delineation of cardiac anatomy. This anatomy is sometimes extraordinarily complex, particularly in the postoperative state. In addition to anatomical detail, however, the choice of medical versus surgical versus catheter-based therapy in this patient population is often determined by ventricular function and hemodynamics, including the degree of left-to-right or right-to-left shunting, cardiac output, and the level of pulmonary arterial pressure, flow, and resistance. The assessment of valvular function is important in most common types of congenital heart disease. Finally, the delineation of the condition of prosthetic materials, including extracardiac conduits, for complex disorders is a goal of imaging in this patient population.

SPECIAL DIAGNOSTIC CONSIDERATIONS

Since the vast majority of congenital heart disorders are amenable to curative or palliative surgical correction, there is a need for comprehensive and quantitative anatomical, physiological, and hemodynamic evaluation. Thus, modalities that demonstrate anatomy and physiology with accuracy and precision sufficient for surgical or catheter-based therapy planning are most useful. Because of the broad age group involved and the likelihood of serial studies, the clinician will wish to avoid or minimize exposure to ionizing radiation. The acutely ill newborn, particularly with cyanosis, requires an expeditious evaluation, often at the bedside in the emergency department or critical care unit. Finally, the ability to recognize cardiac disorders in utero makes fetal examination an additional special consideration in women at increased risk for bearing children with congenital heart disease.

ESSENTIAL DIAGNOSTIC APPROACHES TO CONGENITAL HEART DISEASE

During the initial development of the field of pediatric cardiology, the definitive diagnostic approach to the patient with congenital heart disease was to perform cardiac catheterization and angiography. The cardiac catheterization laboratory is still the standard venue for evaluation of pressures throughout the cardiovascular system as well as vascular resistance. For example, the presence and severity of pulmonary arterial hypertension is an important determinant of the suitability of patients for surgical therapy in a variety of congenital cardiac disorders. In addition to pressure measurement and resistance calculation, cardiac catheterization permits accurate assessment of shunt flow with the use of oximetry and dye curves. Finally, angiography permits detailed anatomical evaluation of chambers, great vessels, and coronary vasculature.

An additional feature of modern practice in congenital heart disease is the growing set of interventional techniques that can be performed in the catheterization laboratory.[2] Balloon valvuloplasty for pulmonary valve stenosis, placement of a closure device for patent ductus arteriosus, and balloon dilation of coarctation of the aorta are three examples of these interventional procedures. These diagnostic and, particularly, therapeutic considerations continue to make cardiac catheterization an important modality in the care of patients with congenital heart disease.

Although cardiac catheterization with angiography remains an important approach to the patient with congenital heart disease, echocardiography has made an enormous impact in this patient population. Two-dimensional echocardiographic imaging permits accurate diagnosis of fetal cardiac anatomy and physiology[3] as well as anatomical and functional abnormalities in newborns, infants, children, and adults. In many cases, the information from echocardiography makes cardiac catheterization unnecessary in patients who do not require catheter-based intervention.[4, 5] The addition of Doppler echocardiography permits accurate determination of hemodynamic variables such as transvalvular gradient,[6] shunt flow,[7] cardiac output, and ventricular[8] and pulmonary arterial pressures.[9] Finally, the more recent introduction of transesophageal echocardiography (TEE)[10, 11] has permitted diagnoses in the minority of cases in which transthoracic examination is not of sufficient quality for definitive diagnosis. Increasingly, transesophageal echocardiography is also being used in the operating room to assist surgical procedures and to evaluate the results prior to closing.[12] Recent studies have emphasized the importance of determining the cost-effectiveness of echocardiography for problems such as evaluating children with heart murmurs,[13] although much more research related to medical outcomes is needed in this group of patients.

In situations in which echocardiography and cardiac catheterization give similar information, the common clinical choice is to utilize echocardiography because of the noninvasive nature of the technique, the lack of ionizing radiation, and the lower cost.

In addition to echocardiography and cardiac catheterization, other imaging modalities are informative in congenital heart disease. Chest roentgenography is still quite useful in identifying many features of cardiac and thoracic anatomy as well as in giving some information on pulmonary blood flow. Although largely supplanted by echocardiography for the assessment of chamber sizes and function, chest roentgenography remains helpful in the initial diagnosis and follow-up of many conditions. While not widely available, fast computed tomography (CT) offers precise and accurate diagnosis,[14] particularly in adults with congenital heart disease. Technical improvements resulting in finer image resolution and smaller image slice thickness may make CT more useful in infants and children. Radionuclide techniques are used in selected patients to assess shunt flow and other functional data. Finally, magnetic resonance imaging (MRI) is of increasing importance, especially in some complex forms of congenital heart disease.[15–17] Particularly after surgery and in patients with extracardiac conduits, MRI adds information.[18] Technical improvements in both CT and MRI may increase the utility of both techniques for goals such as the following: (1) assessing peripheral pulmonary arterial size and flow in cases in which echocardiography cannot visualize these more distal vessels; (2) defining the anatomical details of all portions of the ascending and descending aorta; and (3) recognizing bronchial compression due to mechanisms such as enlargement of the pulmonary arteries or left atrium.

SPECIFIC EXAMPLES

Some specific examples of the use of imaging techniques in the diagnosis of congenital heart disease follow. For the sake of simplicity, the examples are divided into acyanotic and cyanotic diseases.

Acyanotic Diseases

Valvular Disease

The etiology of valvular disease is changing: congenital valvular disorders are becoming a more prominent portion of the spectrum, replacing the now less common rheumatic heart disease. The use of imaging techniques in congenital valvular disease adheres to the principles for valvular heart disease outlined in Chapter 10.

As in other causes of valve disease, echocardiography is the method of choice for diagnosis[6] and serial follow-up. In addition to the physiologic assessment of severity of valvular stenosis and regurgitation required for any etiology of valvular disease, the clinician caring for patients with congenital heart disease also desires to identify the more detailed anatomical characteristics of the valve. For example, balloon valvuloplasty is the primary approach in many patients with pulmonic valve stenosis and is used increasingly in children with aortic stenosis. Those with dysplastic, greatly thickened valves, however, may be more difficult to treat with balloon dilation. Thus, echocardiography has had an impact on the selection of patients for balloon pulmonic valvuloplasty based on assessment of valve anatomy.

Although echocardiography is extremely useful in evaluating patients with congenital valvular disorders, cardiac catheterization is still sometimes needed. In particular, catheterization with angiography is performed when echocardiographic assessment yields equivocal results or, in the adult, when coronary arterial anatomy must be defined.

Shunt Lesions

Shunts at the level of the atria, ventricles, or great arteries are common acyanotic disorders. Imaging techniques are utilized to identify the presence of a shunt, to quantify the amount of shunting (e.g., by calculation of the pulmonary-to-systemic flow ratio [Qp:Qs]), and to estimate pulmonary arterial pressures. Echocardiography with Doppler imaging is the technique of choice for the identification of the source of the shunt, including the demonstration of multiple ventricular septal defects (VSDs); determination of Qp:Qs; and estimation of pulmonary artery pressure. In some patients, the addition of transesophageal echocardiography is necessary for optimal diagnosis.

Although echocardiography is the initial approach in the patient with shunt lesions, at times, cardiac catheterization is still necessary for precise definition of the level of pulmonary arterial pressure and resistance. For example, in cases in which pulmonary artery pressure appears to be elevated but the patient does not have obvious stigmata of inoperable pulmonary hypertension, cardiac catheterization is indicated to assess operability by calculation of pulmonary and systemic resistances.

First-pass radionuclide angiography,[19] CT,[20] and MRI[21] are also useful in assessing the quantity of shunting.

The assessment of the patient with VSD illustrates the use of imaging methods in the diagnosis of patients with shunts. Transthoracic echocardiography is the primary imaging modality in the management of children with VSD. Beyond visualization of the defect, Doppler methods can be used to assess the pressure differential between the ventricles,[8] providing an estimation of pulmonary artery pressure in the absence of pulmonic stenosis. In addition, Doppler flow can be used to estimate Qp:Qs based on calculation of left heart versus right heart cardiac output (e.g., flow in the aorta and pulmonary artery, respectively). Radionuclide angiography, CT, and MRI studies can also quantitate shunt volume, although these techniques often do not add information to that obtained by echocardiography. Color Doppler imaging is also useful for defining the presence and extent of aortic insufficiency, an important consideration for early surgery in children with VSD.

Coarctation of the Aorta

The identification of coarctation is a bedside diagnostic maneuver accomplished during the physical examination, which can also identify the approximate location of the coarctation by noting which extremities are in the high-pressure versus low-pressure zones. Some anatomical aberrations, such as anomalous origin of the right subclavian artery from the distal thoracic aorta, may confound the bedside assessment of coarctation location.

Chest roentgenography is useful in the assessment of coarctation, as rib notching gives evidence of increased collateral flow through intercostal arteries.

Echocardiography precisely defines coarctation location and severity based on gradient estimation through Doppler techniques. Fast CT and MRI also offer excellent delineation of aortic anatomy and, utilizing flow-sensitive MRI pulse sequences, the flow characteristics of the coarctation,[22] including flow in collateral vessels.[23] However, there is no compelling evidence that MRI or CT is generally necessary if high-quality echocardiographic data are available. Computed tomography and MRI may be useful in older children and in adults in determining the length of aortic coarctation and arch size, important factors in surgical planning.

Cyanotic Diseases

A large number of cyanotic disorders are diagnosed in part utilizing imaging techniques. Three examples are tetralogy of Fallot, Ebstein's anomaly, and Eisenmenger's complex.

Tetralogy of Fallot

The most common cyanotic cardiac disease, tetralogy of Fallot, will be increasingly encountered by practitioners caring for children, adolescents, and adults. The anatomical substrate of tetralogy of Fallot is defined precisely and reliably with the use of echocardiography and Doppler techniques. Prior to surgery, cardiac catheterization and angiography are commonly performed to evaluate coronary arterial anatomy (e.g., anomalous origin of the left anterior descending artery from the right coronary artery) and to assess precisely the size of the pulmonary arteries. Although MRI and CT also clearly define the anatomy in tetralogy of Fallot, echocardiography and cardiac catheterization remain the essential methods in this application.

Ebstein's Anomaly

The characteristic apical displacement of tricuspid valve leaflets seen in Ebstein's anomaly is well demonstrated with echocardiography,[24] and the hemodynamic sequelae of tricuspid regurgitation are demonstrable with Doppler methods. Cardiac catheterization and electrophysiologic studies have been utilized in the past in the diagnosis of Ebstein's anomaly. However, echocardiography is currently the most important approach to this diagnosis. The degree of shunting can be evaluated, as noted previously, with the use of echocardiographic or radionuclide methods.

Eisenmenger's Physiology

The patient with a shunt at intracardiac or great artery levels who develops pulmonary arterial hypertension (Eisenmenger's complex) is usually evaluated with chest roentgenography and echocardiography. The chest x-ray shows enlarged central pulmonary arteries with the peripheral "pruning" characteristic of pulmonary hypertension. Echocardiography demonstrates the presence of an intracardiac or a great artery communication, particularly with transesophageal techniques. If any question remains about the operability of the patient, cardiac catheterization is performed to assess pulmonary vascular resistance. Injection of radiopaque dye into the main pulmonary arteries can be accomplished, although the complications are more common with severe pulmonary hypertension.

Postoperative Patients

Perhaps the most rapidly growing segment of the population with congenital heart disease comprises patients who have undergone curative or palliative surgical or catheter interventions. In general, echocardiography is the first approach to the evaluation of these patients. Whether employed in the operating room, immediately postoperatively, or later for serial examinations, echocardiography is extremely useful. Assessment of prosthetic valves and conduits may be difficult with transthoracic approaches, although transesophageal echocardiography has improved the utility of ultrasound in these patients.

Both MRI[25–27] and fast CT[28] can make important contributions to the postoperative follow-up of patients with congenital heart disease. In particular, MRI has proved useful in the assessment of complex postoperative anatomy, such as in patients with extracardiac conduits.[18]

UNANSWERED QUESTIONS

The ultimate roles of invasive versus noninvasive diagnostic methods and of catheter interventional techniques in congenital heart disease remain to be determined. If the recent promise of the interventional procedures is realized, a sizable proportion of simple, acyanotic defects will be corrected in the cardiac catheterization laboratory. If the noninvasive diagnostic methods prove as efficacious in the long run as they appear at this juncture, most diagnosis will be relegated to echocardiography and MRI, and the catheterization laboratory will be used largely for therapy.

Another unanswered question regarding diagnosis in congenital heart disease is the eventual role of MRI techniques, particularly with regard to or combined with echocardiography.[29–31] Magnetic resonance angiographic imaging studies have demonstrated the ability to delineate anatomy as fine as that of the coronary arteries.[32] Further studies have demonstrated important flow information available in phase-sensitive MRI procedures.[22, 23] Finally, MR spectroscopy may offer insight into myocardial metabolism.[33] If the demonstrations of hemodynamic and fine anatomical detail reach their apparent potential, and given the ability of MRI to identify abnormalities of extracardiac conduits and other complex postoperative anatomy, MRI could, in the future, become an essential technique for the diagnosis of congenital heart disease.

CONCLUSIONS

From the perspective of the mid-1990s, cardiac catheterization with angiography and echocardiography are the two predominant techniques in the diagnosis and serial evaluation of congenital heart disease. The technique of first choice for the initial evaluation of most patients is echocardiography, and it is unlikely that any technique will displace it in the foreseeable future. The advent of improvements in MRI may elevate the role of this technique in congenital heart disease.

The catheterization laboratory will probably become increasingly focused on interventional procedures, with echocardiography, CT, and MRI used to make the diagnosis and assess the suitability of catheter or surgical interventions. Thus, the practitioner of the future will need access to these multiple imaging methods to provide optimal management for patients with congenital heart disease.

References

1. Skorton, D. J., Garson, A., Jr. (guest eds.): Congenital Heart Disease in Adolescents and Adults. Cardiol. Clin. 11(4):543–720, 1993.
2. Landzberg, M. J., and Lock, J. E.: Interventional catheter procedures used in congenital heart disease. Cardiol. Clin. 11:569, 1993.
3. Huhta, J. C., Carpenter, R. J., Jr., Moise, K. J., Jr., et al.: Prenatal diagnosis and postnatal management of critical aortic stenosis. Circulation 75:573, 1987.
4. Sharma, S., Anand, R., Kanter, K. R., et al.: The usefulness of echocardiography in the surgical management of infants with congenital heart disease. Clin. Cardiol. 15:891, 1992.
5. Huhta, J. C., Glasgow, P., Murphy, D. J., et al.: Surgery without catheterization for congenital heart defects: Management of 100 patients. J. Am. Coll. Cardiol. 9:823, 1987.
6. Bengur, A. R., Snider, A. R., Serwer, G. A., et al.: Usefulness of Doppler mean gradient in evaluation of children with aortic valve stenosis and comparison to gradient at catheterization. Am. J. Cardiol. 64:756, 1989.
7. Barron, J. V., Sahn, D. J., Valdes-Cruz, L. M., et al.: Clinical utility of two-dimensional Doppler echocardiographic techniques for estimating pulmonary-to-systemic blood flow ratios in children with left-to-right shunting atrial septal defect, ventricular septal defect, or patent ductus arteriosus. J. Am. Coll. Cardiol. 3:169, 1984.
8. Murphy, D. J., Jr., Ludomirsky, A., and Huhta, J. C.: Continuous-wave Doppler in children with ventricular septal defect: Noninvasive estimation of interventricular pressure gradient. Am. J. Cardiol. 57:428, 1986.
9. Musewe, N. N., Smallhorn, J. F., Benson, L. N., et al.: Validation of Doppler-derived pulmonary arterial pressure in patients with ductus arteriosus under different hemodynamic states. Circulation 76:1081, 1987.
10. Ritter, S. B.: Transesophageal real-time echocardiography in infants and children with congenital heart disease. J. Am. Coll. Cardiol. 18:569, 1991.
11. Fyfe, D. A., Ritter, S. B., Snider, A. R., et al.: Guidelines for transesophageal echocardiography in children. J. Am. Soc. Echocardiogr. 5:640, 1992.
12. Roberson, D., Muhuideen, I., Silverman, N., et al.: Intraoperative transesophageal echocardiography in infants and children with congenital cardiac shunt lesions. J. Am. Soc. Echocardiogr., 3:213, 1990.
13. Danford, D. A.: Cost-effectiveness of echocardiography for evaluation of children with murmurs. Echocardiography 12:153, 1995.

14. Husayni, T.: Ultrafast computed tomographic imaging in congenital heart disease. *In* Stanford, W., and Rumberger, J. A. (eds.): Ultrafast Computed Tomography in Cardiac Imaging: Principles and Practice. Mt. Kisco, NY, Futura Publishing, 1992, p. 311.

15. Link, K. M., and Lesko, N. M.: Magnetic resonance imaging in the evaluation of congenital heart disease. Magn. Reson. Q. 7:173, 1991.

16. Fellows, K. E., Weinberg, P. M., Baffa, J. M., et al.: Evaluation of congenital heart disease with MR imaging: Current and coming attractions. A. J. R. 159:925, 1992.

17. Kersting-Sommerhoff, B. A., Diethelm, L., Teitel, D. F., et al.: Magnetic resonance imaging of congenital heart disease: Sensitivity and specificity using receiver operating characteristic curve analysis. Am. Heart J. 118:155, 1989.

18. Martinez, J. E., Mohiaddin, R. H., Kilner, P. J., et al.: Obstruction in extracardiac ventriculopulmonary conduits: Value of nuclear magnetic resonance imaging with velocity mapping and Doppler echocardiography. J. Am. Coll. Cardiol. 20:338, 1992.

19. Maltz, D. L., and Treves, S.: Quantitative radionuclide angiocardiography: Determination of Qp:Qs in children. Circulation 47:1048, 1973.

20. MacMillan, R., Rees, M., Eldredge, W. J., et al.: Quantitation of shunting at the atrial level using rapid acquisition computed tomography with comparison with cardiac catheterization. J. Am. Coll. Cardiol. 7:946, 1986.

21. Brenner, L. D., Caputo, G. R., Mostbeck, G., et al.: Quantification of left-to-right atrial shunts with velocity-encoded cine nuclear magnetic resonance imaging. J. Am. Coll. Cardiol. 20:1246, 1992.

22. Mohiaddin, R. H., Kilner, P. J., Rees, S., et al.: Magnetic resonance volume flow and jet velocity mapping in aortic coarctation. J. Am. Coll. Cardiol. 22:1515, 1993.

23. Steffens, J. C., Bourne, M. W., Sakuma, H., et al.: Quantification of collateral blood flow in coarctation of the aorta by velocity encoded cine magnetic resonance imaging. Circulation 90:937, 1994.

24. Ports, T. A., Silverman, N. H., and Schiller, N. B.: Two-dimensional echocardiographic assessment of Ebstein's anomaly. Circulation 58:336, 1978.

25. Fogel, M. A., Donofrio, M. T., Ramaciotti, C., et al.: Magnetic resonance and echocardiographic imaging of pulmonary artery size throughout stages of Fontan reconstruction. Circulation 90:2927, 1994.

26. Rebergen, S. A., Ottenkamp, J., Doornbos, J., et al.: Postoperative pulmonary flow dynamics after Fontan surgery: Assessment with nuclear magnetic resonance velocity mapping. J. Am. Coll. Cardiol. 21:123, 1993.

27. Rebergen, S. A., Helbing, W. A., Van der Wall, E. E., et al.: MR velocity mapping of tricuspid flow in normal children and patients after Mustard or Senning repair. Radiology 194:505, 1995.

28. Matherne, G. P., Frey, E. E., Atkins, D. L., et al.: Cine computed tomography for diagnosis of superior vena cava obstruction following the Mustard operation. Pediatr. Radiol. 17:246, 1987.

29. Simpson, I. A., and Sahn, D. J.: Adult congenital heart disease: Use of transthoracic echocardiography versus magnetic resonance imaging scanning. Am. J. Card. Imaging 9:29, 1995.

30. Hirsch, R., Kilner, P. J., Connelly, M. S., et al.: Diagnosis in adolescents and adults with congenital heart disease: Prospective assessment of individual and combined roles of magnetic resonance imaging and transesophageal echocardiography. Circulation 90:2937, 1994.

31. Masui, T., Seelos, K. C., Kersting-Sommerhoff, B. A., et al.: Abnormalities of the pulmonary veins: Evaluation with MR imaging and comparison with cardiac angiography and echocardiography. Radiology 181:645, 1991.

32. Manning, W. J., Li, W., and Edelman, R. R.: A preliminary report comparing magnetic resonance coronary angiography with conventional angiography. N. Engl. J. Med. 328:828, 1993.

33. Whitman, J. R., Chance, B., Bode, H., et al.: Diagnosis and therapeutic evaluation of a pediatric case of cardiomyopathy using phosphorus-31 nuclear magnetic resonance spectroscopy. J. Am. Coll. Cardiol. 5:745, 1985.

CHAPTER

13 Pericardial Disease

Bruce H. Brundage, M.D.

ACUTE PERICARDITIS _____ 93
ACUTE PERICARDIAL TAMPONADE _____ 94
CONSTRICTIVE PERICARDITIS _____ 94
EFFUSIVE CONSTRICTIVE PERICARDITIS _____ 94
OTHER PERICARDIAL DISEASES _____ 94
SUMMARY _____ 95

Physical examination and electrocardiography are extremely important in making the diagnosis of pericardial disease, but imaging is also recognized as a critical component. Once the diagnosis is suspected, some form of imaging of the pericardium is almost always employed. Virtually every type of imaging method has been evaluated to determine its usefulness in diagnosing pericardial disease. This chapter identifies which methods are essential, which compete with others, and which are complementary for each of the major categories of pericardial disease to provide the reader with an integrated approach to imaging pericardial disease. Unresolved issues regarding the use of imaging in the diagnosis of pericardial disease are also identified.

ACUTE PERICARDITIS

The diagnosis of acute pericarditis is usually suggested by signs and symptoms, and once the diagnosis is under consideration a chest roentgenogram is almost always obtained. When a large pericardial effusion is associated with the pericarditis, the chest film has the characteristic features of an enlarged cardiac silhouette with a narrow hilum. Occasionally, the lateral chest film detects an anterior fat line within the cardiac silhouette, making the diagnosis of a pericardial effusion highly likely. Unfortunately, this radiographic sign is not very sensitive. The pericardial fat sign is much easier to detect with fluoroscopy, but this technique is not often employed because echocardiography has become widely available. Echocardiography is highly sensitive for detecting even small pericardial effusions and is utilized in virtually all patients suspected of having acute pericarditis.[1] Sometimes the two-dimensional echocardiographic images can also suggest the nature of the effusion by identifying intrapericardial strands or demonstrating increased reflectance from the fluid.[2]

Magnetic resonance imaging (MRI) and conventional and fast computed tomography (CT) are sometimes helpful in the evaluation of the patient with acute pericarditis.[3–5] In particular, the evaluation of suspected pericarditis in a patient after open heart surgery can be problematic.[6] Sometimes the effusion is loculated and, if it is posterior or rightward, may be difficult to detect with transthoracic echocardiography. In this situation, transesophageal echocardiography, however, may be useful. In these cases, the unlimited field of view of MRI and fast CT can also be helpful, especially when the pericarditis is due to invasion by tumor from the adjacent mediastinum. These techniques can define the pericardial involvement and confirm that the pericardial effusion is due to metastatic tumor.[7] Some reports have indicated that alterations in the MRI signal from the pericardial fluid can suggest the nature of the fluid, differentiating among transudate, exudate, hemorrhage, and chyle.[8] However, further investigations are necessary before MRI, as well as other imaging techniques, can be relied on to identify the etiology of effusive pericarditis. One novel approach that uses a flexible optical fiberscope to visualize the pericardial space through a transcutaneously placed sheath has been suggested by Kondos and colleagues.[9] Such an approach, if successful, could guide biopsy and eliminate the need for diagnostic surgery. Further developments in ultrasound and MRI are likely to assist in determining the etiology of acute pericarditis by elucidating the nature of the pericardial fluid.

ACUTE PERICARDIAL TAMPONADE

The clinical signs of pericardial tamponade in a patient who is hemodynamically unstable are sufficient reason to proceed directly to pericardiocentesis. However, many patients are stable enough that the clinician seeks to confirm the diagnosis of pericardial effusion and tamponade. Without question, Doppler echocardiography is the diagnostic test of choice. The presence of right ventricular and atrial diastolic collapse, cardiac oscillation, and alterations in venae cavae, and right- and left-sided transvalvular flow all are useful signs of tamponade.[10, 11] In some cases, some Doppler echocardiographic signs may be present before other clinical signs of tamponade are seen, making early intervention possible. In the past, cardiac catheterization was often employed to diagnose cardiac tamponade by detecting characteristic hemodynamic changes. Today, cardiac catheterization may be used to monitor the hemodynamic state during and after pericardiocentesis but is less often employed to make the initial diagnosis because of the clinician's confidence in the echocardiographic findings. Cardiac fluoroscopy is still widely utilized to guide the performance of pericardiocentesis, but this, too, is increasingly being replaced by echocardiographic guidance.[12] In the future, cardiac fluoroscopic guidance may be reserved for these patients in whom good echocardiographic images are not obtainable.

It has been suggested that even balloon pericardiotomy can be guided with echocardiography.[13] However, others argue that cardiac cinefluoroscopy is required to adequately monitor balloon inflation.[14]

Very occasionally, MRI or fast CT may identify a pericardial effusion not detected by echocardiography or cardiac catheterization in a hemodynamically unstable patient following chest trauma or cardiac surgery and thereby lead to the diagnosis of tamponade.

CONSTRICTIVE PERICARDITIS

Constrictive pericarditis is an insidious disease that can confound the most astute clinician. Advances in cardiac imaging, however, have significantly improved our diagnostic accuracy. In as many as 50 percent of cases, the pericardium calcifies, making detection with chest roentgenography possible. However, pericardial calcification may be easily overlooked on the posteroanterior film, so a lateral view must always be obtained when the diagnosis is suspected. Doppler echocardiography should also be performed in all patients suspected of exhibiting constrictive pathophysiology. High reflectance and thickening of the posterior pericardium may suggest the diagnosis, although these findings are neither highly sensitive nor specific.[15] Alterations in caval, pulmonary vein, and intracardiac Doppler flow during the respiratory cycle are more reliable signs of constriction.[16] An inspiratory increase in velocity of early diastolic transtricuspid flow associated with a decrease in transmitral flow is probably the most reliable sign. A reversal of this pattern is seen during expiration. Cardiac catheterization is often employed to confirm the presence and establish the severity of constrictive pathophysiology. In the past, right atrial angiography to detect straightening of the lateral border, or coronary angiography to define the pericardial thickness by the depth of the arteries within the cardiac silhouette, has been recommended. The advent of tomographic imaging, however, has significantly reduced the

need for their use. Magnetic resonance imaging or fast CT can accurately define the thickness of the pericardium.[17, 18] Conventional CT has also been employed with some success, but the image resolution of this modality is not as good as that of MRI or fast CT because of motion artifact caused by cardiac contraction.[19] Therefore, when Doppler echocardiography and cardiac catheterization have not definitively established the diagnosis, MRI or fast CT should be performed to distinguish between patients with restrictive cardiomyopathy and those with constrictive pericarditis.

Even though the diagnosis of constrictive pericarditis may be secure, diagnosticians and surgeons may be uncertain about the success of surgical treatment. Pericardiectomy is an extremely difficult and tedious operation for even the most experienced surgeon. Adequate removal of the firmly adherent pericardium from the myocardium without injury to the coronary arteries or inadvertently entering the right ventricle or atria is challenging. Surgeons would be greatly aided if they could know how adherent the pericardium is, on a region-by-region basis. Then surgery could be focused on the regions where the likelihood of adequate removal is high; thus, valuable surgical time would not be expended on regions where the fibrotic process has extended deep into the myocardium, making surgical release virtually impossible. The relatively new tomographic techniques, MRI and fast CT, have shown real promise in assisting with this surgical dilemma.

EFFUSIVE CONSTRICTIVE PERICARDITIS

Some cases of acute pericarditis with effusion, usually caused by infection with pyogenic organisms or tuberculosis, may proceed rapidly, over days to weeks, to constrictive pathophysiology. When this sequence of events occurs, the diagnosis of effusive constrictive pericarditis is made. Some patients may also have experienced tamponade during the early stages of the acute pericarditis. Recognition that the patient has progressed from acute pericarditis with or without tamponade to constrictive pathophysiology is not always easy, but the wide availability of Doppler echocardiography has certainly assisted the clinician in earlier recognition of this condition.[20] The ease and safety of serial echocardiography in patients with effusive acute pericarditis is the basis for the improvement in diagnosis. As previously described, there are characteristic echocardiographic and Doppler signs for both tamponade and constriction, so the echocardiographer can track the changes in pathophysiology with serial studies. In cases in which the diagnosis is still in doubt, cardiac catheterization is necessary.

Recently, one investigative group suggested that color flow Doppler imaging of the movement of the intrapericardial fluid during the cardiac cycle may indicate the development of a constrictive state in the patient with an effusion.[21] Occasionally, MRI or fast CT may prove helpful in the patient with effusive constrictive pericarditis when the effusion is loculated posteriorly or over the right atrium. Furthermore, the surgeon may be aided by MRI or fast CT images in planning the removal of the pericardium.

Perhaps in the future, improved tissue characterization with ultrasound or MRI may define attributes of inflamed pericardium that are likely to lead to a constrictive pathophysiology. Likewise, characterization of the nature of the pericardial fluid may also have value in predicting development of a constrictive state.

OTHER PERICARDIAL DISEASES

The chest roentgenogram can often suggest the presence of a pericardial cyst or mass or the absence of the left hemipericardium. However, the high spatial resolution tomographic techniques, MRI and fast CT, have greatly facilitated the diagnosis of these entities and are now the diagnostic methods of choice[22] (see Chapter 57). These methods are also helpful in defining the etiology of pericardial masses, as their origin is often related to other mediastinal pathology. Since pericardial motion is often not great during the cardiac cycle, conventional CT imaging can also be employed in these conditions.[23] Pericardial lipoma is a fairly common etiology among the causes of a pericardial mass. The high signal of fat causes a characteristic image by MRI, and the low density of fat likewise creates a characteristic image by CT. Therefore, both techniques are ideal for diagnosing pericardial lipomas. Similarly, both are the best methods for detecting pericardial lipomatosis.

SUMMARY

Pericardial disease is an uncommon form of heart disease; therefore, clinicians often do not consider its presence. However, the widespread use of echocardiography in many patients with signs and symptoms suspected of being of cardiac origin has led to much earlier detection and more accurate categorization of pericardial disease. Recent development of the high-resolution tomographic imaging methods, MRI and fast CT, has further improved diagnostic accuracy.

References

1. Horowitz, M. S., Schultz, C. S., Stinson, E. B., et al.: Sensitivity and specificity of echocardiographic diagnosis of pericardial effusion. Circulation 50:239, 1974.
2. Martin, R. P., Bowden, R., Filly, K., et al.: Intrapericardial abnormalities in patients with pericardial effusion: Findings by two-dimensional echocardiography. Circulation 61:568, 1980.
3. Stark, D. D., Higgins, C. B., Lanzer, P., et al.: Magnetic resonance imaging of the pericardium: Normal and pathologic findings. Radiology 150:469, 1984.
4. Isner, J. M., Carter, B. L., Bankoff, M. S., et al.: Computed tomography in the diagnosis of pericardial heart disease. Ann. Intern. Med. 97:473, 1982.
5. Grover-McKay, M., Burke, S., Thompson, S. A., et al.: Measurement of pericardial thickness by cine computed tomography. Am. J. Card. Imaging 5:98, 1991.
6. Higgins, C. B., Mattrey, B. F., and Shea, P.: CT localization and aspiration of postoperative pericardial fluid collection. J. Comput. Assist. Tomogr. 7:734, 1983.
7. Stanford, W., Rooholamini, S. A., and Galvin, J. R.: Ultrafast computed tomography in the detection of intracardiac masses and pulmonary artery thromboembolism. In Stanford, W., and Rumberger, J. A. (eds.): Ultrafast Computed Tomography in Cardiac Imaging: Principles and Practice. Mt. Kisco, NY, Futura Publishing, 1992, p. 240.
8. Rokey, R., Vick, G. W., III, Bolli, R., et al.: Assessment of experimental pericardial effusion using nuclear magnetic resonance imaging techniques. Am. Heart J. 121(4 Part 1):1161, 1991.
9. Kondos, G. T., Rich, S., and Levitsky, S.: Flexible fiberoptic pericardioscopy for the diagnosis of pericardial disease. J. Am. Coll. Cardiol. 7:432, 1986.
10. Borganelli, M., Byrd, B. F., III: Doppler echocardiography in pericardial disease. Cardiol. Clin. 8:333, 1990.
11. Schutzman, J. J., Obarski, T. P., Pearce, G. L., et al.: Comparison of Doppler and two-dimensional echocardiography for assessment of pericardial effusion. Am. J. Cardiol. 70:1353, 1992.
12. Sanders, W. H. J., and Lampmann, L. E. H.: Percutaneous ultrasound-guided management of pericardial fluid. Eur. J. Radiol. 12:147, 1991.
13. Vora, A. M., and Lokhandwala, Y. Y.: Echocardiography-guided creation of balloon pericardial window. Cathet. Cardiovasc. Diagn. 25:164, 1992.
14. Ziskind, A. A., and Burstein S.: Echocardiography vs. fluoroscopic imaging. Cathet. Cardiovasc. Diagn. 27:86, 1992.
15. Schnittger, I., Bowden, R. E., Abrams, J., et al.: Echocardiography: Pericardial thickening and constrictive pericarditis. Am. J. Cardiol. 42:388, 1978.
16. Hatle, L. K., Appleton, C. P., and Popp, R. L.: Differentiation of constrictive pericarditis and restrictive cardiomyopathy by Doppler echocardiography. Circulation 79:357, 1989.
17. Sechtem, U., Tscholakoff, D., and Higgins, C. B.: MRI of the abnormal pericardium. A. J. R. 147:245, 1986.
18. Oren, R. M., Grover-McKay, M., Stanford, W., et al.: Accurate preoperative diagnosis of pericardial constriction using cine computed tomography. J. Am. Coll. Cardiol. 22:832, 1993.
19. Isner, J. M., Carter, B., Bankoff, M. S., et al.: Differentiation of constrictive pericarditis from restrictive cardiomyopathy by computed tomographic imaging. Am. Heart J. 105:1019, 1983.
20. Wolf, W. J.: Echocardiographic features of a purulent pericardial peel. Am. Heart J. 111:990, 1986.
21. Lai, L. P., Shyu, K. G., Chang, C. I., et al.: Pericardial color Doppler flow in postpericardiotomy effusive constrictive pericarditis. Cardiology 83:132, 1993.
22. Amparo, E. G., Higgins, C. G., Farmer, D., et al.: Gated MRI of cardiac and paracardiac masses: Initial experience. A. J. R. 143:1151, 1984.
23. Gross, B. H., Glazer, G. M., and Francis, I. R.: CT of intracardiac and intrapericardial masses. A. J. R. 140:903, 1983.

CHAPTER

14 Cardiovascular Trauma

David J. Skorton, M.D.

GOALS OF IMAGING IN CARDIOVASCULAR TRAUMA _____ 95
SPECIAL DIAGNOSTIC CONSIDERATIONS _____ 96
ESSENTIAL GENERAL DIAGNOSTIC APPROACHES TO CARDIOVASCULAR TRAUMA _____ 96
SPECIFIC EXAMPLES _____ 96
Aortic Transection or Rupture _____ 96
Myocardial Contusion _____ 97
Pericardial Injuries _____ 97
Coronary Artery Trauma _____ 97
Valvular Trauma _____ 97
Other Penetrating Chest Trauma _____ 97
UNANSWERED QUESTIONS _____ 97
CONCLUSIONS _____ 98

Trauma to the heart and great vessels is, unfortunately, a problem of growing concern in modern cardiovascular practice. In persons younger than age 40, violent injury accounts for a large proportion of deaths, and, among these deaths, cardiovascular trauma is a leading cause.[1] The wide variety of causes of trauma include, but are not limited to, automobile injuries; falls; blunt and sharp trauma, including stab wounds and lacerations; gunshot wounds; and inadvertent side effects of medical devices. This wide range of etiologies produces an equally wide range of lesions. Thus, virtually the entire spectrum of cardiovascular structures may be involved by traumatic injuries.

GOALS OF IMAGING IN CARDIOVASCULAR TRAUMA

The major goal in evaluating the patient with cardiac trauma is to identify the disorder, with particular attention paid to the recognition of sequelae of trauma that are potentially life threatening. This approach focuses particular attention on entities such as aortic transection or rupture, cardiac tamponade, coronary artery lacerations, severe myocardial contusion, and free wall laceration or rupture. The range of these acutely life-threatening disorders dictates a similar range of diagnostic imaging approaches. Commonly, speed in diagnosis is of the essence; this need to expedite management often dictates which diagnostic modality is employed. It is of note that in nonpenetrating (blunt) cardiovascular trauma, visible thoracic wall injury may not be present despite severe cardiovascular injury.[1] Thus, a high index of suspicion is necessary for optimal management of these patients.

SPECIAL DIAGNOSTIC CONSIDERATIONS

As noted, the range of problems encountered in cardiovascular trauma is broad and includes damage to all cardiac structures and great vessels. Therefore, the clinician must be prepared to diagnose and deal with an unusual variety of disorders, including intrapericardial bleeding (related to laceration of the cardiac chambers, coronary arteries, veins, or other structures) leading to cardiac tamponade; low output from myocardial contusion; acute valvular regurgitation due to avulsion of valvular structures, including chordae tendineae and papillary muscles; and intrathoracic bleeding from damage to the great vessels. The latter problem, transection of the aorta or avulsion of one of its branches, may occur as the result of direct trauma or deceleration injury (e.g., a fall or an automobile accident); it is one of the most common serious injuries from blunt trauma encountered clinically.

Careful attention to logistics is essential so that therapy is not postponed or interrupted because of the need to transport patients to distant sites. An algorithm is needed[2] by which the lesions most likely to be fatal are considered first and the most sensitive diagnostic tests are chosen to identify them before the clinician progresses to an evaluation of less life-threatening problems or to the application of more time-consuming or nonspecific imaging methods that could impede resuscitation.

Finally, disruptions of noncardiac anatomy or other obstacles to imaging are important considerations in the care of the patient with cardiovascular trauma. For example, trauma to the chest wall may preclude transthoracic echocardiography, and intrathoracic foreign bodies may alter the images produced with a variety of imaging methods.

ESSENTIAL GENERAL DIAGNOSTIC APPROACHES TO CARDIOVASCULAR TRAUMA

Echocardiography is a common first-line approach to the patient with known or suspected cardiovascular trauma.[3–9] Echocardiography is portable and, thus, easily applied in any clinical setting. The range of traumatic cardiovascular disease that can be diagnosed with echocardiography encompasses nearly all the diagnoses of interest, with the exception of coronary arterial or venous lacerations. Myocardial contusion, pericardial hematoma and tamponade, aortic rupture, and other great vessel injuries all are amenable to evaluation with transthoracic or transesophageal echocardiography. The well-established ability of echocardiography to define normal and abnormal endocardial motion and ventricular wall thickening makes it an excellent technique for delineating new abnormalities of contraction subsequent to myocardial contusion. Similarly, the ability of echocardiography to identify pericardial effusion and to support the diagnosis of tamponade is useful in the trauma setting where these abnormalities occur as the result of intrapericardial hemorrhage.

One potentially severe limitation of transthoracic echocardiography in trauma is in its application in patients with severe chest wall trauma. Abnormalities such as chest contusion or flail chest may make it nearly impossible to perform adequate transthoracic echocardiographic examination in this setting. Transesophageal echocardiography[10–16] obviates this problem if there is no severe maxillofacial, cervical spinal, mediastinal, or esophageal injury.

Other diagnostic techniques also have important roles in the evaluation of the trauma patient. Chest roentgenography may be useful in identifying rib fracture and pericardial effusion (implying hemopericardium) and in suggesting aortic rupture by the finding of mediastinal widening. Cardiac catheterization with angiography is still the technique of choice for the identification of abnormalities of the coronary arterial and venous system, including vessel lacerations, contusions, or effacement by mediastinal hematoma.

Aortography has long been the standard for the diagnosis of aortic transection and rupture, common serious sequelae of trauma.[1, 17, 18] Computed tomography (CT) has also proved useful in identifying aortic rupture.[19–23] Particularly when patients are already undergoing CT for head or abdominal injuries, this method may also be applied expeditiously to identify aortic rupture. Recently, the advent and widespread availability of transesophageal echocardiographic assessment of aortic dissection and rupture[15] have made it an additional first-line technique for the identification of aortic rupture due to trauma.

There is considerably less experience with the use of magnetic resonance imaging (MRI) in trauma. The lack of portability and the slow speed of this technique make it difficult to utilize in patients with severe trauma, in whom transportation is an important consideration. However, MRI offers superb delineation of great vessel and cardiac chamber anatomy, and newer "ultrafast" methods[24] may prove useful in the emergency setting. Demonstration of MRI angiography of the coronary arteries[25] suggests that in the future this technique may be useful for the identification of coronary abnormalities in trauma as well.

One role of radionuclide methods in the diagnosis of cardiovascular trauma is in the assessment of cardiac function.[26] Further, myocardial contusion may be identified by myocardial scintigraphy, with the use of either perfusion tracers[27] or necrosis-avid tracers.[28]

SPECIFIC EXAMPLES

Although the range of potential problems due to trauma is large, a few examples serve to indicate some approaches to diagnosing these injuries with imaging techniques.

Aortic Transection or Rupture

Rupture or transection of the aorta is an extremely common manifestation of cardiovascular trauma.[1] Rupture most commonly occurs at the isthmus because of the tethering effect of the ligamentum arteriosum. Many patients with aortic rupture do not survive long enough to undergo successful treatment, but some do come to medical care and require rapid evaluation and management. Chest roentgenography is helpful in identifying widening of the superior mediastinum. However, aortography remains the standard approach to the diagnosis of this disorder and is performed in the majority of medical centers as the primary approach to dealing with patients in whom aortic rupture, transection, or laceration is suspected.[1, 17, 18] Aortography has the advantage of visualization of the entire thoracic aorta, including all branches. Computed tomography may also be useful in these patients,[19–23] particularly if it is available in the emergency room and is being used to evaluate injuries of the head or abdomen.

Although echocardiography can identify aortic dissection, transthoracic echocardiography has not emerged as a first-line approach to the assessment of potential aortic rupture in the emergency setting. However, transesophageal echocardiography is showing substantial promise in this regard. Recent studies[15] have suggested excellent sensitivity and specificity for transesophageal echocardiography, which may be applied more rapidly than aortography in the emergency setting. Transesophageal echocardiography is also of use in the operating room.[29] What remains to be proved is whether the technique will be reliable in widespread practice for identifying injuries to aortic vessel branches.

Magnetic resonance imaging is extremely useful for the assessment of chronic disorders of the aorta but has not yet achieved the status of a first-line approach to the diagnosis of acute traumatic aortic rupture.

Myocardial Contusion

Nonpenetrating chest trauma may lead to myocardial contusion,[30] which can be difficult to diagnose. In particular, coexisting gross trauma to the chest wall may mask findings suggestive of myocardial contusion. The assessment of myocardial contusion with imaging or other techniques can be quite challenging. Chest roentgenography generally is not useful except in the identification of other evidence of chest trauma, such as pulmonary contusion and rib fracture. Echocardiography can identify abnormal regional wall motion and chamber enlargement. This ability is most useful in the patient in whom there is no suspicion of pre-existing regional left or right ventricular contractile dysfunction. In such a patient, the presence of a well-demarcated contraction abnormality or aneurysmal bulging is quite suggestive of myocardial contusion. The presence of severe chest wall trauma may make the application of transthoracic echocardiography difficult. However, transesophageal echocardiography is useful in this application and may become the ultrasound procedure of choice in the emergency assessment of patients with suspected myocardial contusion who have coexisting chest wall trauma.

Radionuclide imaging is helpful in the identification of myocardial contusion through at least two different strategies. First, perfusion scintigraphy may show areas of reduced perfusion related to myocardial contusion.[27] Also, technetium-99m–labeled pyrophosphate may be employed to identify acute injury.[28] Antimyosin antibody imaging should be applicable to contusion, but this technique has been little studied in this setting.

Other imaging methods capable of identifying wall motion abnormalities, such as MRI and CT, would probably also be of use in these patients, although the portability of echocardiography makes it the procedure of choice for identifying wall motion abnormalities in suspected contusion.

Cardiac catheterization and angiography are usually not necessary in the setting of suspected acute myocardial contusion.

Pericardial Injuries

Hemopericardium and tamponade may result from nonpenetrating trauma, from laceration of a cardiac chamber or coronary vessel, from delayed cardiac rupture following myocardial contusion, or from late pericarditis. Echocardiography is exquisitely sensitive in identifying the presence and approximate volume of pericardial fluid.[31] Echocardiography may also give indirect evidence of tamponade physiology.[32] Magnetic resonance imaging and fast CT give information on the location and amount of pericardial fluid that is probably superior to that produced by echocardiography. However, the portability of echocardiography usually makes it a procedure of more immediate utility in the emergency assessment of patients with nonpenetrating chest trauma suspected of having pericardial damage.

Coronary Artery Trauma

Contusion or laceration of coronary arteries may lead to myocardial infarction, although the specific role of trauma to the coronary artery versus pre-existing atherosclerosis versus direct myocardial contusion is somewhat controversial.[1] Arteriovenous fistulae, left ventricular aneurysm, and intrapericardial bleeding are sequelae of coronary injury due to blunt or penetrating chest trauma. The chest radiograph is of little use in this situation except in the identification of pulmonary or musculoskeletal complications of the trauma. Echocardiography, either transthoracic or transesophageal, can identify the presence of new abnormalities in regional wall contraction or aneurysm formation secondary to ischemia from coronary artery occlusion due to trauma. As of this writing, however, echocardiography is not capable of identifying specific sites of coronary arterial laceration. Selective coronary angiography is definitive, although some authors advise against employing angiography in the acute setting.[1] The surgeon may be left with the option of exploration of the mediastinum and direct visualization of the major coronary arteries.

Valvular Trauma

The cardiac valves may be injured in nonpenetrating or penetrating trauma. Some of these injuries result from acceleration or deceleration injuries, leading, for example, to rupture of chordae tendineae or papillary muscles. Other sequelae are due to direct damage to the valve structures. Echocardiography, including transesophageal approaches, should be the method of first choice for the assessment of the cardiac valves.[12, 14] If severe chest trauma precludes both the transthoracic and the transesophageal approaches, direct epicardial imaging in the operating room may be useful. Cardiac catheterization and angiography may occasionally be necessary in this patient population, but, in general, echocardiography should be the approach of choice.

Other Penetrating Chest Trauma

Trauma may be due to penetration by a variety of objects; unfortunately, violent chest penetration by bullets, knives, and other objects is becoming increasingly common. As may be suspected, the problems resulting from such penetration are difficult to predict. Echocardiography is valuable in the identification of some sequelae of penetrating cardiac injury,[16] including pericardial bleeding, valve avulsion, and intracardiac foreign bodies. At times, extremely rapid diagnostic decision-making may be required in an unstable patient who needs urgent exploratory thoracotomy because of severe hypotension or other emergent problems. In this setting, transesophageal echocardiography may be extraordinarily useful to the cardiothoracic surgeon in deciding on a therapeutic approach, as it may be performed quickly in the emergency room or even in the operating room during surgery.

UNANSWERED QUESTIONS

A major unanswered question is, What are the relative roles of aortography, transesophageal echocardiography, and CT in suspected aortic rupture? Unsettled issues include the relative sensitivity and specificity of each and their relative cost-effectiveness.

Definitive recognition of involvement of the coronary arteries by trauma necessitates the use of selective coronary angiography. One important unanswered question deals with the eventual role of methods such as transesophageal echocardiography, MRI, or fast CT in the delineation of coronary arterial anatomy. Should these methods prove as capable as their early promise suggests, some coronary arteriograms may be avoided.

Another unanswered question concerns the need for more direct, higher resolution identification of acute myocardial contusion than what is currently possible with radionuclide techniques. In particular, abnormalities of regional ventricular contraction, as demonstrated with echocardiography or other methods, are somewhat nonspecific. Acute injury, chronic ischemic heart disease, and scar from an old injury all may produce similar wall motion disturbances. If the patient is young and, therefore, atherosclerotic disease is not a serious consideration, a regional wall motion disturbance may be considered pathognomonic of acute myocardial contusion. However, in patients older than 40 years of age, in whom atherosclerotic cardiovascular disease is common, the finding of a regional wall motion disturbance may be difficult to interpret.

CONCLUSIONS

Cardiovascular trauma remains an important cause of morbidity and mortality. Imaging techniques are extremely useful in the diagnosis of these patients. Aortic transection or rupture is a common, serious sequela of trauma. Aortography is currently the standard diagnostic procedure, although transesophageal echocardiography and CT may make important contributions to this diagnosis. Pericardial injuries with resultant tamponade may be confidently identified with echocardiography. Myocardial contusion requires a high index of suspicion and the diagnosis may be accomplished with a combination of echocardiography and radionuclide methods. The wide variety of other cardiovascular traumatic disorders requires a similarly wide range of imaging approaches.

References

1. Cohn, P.F., and Braunwald, E.: Traumatic heart disease. *In* Braunwald, E. (ed.): Heart Disease. Philadelphia, W.B. Saunders, 1992, p. 1151.
2. Mattox, K.L., Limacher, M.C., Feliciano, D.V., et al.: Cardiac evaluation following heart injury. J. Trauma 25:758, 1985.
3. Bolton, J.W., Bynoe, R.P., Lazar, H.L., et al.: Two-dimensional echocardiography in the evaluation of penetrating intrapericardial injuries. Ann. Thorac. Surg. 56:506, 1993.
4. Hassett, A., Moran, J., Sabiston, D.C., et al.: Utility of echocardiography in the management of patients with penetrating missile wounds of the heart. J. Am. Coll. Cardiol. 7:1151, 1986.
5. Xie, S.W., and Picard, M.H.: Two-dimensional and color Doppler echocardiographic diagnosis of penetrating missile wounds of the heart: Chronic complications from intracardiac course of a bullet. J. Am. Soc. Echocardiogr. 5:81, 1992.
6. Homma, S., Gillam, L.D., and Weyman, A.E.: Echocardiographic observations in survivors of acute electrical injury. Chest 97:103, 1990.
7. Oh, J.K., Meloy, T.D., and Seward, J.B.: Echocardiography in the emergency room: Is it feasible, beneficial, and cost-effective? Echocardiography 12:163, 1995.
8. Schiavone, W.A., Ghumrawi, B.K., Catalano, D.R., et al.: The use of echocardiography in the emergency management of nonpenetrating traumatic cardiac rupture. Ann. Emerg. Med. 20:1248, 1991.
9. Baxa, M.D.: Cardiac rupture secondary to blunt trauma: A rapidly diagnosable entity with two-dimensional echocardiography. Ann. Emerg. Med. 20:902, 1991.
10. LiMandri, G., Gorenstein, L.A., Starr, J.P., et al.: Use of transesophageal echocardiography in the detection and consequences of an intracardiac bullet. Am. J. Emerg. Med. 12:105, 1994.
11. Brooks, S.W., Young, J.C., Cmolik, B., et al.: The use of transesophageal echocardiography in the evaluation of chest trauma. J. Trauma 32:761, 1992.
12. Turabian, M., and Chan, K.-L.: Rupture of mitral chordae tendineae resulting from blunt chest trauma: Diagnosis by transesophageal echocardiography. Can. J. Cardiol. 6:180, 1990.
13. Shapiro, M.J., Yanofsky, S.D., Trapp, J., et al.: Cardiovascular evaluation in blunt thoracic trauma using transesophageal echocardiography (TEE). J. Trauma 31:835, 1991.
14. Spangenthal, E.J., Sekovski, B., Bhayana, J.N., et al.: Traumatic left ventricular papillary muscle rupture: The role of transesophageal echocardiography in diagnosis and surgical management. J. Am. Soc. Echocardiogr. 6:536, 1993.
15. Smith, M.D., Cassidy, J.M., Souther, S., et al.: Transesophageal echocardiography in the diagnosis of traumatic rupture of the aorta. N. Engl. J. Med. 332:356, 1995.
16. Skoularigis, J., Essop, M.R., and Sareli, P.: Usefulness of transesophageal echocardiography in the early diagnosis of penetrating stab wounds to the heart. Am. J. Cardiol. 73:407, 1994.
17. Fisher, R.G., and Ben-Menachem, J.: Penetrating injuries of the thoracic aorta and brachiocephalic arteries: Angiographic findings in 18 cases. AJR 149:601, 1987.
18. Daniels, D.I., and Maddison, F.E.: Ascending aortic injury: An angiographic diagnosis. AJR 136:812, 1981.
19. Miller, F.B., Richardson, J.D., Hollis, A.T., et al.: Role of CT in the diagnosis of major arterial injury after blunt thoracic trauma. Surgery 106:596, 1989.
20. Brooks, A.P., Olson, L.K., and Shackford, S.R.: Computed tomography in the diagnosis of traumatic rupture of the thoracic aorta. Clin. Radiol. 40:133, 1989.
21. Raptopoulos, V., Sheiman, R.G., Phillips, D.A., et al.: Traumatic aortic tear: Screening with chest CT. Radiology 182:667, 1992.
22. Thompson, B.H., and Stanford, W.: Utility of ultrafast computed tomography in the detection of thoracic aortic aneurysms and dissections. Semin. Ultrasound CT MR 14:117, 1993.
23. Richardson, P., Mirvis, S.E., Scorpio, R., et al.: Value of CT in determining the need for angiography when findings of mediastinal hemorrhage on chest radiographs are equivocal. AJR 156:273, 1991.
24. Pearlman, J.D., and Edelman, R.R.: Ultrafast magnetic resonance imaging: Segmented turboflash, echo-planar, and real-time nuclear magnetic resonance. Radiol. Clin. North Am. 32:593, 1994.
25. Manning, W.J., Li, W., and Edelman, R.R.: A preliminary report comparing magnetic resonance coronary angiography with conventional angiography. N. Engl. J. Med. 328:828, 1993.
26. Skarsgard, E.D., Phang, P.T., Belzberg, A.S., et al.: Effect of cardiac stabbing on ventricular function: Evaluation of radionuclide angiography. Can. J. Surg. 36:425, 1993.
27. Kumar, S.A., Puri, V.K., Mittal, V.K., et al.: Myocardial contusion following nonfatal blunt chest trauma. J. Trauma 23:327, 1983.
28. Chiu, C.L., Roelofs, J.D., Go, R.T., et al.: Coronary angiographic and scintigraphic findings in experimental cardiac contusion. Radiology 116:679, 1975.
29. Ellis, J.E., and Bender, E.M.: Intraoperative transesophageal echocardiography in blunt thoracic trauma. J. Cardiothorac. Vasc. Anesth. 5:373, 1991.
30. Hossack, K.F., Moreno, C.A., Vanway, C.W., et al.: Frequency of cardiac contusion in nonpenetrating chest injury. Am. J. Cardiol. 61:391, 1988.
31. D'Cruz, I.A., Cohen, H.D., Prabbu, R., et al.: Potential pitfalls in quantification of pericardial effusion by echocardiography. Br. Heart J. 39:529, 1977.
32. Singh, S., Wann, S., Schuchard, G.H., et al.: Right ventricular and right atrial collapse in patients with cardiac tamponade: A combined echocardiographic and hemodynamic study. Circulation 68:294, 1983.

CHAPTER

15 Diseases of the Great Vessels

Bruce H. Brundage, M.D.

AORTIC DISSECTION _____ 99
THORACIC AORTIC ANEURYSM _____ 99
OTHER AORTIC DISEASES _____ 99
PULMONARY ARTERY
    EMBOLISM _____ 100

PULMONARY ARTERIOVENOUS
    MALFORMATION _____ 100
OTHER PULMONARY VASCULAR
    DISEASES _____ 100
SUMMARY _____ 100

This chapter examines the relationship among the various imaging modalities used to visualize pathology of the aorta and pulmonary artery. Covered in detail are the major diseases of the great vessels: aortic dissection, thoracic aortic aneurysm, and pulmonary artery embolism. Other less common diseases of the aorta and pulmonary artery are only briefly discussed. For each disease category the essential imaging technique or techniques are presented with the rationale for their importance. Competing and complementary technologies are also identified. Finally, unresolved issues regarding the clinical use of imaging techniques for the diagnosis of the major diseases of the great vessels are discussed. The hope is that this chapter will serve as an introduction to the subsequent chapters in this book that deal with specific imaging modalities and their use in the diagnosis of diseases of the great vessels as well as give the reader some sense of the relative value of these techniques in the diagnostic work-up.

AORTIC DISSECTION

Dissection of the aorta is not a very common disease but occurs frequently enough that every clinician will encounter the entity a number of times in practice. Moreover, the clinical course of the disease is often catastrophic, requiring early diagnosis and aggressive treatment. Advances in cardiac imaging have given the physician a variety of diagnostic tools to assist in its recognition. The problem facing the cardiologist, radiologist, and surgeon is which diagnostic technique(s) to choose.

The chest roentgenogram often provides the first clue that a patient presenting with chest pain has an aortic dissection by demonstrating unusual widening of the mediastinum. Occasionally, displacement of a calcified intima in the aortic knob confirms the diagnosis, but in the majority of patients further imaging studies must be performed before the clinician can be certain.[1] Many patients with aortic dissection are hemodynamically unstable and require close monitoring of vital signs. Therefore, the next imaging test commonly performed—because it can be performed at the bedside—is a transthoracic echocardiogram. This technique has a good sensitivity and specificity for diagnosing type A, or ascending, aortic dissection but is relatively insensitive for type B, or descending, aortic dissection.[2] In many institutions, contrast-enhanced computed tomography is the next study to be performed. Computed tomography has quite good sensitivity and specificity, and in many cases no further studies may be needed.[3] If these studies do not clarify the diagnosis, then aortography is commonly performed. In some institutions, aortography may be the imaging procedure of choice, or when the patient is unstable and emergency surgery is planned it may be the only imaging procedure performed other than a chest roentgenogram.[4] Transesophageal echocardiography is increasingly being used as a front-line imaging modality for the diagnosis of aortic dissection, and certainly it is more sensitive than the transthoracic approach.[5] Many echocardiographers proceed directly to a transesophageal study if there are any questions remaining after the transthoracic evaluation. In other centers, magnetic resonance imaging (MRI) is the next imaging modality to be employed.[6] One study comparing MRI, transesophageal echocardiography, and conventional computed tomography (CT) concluded that MRI was the most sensitive and specific for all types of dissection.[7] However, MRI is limited to patients who are reasonably stable, and this technique certainly has not been accepted in all institutions as the preferred test. Fast CT is available in only about 60 centers worldwide, so the experience with it in the diagnosis of dissection is somewhat limited. In any regard, this imaging modality appears to be very accurate in the diagnosis of all types of dissection and may rival MRI.[8, 9]

Consequently, the diagnostician and the surgeon are faced with a rather wide array of diagnostic tools and must decide which ones are necessary for each patient. Institutional experience plays a major role in the decision. In some centers, transesophageal echocardiography may be preferred over CT or MRI, while in others aortography may still be the first choice.[10] The stability of the patient also influences which techniques are chosen. A very stable patient may have contrast-enhanced CT as the initial imaging evaluation or, possibly in some centers, MRI. The certainty of the diagnosis also influences which imaging modalities are employed. In some patients, several different studies may be required because aortic dissection is a disease that requires absolute certainty about the diagnosis. In the future, when there is more experience with transesophageal echocardiography, MRI, and fast CT, diagnostic algorithms are likely to be developed that will take into consideration the stability of the patient, the relative diagnostic accuracies of the various techniques, and cost to guide the diagnostician and the surgeon in the appropriate use of one or more imaging modalities.

After successful treatment of acute aortic dissection, medical or surgical, follow-up is required with some form of imaging to confirm that there is anatomical stability. Conventional contrast-enhanced CT and MRI are the two most commonly employed methods.[11, 12] Fast CT will probably be a very satisfactory method as well. The role of transesophageal echocardiography for this purpose is less well established but promising.[13]

THORACIC AORTIC ANEURYSM

Aneurysms of the thoracic aorta are of multiple etiologies, including atherosclerosis, aortic root disease, trauma, infection, and inflammatory disease of unknown etiology. Consequently, the etiology may define which imaging modalities are most appropriate for diagnosis.

Whatever the etiology of thoracic aortic aneurysms, the chest roentgenogram is always appropriate as the first step in the imaging evaluation. Indeed, the diagnosis is often first suspected after the physician views the chest film. On occasion, aortic root disease may not be apparent on the chest roentgenogram. Aortography is the diagnostic procedure of choice in atherosclerotic, traumatic, and syphilitic aneurysms because it defines the limits of the aneurysm and its relation to major aortic branch vessels.[14] However, there is some risk of embolism with invasive aortography, albeit small. Continued development of transesophageal Doppler echocardiography, MRI, and CT, particularly fast CT, is making these techniques increasingly attractive alternatives to aortography.[15–17] These modalities are noninvasive or minimally invasive, provide much better definition of any intra-aneurysm pathology, such as thrombus, and provide a better understanding of three-dimensional relationships. As these techniques become better at defining branch vessels, they could one day replace invasive iodinated contrast aortography.

Aortic root disease is often detected with transthoracic echocardiography, which can also assess the degree of associated aortic valve regurgitation.[18] Transesophageal echocardiography has also been used.[19] In cases not requiring surgery, a chest roentgenogram and an echocardiogram may complete the imaging evaluation. If surgery is under consideration, cardiac catheterization is usually performed to define precisely the size of the aorta, quantitate the aortic regurgitation, and define the coronary anatomy. In the future, MRI and fast CT may also find a role in the assessment of this disease.[8, 20] They already provide precise measurement of the aortic root size and quantitate the amount of aortic regurgitation by comparing left and right ventricular stroke volume; someday, they may be able to provide adequate resolution of the coronary arteries.

The many advances in echocardiography, MRI, and CT have given the clinician more choices for imaging the aorta. While iodinated contrast aortography remains the first choice for most, it is likely that the less invasive techniques will become increasingly popular, and one day they may supplant standard angiography. Hopefully, cost-effective algorithms will be developed for each type of aortic aneurysm to help guide the diagnostician and the surgeon in choosing the most appropriate imaging tests.

OTHER AORTIC DISEASES

Congenital diseases of the aorta, including coarctation and arteritides such as Takayasu arteritis, are usually evaluated with aortography, but as transesophageal Doppler echocardiography, MRI, and fast CT evolve, they may play a larger role in the future.

The increasing use of transesophageal echocardiography has led to the recognition of a new entity, complex aortic wall plaque.[21] When present in the aortic arch, this intimal pathology can be an important cause of embolic stroke. One may expect that as more clinical experience is gained with the evolving tomographic imaging techniques, further insights into the pathology of aortic disease will occur.

PULMONARY ARTERY EMBOLISM

Until very recently, little had changed in the imaging approach to diagnosing pulmonary embolism. A chest roentgenogram is performed initially and is helpful in excluding other pulmonary pathology as the cause of the patient's signs and symptoms. Occasionally, there are radiographic signs, such as a Hampton hump, that strongly suggest the diagnosis, but in most patients the chest film is unrevealing or nonspecific. Clinicians are trained to have a low threshold for considering the diagnosis and to employ pulmonary ventilation ($\dot{V}$) and perfusion ($\dot{Q}$) scintigraphy in any patient with suspicious symptoms, signs, or clinical circumstances. The test has a sensitivity of 98 percent for pulmonary emboli but only a low specificity of 10 percent. Therefore, approximately one third of patients have an intermediate-probability $\dot{V}/\dot{Q}$ scan, and pulmonary angiography is required to clarify the diagnosis. A multicenter study also indicates that a low-probability scan is associated with a 12 percent incidence of pulmonary emboli and a high-probability scan is not associated with pulmonary embolism in 59 percent of patients.[23] Pulmonary angiography remains the gold standard but is associated with some risk and errors in diagnosis.[24] Now, advances in MRI, fast CT, and spiral CT imaging have produced sufficient resolution of the pulmonary vessels that these techniques are being given serious consideration as alternatives to lung scintigraphy and conventional pulmonary angiography.[25-27] Further clinical trials are needed, however, before these methods can be recommended for routine clinical use.

PULMONARY ARTERIOVENOUS MALFORMATION

Arteriovenous malformations of the lung are uncommon and, when seen, are often associated with hereditary hemorrhagic telangiectasia. The diagnosis may be suggested by a chest roentgenogram that defines the presence of two vascular shadows associated with a nodular lung density. Classically, the diagnosis is made with cardiac catheterization and pulmonary angiography. A number of centers have reported the evaluation of these arteriovenous malformations with conventional CT.[28, 29] Fast CT may prove even more successful in imaging these lesions than conventional or spiral CT because of the elimination of vascular motion.[30] Investigators have suggested that tomographic techniques may be more successful in detecting small multiple arteriovenous malformations than pulmonary angiography. This information is important in planning surgical therapy. In some centers, CT or fast CT is on the verge of replacing pulmonary angiography.

OTHER PULMONARY VASCULAR DISEASES

A variety of pathophysiologic states lead to occlusive disease of the small pulmonary vessels, such as long-standing intracardiac shunts, collagen vascular disease, some hepatic conditions, human immunodeficiency virus (HIV) infection, and idiopathic causes. In advanced stages, vascular abnormalities can be recognized with chest roentgenography and pulmonary angiography. Earlier stages of the disease can be inferred only by noting changes in pulmonary hemodynamics. Doppler echocardiography has become the standard for noninvasive assessment of pulmonary artery pressure.[31] Several investigators have begun to use intravascular ultrasound to evaluate these vessels in patients.[32] Apparently, changes in the pulmonary vessel wall can be seen in patients with elevated pulmonary artery pressure. Further research of this type is likely to lead to a better understanding of small pulmonary vessel pathology in the living human that is not possible with the other imaging techniques.

SUMMARY

Chest roentgenography and conventional angiography have been the cornerstone of the evaluation of diseases of the great vessels. Significant advances in Doppler echocardiography, MRI, and CT in the past several years have opened the door to a whole set of new options for diagnosis. It is in the realm of possibility that invasive angiography of the great vessels will be replaced by these imaging techniques in the next few years. Intravascular ultrasound may also find a place in the evaluation of small pulmonary and systemic vessels.

References

1. Hartnell, G.G., Wakeley, C.J., Tottle, A., et al.: Limitations of chest radiography in discriminating between aortic dissection and myocardial infarction: Implications for thrombolysis. J. Thorac. Imaging 8:152, 1993.
2. Cigarroa, J.E., Isselbacher, E.M., DeSanctis, R.W., et al.: Diagnostic imaging in the evaluation of suspected aortic dissection. N. Engl. J. Med. 328:35, 1993.
3. Goodwin, J.D.: Conventional CT of the aorta. J. Thorac. Imaging 5:18, 1990.
4. Mast, H.L., Gordon, D.H., and Kantor, A.M.: Pitfalls in diagnosis of aortic dissection by angiography: Algorithmic approach utilizing CT and MRI. Comput. Med. Imaging Graph. 15:431, 1991.
5. Ballal, R.S., Nanda, N.C., Gatewood, R., et al.: Usefulness of transesophageal echocardiography in assessment of aortic dissection. Circulation 84:1903, 1991.
6. Nienaber, C.A., Spielmann, R.P., Kodolitsch, Y.V., et al.: Diagnosis of thoracic aortic dissection: Magnetic resonance imaging versus transesophageal echocardiograph. Circulation 85:434, 1992.
7. Nienaber, C.A., Kodolitsch, Y.V., Nicolas, V., et al.: The diagnosis of thoracic aortic dissection by noninvasive imaging procedures. N. Engl. J. Med. 328:1, 1993.
8. Stanford, W., Rooholamini, S.A., and Galvin, J.R.: Ultrafast computed tomography in the diagnosis of aortic aneurysms and dissections. J. Thorac. Imaging 5:32, 1990.
9. Hamada, S., Takamiya, M., Kimura, K., et al.: Type A aortic dissection: Evaluation with ultrafast CT. Radiology 183:155, 1992.
10. Naidich, J.B., and Crystal, K.S.: Diagnosis of dissecting hematoma of the aorta: A choice between good and better. Radiology 190:16, 1994.
11. Rofsky, N.M., Weinreb, J.C., Grossi, E.A., et al.: Aortic aneurysm and dissection: Normal MR imaging and CT findings after surgical repair with the continuous-suture graft-inclusion technique. Radiology 186:195, 1993.
12. Di Cesare, E., Di Renzi, P., Pavone, P., et al.: Postsurgical follow-up of aortic dissections by MRI. Eur. J. Radiol. 13:27, 1991.
13. Roudaut, R.P., Marcaggi, X.L., Deville, C., et al.: Value of transesophageal echocardiography combined with computed tomography for assessing repaired type A aortic dissection. Am. J. Cardiol. 70:1468, 1992.
14. Sanders, C.: Current role of conventional and digital aortography in the diagnosis of aortic disease. J. Thorac. Imaging 5:48, 1991.
15. Revel, D., Loubeyre, P., Delignette, A., et al.: Contrast-enhanced magnetic resonance tomoangiography: A new imaging technique for studying thoracic great vessels. Magn. Reson. Imaging 11:1101, 1993.
16. Costello, P., Ecker, C.P., Tello, R., et al.: Assessment of the thoracic aorta by spiral CT. A.J.R. 158:1127, 1992.
17. Thompson, B.H., and Stanford, W.: Utility of ultrafast computed tomography in the detection of thoracic aortic aneurysms and dissections. Semin. Ultrasound CT MRI 14:117, 1993.
18. Come, P.C., Fortuin, N.J., White, R.I., et al.: Echocardiographic assessment of cardiovascular abnormalities in the Marfan syndrome. Am. J. Med. 74:465, 1983.
19. Simpson, I.A., de Belder, M.A., Treasure, T., et al.: Cardiovascular manifestations of Marfan's syndrome: Improved evaluation by transesophageal echocardiography. Br. Heart J. 69:104, 1993.
20. Schaefer, S., Peshock, R.M., Malloy, C.R., et al.: Nuclear magnetic resonance imaging in Marfan's syndrome. J. Am. Coll. Cardiol. 9:70, 1987.
21. Karalis, D.G., Chandrasekaran, K., Victor, M.F., et al.: Recognition and embolic potential of intraaortic atherosclerotic debris. J. Am. Coll. Cardiol. 17:73, 1991.
22. Fraser, R.G., and Paré, J.A.P. (eds.): Embolic and thrombotic diseases of the lungs in diagnosis of diseases of the chest. In Diagnosis of Diseases of the Chest. Philadelphia, W.B. Saunders, 1978, pp. 1135–1200.
23. A Collaborative Study by the PIOPED Investigators: Value of the ventilation/perfusion scan in acute pulmonary embolism: Results of the Prospective Investigation of Pulmonary Embolism Diagnosis (PIOPED). J.A.M.A. 263:2753, 1990.
24. Stein, P.D., Athanasoulis, C., Alavi, A., et al.: Complications and validity of pulmonary angiography in acute pulmonary embolism. Circulation 85:462, 1992.
25. Loubeyre, P., Revel, D., Douek, P., et al.: Dynamic contrast-enhanced MR angiography of pulmonary embolism: Comparison with pulmonary angiography. A.J.R. 162:1035, 1994.
26. Teigen, C.L., Maus, T.P., Sheedy, P.F., II, et al.: Pulmonary embolism: Diagnosis with contrast-enhanced electron-beam CT and comparison with pulmonary angiography. Radiology 194:313, 1995.
27. Remy-Jardin, M., Remy, J., Wattinne, L., et al.: Central pulmonary thromboembolism: Diagnosis with spiral volumetric CT with the single-breath-hold technique; comparison with pulmonary angiography. Radiology 185:381, 1992.
28. Remy, J., Remy-Jardin, M., Wattinne, L., et al.: Pulmonary arteriovenous malformations: Evaluation with CT of the chest before and after treatment. Radiology 182:809, 1992.

29. White, R.I., Jr.: Pulmonary arteriovenous malformations: How do we diagnose them and why is it important to do so? Radiology 182:633, 1992.

30. Love, B.B., Biller, J., Landas, S.K., et al.: Diagnosis of pulmonary arteriovenous malformation by ultrafast chest computed tomography in Rendu-Osler-Weber syndrome with cerebral ischemia: A case report. Angiology 43:522, 1992.

31. Schiller, N.B.: Pulmonary artery pressure estimation by Doppler and two-dimensional echocardiography. Cardiol. Clin. 8:277, 1990.

32. Pandian, N.G., Weintraub, A., Kreis, A., et al.: Intracardiac, intravascular, two-dimensional, high-frequency ultrasound imaging of pulmonary artery and its branches in humans and animals. Circulation 81:2007, 1990.

CHAPTER

16 Principles and Instrumentation for Radiography

James S. Whiting, Ph.D.

PROPERTIES OF X-RAYS ____ 102
Interactions of X-Rays With Matter ____ 103
Attenuation ____ 103
X-RAY PRODUCTION AND CONTROL ____ 103
X-Ray Tube ____ 103
Filtration ____ 105
Collimation ____ 105
X-Ray Generators and Exposure
  Control ____ 105
IMAGE FORMATION ____ 105
Image Geometry ____ 105
Resolution ____ 106
Contrast ____ 107
Noise ____ 110
THE IMAGE INTENSIFIER ____ 110
Components and Basic Operation ____ 110
Magnification Modes ____ 110
Intensification Gain ____ 111
Detective Quantum Efficiency ____ 111
Resolution ____ 111
Contrast ____ 111
Distortion ____ 111
FLUOROSCOPY ____ 111
X-Ray Technique ____ 111
Videocamera ____ 112
CINEANGIOGRAPHY ____ 113
X-Ray Technique ____ 113

Biplane Cineangiography ____ 114
Cine Camera ____ 114
Cine Film ____ 114
Analog Videorecording Devices ____ 115
GENERAL PRINCIPLES OF DIGITAL
  IMAGING ____ 115
Conversion of Images to Digital Form ____ 115
DIGITAL IMAGE STORAGE ____ 116
On-Line Storage ____ 117
Archival Storage ____ 117
DIGITAL IMAGE VIEWERS AND
  WORKSTATIONS ____ 118
DIGITAL IMAGE PROCESSING ____ 118
Gray-Scale Transformations ____ 118
Image Processing Filters ____ 118
Digital Subtraction Angiography ____ 120
IMAGE DATA COMPRESSION ____ 120
APPLICATIONS OF DIGITAL IMAGING ____ 120
Processing and Display ____ 120
Quantification ____ 121
RADIATION PROTECTION ____ 122
Maximum Permissible Dose and the ALARA
  Principle ____ 122
Intensity, Area, Time, Distance, and
  Shielding ____ 122
Technical Dose Reduction Methods ____ 123
SUMMARY ____ 124

Modern radiographic coronary angiography systems are highly automated to provide good quality fluoroscopic, cine film, and digital images under a wide range of conditions. Automation insulates the angiographer from many of the technical details of the x-ray imaging process, allowing angiography and interventional procedures to be performed with smaller staffs and with fewer distractions. Nevertheless, angiographers who have a firm understanding of radiographic physical principles and instrumentation can obtain better quality images at lower radiation dose to the patient, the staff, and themselves. This understanding is essential for building and maintaining a high-quality catheterization laboratory.

There are a number of good texts covering the physics of diagnostic radiology,[1-3] most designed as required reading for a one-year radiology residents' physics course. These texts cover fluoroscopy, cineangiography, ultrasound, computed tomography, magnetic resonance imaging, film processing, quality assurance, and radiation protection at a depth appropriate for cardiologists with major cardiac imaging activity. In addition to these general sources, the American College of Cardiology/American Heart Association (ACC/AHA) Ad Hoc Task Force on Cardiac Catheterization has published guidelines for cardiac catheterization[4] that include a succinct description, minimum specifications, and recommenda-

tions for radiographic equipment. These guidelines (or their most recent update) should be required reading for angiographers and laboratory directors.

This chapter covers the principles and instrumentation for x-ray fluoroscopy and cardiac angiography with an emphasis on those factors that influence image quality or radiation dose and are under the direct control of the angiographer or that influence equipment selection or maintenance.

PROPERTIES OF X-RAYS

X-rays may be thought of as infinitely small particles, called photons, which emanate from a source and move in straight lines at the speed of light until they interact with the atoms in the patient or the image receptor. Each photon carries a specific amount of energy. During interaction, a photon may be completely absorbed, transferring all of its energy to the interacting matter, or it may be "scattered" (deflected) by an atom or electron, giving up part of its energy and changing direction. The probability that a photon passing through matter will interact is determined by the density and thickness of the matter (i.e., how many atoms the photon is likely to approach closely or hit during passage through the matter), by the atomic number of the atoms (which determines the number of electrons per atom and how tightly each electron is bound to the nucleus), and by the energy of the photon. An understanding of the interplay between these factors is essential to understanding x-ray image formation and image quality.

Interactions of X-Rays With Matter

Of the several possible mechanisms of interaction between x-rays and matter, only two, the photoelectric effect and Compton scattering, play a significant role in cardiac angiography. The probability of interaction depends on x-ray photon energy for both mechanisms, but in different ways. Because the relative contributions of these two interactions to the x-ray image differ significantly and because they depend on angiographic factors partly under the control of the angiographer, each mechanism is discussed separately here.

Photoelectric Effect

The photoelectric effect is an interaction in which the x-ray photon is completely absorbed by an atom and its energy is transferred entirely to one of the atom's electrons (hence the name), which is then ejected from the atom. The complete removal of the initial (or "primary") x-ray photon is highly desirable for x-ray image formation. An object that interacts primarily by photoelectric effect casts a high-contrast shadow on the image receptor.

Conservation of energy requires that the x-ray photon energy be greater than the binding energy of the ejected electron. The probability of photoelectric effect interaction increases sharply at each electron binding energy (i.e., for each electron shell), in order of decreasing energy. Only the K-shell electron binding energy is high enough to be of importance. The sharp increase in attenuation at the K-shell binding energy is often referred to as the "K edge." Above the K edge, the photoelectric interaction probability again decreases as the inverse of the photon energy raised to the third power. At a fixed photon energy, the probability for photoelectric interaction is roughly proportional to the third power of the atomic number, so elements with high atomic number (e.g., iodine [atomic number 53]) absorb x-rays by photoelectric effect much more strongly than do elements of low atomic number, such as hydrogen, carbon, and oxygen (atomic numbers 1, 12, and 16, respectively). This difference is maximum when the photon energy is just above the K edge for the heavier element (33.2 keV for iodine).

The products of photoelectric absorption are the ejected photoelectron and the new x-ray photon emitted by the atom at an energy slightly below the binding energy of the ejected photoelectron. Because this energy is characteristic to the specific type of atom, the new photon is called a characteristic x-ray. The ejected photoelectron is absorbed by tissue very close to its site of origin. Its energy contributes to patient radiation dose but not to image formation. The direction of the characteristic x-ray is completely random in relation to the direction of the primary x-ray. Therefore, only a small fraction is emitted toward the image receptor. Those photons that do reach the image receptor land in random locations and therefore add a contrast-reducing haze to the image.

Compton Scattering

Compton scattering is an interaction in which the photon is deflected by a collision with a loosely bound electron, with only some of the energy of the incident photon transferred to the electron. This interaction differs from the photoelectric effect in three important ways. First, unlike the characteristic x-rays emitted by the photoelectric effect, photons that scatter are almost twice as likely to continue in the general direction of the image intensifier, retaining most of their original energy. Compton-scattered photons are therefore much more likely to reach the image intensifier, reducing image contrast. Compton scatter from the patient is also the main source of radiation exposure to the angiographer and staff. Second, the probability of Compton scattering is not a strong function of atomic number; iodinated contrast material produces about the same amount of Compton scattering as tissue does, so this interaction contributes little to angiographic contrast. Third, Compton scattering decreases inversely with only the first power of the photon energy, compared with the third power of energy for the photoelectric effect. Therefore, the probability of Compton scattering relative to photoelectric effect increases as the square of the photon energy.

Because Compton scattering produces negligible contrast itself and the scattered x-rays reduce contrast, image quality is optimized by keeping photon energy low, to minimize Compton scattering, but above the K edge of iodine, to maximize attenuation by contrast material.[5] Patient dose, on the other hand, is reduced by increasing energy, to minimize the attenuation of photons by the patient. The choice of tube voltage is therefore a tradeoff between image quality and patient dose. Both optimal image quality and acceptable dose can be achieved with a tube voltage of about 70 kV for thin patients, but for thicker patients the voltage must be increased to avoid unacceptably high dose (and excessive heating of the x-ray tube).

Attenuation

X-ray photons traveling directly from the x-ray tube through the patient to the image intensifier without interaction are called the *primary beam*. Interactions within the patient that either absorb or scatter these photons attenuate the primary beam. The differential attenuation of the primary beam between arteries and their surroundings produces object contrast. Primary beam intensity (I) is an inverse exponential function of the distance, x, traveled through an attenuator:

$$I = I_0 \exp(-\mu x) \qquad \text{(Eq. 1)}$$

where I_0 is the x-ray intensity with no attenuation, and μ is the *linear attenuation coefficient* of the attenuating material, which is essentially the sum of the probabilities per unit distance for photoelectric effect and Compton scattering. In general, attenuation coefficients are lower for higher energy photons, which means there is less attenuation (the photons are more penetrating) at higher energies. At the K-edge energy, the attenuation coefficient increases discontinuously. The difference between the attenuation coefficients of iodinated contrast material and human soft tissue (which is mostly water) is greatest at an energy just above the K edge for iodine, 33.2 keV.

X-RAY PRODUCTION AND CONTROL

X-Ray Tube

X-rays for diagnostic radiology are produced by bombarding a tungsten anode with high-voltage electrons within a vacuum tube, in a physical process called Bremsstrahlung ("braking radiation"). The voltage applied to the x-ray tube (called the *tube voltage*, or often just "the *kV*") determines the maximum energy of the individual x-ray photons produced, although photons with a wide range of energies up to this maximum are always produced. As described previously, photon energy determines the degree of penetration through human tissue and angiographic contrast material and is the major determinant of image quality and radiation dose. Therefore, it is said that tube voltage determines the "quality" of the x-ray beam. Tube voltages used in cardiac cineangiography and fluoroscopy range from 60 to 120 kV, depending on patient thickness.

The number of high-voltage electrons striking the anode per unit time (measured in milliamperes) is called the *tube current*, the anode current, or simply "the *mA*." The tube current determines the intensity, or "quantity" of the x-ray beam for a given tube voltage but does not affect beam quality. Tube current ranges from a few milliamperes during fluoroscopy up to as high as 1000 mA during cineangiography. Beam quantity, or intensity, is most often expressed as the exposure per unit time, measured by a suitably calibrated radiation exposure meter at the center of the beam a fixed distance from the x-ray tube. For a given tube voltage, the intensity of the x-ray beam is directly proportional to the tube current. Tube voltage strongly affects both beam quantity and beam quality, because the number of x-ray photons produced by each electron increases more than proportionally with voltage, owing to the increased yield of the Bremsstrahlung process at higher voltage. In summary, tube voltage determines beam quality and strongly affects beam quantity, whereas tube current affects only beam quantity.

The most convenient unit of energy for individual electrons or photons is the electron volt (eV), defined as the energy an electron receives when it is accelerated through a potential of 1 volt. The electrons' energy when they strike the anode is numerically equal to the tube voltage, expressed in keV (1 keV = 1000 eV). Although all the electrons striking the anode have a single energy, the x-ray photons produced by their collisions with tungsten nuclei have all possible energies from zero to the electrons' energy.

Cathode and Focusing Cup

Electrons are supplied by heating the *cathode*, a tungsten filament similar to that in an incandescent light bulb, by passing a current through it. This current, called the *filament current*, determines the temperature of the cathode, which in turn determines the rate at which electrons are ejected into the vacuum and accelerated toward the anode (defined as the tube current). For a given tube voltage, x-ray intensity is proportional to tube current, which is determined by (but *not* proportional to) the filament current. This dependence on filament temperature is the reason tube current cannot be adjusted as quickly as tube voltage or exposure time by the x-ray generator's automatic exposure control—it takes time for the filament to be heated or to cool off. It is also one of the reasons for the delay of about 1 second after the operator steps on the cine–foot pedal before exposures begin. During fluoroscopy, the filament is relatively cool; it must be heated to a much higher operating temperature before the first cine exposure is made.

Surrounding the filament on one side is a hemicylindrical electrode called the *focusing cup*; it is negatively charged to repel the electrons and direct them toward a small area on the anode, called the target or focal spot, where the x-rays are actually produced. The apparent size of the x-ray source, called the *focal spot size*, significantly affects image quality. X-ray tubes have two filaments, one small and one large, to provide a choice of two focal spot sizes. The small focal spot provides the best image resolution, because a smaller x-ray source casts a sharper silhouette. The larger focal spot allows exposures to be made with higher average power, for penetration of thick patients. The power rating for a given focal spot size can be increased by decreasing the angle the anode makes with the central ray of the x-ray beam (the "anode angle"). Reducing this angle foreshortens the focal spot, allowing the electron beam to be spread over a larger area for the same apparent focal spot size. The target angle must be greater than half the angle subtended by the largest desired field of view, because the anode absorbs all x-rays emitted at an angle less than 0° (tangent to the anode). Maximum field of view may be estimated from simple trigonometry: FOV = 2 SID tan (θ), where FOV is the field of view and SID is the source–to–image intensifier distance. Target angles of 6° to 9° provide maximum power rating with adequate field of view for cardiac angiography.

X-Ray Tube Ratings

The energy carried by the electrons per unit time as they strike the anode is called the *power*. It is measured in watts and is equal to the product of tube voltage times tube current. A typical power for fluoroscopy is 160 W (80 kV × 2 mA), about the same as a light bulb. During a cineangiographic exposure, the instantaneous power is typically 32,000 W (80 kV × 400 mA), or 32 kW, and it may go as high as 65 kW. Because x-ray production is less than one percent efficient, most of the electric power applied to the tube is converted to heat at the focal spot. This heat is responsible for several important technical constraints on x-ray tube operation. First, the temperature of the focal spot must be kept below the melting point of tungsten (3370° C). For this reason, the anode is actually a disk that is rotated at high speed during exposures. The focal spot is located near the edge of the disk so that the heat is distributed along a circumferential "focal track." Second, the entire anode assembly must not be heated so much that thermal expansion damages the precision bearings on which it rotates. Third, the tube housing as a whole must not become so hot that it is damaged by the high temperature or by thermal expansion. These three constraints set limits on individual exposures, on individual cine image sequences, and on the average tube loading rate during procedures, respectively. Although these constraints are met automatically by modern x-ray generators, it is important to understand them because they determine the interrelation between image quality, dose, and selections made by the angiographer, such as image intensifier magnification mode.

Focal Track Power Ratings

Tubes for cardiac angiography are designed for an anode rotational rate during cine exposures of 10,000 rpm, corresponding to one complete rotation during a each typical 6-msec exposure. Even with a high-speed rotating anode, heating of the focal track limits the maximum power that can be applied to the x-ray tube to 20 to 35 kW for the small focal spot and 50 to 65 kW for the large focal spot.

Anode Heat Capacity and Cooling Curves

Regardless of focal spot size, the total energy applied to the x-ray tube in a single sequence is limited by the anode heat capacity. Total energy (in joules) is the product of the average power and the cine run time. Average power is calculated by multiplying the instantaneous power times the pulse width (in seconds) times the frame rate (in frames per second, or fps). For historical reasons, the anode heat capacity is usually specified in "heat units" rather than joules, with 1 J equal to 1.35 HU. X-ray tubes for diagnostic angiography should have an anode heat capacity of at least 400,000 HU, and interventional laboratories should have a capacity at least double that, preferably over 1 million HU. The anode heating for a typical 6-second cine sequence at 30 fps, 80 kV, 400 mA, and a 5-msec pulse width is [(6)(30)(80)(400)(0.005)(1.35)], or 38,880 HU, so at least 10 such cine runs can be acquired in rapid sequence without anode overheating. For a heavy patient requiring twice the power and an 8-msec pulse width, the anode would receive more than three times this much heat and would require time to cool between runs to avoid overheating a 400,000-HU tube. Larger anodes have higher heat capacity and higher focal spot power ratings but may require excessively long times to come up to speed. Rapid cooling time is important regardless of anode heat capacity, and the anode should take no longer than 4 minutes to cool from maximum to 50 percent capacity. Angiography x-ray generators should be equipped with a "heat integrator" to automatically prevent anode overheating.

Tube Housing Heat Capacity and Cooling Curves

Although the maximum temperature of the tube housing is lower than that of the anode, its much greater mass gives it a typical heat capacity of 1.5 to 2 million HU. However, because of its lower temperature, its cooling rate is considerably slower than that of the anode, unless it is equipped with either forced air or circulating liquid cooling. The latter cooling system is highly recommended for busy interventional laboratories to avoid long waiting periods caused by heat buildup in the housing.

Filtration

Figure 16–1 is a graph of x-ray intensity versus energy, called the x-ray spectrum, for a tube voltage of 90 kV. The solid line is the spectrum as the photons emerge from the x-ray tube. This spectrum is unacceptable for clinical angiography because more than 50 percent of the intensity is below 33 keV, where the difference between tissue and iodine attenuation is small, and a high fraction of the beam will be absorbed by the patient, resulting in a very high radiation dose. In practice (and by law), a metallic "filter" is mounted where the beam exits the x-ray tube to absorb these low-energy photons and shape the spectrum so that it is most intense in the energy range above 30 keV, where iodine contrast relative to patient dose is the highest (dashed lower curve in Figure 16–1). The legal minimum thickness total filtration for coronary angiography is the equivalent of 2.5 mm of aluminum, including the filtration by the x-ray tube and housing. Additional filtration would further reduce patient dose but would also require higher tube power to compensate for unavoidable attenuation of some of the desired photon energies. Excessive filtration therefore increases the heat loading of the tube, decreasing tube life and possibly reducing image quality by requiring some combination of higher tube voltage, longer exposure, and larger focal spot. The same is true for heavy metal "K-edge filters" such as gadolinium or erbium, and these filters are not recommended except for angiography in the thinnest pediatric patients.[6, 7]

Collimation

Collimators allow the angiographer to restrict the x-ray beam to the desired field of view. By reducing the beam area, the angiographer can significantly improve image contrast while reducing x-ray exposure to the patient and scatter radiation exposure to the staff. Careful collimation and patient positioning ("panning") are the most important means the angiographer has of controlling image quality. Collimators may be circular, rectangular, or both. Circular collimators are the simplest to operate, having a single control for diameter, and are a natural choice if the entire circular output phosphor is to be displayed on the video monitor or recorded on cine film ("exact framing"). Rectangular collimators usually have separate controls for width and height, providing greater flexibility for matching the field shape to the anatomy, and are a better match if the image is to be expanded to fill the entire rectangular video, digital, or cine film frame ("total overframing"). Systems with both

collimator shapes allow the angiographer to more completely confine scatter-producing radiation to the area of interest.

Some systems have an additional set of curved, partially-absorbing collimators that can be rotated and positioned along the heart-lung margin to reduce the intense radiation that penetrates the lung and prevent overexposure of coronary arteries near the margin. Careful use of these "cardiac" or "lung" filters can significantly improve image quality in some views, but they should be used as a supplement and not a substitute for careful, tight collimation.

X-Ray Generators and Exposure Control

The system that provides the high voltage and controls the x-ray tube is called the x-ray generator. X-rays are produced only at the instant the electrons strike the target, so the generator can produce brief pulses of x-rays by electronically switching on and off the voltage to the x-ray tube. The short, high-intensity exposures used in cardiac angiography require that the x-ray generator be rated to deliver a power of up to 100 kW to the tube at all voltages from 70 kV to 125 kV.

The generator automatically adjusts tube voltage, tube current, and exposure time to maintain a constant image intensifier light output in response to changes in patient absorption caused by panning, respiration, or injection of contrast material. Because tube current can be changed only relatively slowly (taking about 1 second), rapid adjustments are made by changing voltage or pulse width, and tube current is varied as needed to keep the average tube voltage and pulse width near the optimal values of 70 to 90 kV and 4 to 6 msec, respectively. The programmed combinations of tube voltage, tube current, and pulse width as a function of patient thickness have a significant effect on image quality but are seldom adjustable by the operator. Some systems allow the angiographer to select starting, minimum, or maximum limits for tube voltage or pulse width, or to select different programs for pediatric patients (e.g., programs favoring shorter pulse widths that can stop the motion at higher heart rates). Some systems leave focal spot size as a manual selection, and others automatically switch to the large focal spot only if tube voltage is driven higher than 90 kV by a large patient or a highly angulated view. Usually, sharper images, lower patient dose, and longer tube life are achieved by use of the small focal spot, because the generator uses lower tube current and higher voltage at that setting. For digital recording, some generators allow selection of reduced exposure modes that can be used for ventriculography without significant loss of diagnostic information. A special mode for digital densitometric studies is available on some generators; it keeps exposure factors constant throughout each cine run and bypasses any digital signal processing, facilitating quantitative processing of the image after acquisition.

If an x-ray exposure reaching the image intensifier is too low at the maximum power allowable for the small focal spot (because of a thick patient or an angulated projection), the generator automatically increases tube voltage and lowers tube current so that x-ray output and penetration are increased, without increasing electric power, until an adequate exposure is received at the image intensifier. If the required tube voltage exceeds about 90 kV, the large focal spot should be used to avoid significant loss of contrast from increased Compton scattering. As a rule of thumb, the tube current must be doubled to compensate for every 10 kV decrease in tube voltage.

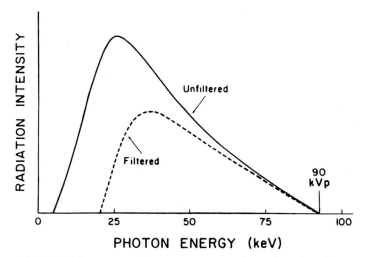

FIGURE 16–1. Bremsstrahlung x-ray spectrum for 90 kV tube voltage, with *(dashed curve)* and without *(solid curve)* added aluminum filtration. (From Curry, T.S., Dowdey, J.E., and Murry, R.C.: Christensen's Physics of Diagnostic Radiology. 4th ed. Philadelphia, Lea & Febiger, 1990, p. 89, with permission.)

IMAGE FORMATION

Image Geometry

The angiographic imaging process consists of casting shadows from a "point source" of radiation onto an image intensifier. Shadows are always larger than the objects that cast them. Figure 16–2 shows how the magnification factor (M) is calculated (by similar triangles) as the distance from the source to the image (SID) divided by the distance from the source to the object (SOD): M = SID/SOD. The size of the image of an object is equal to M times the true diameter. Placing the image intensifier directly against the patient minimizes magnification but, because the coronary arteries are still some distance from the image, their magnification is still typically between 1.05 and 1.1. The effect of geometric magnification on image quality is complex and affects resolution, contrast, and noise.

Resolution

Spatial resolution denotes the ability to depict fine detail in an image. There are different ways of defining resolution. Each definition has its own precise method of measurement, but because they measure different aspects of image quality, conversion from one measure of resolution to another is not always possible.

Probably the most intuitive definition of resolution is the expression of the finest detail that can be detected in an image, often called "*limiting resolution.*" Limiting resolution may be measured subjectively by viewing the image of a lead (Pb) test pattern like that in Figure 16–11. The *spatial frequency* of the pattern is the number of bars per millimeter. This is usually expressed as line-pairs per millimeter (lp/mm), with a bar and its adjacent space forming a pair of "lines," one dark and one light, like a complete cycle of a sine wave. Limiting resolution is expressed as the highest spatial frequency at which any intensity variation, or "modulation," can be detected. Because this is such a quick and easy procedure, measurement of limiting resolution is often performed as part of a routine quality control program.[2, 8] However, it is an incomplete

description of resolution because it expresses only the highest spatial frequency that can be barely seen; it provides no information about how well patterns are seen at lower spatial frequencies, an important property that can and does differ significantly between imaging systems that have identical limiting resolutions.

Another intuitive, but harder to obtain, measure of resolution is the *point spread function* (PSF)—defined as the pattern of blurring that occurs when the object imaged is a mathematically sharp point—and the closely related *line spread function.* As rough rule of thumb, limiting resolution is approximately half the reciprocal of the full width at half maximum of the line spread function. Although special equipment is required to measure it, the PSF is an attractive measure of resolution because it is intuitively related to the physical processes that produce the blurring. For this reason, the width of the PSF is used in the discussion of sources of system blur in the following sections. Unlike limiting resolution, the PSF contains a complete description of the resolving capabilities of the imaging system. However, the relation between the PSF and the visibility of image details is not intuitive. The relation can be made more direct by recognizing that reproduction of a mathematical point requires that the imaging system record all spatial frequencies equally well. The specific shape of the PSF is determined by how well the imaging system reproduces intensity variations (called "modulation") at different spatial frequencies. A plot of the percent modulation that is recorded in the image as a function of spatial frequency is called the *modulation transfer function* (MTF) of the imaging system. The MTF is easily obtained from the PSF by taking the absolute value of the Fourier transform, a simple operation on a computer. One advantage of the MTF is that is expresses how well the system preserves the contrast of objects with different spatial frequencies. The limiting resolution roughly corresponds to the spatial frequency for which the MTF approaches zero. In practice, test grids are typically just visible at an MTF of 10 percent, although the exact number depends on many factors in a complex way. At spatial frequencies lower than that corresponding to the limiting resolution, the MTF describes how well the imaging system preserves the original contrast of larger objects, a feature that may be more important than limiting resolution for detection of low-contrast angiographic features. The simple line ratio measurement of percent contrast, described in the section on image intensifiers, is an index of the MTF at very low spatial frequency. Thus, the two most important measurements that can be made in the field for image intensifier acceptance and quality assurance testing, line ratio and limiting resolution, are directly related to the MTF curve at its low and high spatial frequency limits.

Imaging System Blur

The system that detects and records the x-ray image introduces some blurring, or "unsharpness," that reduces image resolution. In cine film angiography, the main source of this blur is the spreading of light in the image intensifier input phosphor. This phenomenon causes light emitted by the absorption of x-ray photons at a point to spread out into an approximately Gaussian PSF, as shown by the outside curve in Figure 16–3. The width at half maximum of the image intensifier PSF is on the order of 0.14 mm, corresponding to a limiting resolution of 3.6 lp/mm. In fluoroscopy and digital angiography, the system PSF is mainly determined by the resolution of a 525-line video image or by the pixel size. For example, the pixel size for a 512 by 512 matrix used to digitize a 15.2 cm (6-inch) image intensifier is 152 mm divided by 512, or 0.3 mm, corresponding to a limiting resolution of 1.7 lp/mm (Table 16–1).

Focal Spot Blur

The focal spot is not a true "point source" of radiation but has width of about 0.6 mm for the small focal spot, or 0.9 mm for the large focal spot. These are nominal sizes; the actual sizes are frequently 50 percent larger. Each true point within the focal spot casts a truly sharp shadow of the cardiac anatomy onto the image

RADIOGRAPHIC MAGNIFICATION

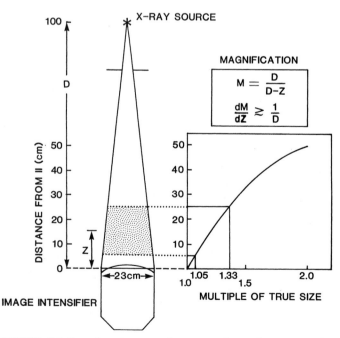

FIGURE 16–2. *Left,* Schematic of geometry for cardiac angiography. Shading shows typical location of coronary arteries. D is the source-to-image distance and Z is the source-to-object distance. The relative object position plotted in Figure 16–5 is s = Z/D. *Right,* Relation between Z and geometric magnification for D = 100 cm. (From Whiting, J.S., Pfaff, J.M., and Eigler, N.L.: Effect of radiographic distortions on the accuracy of quantitative angiography. Am. J. Card. Imaging 2:239, 1988, with permission.)

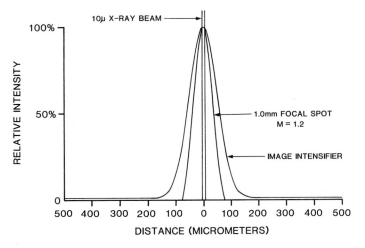

FIGURE 16-3. Idealized image intensifier and focal spot line spread functions. (From Whiting, J.S., Pfaff, J.M., and Eigler, N.L.: Effect of radiographic distortions on the accuracy of quantitative angiography. Am. J. Card. Imaging 2:239, 1988, with permission.)

intensifier, but at a slightly different place than all the other points. The result is a blurring of the image by an amount that is directly proportional to the size of the focal spot. The constant of proportionality is $M - 1$, which is zero when the object is directly on the image receptor ($M = 1$) and unity when the object is halfway between the focal spot and the image ($M = 2$), as shown in Figure 16-4. Keeping in mind that when $M = 2$ the image is twice as large as the object, the focal spot blur or unsharpness in the object plane is effectively only half the focal spot size.

The combined effects of magnification and increased blur on object resolution are summarized in the nomogram in Figure 16-5. The effects of geometric magnification on receptor (image intensifier) blur and focal spot blur are given by straight lines when they are plotted as functions of the fractional distance of the object from the image intensifier, [(SID − SOD)/SID]. The overall resolution is the root squared sum of these contributions (dashed line in Fig. 16-5). If P is the receptor blue, F is the focal spot blur, and s is the relative object position (fraction of SID), the minimum effective blur (best resolution) is equal to $PF/(F^2 + P^2)^{1/2}$, and occurs at $s = P^2/F^2 + P^2)$, corresponding to a magnification of $1 + P^2/F^2$. For magnifications, overall blurring begins to increase, so that at a magnification of $M = (F^2 + P^2)/(F^2 - P^2)$ the resolution is equal again to that at $M = 1$; beyond this, resolution degrades rapidly because of focal spot blur. For example, for a focal spot size of 0.9 mm and pixel size of 0.3 mm, effective blur is equal to or greater than 0.3 mm between $M = 1$ and $M = 1.25$, with an optimum effective blur of 0.28 mm at a magnification of $M = 1.11$. For a typical SID of 100 cm, this corresponds to an object located at a distance from the image intensifier input of 0 to 20 cm, with an optimum distance of 9.9 cm.

Motion Blur

The coronary arteries are blurred by the distance they move in the plane of the image during each exposure. This motion unsharpness is minimized by the use of very brief exposures. For adult coronary angiography, pulse widths of 4 to 6 msec usually produce acceptable blurring, but pulse widths of 2 to 4 msec may be necessary to avoid excessive blurring of rapidly moving coronary arteries in pediatric angiography. Fortunately, sufficient exposures can be delivered in these times for most patients without operating the x-ray tube at excessive power. For very heavy patients, some systems allow the pulse width to increase to 7 or 8 msec in a tradeoff between motion unsharpness and an adequate exposure at a reasonable tube voltage. Magnification has no effect on relative motion unsharpness because the arteries and the blur are both magnified equally.

Contrast

Contrast in angiography is the result of the differential absorption of x-rays by blood or tissue and by the iodine in contrast

TABLE 16-1. EFFECT OF FRAMING AND MAGNIFICATION MODE ON FIELD OF VIEW (FOV), ON DIGITAL MATRIX SIZE FOR DIGITAL RESOLUTION EQUAL TO THE 3.5 lp/mm RESOLUTION OF THE IMAGE INTENSIFIER, AND ON PIXEL SIZE AND MAXIMUM RESOLUTION OBTAINED WITH A 512 × 512 MATRIX*

	Image Intensifier Mode in cm (inches)		
	22.9 (9.0)	**15.2 (6.0)**	**11.4 (4.5)**
EXACT FRAMING (CIRCULAR IMAGE)			
Diagonal FOV (cm)	22.9	15.2	11.4
Horizontal/Vertical FOV (cm)	22.9	15.2	11.4
Required matrix size for 3.5 lp/mm	1603	1064	798
Pixel size (mm)	0.45	0.30	0.22
Maximum resolution† (lp/mm)	1.12	1.68	2.25
TOTAL OVERFRAMING (SQUARE IMAGE)			
Diagonal FOV (cm)	22.9	15.2	11.4
Horizontal/Vertical FOV (cm)	16.2	10.8	8.1
Required matrix size for 3.5 lp/mm	1134	756	567
Pixel size (mm)	0.32	0.21	0.16
Maximum resolution† (lp/mm)	1.58	2.37	3.16

*For geometric magnification M less than 1.2, the FOV is reduced by 1/M and resolution increased by M. Focal spot blur reduces resolution for higher geometric magnification.

†Maximum theoretical resolution in horizontal and vertical directions. Actual resolution is typically lower than this value by a factor of about 0.70 (the Kell factor).

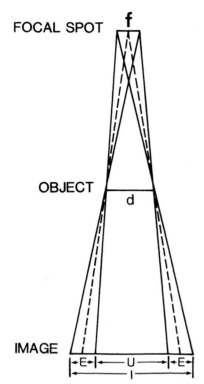

FIGURE 16–4. Focal spot unsharpness with a geometric magnification of M = 2. Edge blurring (E) in the image plane is equal to the focal spot size (f), but its effective size relative to the object plane is f/M because the object's image is magnified by M. (From Curry, T.S., Dowdey, J.E., and Murry, R.C.: Christensen's Physics of Diagnostic Radiology. 4th ed. Philadelphia, Lea & Febiger, 1990, p. 227, with permission.)

material injected into the arteries. It is helpful to separate angiographic contrast into three components. *Object contrast*, or primary radiation contrast, refers to the relative difference in primary beam intensity transmitted through different objects in the patient, such

as opacified arteries; *recorded contrast* refers to contrast in the recorded image data, including the contrast-reducing effects of x-ray scatter and the imaging system; *displayed contrast* refers to the image contrast as viewed by the human observer, including the effects of any image processing and the effect on contrast of the display device.

Object Contrast

Angiographic object contrast is determined by the thickness of the object and the difference between its attenuation coefficient and that of the background tissue. Referring to Figure 16–6, object contrast is equal to the change in the primary beam intensity, ΔP, caused by the object detail, divided by the background primary intensity, P. Using Equation 1 and the fact that the attenuation of superimposed materials is multiplicative,

$$P(x,T) = I_0 \exp[-T\mu_T] \exp[-x(\mu_I - \mu_T)]$$

and

$$\Delta P/P = \frac{P(0,T) - P(x,T)}{P(0,T)} = 1 - \exp[-x(\mu_I - \mu_T)] \quad \text{(Eq. 2)}$$

where x and μ_I are the thickness and attenuation coefficient of iodinated contrast material, respectively, and T and μ_T are the patient tissue thickness and attenuation coefficient. Here it is assumed that the x-ray beam is monoenergetic. The object contrast, ΔP divided by P, depends only on the object thickness and the difference between tissue and iodine attenuation coefficients; it is independent of patient thickness because both ΔP and P depend on patient thickness in the same way. This is reflected on the right side of Figure 16–6 (*dashed line*), which is a graph of the logarithm of the primary beam intensity:

$$\log[P(x,T)] = \log(I_0) - T\mu_T - x(\mu_I - \mu_T) \quad \text{(Eq. 3)}$$

indicating that an object of thickness x reduces the log intensity by the same absolute amount, $x(\mu_I - \mu_T)$, regardless of patient thickness. This is the basis of the measurement of object thickness by

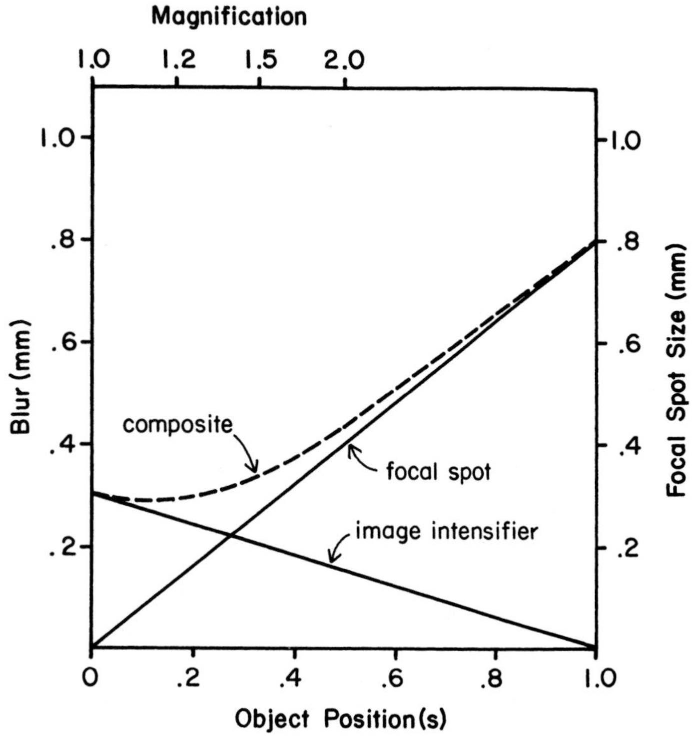

FIGURE 16–5. Image receptor blur *(left axis)* and focal spot blur *(right axis)* versus relative distance from image intensifier (as fraction of source-to-image distance) and geometric magnification *(top scale)*. (From Whiting, J.S., Pfaff, J.M., and Eigler, N.L.: Effect of radiographic distortions on the accuracy of quantitative angiography. Am. J. Card. Imaging 2:239, 1988, with permission.)

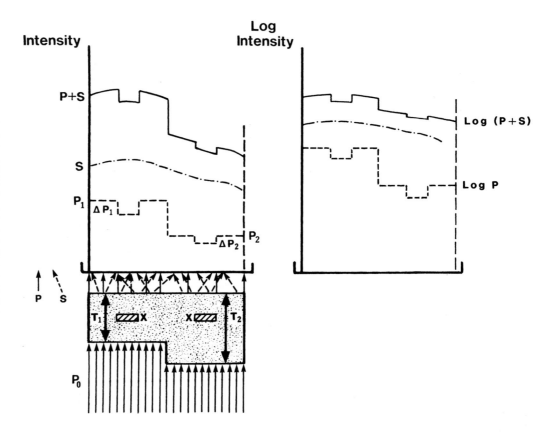

FIGURE 16–6. Illustration of factors determining detected contrast. X-rays transmitted without scattering through tissue thicknesses T_1 and T_2 produce primary intensities P_1 and P_2, respectively. Identical absorbers of thickness x produce changes in primary intensity ΔP_1 and ΔP_2, which are directly proportional to P_1 and P_2 by the Lambert-Beers Law. Thus, the change in the logarithm of the primary intensity is the same for both absorbers. Scattered radiation produces a substantial additive intensity contribution that results in differences between the log ΔP in spite of equal absorber thicknesses.

x-ray densitometry. Because the human visual system perceives equal changes in log intensity as equal contrasts, Figure 16–6 indicates that in an ideal primary x-ray image the contrast of an object is proportional to its thickness regardless of the thickness of tissue in which it is embedded. There are two ways to maximize the difference between tissue and contrast material attenuation coefficients: by using a contrast material with the highest possible concentration of iodine, typically 320 to 370 mg/mL unless clinically counterindicated, and by maintaining tube voltage between 70 and 90 kV with at least 3 mm aluminum equivalent total filtration, so that the Bremsstrahlung energy spectrum peaks just above 33.2 keV, the iodine K-edge energy. In addition to object contrast, several other important factors contribute to the contrast of the final displayed image.

Recorded Contrast

Object contrast is degraded by radiation scatter and light glare in the imaging system, which add no information but are recorded along with the primary image. Figure 16–6 illustrates how the addition of this spurious background scatter (S) increases the recorded intensity from P to P + S without changing ΔP (left), resulting in a loss of contrast from Δ/P down to $\Delta P/(P + S)$. If the contribution of scatter and glare is equal to the primary intensity (which is typical), the contrast is reduced by half. Scatter reduces contrast the most in dense areas adjacent to lung, because that is where the ratio of scatter to primary intensity, S/P, is the highest. The effect of scatter on contrast is seen graphically in the log intensity plot (see Fig. 16–6, *right*), approximately as it would be visually perceived in an image. Minimization of scatter and glare can contribute significantly to better image quality. X-ray scatter reduction techniques are discussed in the next section. Glare is discussed in the section on image intensifiers.

Scatter Reduction

Antiscatter grids selectively transmit photons that have traveled directly from the x-ray tube focal spot (i.e., the primary beam) and absorb photons that arrive from other directions. This is accom-

plished by a series of thin lead foil strips separated by relatively radiolucent spacer strips, arranged like a miniature venetian blind. The parallel lead strips corresponding to the vanes of the blind are angled slightly so that radiation emanating from a point source a certain distance away, called the focal distance for the grid, can pass through the spacer material parallel to each lead strip. Grids can be made more selective by increasing the ratio of the height of the strips to the width of the spacer material, called the grid ratio, but higher-ratio grids also require higher patient dose. For adult coronary angiography, a grid ratio of 8:1 or 10:1 represents a good compromise between scatter reduction and increased patient dose for equal input exposure. A 10:1 grid with carbon fiber spacer material rejects roughly 90 percent of the scatter radiation but requires about double the patient dose. Dedicated pediatric systems can use lower grid ratios of 5:1 or 6:1 to obtain acceptable image contrast with lower dose because these thinner patients produce less radiation scatter.

A second important method for minimization of scatter is collimation of the x-ray beam to as small a beam area as possible, because scatter is roughly proportional to irradiated volume, which is proportional to field size. Figure 16–7 shows a plot of scattered and direct primary photons reaching the image intensifier as a function of the diameter of a circular field of view, assuming a uniform object. The primary intensity is independent of field size, but the scatter component increases by 50 percent for a 9-inch field compared with a 4.5-inch field. Inclusion of high-intensity lung areas in the larger field of view adds significant scatter, so careful collimation of lung can further increase recorded contrast.

Displayed Contrast

The characteristics of the display system further modify the contrast of the final image. These characteristics include cine film contrast, projector brightness, digital processing, and videocamera or monitor response functions. The relation between recorded intensities and displayed intensities is called the characteristic curve for the display device or medium. All display devices have a limited range of displayed intensities; to preserve information, it is important that the mapping from recorded to displayed intensities

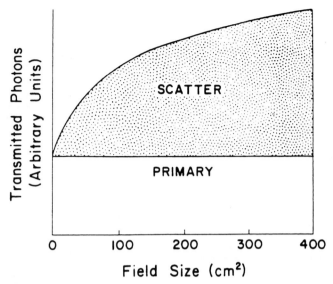

FIGURE 16–7. Idealized plot of primary and total radiation striking the image intensifier as a function of beam area. The 200 cm² area corresponds to a 6-inch image intensifier field of view. (From Curry, T.S., Dowdey, J.E., and Murry, R.C.: Christensen's Physics of Diagnostic Radiology. 4th ed. Philadelphia, Lea & Febiger, 1990, p. 98, with permission.)

not exceed this range. This consideration dictates that cine film for cardiac angiography must have relatively wide latitude, implying low contrast, as discussed in the section on film characteristics. Video display devices should be adjusted to maximize contrast without saturation in either the brightest or darkest areas. Displayed contrast can be adjusted to higher levels if careful collimation and cardiac filters are used to limit the dynamic range of the recorded image.

Noise

Quantum Noise

Radiographic image intensity is built up of individually detected x-ray photons, or "quanta." Because the individual photons arrive randomly, the number of photons detected in any given area of the image, and thus the intensity, has a random uncertainty exactly like the uncertainty in the counts from a radioactive source—that is, the standard deviation is equal to the square root of the number of photons detected. Random intensity fluctuations give radiographic images a mottled appearance, called *quantum noise* or *quantum mottle*, that interferes with the perception of low-contrast features. For a fixed photon energy spectrum (beam quality), the absolute magnitude of quantum noise is proportional to the square root of the exposure at the image intensifier input phosphor, called the *input exposure*.

The relative magnitude of quantum mottle is equal to intensity standard deviation divided by intensity, which is inversely proportional to the square root of radiation exposure. At a typical input exposure of 30 μR for coronary angiography, there are roughly 2400 photons per square millimeter, or only 150 photons per pixel for a 512 by 512 matrix with exact framing in the 6-inch mode (see Table 16–1). Therefore, the percent intensity fluctuation of a single pixel that results from quantum noise at this exposure is $1/(150)^{1/2}$, or about 8 percent. Rose[9] found that, to be detected by a human observer, a feature's displayed contrast must be five to seven times greater than the relative quantum noise for the same area as the feature. For detection of a feature of 1 mm² (16 pixels), the quantum noise would be $1/(2400)^{1/2}$ or about 2 percent. The Rose model implies that quantum noise in the coronary angiogram limits detectability to those features of 1 mm² with contrast greater than about 5 × .02, or 10 percent. Smaller features require higher

contrast to be detected and larger ones, lower contrast. Visual detectability during fluoroscopy, which uses about one tenth the dose per image, requires $(10)^{1/2}$ or 3.2 times the contrast, or features 3.2 times larger in area. This fact limits the advantage to be gained by the use of high spatial resolution fluoroscopy.

The human visual system is able to perform temporal integration when viewing fluoroscopic or cine sequences, so that the perceived magnitude of quantum noise for an angiogram viewed dynamically is significantly lower than it is for a single frame.[10, 11] Subtle details are usually better perceived by viewing an angiogram in motion at the highest possible frame rate, but this effect is reduced or reversed if there is rapid arterial motion.[12]

Structured Noise

Noise that is fixed or almost constant from frame to frame is called *structured noise*. The most important source of this noise is the patient; any structure that interferes with the visibility of the artery of interest is considered noise, including ribs, the textured appearance of the lungs and pulmonary vasculature, and even other overlapping coronary arteries. Because structured noise is not reduced by increasing the dose, it places an upper limit on the improvement of image quality that can be achieved by reducing quantum noise. Sources of structured noise that should not be visible in angiograms from a high-quality catheterization laboratory include cutoff from a misaligned antiscatter grid, contrast material on the support table or image intensifier input, mottle from a damaged or defective image intensifier tube, and dust or dirt on the image intensifier output phosphor or videocamera target.

THE IMAGE INTENSIFIER

Components and Basic Operation

The image intensifier is a vacuum tube device that converts the pattern of x-ray energy absorbed at its input into a bright, visible-light image at its output. X-rays are absorbed by a large-diameter cesium iodide phosphor on the inside of the front surface of the vacuum tube. Diameters of 7 to 10 inches are typical for cardiac angiography. Light emitted by the *input phosphor* ejects electrons from the *photocathode*, a thin layer of metal coating the vacuum side of the phosphor. Because the number of electrons ejected is proportional to the absorbed x-ray energy, they form an electron density "image" corresponding to the received x-ray intensity pattern. Inside the vacuum, these electrons are accelerated by a 30,000-volt potential and focused onto a thin, small-diameter (approximately 1-inch) *output phosphor* coated on the vacuum side of an optical quality glass window. The accelerated photons produce a fluorescent image bright enough to record on cine film with a videocamera, much brighter than the fluorescence that could be produced by x-rays alone. This fact gives the x-ray image intensifier its name.

Magnification Modes

Image intensifiers designed for cardiac angiography typically have a maximum field of view of 7 to 10 inches diameter, determined by the size of the input phosphor. These systems also provide one or two smaller fields of view, or *magnification modes*, in which a reduced area of the input phosphor is electronically focused onto the full output phosphor area, resulting in an image with magnified details. Triple-mode image intensifiers are most common, with typical magnification mode combinations of 10, 7, and 5 inches, or 9, 6, and 4.5 inches, corresponding to full, half, and quarter input image area sizes, respectively. Selection of an increased magnification mode also increases the x-ray dose, which in general improves image quality by reducing x-ray quantum noise.

Intensification Gain

The brightness of the output phosphor per unit input exposure rate is called the *conversion factor*, and it is usually specified in units of candelas per square meter per milliroentgen per second (cd/m²/mR/s). The conversion factor depends on several fixed properties of image intensifier design, including the input phosphor thickness and the acceleration voltage; it also depends on the magnification mode selected by the angiographer. The image intensity at the output phosphor is directly proportional to the area of the input field view. Therefore, the 7-inch and 5-inch magnification modes have conversion factors of about one half and about one quarter, respectively, of that of the 10-inch field of view. Because most x-ray generators are designed to keep the output phosphor image brightness constant for all magnification modes, the 7-inch and 5-inch modes require about two and about four times, respectively, the x-ray exposure rate of the 10-inch mode.

Detective Quantum Efficiency

Because visual detection of low-contrast features is determined by the signal-to-noise ratio, the ability of an image intensifier to preserve the signal-to-noise ratio presented to it in the x-ray image is an important measure of performance. The *detective quantum efficiency*, DQE, (sometimes called "quantum detection efficiency," or QDE) is defined as the squared ratio of quantum signal to noise for the input x-ray image divided by that for the output image. Because quantum noise is proportional to the square root of dose, DQE is, roughly speaking, the dose efficiency of the image intensifier tube: It is a measure of how completely the image intensifier absorbs the incident x-ray quanta and converts them into an output image. Image intensifier DQE depends primarily on the thickness and composition of the input phosphor and on the x-ray transparency of the input window. High DQE allows dose to be reduced, increasing quantum noise. In the 1970s, image intensifier DQE improved dramatically after cesium iodide replaced less efficient input phosphor materials, and further gains have been achieved by replacing the thick glass *input window* with a thinner, less absorbent metal input window. With these factors optimized, DQE may now be increased only by increasing the input phosphor thickness, which results in a reduction of spatial resolution. Selection of an image intensifier now involves a tradeoff between dose and resolution.

Resolution

Image intensifier spatial resolution is primarily determined by the lateral spreading of light within the input phosphor, the extent of which increases with phosphor thickness. Secondarily, electron focusing in the image intensifier and output phosphor blur also contribute to overall unsharpness. Standard image intensifiers for diagnostic coronary angiography have a limiting resolution greater than 4 lp/mm. High-DQE image intensifiers with thicker input phosphors sacrifice some spatial resolution for reduced radiation dose but should still resolve at least 3.6 lp/mm. Because resolution is primarily limited by the input phosphor, image intensifier magnification mode has only a small effect on how many line pairs can be resolved at the output phosphor, even though the test pattern image is magnified. However, if the viewing or recording system has lower resolution than the input phosphor, magnification improves the overall resolution (up to the limiting input phosphor resolution) by enlarging the image to be recorded. Resolution displayed on a video monitor or recorded on a 512 by 512 pixel digital system can be increased significantly by use of the image intensifier magnification modes, but resolution on cine film, which has better spatial resolution than the input phosphor, is not affected (see Table 16–1). It is important to distinguish between the spatial resolution of high-contrast test objects and the detectability of low-contrast features.[13] The latter depends on the feature's signal-to-noise ratio, which depends more on contrast, DQE, and radiation dose than on spatial resolution.[14, 15] For this reason, image intensifiers for interventional coronary angiography should be selected for high contrast and high DQE, rather than for highest limiting resolution. Nevertheless, limiting resolution, even in high-DQE tubes, should be at least 3.6 lp/mm in the 7-inch mode.

Contrast

An ideal image intensifier would produce an exact replica of the input x-ray image as a light image at its output. In addition to the loss of contrast caused by scattered radiation, the "veiling glare" produced by scattering of the bright light in the output phosphor also results in loss of contrast.[16] A measure of maximum image intensifier contrast can be obtained in the catheterization laboratory by blocking 10 percent of the field of view diameter with a lead bar and calculating the "line ratio," defined by Moore[2] as the ratio of brightness next to the bar to brightness in the shadow of the bar. Line ratios measured in this way can exceed 20:1 and should be at least 12:1 for interventional coronary angiography.

Distortion

The spherical input surface of the image intensifier produces a radial exaggeration of the size of objects near the edge of the output image, known as pincushion distortion. The degree of distortion is relatively insignificant in modern image intensifiers,[17, 18] particularly in magnification modes, which use only the central area of the input phosphor. For highly accurate measurement of absolute coronary artery dimensions, pincushion distortion can be measured and corrected with a calibration grid.[17, 19–21]

FLUOROSCOPY

X-ray fluoroscopy provides live ("real-time") imaging for placing of catheters and manipulation of devices such as pacemaker electrodes, angioplasty balloons, and stents. Because these devices are usually easy to visualize well enough to position them, and because fluoroscopy often must be performed for extended periods, image quality is intentionally sacrificed to keep the radiation dose rate as low as possible; image intensifier input exposure rates are typically less than 10 percent of those used for cine recording.

X-Ray Technique

X-ray technique for fluoroscopy is designed to provide adequate real-time visual guidance during procedures while minimizing radiation dose to patient and operator. Image quality can be sacrificed for lower dose by reducing the input exposure per frame by increasing tube voltage, or by reducing frame rate.

Exposure per Frame

Image intensifier input exposure rate determines image noise. Image noise quality is acceptable at 50 to 100 μR per second (1.7 to 3.3 μR per frame at 30 fps) for the 6- or 7-inch field of view, but it should be adjusted as low as possible to minimize patient and staff exposure. This exposure rate is about one tenth of that required for acceptable cineangiography. Skin entrance dose rate depends on patient thickness and projection but is limited by law to 10 R per minute. If a boost mode is available for recording high-dose fluoroscopy,[22] then normal automatic exposure is limited to 5 R per minute. If the generator allows manual selection of lower than normal fluoroscopic dose (sometimes labeled "fluoro detail" or "video gain"), the lowest dose that allows adequate device manipulation should be chosen.

Videocamera

The output phosphor image is focused onto the videocamera target by two lenses. A large objective lens is located at its focal length from the output phosphor (i.e., it is focused at infinity) to collect as much light as possible. A camera lens, also focused at infinity, produces a sharp image on the videocamera input target. The size of the image on the videocamera target is equal to the output phosphor image size times the ratio of the objective and camera lens focal lengths. The camera lens focal length is chosen to produce the desired mapping of the circular output phosphor image onto the square scanned area of the videocamera, known as the *framing*. Figure 16–8 shows two possible choices, exact framing and total overframing. To achieve total overframing, the circular output phosphor is optically magnified so that it entirely fills the frame, as shown on the right. The diagonal field of view *(arrows)* is the same for both framing methods, but it is displayed 41 percent larger with total overframing. Subtotal overframing on cine film, also shown on the right, matches the vertical field of view of the digital image. The x-ray collimators used must match the displayed or recorded image shape *(shaded area)*—circular for exact framing, rectangular or square for total overframing.

Spatial resolution in fluoroscopy is limited by the resolution of the television camera and monitor rather than that of the image intensifier tube. In addition to video system resolution, overall resolution in the object plane also depends on geometric magnification, image intensifier magnification mode, and the choice of framing.

Using the number of displayed lines as the ideal, actual measured resolution is typically lower by a factor of about 0.7, sometimes referred to as the Kell factor. A 525-line videocamera and monitor system typically has a resolution of about 370 lines, or 165 line pairs. The resolutions listed in Table 16–1 must therefore be considered very optimistic upper limits.

Basics of Operation

Videocameras for medical fluoroscopy are of the vidicon type, consisting of a vacuum tube with a light-sensitive, photoconducting input target. The image on the target is scanned by an electron beam in lines from left to right, top to bottom, but the lines are not necessarily scanned in order. The signal produced by the scanning electron beam is sent to the video monitor, where it controls the intensity of another electron beam that writes the image onto the display screen. The videocamera and monitor must be synchronized in order to produce an image. This synchronization is achieved by requiring that the camera, monitor, and any other equipment in the system (e.g., videotape recorders) conform to the same precise protocol for generation and interpretation of the video signal. The protocol most commonly used for medical

fluoroscopy is based on the Electronics Industries Association RS-170 video signal standard that was developed for black and white commercial television, making it possible to combine cameras, recorders, videoprocessors, and monitors from many different manufacturers.

Standard videocameras were developed to meet four competing technical criteria: frame rate adequate to smoothly depict motion, adequate resolution in vertical and horizontal directions, unobjectionable display flicker, and limited bandwidth for broadcast and videotape recording. Although many combinations of scanning parameters are possible, the compromise established as the standard in the early days of television was a frame rate of 30 fps and a line rate of 525 lines per frame, with a 2:1 interlaced scanning order. The reasons for the choice of line rate and 2:1 interlace are related to the second and fourth criteria in a somewhat complicated way that is relevant for understanding why and how modern video systems are now diverging from this standard. First, bandwidth refers to the maximum electrical signal frequency required to transmit or record the live video image. The bandwidth required (cycles per second) is approximately equal to the product of frame rate (frames per second), scan lines (lines per frame), and horizontal resolution (cycles per line). For equal horizontal and vertical resolution, the horizontal resolution must equal one half the number of lines (assuming a square image, as used in medical imaging—broadcast television has a 5:4 aspect ratio, requiring horizontal resolution equal to 25 percent of the number of line pairs). The bandwidth required is, therefore, equal to the frame rate times half the squared number of lines.

For a system of 30 fps and 525 lines, the minimum bandwidth is 4.1 MHz (4100 cycles per second), which was only slightly above the design limit for early television. Unfortunately, a scan rate of 30 Hz is too low to hide the appearance of flicker, which is detectable when the intensity of a display oscillates at rates below about 45 Hz. A clever method called 2:1 interlaced scanning was invented that allowed the monitor to be scanned at twice the frame rate without increasing the bandwidth or reducing the number of lines. Each frame is scanned in two passes of alternating lines, as shown in Figure 16–9; each scan produces an image called a field, and each field contains half the lines of the full frame. The field scan rate of 60 Hz is high enough that flicker is not objectionable, and visual persistence integrates sequential fields, producing a perceived full-frame image.

Standard videocameras work well for constantly illuminated, slowly changing scenes for which the effective exposure time of 1/30 second is sufficient to avoid motion blurring. More rapidly moving objects may still appear sharp in each field, owing to the shorter field "exposure time" of 1/60 second, but with only half the vertical resolution. If there is either horizontal or vertical motion between fields, the images in the two half-resolution fields will not visually align, causing a loss of resolution. Very rapid motion, such as that of the coronary arteries during systole, produces significant blurring within each field during the 1/60-second exposure time. Some fluoroscopic systems are capable of producing pulsed x-ray exposures of less than 1/200 second (5 msec), which is short enough to eliminate most motion blurring. However, the loss of resolution caused by object motion between interlaced fields occurs even in the absence of motion blur in each field. This is because separate exposures, at different times, are used to produce each field. The problem could be avoided by pulsing the x-ray beam just once per frame, as is done during cineangiography, but this method is not satisfactory because of a technical problem: the latent image for the second field is partially erased when the first field is scanned, resulting in a significant intensity difference between the two fields. This difference is responsible for the flicker seen with conventional fluoroscopic systems during cine filming.

Progressive Scan Video

The best solution to both the resolution and flicker problems is not to use interlaced scanning. Pulsed-exposure, progressive scan video, in which all 525 lines of the image are scanned in natural

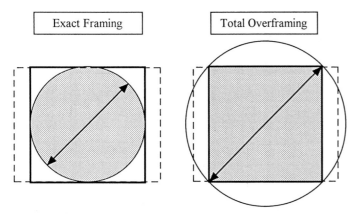

| Exact Framing | Total Overframing |

FIGURE 16–8. Framing for square video and digital display *(solid squares)* and for 4:3 aspect ratio cine film with equal vertical field of view *(dashed rectangles)*. The solid circle represents the output phosphor.

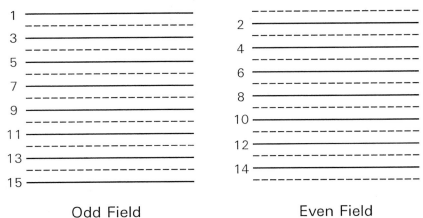

FIGURE 16–9. Interlaced scanning. During the first field scan *(left)*, only the odd numbered lines are scanned by the electron beam *(solid lines)*. The unscanned even lines *(dashed)* are scanned during the second pass, as shown on the right. Unless additional light reaches the target after the first field is scanned, the second field will be less intense because of partial charging from the even numbered scan lines.

order after a brief x-ray exposure, eliminates both motion blur and interfield misalignment. Progressive scan without flicker can be achieved by the use of digital technology or increased bandwidth, or both. One common method is to use a digital scan converter that stores each 525-line progressive scan image into its memory and reads it out as a 525-line, 2:1 interlaced image (with an imperceptible one-frame delay). Alternatively, each complete 525-line frame can be read out twice as both fields of an interlaced 1049-line video signal, in which case the scan converter is called an upscanner. The doubled number of lines per field produces an image with less residual flicker than standard 525-line video, because all 525 lines are refreshed at 60 Hz,[23] and the half-line shift between "fields" produces a smooth image with no perceivable dark lines between scan lines. Upscanning requires high-line monitors. This is one application of high-line video systems that is compatible with 512 by 512 digital acquisition.

Brightness Linearity

Several of the important properties of a videocamera are determined by the photoconducting target material.[24] Videocamera tubes such as Plumbicons° (lead oxide), Saticons,† Chalnicons,‡ and Neuvicon or Primicon§ produce a linear response between light intensity and output signal. This eliminates a source of nonlinearity that would otherwise have to be corrected for digital quantitative applications. In general, the response curve of videocameras is $V = I^\gamma$ where V is the output signal voltage, I is the input brightness, and γ ("gamma") is the power factor. A gamma less than 1 produces increased contrast in darker areas of the image and decreased contrast in brighter areas. This complements the video display monitor's gamma of about 2, which reduces contrast in the dark areas and enhances contrast in the bright areas. A videocamera with a gamma less than 1 therefore produces a better video monitor image, with about equal contrast in the light and dark areas. A linear videocamera ($\gamma = 1$) is required for digital subtraction and quantitation, but digital enhancement with the equivalent of a gamma of about 0.6 is usually applied to linearly acquired images before display. Some systems with linear cameras have an electronic logarithmic filter that can be switched on to produce the rough equivalent of a gamma of 0.6 for live fluoroscopic viewing; it is switched off for quantitative digital acquisitions.

Lag

Lag is produced whenever more than one scan is required to completely erase the image on the target. Cameras with relatively high lag are frequently used for general fluoroscopy because the lag reduces the quantum noise in each frame by integrating several

°Philips Medical Systems, Inc., Shelton, CT.
†Siemens Medical Systems, Inc., Erlangen, Germany.
‡Toshiba Medical Systems Co., Ltd., Tokyo, Japan.
§GE Medical Systems, Milwaukee, WI.

video frames. However, this temporal integration is unacceptable for coronary angiography because it produces multiple ghost images or blurring of rapidly moving objects.[24, 25] Lead oxide and several other videocamera target materials have frame-to-frame image retention of less than 10 percent, which is considered the maximum acceptable lag for cardiac imaging.[25] Lag increases with camera tube age and should be checked as part of a regular imaging chain quality control program.[2, 8] Lag also depends on input light level. During calibration of the fluoroscopic imaging chain, and before a videocamera tube is replaced because of excessive lag, it is important to verify adequate input light intensity.

Monitors

Monitors for cardiac angiography should be located as close to the operator as possible and should have a diagonal screen size equal to about one fourth of the distance between monitor and operator for the best combination of image size, scan line visibility, and perceived brightness. Although standard 525-line interlaced display is adequate, image quality is subjectively improved by using an upscanner to convert to a 1049-line interlaced display. The upscanner treats the 525-line frame as both fields of a 1049-line interlaced display, and the fields are displayed one after the other offset by one line, producing a display with the same actual spatial resolution but with no detectable scan lines. The monitors must be high-line monitors. Alternatively, the videocamera can be operated in 1023 or 1049 interlaced mode directly, obviating the need for a scan converter. Although in principle this approach doubles the vertical resolution, compared with the upscanned 525-line video, the increased spatial resolution does not produce an improvement in the perception of intracoronary features, wires, or devices because of the high noise and low contrast produced in fluoroscopy. A disadvantage of using a high-line camera is that it requires high-line recording devices.

Videorecording Devices

Fluoroscopy is not routinely recorded during cardiac angiography because the normal fluoroscopic dose rate produces image quality only good enough for manipulation of devices such as catheters. Videorecording of high-dose fluoroscopy and cineangiography are discussed in the next section.

CINEANGIOGRAPHY

X-Ray Technique

Frame Rate

Cardiac angiography is conventionally performed at 30 fps for adults and 60 fps for many pediatric studies. Although higher acquisition rates of 45 or 60 fps are possible and produce very smooth slow motion when viewed at the standard 24 fps, the consensus appears to be that this advantage is not worth the increase in radiation dose (50 or 100 percent, respectively, compared with the conventional rate) in addition to the increased film cost and processing time. Frame rates lower than 30 fps produce rough, jerky motion with higher perceived quantum noise when viewed dynamically, unless the input exposure per frame is increased.

Exposure per Frame

X-ray technique for cineangiography is designed to provide definitive diagnosis of cardiac anatomy and pathology, so exposure factors are chosen to produce the best possible image quality within the technical constraints of the x-ray tube; patient dose is a secondary, but still important, concern. The quantum noise in the cineangiogram is determined by the radiation exposure per frame at the image intensifier input phosphor. Over the past 20 years, a consensus has evolved (and a joint ACC/AHA task force has recommended[4]) that an input exposure of 30 μR ± 50 percent per frame in the 6-inch magnification mode is adequate for coronary angiography. Input exposures for 9- or 10-inch modes and for 4.5- or 5-inch modes are about half and double this exposure, respectively, with the same output image brightness. Quantum noise is significantly reduced as magnification is increased because of the increased dose per frame. Input exposures lower than those recommended produce images that most angiographers judge to be excessively noisy, and higher exposures lead to excessive patient dose and x-ray tube heat loading.

At the recommended input exposure, each still frame contains significant quantum noise, but the perception of this noise is reduced when the angiogram is viewed dynamically. Although a higher dose per frame would reduce quantum noise, the signal-to-noise ratio is ultimately limited by the structured noise produced by noncardiac patient anatomy, which is independent of dose. In addition, currently available x-ray tubes are not capable of significantly increased dose per frame without unacceptable increases in exposure duration (leading to increased motion blurring), in tube voltage (leading to loss of iodine contrast), or in focal spot size (leading to increased focal spot unsharpness). The recommended input exposure optimally balances available technology and image quality for coronary angiography.

X-Ray Tube Voltage, Tube Current, and Pulse Width

For adult coronary angiography, tube voltage should be between 70 and 90 kV to optimize iodine contrast for a given patient radiation dose. Thicker patients may require higher tube voltage to achieve adequate input exposure within the power limits of the x-ray tube. The exposure control systems of modern x-ray generators ("automatic brightness control" units) keep input exposure constant by automatically adjusting tube voltage, tube current, and exposure time (pulse width) according to a program designed to optimize image quality within the power limits of the x-ray tube focal spots. Typically, tube voltage, pulse width, and tube current are all low for thin patients. Cineangiographic exposures times in the range of 2 to 7 msec are required to "freeze" the motion of rapidly moving coronary arteries. As patient thickness increases, current is increased first, then pulse width is increased up to a maximum set at about 7 msec, and finally tube voltage is increased. When tube voltage reaches about 90 kV, some systems automatically switch to the large x-ray tube focal spot, allowing higher tube current. Only as a last resort is tube voltage increased above 90 kV. Some systems use a fixed pulse width, and the exact algorithm used to adjust voltage, current, and time differs between systems. Some systems allow minimum or maximum thresholds for pulse width and tube voltage to be set by the angiographer in order to fine tune operation for specific purposes. For example, a lower pulse width threshold may be desirable for patients in whom rapid heart rates produce greater than normal motion blurring.

Biplane Cineangiography

Biplane cineangiography provides three advantages over single plane angiography: two views can be acquired during a single contrast injection, reducing the patient's contrast material burden; during interventions, the angiographer can switch rapidly between two projections to check the positioning of intracoronary devices without moving the imaging system; and recording of simultaneous (or almost simultaneous) views allows exact determination of geometric magnification[26] and three-dimensional reconstruction of the coronary arteries.[27-31] Only the first two of these applications appear to be in current clinical use. The disadvantages of biplane cineangiography are that equipment and service costs are substantially higher, the additional equipment requires more space and reduces access to the patient, and x-ray exposure to the operator and staff may be higher because of the difficulty of optimally positioning radiation shields for both projections. Biplane coronary angiography is significantly more efficient with the use of an autopositioning system to quickly move the imaging planes into a sequence of standard biplane views.

The imaging systems for both planes are essentially identical and work independently, except that x-ray exposures alternate between planes. This allows one generator to power both tubes, but, more importantly, it eliminates contrast-reducing interplane radiation scatter by preventing simultaneous exposures.

Cine Camera

The cine camera used almost universally for cardiac cineangiography today is the Arritechno* 35/90. Filming rates of 15, 30, 45, 60, and 90 fps are available, although 30 and 60 fps are only speeds commonly used. For cardiac angiography, the camera uses a so-called half-frame image format measuring 24 mm in width (across the film) and 18 mm in height (along the film). The camera is equipped with a rotating shutter that blocks all light from the image intensifier during film motion; this is especially important during biplane angiography to prevent fogging of the film by scattered radiation from the opposite plane. As in the case of the videocamera, framing of the circular output phosphor on the rectangular film format is determined by the cine camera lens focal length. Maximum horizontal framing or subtotal overframing (see Fig. 16–8, *dashed rectangle, right*) is recommended for coronary angiography.[4] The latter matches the fluoroscopic field of view when total overframing is used for the videocamera. This ensures that the entire visible fluoroscopic image is recorded on cine film and encourages tight collimation.

Cine Film

The 35-mm cine film used in cardiac angiography can resolve about 80 lp/mm on the film itself, corresponding to more than 12 lp/mm at the patient with an image intensifier in the 6-inch magnification mode. Cine film projectors typically can resolve only about 48 lp/mm, but this still corresponds to more than 7 lp/mm at the image intensifier input, well above the resolution of the image intensifier itself. Projector performance for both still frames and dynamic display at all available speeds should be checked periodically with a precision alignment test film (such as SMPTE test film 35-PA, Society of Motion Pictures and Television Engineers, White Plains, NY).

Film Characteristics

Cine film selection and processing has a major effect on image quality. Cine film for coronary angiography should have low to medium contrast to allow a wide range of image intensities at the output phosphor to be recorded and adequately displayed. This is particularly important with modern, high–contrast ratio image

---

*Arnold & Richter Cine Technik GMBH & Co., Munich, Germany.

intensifiers. High-contrast cine film can produce impressive images if the range of intensities in the image (the "dynamic range") is small and the exposure is just right, but images with wider dynamic range, including most coronary angiograms, tend to suffer from overexposed or underexposed areas with significant loss of detail. Cine film with a relatively low average gradient of 1.2 to 1.7 is optimal for coronary angiography.

Film speed refers to the relative sensitivity of film to light in relation to production of a standard optical density: a "fast" film requires a lower light exposure than a "slow" film. Image intensifier input exposure (and thus the output phosphor light exposure) is fixed on the basis of quantum noise and patient dose considerations, not cine film sensitivity. Accommodation of different film sensitivities is made by adjusting the optical aperture of the cine camera lens. Because the lens produces a sharper, higher-contrast image with a smaller aperture, there is an advantage to faster cine film. On the other hand, very fast films have larger grain size, which in extreme cases can contribute to image noise. Therefore, the cine film used should be fast enough to allow stopping down the camera aperture at least two "f/stops" (each "stop" reduces aperture area by a factor of 2) but not so fast that film grain becomes visible under normal viewing conditions. Under no circumstances should cine film density be adjusted by changing the x-ray input exposure, which, as discussed, would produce suboptimal image quality or excessive patient radiation dose, or both.

Processing

Several excellent commercial processors for 35-mm cine film are available for laboratories with light or heavy workloads. The processor must maintain tight control of developing time, temperature, developer replenishment, fixing, washing, and drying. Because an error in any one of these steps can result in an inferior or unusable film, processing can easily become the weakest link in the imaging procedure without a meticulous daily quality control program.[2, 4, 8] At minimum, such a program must expose and develop a test strip to measure film base, fog, speed, and contrast index. These values must be recorded at least daily (many busy laboratories run a strip with every film) so that problems can be found and corrected before a clinical film is damaged or lost. Films should routinely be examined critically for processor artifacts such as streaks, stickiness, or mottle. Special attention should be paid to test strips after any change, such as starting a new lot number of film or mixing a new batch of developer. Film speed, in particular, varies significantly from lot to lot, and adjustment of cine camera apertures or *minor* adjustment of processing time should be made to keep on-frame film density constant.

Analog Videorecording Devices

Videotape

The use of analog videotape is unacceptable as a primary archive for coronary angiograms. Although videotape is widely accepted for medical ultrasonography and has the advantages that the equipment for recording and playback are standard, widely available, and inexpensive, even S-VHS videocassette recorders unacceptably degrade the resolution and signal-to-noise ratio of coronary angiograms. Image quality is further degraded each time the tape is viewed, as well as by the passage of time. Until recently videotape was used to provide instant playback during coronary angiography, but it has largely been replaced by digital recording devices, especially in interventional laboratories where the superior cine loop replay and still frame performance of digital equipment is a major advantage.

Analog Optical Disk

The analog optical disk is a write-once, nonerasable medium for recording and playback of video signals. Twelve-inch diameter analog optical disks have a capacity of about 20 minutes for video signals of 525 lines and 30 fps; this is equivalent to 36,000 frames and is sufficient for about 20 complete coronary angiograms. Video bandwidth is 8 MHz, adequate to provide horizontal resolution of about 650 lines (for standard videocameras). The signal-to-noise ratio is specified at better than 45 dB, or 178:1 (see the section on noise), which would add less than 4 percent to the quantum noise in a cineangiogram. Analog optical disk systems are usually integrated with a desktop computer that keeps an index of patients and runs, allowing rapid random access to any patient sequence, a major advantage over videotape. Another significant advantage over tape is the ability of video disks to rapidly replay a single sequence in an endless loop format. However, analog optical disks are not reusable and cost significantly more than videotape, so they would be an expensive alternative to videotape or digital recording solely for instant replay during procedures.

At least one manufacturer has developed an economical archival system using analog optical disks to replace cine film. The media are claimed to be stable for at least 10 years. However, given the enormous push in consumer electronics (and medical imaging) for all-digital video media, devices to *play* analog optical disks may not be available in 10 years. There are some other disadvantages of this medium as a primary archival medium. Image quality is adequate for analog recording and replay of images acquired from a 512 by 512 digital system, but redigitization of the signal to perform analysis or image enhancement does not recover the original digital image. The extent of degradation depends on how the signal is filtered before and after recording and on the alignment of the samples (pixels) between the first and second digitizations. If enhanced images are stored, some kinds of quantitative analysis or re-enhancement may not be possible. Nevertheless, the relatively low equipment and media costs and high speed compared with digital archival systems currently make this medium an attractive possibility for some laboratories.

GENERAL PRINCIPLES OF DIGITAL IMAGING

The basic concept of digital imaging is that an image is converted to numbers, the numbers are stored and possibly manipulated or analyzed by a computer, and then the numbers are converted back into a visual image for viewing. All current digital cardiac angiography systems use a videocamera to provide an electronic video image from a conventional x-ray image intensifier. It is the analog signal from this video system that is viewed on the video monitor during conventional fluoroscopy. In digital imaging systems, the analog video signal is intercepted before it is displayed on the monitor. The signal is converted into a digital or numerical form and stored or manipulated by a computer before being reconverted to an analog video signal for display. Figure 16–10 is an overview of a typical system, showing the major components.

Conversion of Images to Digital Form

Conversion of an image into a finite set of numbers is called digitization. In all currently available digital angiography systems, digitization consists of three steps: scanning, sampling, and quantization.

Sampling

The intensity along each raster scan is measured, or sampled, at evenly spaced points. Each of these measured values represents the brightness at one location in the image, known as a picture element or pixel. A digitized image consists of rows and columns of pixels, and the brightness of each pixel is represented by an intensity value. The maximum resolution of a digital image is limited by the pixel size in accordance with the Nyquist sampling theorem, which states that a sinusoidally varying intensity can be accurately reproduced from sampled data only if the pixel size is

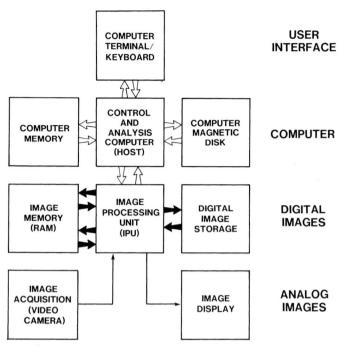

FIGURE 16–10. Overview of typical digital imaging system components and signal pathways. Large open arrows represent digital data, large solid arrows represent digital image data, and solid lines represent analog video signals. As the speed and memory of standard computers have increased, the separation between computer and image memory and the need for a separate image processing unit, have diminished. Desktop workstations based on personal computers can now perform most image processing and analysis functions that formerly required special hardware, although they are still too slow to perform filtering procedures in real time.

less than half the wavelength.[32] The effective pixel size is determined by mapping the pixel array onto the field of view in the object plane, and the effective size depends on geometric magnification, image intensifier mode, framing, and matrix size (see Table 16–1). For example, a 512 by 512 digital image of an inscribed 15.2 cm (6-inch) diameter image intensifier (total overframing) has pixel spacing of (152 mm)/512, or 0.30 mm, so the shortest wavelength that can accurately be represented is 0.59 mm, corresponding to a maximum spatial frequency of 1/(0.59 mm), or 1.7 mm^{-1}. The resolution of modern image intensifier tubes is greater than 3.5 lp/mm, requiring a pixel spacing of 0.14 mm at the input phosphor, or a matrix size of 1064 by 1064 for the 6-inch mode with exact framing.

Quantization

Each pixel intensity is converted to an integer between 0 and $(N_g - 1)$, where N_g is the number of gray levels in the digital image. This conversion of a continuous range of intensities to a set of discrete gray levels is called quantization.

Both horizontal sampling and quantization are performed by the analog-to-digital converter. Because a binary digital computer stores and manipulates these image data, it is efficient to choose the number of gray levels and the number of rows and columns to be powers of 2. For reasons having nothing to do with digital imaging, video standards developed long ago call for 525 horizontal raster lines; all but 13 lines of a standard video frame can be stored in a digital image with 512, or 2^9, rows. In most digital angiography applications, the number of rows is chosen to be equal to the number of columns. Thus, the de facto standard digital image size for cardiac digital angiography is 512 rows by 512 columns.

Bit Depth

The number of gray levels determines the precision with which the original image intensities are represented in the digital image;

it also determines the number of binary digits (bits) the analog-to-digital converter (and the image memory) must use to represent the intensity. The number of bits is equal to the power of 2 that is equivalent to the number of gray levels. The difference between a quantized gray level and the original intensity is at most half of the increment between gray levels. For a typical angiographic image, the mean square quantization error is equal to one twelfth of the gray scale increment.[33] Correct choice of the number of bits depends on the range and precision of intensities in the original image; that is, on its signal-to-noise ratio.

Noise

Image noise refers to random image intensity variations; it is a critically important measure of image quality because it fundamentally limits the detection of small, low-contrast features.[14, 15, 34] The primary sources of noise in digital cardiac angiography are quantum noise (which results from the detection of a finite number of x-ray photons in each pixel), electronic noise (which is added by the preamplifier of the video camera), and digitization noise (which is caused by the discrete increment between gray levels in a digital image). In a properly designed and operated imaging system, the total image noise should be dominated by quantum noise, because otherwise the patient x-ray dose could be reduced without sacrificing image quality. Low-noise videocameras are used in digital coronary angiography to keep electronic noise well below quantum noise. Quantization error can be made small compared with overall noise by choosing the increment between gray levels to be less than twice the quantum noise.[35–37]

The imaging system signal-to-noise ratio (SNR) can be defined as the range of intensities to be digitized (the signal), divided by the root-mean-square deviation of intensity (the noise). System SNR is frequently expressed using the logarithmic decibel (dB) scale: the ratio in decibels is equal to $20 \log_{10}(SNR)$. Thus, 60 dB corresponds to a SNR of 1000:1, and 48 dB represents a SNR of 250:1. The number of gray levels must be sufficient to cover the range of intensities within the original image. The minimum number of gray levels needed is the SNR divided by the increment between gray levels. As an important example, cardiac angiography can be satisfactorily performed using an x-ray exposure of 30 μR per image.[4] This exposure produces an SNR of about 100:1, which, using an increment of twice the quantum noise, would require about 50 gray levels. However, this rule is complicated by the fact that the magnitude of the quantum noise is proportional to the square root of exposure. In a cardiac angiogram, the least intense area of the image typically receives one sixteenth the exposure and therefore has one fourth the quantum noise standard deviation, so the gray level increments must be made one fourth as large. Thus, 200 gray levels are needed to digitize a 30 μR exposure image with a 16:1 intensity range, requiring a minimum of 8 bits (256 gray levels).

DIGITAL IMAGE STORAGE

After an angiogram has been digitized, it must be stored for later processing or display. There are four general classes of storage: display buffer memory, which contains the image currently displayed on the video monitor; high-speed image memory, from which images are transferred to the display buffer at rates of up to one image every 1/30 second ("real time" for standard video); on-line mass storage, which may contain image series from several patient examinations for direct access, but often at a rate slower than real time; and archival storage, for long-term, off-line storage. The space required to store a digital image depends on the number of pixels and the bits per pixel. An image array of 512 rows by 512 columns has 512 × 512 or 262,144 pixels. When working with large powers of 2, it is convenient to define a slight modification of the standard scientific prefixes for powers of 10, making use of the fact that 2^{10} (or 1024) is close to 10^3 (or 1000), as shown in

Table 16–2. Using this notation, a 512 by 512 digital image is said to contain 256 kilopixels. If each pixel is quantized to 8 bits (1 byte), the required storage space is 256 kilobytes.

On-Line Storage

On-line image storage refers to storage of images for immediate access. There are several types of on-line storage, and they differ in cost, capacity, and speed.

Solid State Memory

The fastest and most expensive (per image) memory is solid state *Random Access Memory* (RAM). Digital angiography systems differ widely in amount of image RAM—from 256 kilobytes (a single image) to 80 megabytes (320 images) and more—and in the ways in which the memory is used. Some common uses are described here.

The display buffer consists of RAM connected directly to the digital-to-analog converter that drives the video monitor. Many systems are designed with space for more than one image in the display buffer, allowing an image to be displayed from one area of the buffer while a new image is being transferred to another area. After the transfer is complete, the system can cause the area containing the new image to be displayed, so that the display instantaneously switches from one image to the next.

In some systems, the image RAM is used as a buffer for recording cine image sequences. Images are stored at real-time rates in RAM (the buffer memory) and transferred to another storage medium such as magnetic disk at a different rate, relaxing the requirement for rigid synchronization of the electromechanical disk drive with real-time digital-electronic image acquisition. If the buffer is large enough to hold an entire cine sequence, the magnetic disks can operate at a much slower rate, because the time between cine runs can be used to transfer the images. The extra time allowed for disk storage can also be used to perform lossless image data compression (discussed in a later section), which can increase disk capacity by a factor of two to four times that of uncompressed data. Sufficient RAM to store an entire sequence is also an advantage for image analysis workstations because it allows display of the sequence so that frames can be selected for analysis, and it is a necessity for multiple image analysis algorithms.

Real-Time Digital Magnetic Disk

On-line mass storage systems for cardiac digital angiography usually consist of special high-speed digital magnetic disk drives capable of recording 512 by 512 images at a rate of 30 per second. A system with such a disk does not need a separate, large image memory because images can be loaded directly from disk to the display buffer in real time.

Archival Storage

Because of the large number of images created during cineangiography, long-term storage has been one of the major problems that have kept digital angiography from replacing film as the primary recording medium.

Owing to the rapid pace of technological development, digital media standards are likely to change much more often than the cine film standard, which has been in use in its present form for more than 20 years. As a result, single-patient physical media such as the CD-R described in a later section, will become obsolete several times over the archival lifetime of digital angiograms. Single-patient or "unit-record" physical media are expensive and difficult to manage in large numbers and are subject to damage, misfiling, loss, and theft; in the future, they should only rarely need to be used for data exchange outside the laboratory to places to which networks do not extend. The ideal digital replacement for the cine film archive will be a "black box" that is as invisible to the user as the warehouse containing last year's cine films but is instantly accessible from the review station by high-speed network. The physical inner workings of the "black box" archive, whether magnetic tape, optical disk, or three-dimensional holographic storage, will change and improve many times, but this should not be a concern: when the vendor maintaining the "box" decides to upgrade, the data will simply be transferred before the old medium is taken off line. The characteristics that matter to the users are storage capacity, data integrity, security (both physical and legal), access speed, and the stability of the standard protocols for storing and retrieving data to assure continuity of access over archival time periods. Networks, media, and storage systems are rapidly approaching the speed, reliability, and scalability needed for an all-digital data archive for cardiac angiography. The standard formats and protocols for data storage and access are being addressed by the ACR/ACC/NEMA DICOM standard described in this chapter. These protocols and the software needed to implement them on a large scale are much more difficult and critical issues than the hardware or media. Until these issues stabilize, caution is advised before proven cine film technology is abandoned.[38]

Cine Film

Most laboratories that acquire and read all studies digitally still continue to use 35-mm cine film as the primary recording, transfer, and archival medium because of its superior spatial resolution, universal format, convenience of playback (including the ability to project on the wall for conferences), and guaranteed stability of the physical medium and format over an archival lifetime of at least 10 years. The cost is about $80 per patient study for film, processing, and storage.

Magnetic Tape

Digital audiotape (4-mm DAT) and 8-mm exabyte tape are now commonly used for computer data backup and have sufficient capacity for digital angiography archiving. Many laboratories dump each day's studies to an Exabyte tape as a cine film backup or for future digital analysis. Autoloading "jukebox" devices exist that provide software-controlled access to a large library of tapes, and a "black box" archiving method could be designed based on this technology. However, the data access and transfer rates for these media are too slow for routine clinical access in a busy laboratory.

Another tape medium, which has been developed into a completely automated archive, is the D2 digital videotape system,° originally designed for broadcast real-time videorecording and playback. Storage capacity is very high (up to 30 patient studies per tape, 30,000 studies total archive on-line with a robotic tape library), and mean access time to any stored study is claimed to be less than 1 minute. D2 was designed to record and replay analog

---

°Song Corporation, Tokyo, Japan.

TABLE 16–2. DECIMAL AND BINARY PREFIXES FOR LARGE NUMBERS

Prefix	Decimal Values			Binary Values
kilo-(K)	10^3 (thousand)	1000	2^{10}	1024
mega-(M)	10^6 (million)	1000 thousand = 1,000,000	2^{20}	1024 K = 1,048,576
giga-(G)	10^9 (billion)	1000 million = 1,000,000,000	2^{30}	1024 M = 1,073,741,824
tera-(T)	10^{12} (trillion)	1000 billion	2^{40}	1024 G

video, which it does very well. Some degradation occurs, however, if the video signal from the x-ray imaging system has already been digitized before it is recorded on D2. In its standard configuration, correction of this problem would require conversion of the digital image to analog, to be redigitized at the D2. If the images stored on D2 are to be digitally enhanced or analyzed later, they must again be converted to analog and redigitized by the workstation. Each of these transcriptions can introduce errors that may or may not affect visual perception or quantitative analysis. Nevertheless, D2 appears to be an excellent candidate for the "inner workings" of a full-featured digital angiography archive system.

Image data integrity, security, access time (with multiple users and simultaneous real-time acquisition), and long-term stability are complex issues that must be field-verified over time for any archival system. It seems likely that the interactive entertainment and digital communications industries will continue to drive rapid development of digital image communications and display and that the future lies with all-digital imaging directly to the display station. However, this prospect need not prevent an appropriate investment in currently available systems, because the need to periodically upgrade the media and technology inside a central digital archive should be expected.

Digital Compact Disk

Digital compact disk, or CD-ROM, is now a widely established standard medium for mass distribution of software and data at the consumer level. A newer technology called CD-R (Compact Disk–Recordable) allows "write-once" recording on a nonerasable medium that is physically similar to the CD-ROM (i.e., a 5.25-inch optical disk). Hardware and software for recording and reading CD-R are rapidly improving in ease of use, speed, cost, and compatibility among manufacturers. The medium itself has a single-side capacity of 680 megabytes, which is equivalent to 4800 frames with a resolution of 512 by 512 by 8 and 2:1 lossless compression, sufficient to record almost any angiographic procedure on a single disk. The fastest currently available readers (called "6X" readers because they operate at 6 times the speed of a standard audio CD) can transfer 2:1 compressed images at 8 fps, two to four times slower than desired for viewing, and they require about 5 minutes to transfer an average study to a digital viewer. The CD-R is much more compact and physically robust than magnetic media, making it a good choice for exchanging digitally recorded coronary angiograms between laboratories.

The American College of Cardiology, the American College of Radiology, and the National Electrical Manufacturers Association (ACC/ACR/NEMA) have developed a standard format for digital angiogram exchange, DICOM (Digital Imaging and Communication in Medicine), that includes CD-R as the exchange medium. The question of a digital archival medium to replace cine film was deliberately not addressed in the standard. Although CD-R is appropriate for image exchange, which is by nature transient, there is no guarantee that the technology (or the medium) will remain stable over the 5 to 10 years required for archival storage. It seems certain that much faster and more compact mass storage solutions will continue to emerge.

DIGITAL IMAGE VIEWERS AND WORKSTATIONS

Digital angiograms are not as convenient to review as cine film angiograms because of the lack of digital media with fast enough reading and writing rates and the lack of inexpensive display devices analogous to cine film projectors with which to view them. Review and analysis of digital angiograms may be done on the digital angiography system itself, but this is suboptimal in busy laboratories because analysis, acquisition, and review cannot be done simultaneously. For in-lab review, there appear to be two good choices: a network of review stations connected to a central

server, or a unit-record digital medium fast enough for direct real-time replay. A workstation with full analysis and display facilities networked with the acquisition or on-line archiving system has the advantage that storage media need not be physically transported and mounted on the workstation. The workstation can also be equipped to read any of the archival image storage media (e.g., CD-R optical disks). In either case, the original digital data is available for viewing and analysis with no degradation. After a standard format has been adopted and the new equipment universally installed, digital media allows the same easy interchange of images that 35-mm cine film currently provides.

Another approach to the non-film review problem has been to make an analog videotape recording for review. Low-noise, high-bandwidth videocassette technology can record images with little apparent degradation[39] so long as they are viewed at normal speed, and particularly if optimal image enhancement is performed before recording. However, the image quality of still frames and slow motion is significantly degraded. Another disadvantage of this approach is that the videotaped images cannot be manipulated or analyzed quantitatively. Redigitizing the recorded images or copying them to another tape results in significant degradation. As a result, coronary angiograms recorded on videotape are widely considered substandard.

The vastly increased power of personal computers and desktop workstations now makes them fully capable of performing sophisticated image analysis and display that formerly would have required specialized equipment.

DIGITAL IMAGE PROCESSING

Gray-Scale Transformations

The simplest digital image processing method is to change each original gray level to some other level based on a table of correspondence called an intensity transformation table or "look-up table." This process is the basis for window and level adjustments to optimize displayed contrast and brightness. It is also used to invert image contrast in order to display a "negative" image, with white arteries on a black background, as in a cine film. More subtle adjustments of the gray scale, such as the logarithm transformation, are used to allow equal feature contrast to be displayed equally in dark and light areas even though the video monitor contrast is higher in the bright areas. As simple as these controls are, they are useful, and they are not available with cine film (except prospectively, to a limited extent, by choice of film type).

Image Processing Filters

Image manipulations may also be divided into point operations, such as contrast enhancement or subtraction, which are performed on a pixel-by-pixel basis; "neighborhood" operations, in which the intensity of a given pixel depends on the pixel intensities in the neighborhood of the original pixel;[40] and multiple image operations. Examples of neighborhood operations are edge enhancement, smoothing or blurring, and zooming a portion of an image to make it appear larger on the screen. An example of a multiple-image operation is digital subtraction angiography, in which a new image is formed by subtracting two original images. Some important image processing procedures are categorized in Table 16–3 according to the information used to calculate each pixel.

Spatial Filtration

Spatial filtration, or convolution, is a neighborhood operation in which the intensity of each pixel is replaced by some function of the intensities of other pixels, usually those in its immediate neighborhood. The most common class of spatial filter replaces each pixel with a weighted average of its original intensity and that of the pixels surrounding it. The effect of the filter on the image

TABLE 16–3. CLASSIFICATION OF IMAGE PROCESSING PROCEDURES

	Point Operations	Neighborhood Operations
Single image	Window, level Logarithmic transform Histogram equalization Pseudocolor display	Convolution 　Edge enhancement 　Smoothing Median filter noise 　reduction
Multiple images	Subtraction 　Mask mode 　Time interval Time-domain filtration 　Recursive 　Matched filter Functional imaging	

can be varied by selecting the size of the neighborhood to be averaged and the pattern of weights to be applied to each pixel within the neighborhood. The same pattern of weights, called a kernel, is applied equally to each pixel in the image. Figure 16–11 shows the effects of three simple kernels *(top row)* on a coronary angiogram *(middle row)* and a resolution pattern *(bottom row)*. The first kernel specifies that each pixel shall be replaced by itself plus zero times the sum of its eight nearest neighbors. This is a trivial filter because it reproduces the original image. The second kernel specifies that each pixel be replaced by an evenly-weighted average of itself and its eight nearest neighbors. This filter has two noticeable effects on the images: it reduces random pixel-to-pixel fluctuations (noise), and it blurs image detail. Both effects are directly proportional to the size of the kernel. An evenly-weighted kernel with 5 by 5 elements will produce more smoothing and blurring than this 3 by 3 kernel, but both processed images will

have the same overall intensity as the original, because the sum of the kernel elements is 1.0. The third kernel specifies that each pixel be replaced by nine times the original pixel intensity minus the intensities of its eight nearest neighbors. If all nine pixels have the same intensity, this kernel has no effect. However, if the original pixel is just *outside* a region of increased intensity, so that several of its nearest neighbors have higher values, the original pixel is replaced by a lower value. Pixels just *inside* a region of increased intensity are replaced by higher values. The result is edge enhancement. This filter noticeably enhances the contrast of the edges of the coronary arteries, the resolution pattern, and the quantum noise.

The action of spatial filters is often described by the language of time-domain signal filtration: the second filter in Figure 16–11 is a "low-pass" filter because it preserves the contrast of large areas (low spatial frequencies) while reducing the contrast of small details (high spatial frequencies); the overall "gain" is equal to the sum of the weights in the kernel. The highly developed theory of time-domain signal filtration carries over in a straightforward way to two-dimensional spatial images. For example, a high-pass filter can easily be designed that would suppress large area intensity differences while enhancing sudden changes in spatial intensity such as those occurring at the edges of the coronary arteries.

Noise Reduction

Filters that reduce quantum noise can be designed, but they have not yet found wide use in coronary angiography. The simplest of these, spatial smoothing, merely blurs the image, reducing the noise but also reducing the spatial resolution needed to see important detail. Temporal smoothing, the digital averaging of several sequential frames, is frequently used for fluroscopy of stationary body parts, but it has the same adverse effect as spatial smoothing on moving coronary arteries. More sophisticated noise reduction techniques, such as the median filter, are more computationally expensive (i.e., they require more steps), and they are currently

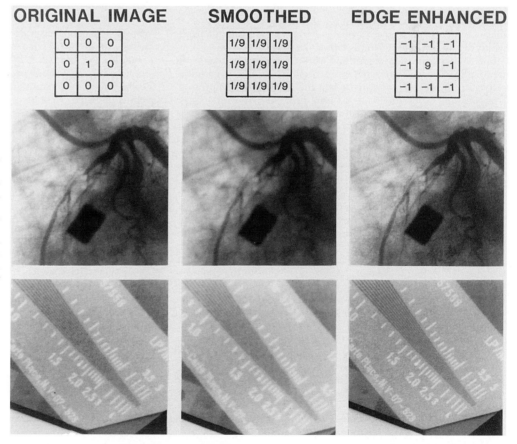

FIGURE 16–11. Examples of image enhancement with a 3 by 3 filter kernel. Each pixel of the processed image is the weighted sum of the original pixel and its eight nearest neighbors. The weights, specified by the "kernels" shown at the top, determine the effect of the convolution, as shown in the processed angiograms and resolution grids below. The kernel on the left reproduces the original image because each pixel is replaced by its own original value.

too slow to be performed in real time without costly specialized equipment. Whether such filters can actually improve observer performance has not yet been determined.

Digital Subtraction Angiography

Subtraction is a powerful technique for detecting subtle differences between two almost identical images. In cardiology, the image of the heart without contrast material (the mask) is subtracted from the image made after injection of contrast material, resulting in two potential benefits. First, the range of intensities in the final, subtracted image is typically reduced by a factor of eight because the image consists only of intensity changes that result from the addition of contrast material. This allows the subtracted image to be contrast-enhanced by a similar factor. Second, after subtraction of stationary structures from the image, features of the opacified cardiac anatomy become more conspicuous.[41] Subtraction is therefore a method for removing a significant source of noise from angiographic images—the structured noise caused by overlying bone and soft tissues. Unfortunately, subtraction cannot reduce random noise, such as quantum mottle, because this noise varies from one frame to another. In fact, the quantum noise in a subtracted image is actually greater than that in the original images; it is equal to the square root of the sum of the squared quantum noise in the mask and in the raw image.[42]

Digital subtraction has not been found to be useful for routine cardiac angiography. Its main disadvantage is that patient motion occurring between the capture of the mask and the contrast image results in enhanced "misregistration" artifacts, which may obscure the angiogram more than the original, unenhanced patient structures.

IMAGE DATA COMPRESSION

The large volume and high rate of data produced by digital coronary angiography is a problem both for storage and for transmission over networks. Digital image compression techniques exist that can reduce the storage space and transmission time or bandwidth required. Compression is either "lossless" or "lossy."

Lossless compression algorithms work by converting images to more efficient data representations with no loss of information; the original data is exactly restored when the image is decompressed. Compression ratios of about 3:1 can be achieved with lossless compression of coronary angiograms.

Lossy compression works by approximating or simply not storing part of the data, so that some information is irretrievably lost. A simple and common example of lossy compression is the use of a 512 by 512 matrix for digital angiography, which results in greater than 4:1 compression of the 1064 by 1064 matrix required to record the full image resolution (see Table 16–1, 6-inch mode, exact framing). Lossy compression is successful if only "useless" information is lost and all the *useful* information can be restored. Lossy image compression algorithms, such as the type developed by the Joint Picture Experts Group, work by approximating data in ways designed to minimize the impact of errors on image quality (i.e., on the useful information). There is no limit to the compression ratio achievable with lossy compression, but the higher the compression ratio for a given compression algorithm, the greater the loss of information. The definition of what is useful information depends strongly on the purpose of the image—on what the viewer needs to see. In the jargon of image perception, image quality is defined by observer performance for specific relevant visual tasks.[43] Coronary angiography clearly involves many different visual tasks of some subtlety, making the definition of angiographic image quality complex. Nevertheless, there are strong economic and practical motivations for using both lossless and lossy compression in digital angiography. A consensus on the acceptable type and amount of compression error will eventually emerge, just as a

consensus has been reached on the acceptable level of quantum noise. The difference is that accepting higher quantum noise reflects a desire to minimize radiation dose to the patient, whereas accepting lossy compression primarily reflects a desire to reduce the cost of digital angiography.

APPLICATIONS OF DIGITAL IMAGING

Processing and Display

Digital imaging provides superior playback image quality and display flexibility, including scan conversion for progressive videocamera readout, real-time edge enhancement, and high-quality display of reference and roadmap images. Interventional laboratories in particular should be equipped with at least a minimal digital system to take advantage of these features.

Progressive scan fluoroscopy improves fluoroscopic resolution and allows radiation dose to be reduced without loss of image quality.[44, 45] These advantages require a minimal digital imaging system consisting of digital scan converter, pulsed x-ray fluoroscopic exposures at 30 fps, and 30-Hz progressive scan mode videocamera operation. The same relatively inexpensive system completely removes flicker during 30 fps cine filming, producing a dynamic image that is much smoother and easier to interpret. Recorded video still frames with progressive scan have resolution superior to standard 2:1 interlaced video because the entire frame is recorded from a single short x-ray exposure rather than from two separate exposures made $\frac{1}{60}$ second apart.[46]

Digital images can be enhanced to sharpen edges and improve contrast, manipulations that have been found to improve detectability of simple patterns in radiographic noise[47, 48] and that may also improve detectability of atherosclerotic plaque morphology.[49] Edge enhancement seems to work by approximately restoring the image to its unblurred condition, increasing the contrast of small features such as guidewires. Real-time image enhancement can be performed by a relatively inexpensive add-on video processor or as part of a more elaborate digital system.

A principal advantage of digital coronary angiography is the ease with which cine runs can be rapidly recalled and smoothly displayed as an endlessly repeating loop or in a back-and-forth "palindromic" format.[12] With sufficient digital memory, all sequences can be instantly available for display, either as still frames or cine loops, in a manner that is much quicker and smoother than is possible with videotape recorders. A series of representative still frames documenting a procedure can be printed for inclusion in the patient report.

Digital systems provide a variety of visual aids for guiding interventions. The simplest is the reference image or loop, a high-quality still frame or dynamic loop of the target lesion displayed adjacent to the live fluoroscopic image, usually on a separate monitor. A roadmap is a reference image displayed on the live image monitor in such a way that both the reference image and the devices being manipulated under fluoroscopy can be seen superimposed. Static roadmap images are commonly used for interventions outside the heart, but cardiac motion makes them less useful for coronary angioplasty. A synchronized dynamic roadmap uses the electrocardiogram to synchronize the replay of the superimposed reference loop with the live fluoroscopic image, so that intracoronary devices appear to move with the roadmap image.[50]

It is well known that dynamic display of an image sequence produces better apparent image quality because temporal integration in the visual system reduces quantum noise. On the other hand, rapid movement of the coronary arteries in a dynamic display reduces visual detectability of subtle arterial features. A digital display workstation can be programmed to track the motion of a coronary artery segment and redisplay the sequence with the artery stabilized at a fixed location on the screen. Observer performance studies[12] have shown that this "stenosis-stabilized" display improves detectability of intracoronary features by an amount equivalent to a 60 to 70 percent increase in feature contrast; the procedure reduces observer uncertainty and reduces the time required to detect a known feature by more than 50 percent. Advanced optimal display techniques such as this may have a significant impact on clinical coronary angiographic interpretation. A combination of stenosis stabilization and dynamic roadmapping should eventually allow angiographers to have a stationary, rather than constantly moving, field of view, perhaps allowing finer control over the manipulation and positioning of intracoronary devices.

Quantification

Next to immediate, flexible display, quantification is digital angiography's strongest advantage over film. Left ventricular wall motion analysis and quantitative coronary angiography are more easily and objectively performed with the aid of digital image processing. Many of the subjective steps, such as tracing of edges, can be completely automated, increasing accuracy and reproducibility and decreasing analysis time.

Quantitative analysis of angiographic data requires, at a minimum, that the system have frame-storage capability, and for most useful work storage of at least a full cine run is required so that a frame can be chosen for analysis at peak opacification and at the optimum point in the cardiac cycle. Enough memory to store a cine run is an absolute requirement for analysis of density versus time data.

The digital acquisition systems provided by x-ray equipment manufacturers all have some basic quantification tools, usually including vessel sizing (manual or automatic) and ejection fraction calculation. The sophistication and accuracy of these systems vary and should be validated as part of the acceptance testing of a new system.

Spatial Measurement

Spatial dimensions are easily measured in digital images because each pixel has unique coordinates. With the use of a trackball or mouse as a pointer, features such as the ventricular wall may be outlined and ventricular volumes, stroke volume, and ejection fraction automatically calculated based on the desired algorithm. Outlining of the ventricle and tracing of coronary artery stenoses can be automated with the use of edge detection algorithms. This eliminates subjective variability and may improve absolute accuracy. The fundamental bases for these methods are discussed in this section.

Accuracy and Calibration

The pixels of a digital image form a highly accurate rectilinear array, so that the x and y coordinates of a pixel are exact multiples of the pixel size. The distance in the image plane between any two pixels is easily calculated by the theorem of Pythagoras. Although the shortest distance that can be measured is the pixel size, the actual limit of accuracy often is determined by unsharpness, noise, and distortions that occur in the radiographic imaging process before digitization[51] rather than by the pixel size itself.

Magnification

The pixel size is defined by the size of the object that maps exactly into one pixel of the image. This size depends on the radiographic magnification of the object, the electronic minification of the image by the image intensifier tube, the magnification of the image intensifier output by the videocamera optics, and the way in which the videocamera image is scanned and the signal digitized. The overall effect of these magnifications can be calibrated by determining the number of pixels corresponding to an object of known size, for a given radiographic magnification and image intensifier mode. The error introduced by the finite pixel size can be minimized by use of an object whose size corresponds to many pixels.

Pincushion Distortion

Pincushion distortion is an exaggeration of the distances measured from the center of the image as a result of the curvature of the input phosphor of the image intensifier. The pincushion distortion of most modern image intensifier tubes used for cardiac angiography is in the range of 1 or 2 percent,[17, 18] considerably less than those of a decade ago,[19] and for most routine measurements it is not a significant source of error. Distance measurements can be automatically corrected for pincushion distortion in a digital image by converting to polar coordinates and correcting the radial distances with the use of calibration data obtained from a test pattern.[17, 19, 20] This technique is fast and easy to implement because only the coordinates being measured are corrected. An alternative approach is to warp the entire image to remove pincushion distortion before measurement.[21] Because all pixels in the image are affected, this correction takes longer, but it is practical for single frames.

Edge Detection

Because of the unsharpness of the borders of objects such as coronary arteries and the left ventricle on angiographic imaging, measurement accuracy is affected by subjective determination of the precise location of edges. Digital edge detection methods define these edges objectively. At the fundamental level, computer edge detection methods used in digital angiography identify edges along a single one-dimensional profile at a time. A variety of edge-selective criteria have been used to design edge detection algorithms.[52-54] Some of these are discussed in Chapter 23 on quantitative coronary angiography. A common element in many of these methods is the first derivative criterion. In this method, the edge is identified by the maximum change in image intensity between adjacent pixels along a profile. A maximum second derivative criterion has also been used. All edge detection methods depend on an assumed relation between the shape of the edge intensity profile in the image and the true projected border of the object. The principal sources of systematic error in measurements of relative coronary artery diameter are related to the dependence of profile shape on coronary artery cross-sectional shape and to the image system blur function.[55] Random error primarily consists of false edge detections caused by quantum and structured noise. Methods for minimizing these errors by combining information from multiple adjacent profiles[56, 57] are used by most of the commercially available quantitative coronary angiography and ventriculographic analysis systems.

Densitometry

The basis of x-ray densitometry is calculation of the amount of contrast material along each ray through the patient from the x-ray intensity information recorded in the angiogram. In principle, densitometry can be used to measure the thickness of any object containing a known concentration of contrast material or to measure the concentration of contrast material if the thickness is known. Densitometry provides a way to measure vessel cross-sectional area and chamber volumes that is almost independent of imaging system unsharpness or motion blurring.[58, 59] Most applications of densitometry require only relative measurement of contrast material. Some measurements, such as absolute cross-sectional areas of coronary arteries, that would seem to require absolute densitometry can often be made relative to a calibration object. Relative densitometry is much easier because it does not require knowledge of absolute contrast material concentration and because some of the densitometric errors cancel out in the ratio of two measurements. However, several important errors are nonlinear and do not cancel out, even in relative measurements. Furthermore, most error sources are spatially or temporally variant and produce error in ratios of measurements that are separated in time or space, even if the error at each point is linear.

The most important error sources are x-ray scatter and image intensifier veiling glare. Both add a spatially variant bias to the image, reducing contrast, and together they are typically equal to or greater than the primary intensity. Failure to subtract scatter and veiling glare results in gross underestimation of absolute contrast material density and a nonlinear relation between pixel intensity and relative contrast material density.

Densitometric quantitative coronary angiography (QCA) measurements available on most commercially-available QCA systems provide no correction for beam hardening, x-ray scatter, or veiling glare, even though effective methods for measuring and correcting the major errors are available.[60-63]

Time-Density Analysis

Time-density analysis refers to the measurement of the arrival or washout of contrast material by digital angiography. Time-density analysis is subject to the same densitometric errors as those that limit the accuracy of densitometric QCA. Nonlinear densitometry produces errors in most parameters derived from the time-density curves, including mean transit time, washout rate, full-width half maximum, and area under the curve. Scatter and veiling glare are time-dependent owing both to patient-related factors such as respiration and to the reduced scatter and veiling glare that occurs because the injected contrast material attenuates the primary beam. This is an often-overlooked source of error. Failure to correct for attenuation of the primary beam can produce overestimation of rates of appearance and washout of as much as 20 percent.[51]

Additional major sources of error include change in patient thickness caused by respiratory motion and problems related to the suitability of the contrast material as a blood flow tracer,[64, 65] such as its physiologic effect on cardiac function and the circulatory system, high viscosity and density, and incomplete mixing with blood. Despite the many potential sources of error, angiographic time-density analysis has successfully been applied to measurement of coronary artery blood flow[66] and flow reserve,[67-73] left ventricular ejection fraction,[74, 75] mitral and aortic valve regurgitation,[76] and myocardial perfusion.[77-82]

RADIATION PROTECTION

Maximum Permissible Dose and the ALARA Principle

Radiation exposure is a known health hazard, both to patients and to catheterization laboratory personnel. After almost 100 years of experience and research, the types and magnitudes of risk are perhaps better understood than those of any other environmental or medical biohazard. Risk of cancer from radiation exposure levels encountered in cardiac catheterization are too low to be detected by epidemiological studies. However, the risk from low-level exposure has been derived by extrapolation from data in populations exposed to high radiation levels. Table 16–4 gives the estimated lifetime cancer risks per rem based on extrapolation from increased cancer incidence in high-dose groups. The maximum permissible

TABLE 16–4. ESTIMATED LIFETIME CANCER RISKS (CHANCES IN 1 MILLION PER REM)

Type of Cancer	Fatal Cancer		Curable Cancer	
	Male	*Female*	*Male*	*Female*
Lung	20	20	1	1
Leukemia	24	16	1.2	0.8
Thyroid	3.3	6.7	63	127
Breast		50		30
Other	50	50	15	15

Adapted from the Handbook of Selected Tissue Doses for Projections Common in Diagnostic Radiology, DHHS Publication 89–8031, December 1988.

TABLE 16–5. MAXIMUM PERMISSIBLE DOSE (MPD) FOR RADIATION WORKERS

Organ or Tissue	MPD (rem/year)
Whole-body exposure	5
Lens of eye, gonads, red bone marrow	5
Hands	75
Forearms	30
Other organs (including thyroid)	15

dose (MPD) for radiation workers established by the National Council on Radiation Protection and Measurements (NCRP) is based on such estimates and is designed to keep the recognized radiation risks well below statistical significance (Table 16–5). The NCRP Report No. 91, June 1987, recommended that the cumulative lifetime whole-body MPD be reduced to 1 rem per year of life, down from the previous recommendation of 5 rem per year after 18 years of life. Although this recommendation has not yet become law, it should inspire continued dedication to the principle of keeping radiation exposure as low as reasonably achievable ("ALARA") for angiographers, whose careers may span 30 or more years. Although all the risks in Table 16–4 are small per rem relative to the natural incidence of cancer, any avoidable radiation exposure is an avoidable risk. Therefore, it is the legal and ethical responsibility of the angiographer to maintain the ALARA principle. Exposure levels in cardiac catheterization laboratories are significant for both patient and staff, as shown in Table 16–6. The remainder of this section describes how to minimize radiation exposure to both patient and staff.

Intensity, Area, Time, Distance, and Shielding

The keys to ALARA in the cardiac catheterization laboratory are to use minimum x-ray tube output rate consistent with minimum required image quality; to minimize field of view; to minimize the time during which the x-ray tube is energized; to maximize distance between the x-ray tube and the patient and between patient and staff; and to effectively use radiation shields.

Exposure Rate

The calibration of the fluoroscopic and angiographic automatic exposure controls directly affects both patient and staff radiation dose rate.[83] The operation of the automatic exposure system represents a complex balancing of many factors affecting both image quality and dose. Its calibration must be carefully reviewed as part of the comprehensive quality assurance program that is essential for the operation of a cardiac catheterization laboratory. Image intensifier input exposure rates for fluoroscopy and cineangiography must conform to the guidelines established by the ACC/AHA Inter-Society Commission for Heart Disease Resources.[4] Patient skin entrance exposure rate must meet the legal limits for fluoroscopy. Some fluoroscopic systems allow the angiographer to manually select reduced exposure rates. This should be done whenever

TABLE 16–6. TYPICAL EXPOSURE RATES DURING CARDIAC ANGIOGRAPHY IN STRAIGHT ANTERIOR VIEW*

	Patient Skin Entrance Exposure (R/min)	Waist-Level Scatter at 4 Feet From Table Center (mR/hr)
Fluoroscopy	5 R/min	34 mR/hr
Cineangiography	50 R/min	340 mR/hr

*Rates are significantly higher for lateral and angulated views.
Data from Moore, R. J.: Imaging Principles in Cardiac Angiography. Rockville, Md., Aspen Publishers, Inc., 1990, p. 230.

possible, consistent with the actual clinical imaging task. Image quality for a given x-ray exposure is a function of image intensifier DQE. For laboratories doing many interventions, high-DQE image intensifiers should be specified to provide the best contrast-to-noise ratio at the expense of a small loss of spatial resolution. The loss of spatial resolution is not great enough to be detected in fluoroscopic or digital angiography images, although it is measurable with the use of high-contrast test objects on cine film.

Field of View

For a given image intensifier magnification mode, patient dose and staff exposure from scattered radiation are approximately proportional to the collimated field of view. Collimating a 10-inch field to a 7-inch diameter reduces exposure rate by about half. Reducing the field of view by changing the magnification mode increases x-ray tube output and patient exposure, as described in the image intensifier section, but because the exposure rate is approximately inversely related to field of view, the scattered radiation exposure rate is approximately constant. The dose-volume product (dose times volume of tissue irradiated) may actually be smaller in magnification mode if the automatic exposure control system increases x-ray tube output by increasing tube voltage. A good rule of thumb is that the more the collimators are visible on the monitor, the lower the patient and staff exposure. Reduced field of view also generally improves image contrast by reducing the amount of scattered radiation that reaches the image intensifier.

Time

Because radiation exposure is directly proportional to the time the x-ray beam is on, judicious use of the fluoro– and cine–foot pedals is an effective means of reducing patient and staff radiation dose. With practice and conscious effort, it is possible to perform catheterization with a fraction of the fluoroscopic exposure time by using a series of brief exposures at just those moments when there is a "need to see." The exposure rate during cine (or digital) recording is typically 10 times that of fluoroscopy, so limiting the number and length of cine views can significantly reduce overall exposure for diagnostic examinations. However, because total cine times are typically less than 1 minute, the exposure from fluoroscopy actually predominates when fluoroscopic exposure times exceed about 10 minutes, as is common for interventional procedures.[84] In this setting, it is especially efficacious to minimize fluoroscopic exposure rate and field of view. Newer technical fluoroscopic dose reduction methods, described in the following sections, may also be employed.

Distance

X-ray intensities obey an approximate inverse square relation with distance from a point source of radiation. This affects staff dose (distance from the source of scatter—the patient) and patient dose (distance from the x-ray tube). For a fixed image intensifier input exposure, patient skin entrance exposure is inversely proportional to the distance from the x-ray tube focal spot to the patient's skin. The mechanical flexibility of isocentric angiography positioners puts responsibility for maintaining maximal source-to-skin distance in the hands of the angiographer. Distances longer than 50 cm (20 inches) can often be achieved by using a source-to-detector distance of 100 cm and keeping the patient as close to the image intensifier as possible. The worst case is for highly angulated views that force both the x-ray tube and the image intensifier to be close to the patient and require very high x-ray tube output because of the long path length through the patient. Under these conditions, the skin exposure rate can be 10 to 20 times that of a straight anterior view. Image quality is also severely degraded by increased tube voltage and scatter in these views, and they should be avoided if possible, particularly for procedures requiring extended fluoroscopy time.

As a rough rule of thumb, the table-level scatter exposure rate 1 meter (3 feet) from the beam center is about $\frac{1}{1000}$ of the skin entrance exposure rate. For fluoroscopy, this implies that a typical measured scatter for 5 R per minute fluoroscopy would be about 30 mR per hour at waist height 1 meter from the center of the table for a straight anterior view. The angiographer's exposure rate is approximately inversely proportional to the distance from the source of scattered radiation, the intersection of the x-ray beam and the patient. A decrease in distance from the center of the beam from 3 feet to 2 feet doubles the angiographer's exposure rate, all else being equal. The source of scattered radiation is primarily the point at which the x-ray beam enters the patient. The angiographer's exposure is greatest when this area is nearest, as in lateral views with the beam entrance on the angiographer's side of the table, and it is in these situations that stepping back even a small distance has the greatest effect on dose reduction.[85, 86]

One of the most effective means for reducing staff radiation exposure is to ensure that personnel perform their duties no closer to the x-ray beam than necessary during imaging. Some laboratories have found that staff awareness has improved and film badge readings have significantly declined after the floor has been clearly marked with exposure zones measured by the radiation safety officer.

Shielding

The high levels of scatter radiation in the catheterization laboratory[87] require the use of protective shielding, in addition to time and distance, to reduce exposure.[88] Rubberized lead aprons with lead-equivalent thickness[89] of 0.5 mm should be worn by tableside personnel to reduce scatter exposure by a factor of about 50. Lighter aprons with lead-equivalent thickness of 0.25 mm and an exposure reduction factor of about 25 may be worn by in-room staff stationed farther from the x-ray beam, balancing the reduced risk from radiation with the real risk of back problems caused or exacerbated by wearing heavy lead aprons all day. Back strain can be significantly reduced by the use of two-piece lead garments consisting of a skirt and a jacket.

The protection of the lead apron may be extended to the lower neck by using a 0.5 mm lead-equivalent thyroid shield; this is desirable because of the relatively high sensitivity of the thyroid for radiation-induced cancer (see Table 16–4). In addition, radiation exposure to the lens of the eye is known to induce cataracts, with a latent period of up to 20 years. Unlike carcinogens, for which a finite increased risk is associated with any exposure no matter how small, cataract induction appears to have a threshold dose of well over 2.5 Gy (some estimates are as high as 7.5 Gy for protracted exposures), below which risk for cataracts is not increased by x-radiation. Although cardiac angiographers are unlikely to reach a threshold dose for cataract induction over even a long career, protective eyeglasses with leaded lenses are available. To be effective, these glasses must have side shields, because the angiographer usually faces the video monitor rather than the patient during imaging.

A very effective means for reducing angiographer head and neck exposure is a ceiling-suspended leaded glass or acrylic x-ray shield. If possible, this shield should be positioned between the angiographer's head and scattered x-rays from both the beam entrance (tube side) and beam exit (image intensifier side) areas. For views in which the x-ray tube is on the same side as the angiographer, it is particularly important to shield the area where the beam enters the patient. Other shielding devices that angiographers may wish to consider include tableside drapes to reduce scatter radiation to the legs and feet and full-length floor-standing shields. In the spirit of ALARA, such devices should be used if they do not interfere with patient care, particularly in high-volume interventional laboratories.

Technical Dose Reduction Methods

A number of technical means for reducing radiation exposure during fluoroscopy or coronary angiography are under development. Careful collimation and the use of cardiac contour "lung filters" are well established methods of reducing scatter radiation dose. Labbe and associates[90] and Rudin and Bednarek[91] have developed devices to extend these methods by severely reducing the x-ray beam intensity except at the center of the image. A real-time image processor compensates for the attenuation and results in a full-field image with lower exposure to the patient and the operator and improved contrast in the central "foveal" area owing to reduction of scatter and veiling glare.

Studies suggest that a lower fluoroscopic dose rate is produced for equal image quality with 30-Hz x-ray pulses with progressive scanning versus 60-Hz x-ray or continuous x-ray exposure with interlaced scanning.[44, 45, 92] Reducing fluoroscopic dose by reducing the frame rate to 15 or even 7.5 fps has been found by some investigators to be acceptable for catheter manipulation,[93, 94] but the resulting jerkiness of motion would be objectionable to many angiographers. For stationary disks, Aufrichtig and colleagues[95] have found that dose reductions of 22 and 49 percent are achievable for rates of 15 and 7.5 fps, respectively. These results must be interpreted with care, however, because the increased jerkiness of coronary artery motion at reduced frame rates is almost certain to reduce observer performance. For pediatric fluoroscopy, Rossi and co-workers[96] found that simply reducing the dose per frame is a better alternative for dose reduction than reducing the frame rate.

Eigler and colleagues[12] have described a new method that may allow the combination of both these approaches to dose reduction. In this digital cine display method, a lesion of interest is "stabilized" by digitally translating each frame so that the lesion is always centered in the display. Their results suggest that this new display method may improve detection of subtle morphologic features in coronary angiograms and may permit lower dose or frame rate without loss of feature detectability.

SUMMARY

Everyone interested in cardiac imaging must understand the principles of x-ray imaging in order to produce the best possible pictures. Furthermore, x-ray imaging is moving toward digital acquisition and display, so those interested in cardiac imaging should understand the general principles of digital imaging as well. Finally, all x-ray techniques are potentially harmful to the patient and the imaging team, so an in-depth understanding of how to minimize the risk to both is mandatory.

References

1. Curry, T.S., III, Dowdey, J.E., and Murry, R.C., Jr.: Christensen's Physics of Diagnostic Radiology. Philadelphia, Lea & Febiger, 1990, p. 1.
2. Moore, R.J.: Imaging Principles in Cardiac Angiography. Rockville, Md., Aspen Publishers, 1990.
3. Kelsey, C.A.: Essentials of Radiology Physics. St. Louis, Warren H. Green, 1985.
4. Friesinger, G.C., Adams, D.F., et al.: Optimal resources for examination of the heart and lungs: Cardiac catheterization and radiographic facilities. Circulation 68:893A, 1983.
5. Lumbroso, P., and Dick, C.E.: X-ray attenuation properties of radiographic contrast media. Med. Phys. 14:752, 1987.
6. Heggie, J.C.: The usefulness of K-edge filters in automatic brightness controlled fluoroscopy and digital subtraction angiography. Australas. Phys. Eng. Sci. Med. 15:9, 1992.
7. Gagne, R.M., Quinn, P.W., et al.: Comparison of beam-hardening and K-edge filters for imaging barium and iodine during fluoroscopy. Med. Phys. 21:107, 1994.
8. Gray, J.E., Winkler, N.T., et al.: Quality Control in Diagnostic Imaging. Baltimore, University Park Press, 1983.
9. Rose, A. (ed.): Comparative noise properties of vision, television, and photographic film. In Vision: Human and Electronic. New York, Plenum Press, 1973, p. 95.
10. Whiting, J.S., and Eckstein, M.P., et al.: Human performance and response time for signal detection in noisy cine image sequences. Med. Phys. 1995 (in press).
11. Wilson, D.L., Xue, P., et al.: Perception of fluoroscopy last-image hold. Med. Phys. 21:1875, 1994.
12. Eigler, N.L., Eckstein, M.P., et al.: Improving detection of coronary morphologic features from digital angiograms: Effect of stenosis stabilization display. Circulation 89:2700, 1994.
13. Wagner, A.J., Barnes, G.T., et al.: Assessing fluoroscopic contrast resolution: A practical and quantitative test tool. Med. Phys. 18:894, 1991.
14. Motz, J.W., and Danos, M.: Image information content and patient exposure. Med. Phys. 5:8, 1978.
15. Wagner, R.F., and Brown, D.G.: Unified SNR analysis of medical imaging systems. Phys. Med. Biol. 30:489, 1985.
16. Roehrig, H., Nudelman, S., et al.: Electro-optical devices for use in photoelectronic-digital radiology. In Fullerton, G.D. (ed.): Electronic Imaging in Medicine. AAPM Monograph No. 11. New York, AIP Press, 1984.
17. Chakraborty, D.P.: Image intensifier distortion correction. Med. Phys. 14:249, 1987.
18. Rudin, S., Bednarek, D.R., et al.: Accurate characterization of image intensifier distortion. Med. Phys. 18:1145, 1991.
19. Brown, B.G., Bolson, E., et al.: Quantitative coronary arteriography: Estimation of dimensions, hemodynamic resistance, and atheroma mass of coronary artery lesions using the arteriogram and digital computation. Circulation 55:329, 1977.
20. Blanc, S., and Liénard, J.: Geometric distortion in x-ray image intensifiers and its modelling. Thompson-CGR Technical Report, 1986.
21. Tehrani, S., LeFree, M.T., et al.: High-speed digital radiographic pincushion distortion correction using an array processor. I.E.E.E. Trans. 0276–6574:615, 1987.
22. Sagawa, K., and Takeichi, K.: Spectral luminous efficiency functions in the mesopic range. J. Opt. Soc. Am. [A] 3:71, 1986.
23. Suddarth, S.A., and Johnson, G.A., et al.: Performance of high-resolution monitors for digital chest imaging. Med. Phys. 14:253, 1987.
24. Sandrik, J.M.: The video camera for medical imaging. In Fullerton, G.D. (ed.): Electronic Imaging in Medicine. AAPM Monograph 11. New York, AIP Press, 1984.
25. Gray, J.E., Stears, J.G., et al.: Fluoroscopic imaging: Quantitation of image lag or smearing. Radiology 150:563, 1984.
26. Wollschläger, H., Lee, P., et al.: Improvement of quantitative angiography by exact calculation of radiological magnification factors. I.E.E.E. Trans. 276:483, 1985.
27. Pope, D.L., van Bree, R.E., et al.: Cine 3-D reconstruction of moving coronary arteries from DSA images. Comput. Cardiol. 0276–6574:277, 1987.
28. Seiler, C., Kirkeeide, R.L., et al.: Measurement from arteriograms of regional myocardial bed size distal to any point in the coronary vascular tree for assessing anatomic area at risk. J. Am. Coll. Cardiol. 21:783, 1993.
29. Metz, C.E., and Fencil, L.E.: Determination of three-dimensional structure in biplane radiography without prior knowledge of the relationship between the two views: Theory. Med. Phys. 16:45, 1989.
30. Robert, N., Peyrin, F., et al.: Binary vascular reconstruction from a limited number of cone beam projections. Med. Phys. 21:1839, 1994.
31. Rake, S.T.: Three-dimensional reconstruction of arteries from biplane angiograms. Med. Inform. 16:195, 1991.
32. Pratt, W.K.: Digital Image Processing. New York, John Wiley & Sons, 1991.
33. Widrow, B.: A study of rough amplitude quantization by means of Nyquist sampling theory. I.E.E.E. Trans. Circuit Theory CT 3:266, 1956.
34. Wagner, R.F.: Toward a unified view of radiological imaging systems: Part II. Noisy images. Med. Phys. 4:279, 1977.
35. Kruger, R.A., Mistretta, C.A., et al.: Physical and technical considerations of computerized fluoroscopy difference imaging. I.E.E.E. Trans. Nucl. Sci. 28:205, 1981.
36. Shroy, R.E., Jr.: Dependence of noise on array width and depth in digital radiography. Med. Phys. 15:64, 1988.
37. Burgess, A.E.: Effect of quantization noise on visual signal detection in noisy images. J. Opt. Soc. Am. [A] 2:1424, 1985.
38. Nissen, S.E., Pepine, C.J., et al.: Cardiac angiography without cine film: Erecting a "Tower of Babel" in the cardiac catheterization laboratory. J. Am. Coll. Cardiol. 24:834, 1994.
39. Gray, J.E., Wondrow, M.A., et al.: Technical considerations for cardiac laboratory high-definition video systems. Cathet. Cardiovasc. Diagn. 10:73, 1984.
40. Castleman, K.R., Selzer, R.H., et al.: Vessel edge detection in angiograms: An application of the Wiener filter. In Castleman, K.R. (ed.): Digital Signal Processing. Englewood Cliffs, NJ, Prentice-Hall, 1979.
41. Revesz, G.: Conspicuity and uncertainty in the radiographic detection of lesions. Radiology 154:625, 1985.
42. Kruger, R.A., and Riederer, S.J.: Basic Concepts of Digital Subtraction Angiography. Boston, G.K. Hall Medical Publishers, 1984.
43. Barrett, H.H.: Objective assessment of image quality: Effects of quantum noise and object variability. J. Opt. Soc. Am. [A] 7:1266, 1990.
44. Holmes, D.R., Jr., Wondrow, M.A., et al.: Effect of pulsed progressive fluoroscopy on reduction of radiation dose in the cardiac catheterization laboratory. J. Am. Coll. Cardiol. 15:159, 1990.
45. Wondrow, M.A., Bove, A.A., et al.: Technical consideration for a new x-ray video progressive scanning system for cardiac catheterization. Cathet. Cardiovasc. Diagn. 14:126, 1988.
46. Seibert, J.A., Barr, D.H., et al.: Interlaced versus progressive readout of television cameras for digital radiographic acquisitions. Med. Phys. 11:703, 1984.
47. Ishida, M., Doi, K., et al.: Digital image processing: Effect on detectability of simulated low-contrast radiographic patterns. Radiology 150:569, 1984.
48. Loo, L.N., Doi, K., et al.: Investigation of basic imaging properties in digital radiography: 4. Effect of unsharp masking on the detectability of simple patterns. Med. Phys. 12:209, 1985.
49. Whiting, J.S., Eigler, N.L., Pfaff, J.M., et al.: Improved angiographic detection of coronary morphology in spatially filtered images. (Abstract.) Circulation 80:II, 1989.
50. Elion, J.L., Fischer, P.L.C., et al.: Time stretching strategies for optimal temporal alignment of image sequences of unequal duration. I.E.E.E. Trans. 0276–6574:619, 1987.

51. Whiting, J.S., Pfaff, J.M., et al.: Effect of radiographic distortions on the accuracy of quantitative angiography. Am. J. Card. Imaging 2:239, 1988.
52. Fleagle, S.R., Johnson, M.R., et al.: Geometric validation of robust method of automated edge detection in clinical coronary arteriography. Comput. Cardiol. 1986, pp. 197–200.
53. Fujita, H., Doi, K., et al.: Image feature analysis and computer-aided diagnosis in digital radiography: 2. Computerized determination of vessel sizes in digital subtraction angiography. Med. Phys. 14:549, 1987.
54. Reiber, J.H.C., Kooijman, C.J., et al.: Coronary artery dimensions from cineangiograms: Methodology and validation of a computer-assisted analysis procedure. I.E.E.E. Trans. Med. Imaging 3:131, 1984.
55. Weber, D.M.: Absolute diameter measurements of coronary arteries based on the first zero crossing of the Fourier spectrum. Med. Phys. 16:188, 1989.
56. van der Zwet, P.M., and Reiber, J.H.: A new approach for the quantification of complex lesion morphology: The gradient field transform. Basic principles and validation results. J. Am. Coll. Cardiol. 24:216, 1994.
57. Sonka, M., Wilbricht, C.J., et al.: Simultaneous detection of both coronary borders. I.E.E.E. Trans. Med. Imaging 12:588, 1993.
58. Kruger, R.A.: Estimation of the diameter of and iodine concentration within blood vessels using digital vessels using digital radiography devices. Med. Phys. 8:652, 1981.
59. Parker, D.L., Clayton, P.D., et al.: The effects of motion on quantitative vessel measurements. Med. Phys. 12:698, 1985.
60. Shaw, C.G., and Plewes, D.B.: Quantitative digital subtraction angiography: Two scanning techniques for correction of scattered radiation and veiling glare. Radiology 157:247, 1985.
61. Maher, K.P.: Comparison of scatter measurement techniques in digital fluoroscopy. Phys. Med. 9:1977, 1993.
62. Love, L.A., and Kruger, R.A.: Scatter estimation for a digital radiographic system using convolution filtering. Med. Phys. 14:178, 1987.
63. Molloi, S.Y., and Mistretta, C.A.: Scatter-glare corrections in quantitative dual energy fluoroscopy. Med. Phys. 15:289, 1988.
64. Bassingthwaighte, J.B.: Physiology and theory of tracer washout techniques for the estimation of myocardial blood flow: Flow estimation from tracer washout. Prog. Cardiovasc. Dis. 20:165, 1977.
65. Bassingthwaighte, J.B., Strandell, T., et al.: Estimation of coronary blood flow by washout of diffusible indicators. Circ. Res. 23:259, 1968.
66. Hoffmann, K.R., Doi, K., et al.: Determination of instantaneous and average blood flow rates from digital angiograms of vessel phantoms using distance-density curves. Invest. Radiol. 26:207, 1991.
67. Hangiandreou, N.J., Folts, J.D., et al.: Coronary blood flow measurement using an angiographic first pass distribution technique: A feasibility study. Med. Phys. 18:947, 1991.
68. Eigler, N.L., Schühlen, H., et al.: Digital angiographic impulse resonance analysis of regional myocardial perfusion: Estimation of coronary flow, flow reserve and distribution volume by compartmental transit time measurement in a canine model. Circ. Res. 68:870, 1991.
69. Schühlen, H., Eigler, N.L., Pfaff, J.M., et al.: Effect of subcritical stenosis on coronary and myocardial flow reserve in territory supplied by other non-stenotic arteries. (Abstract.) J. Am. Coll. Cardiol. 13:7A, 1989.
70. Vogel, R.A., LeFree, M.T., et al.: Application of digital techniques to selective coronary arteriography: Use of myocardial contrast apperance time to measure coronary flow reserve. Am. Heart J. 107:153, 1984.
71. de Bruyne, B., Dorsaz, P.A., et al.: Assessment of regional coronary flow reserve by digital angiography in patients with coronary artery disease. Int. J. Card. Imaging 3:47, 1988.
72. Cusma, J.T., Toggart, E.J., et al.: Digital subtraction angiographic imaging of coronary flow reserve. Circulation 75:461, 1987.
73. Pijls, N.H.J., Aengevaeren, R.M., et al.: Concept of maximal flow ratio for immediate evaluation of percutaneous transluminal coronary angioplasty result by videodensitometry. Circulation 83:854, 1991.
74. Chappuis, F., Widmann, T., et al.: Quantitative assessment of regional left ventricular function by densitometric analysis of digital-subtraction ventriculograms: Correlation with myocardial systolic shortening in dogs. Circulation 77:457, 1988.
75. Chappuis, F., Widmann, T.F., et al.: Densitometric regional ejection fraction: A new three-dimensional index of regional left ventricular function. Comparison with geometric methods. J. Am. Coll. Cardiol. 11:72, 1988.
76. Grayburn, P.A., Nissen, S.E., et al.: Quantitation of aortic regurgitation by computer analysis of digital subtraction angiography. J. Am. Coll. Cardiol. 10:1122, 1987.
77. Kirkeeide, R.L., Lance, G., et al.: Assessment of coronary stenoses by myocardial perfusion imaging during pharmacologic coronary vasodilation: VII. Validation of coronary flow reserve as a single integrated functional measure of stenosis severity reflecting all its geometric dimensions. J. Am. Coll. Cardiol. 7:103, 1986.
78. Whiting, J.S., Eigler, N.L., et al.: Coronary angiographic determination of myocardial perfusion and flow reserve. Am. J. Card. Imaging 7:294, 1993.
79. Eigler, N.L., Pfaff, J.M., et al.: Digital angiographic impulse response analysis of regional myocardial perfusion: Linearity, reproducibility, accuracy, and comparison with conventional indicator dilution curve parameters in phantom and canine models. Circ. Res. 64:853, 1989.
80. Dubois, E., and Shaker, S.: Noise reduction in image sequences using motion-compensated temporal filtering. I.E.E.E. Trans. Commun. 32:826, 1984.
81. Whiting, J.S., Drury, J.K., et al.: Digital angiographic measurement of radiographic contrast material kinetics for estimation of myocardial perfusion. Circulation 73:789, 1986.
82. Schühlen, H., Eigler, N.L., et al.: Digital angiographic impulse response analysis of regional myocardial perfusion: Detection of autoregulatory changes in nonstenotic coronary arteries induced by collateral flow to adjacent stenotic arteries. Circulation 89:1004, 1994.
83. Boone, J.M., Pfeiffer, D.E., et al.: A survey of fluoroscopic exposure rates: AAPM Task Group No. 11 Report. Med. Phys. 20:789, 1993.
84. Bell, M.R., Berger, P.B., et al.: Balloon angioplasty of chronic total coronary artery occlusions: What does it cost in radiation exposure, time, and materials? Cathet. Cardiovasc. Diagn. 25:10, 1992.
85. Grant, S.C., Bennett, D.H., et al.: Reduction of radiation exposure to the cardiologist during coronary angiography by the use of a remotely controlled mechanical pump for injection of contrast medium. Cathet. Cardiovasc. Diagn. 25:107, 1992.
86. Pitney, M.R., Allan, R.M., et al.: Modifying fluoroscopic views reduces operator radiation exposure during coronary angioplasty. J. Am. Coll. Cardiol. 24:1660, 1994.
87. Boone, J.M., and Levin, D.C.: Radiation exposure to angiographers under different fluoroscopic imaging conditions. Radiology 180:861, 1991.
88. Marshall, N.W., Faulkner, K., et al.: An investigation into the effect of protective devices on the dose to radiosensitive organs in the head and neck. Br. J. Radiol. 65:799, 1992.
89. Murphy, P.H., Wu, Y., et al.: Attenuation properties of lead composite aprons. Radiology 186:269, 1993.
90. Labbe, M.S., Chiu, M., et al.: The x-ray fovea, a device for reducing x-ray dose in fluoroscopy. Med. Phys. 21:471, 1994.
91. Rudin, S., and Bednarek, D.R.: Region of interest fluoroscopy. Med. Phys. 19:1183, 1992.
92. Seibert, J.A.: Improved fluoroscopic and cine-radiographic display with pulsed exposures and progressive TV scanning. Radiology 159:277, 1986.
93. Grollman, J.H., Jr., Klosterman, H., et al.: Dose reduction low pulse-rate fluoroscopy. Radiology 105:293, 1972.
94. Fritz, S.L., Mirvis, S.E., et al.: Phantom evaluation of angiographer performance using low frame rate acquisition fluoroscopy. Med. Phys. 15:600, 1988.
95. Aufrichtig, R., Xue, P., et al.: Perceptual comparison of pulsed and continuous fluoroscopy. Med. Phys. 21:245, 1994.
96. Rossi, R.P., Wesenberg, R.L., et al.: A variable aperture fluoroscopic unit for reduced patient exposure. Radiology 129:799, 1978.

17 The Chest Radiograph in the Adult Patient

Melvin D. Cheitlin, M.D.

TECHNICAL CONSIDERATIONS _____ 126
SYSTEMATIC EXAMINATION OF THE CHEST
   FILM _____ 127
NORMAL CHEST RADIOGRAPH _____ 128
SPECIFIC CHAMBER ENLARGEMENT _____ 128
Left Ventricle _____ 128
Left Atrium _____ 128
Superior Vena Cava _____ 128
Right Atrium _____ 128
Right Ventricle _____ 131

The Aorta _____ 131
Pulmonary Arteries and Veins _____ 134
CONGESTIVE HEART FAILURE _____ 134
THE PERICARDIUM _____ 139
CALCIFICATIONS _____ 141
Intracardiac Calcifications _____ 141
Extracardiac Calcifications _____ 143
PARACARDIAC DENSITIES _____ 143
POSITIONAL ABNORMALITIES _____ 143
SUMMARY _____ 143

The chest roentgenogram was the first imaging technique introduced for the evaluation of a patient with suspected heart disease. It and the later electrocardiogram were the most important and literally the only noninvasive imaging techniques available in cardiology until the middle 20th century.

The chest radiograph provides information as to the overall size of the cardiac silhouette, hints as to which chambers are enlarged, and indicates cardiac functional disability by the presence of pulmonary vascular redistribution, interstitial edema, or frank pulmonary edema. The limitations of the chest radiograph are well known. There are only four densities discriminated by the usual chest roentgenogram: air, tissue or water density, bone, and fat. The silhouette of the heart, a three-dimensional structure, is projected against a two-dimensional plane. Because all the chambers are of the same density, enlargement of individual chambers can be inferred only by the way the enlargement distorts the outline of the cardiac silouhette. Considerable chamber enlargement can occur without such distortion, and enlargement of one chamber can displace another, resulting in a simulated enlargement of the displaced chamber. With the development of echocardiography, Doppler techniques, radionuclide angiography, computed tomography, and magnetic resonance imaging, a detailed, chamber-specific evaluation of cardiovascular structure and function is possible. In the last decade of the 20th century, it is therefore important to ask whether there is still any use for the chest radiograph in the evaluation of the patient with heart disease, now that more specific and more accurate ways of defining intercardiac anatomy and pathology are available. This chapter details what can be learned from the chest radiograph. A few specific answers are immediately available regarding the continuing usefulness of this established technique.

1. The chest radiograph, even with multiple views, is magnitudes less expensive than any of the more sophisticated tests. In an era in which cost containment in the delivery of medical care is an important problem to be solved, this characteristic is extremely important.

2. The chest radiograph can demonstrate important pathology that would be missed by transthoracic echocardiography. This is especially true with pathology of the ascending aorta, the pulmonary vessels, and the paracardiac structures. Pathology such as pericardial calcification, abnormal vascular structures, right-sided aortic arch, pericardial cyst, pulmonary arteriovenous fistula, aortic dilatation or aneurysm, aortic coarctation, coronary calcification, calcification of patent ductus arteriosus, dextroposition of the heart with pulmonary sequestration in patients with the scimitar syndrome, and total or partial anomalous pulmonary venous drainage is readily recognizable. Evidence of pulmonary venous congestion, interstitial edema, or pulmonary edema is easily seen on the plain chest film because of vascular redistribution, Kerley's B lines, peribronchial cuffing, and alveolar fluid.

3. The clinical radiograph can reveal skeletal abnormalities that may help the physician make a diagnosis in a patient with suspected cardiovascular disease. The radiograph yields good visualization of the narrow anteroposterior diameter of the chest that, together with a straight spine, suggests a diagnosis of "pancake heart" in a patient with a loud systolic ejection murmur, or pectus excavatum as an explanation for systolic murmur. Also, bony metastasis can be seen, suggesting the etiology of a pericardial effusion, as can rib notching as a clue to coarctation of the aorta, and so forth.

4. The chest radiograph may provide information on the overall size of the cardiac silhouette, which may be more predictive of prognosis than the detailed information concerning the size of any specific chamber.[1]

5. The findings on chest radiography can help suggest the need for a more specific noninvasive or invasive test in the definitive workup of the patient's problem. Any questions of which chambers are enlarged that are raised by the chest radiograph are answered by two-dimensional echocardiography. The typical radiographic findings of mitral stenosis can provide clues to the severity of the disease process. Calcification of the pericardium is a good clue to the presence of constrictive pericarditis in a patient presenting with the clinical picture of right-sided heart failure.

6. Many cardiovascular diagnoses can be made with only a history, a physical examination, and a chest radiograph, a relatively inexpensive workup that can lead to an appropriate plan for management without the need for more expensive evaluations. This is true of mitral and aortic stenosis, severe aortic regurgitation, mitral regurgitation, and some other common congenital heart defects, such as atrial septal defect, ventricular septal defect, patent ductus arteriosus, and right-sided aortic arch.

TECHNICAL CONSIDERATIONS

The heart in the mediastinum is a three-dimensional structure. Consequently, multiple views are necessary to form an idea of the three-dimensional shape of the heart. The usual views are the posteoanterior (PA) view and the lateral view, usually the left lateral view. Less commonly, the 30-degree right anterior oblique (RAO) and 60-degree left anterior oblique (LAO) views are taken. Because all the cardiac chambers and the blood have the same radiographic density and all are located within a single structure, the only cardiac borders visible are those outlined against the lesser density of air-filled lung. It follows that only the outside contour of the cardiac, aortic, and mediastinal structures can be seen. Any enlargement or dilatation that occurs within the structure is not visible on the plain chest radiograph if it does not distort the outline of the cardiac silhouette. Also, intracardiac abnormalities, including septal defects, papillary muscle defects, valvular defects, and intracardiac masses such as tumor or thrombi, all have the same density as the cardiohemic structure and therefore are indistinguishable unless they are calcified. Metallic foreign bodies are also visible on chest radiography.

The x-rays are generated from the x-ray cathode, with a source of some discrete small size, and diverge from this source. The closer the object of interest is to the cathode, the more likely the x-rays are to diverge after passage through the object and to magnify the apparent size of the object of interest before striking the film. Therefore, the object of interest on the x-ray film is placed a distance from the source, by convention 6 feet, at which the x-rays passing through the body are parallel and therefore cause no magnification.

In addition, the heart is in an eccentric position in the chest, more anterior than posterior in the mediastinum. A PA projection, in which the anterior chest is pressed against the film, magnifies the heart less than does an AP position, in which the back is against the film and the heart is close to the cathode source.

The heart is a regular structure with an irregular outline, so the AP leaning of the chest against the film can foreshorten the heart and change its shape. A lordotic film, in which the beam enters the back at a more superior position than that at which it leaves the anterior chest, makes the root of the heart appear narrower and the cardiac silhouette more spherical.

A similar problem occurs with angulation of the chest away from the direct AP position. As the chest turns to the right (the LAO position), different surfaces of the heart are silhouetted, compared with the PA view. If the chest is turned to the left (RAO position), still other chambers from the cardiac silhouette on the film. Therefore, different positions are useful in evaluating the different chambers.

Finally, the degree of x-ray penetration depends on the technique used to obtain the chest radiograph. Films that are overpenetrated tend to burn out the subtle differences in contrast density between structures that would be seen on a properly exposed film. If penetration is insufficient, structures that have subtle differences in x-ray absorption are again difficult to differentiate. Therefore, proper positioning as well as proper x-ray technique is necessary for obtaining most accurate information from the chest radiograph.

A chest radiograph taken with proper technique should allow the intervertebral spaces and the descending aorta to be just distinguishable behind the cardiac silhouette. If the spine and intervertebral spaces are clearly seen behind the entire cardiac silhouette, then the film is overpenetrated and the film looks "burned out." The AP position is proper when the clavicles are below the inferior border of the first rib and an inspiration is of sufficient degree to put the diaphragm in the right chest at the level of the ninth rib. The proper PA position occurs when the two proximal ends of the clavicle are equidistant from the middle, defined by the dorsal spinous process of the vertebral bodies. Furthermore, about one third of the heart should be to the right of the midline, and two thirds to the left. If the heart is too central, either there is some degree of dextropositioning of the heart or the patient is turned to the right (i.e., in some degree of left anterior obliquity). Also, left-sided tension pneumothorax or hyperinflation can push the heart to the right. If the heart is more to the left, with less than a third of the cardiac silhouette to the right of the midline, either the

heart is moved into the left chest—which can be seen with absence of the left hemipericardium, left-sided atelectasis, right-sided tension pneumothorax, or hyperinflation—or the patient is turned to the left and is therefore in some degree of right anterior obliquity.

SYSTEMATIC EXAMINATION OF THE CHEST FILM

To avoid overlooking important information, a systematic routine for examination of the chest radiograph should be followed. The following order of examination is suggested.

First, evaluate the degree of penetration, the position of the patient, whether the film is a true PA film or off-center, and whether there is a degree of right or left obliquity. Look at the right and left film markers so as not to miss dextrocardia.

Second, examine the bony skeleton for abnormal radiolucencies. Assess the ribs and clavicles for fractures. Look for extra or missing ribs and for rib notching. Examine the lateral film for the lack of the normal lordosis of the spine (straight back), for the depth of the posteroanterior diameter of the chest, for kyphoscoliosis, and for pectus excavatum and carinatum.

Third, examine the depth of inspiration and the height of the diaphragm. Normally, the diaphragm on which the mass of the heart lies is lower, and usually this is the left hemidiaphragm. With proper inspiration, the right hemidiaphragm should be at the level of the ninth rib posteriorly. A poor inspiration changes the penetration of the lungs, and an expiratory film can simulate pulmonary edema.

Fourth, examine the image of the trachea, noting whether it is midline, the side on which the aortic knob is located, and the angle of branching of the right and left bronchi.

Fifth, examine both lungs for abnormalities, including densities such as masses or cavities. Examine the minor fissure in PA chest film and the major fissures in the lateral film for position and prominence. With pleural effusion, these fissures become more prominent, and, at times, a loculated pleural effusion can look like a pulmonary mass. Examine the pulmonary vascular film markings. Normally, they are largest at the hilum and rapidly decrease in diameter as they divide peripherally. The upper limit of normal in width of the right descending lower pulmonary artery lateral to the cardiac silhouette is 15 mm in men and 14 mm in women.[2] The ratio of the width of the central pulmonary arteries to the segmental arteries at the base of the lung varies from 3:1 to 5:1. With pulmonary hypertension or increased pulmonary blood flow, these pulmonary hilar vessels increase in size. In the upright position, the pulmonary vessels, including arteries and veins equidistant from the hilum, are larger in the lower lobe of the lung than in the upper lobe. With increased pulmonary venous pressure, the blood is directed away from the lower lobe to the upper lobes of the lung, reversing the usual pattern (so-called vascular redistribution). Pulmonary vascular congestion leads to increased fluid in the pulmonary interstitium, which can be seen in the interlobular fissures as Kerley's B lines, as cuffing around small airways or vessels, as thickening of the paratracheal stripe, or as alveolar edema and pulmonary edema. Examine the costophrenic angles for signs of fluid or pleural effusion. Also note densities that obliterate the normal border of the heart, suggesting consolidation of the lung next to the heart, such as occurs with collapse of the right middle lobe. Look for retrocardiac densities caused by pulmonary consolidation and pneumonitis. Look for calcification in pulmonary parenchyma, pericardium, and pleura. If abnormal pulmonary densities are seen, note the sharpness of borders, whether there are calcifications or fluid or air levels in the densities, and whether there are vessels stranding toward the cardiac silhouette.

Sixth, examine the vascular shadows. Trace the ascending aorta, the transverse arch, the aortic knob, and the descending aorta. Determine the existence of any calcification as well as which bronchus the aortic knob passes over and whether the right pulmonary artery is above or below the right bronchus. Observe the sharpness of the aortic knob, the position and shape of the descending aorta, and any aneurysms or dilatations. Look at the superior mediastinum for abnormal widening or masses, which could be thymus, substernal thyroid, or tumor.

Seventh, examine the cardiac silhouette. Note any paracardiac masses and their position. Trace the cardiac silhouette from the right cardiodiaphragmatic junction, superior and around to the left cardiodiaphragmatic junction. Evaluate the prominence of the right atrium and its junction with the inferior and superior venae cavae, the prominence of the right atrium, the ascending aorta and knob, the main pulmonary artery segment, the area just below where the left atrial appendage can be seen if it is enlarged, and the sweep of the left ventricle to the diaphragm. In the lateral film, again look at each surface of the heart, anteriorly at the right ventricle and the ascending aorta, and posteriorly at the aortic window with the left atrium above and the left ventricle below. Look specifically for calcification within the cardiac silhouette. Frequently, especially in the lateral and oblique films, calcification can be seen in the aortic valve or the mitral valve. Also with careful inspection, especially along the left cardiac border in the PA film, parallel lines of calcification can be seen in the left anterior descending coronary artery. Occasionally in the lateral film, the entire right coronary artery and left coronary artery can be seen to be calcified. Calcification of a left ventricular aneurysm and, occasionally, intracardiac masses, tumor, or thrombi can be seen.

Eighth, look at the neck and the subdiaphragmatic areas, which are not well seen on chest radiographs. Identify the stomach bubble properly on the left. At times, calcification of the carotid arteries, calcification of the spleen, a calcified abdominal aortic aneurysm, or a calcified splenic artery aneurysm can be seen, as can gallstones and air under the hemidiaphragm.

NORMAL CHEST RADIOGRAPH

With a proper inspiration, the right hemidiaphragm should be seen to descend down to the ninth rib posteriorly. Normally, the left hemidiaphragm is lower than the right because of the presence of the heart. The pulmonary vessels in the lower lung should be more prominent than the upper vessels. There should be no cuffing around the airways, no Kerley's B lines, and no pleural effusion.

The overall size of the cardiac silhouette can be described in several ways. The classic cardiothoracic ratio is still a good way of assessing the overall cardiac size.[3] This is done by dividing the largest transverse diameter of the heart by the largest transthoracic diameter.[3] Normally, the cardiothoracic ratio is 0.5 or less. In normal infants, it can be as large as 0.6. The ratio can be abnormally large in a normal person who does not make a good inspiratory effort.

Another technique, much less used, is to calculate a rough cardiac volume by multiplying three diameters of the heart that represent the three dimensions. If A is equal to the distance from the right cardiodiaphragmatic junction to the place on the left heart border at which the main pulmonary artery segment and left atrial appendage meet in the PA film, B is equal to the distance from the right atrial superior vena caval junction to the apex of the left ventricle in the PA film, and C is equal to the largest AP diameter of the cardiac silhouette in the lateral film, then

$$\text{Relative cardiac volume} = \frac{A \times B \times C \times K}{\text{body surface area}}$$

where K is equal to a constant related to the 6-foot difference between film and x-ray tube (K = 0.42). A volume of less than 450 mL/m^2 for women or 500 mL/m^2 for men is considered normal, with a volume greater than 490 mL/m^2 for women or 540 mL/m^2 for men being definitely abnormal.[4]

The cardiac silhouette itself is shown in Figure 17–1. The outlines in the PA and left lateral views are shown, with the chambers that form the borders indicated.

SPECIFIC CHAMBER ENLARGEMENT

Left Ventricle

Concentric left ventricular hypertrophy affects the overall size of the left ventricle little enough so as not to be obvious in the chest radiograph. With dilatation of the left ventricle, eccentric hypertrophy occurs and there is enlargement of the cardiac silhouette (Fig. 17–2). The left ventricle usually enlarges to the left and posteriorly. The apex of the heart is displaced inferiorly and to the left, increasing the cardiothoracic ratio (see Fig. 17–2A). In the left lateral film, the left ventricle bulges posteriorly, so with a good inspiration the left ventricle crosses the shadow of the inferior vena cava less than 2 cm above the hemidiaphragm or even below the diaphragm (see Fig. 17–2B). In the 60-degree LAO view with a deep inspiration, normally the left ventricle should clear the spine; with left ventricular enlargement, it fails to do so. The best examples of left ventricular dilatation are seen with severe chronic mitral or aortic regurgitation or congestive cardiomyopathy.

Left Atrium

The left atrium is a posterior structure in the cardiac silhouette. With enlargement, in the PA film, the left atrial appendage (the left auricle) enlarges to the left and appears as a bulge just under the shadow of the main pulmonary artery (Fig. 17–3). Normally, this area is flat and indistinguishable from the superior part of the left ventricle. The body of the left atrium enlarges posteriorly and to the right (Fig. 17–4B; see Fig. 17–3B). It displaces the esophagus posteriorly and to the right. This displacement is easily seen with a barium swallow to opacify the esophagus. As the left atrium enlarges, it displaces the left mainstem bronchus posteriorly (see Figs. 17–3B and 17–4B) and superiorly, increasing the angle between the right and the left main bronchi (see Fig. 17–4A). In the PA film with a large atrium, the left mainstem bronchus becomes horizontal (see Fig. 17–4A).

As the body of the left atrium enlarges to the right, it often appears as a double density behind the right atrial shadow in the PA film (see Figs. 17–3A and 17–4A) and finally bulges to the right beyond the cardiac shadow.

In some patients with mitral regurgitation, the left atrium can become gigantic, expanding all the way to the right chest wall. As it massively enlarges, it can collapse the lung, causing atelectasis. Left atrial enlargement occurs with left ventricular failure, mitral stenosis, and mitral regurgitation (see Fig. 17–4). The left atrium also enlarges whenever the left atrial pressure increases and therefore can be seen when there is diastolic dysfunction of the left ventricle without systolic dysfunction, as in hypertrophic cardiomyopathy.

Superior Vena Cava

Normally, the superior vena cava may form the right superior contour of the mediastinal shadow. When the superior vena cava is enlarged in right-sided heart failure, the azygous vein enlarges as it joins the superior vena cava. Anomalously draining pulmonary veins at times can be seen in the lung as they enter into the cardiac silhouette. The persistent left superior vena cava can be seen in the left upper mediastinum, forming an arc medial and superior to the left lung.

Right Atrium

The right atrial border appears on the right border of the heart in the PA view and at the upper left border of the heart in the

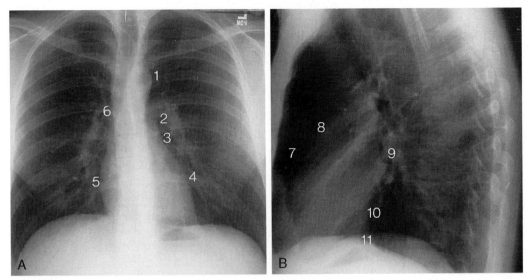

FIGURE 17-1. Normal cardiac silhouette. *A,* Posteroanterior (PA) view. 1 = Aortic knob. 2 = Main pulmonary artery segment. 3 = Segment of left atrial appendage. 4 = Left ventricle. 5 = Right atrial border. 6 = Ascending aorta. *B,* Left lateral view. 7 = Right ventricle. 8 = Right ventricular outflow tract. 9 = Left atrium. 10 = Left ventricle. 11 = Inferior vena cava.

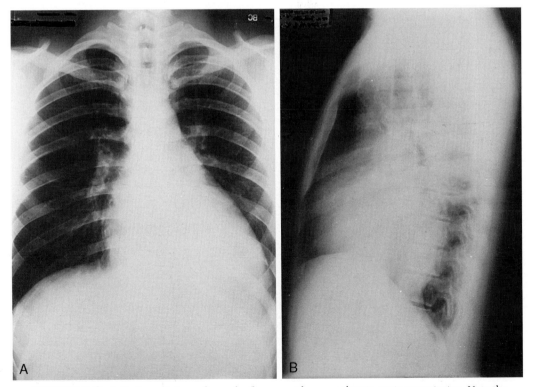

FIGURE 17-2. *A,* Posteroanterior radiograph of a man with severe chronic aortic regurgitation. Note the enlarged left ventricle with the apex displaced to the left and inferiorly. *B,* Left lateral chest radiograph in same patient as in *A.* Note the large left ventricle, which extends markedly posterior, far behind the vena cava shadow.

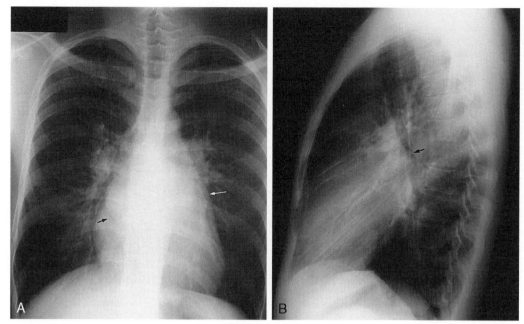

FIGURE 17–3. *A,* Posteroanterior chest radiograph of a 40-year-old man with severe mitral stenosis. Note the double density of the enlarged left atrium behind the right atrium *(black arrow),* the increased upper lobe vascularity, and the bulge along the left cardiac border caused by left appendage enlargement *(white arrow).* *B,* Left lateral chest radiograph. Note the left atrial enlargement displacing the left mainstem bronchus posteriorly *(arrow).*

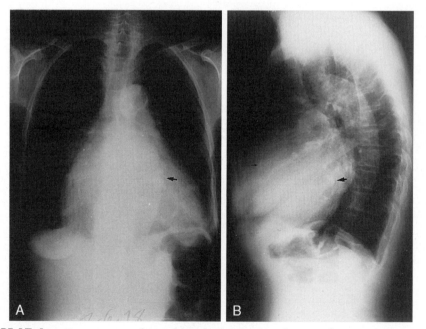

FIGURE 17–4. *A,* Posteroanterior chest radiograph of a woman with severe chronic mitral regurgitation with right heart failure. Note the markedly enlarged cardiac silhouette with increased cardiothoracic ratio. There is right atrial enlargement, a double density behind the right atrium and elevated left mainstem bronchus caused by left atrial enlargement, and an uncoiled descending aorta. The calcification in the mitral annulus is seen as a reversed C-shaped calcification *(arrow).* *B,* Left lateral chest radiograph of the same patient as in *A.* Note the enlarged left ventricle and the left atrium posteriorly, the posteriorly displaced left bronchus, and the calcification in the mitral annulus *(large arrow).* Anteriorly over the right ventricle there is a curvilinear line calcification, probably in the right coronary artery *(small arrow).*

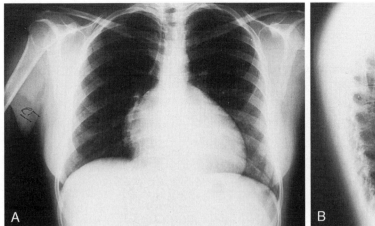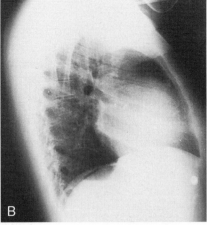

FIGURE 17–5. *A,* Posteroanterior chest radiograph of a patient with the Ebstein anomaly. Note the long sweep of the right atrium, the globular-shaped heart, the small pulmonary arteries, and the clear lung fields. In this congenital disease, there is a displacement of the septal and posterior leaflet into the right ventricle, so part of the anatomical right ventricle is above the tricuspid valve, forming an "atrialized" portion of the right ventricle. There is often a right-to-left shunt through a blown-open foramen ovale or atrial septal defect and, therefore, arterial desaturation and a decrease in pulmonary blood flow. *B,* Right lateral chest radiograph of same patient as in *A.* Note the retrosternal filling caused by the displacement of the outflow tract of the right ventricle by the "right atrium," which is enlarged by the atrialized portion of the right ventricle.

LAO view. If the right atrium enlarges, the arc from the diaphragm to the junction of the superior vena cava increases in size, and the right atrium enlarges to the right (Fig. 17–5; see Fig. 17–4A). This is best seen in the PA film (Fig. 17–6). Such patients may also have right ventricular failure (see Fig. 17–4A). Patients with severe tricuspid regurgitation develop large right atria, especially those with right ventricular dilatation without left atrial enlargement (see Fig. 17–6). In Ebstein disease, in which the posterior and septal leaflets of the right tricuspid valve are displaced into the right ventricle, the right atrial chamber enlarges (see Fig. 17–5A). With tricuspid stenosis, there is isolated dilatation of the right atrium.

Right Ventricle

The right ventricle is an anterior structure. With dilatation, this chamber enlarges anteriorly and to the left, pushing the left ventricle leftward and posteriorly. In the PA film, right ventricular enlargement may look indistinguishable from left ventricular enlargement (Figs. 17–7 and 17–8). With right ventricular hypertrophy without chamber enlargement, there is rounding out of the left border of the heart, raising the apex of the heart off the diaphragm (Fig. 17–9). In the left lateral position, the right ventricle encroaches on the retrosternal space, filling more than the lower third of that space (Fig. 17–10). The best examples of right ventricular hypertrophy are seen with pulmonary valve stenosis, primary or secondary pulmonary hypertension (Fig. 17–11; see Fig. 17–8), tetralogy of Fallot (see Fig. 17–9), mitral stenosis, and cor pulmonale (Fig. 17–12). Right ventricular dilatation is seen with right ventricular failure and atrial septal defects.

The Aorta

The aorta arises at the aortic annulus, which is within the cardiac silhouette on chest radiographs. Therefore, the root of the aorta is within the cardiac silhouette and can enlarge without distorting the cardiac silhouette. The ascending aorta passes to the right, somewhat anteriorly and superiorly, and usually forms the right border of the upper mediastinum (see Fig. 17–1A). As it passes superiorly, the aortic arch bends posteriorly and to the left over the left mainstem bronchus, gives off the great vessels, and forms the aortic knob seen in the PA film. The aorta then goes inferiorly to the left of the spine and passes through the diaphragm at the diaphragmatic hiatus.

With age and developing atherosclerosis, the aorta stiffens, dilates, and elongates. Because it is attached at the aortic ring and at the diaphragmatic hiatus, the aorta uncoils (see Fig. 17–12). The ascending aorta bulges to the right as a prominent curved shadow of the mediastinum, and the descending aorta bends more prominently to the left. With elongation of the aorta, the great vessels are pushed superiorly.

FIGURE 17–6. Posteroanterior chest radiograph of a woman with severe tricuspid regurgitation. Note the enlarged right atrium, enlarging to the right. The pulmonary vessels are normal.

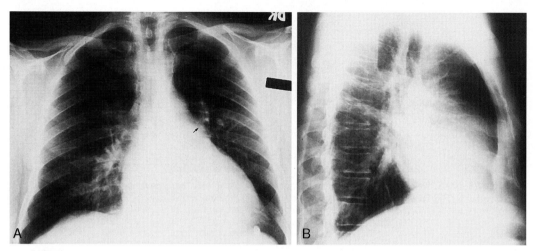

FIGURE 17–7. *A*, Posteroanterior chest radiograph of a patient with a secundum atrial septal defect. The cardiac silhouette is enlarged owing to a dilated right ventricle, although this could look like left ventricular enlargement. The main pulmonary artery segment *(arrow)* is not as large as is usually seen, but the right hilar vessels are prominent. *B*, Right lateral chest radiograph of same patient as in *A*.

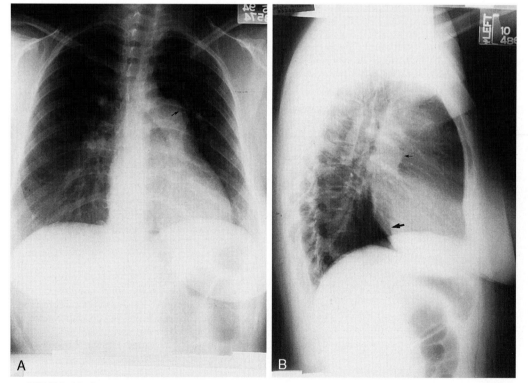

FIGURE 17–8. *A*, Posteroanterior chest radiograph of a woman with primary pulmonary hypertension. Note the very large main pulmonary artery *(arrow)* and the large primary branches of the right and left pulmonary arteries. The cardiac silhouette is at the upper center of normal in this projection. *B*, Right lateral chest radiograph in the same patient as in *A*. The circular shadow of the large right pulmonary artery is seen in the middle mediastinum behind the ascending aorta *(small arrow)*. The enlarged right ventricle has displaced the left ventricle posteriorly so that it crosses the inferior vena cava below the diaphragm *(large arrow)*. This could be mistaken for left ventricular enlargement.

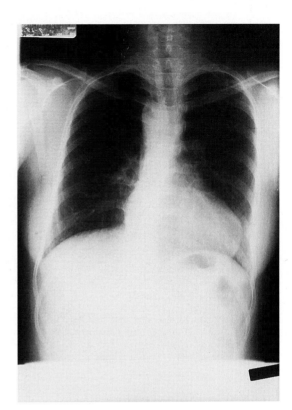

FIGURE 17–9. Posteroanterior chest radiograph of patient with tetralogy of Fallot. Note the right-sided aortic arch with the right-sided descending aorta. The apex of the heart is lifted off the left hemidiaphragm because of right ventricular hypertrophy. The pulmonary arterial vessels are normal to small, as is the area of the main pulmonary artery along the left cardiac silhouette.

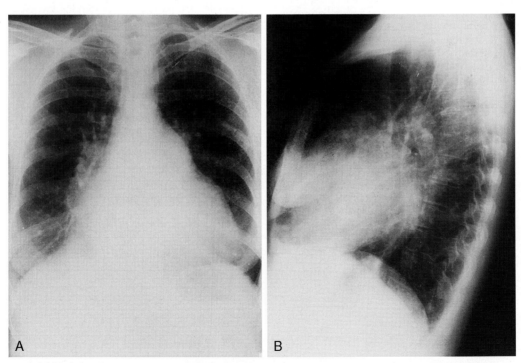

A

B

FIGURE 17–10. *A*, Posteroanterior chest radiograph in a woman with severe mitral stenosis and pulmonary hypertension. Note the enlarged main pulmonary artery segment. Below the main pulmonary artery there is a second bulge resulting from an enlarged left atrial appendage. The prominent upper lobe vascularity and the enlarged cardiac silhouette are caused by pulmonary venous hypertension and right ventricular dilatation. *B*, Left lateral chest radiograph in the same patient as in *A*. There is prominence of the right ventricle, which fills half the retrosternal space. The left atrium is enlarged posteriorly.

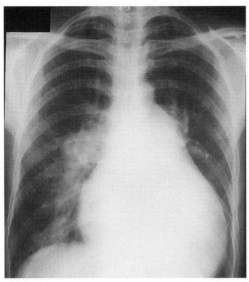

FIGURE 17–11. Posteroanterior chest radiograph in a patient with atrial septal defect and pulmonary vascular disease with pulmonary hypertension. Note the enlarged cardiac silhouette resulting from the enlarged right ventricle and right atrium and the giant right main pulmonary artery and right pulmonary artery with marked tapering. The aortic knob is small, and the lateral lung fields are relatively clear ("pruning").

Aortic aneurysms can be seen as bulges along this aortic silhouette, and they occur most frequently in the low ascending aorta and in the high descending aorta (Figs. 17–13 and 17–14). Intimal calcification is common with advancing age (see Fig. 17–13). It becomes visible in the arch as it passes posteriorly, causing the calcification of the aortic knob in the PA film (see Fig. 17–4). With aortitis, ascending aorta calcification is seen, and with atherosclerosis, increasing descending aortic calcification is seen. With aortic dissection, although the aorta can appear normal, there is usually widening of the mediastinum, bulging of the aorta, and a loss of definition of the aortic knob or descending aorta as bleeding occurs into the adventitia and periaortic areas (Figs. 17–15 and 17–16). Widening occurs with bleeding into the mediastinum, and frequently a cap appears over the left lung and the aortic knob becomes obscured. There may be left pleural effusion and, occasionally, right pleural effusion.

Pulmonary Arteries and Veins

The main pulmonary artery is seen just under the aortic knob (see Fig. 17–1). Its diameter is normally about the same as that of the aortic knob. The right pulmonary artery passes at right angles to the main pulmonary artery, behind the ascending aorta and superior to the left atrium, and divides at the right hilum into an upper and lower pulmonary artery. As the pulmonary artery passes into the lung from the hilum, it narrows in diameter and repeatedly bifurcates, with the distal vessels becoming progressively smaller. In men, the right lower pulmonary artery at the level of the cardiac silhouette is 15 mm or less in diameter, and in women it is 14 mm or less.[2]

As the pulmonary artery enlarges owing to pulmonary hypertension or increased pulmonary blood flow, the diameter of the main pulmonary artery becomes larger than that of the aortic knob (Fig. 17–17; see Fig. 17–11). The main pulmonary artery bulges beyond the left border of the heart. The primary branches can enlarge and become aneurysmal with pulmonary hypertension (Fig. 17–18). Calcification of the primary branches of the pulmonary artery occurs with long-standing pulmonary hypertension (see Fig. 17–18). With severe increases in pulmonary vascular resistance, the lateral third of the lung has fewer small branches of the pulmonary artery and becomes clear, so-called "pruning" (see Figs. 17–11 and 17–18). With decreased pulmonary blood flow, the pulmonary vessels become small (Fig. 17–9). With pulmonary embolism, segments of the lung supplied by the obstructed pulmonary artery appear devoid of pulmonary vascular markings (see Fig. 17–19). In the PA film, the right pulmonary artery is normally superior to the right mainstem bronchus, and the left is inferior to the left mainstem bronchus.

The pulmonary veins pass from the lung into the posterior aspect of the left atrium at the right and left upper and lower borders of the left atrium. They normally increase in size as they approach the cardiac silhouette, and they are more horizontal near the hilum than are the pulmonary arteries. In congestive heart failure or when left atrial pressure is elevated for any reason, increased pulmonary vascular resistance in the lower lung causes diversion of blood to the upper lobes, resulting in prominence of the upper lobe vasculature, including the pulmonary veins (see Figs. 17–3A and 17–10A).

CONGESTIVE HEART FAILURE

With systolic left ventricular dysfunction, compensation occurs as the result of an increase in the left ventricular volume and the

Text continued on page 139

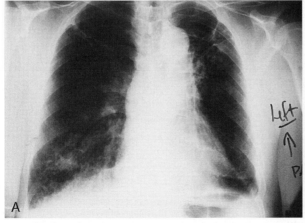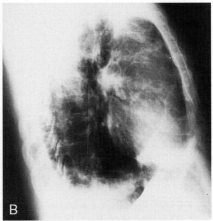

FIGURE 17–12. *A*, Posteroanterior chest radiograph of a patient with chronic obstructive pulmonary disease and aortic regurgitation. Note the increased interstitial lung markings and fibrosis, especially in right lower lung and left upper lobe, with interstitial infiltrate obscuring the right hemidiaphragm. The diaphragms are depressed. In the right lung, there are radiolucencies consistent with air blebs. The ascending aorta is prominent, and the descending aorta is uncoiled. *B*, Right lateral chest radiograph of the same patient as in *A*. The increased pulmonary interstitial markings are more noticeable here. The left ventricle is dilated posteriorly but still crosses the inferior vena cava 2 cm above the left hemidiaphragm because it is so depressed by the chronic lung disease. The right ventricle fills the retrosternal space.

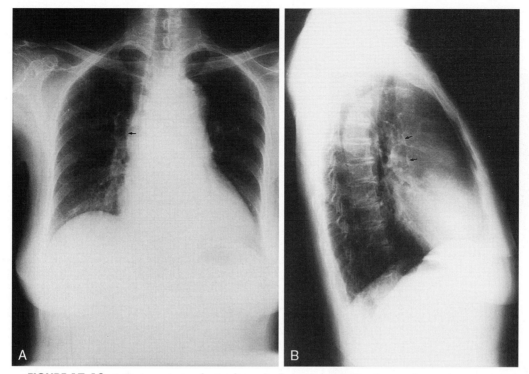

FIGURE 17–13. *A*, Posteroanterior chest radiograph of a patient with chronic ascending aortic aneurysm. Note the prominence of the right upper mediastinum where the aorta bulges to the right *(arrow)*. The aortic knob is enlarged, and calcification is seen in the knob. *B*, Right lateral chest radiograph of the same patient as in *A*. Note the calcification of the posterior ascending aorta extending into the arch *(arrows)*. The calcification permits the measurement of the ascending aorta, which is enlarged and therefore aneurysmal. Calcifications in the arch and descending aorta make the entire aorta visible.

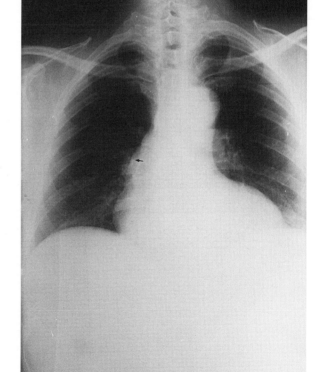

FIGURE 17–14. Posteroanterior chest radiograph. The patient has enlargement of the base of the ascending aorta as a result of a chronic ascending aortic aneurysm *(arrow)*.

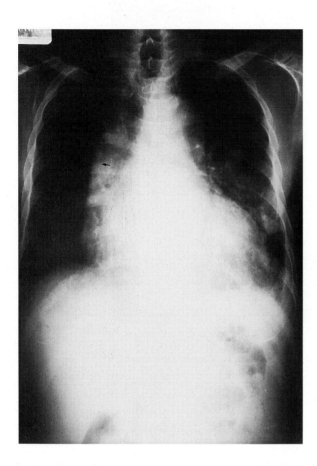

FIGURE 17–15. Posteroanterior chest radiograph of a patient with type I aortic dissection. The film is overpenetrated. Note the density along the upper right mediastinum as the dissected ascending aorta dilates *(arrow)* and the bowed, uncoiled descending aorta. The aortic knob is indistinct. There is cardiac enlargement owing to the presence of long-standing hypertension.

FIGURE 17–16. Posteroanterior chest radiograph of a patient with type I aortic dissection. There is prominence of the aortic knob with an uncoiled descending aorta. The ascending aorta shadow is enlarged to the right *(arrow)*. There is left ventricular enlargement owing to hypertensive cardiovascular disease.

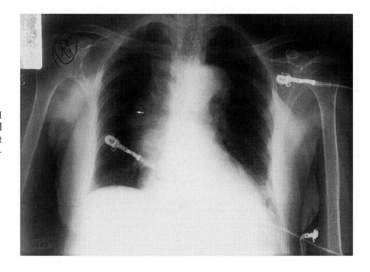

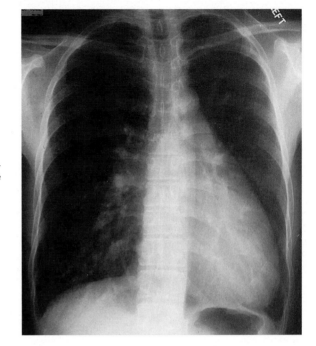

FIGURE 17-17. Posteroanterior chest radiograph of a 20-year-old man with a secundum atrial septal defect. Note the enlarged cardiac silhouette caused by right ventricle dilatation and the increased pulmonary vascularity.

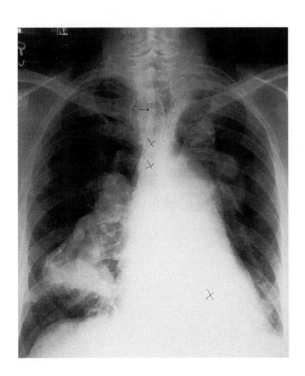

FIGURE 17-18. Posteroanterior radiograph of a 62-year-old man with pulmonary hypertension secondary to an atrial septal defect with severe pulmonary vascular disease. Note the dilated right ventricle and the massively dilated main pulmonary artery and primary and secondary pulmonary artery branches. There is calcification in the right pulmonary artery. The lateral lung fields are remarkably devoid of pulmonary vascular markings ("pruning").

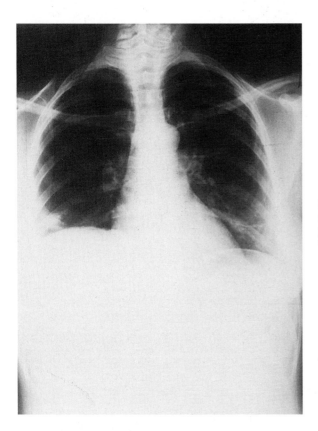

FIGURE 17–19. Posteroanterior chest radiograph of a woman with right-sided pulmonary embolism. There is a density in the right lung at the costophrenic angle. The right pulmonary artery is dilated without normal tapering of the pulmonary artery and with decreased vascularity of the right lung.

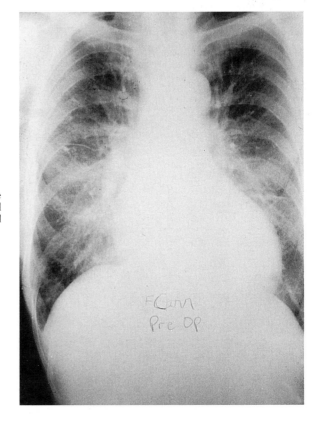

FIGURE 17–20. Posteroanterior chest radiograph of a 75-year-old man with severe aortic stenosis, a dilated left ventricle, and congestive heart failure. Note the increased pulmonary vascular markings, the prominent upper lobe vascularity, and the interstitial edema.

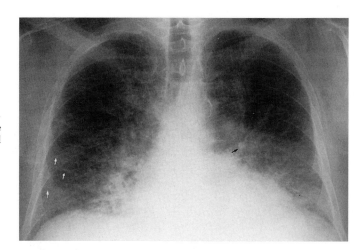

FIGURE 17–21. Posteroanterior view of a patient with dilated cardiomyopathy and severe left-sided heart failure and pulmonary edema. Note the Kerley's B lines *(white arrows)* in the costophrenic angles, the cuffing of fluid around the small airways *(black arrow)*, and the alveolar pulmonary edema.

development of eccentric hypertrophy. Therefore, with congestive heart failure, left ventricular dilatation is commonly seen in the chest radiograph. With an increase in left ventricular filling pressure, the left atrium also enlarges. The increase in pulmonary venous pressure enlarges the pulmonary veins. With pulmonary congestion, there is redistribution of blood flow to the upper lobes, causing prominence of upper lobe arteries and veins compared with those in the lower lobe (Fig. 17–20). Interstitial fluid is seen as densities around vessels and small airways (cuffing) and as Kerley's B lines, caused by interstitial fluid in interlobular fissures (Fig. 17–21). These fissures are seen as straight, horizontal, linear markings, 1 to 2 cm in length, usually in the costophrenic angles on the PA film (Fig. 17–22; see Fig. 17–21). Finally, alveolar edema and pulmonary edema are seen (see Figs. 17–21 and 17–22).

With left-sided heart failure and elevation of left atrial pressure, there is elevation of pulmonary artery pressure and right ventricular failure. The right ventricle and right atrium dilate. With an elevation in systemic venous pressure, the azygous vein may dilate and is then seen as a rounded density along the right mediastinal border. Pleural effusions usually do not occur without the develop-

ment of both right-sided and left-sided heart failure. In congestive heart failure, the pleural effusion may be right-sided or bilateral. Isolated left-sided pleural effusion is rare in congestive heart failure and should raise the question of some other cause, such as pulmonary embolism, pneumonia, malignancy, or left-sided subdiaphragmatic disease.

THE PERICARDIUM

Usually, the pericardium is indistinguishable from the cardiac silhouette on the chest radiograph. With disease, the pericardium can become calcified and therefore visible, especially in the LAO and left lateral views, both anteriorly and posteriorly (Fig. 17–23). In the PA film, frequently calcium can be seen only in the left atrioventicular sulcus.

With pericardial effusion, the cardiac silhouette enlarges, the various indentations between the aortic knob and the pulmonary artery and between the pulmonary artery and the left ventricle

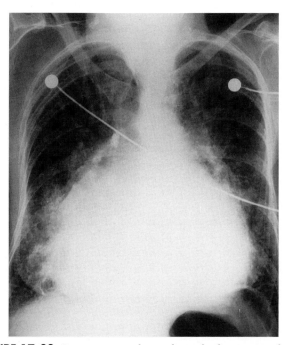

FIGURE 17–22. Posteroanterior chest radiograph of a patient with aortic stenosis and regurgitation, mitral stenosis, and severe mitral regurgitation. Note the very large left atrium, valvular redistribution, Kerley's B lines, and pulmonary edema.

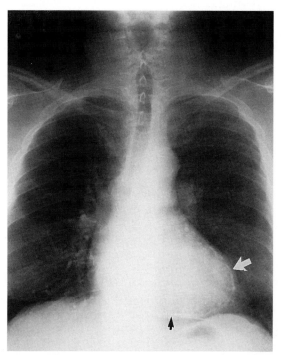

FIGURE 17–23. Posteroanterior view of a patient with constrictive pericarditis. Note the calcification seen in the pericardium *(white arrow)*. The calcification also includes the diaphragmatic pericardium *(black arrow)*.

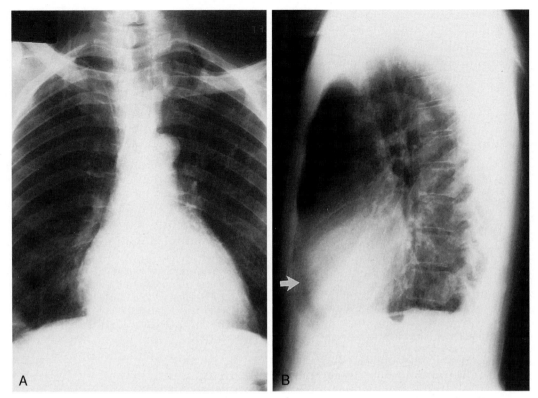

FIGURE 17–24. *A,* Posteroanterior view of a patient with idiopathic pericarditis and pericardial effusion. Note the enlargement of the cardiac silhouette and the lack of increase in pulmonary vascular markings. *B,* Left lateral view of the same patient as in *A.* Note the apparent enlargement of the cardiac silhouette and the radiolucent line in the anterior part of the cardiac silhouette, separated from the retrosternal area *(arrow).* Epicardial fat is seen, separated from the retrosternal area by fluid.

become less obvious, and the silhouette becomes smoother (Figs. 17–24 and 17–25). The lateral wings of the pericardium fill out laterally and posteriorly. In the lateral film, the fluid separates the retrosternal region from the epicardial fat, and the radiolucent fat, which is usually against the posterior sternum, is displaced posteri-

orly with apparent enlargement of the cardiac silhouette (see Fig. 17–24B). This is good evidence for a pericardial effusion.

With congenital absence of the left hemipericardium, the cardiac silhouette is displaced into the left chest, and the amount of cardiac silhouette to the right of the midline in the PA film is decreased

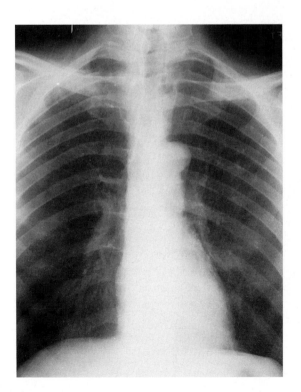

FIGURE 17–25. Posteroanterior chest radiograph of the same patient as in Figure 17–24, 6 months after pericardial effusion resolved.

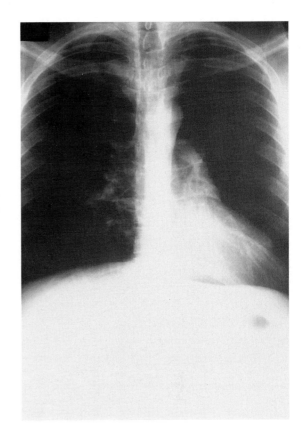

FIGURE 17–26. Posteroanterior view of a 24-year-old man with congenital absence of the left hemipericardium. Note the displacement of the heart to the left and the sharp delineation of the aortic knob from the main pulmonary artery by interposed lung.

(Fig. 17–26). Also, the lung expands directly against the heart, so air-filled lung is inserted between the aortic knob and the main pulmonary artery and between the left ventricle and the diaphragm (see Fig. 17–26). If there is only partial absence of the left hemipericardium, the left atrial appendage may be the only structure to herniate through the defect, and this herniation forms an isolated bulge along the left border of the cardiac silhouette under the main pulmonary artery segment.

CALCIFICATIONS

Intracardiac Calcifications

Valve rings and valve leaflets can calcify (Fig. 17–27; see Fig. 17–4). All the valves are central structures and overlie the spine in the PA film. Therefore, even heavily calcified valves can be missed in the PA film, and the calcification is better seen in the oblique

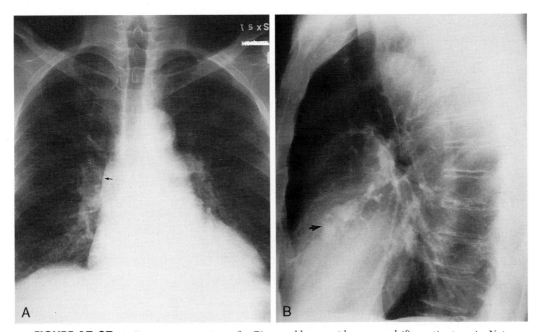

FIGURE 17–27. A, Posteroanterior view of a 70-year-old man with severe calcific aortic stenosis. Note the poststenotic dilated ascending aorta (arrow). B, Left lateral view of the same patient as in A. Note the heavily calcified aortic valve within the cardiac silhouette (arrow).

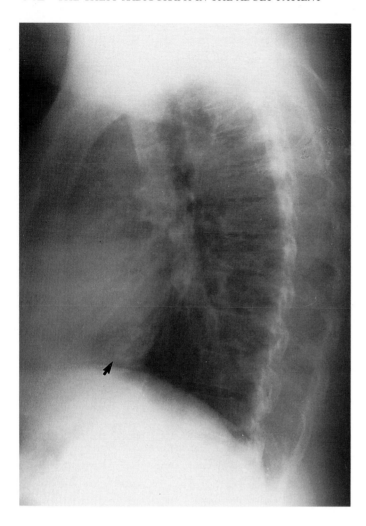

FIGURE 17–28. Left lateral radiograph of a 55-year-old man with a mobile mass in the left ventricle just under the septal leaflet of the mitral valve (*arrow*). He has had a diaphragmatic wall myocardial infarction, and the calcified mass is probably a calcified thrombus.

and lateral views (see Fig. 17–27). Especially important is aortic valve calcification, which can be prominent. Mitral valve calcification is much less frequent because it occurs exclusively in mitral stenosis, which is decreasing in incidence in the United States. Also, most patients with severe mitral stenosis undergo surgical treatment; because the mitral stenosis does not persist chronically, it is less likely to calcify. Calcification of the tricuspid and pulmonic valves is extremely rare. Calcification of leaflets can become more

obvious with motion, and therefore calcification is better seen on fluoroscopy.

Calcification of the mitral annulus (see Fig. 17–4) is common in elderly patients and frequently is associated with mitral regurgitation. With some patients, it is associated with conduction system disease and is called Lev disease. It is also seen in connection with other diseases, such as Marfan disease.

Other intracardiac structures can be calcified, such as left atrial

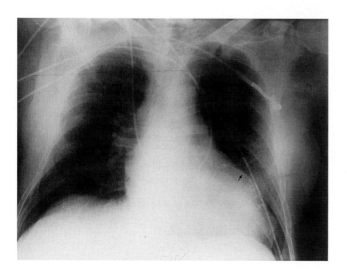

FIGURE 17–29. Posteroanterior chest radiograph in a patient with calcified left ventricular aneurysm. The patient has an old anteroseptal myocardial infarction. Note the enlarged left ventricle and the curvilinear density near the electrode wire next to the left ventricle, which is calcification in a ventricular aneurysm (*arrow*).

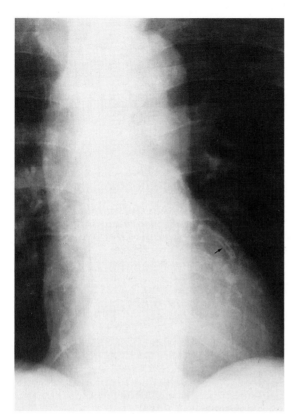

FIGURE 17-30. Posteroanterior view of a 70-year-old man with severe coronary artery disease. Note the calcification in the left anterior descending coronary artery *(arrow)*.

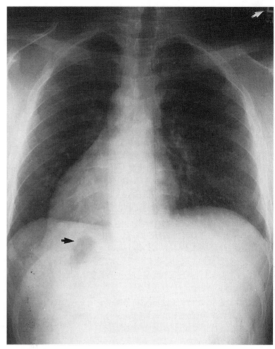

FIGURE 17-31. Posteroanterior view of a 24-year-old man with dextrocardia and situs inversus. Note the stomach bubble at the left *(black arrow)* and the marker accurately identifying the left side ("L") *(white arrow)*.

myxomas, other cardiac tumors, and intrachamber thrombi (Fig. 17–28). Calcification of a left ventricular aneurysm is common (Fig. 17–29).

Extracardiac Calcifications

Calcification of the pericardium occurs in pericardial disease with and without constrictive pericarditis (see Fig. 17–23). Calcification of the coronary arteries is also common (see Fig. 17–29) and is best detected with fluoroscopy (Fig. 17–30) or with fast computed tomography. Calcification in the pulmonary artery is always associated with pulmonary hypertension and atherosclerosis of the pulmonary artery (see Fig. 17–18). Calcifications in the aorta and in aortic aneurysms have already been mentioned.

PARACARDIAC DENSITIES

Abnormal densities immediately adjacent to the cardiac silhouette are sometimes seen. Such abnormalities include pericardial cysts, aneurysms of the pulmonary veins (pulmonary venous varicosities), discrete coronary artery aneurysms, and aneurysmal coronary arteries, as seen with very large coronary cameral and coronary arteriovenous fistulas. Aneurysms of the aorta, massively enlarged pulmonary arteries, and pulmonary arteriovenous fistulas can be mistaken for pulmonary masses.

POSITIONAL ABNORMALITIES

When the heart is on the right side of the chest, this abnormality is called dextrocardia. This condition can result from dextroposi-

tion, when the normal d-loop ventricle in the embryo does not rotate into the left chest, or from an l-loop ventricle that rotated into the right chest—true dextrocardia. True dextrocardia is frequently associated with situs inversus, in which the atria and the viscera are also reversed right to left. With situs inversus, the stomach bubble is on the right and the liver is on the left (Fig. 17–31).

SUMMARY

The chest radiograph is one of the first noninvasive imaging techniques available for the diagnosis of pulmonary and cardiac disease. Even with the sophisticated noninvasive imaging techniques now available, which can better delineate chamber size and intracardiac abnormalities, the information obtained from the plain chest film is still important. The chest film can aid in the recognition of paracardiac and intracardiac abnormalities that may not be apparent on an echocardiogram and in the selection of other, more expensive imaging techniques to more definitively diagnose the patient's problem. Cardiac imagery should start with the plain chest radiograph.

References

1. Hammermeister, K.E., Chikos, P.M., Fisher, L., et al.: Relationship of cardiothoracic ratio and plain film heart volume to late survival. Circulation 59:89, 1979.
2. Chen, J.T., Behar, V.S., Morris, J.J., Jr., et al.: Correlation of roentgen findings with hemodynamic data in pure mitral stenosis. AJR 102:280, 1968.
3. Glover, L., Baxley, W.A., and Dodge, H.T.: A quantitative evaluation of heart size measurements from chest roentgenograms. Circulation 47:1289, 1973.
4. Keats, T.E., and Enge, I.P.: Cardiac mensuration by the cardiac volume method. Radiology 85:850, 1965.

18 Radiographic Contrast Agents

John W. Hirshfeld, Jr., M.D.

**THE PHYSICS OF DIAGNOSTIC X-RAY
IMAGING** _____ 144
**PERFORMANCE CRITERIA FOR INTRAVASCULAR
RADIOGRAPHIC CONTRAST AGENTS** _____ 144
HISTORICAL BACKGROUND _____ 145
**ANGIOGRAPHIC CONTRAST AGENTS CURRENTLY
MARKETED IN THE UNITED STATES** _____ 148
Importance of Iodine Concentration _____ 148
    1.5 Ratio Ionic Agents _____ *148*
    3.0 Ratio Ionic Agent _____ *149*
    3.0 Ratio Nonionic Agents _____ *149*
    6.0 Ratio Nonionic Agent _____ *149*
**PHARMACOLOGIC EFFECTS OF ANGIOGRAPHIC
CONTRAST AGENTS** _____ 149
Acute Toxicity _____ 149
Effects of Intravascular Bolus Injection _____ 150
    Effect on Intravascular Volume _____ *150*
    *Effect on Systemic Vascular
Resistance* _____ *151*
    Effect on Systemic Arterial Pressure _____ *151*
    Effect on Ventricular Filling Pressure _____ *151*

    Effect on Cardiac Output _____ *152*
**Effects of Selective Intracoronary
Injection** _____ 153
    *Effects on Myocardial Performance and
Systemic Arterial Pressure* _____ *153*
    Cardiac Electrophysiologic Effects _____ *154*
Other Noncardiovascular Effects _____ 156
    *Immediate Generalized, or Anaphylactoid,
Reaction* _____ *157*
    Effects on Renal Function _____ *158*
    Effects on Pulmonary Function _____ *159*
    Gastrointestinal Effects _____ *159*
    Hematologic Effects _____ *159*
    Effects on Blood Vessels _____ *159*
**CRITERIA FOR SELECTION OF CONTRAST AGENTS
FOR CARDIAC ANGIOGRAPHY** _____ 159
The Contrast Agent Selection Problem _____ 159
**Clinical Trials Comparing Different Classes of
Contrast Agents** _____ 160
**Strategy for Selective Use of Low-Osmolality
Contrast Agents** _____ 162

THE PHYSICS OF DIAGNOSTIC X-RAY IMAGING

All imaging techniques that use diagnostic x-rays rely on regional differences in the absorbance of x-ray photons. The conventional radiographic image is a two-dimensional analogue display of the spatial variations in x-ray absorbance of the three-dimensional structure being imaged. In the display, a large transmitted signal (black on a conventional x-ray film) represents a comparatively small x-ray absorbance or radiographic density, and a small signal (white) represents a greater density. For a structure to be differentiated from its surrounding tissues, its x-ray absorbance must be either greater than or less than that of the surrounding tissues. The amount of difference, or image contrast, required is related inversely to the size of the structure.

Conventional radiographic imaging employs x-ray photon energies in the so-called "diagnostic" range of 60 to 125 kilovolts peak, or kV(p). The ability of a material to absorb these photons is determined predominantly by two properties: (1) the atomic number of the elements of which the structure is composed and (2) the density of the atoms in the structure. Most body tissues are solid- or liquid-phase structures composed predominantly of hydrogen, carbon, and oxygen, which have atomic numbers of 1, 6, and 8, respectively. Bones are solid-phase structures that are easily resolved from surrounding structures because they contain large quantities of calcium (atomic number 20). Lungs contain predominantly gases that are composed of nitrogen (atomic number 7), oxygen, hydrogen, and carbon. These gases are distinguished from surrounding liquid and solid structures by the smaller elemental densities of their atoms.

Diagnostic x-ray techniques cannot produce resolution of internal cardiac structures and blood vessels because the x-ray absorbance of these structures is identical to that of the blood contained within them. Thus, they have no radiographic contrast and cannot be imaged by means of conventional radiographic tech-

niques. Radiographic contrast can be created, however, by transiently replacing the blood within these structures with a contrast agent with greater radiographic density.

PERFORMANCE CRITERIA FOR INTRAVASCULAR RADIOGRAPHIC CONTRAST AGENTS

Intravascular radiographic contrast agents make cardiac and vascular structures visible by increasing the x-ray absorbance of the fluid inside them, thus increasing the radiographic density of a structure's lumen. Theoretically, cardiovascular structures can also be imaged by decreasing their x-ray density. This approach has been tried to a limited extent with the use of gases such as carbon dioxide as contrast agents. However, the image quality of such techniques is poor because even with rapid intravascular injection of large volumes of gas, it is difficult to replace the blood completely by the gas, and layering of blood within the vessel distorts the image. Consequently, all current techniques employ fluid-contrast agents, which increase x-ray absorbance.

The image contrast needed to resolve an object 1 mm in diameter (the diameter of a small coronary branch) requires that the object's x-ray absorbance be roughly 10 percent greater than that of the surrounding structures.[1] Larger structures require less image contrast. Accordingly, the x-ray absorbance of an intravascular contrast agent must be sufficiently greater than that of blood to increase the vessel's radiographic density to a value 10 percent greater than that of the entire thickness of the tissues traversed by the x-ray beam.

A suitable angiographic contrast agent must meet several criteria: First, it must be a liquid at body temperature, with a viscosity similar to that of blood. To be suitable for intravascular injection, it probably should be an aqueous solution, like blood plasma. Second, it must contain an element that has a sufficiently high atomic number in a concentration adequate to provide an x-ray absorbance that is at least 10 percent greater than that of blood. Third, the constituents of the suitable contrast agent must be biocompatible, have minimal deleterious effects in the required concentrations, and be easily eliminated from the body. No currently available x-ray contrast agent fully satisfies all these criteria completely, although considerable progress has been made toward that goal.

HISTORICAL BACKGROUND

Roentgen discovered x-rays in 1895.[2] Excited endeavors to image internal body structures ensued rapidly thereafter. The need for contrast agents to image blood vessels became promptly apparent, but most of the elements with high atomic numbers proved to be too toxic for intravascular administration in the concentrations needed to generate sufficient image contrast. Early workers investigated a number of potential contrast agent preparations. The first vascular images of diagnostic quality in a living human were obtained in 1923 by Berberich and Hirsch, who used injection of a 20 percent solution of strontium bromide (atomic numbers 38 and 35, respectively).[3] Iodine (atomic number 53) soon emerged as the element with the best combination of physical, chemical, and pharmacologic properties for intravascular imaging. In 1924, Brooks reported vascular imaging with intra-arterial injection of sodium iodide.[4] Taking advantage of sodium iodide's high aqueous solubility, he prepared a solution that was approximately 40 percent iodine by weight (and that had a sodium concentration of approximately 7 mol/L!) by dissolving 100 g of sodium iodide in 100 mL of water. His description of the angiographic procedure makes clear that this preparation was less than ideal as an arteriographic agent:

The entire thigh is prepared for operation. A sterile tourniquet is placed around the thigh as high as possible, but is not tightened. With a local anesthetic of 0.5 percent procaine, the femoral artery is exposed in the proximal end of Hunter's canal. Only enough of the artery is exposed to permit the application of a Crile artery clamp, which is not tightened. The roentgen-ray tube is placed over the knee region, and a large photographic film with a screen is placed under the knee and leg. The patient is now given nitrous oxid gas. It has been found that there is pain during the period the solution is in the artery, and the patient cannot be kept still enough to get a good roentgenogram unless a general anesthetic is used. The tourniquet proximal to the exposed artery is tightened enough to produce a filling of the veins. When the veins are full, the clamp on the artery is tightened enough to occlude the artery completely. A short interval is then allowed to elapse for the artery distal to the clamp to empty its blood. A medium sized needle is introduced into the lumen of the artery, and 10 c.c. of the sodium iodid solution is injected. The roentgen-ray tube is then operated for the briefest period possible to secure a good plate. A second plate may be taken of the distal third of the leg and foot. The tourniquet is released, the clamp removed from the artery, and the gas anesthetic discontinued. The wound is then closed.[4]

Brooks' experience demonstrated the feasibility of arteriography using iodine as the contrast agent element. It also demonstrated that the iodide ion itself was unacceptable in this role because of its absolute physiochemical limitations. The molar concentrations of iodide ion required to achieve adequate image contrast are 70 times greater than the molar concentration of ions in body fluids, and the quantities of iodine needed to perform the typical angiographic examination are enormous compared with either total body stores or the normal daily intake (Fig. 18–1).

An improved method for delivering large quantities of highly concentrated iodine was needed. Fortunately, iodine is readily incorporated into organic molecules. The history of the molecular evolution of iodinated radiographic contrast agents is illustrated in Figure 18–2. The first attempt to use organified iodine as a contrast agent employed a complex of sodium iodide and urea.[5] This complex, however, also proved to be unacceptably toxic. Selectan, the first iodinated organic molecule that was successfully administered to humans, was introduced in 1928; it had been synthesized originally as a potential antibiotic by Binz and Rath.[6] It was studied and found to be effective as a urographic contrast agent by Swick.[7] It also proved to be unacceptably toxic, however (the maximum tolerated human dose was 18 g), and it was not adequately soluble in water. Two years later, in 1930, the substitution of the methyl moiety with a carboxyl group produced Uroselectan (Schering, AG). Development of this compound represented a true breakthrough. Its toxicity was one tenth that of Selectan, and it was substantially more water soluble.[8] Although Swick studied it primarily as a urographic agent,[7] other investigators, including Forssman, who used it to opacify the right heart in animals,[9] recognized its potential as a vascular and cardiac contrast agent.

Once organified iodine was established as a successful intravascular contrast agent, work was directed toward developing improved molecules. Investigators rapidly realized that a satisfactory intravascular contrast agent formulation required an iodine content of at least 20 percent by weight, and that better opacification and detail resolution required even greater concentrations. This fundamental physical problem required that the formulations of intravascular contrast agent molecules be highly concentrated in comparison with the solute concentrations of body fluids. The problem was to

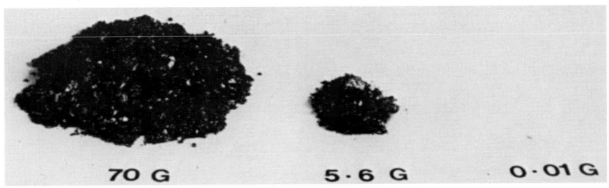

FIGURE 18–1. The relationship between the quantities of iodine employed in angiographic examinations and those in total body stores. The 70-g pile of crystalline iodine on the left represents the amount of iodine in 200 mL (a representative total patient dose for a complex angiographic procedure) of a contrast agent containing 350 mg/mL of iodine. The 5.6-g pile in the center represents the amount of iodine contained in 16 mL of contrast agent. The 0.01-g pile on the right represents the normal total body content of iodine. (From Grainger, R.G.: Osmolalities of intravascular radiological contrast media. Br. J. Radiol. 53:739–746, 1980, with permission.)

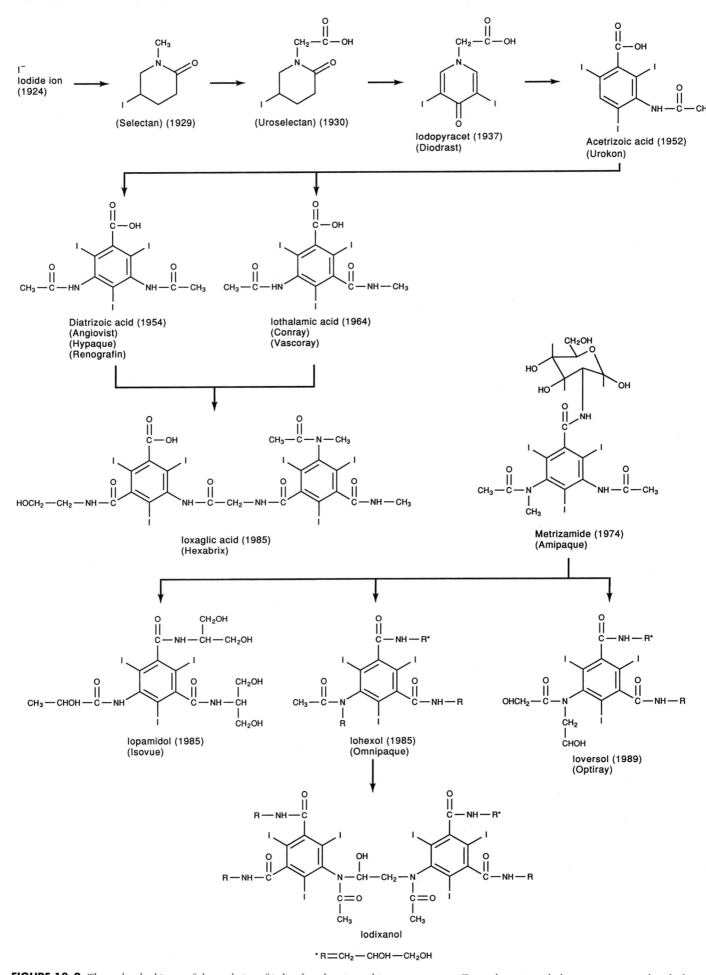

FIGURE 18-2. The molecular history of the evolution of iodine-based angiographic contrast agents. For each compound, the generic name is listed, along with common trade names and the year of introduction into clinical use.

design molecules that had physical and biochemical properties compatible with intravascular administration, which incorporated an adequate elemental density of iodine into solution.

A molecule's ability to deliver iodine is characterized by its *iodine ratio*, the ratio of the number of iodine atoms in a molecule to the number of osmotically active particles that the molecule produces in solution. Uroselectan contains one iodine atom per two osmotically active particles. Thus, it has an iodine ratio of 0.5. Since 1930, the focus of contrast-agent molecule "horsepower race" has been to increase the iodine ratio, which correspondingly reduces the toxicity of contrast agent molecules. Many contrast agent molecules are organic acids that achieve water solubility by ionization of the carboxyl moiety. Whereas this approach simplifies the problems of creating water-soluble organic molecules, the obligatory cation, which accompanies the iodine-bearing anion, doubles the number of osmotically active particles in solution.

Development focused initially on increasing the iodine content of the contrast agent molecule. If a molecule contained more iodine atoms, a lower molar concentration would be required to achieve a given iodine density. The first major improvement occurred in 1931 with the synthesis of iodopyracet (Diodrast [Winthrop]) and Neo-Iopax (Uroselectan B), which have two iodine atoms per molecule and, accordingly, are 1.0 ratio agents.[10] These molecules were used actively for 20 years, and considerable research that laid the groundwork for cardiac angiography was performed with these molecules. The next significant advance was the synthesis of acetrizoic acid (Urokon [Mallinckrodt]) by Wallingford, which was introduced into clinical radiology in 1952. This material added a third iodine atom, producing a 1.5 ratio agent, which carried the halogen-substituted benzene ring to its maximum achievable iodine content.[11] This accomplishment was the culmination of 20 years of work (slowed somewhat by World War II) in an effort to overcome the organic synthetic problems of creating 2,4,6-tri-iodinated aromatic molecules and to reduce the substantial toxicity of the first molecules synthesized in this class.

The acetrizoic acid class of contrast agents was further refined by substituting the 5 position with an amide. The first and prototypical member of this class is diatrizoic acid (Hypaque, MD-76, Renografin), which was introduced into clinical use in 1954 and, until the late 1980s, was the most widely used of all intravascular contrast agent molecules.[12] Iothalamic acid (Conray) was subsequently developed as a derivative of diatrizoic acid and was found to have similar pharmacologic properties.

By 1960, investigators had established that, despite substantial improvements in radiographic equipment, an angiographic contrast agent required at least 30 percent iodine by weight to produce satisfactory opacification of small vessels. Even the tri-iodinated molecules required very large molar concentrations to achieve iodine contents at this level. To maintain the required high degree of aqueous solubility, all the previously synthesized contrast agent molecules relied on an ionizing functional group at the 1 position. The ionic property caused two problems.

The first problem was that the cation associated with the contrast agent molecule was present in such large concentrations that its pharmacologic, electrophysiologic, and physiochemical properties became an important determinant of the properties of the contrast agent formulation. The simplest formulation of an ionic contrast agent would use an inorganic biocompatible cation, such as sodium. However, to achieve a satisfactory concentration of the iodine-containing anion requires a cation concentration of approximately 1000 mEq/L (more than six times the normal concentration of sodium in plasma). A solution with this high a sodium concentration is electrophysiologically unacceptable for direct injection into coronary arteries. Consequently, a cation was needed that is not electrophysiologically active. Methylglucamine (meglumine), an organic cationic molecule, has such properties and is the cation in most currently used ionic contrast-agent formulations. A shortcoming of methylglucamine, however, is that, compared with sodium, it increases the solution viscosity, making extremely concentrated solutions difficult to inject through catheters. Therefore, the currently used formulations represent a compromise: they contain a concentration of sodium approximating that of blood plasma, and the remaining cation space is filled with methylglucamine. Thus, a typical diatrizoate-based contrast agent formulation contains 10 percent sodium diatrizoate and 66 percent methylglucamine diatrizoate by weight. The sodium concentration of such a formulation is 160 mEq/L.[13]

The second problem of the previously synthesized contrast agent molecules is that the ionic nature of the compound requires that the associated cation be in solution, which doubles the number of osmotically active particles associated with the contrast agent molecule. As a consequence, the solution osmolalities, clinically useful formulations of the ionic tri-iodinated contrast agent molecules, exceed 2000 mOsm/kg—more than seven times the osmolality of blood plasma.

The tri-iodinated ionic contrast agents, although substantially improved over the molecules used earlier, still have toxicities that limit the volume that can be administered, particularly to hemodynamically fragile patients (see later discussion). In 1969, Almen reasoned that a major component of the toxicity was not the contrast agent molecule itself, but the high osmolality of the solution of the contrast agent formulation.[14] He identified several potential approaches to reducing contrast agent osmolality (by increasing the iodine ratio). One approach was the replacement of the ionizable functional group with a polar nonionizing functional group that would maintain aqueous solubility but, because of the absence of an associated cation, would reduce the osmolality of a formulation by a factor of two.[14] This reasoning led to the synthesis of metrizamide, a tri-iodinated aromatic molecule in which the carboxyl group of the ionic molecules is replaced by a sugar.[15]

Metrizamide, the first 3.0 ratio agent, was introduced into clinical radiology in 1974. Because of aggregation of contrast agent molecules in solution, it proved to have a measured osmolality that is actually lower than that predicted from theoretical calculations.[16] Experimental and clinical studies showed that, compared with the ionic acetrizoic acid derivatives, it was less toxic, and that it caused fewer hemodynamic and electrophysiologic changes.[17] Unfortunately, metrizamide is extremely expensive to synthesize, lacks thermostability, and is not stable in solution. These shortcomings make it cumbersome to use and have limited its usefulness in procedures that require large quantities of contrast agent, such as cardiac angiography. It proved to be extremely successful, however, as a myelographic agent and clearly demonstrated the value of reducing contrast agent osmolality to improve tolerance.

Once metrizamide had demonstrated the benefit of the nonionic approach to reducing osmolality, subsequent research focused on developing compounds that would achieve osmolality reduction and were practical to use. Two of the approaches proposed by Almen were used. The first was the synthesis of other 3.0 ratio nonionic compounds. This led to the introduction of iohexol[18] and iopamidol[19] in 1985 and ioversol[20] in 1989. All three of these compounds are 3.0 ratio agents that are thermostable and less expensive to synthesize than metrizamide. Their pharmacologic properties and toxicities are similar to those of metrizamide.

Almen's second approach was the synthesis of an ionic agent with six iodine atoms per molecule, which was accomplished by linking two 1.5 ratio ionic molecules together and converting one of the carboxyl groups to an amide. This class of molecules, termed monoacid dimers, which also have a 3.0 iodine ratio, is represented by ioxaglate, which was introduced in 1984.[21] Ioxaglate proved to have a rate of hemodynamic performance comparable to that of the 3.0 ratio nonionic agents, but a frequency of minor adverse reactions (chiefly nausea) that was intermediate between the 1.5 ratio ionic agents and the 3.0 ratio nonionic agents.[22]

Subsequent radiographic contrast agent development has focused on reducing osmolality further. The outcome of this research has been to apply the dimer approach to nonionic molecules. This strategy has led to the synthesis of several nonionic dimers that have iodine ratios of 6.0. These molecules offer the possibility of a formulation isotonic to plasma with an iodine concentration that is suitable for angiography. Iodixanol is one such molecule released for clinical use in several European countries and that researchers are anticipating for release in the United States in late 1995.[23, 24] Solutions of iodixanol are considerably more viscous (18.9 mPa per second at 20° C for 300 mg of iodine per mL) than comparably concentrated solutions of 3.0 ratio nonionic agents (iohexol viscosity is 11.6 mPa per second at 20° C for 300 mg of iodine per mL).[25] This property has limited iodixanol's maximum iodine concentration to 32 percent and has precluded the clinical development of some other 6.0 ratio molecules, which proved to have unacceptable solution viscosity. At a 32 percent iodine concentration, solutions of iodixanol are hypotonic to plasma, and, accordingly, the clinical formulations have added quantities of inorganic ions to achieve an osmolality of 285. The opportunity to add electrolytes to the formulation prompted a study to determine the formulation's optimal inorganic ion composition. Extensive studies of different inorganic ionic compositions demonstrated that the optimal composition was a total ionic composition that made the solution osmolality isotonic to plasma, which contained sodium and calcium ions in the same ratio as is present in normal plasma.[26] The formulation, which will be marketed for cardiac angiographic use, contains 32 percent iodine and contains added sodium and calcium chloride in the ratios described previously.

Animal studies indicate that iodixanol has the highest intravenous median lethal dose (LD_{50}) observed for an iodinated contrast agent and that it causes less hemodynamic disturbance than do formulations of the 3.0 ratio nonionic agents with comparable iodine concentrations.[24] It is logical to expect that the lower osmolality of iodixanol would confer even lower toxicity and superior clinical performance. Currently, limited data are available to characterize the clinical performance of iodixanol relative to 3.0 ratio agents. The available data indicate clinical performance that is at least comparable to and may be superior to that of 3.0 agents.[27] Currently, however, insufficient data are available to allow a rigorous comparison of the clinical performance of iodixanol with the currently marketed 3.0 ratio agents.

ANGIOGRAPHIC CONTRAST AGENTS CURRENTLY MARKETED IN THE UNITED STATES

Importance of Iodine Concentration

As discussed earlier, an angiographic contrast agent must deliver to the vascular structure being imaged an elemental density of iodine that is adequate to resolve that structure. The lowest iodine concentration that is adequate to resolve small vessels, such as coronary arteries in large, heavy patients, is 300 mg/mL. All the contrast agents marketed in the United States for cardiac angiography meet this criterion, with iodine concentrations ranging from 320 to 400 mg/mL. All these agents provide acceptable opacification. In fact, differences between the levels of opacification provided by the different marketed iodine concentrations are essentially imperceptible in clinical use (Fig. 18–3). Thus, a preparation with an iodine concentration of 370 mg/mL does not provide vascular opacification that is superior clinically to that provided by a preparation with an iodine concentration of 320 mg/mL. Some of the relevant properties of contrast agents that are currently marketed for cardiac angiography are compiled in Table 18–1.

1.5 Ratio Ionic Agents

The diatrizoate anion is the basis of virtually all the 1.5 ratio ionic agents used for cardiac angiography in the United States. An iothalamate-based agent is also marketed and is used principally for cerebral angiography but has seen limited use for cardiac angiography. Diatrizoate is available in many formulations and concentrations for different intravascular applications and is marketed in the United States under three different trade names. All

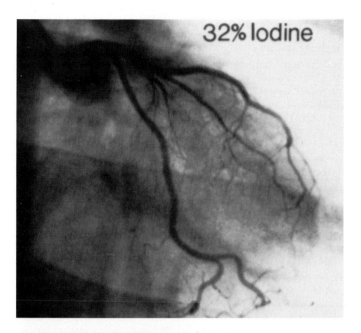

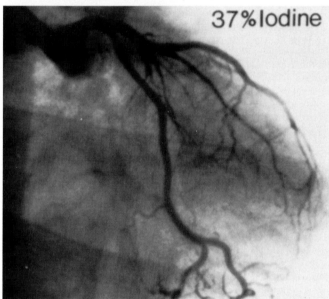

FIGURE 18–3. Frames from two left coronary angiograms from the same patient (height, 70 inches; weight, 225 lb) exposed in the same radiographic projection. The upper frame was obtained with a contrast agent containing 320 mg of iodine per mL and the lower frame was obtained with an agent containing 370 mg of iodine per mL.

preparations used for cardiac angiography contain 76 percent contrast agent by weight, with a ratio of methylglucamine cation to sodium cation of 6.6:1.0. Because of differences in other additives, the sodium concentration of the different formulations varies from 160 to 190 mEq/L. This range of sodium concentration has been found to be optimal in terms of minimizing cardiac electrophysiologic effects during selective coronary injection.[13, 28–30] Higher or lower sodium concentrations cause a greater frequency of ventricular fibrillation during selective intracoronary injection.

The diatrizoate formulations also differ in their calcium-binding properties. All the formulations contain ethylenediaminetetraacetic acid (EDTA), but in one of the formulations (Hypaque-76), the EDTA is enriched with calcium. The other two formulations (MD-76 and Renografin-76) contain EDTA that is not calcium-enriched. In addition, these latter two formulations contain citrate ion, originally included for the purpose of chelating trace quantities of heavy

TABLE 18–1. CHEMICAL COMPOSITIONS AND SELECTED PHYSICAL AND PHARMACOLOGIC PROPERTIES OF INTRAVASCULAR IODINATED CONTRAST AGENTS

	Hypaque-76	Renografin-76	MD-76	Vascoray	Isovue	Omnipaque	Optiray	Hexabrix	Visipaque
Iodine concentration (mg/mL)	370	370	370	400	370	350	320, 370	320	320
Iodine-containing molecule	Diatrizoate	Diatrizoate	Diatrizoate	Iothalamate	Iopamidol	Iohexol	Ioversol	Ioxaglate	Iodixanol
Cations	Methyl-glucamine, sodium	Methyl-glucamine, sodium	Methyl-glucamine, sodium	Methyl-glucamine, sodium	None	None	None	Methyl-glucamine, sodium	None
Intravenous LD$_{50}$ (g iodine/kg)	7.5	7.5	7.5	6.2	21.8	24.2	17.0	11.2	>20.9
Measured osmolality (mOsm/kg)	2016	1940	2140	2400	796	844	702	600	290
Viscosity (37°C)	8.32	8.4	9.1	9.0	9.4	10.4	5.8	7.5	11.8
Sodium concentration (mEq/L)	160	190	190	408	Trace	Trace	Trace	150	31
Other additives	0.01% sodium calcium EDTA	0.32% sodium citrate, 0.04% sodium EDTA	0.32% sodium citrate, 0.04% sodium EDTA	0.0125% NaH$_2$PO$_4$, 0.0125% sodium calcium EDTA	0.05% disodium calcium EDTA, 0.02% tro-methamine	0.01% disodium calcium EDTA, 0.02% tro-methamine	0.02% disodium calcium EDTA, 0.02% tro-methamine	0.02% disodium calcium EDTA, 0.02% tro-methamine	0.01% sodium dicalcium EDTA, 0.011% sodium chloride, 0.0044%, 0.012% tro-methamine

metals to enhance shelf life. The significance of the differences in calcium-binding properties and sodium concentration is examined in the discussion of cardiac electrophysiologic effects of selective intracoronary injection, which is found later in this chapter.

The iothalamate molecule is marketed in the United States for cardiac use under the trade name of Vascoray. Its formulation by weight contains 26 percent sodium salt and 52 percent methylglucamine salt, and it has an iodine content of 400 mg/mL. Its formulation also contains calcium-enriched EDTA and does not contain citrate.

3.0 Ratio Ionic Agent

Ioxaglate is marketed in the United States as Hexabrix. Unlike the other agents, its formulation is somewhat less concentrated, containing 32 percent iodine. This lower concentration was selected as a consequence of the molecule's physical properties. A concentration that would contain 37 percent iodine would have an unacceptably high viscosity. Its formulation by weight includes 39.3 percent methylglucamine salt and 19.6 percent sodium salt. It contains calcium-enriched EDTA and does not contain citrate.

3.0 Ratio Nonionic Agents

Three 3.0 ratio nonionic agents are currently marketed in the United States: iohexol (Omnipaque), iopamidol (Isovue), and ioversol (Optiray). These three molecules have similar structures. The formulations are also similar, except for the concentrations of the contrast agent molecule: iohexol, 35 percent iodine; iopamidol, 37 percent iodine; and ioversol, 32 percent iodine. Only trace quantities of sodium are present in the formulations of the nonionic agents.

6.0 Ratio Nonionic Agent

Iodixanol is marketed in several European countries and is expected to be approved in the United States in mid-1995 under the trade name Visipaque. The formulation of iodixanol contains 32 percent iodine. Pure solutions at the concentration of 320 mg of iodine per mL are hypotonic to blood (osmolality 207 mOsm/kg). Consequently, additional osmotically active constituents are added to raise the solution osmolality to 290: 0.044 mg/mL CaCl$_2$; 1.11

mg/mL NaCl; and 0.1 mg/mL edetate calcium disodium.[31] A comparison of the performance of the currently marketed contrast agents is discussed in detail in the next section.

PHARMACOLOGIC EFFECTS OF ANGIOGRAPHIC CONTRAST AGENTS

An overall summary of the cardiovascular and noncardiovascular actions of radiographic contrast agents is provided in Tables 18–2 and 18–3.

Acute Toxicity

The ideal contrast agent would be biologically inert. The agents currently used are not inert but have remarkably little toxicity. This characteristic results, in part, from their lack of protein-binding affinity, high water solubility, and large molecular size and the lack of existence of transport mechanisms to facilitate their entry into cell interiors. These properties minimize their penetration of the intercellular space as long as the cell membrane structure is intact.

Because the purpose of these molecules is to deliver iodine, their toxicity is most meaningfully expressed as the LD$_{50}$ in terms of grams of iodine delivered per kilogram of body weight. This value expresses the pharmacologic toxicity in terms of the molecule's functional role.

Published LD$_{50}$ values vary somewhat from study to study, because the actual value is highly influenced by particular experimental conditions (e.g., the injection rate), and not all LD$_{50}$ determinations are made with the use of the same experimental protocol. For example, published LD$_{50}$ values for diatrizoate vary from 4.6 to 8.0 g of iodine per kg.[32, 33] The data cited here and in Table 18–1 are taken from the manufacturers' published data, as approved by the U.S. Food and Drug Administration. Thus, they may be considered to represent roughly comparable experimental protocols and provide an approximate basis for comparing the toxicities of the different agents. The intravenous mouse LD$_{50}$ for bolus injection varies from 7.5 g of iodine per kg for diatrizoate, to 14 g of iodine per kg for iohexol, to 21 g of iodine per kg for iodixanol.[32] For a

TABLE 18–2. CARDIOVASCULAR ACTIONS OF RADIOGRAPHIC CONTRAST AGENTS*

Action	1.5 Ratio Ionic Agents†	3.0 Ratio Ionic Agent	3.0 Ratio Nonionic Agents	6.0 Ratio Nonionic Agent
Acute expansion of intravascular volume	+ + +	+	+	+
Transient systemic arteriolar vasodilation	+ + +	+	+	0
Transient depression of myocardial contractile function	+ +	+	0	0
Alteration of myocardial metabolism	+ +	?	+	?
Transient increase in cardiac filling pressure	+ + +	+	+	+
Transient increase in cardiac output	+ + +	+	+	+
Transient decrease in arterial pressure	+ + (Ca^{2+} binding) + (non-Ca^{2+} binding)	+	0	0
Bradycardia after intracoronary injection	+ + + (Ca^{2+} binding) + (non-Ca^{2+} binding)	+	0	0
Prolongation of ventricular repolarization	+ + + + (Ca^{2+} binding) + + (non-Ca^{2+} binding)	+ +	+	+
Decrease in ventricular fibrillation threshold	+ + + (Ca^{2+} binding) + (non-Ca^{2+} binding)	+	+	+

*Administered via intravascular bolus or intracoronary injection.
†Where appropriate, the effects of these agents are subdivided into formations with and without calcium-binding properties.

solution containing 37 percent iodine, this range represents an injection volume range of 21.6 to 65.4 mL/kg. Because total blood volume is approximately 70 mL/kg, the LD_{50} for an intravenous bolus dose of these agents ranges from 31 to 93 percent of total blood volume.

Animals given lethal intravenous boluses of contrast agents die of respiratory distress due to pulmonary edema. This phenomenon is not surprising when one considers the total quantity of agent injected. The LD_{50} of each of the currently used agents, when expressed in terms of the quantity of osmotically active solute, is comparable to the total intravascular volume.

Generalization of these data to humans indicates that for a 70-kg subject, the intravenous bolus LD_{50} for these agents ranges from 1400 mL for diatrizoate to 4500 mL for iodixanol. Average contrast-agent doses for diagnostic cardiac angiographic procedures range from 145 mL[34] to 200 mL.[35] Thus, in healthy subjects, the therapeutic index for these compounds probably ranges from 10 to 31. Obviously, in seriously ill patients, particularly those with severe and unstable cardiac disease, the therapeutic index is smaller.

Effects of Intravascular Bolus Injection

Cardiac angiography involves intravascular bolus injection of contrast agents. Typical injection volumes vary from 3 to 9 mL for selective coronary opacification and from 45 to 60 mL for cardiac and great vessel opacification. The effects of bolus injection may be separated into three groups: (1) effects on intravascular volume, (2) effects on the systemic vasculature, and (3) direct myocardial effects. The direct myocardial effects are discussed in detail in later sections on selective intracoronary injection and myocardial performance.

Effect on Intravascular Volume

In the rapid intravascular injection of 50 mL of a contrast agent, the same quantity of osmotically active solute is administered as is present in 50 to 250 mL of plasma, depending on which contrast agent is used. When hypertonic agents are used, the large quantity of osmotically active solute rapidly draws water into the intravascular compartment. Some of this water is drawn from red blood cells, but the majority comes from the extravascular compartment. The magnitude of this effect is directly related to the osmolality of the particular contrast agent molecule and to the volume injected. The effect is reflected in a transient decrease in blood hemoglobin concentration (Fig. 18–4), which is caused by red blood cell dilution by the acute expansion of intravascular plasma volume.

The contrast agent molecule is initially confined to the intravascular compartment, but it gains access to the entire extracellular

TABLE 18–3. NONCARDIOVASCULAR ACTIONS OF RADIOGRAPHIC CONTRAST AGENTS*

Action	1.5 Ratio Ionic Agents	3.0 Ratio Ionic Agent	3.0 Ratio Nonionic Agents	6.0 Ratio Nonionic Agent
Frequency of immediate generalized (anaphylactoid) reaction. (Severe form is rare with all agents)	+ +	Inadequate data	+	+
Frequency of nephrotoxicity				
Low-risk patients	Rare	Inadequate data	Rare	Rare (related to volume injected) Inadequate data
High-risk patients (renal disease, diabetes, myeloma)	+ + (Related to volume injected)	Inadequate data	+ (Related to volume injected)	
Effects on lung airway dynamics (effect is greater in asthmatics)	+	Inadequate data	0	Inadequate data
Effect on vascular endothelium (disruption by large concentrations)	+ + +	+	+	Inadequate data
Anticoagulant activity	+ + + +	+ + +	+ +	+ +
Effect on red blood cell morphology (RBC crenation)	+ + +	Inadequate data	+	+
Frequency of nausea and vomiting	+ + +	+ +	Rare	Rare
Severity of pain during extracardiac selective intra-arterial injection	+ + +	+	+	0

*Administered via bolus or selective intracoronary injection.

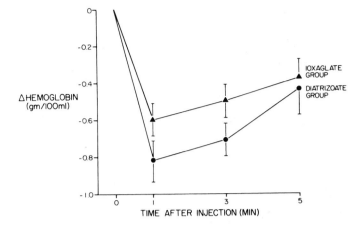

FIGURE 18–4. The time-related change in whole-blood hemoglobin concentration that occurs after a bolus injection of 45 mL of a 1.5 ratio ionic agent (diatrizoate, 370 mg/mL iodine concentration), compared with the changes caused by a 3.0 ratio ionic agent (ioxaglate, 320 mg of iodine per mL concentration). The decrease in hemoglobin concentration reflects the degree of the acute expansion of plasma volume caused by the contrast agent. The magnitude of the change is less with the 3.0 ratio agent. (From Hirshfeld, J.W., Jr., Laskey, W.K., Martin, J.L., et al.: Hemodynamic changes induced by cardiac angiography with ioxaglate: Comparison with diatrizoate. J. Am. Coll. Cardiol. 2:954, 1983. Reprinted with permission from the American College of Cardiology.)

fluid compartment fairly rapidly.[36, 37] The typical elimination half-life from the intravascular compartment is 24.4 ± 6.3 minutes.[25] This elimination is a combination of movement out of the intravascular compartment into the extracellular fluid and excretion, predominantly renal. Little, if any, of the contrast agent molecule enters the intracellular compartment when cell membrane structure is intact.

Effect on Systemic Vascular Resistance

Contrast agents all produce acute arteriolar vasodilation, causing a transient reduction in systemic vascular resistance shortly after injection. The onset of the vasodilation coincides with the arrival of the contrast agent molecule at the systemic arterioles, and the magnitude is related to the concentration of the agent as it reaches the systemic arterioles. This vasodilation is mediated by a physicochemical, rather than a pharmacologic, process and is related predominantly to the osmolality of the solution that reaches the systemic vasculature. Similar responses to the injection of other hypertonic solutions have been observed, and the magnitude of the response is related to the osmolality of the solution[38, 39] (Fig. 18–5). Possibly, the transient vasodilation is caused by the osmotically driven extraction of water from the cells of the systemic microvasculature.[40]

Thus, the magnitude of the vasodilator effect is related to three variables: (1) the injection volume (the larger the volume, the greater the vasodilation); (2) the osmolality of the injected agent (high-osmolality agents cause a greater vasodilation than low-osmolality agents); and (3) the site of injection (injections on the arterial side of the circulation produce greater effects than injections on the venous side).

Effect on Systemic Arterial Pressure

The vasodilation caused by contrast agents causes a transient reduction in arterial pressure that begins within 10 seconds following injection. The arterial pressure usually reaches its nadir by 30 to 45 seconds after injection and returns to the baseline value within 60 to 90 seconds[20, 21] (Fig. 18–6). It is common for arterial pressure to subsequently overshoot to a level above the preinjection pressure for a variable period. Because the drop in arterial pressure is mediated principally by the osmotically induced systemic vasodilation, the magnitude and duration of the decrease are related to the osmolality of the injected contrast agent. The 3.0 and 6.0 ratio agents cause less change than the 1.5 ratio agents.

Effect on Ventricular Filling Pressure

Contrast agents cause acute expansion of intravascular volume and a late increase in arterial pressure. Some contrast agents also depress myocardial contractile performance (see later discussion). These effects combine to produce a transient elevation of cardiac filling pressures.[41] This phenomenon occurs on both the left and the right sides of the heart, but because most cardiac disease predominantly affects the left side of the heart, and because elevation of filling pressure of the left side of the heart has greater immediate clinical consequences, the changes on the left side are both greater in magnitude and of greater clinical importance (Figs. 18–7 and 18–8).

For a typical bolus injection, such as 45 mL for ventriculography, the magnitude of the increase in left ventricular end-diastolic pressure varies with the osmolality of the contrast agent injected and with the nature of the particular patient's heart disease. The increases are the smallest in healthy individuals and are greatest in

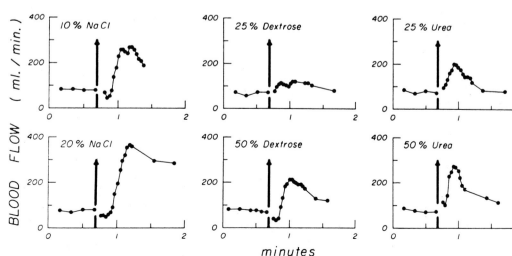

FIGURE 18–5. The vasodilatory response to the injection of several solutions of different solute concentrations into the femoral artery of a dog. Note that all the solutions produce vasodilation and that the magnitude of vasodilation is related to the concentration of the solution. (From Marshall, R.J., and Shepherd, J.T.: Effects of injections of hypertonic solutions on blood flow through the femoral artery of the dog. Am. J. Physiol. 197:951, 1959, with permission.)

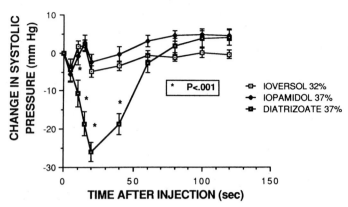

FIGURE 18–6. The time-related change in systemic arterial pressure after left ventriculography with 45 mL of 1.5 ratio ionic contrast agent (diatrizoate, 370 mg of iodine per mL concentration) and two 3.0 ratio nonionic contrast agents (ioversol, 320 mg of iodine per mL concentration; iopamidol, 370 mg of iodine per mL concentration). The magnitude of the decrease is greater with the 1.5 ratio ionic contrast agent. (From Hirshfeld, J.W., Jr., Wieland, J., Davis, C.A., et al.: Hemodynamic and electrocardiographic effects of ioversol during cardiac angiography comparison with diatrizoate. Invest. Radiol. 24:138, 1989, with permission.)

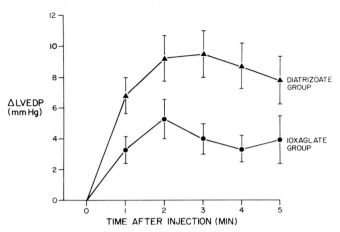

FIGURE 18–8. The time-related change in left ventricular end-diastolic pressure (LVEDP) after left ventriculography with 1.5 ratio ionic and 3.0 ratio ionic contrast agents. The format of this figure is identical to that of Figure 18–7. The change caused by the 1.5 ratio agent is greater. (From Hirshfeld J.W., Jr., Laskey, W.K., Martin, J.L., et al.: Hemodynamic changes induced by cardiac angiography with ioxaglate: Comparison with diatrizoate. J Am. Coll. Cardiol. 2:954, 1983, with permission.)

individuals whose ventricular compliance is reduced by hypertrophy and in individuals with impaired left ventricular function who are on the steep portion of their diastolic pressure-volume relationship. An early report suggested that the degree of increase in left ventricular end-diastolic pressure was related to the presence and severity of coronary artery disease,[42] but more recent studies have shown no such relationship.[43] The average increase in left ventricular end-diastolic pressure after injection of a 1.5 ratio ionic agent is 9 mm Hg, whereas the average increase after injection of a 3.0 ratio ionic or nonionic agent is 4 mm Hg (Fig. 18–9; see Fig. 18–8).[20, 21]

Although one might anticipate that the lower osmolality of the 6.0 ratio agent iodixanol might result in an even smaller increase in left ventricular end-diastolic pressure following left ventriculography, clinical studies comparing iodixanol to the 3.0 ratio agent iohexol have not demonstrated a difference.[24] This may be because the change caused by iohexol is so small that substantial statistical power may be required to detect a difference, or that a detectable difference exists only in patients with greatly impaired left ventricular function.

The clinical importance of an increase in left ventricular filling pressure is determined by the magnitude of the increase and the level from which it began. Obviously, an increase of 9 mm Hg in a healthy individual with a baseline value of 12 mm Hg is of no clinical consequence; however, a comparable, or possibly greater, increase from a baseline value of 35 mm Hg in a precariously ill patient with severe aortic stenosis and coronary disease may cause serious clinical deterioration.

Effect on Cardiac Output

In most patients, the increased intravascular volume and the systemic arteriolar vasodilation increase cardiac output transiently (Fig. 18–10). The magnitude of the increase in cardiac output is determined by the nature of the patient's heart disease and by the osmolality of the injected contrast agent. Because the 3.0 and 6.0 ratio agents increase intravascular volume less than the 1.5 ratio agents, they cause less of a change in cardiac output. The cardiac output peaks approximately 2 minutes after injection and usually returns to the preinjection value within 5 minutes.[20, 21] As is the case with ventricular filling pressures, the changes in cardiac output

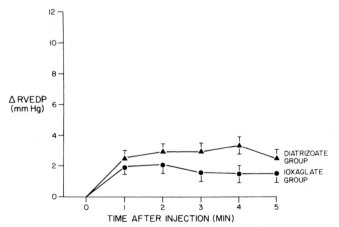

FIGURE 18–7. The time-related change in right ventricular end-diastolic pressure (RVEDP) after left ventriculography with 1.5 ratio ionic and 3.0 ratio ionic contrast agents. The increase caused by the 3.0 ratio agent is less than that caused by the 1.5 ratio agent. (From Hirshfeld J.W., Jr., Laskey, W.K., Martin, J.L., et al.: Hemodynamic changes induced by cardiac angiography with ioxaglate: Comparison with diatrizoate. J Am. Coll Cardiol. 2:954, 1983, with permission.)

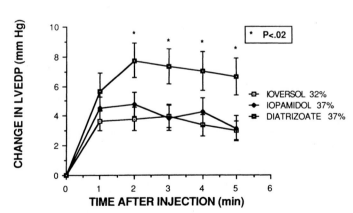

FIGURE 18–9. The time-related change in left ventricular end-diastolic pressure after left ventriculography with a 1.5 ratio ionic and two 3.0 ratio nonionic contrast agents. The format of this figure is identical to that of Figure 18–6. The increase caused by the 1.5 ratio ionic agent is greater. (From Hirshfeld, J.W., Jr., Wieland, J., Davis, C.A., et al.: Hemodynamic and electrocardiographic effects of ioversol during cardiac angiography. Comparison with diatrizoate. Invest. Radiol. 24:138–144, 1989, with permission.)

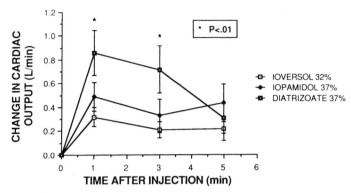

FIGURE 18–10. The time-related change in cardiac output after left ventriculography with a 1.5 ratio ionic and two 3.0 ratio nonionic contrast agents. The increase caused by the 1.5 ratio ionic agent is greater. (From Hirshfeld, J.W., Jr., Wieland, J., Davis, C.A., et al.: Hemodynamic and electrocardiographic effects of ioversol during cardiac angiography. Comparison with diatrizoate. Invest. Radiol. 24:138–144, 1989, with permission.)

caused by left ventriculography with the 6.0 ratio agent iodixanol are similar to the changes caused by 3.0 ratio agents.[24]

Effects of Selective Intracoronary Injection

Coronary arteriography involves the selective intracoronary injection of 3 to 9 mL of contrast agent. During each injection, the blood passing through the coronary vascular bed is replaced for approximately 5 seconds with nearly undiluted contrast agent. The effects of this intervention are attributable to the properties of the contrast agent molecule, to the other constituents of the contrast agent formulation, and to the osmolality of the formulation. Most experimental studies of the response to selective intracoronary injection attempt to replicate clinical coronary arteriography. They use bolus intracoronary injections of contrast agent in volumes and durations that are comparable to those achieved in clinical coronary arteriography.

Effects on Myocardial Contractile Performance and Systemic Arterial Pressure

There are substantial differences in the responses to selective intracoronary injection of the different classes of clinically available contrast agents (Fig. 18–11). These changes in myocardial contractile performance are not merely due to the transient replacement of blood by a fluid that does not transport oxygen. Injection of a solution with a physiologic ionic composition that does not transport oxygen, such as Hartman solution, produces little change in left ventricular systolic performance.[44] Rather, the changes are attributable to actual metabolic actions of the formulations.

The injection of 1.5 ratio ionic agents transiently depresses left ventricular contractile function. Following injection, there is a transient decrease in left ventricular peak systolic pressure that is maximal 10 seconds after the onset of the injection and resolves within 45 to 60 seconds. This decrease occurs in association with a decrease in the maximum rate of increase of left ventricular pressure (peak dP/dt) and an increase in left ventricular end-systolic and end-diastolic diameter, indicating that there is an actual decrease in myocardial inotropic state.[45, 46] The magnitude of the evoked changes is modest (see Fig. 18–11) and is of no clinical significance in an individual with normal or moderately impaired cardiac function. Intracoronary injection of ioxaglate, a 3.0 ratio ionic agent, causes changes that are qualitatively similar to but smaller in magnitude than those of the 1.5 ratio ionic agents.[42]

On the other hand, the response to injection of a 3.0 ratio nonionic agent is quite different. Instead of depressing left ventricular systolic performance, a 3.0 ratio nonionic agent actually transiently increases the myocardial inotropic state, resulting in an increase in left ventricular systolic shortening. This phenomenon is

not due to an intrinsic positive ionotropic property of the 3.0 ratio nonionic agent molecules but instead is attributable to the absence of sodium in their formulations, probably mediated by enhanced sodium-calcium exchange.[47]

The response to intracoronary injection of the 6.0 ratio agent iodixanol is similar to that evoked by 3.0 ratio nonionic agents, although the degree of increase of the myocardial inotropic state is slightly less, most likely because the iodixanol formulation is not sodium-free.[48]

The calcium-binding property of a contrast agent's formulation is a major contributor to its effect on myocardial contractile function. None of the 3.0 or the 6.0 ratio agents have calcium-binding formulations. However, the formulations of two of the 1.5 ratio ionic agents (MD-76 and Renografin-76) have calcium-binding properties. Following intracoronary injection of calcium-binding contrast agents, the coronary venous effluent calcium ion concentration falls transiently.[49-51] This transient regional hypocalcemia transiently decreases myocardial contractile force until the contrast agent washes out of the vascular bed and normal myocardial concentrations of calcium are restored. The reduction in left ventricular contractile performance correlates temporally with the reduction in calcium ion concentration in the coronary sinus effluent (Fig. 18–12).[52]

The magnitude of myocardial contractile depression caused by the ionic agents is also related to the osmolality of the solution.[53] The 1.5 ratio ionic agents also cause longer lasting effects on myocardial metabolism. After injection, myocardial uptake of free fatty acids increases, and uptake of lactate and of glucose decreases. The clinical and functional significance of this observation has not been defined.[54]

The net clinical consequence of all these effects is that selective coronary arteriography with ionic 1.5 ratio agents causes a transient

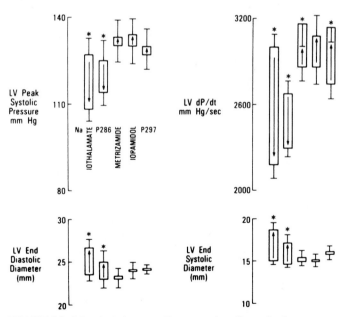

FIGURE 18–11. Block diagrams illustrating the effects of selective intracoronary injection of 1.5 ratio ionic (iothalamate), 3.0 ratio ionic (P-286 = ioxaglate), and 3.0 ratio nonionic contrast agents (metrizamide, iopamidol, and P-297) in volumes comparable to those used in clinical coronary arteriography. The data presented are for left ventricular peak systolic pressure, peak systolic dP/dt, and end-diastolic and end-systolic diameters. One end of each block indicates the average value and the standard error of the mean (SEM) during the control period, and the other end indicates the average value and SEM at the peak of the response. The direction of the change is indicated by the arrow in each block. The ionic agents depress left ventricular myocardial performance, whereas the nonionic agents enhance it. (From Higgins, C.B., Sovak M., Schmidt, W.S., et al.: Direct myocardial effects of intracoronary administration of new contrast materials with low osmolality. Invest. Radiol. 15:39, 1980, with permission.)

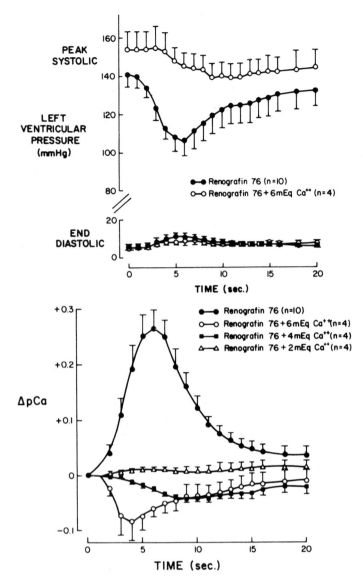

FIGURE 18–12. The time-related changes in left ventricular pressure *(left panel)* and the negative log of coronary sinus ionized calcium pCa *(right panel)* following selective left coronary injection of Renografin-76 with and without calcium enrichment. (An increase in pCa represents a decrease in calcium ion concentration.) Note that calcium enrichment increases coronary sinus calcium concentration and attenuates the contrast agent–induced depression of myocardial contractile performance. (From Bourdillion, P.D., Bettmann, M.A., McCracken S., et al.: Effects of a new nonionic and a conventional ionic contrast agent on coronary sinus ionized calcium and left ventricular hemodynamics in dogs. J. Am. Coll. Cardiol. 6:845–853, 1985. Reprinted with permission from the American College of Cardiology.)

decrease in systemic arterial pressure, whereas injections of 3.0 ratio and 6.0 ratio nonionic agents produce little or no change. Of the 1.5 ratio ionic agent formulations, calcium-binding formulations cause a greater drop than non–calcium-binding formulations.[55] In general, the overall magnitude of the effect of any particular contrast agent on arterial pressure, however, is modest and of little clinical importance. The effect of the contrast agent itself is typically overshadowed by the effect of the voluntarily held inspiration that the patient performs during the injection (Fig. 18–13).

Cardiac Electrophysiologic Effects

Not surprisingly, contrast agents affect several cardiac electrophysiologic properties. Many contrast agent–induced adverse reactions are due to alterations in these properties. Indeed, until Sones

serendipitously observed that inadvertent selective coronary injection of a diatrizoate contrast agent did not cause cardiac arrest, the prevailing belief was that the heart could not tolerate selective intracoronary injection of iodinated contrast agents.

The cardiac electrophysiologic effects of contrast agents may be divided into those of impulse formation and conduction, repolarization, and arrhythmias.

Impulse Formation and Conduction

A transient reduction in sinus node rate of depolarization accompanies selective coronary injection of 1.5 ratio ionic contrast agents. Typically, the reduction in heart rate is greatest 10 to 15 seconds after injection, and the heart rate returns to baseline values within 30 seconds (Fig. 18–14). The degree of slowing evoked by right coronary injection is greater than that caused by left coronary injection, presumably because the arterial supply to the sinoatrial and atrioventricular nodes is most commonly derived from the right coronary artery.[56] Because bradycardia also follows selective left coronary injection, however, the mechanism is clearly more complex than simply a direct effect on the sinoatrial node. The response may also be evoked by superselective infusion of contrast agents into the sinoatrial nodal artery. It is attenuated but not abolished by pharmacologic autonomic blockade.[57] On the other hand, the bradycardia caused by injection into an artery that does not supply the sinoatrial node is completely blocked by atropine.[58] These observations show that the bradycardia is due to a combination of a direct depression of impulse formation in the sinoatrial node and an autonomically mediated reflex. The degree of slowing caused by 3.0 ratio nonionic and ionic agents and 6.0 ratio agents is less than that evoked by 1.5 ratio ionic agents.[59, 60]

In general, this slowing is of little clinical significance, because it may be minimized with use of proper operator technique. The slowing is more pronounced when the impulse-forming cells are allowed to remain in contact with the contrast agent for a longer period of time. Such circumstances occur when the duration of the intracoronary injection is excessive, when the injection is made after a period of obstruction of coronary flow by a catheter tip wedged in the coronary orifice, or when a wedged catheter tip is not promptly removed from a coronary orifice to allow washout of the contrast agent.[61]

Selective intracoronary injection of contrast agents also prolongs atrioventricular conduction by slowing conduction through the atrioventricular node without affecting infranodal conduction.[62] In contrast with the effect on the sinoatrial node, the effect on the atrioventricular node has no autonomic component, and the degree of impairment of its conduction is not influenced by pharmacologic autonomic blockade.[57] The degree of impairment of atrioventricular nodal conduction evoked by 3.0 ratio and 6.0 ratio nonionic agents is less than that evoked by 1.5 ratio ionic agents.

Repolarization

Prolongation of ventricular myocardial repolarization occurs in response to selective intracoronary injection of all contrast agents and is reflected in a prolongation of the QT interval on the body surface electrocardiogram.[63] This effect is the result of three properties of a contrast agent formulation, which combine to delay repolarization. These properties are (1) the specific contrast agent molecule; (2) the osmolality of the contrast agent formulation; and (3) the ionic composition, including calcium-binding properties, of the contrast agent formulation.

The 1.5 ratio ionic agents evoke a greater prolongation of the QT interval than either the 3.0 ratio ionic agent, which is intermediate, or the 3.0 ratio nonionic agents, which prolong it the least.[17, 20, 55, 64-66] The maximum prolongation of the QT interval after selective intracoronary injection of a 3.0 ratio nonionic agent is approximately 20 msec, as opposed to 30 msec for the 3.0 ratio ionic agent. The prolongation evoked by 1.5 ratio ionic agents, however, not only is considerably greater but also varies substantially in relation to the calcium-binding properties of the different

LEFT CORONARY ARTERIOGRAPHY WITH HYPAQUE-76™

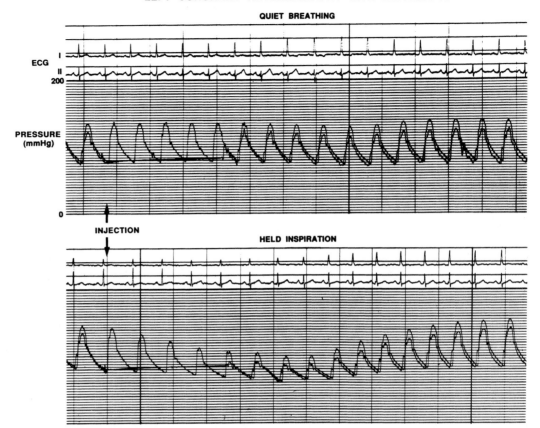

FIGURE 18–13. Comparison of the time-related changes in arterial pressure during clinical coronary arteriography with a 1.5 ratio ionic contrast agent during quiet breathing and during the customary held inspiration. Note that the majority of the decrease in arterial pressure is caused by the hemodynamic effect of breath holding.

formulations. Formulations that are not enriched with calcium, such as MD-76 and Renografin-76, prolong the QT interval by as much as 160 msec. On the other hand, calcium-enriched formulations such as Hypaque-76 prolong the QT interval by only 50 msec,[55, 67] a duration longer than that of the nonionic 3.0 ratio agents but similar to that of the 3.0 ratio ionic agent (Fig. 18–15).

Ventricular Fibrillation Threshold

Ventricular fibrillation is a dramatic adverse reaction to selective coronary arteriography. It occurs as a consequence of both the inherent properties of the contrast agent and the operator technique. All contrast agents decrease the heart's resistance to ventricular fibrillation, as measured by the ventricular fibrillation threshold, the square-wave current required to induce ventricular fibrillation. This effect persists for approximately 60 seconds after selective coronary injection (Fig. 18–16). The degree of reduction of ventricular fibrillation threshold by contrast agents is influenced by the quantity of contrast agent injected, the duration of injection, and the properties and formulation of the particular contrast agent molecule.[61] The ventricular fibrillation threshold is also reduced by myocardial ischemia.[68] The combination of ischemia and contrast agent injection reduces the threshold even further.[61] Both the 3.0 ratio nonionic agents and the 3.0 ratio ionic agent cause less reduction of ventricular fibrillation threshold than do the 1.5 ratio ionic agents.[69]

Also, significant differences among the ionic compositions of the different formulations of the 1.5 ratio ionic agents affect their fibrillatory propensity. These differences are in the content of two important ions—sodium and calcium.[70]

Early experience with coronary angiography, in which ionic diatrizoate-based contrast agents were used, involved considerable work to determine the optimal composition of the cationic component of the solution. If sodium was used to fill the entire cation space, the resulting formulation would have a sodium concentration of 1000 mEq/L, a concentration that would certainly have detrimental electrophysiologic effects when injected selectively into the coronary arteries. Consequently, a portion of the cation space was filled with methylglucamine, a cation that is not electrophysiologically active. Reducing the sodium concentration below 118 mEq/L, however, was found to increase the fibrillatory propensity of an ionic contrast agent formulation.[71] A sodium concentration between 150 and 190 mEq/L was found to cause the least ventricular fibrillation in experimental and clinical studies.[29, 40, 72, 73] Thus, although diatrizoate is marketed in many formulations with different sodium concentrations, the formulations that are appropriate for

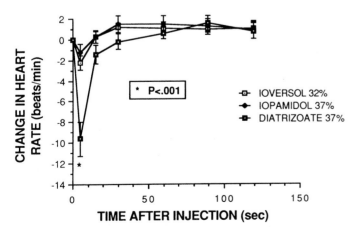

FIGURE 18–14. The time-related change in heart rate after left coronary arteriography with 1.5 ratio ionic and two 3.0 ratio nonionic contrast agents. The decrease caused by the 1.5 ratio ionic contrast agent is greater. (From Hirshfeld, J.W., Jr., Wieland, J., Davis, C.A., et al.: Hemodynamic and electrocardiographic effects of ioversol during cardiac angiography: Comparison with diatrizoate. Invest. Radiol. 24:138–144, 1989, with permission.)

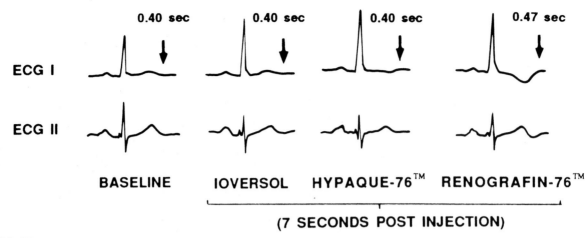

FIGURE 18–15. A comparison of the electrocardiographic changes caused by left coronary arteriography with 1.5 ratio ionic contrast agents with (Renografin-76) and without (Hypaque-76) calcium-binding activity and a 3.0 ratio nonionic agent (ioversol). Representative complexes from ECG leads I and II are shown. The preinjection complexes are shown on the left. The corresponding complexes recorded at the peak effect (7 seconds after injection) are shown on the right. The changes are most marked after the injection of a calcium-binding 1.5 ratio ionic contrast agent.

use in coronary arteriography have a sodium concentration between 160 and 190 mEq/L.

The other important property of a contrast agent formulation that influences its electrophysiologic activity is its calcium-binding activity. The formulations of all contrast agents contain EDTA as a chelating agent to sequester trace quantities of heavy-metal contaminants left in the preparation from manufacturing. EDTA is an avid calcium chelator. In one diatrizoate preparation (Hypaque-76), the EDTA is enriched with calcium to reduce its calcium-binding potential. In the other two preparations (MD-76 and Renografin-76), the EDTA is not calcium-enriched, and, in addition, sodium citrate (another calcium-chelating agent) is added to the formulation. Thus, the latter two formulations have considerably greater calcium-binding activity than the former two.

The difference between the calcium-enriched and the calcium-binding formulations is clearly detectable clinically and is clinically important. Hypocalcemia delays ventricular repolarization, which prolongs the QT interval. Also, because myocardial contractile force depends on calcium-mediated actin-myosin interaction, hypocalcemia can reduce myocardial contractile force. Ionic contrast agent formulations with calcium-binding activity cause a greater prolongation of the QT interval than do otherwise identical formulations that do not bind calcium (see Fig. 18–15).[55, 69] In addition, they cause a greater decrease in arterial pressure after intracoronary injection (Fig. 18–17; see Fig. 18–12).[55]

In 1978, Thompson and colleagues and Violante and associates

showed that the frequency of ventricular fibrillation caused by experimental intracoronary injection of Renografin-76 in dogs was reduced by the addition of calcium ions.[49, 74] Subsequently, Wolf found that the reduction in ventricular fibrillation threshold caused by Renografin-76 was attenuated by the addition of 5 mEq of calcium chloride per L.[61] Wolf and colleagues also found that under identical experimental conditions, Hypaque-76 caused less reduction in ventricular fibrillation threshold than did Renografin-76.[69] In subsequent clinical studies, investigators have observed a reduction in the frequency of episodes of ventricular fibrillation during clinical coronary arteriography, from 0.5 to 2.4 percent in patients studied with Renografin-76 to 0 to 0.1 percent in patients studied with Angiovist, a non–calcium-binding diatrizoate agent.[75-77] (*Note*: Angiovist is no longer marketed in the United States. However, it is identical to Hypaque-76, which is marketed in the United States.)

The 3.0 ratio nonionic agents and the 3.0 ratio ionic agents have been shown experimentally to have less fibrillatory propensity than calcium-binding formulations of 1.5 ratio ionic agents.[61] Differences in fibrillatory propensity between the 3.0 ratio agents and the non–calcium-binding formulations of 1.5 ratio ionic agents have not been demonstrated, however.

Because ventricular fibrillation is such a rare event in cardiac angiography,[76, 78, 79] demonstration of a statistically significant difference in the frequency of ventricular fibrillation between two contrast agents would require a large study population (more than 1000 patients per group). One study compared the frequency of ventricular fibrillation in patients randomized to receive either Renografin-76 or iopamidol during coronary angioplasty, a circumstance in which myocardial ischemia is often provoked. In this study, the Renografin-76 group had a 2.3 percent frequency of ventricular fibrillation, whereas the iopamidol group had a 0.7 percent frequency.[80] If a non–calcium-binding formulation of diatrizoate had been used instead of Renografin-76, the frequency of ventricular fibrillation in the diatrizoate group would probably have been lower. In a trial in diagnostic cardiac angiography involving 2166 patients randomized between Hypaque-76 and iohexol, only one episode of ventricular fibrillation occurred (in the Hypaque-76 group).[34] Thus, because the frequency of ventricular fibrillation caused by non–calcium-binding formulations of 1.5 ratio agents is so low in clinical use, the 3.0 ratio agents do not offer any clinically important advantage over non–calcium-binding 1.5 ratio agents with respect arrhythmia generation.

Other Noncardiovascular Effects

Most studies of the noncardiovascular effects of angiographic contrast agents have been performed with the use of intravenous

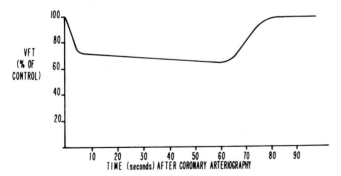

FIGURE 18–16. The time-related change in ventricular fibrillation threshold after left coronary injection of a 1.5 ratio ionic contrast agent. The curve is a smoothed compilation of many determinations. The heart's vulnerability to ventricular fibrillation increases after injection. The increased vulnerability persists for nearly a minute after injection. (From Wolf, G.L.: The fibrillatory properties of contrast agents. Invest Radiol. 15:s208, 1980, with permission.)

(QUIET BREATHING)

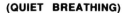

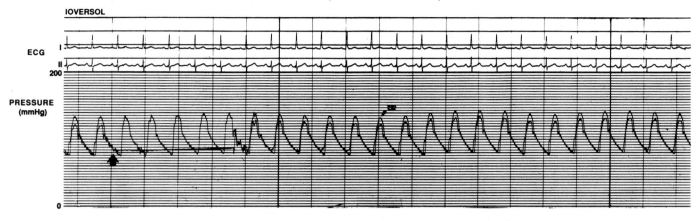

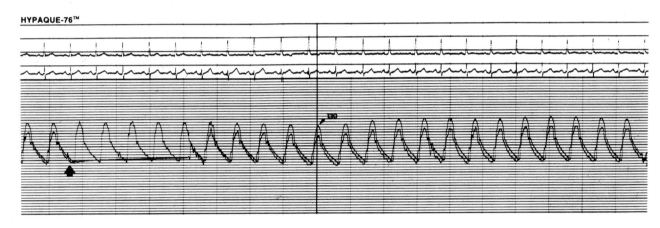

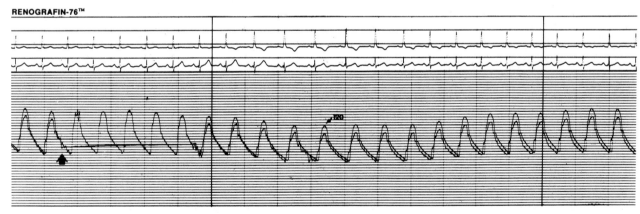

FIGURE 18–17. The time-related changes in systolic arterial pressure and electrocardiography caused by left coronary arteriography with 1.5 ratio ionic contrast agents with (Renografin-76) and without (Hypaque-76) calcium-binding activity and a 3.0 ratio nonionic agent (ioversol). The recordings were made during quiet breathing to isolate the effect of the contrast agent. Note that the decrease in arterial pressure is greatest with the calcium-binding 1.5 ratio ionic agent and is least with the nonionic agent.

injections for other radiographic procedures, such as intravenous urography and computed tomography. Thus, they do not strictly replicate the circumstances occurring in cardiac angiography. Nevertheless, they do provide some useful information concerning other effects of these agents.

Immediate Generalized, or Anaphylactoid, Reaction

The immediate generalized reaction has been termed the *anaphylactoid reaction* because it mimics γ-E immunoglobulin (IgE)–mediated anaphylaxis. This reaction is perhaps the most feared of all reactions, because it can be life threatening. The fully developed

reaction is caused by the release of large quantities of histamine. It typically occurs after the initial injection of contrast agent and is not related to the volume of contrast agent injected. Such reactions include varying severities of urticaria; angioedema, including laryngeal edema; bronchospasm; vasodilation; and increased capillary permeability. Severe immediate generalized reactions can produce life-threatening circulatory collapse or airway obstruction.

These reactions do not appear to be immunologically mediated. No IgE antibody to any contrast agent has ever been identified, and the reactions can occur during a patient's first-ever exposure to a contrast agent.[81] The final common pathway of the immediate generalized reaction is the activation of the complement pathway, leading to mast cell degranulation. The mechanism by which the reaction is initiated is not known.[82]

The frequency of all immediate generalized reactions, including minor urticaria, to 1.5 ratio ionic agents is approximately 5 percent.[83] The frequency of life-threatening immediate generalized reactions to 1.5 ratio ionic agents is approximately 0.1 percent.[84] No diagnostic test is available to detect patients at risk for an immediate generalized reaction.

The severe immediate generalized reaction has long been known to occur after injection of 1.5 ratio ionic agents. Severe immediate generalized reactions to 3.0 ratio nonionic agents have also been reported.[82] Investigators believe, but have not yet proved, that the frequency of severe immediate generalized reactions to 3.0 ratio nonionic contrast agents is less than the frequency of such severe reactions to 1.5 ratio ionic agents. Data that support this idea include a reduced overall fatality rate after exposure to contrast agent[85] and a small frequency of repeat reactions when 3.0 ratio nonionic agents are used in patients who have previously had an immediate generalized reaction to 1.5 ratio ionic agents.[86, 87] Also, the frequency of cutaneous reactions to the 3.0 ratio nonionic contrast agents is less than the frequency of such reactions to the 1.5 ratio agents.

On the other hand, Lasser and associates have reported that pretreatment with two doses of 32 mg of methylprednisolone 12 hours and 2 hours before contrast agent administration causes a substantial reduction in the frequency of all adverse reactions to 1.5 ratio ionic contrast agents (9.5 to 6.4 percent), including severe, life-threatening reactions (0.7 to 0.2 percent).[88] Investigators have not compared the clinical efficacy of corticosteroid pretreatment with that of substitution of a 3.0 ratio nonionic contrast agent for prevention of immediate generalized reactions in patients who have had a previous reaction.

Effects on Renal Function

Renal excretion is essentially the sole means of elimination of contrast agents. The quantity of contrast agent molecules administered is often quite large (more than 100 g). This material functions as an osmotic diuretic and probably also causes transient mild renal dysfunction. This dysfunction is not detectable with routine screening tests in individuals with normal renal function because it is obscured by the renal reserve capacity. In individuals with pre-existing renal disease, diabetes mellitus, or reduced cardiac output, however, the risk and severity of renal injury increase substantially.[89–92]

Clinically important renal failure is extremely rare in patients who undergo cardiac angiography with 1.5 ratio ionic agents, who have no diabetes or pre-existing renal disease, and who receive a total contrast-agent dose less than 125 mL. On the other hand, patients with the combination of pre-existing renal insufficiency and low cardiac output, or pre-existing renal insufficiency and diabetes mellitus, have approximately a 40 percent chance of developing a detectable increase in serum creatinine after exposure to 1.5 ratio ionic contrast agents. In fewer than 10 percent of these high-risk patients who develop measurable changes in renal function, however, is the renal failure severe enough to require dialysis.[92]

The mechanism of contrast agent–induced renal injury is probably a combination of medullary ischemia, which is due to vasoconstriction caused by the contrast agent, and a direct toxic effect of high concentrations of contrast agent on renal tubular cells.[93, 94] A recently reported randomized trial compared a 1.5 ratio agent (Renografin-76) to a 3.0 ratio nonionic agent (iohexol) in terms of the frequency of contrast agent–induced nephropathy following cardiac angiography.[95] The four study groups included patients with and without diabetes mellitus and with and without renal insufficiency (serum creatinine ≥1.5). Renal function was quantified by measurement of serum creatinine before and 24 and 48 hours after contrast agent exposure. The end point was an increase in serum creatinine of at least 1.0 mg/dL within 48 hours. The end-point frequencies are shown in Figure 18–18. Contrast nephropathy was extremely rare (2 of 674) in patients without renal insufficiency. In patients with renal insufficiency, contrast nephropathy occurred more commonly but was less frequent with iohexol than with diatrizoate. The presence of diabetes did not increase the risk of contrast nephropathy in patients without renal insufficiency, whereas diabetic patients with renal insufficiency were more likely to develop contrast nephropathy. Many of the episodes coded as contrast nephropathy were, in fact, asymptomatic transient increases of serum creatinine that had no clinical consequence. However, a smaller number of patients (15 of 1196) had a clinically severe episode with either oliguria (7) or requirement for dialysis (8). These patients, as a group, had more advanced renal insufficiency (mean serum creatinine 2.7 ± 1.2 mg/dL) and received relatively large volumes of contrast agent (mean volume 144 ± 52 mL). Of the patients who required dialysis, five received iohexol and three received diatrizoate.[95]

Clinicians have believed that the frequency and severity of contrast agent–induced renal injury can be minimized in susceptible patients by paying careful attention to maintenance of optimal hydration and cardiac output, concurrent furosemide diuresis, and, perhaps, concurrent administration of mannitol.[94] The efficacy of such strategies has been studied only recently.[96] Solomon and colleagues compared pretreatment with mannitol to furosemide-induced diuresis in the prevention of contrast agent nephropathy.

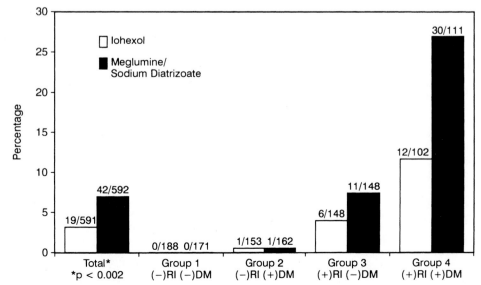

FIGURE 18–18. The percentage of patients who developed contrast agent–induced nephropathy after cardiac angiography segregated by contrast agent type, renal insufficiency, and diabetes mellitus. Nephropathy is defined as an increase in serum creatinine ≥1.0 mg/dL from baseline within 48 to 72 hours after contrast administration. Renal insufficiency is defined as a baseline serum creatinine ≥1.5 mg/dL. The number of patients in each group and the number who developed nephropathy are displayed at the top of each bar. RI = renal insufficiency; DM = diabetes mellitus. Open bars = iohexol; solid bars = diatrizoate. Note that nephropathy is essentially absent in the two groups without renal insufficiency, and that in the groups with renal insufficiency, iohexol causes less nephropathy than diatrizoate. (From Rudnick M.R., Goldfarb, S., Wexler, L., et al.: Nephrotoxicity of ionic and nonionic contrast media in 1196 patients: A randomized trial. Kidney Int. 47:254–261, 1995, with permission.)

Unfortunately, there was no control over either contrast agent volume or contrast agent type in the study, and all patients received intravenous hydration. They found no advantage of either furosemide diuresis or mannitol treatment over hydration alone in protecting against contrast agent nephropathy.[94]

The frequency of contrast agent–induced renal failure may have decreased in recent years. Parfrey and associates recently reported the experience of administering large volumes of contrast agent (both 1.5 ratio and 3.0 ratio agents) to 135 patients with renal insufficiency. The patients had serum creatinine levels between 2 and 5 mg/100 mL, and some had coexisting diabetes. The frequency of clinically significant renal injury (defined as an increase in serum creatinine levels greater than 50 percent) was 7 percent, whereas a comparable control group of hospitalized patients who did not receive contrast agents exhibited a 1.5 percent frequency of deterioration of renal function.[97] No difference in the frequency of renal injury was observed between patients studied with 1.5 ratio agents and those studied with 3.0 ratio agents. However, it is important to point out that the average volume of contrast agent administered was 110 mL. Such experience suggests that careful attention to the patient's hydrational status and limitation of the quantity of contrast agent administered enhance the safety of the use of both 1.5 and 3.0 ratio contrast agents in patients with previously existing renal disease.

Effects on Pulmonary Function

All contrast agents affect airway dynamics, causing a decrease in the 1-second forced expiratory volume.[98] In healthy individuals, this change is modest (0.21 L per second, or 7.5 percent) and is not clinically apparent unless measured. In patients with underlying airway obstruction, such as asthma, however, such a decrease could be clinically important. The decrease in 1-second forced expiratory volume caused by the 3.0 ratio nonionic agents (0.03 L per second, or 0.8 percent) is less than that caused by the 1.5 ratio ionic agents.[99]

Coughing frequently accompanies injections of contrast agents into the right side of the heart and into the pulmonary artery. Not only is this side effect unpleasant for the patient, but also it can compromise the quality of the examination. Presumably, the coughing is caused by irritation of the lungs by the contrast agent as it passes through the pulmonary microcirculation. It occurs in two thirds of studies with 1.5 ratio agents. In one study comparing 1.5 ratio agents with ioxaglate, the frequency of cough evoked by ioxaglate during selective pulmonary angiography was only 0.4 percent.[100]

Gastrointestinal Effects

The most frequent adverse reactions to 1.5 ratio ionic contrast agents are nausea and vomiting, which occur in 5 to 15 percent of patients. This response typically occurs only during the first injection of contrast agent and does not recur with subsequent injections. The frequency of nausea is somewhat less with the 3.0 ratio ionic agents[20, 22] and is virtually eliminated with the 3.0 ratio nonionic agents.[22, 49, 101]

Hematologic Effects

Contrast agents have several measurable effects on blood cells and blood coagulation that are of potential clinical importance. In clinically used concentrations, all contrast agent molecules cause red blood cell deformation. This deformation occurs both through a direct toxic effect on the cell membrane, which produces a crenated echinocyte,[102] and through osmotic extraction of water from the interior of the red cell, which produces a "desiccocyte."[103] Of the two effects, the osmotic effect is more important; as a result, the effect of the 3.0 ratio agents is less than the effect of the 1.5 ratio ionic agents.[104] Although such actions can potentially affect blood viscosity and the rheology of flow through the microcirculation, the clinical significance of these effects has not been established. Nor has the clinical importance of the measurable

differences between the 1.5 ratio agents and the 3.0 ratio agents been established.

The antithrombotic properties of the different contrast agents have received considerable attention in recent years. Interest in this area has been prompted by reports of coronary embolization of thrombi that formed at the tips of angioplasty guide catheters when nonionic contrast agents were used.[105] This has led to the concern that nonionic contrast-agent formulations are, in some way, prothrombotic.

All intravascular contrast agents have inherent anticoagulant properties. If blood is mixed with clinically used concentrations of contrast agents, its clotting time is prolonged. The magnitude of this effect is greatest for the 1.5 ratio ionic agents, particularly for those containing citrate in their formulations, and for ioxaglate, the 3.0 ratio ionic agent. Both diatrizoate and ioxaglate prolong the whole-blood clotting time from 15 minutes to more than 330 minutes. The 3.0 ratio nonionic agents also prolong the clotting time, but to a lesser degree (from 15 minutes to 160 minutes).[106, 107]

In addition, compared with the nonionic agents, ionic contrast agents appear to impair thrombus formation on cardiac catheters and guidewires. Scanning electron micrographic studies of angioplasty guidewires and guide catheters show considerably greater deposition of fibrin and platelets on the guidewires and in the catheter lumina when ionic contrast agents are used than when nonionic agents are used.[108]

The anticoagulant property of contrast agents provides a margin of antithrombotic safety that can partially compensate for shortcomings of operator technique, such as allowing blood to mingle with contrast agent in catheters and syringes.[109] Clearly, the reduced anticoagulant activity of the nonionic 3.0 ratio agents provides less margin for safety in this regard. Ideally, these differences should be clinically unimportant if operators adhere to proper technique. Systemic heparinization, which is employed in many cardiac angiographic studies, should further reduce the risk of thrombus formation. Arterial embolization has occurred, however, during coronary angiography in heparinized patients studied with 3.0 ratio nonionic agents.[104]

Effects on Blood Vessels

All contrast agents exert toxic effects on endothelium. Ultrastructural changes are visible in the aortic endothelium for up to 4 hours after the intravenous injection (1 mL/kg) of 1.5 ratio agents having an iodine concentration of 370 mg/mL.[110] The significance of these observations has not been determined, however. Similar evidence of endothelial damage done by contrast agents has been derived from silver-staining studies of the aorta after contrast agent exposure.[111] This damage appears to be predominantly an osmotically mediated effect, with the effects of the 1.5 ratio ionic agents the most pronounced and the effects of the 3.0 ratio ionic and nonionic agents equivalent to each other and less than those of the 1.5 ratio ionic agents. The significance of these observations for cardiac angiography is also undetermined. The silver-staining studies involve 5-minute applications of undiluted contrast agent to isolated aorta, a condition considerably harsher than that occurring in arterial and cardiac angiography in vivo. On the other hand, these observations may be relevant for phlebography, in which undiluted contrast agent remains in contact with the veins for a longer period of time.

CRITERIA FOR SELECTION OF CONTRAST AGENTS FOR CARDIAC ANGIOGRAPHY

The Contrast Agent Selection Problem

The creation of the 3.0 and the 6.0 ratio contrast agents has presented cardiac angiographers with both an opportunity and a dilemma. The opportunity derives from the low-osmolality agents' clear-cut hemodynamic and electrophysiologic superiority and associated reduced adverse reaction rates. The dilemma derives from the substantial price disparity between the 1.5 ratio agents and the low-osmolality agents. In the United States, the price disparity varies between 12- and 25-fold, depending on locally negotiated purchasing agreements. At the time of this writing, iodixanol had not been released in the United States, and its pricing is unknown but is expected to be somewhat higher than the price of 3.0 ratio agents. (In Europe, the price disparity is smaller, because 1.5 ratio agents are more expensive than in the United States, and the 3.0 ratio agents are cheaper.)

The dilemma is entirely economically driven, as there is no reason to postulate any performance superiority for the 1.5 ratio agents. Thus, the issue is purely one of comparison of the increased cost of the low-osmolality agents with their performance benefit. The financial impact of choosing between 1.5 and 3.0 ratio agents is substantial—at the levels of both the individual laboratory and society. If a laboratory that used 1.5 ratio agents exclusively was to switch completely to using low-osmolality agents, the expense increment would most likely exceed the facility's total expense for technical personnel. The aggregate increment in expense over 2 years for a moderately large-volume laboratory (performing 2000 procedures per year) is equivalent to the purchase price of a complete cineradiographic x-ray unit. At the societal level, Jacobson and Rosenquist estimate that universal adoption of 3.0 ratio contrast agents for all radiologic examinations requiring intravascular contrast agents would cost the United States' health care system $1.1 billion.[112] This calculation includes the incremental savings derived from the reduced costs of treating the expected smaller number of severe contrast-agent reactions that would occur if only 3.0 ratio agents were used. The authors calculated that the universal use of 3.0 ratio contrast agents in the United States would avoid 293 contrast agent–related fatalities per year, at a cost of $3.4 million per death averted, or $106,000 per year of life saved. This monetary value is large compared with the prices that society is willing to pay for other life-prolonging procedures.[111]

The issue is particularly important in adult cardiac angiography because large volumes of contrast agent are used in a typical procedure and a large number of procedures (1.3 million annually in the United States) are performed. The price disparity compels physicians to assess the clinical importance of the superior properties of the low-osmolality agents and to confront the issue of assigning a monetary value to the performance difference. In addition, with the release of 6.0 ratio agents, the relative price-performance benefit of 6.0 ratio agents to that of 3.0 ratio agents must be considered.

A priori, one would expect that the superior hemodynamic and cardiac electrophysiologic properties of the low-osmolality agents would confer greater safety and, as a consequence, better efficacy than that of the 1.5 ratio ionic agents. Furthermore, one might expect that the 6.0 ratio agents would offer even greater safety and efficacy than the 3.0 ratio agents. On the other hand, it is also possible that only a subset of all patients undergoing cardiac angiography actually derive clinically important benefits from low-osmolality agents compared with 1.5 ratio agents. This issue has been addressed by several clinical trials conducted in recent years.

Clinical Trials Comparing Different Classes of Contrast Agents

In 1988, DiBattiste and associates reported a 5000-patient observational registry of cardiac angiographic procedures performed exclusively with 1.5 ratio agents.[78] This study found that the frequency of adverse events increased as the severity of heart disease (assessed clinically by New York Heart Association functional class, hemodynamically by left ventricular end-diastolic pressure, or angiographically by the extent of coronary artery disease) increased (Fig. 18–19). These observations suggested that for less severely ill patients, the risk of an adverse reaction with 1.5 ratio agents was so small that low-osmolality agents might confer little additional benefit.

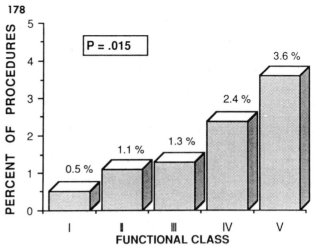

178

FIGURE 18–19. The relationship of the frequency of major contrast agent–related adverse reactions during cardiac angiography to New York Heart Association clinical functional class. (Class V represents patients who were in extreme circulatory failure at the time of the procedure.) Note that the frequency of adverse reactions is increased in the more seriously ill patients. (From DiBattiste, P.M., Kussmaul, W.G., Hirshfeld, J.W.J., et al.: The safety of cardiac angiography with conventional contrast agents. Am. J. Cardiol. 1988; 66(3):355–361. Reprinted with permission.)

Two large observational studies of intravenous administration were reported in 1988 and 1990. These studies also supported the concept that rates of contrast agent–related adverse events were decreased by 3.0 ratio nonionic agents. These trials were not blind or randomized and involved predominantly noncardiac procedures. In Australia, 109,546 procedures were evaluated. Of these, 79,278 procedures were performed with 1.5 ratio ionic agents, resulting in a severe adverse reaction frequency of 0.09 percent and two deaths. The 3.0 ratio nonionic agents were used in 32,268 procedures, which resulted in a severe adverse reaction frequency of 0.02 percent and no deaths.[113] In Japan, 337,647 procedures were evaluated. Of these, 169,284 procedures were performed with 1.5 ratio agents, which resulted in a "severe" adverse reaction frequency of 0.22 percent and one death; 168,363 procedures were performed with 3.0 ratio agents with a 0.04 percent frequency of severe adverse reactions and one death.[114] Although there are differences between the two studies in the overall frequencies of severe adverse reactions, these probably reflect differences in definitions. In both studies, the rates of severe adverse reactions in procedures performed with 3.0 ratio nonionic agents were statistically significantly lower than the corresponding rates for procedures performed with 1.5 ratio agents. On the other hand, because contrast agent–related deaths were so rare, no statistically significant difference between the two classes of agents could be detected for death.

In a study of the adverse reactions to contrast agent administration, Wolf and colleagues surveyed a group of more than 13,000 patients who received either 1.5 ratio ionic agents or 3.0 ratio nonionic agents for intravenous examinations.[115] They observed similar differences in the frequency of minor adverse reactions (2.5 percent in the 1.5 ratio ionic agent group and 0.6 percent in the 3.0 ratio nonionic agent group) and in the frequency of reactions requiring treatment (1.3 percent in the 1.5 ratio ionic agent group and 0.2 percent in the 3.0 ratio nonionic agent group). No deaths occurred in either contrast agent group. They also observed a slightly greater frequency of aftereffects in patients who received the 1.5 ratio ionic agents. Forty percent of patients who received a 1.5 ratio agent reported not feeling completely well for at least 24 hours after the procedure, compared with 32 percent of patients who received a 3.0 ratio nonionic agent.[115]

In 1992 two randomized trials were reported that compared 1.5 ratio agents with 3.0 ratio nonionic agents in cardiac angiography. One trial used Renografin-76 (a calcium-binding formulation),[116] and the other used Hypaque-76 (a non–calcium-binding formulation).[117] Both trials showed an increased frequency of adverse events in patients with more severe heart disease, and both trials showed a lower frequency of mild to moderate adverse events with 3.0 ratio agents but no difference in severe adverse events.

In 1994, Matthai and colleagues reported a single-center, randomized, blind trial of 2166 patients comparing Hypaque-76 to iohexol in cardiac angiography.[34] The patient population of this trial was nearly all inclusive in that only the most ill 3 percent of the laboratory's patient population was excluded from randomization, and all but five eligible patients were successfully randomized. This study again found a low overall incidence of clinically important contrast agent–related adverse events, with a reduced incidence in the group treated with iohexol (iohexol, 2.6 percent; diatrizoate, 4.6 percent; $P = .02$). The study also found that the adverse event rate and the disparity between the event rate for iohexol versus that for diatrizoate increased as the severity of cardiac disease increased. With the use of multiple markers of cardiovascular disease severity, the patient population was stratified into quartiles according to the risk of an adverse event, and the rates of adverse events were compared for the two contrast agent classes. The highest-risk quartile had an adverse event rate that was six times greater than that of the lower risk three quartiles (9 percent versus 1.5 percent). Also, in the high-risk quartile, the risk of an adverse event with diatrizoate was double that for iohexol (12 percent versus 6 percent; $P = .01$). In the three low-risk quartiles, the risk of an event was small, and there was no statistically significant difference between event rates for the two types of contrast agents. These observations suggest that low-osmolality contrast agents provide a substantial benefit to seriously ill patients but have little or no benefit for less ill low-risk patients.

The variables that predicted risk were combined to create a risk-predicting algorithm. This algorithm classifies patients as high risk when they have had a previous adverse reaction to contrast agents or when they have two of the following three characteristics: age greater than 65 years, New York Heart Association functional class equal to IV, or left ventricular end-diastolic pressure greater than 18 mm Hg. This algorithm classified one third of the laboratory's patient population as high risk. Retrospective application of a selective-use strategy by assigning high-osmolality contrast to low-risk patients and low-osmolality agents to high-risk patients yielded an overall adverse event rate that was indistinguishable from that expected for universal use of low-osmolality agents for all patients. However, the selective-use strategy reduced the expense for contrast agent threefold compared with the universal use of low-osmolality contrast.[34]

TABLE 18–4. SUGGESTED INDICATIONS FOR SELECTING LOW-OSMOLALITY CONTRAST AGENTS OVER 1.5 RATIO CONTRAST AGENTS FOR CARDIAC ANGIOGRAPHY

Indication	Rationale	Documentation of Effectiveness
Previous Adverse Reaction to Contrast Agents	Substitution of low-osmolality agent will minimize the likelihood of a reaction.	In this group, the reaction rate to 1.5 ratio agents is 7 × the reaction rate to 3.0 ratio agents.
Clinical-Hemodynamic Criteria At least two of the following: • Age ≥65 yr • Left ventricular end-diastolic pressure ≥16 mm Hg • New York Heart Assn. functional class = IV	The reduced circulatory stress associated with low-osmolality agents enables these patients with impaired cardiac performance to better tolerate the procedure.	In this group, the reaction rate to 1.5 ratio agents is 2 × the reaction rate to 3.0 ratio agents.
Impaired Renal Function • Serum creatinine ≥2.0 mg/dl	The slightly reduced renal stress associated with low-osmolality agents enables patients with renal insufficiency to tolerate the contrast agent better. However, the volume of contrast agent administered is a much more important determinant of renal injury than the type of contrast agent used.	In this group, the rate of detectable decrease in renal function with 1.5 ratio agents is 2 × the rate with 3.0 ratio agents. However, there is no difference between contrast agents in the rate of clinically important (oliguria or dialysis) adverse events.

Extremely High Cardiac Risk
Precarious hemodynamic state
• Left ventricular end-diastolic pressure >40 mm Hg
• Pulmonary capillary wedge pressure >30 mm Hg
• Arteriovenous oxygen difference >7.0 vol.%
• Requirement for pressor or other circulatory support
Severe or unstable coronary disease
• Ongoing acute myocardial infarction
• Severe unstable angina
• Rest angina with reversible ST segment changes
• Strongly positive exercise test
  ≥3-mm ST segment depression at low workload
  Extensive ischemia on thallium scanning
  Left ventricular dilation and lung uptake after exercise
Severe valvular heart disease
• Aortic valve area <0.7 cm²
• Mitral valve area <1.25 cm²
	The reduced circulatory stress associated with low-osmolality agents enables these critically ill patients (who constitute a small fraction of the total population of cardiac angiography patients) to tolerate the procedure better. In these fragile patients, limiting contrast agent volume is an important adjunct to procedure safety.	Based on clinical intuition. There are no rigorous randomized trials studying such patients.

Strategy for Selective Use of Low-Osmolality Contrast Agents

The problem of selecting the most appropriate contrast agent has stimulated considerable debate. Some individuals believe that the benefits of the 3.0 ratio agents outweigh their financial cost and that, accordingly, they should be used universally.[118] Others think that the 3.0 agents should be reserved for certain subsets of patients, but they have difficulty in identifying criteria to distinguish high-risk patients from low-risk ones.[119, 120]

The issue is brought to a particular focus in cardiac angiography, an expensive, widely used procedure that requires large volumes of contrast agent, which is performed in patients, many of whom have severe heart disease—the type of patient who may benefit the most from the advantages of 3.0 ratio agents. On the other hand, cardiac angiography is carried out in a highly controlled and monitored environment and is performed by physicians who are specifically trained to recognize and treat cardiovascular problems. Thus, an adverse event that might lead to severe problems in other environments is often promptly recognized, is preemptively treated, and resolves promptly with no residua. In addition, physicians can enhance the safety of cardiac angiography with 1.5 ratio agents by tailoring the conduct of the procedure to the patient's condition.

Currently available data indicate that in the high-risk one third of patients who undergo cardiac angiography, the superior properties of the 3.0 ratio agents clearly enhance the safety of the procedure. The use of a 3.0 ratio agent is important in these patients. However, in the low-risk two thirds of patients, a diagnostic-quality study can be obtained safely, without adverse reactions, with the use of a non–calcium-binding 1.5 ratio agent.

A framework for identifying high-risk patients who benefit from the use of 3.0 ratio agents is outlined in Table 18–4. The rationale behind each criterion and the documentation of its validity, if available, are also listed in the table.

The proposed indications fall into four categories, based on different rationales.

PRIOR ADVERSE REACTION TO CONTRAST AGENT. If a patient has had a *clearly documented* prior adverse reaction to intravascular contrast (generally either anaphylactoid or hemodynamic), such a patient has a sevenfold greater likelihood of a repeat reaction, and this likelihood is reduced by the substitution of a low-osmolality contrast agent. Such patients constitute approximately 2 percent of a laboratory's patient population. Thus, the use of low-osmolality contrast agents in these patients provides an important safety benefit and does not have a major financial impact on the overall contrast agent usage.

CLINICAL AND HEMODYNAMIC CRITERIA. These criteria identify patients who have a greater likelihood of having advanced heart disease—either advanced coronary disease or severe impairment of hemodynamic cardiac performance. Such patients, compared with low-risk patients, have a sixfold greater likelihood of an adverse event and enjoy a twofold reduction in risk when low-osmolality agents are substituted for high-osmolality agents.

IMPAIRED RENAL FUNCTION CRITERION. The problem of contrast agent nephropathy is confined to the subgroup of patients with baseline impaired renal function. Animal studies and a large randomized trial indicate that 3.0 ratio nonionic agents cause slightly less renal injury than a comparable dose of a 1.5 ratio agent. Clinical studies also clearly show that the risk of contrast agent nephropathy is strongly related to dose, with clinically important renal injury rare at total contrast-agent doses less than 100 mL. Consequently, there is a good rationale for using 3.0 ratio nonionic agents in all patients with significantly impaired renal function. It is important to point out, however, that limitation of dose is the most important way of protecting a patient from contrast agent–induced renal injury and that the use of a 3.0 ratio nonionic agent does not enable one to administer a large volume of contrast agent without risk.

EXTREMELY HIGH-RISK CATEGORY. Patients with the characteristics listed under this category are the most critically ill 3 percent of patients undergoing cardiac angiography. They have very little cardiovascular reserve, and their procedures should be performed with a minimum of cardiovascular stress. As is the case with patients with impaired renal function, a key strategy for minimizing procedure-related stress is, again, minimizing the dose of contrast agent. Omitting ventriculography and minimizing the number of coronary injections are good strategies for curtailing the total dose of contrast agent.

It is clear that current and future economic pressures will cause cardiologists and laboratory directors to consider the cost-benefit issue of contrast agent selection.[121] Universal adoption of 3.0 ratio agents for cardiac angiography is unwarranted. It is clear that diagnostic-quality studies can be obtained safely with 1.5 ratio agents in two thirds of the cardiac angiography patient population. What is not yet clear is whether the safety of the procedure can be further enhanced for high-risk patients by substituting 6.0 ratio agents for 3.0 ratio agents. This question is an important one for future clinical research in cardiac angiography.

References

1. Morgan, R.H.: Physical foundations of radiology. *In* Goodwin PN, et al. (eds.): Physical Foundations of Radiology. New York, Harper & Row, 1970.
2. Roentgen, W.C.: On a new kind of rays. Erst. Mitt. Sitzber. Phys.-Med. Ges. 1895, p. 137.
3. Berberich, J., and Hirsch, S.: Die rontgenographische Darstellum der Arterien und Venenam Lebenden. Klin. Wochenschr. 49:2226, 1923.
4. Brooks, B.: Intraarterial injection of sodium iodid. JAMA 82:1016, 1924.
5. Roseno, A.: Die intravenose Pyelographie. II. Mitteilung klinische Ergebnisse. Klin. Wochenschr. 8:1165, 1929.
6. Binz, A., and Rath, C.: Uber biochemische Eigenschaften von Derivaten des Pyridins und Chinolins. Biochem. Z. 203:218, 1928.
7. Swick, J.: Darstellum der Nierne und harnwefe in Rontgenbild durch intravenose Einbringung eines neuen Kontraststoffes des Uroselectans. Klin. Wochenschr. 8:2087, 1929.
8. Swick, M.: Intravenous urography by means of Uroselectan. Am. J. Surg. 8:405, 1930.
9. Forssman, W.: Uber Kontrastdarstellun der Hohlen des levenden rechten Herzens und der Lungenschlagader. Muench. Med. Wochenschr. 78:489, 1931.
10. Castellanos, A., Pereiras, R., and Garcia, A.: La angiocardiografica radio-opaca. Arch. Estud. Clin. 31:523, 1937.
11. Hoppe, J.O., Larsen, H.A., and Coulston, F.J.: Observations on the toxicity of a new urographic contrast medium, sodium 3,5-diacetamido-2,4,6 tri-iobenzoate (Hypaque sodium) and related compounds. J. Pharmacol. Exp. Ther. 116:394, 1956.
12. Hoppe, J.O.: Some pharmacological aspects of radiopaque compounds. Ann. N.Y. Acad. Sci. 78:727, 1959.
13. Hildner, F.J., Scherlag, B.J., and Samet, P.: Evaluation of Renografin M 76 as a contrast agent for angiocardiography. Radiology 100:329, 1971.
14. Almen, T.: Contrast agent design. J. Theor. Biol. 24:216, 1969.
15. Anonymous: Metrizamide: A non-ionic water-soluble contrast medium. Acta Radiol. Suppl. 1973.
16. Grainger, R.G.: Osmolalities of intravascular radiological contrast media. Br. J. Radiol. 53:739, 1980.
17. Tragardh, B., Lynch, P.R., and Vinciguerra, T.: Effects of metrizamide, a new non-ionic contrast medium, on cardiac function during coronary arteriography in the dog. Radiology 115:59, 1976.
18. Lindgren, E.: Iohexol: A non-ionic contrast medium: Pharmacology and toxicology. Acta Radiol. Suppl. 362, 1980.
19. Thompson, K.R., Evill, C.A., Fritzche, J., et al.: Comparison of iopamidol, ioxaglate, and diatrizoate during coronary angiography in dogs. Invest. Radiol. 15:234, 1980.
20. Hirshfeld, J.W., Jr., Wieland, J., Davis, C.A., et al.: Hemodynamic and electrocardiographic effects of ioversol during cardiac angiography comparison with diatrizoate. Invest. Radiol. 24:138, 1989.
21. Hirshfeld, J.W., Jr., Laskey, W.K., Martin, J.L., et al.: Hemodynamic changes induced by cardiac angiography with ioxaglate: Comparison with diatrizoate. J. Am. Coll. Cardiol. 2:954, 1983.
22. Wisneski, J.A., Gertz, E.W., Dahlgren, M., et al.: Comparison of low osmolality ionic (ioxaglate) versus nonionic (iopamidol) contrast media in cardiac angiography. Am. J. Cardiol. 63(7):489, 1989.
23. Almen, T.: Effects of iodixanol, iopentol, and metriozate on femoral blood flow after injection into the femoral artery of the dog. Acta Radiol. Suppl. 370:69, 1987.
24. Renaa, T., and Jacobsen, T.: Contrast media research: An investment for the future. Acta Radiol. Suppl. 370:9, 1987.
25. Aulie, M.A.: Effects of intravascular contrast media on blood-brain barrier: Comparison between iothalamate, iohexol, iopentol, and iodixanol. Acta Radiol. 28:329, 1987.
26. Jynge, P., Holten, T., Gronas, T., et al.: Nonionic x-ray contrast media and ions: Inotropic effects of calcium addition to iodixanol. (Abstract.) J. Mol. Cell. Cardiol. 1991;23(Suppl. 5):S86.

27. Hill, J.A., Cohen, M.B., Kou, W.H., et al.: Iodixanol, a new isosmotic nonionic contrast agent compared with iohexol in cardiac angiography. Am. J. Cardiol. 74(1):57, 1994.

28. Almen, T.: Effects of metrizamide and other contrast media on the isolated rabbit heart. Acta Radiol. Suppl. 335:216, 1973.

29. Simon, A.L., Shabetai, R., Lang, J.H., et al.: The mechanism of production of ventricular fibrillation in coronary angiography. A.J.R. 114:810, 1972.

30. Snyder, C.F., Formanek, A., Frech, R.S., et al.: The role of sodium in promoting ventricular arrhythmia during selective coronary arteriography. AJR 113:567, 1971.

31. Nycomed Inc.: Draft package insert for iodixanol 320. New York, 1995.

32. Shaw, D.D., and Potts, D.G.: Toxicity of iohexol. Invest. Radiol. 20:S10, 1984.

33. Nycomed Pharmaceuticals, Inc.: Upper range of mouse intravenous LD_{50} for Hypaque 76 as published in the package insert in ref. 31.

34. Matthai, W.H., Kussmaul, W.G., Krol, J., et al.: A comparison of low- with high-osmolality contrast agents in cardiac angiography. Identification of criteria for selective use. Circulation 89(1):291, 1994.

35. Steinberg, E.P., Moore, R.D., Gopalan, R., et al.: Safety and cost effectiveness of high-osmality as compared with low osmolality contrast material in patients undergoing cardiac angiography. N. Engl. J. Med. 326:425, 1992.

36. Dean, P.B., Kivisaari, L., and Kormano, M.: The diagnostic potential of contrast enhancement pharmacokinetics. Invest. Radiol. 13:533, 1978.

37. Newhouse, J.H.: Fluid compartment distribution of intravenous iothalamate in the dog. Invest. Radiol. 12:364, 1977.

38. Marshall, R.J., and Shepherd, J.T.: Effects of injections of hypertonic solutions on blood flow throughout the femoral artery of the dog. Am. J. Physiol. 197:952, 1959.

39. Read, R.C., Johnson, J.A., Vick, J.A., et al.: Vascular effects of hypertonic solutions. Circ. Res. 8:538, 1960.

40. Hilal, S.: Hemodynamic changes associated with intra-arterial injection of contrast media. Radiology 86:615, 1966.

41. Higgins, C.B., Gerber, K.H., Mattrey, R.F., et al.: Evaluation of the hemodynamic effects of intravenous administration of ionic and nonionic contrast materials. Radiology 142:681, 1983.

42. Gensini, G.G., Dubiel, J., Huntington P.P., et al.: Left ventricular end-diastolic pressure before and after coronary arteriography. Am. J. Cardiol. 27:453, 1971.

43. Wolfe, C.L., Winniford, M.D., Wheelan, K.R., et al.: Relation of coronary artery disease and left ventricular systolic dysfunction to left ventricular end-diastolic pressure after left ventriculography. Am. J. Cardiol. 55:1622, 1985.

44. Thompson, K.R., Evill, C.A., Fritzche, J., et al.: Comparison of iopamidol, ioxaglate, and diatrizoate during coronary angiography in dogs. Invest. Radiol. 15:234, 1980.

45. Higgins, C.B., Sovak, M., Schmidt, W.S., et al.: Direct myocardial effects of intracoronary administration of new contrast agent materials with low osmolality. Invest. Radiol. 15:39, 1980.

46. Thompson, K.R., Violante, M.R., Kenyon, T., et al.: Reduction of ventricular fibrillation using calcium-enriched Renografin-76. Invest. Radiol. 13:238, 1978.

47. Kozeny, G.A., Murdock, D.K., Euler, D.E., et al.: In vivo effect of acute changes in osmolality and sodium concentration in myocardial contractility. Am. J. Heart 109:290, 1985.

48. Baath, L., and Almen, T.: Reduction of the risk of ventricular fibrillation in the isolated rabbit heart by small additions of electrolytes to non-ionic monomeric contrast media. Acta. Radiol. 30(3):327, 1989.

49. Caulfield, J.B., Zir, L., and Hawthorne, J.W.: Blood calcium levels in the presence of arteriographic contrast material. Circulation 52:119, 1975.

50. Mallette, L.E., and Gomez, L.S.: Systemic hypocalcemia after clinical injections of radiographic contrast media: Amelioration by omission of calcium chelating agents. Radiology 147:677, 1983.

51. Morris, T.W., Sahler, L.G., and Fischer, H.W.: Calcium binding by radiopaque media. Invest. Radiol. 17:501, 1982.

52. Bourdillion, P.D., Bettmann, M.A., McCracken, S., et al.: Effects of a new nonionic and a conventional ionic contrast agent on coronary sinus ionized calcium and left ventricular hemodynamics in dogs. J. Am. Coll. Cardiol. 6:845, 1985.

53. Popio, K.A., Ross, A.M., Oravec, J.M., et al.: Identification and description of separate mechanisms for two components of Renografin cardiotoxicity. Circulation 58:520, 1978.

54. Wisneski, J.A., Gertz, E.W., Reese, R., et al.: Myocardial metabolic alterations after contrast angiography. Am. J. Cardiol. 50:239, 1982.

55. Matthai, W.H., Groh, W.C., Waxman, H.L., et al.: Adverse effects of calcium binding contrast agents in diagnostic cardiac angiography: A comparison between formulations with and without calcium binding additives. J. Am. Coll. Cardiol. (in press). 1995.

56. MacAlpin, R.N., Widner, W.A., Kattus, A.A., Jr., et al.: Electrocardiographic changes during selective cinearteriography. Circulation 34:627, 1966.

57. Higgins, C.B., and Feld, G.K.: Direct chronotropic and dromotropic actions of contrast media: Ineffectiveness of atropine in the prevention of bradyarrhythmias and conduction disturbances. Radiology 212:205, 1976.

58. Frink, R.J., Merrick, F., and Lowe, H.M.: Mechanism of the bradycardia during coronary angiography. Am. J. Cardiol. 35:17, 1975.

59. Partridge, J.B., Robinson, P.J., Turnbull, C.M., et al.: Clinical cardiovascular experiences with iopamidol: A new non-ionic contrast medium. Clin. Radiol. 32:451, 1981.

60. Sullivan, I.D., Wainwright, R.J., Freidy, J.F., et al.: Comparative trial of iohexol 350, a non-ionic contrast medium with diatrizoate (Urografin 370) in left ventriculography and coronary arteriography. Br. Heart J. 51:643, 1984.

61. Wolf, G.L.: The fibrillatory properties of contrast agents. Invest. Radiol. 15:s208, 1980.

62. Nahkjavan, F.K.: Continuous recording of His bundle electrogram during selective coronary cineangiography in man. J. Electrocardiol. 5:233, 1972.

63. Shabetai, R., Surawicz, B., and Hammill, W.: Monophasic action potential in man. Circulation 38:341, 1968.

64. Bjork, L., Eldh, P., and Paulin, S.: Non-ionic and dimeric contrast media in coronary angiography. Acta Radiol. 18:235, 1976.

65. Wisneski, J.A., Gertz, E.W., Dahlgren, M., et al.: Double-blind comparison of low osmolality ionic (ioxaglate) versus nonionic (iopamidol) contrast media in cardiac angiography. Am. J. Cardiol. 63(7):489, 1989.

66. Wolpers, H.G., Boller, D., Hoeft, A., et al.: The effect of composition on cellular membrane potentials during selective coronary arteriography. Invest. Radiol. 19:291, 1984.

67. Wolf, G.L., and Hirshfeld, J.W., Jr.: Changes in QTc interval with Renografin-76 and Hypaque-76 during coronary arteriography. J. Am. Coll. Cardiol. 1:1489, 1983.

68. Lazarra, R., El-Sherif, N., Hope, R.R., et al.: Ventricular arrhythmias and electrophysiological consequences of myocardial ischemia and infarction. Circ. Res. 1974;35:391.

69. Wolf, G.L., Mulry, C.C., Kilzer, K., et al.: New angiographic agents with less fibrillatory propensity. Invest. Radiol. 16:320, 1981.

70. Wolf, G.L., LeVeen, R.F., Mulry, C., et al.: The influence of contrast media additives upon ventricular fibrillation threshold during coronary angiography in ischemic and normal canine hearts. Cardiovasc. Intervent. Radiol. 4:145, 1981.

71. Almen, T.: Effects of metrizamide and other contrast media on the isolated rabbit heart. Acta Radiol. Suppl. 235:216, 1973.

72. Paulin, S., and Adams, DF.: Increased ventricular fibrillation during coronary arteriography with a new contrast medium preparation. Radiology 1971;101:45.

73. Snyder, C.F., Formanek, A., Frech, R.S., et al.: The role of sodium in promoting ventricular arrhythmia during selective coronary arteriography. Am. J. Roentgenol. 113:567, 1971.

74. Violante, M.R., Thompson, K.R., Fischer, H.W., et al.: Ventricular fibrillation from diatrizoate with and without chelating agents. Radiology 128:497, 1978.

75. Bashore, T.M., Davidson, C.J., Mark, D.B., et al.: Iopamidol use in the cardiac catheterization laboratory: A retrospective analysis of 3313 patients. Cardiology 5:6, 1988.

76. Murdock, D.K., Johnson, S.A., Loeb, H.S., et al.: Ventricular fibrillation during coronary angiography: Reduced incidence in man with contrast media lacking calcium binding additives. Cathet. Cardiovasc. Diagn. 11:153, 1985.

77. Zuckerman, L.S., Friehling, T.D., Wolf, N.M., et al.: Effect of calcium-binding additives on ventricular fibrillation and repolarization changes during coronary arteriography. J. Am. Coll. Cardiol. 10:1249, 1987.

78. DiBattiste, P.M., Kussmaul, W.G., and Hirshfeld, J.W.J.: The safety of cardiac angiography with conventional contrast agents. Am. J. Cardiol. 66(3):355, 1988.

79. Kennedy, J.W.: Complications associated with cardiac catheterization and angiography. Cathet. Cardiovasc. Diagn. 8:5, 1982.

80. Lembo, N.J., Roubin, G.S., Chin, H.K., et al.: Does non-ionic contrast media decrease the incidence of PTCA related complications? Circulation 78(Suppl. II) II-378, 1988.

81. Greenberger, P.A.: Contrast media reactions. J. Allergy Clin. Immunol. 74:600, 1984.

82. Greenberger, P.A., and Patterson, R.: Adverse reactions to radiocontrast media. Prog. Cardiovasc. Dis. 31:239, 1988.

83. Greenberger P.A., Meyers S.N., Kramer B.L., et al.: Effects of beta-adrenergic and calcium antagonists on development of anaphylactoid reactions from radiographic contrast media during cardiac angiography. J. Allergy Clin. Immunol. 80:698, 1987.

84. Shehadi, W.H.: Contrast media adverse reactions: Occurrence, recurrence, and distribution patterns. Radiology 143:11, 1982.

85. Bettmann, M.A., and Morris, T.W.: Recent advances in contrast agents. Radiol. Clin. North Am. 24:347, 1986.

86. Holtas, S.: Iohexol in patients with previous adverse reactions to contrast media. Invest. Radiol. 19:563, 1984.

87. Lalli, AF.: Urography, shock reaction, and repeat urography (editorial). A.J.R. 125:264, 1975.

88. Lasser, E.C., Berry C.C., Talner L.B., et al.: Pretreatment with corticosteroids to alleviate reactions to intravenous contrast material. N. Engl. J. Med. 317:845, 1987.

89. Cochran, S.T., Wong, W.S., and Roe, D.J.: Predicting angiography induced acute renal impairment: Clinical risk model. Am. J. Roentgenol. 141:1027, 1983.

90. D'Elia, J.A., Gleason, R.E., Alday, M., et al.: Nephrotoxicity from angiographic contrast material: A prospective study. Am. J. Med. 72:719, 1982.

91. Port, F.K., Wagoner, R.D., and Fulton, R.E.: Acute renal failure after arteriography. AJR. 121:544, 1974.

92. Taliercio, C.P., Vlietstra, R.E., Fisher, L.D., et al.: Risks for renal dysfunction with cardiac angiography. Ann. Intern. Med. 104:501, 1986.

93. Schwab, S.J., Hlatky, M.A., Pieper, K.S., et al.: Contrast nephrotoxicity: A randomized controlled trial of a nonionic and an ionic radiographic contrast agent. N. Engl. J. Med. 320(3):149, 1989.

94. Messina, J.M., Cieslinski, D.A., Nguyen, V.D., et al.: Comparison of the toxicity of the radiocontrast agents, iopamidol and diatrizoate, to rabbit renal proximal tubule cells in vitro. J. Pharmacol. Exp. Ther. 244(3):1139, 1988.

95. Rudnick, M.R., Goldfarb, S., Wexler, L., et al.: Nephrotoxicity of ionic and nonionic contrast media in 1196 patients: A randomized trial. Kidney Int. 47:254, 1995.

96. Solomon, R., Werner, C., Mann, D., et al.: Comparison of saline, mannitol, and

furosemide to prevent acute decreases in renal function induced by radiocontrast agents. N. Engl. J. Med. 331(21):1416, 1994.

97. Parfrey, P.S., Griffiths, S.M., Barrett, B.J., et al.: Contrast material-induced renal failure in patients with diabetes mellitus, renal insufficiency, or both: A prospective controlled study. N. Engl. J. Med. 320:143, 1989.

98. Littner, M.R., Rosenfield, A.T., Ulreich, S., et al.: Evaluation of bronchospasm during excretory urography. Radiology 124:17, 1977.

99. Dawson, P., Pitfield, J., and Britton, J.: Contrast media and bronchospasm: A study with iopamidol. Clin. Radiol. 34:227, 1982.

100. Smith, D.C., Luis, J.F., Gomes, A.S., et al.: Pulmonary arteriography: Comparison of cough simulation effects of diatrizoate and ioxaglate. Radiology 162:617, 1987.

101. Peck, R.J., Bull, M.J., and Cumberland, D.C.: Comparison of low-osmolar contrast media in cardiac angiography. Br. J. Radiol. 1177, 1985.

102. Bessis, M., Weed, R.J., and LeBlond, P.F.: Red Cell Shape: Physiology, Pathology, and Ultrastructure. New York, Springer-Verlag, 1973.

103. Nathan, D.G., and Shohet, S.B.: Erythrocyte ion transport and hemolytic anemia: Hydrocytosis and desiccocytosis. Semin. Hematol. 7:381, 1970.

104. Aspelin, P.: Effect of ionic and non-ionic contrast media on morphology of human erythrocytes. Acta Radiol. 19:675, 1978.

105. Grollman, J.H.J., Liu, C.K., Astone, R.A., et al.: Thromboembolic complications in coronary angiography associated with the use of nonionic contrast medium. Cathet. Cardiovasc. Diagn. 14(3):159, 1988.

106. Englehart, J.A., Smith, D.C., Maloney, M.D., et al.: A technique for estimating the probability of clots in blood/contrast agent mixtures. Invest. Radiol. 23:923, 1988.

107. Rasuli, P., McLeish, W.A., and Hammond, D.T.: Anticoagulant effects of contrast materials: In vitro study of iohexol, ioxaglate, and diatrizoate. AJR 152:309, 1989.

108. LeFevre, T., Bernard, A., Bertrand, M.E., et al.: Comparison by scanning electron microscopy of the antithrombogenic potential of two low osmolality iodine contrast media during percutaneous transluminal coronary angioplasty. Arch. Mal. Coeur Vaiss. 87:225, 1994.

109. Robertson, H.J.F.: Blood clot formation in angiographic syringes containing nonionic contrast media. Radiology 163:62, 1987.

110. Parvez, Z., Kahn, T., and Moncada, R.: Ultrastructural changes in rat aortic endothelium during contrast media infusion. Invest. Radiol. 20:407, 1985.

111. Nyman, U., and Almen, T.: Effect of contrast agent media on aortic endothelium. Acta Radiol. Suppl. 362:65, 1980.

112. Jacobson, P.D., and Rosenquist, C.J.: The introduction of low-osmolar contrast agents in radiology: Medical, economic, legal, and public policy issues. JAMA 260:1586, 1988.

113. Palmer, F.: The RACR survey of intravenous contrast media reactions: Final report. Australas. Radiol. 32:426, 1988.

114. Katayama, H., Yamaguchi, K., Kozuka, T., et al.: Adverse reactions to ionic and nonionic contrast media. A report from the Japanese Committee on the Safety of Contrast Media. Radiology 175:621, 1990.

115. Wolf, G.L., Arenson, R.L., and Cross, A.P.: A prospective trial of ionic versus nonionic contrast agents in routine clinical practice: Comparison of adverse effects. AJR 152:939, 1989.

116. Barrett, B.J., Parfrey, P.S., Vavasour, H.M., et al.: A comparison of nonionic, low-osmolality radiocontrast agents with ionic, high-osmolality agents during cardiac catheterization. N. Engl. J. Med. 326:431, 1992.

117. Steinberg, E.P., Moore, R.D., Powe, NR, et al.: Safety and cost effectiveness of high-osmality as compared with low-osmolality contrast material in patients undergoing cardiac angiography. N. Engl. J. Med. 326:425, 1992.

118. Wolf, G.L.: Safer, more expensive iodinated contrast agents: How do you decide? Invest. Radiol. 159:557, 1986.

119. White, R.I., Jr., and Holden, W.J.J.: Liquid gold: Low osmolarity contrast media. Radiology 159:559, 1986.

120. Fischer, H.W.: The use of low-osmolar contrast media. JAMA 260:1614, 1988.

121. Brinker, J.A.: Low osmolal contrast: Is it a luxury we can no longer afford? Cathet. Cardiovasc. Diagn. 33(1):20, 1994.

CHAPTER

19 Principles and Practice of Contrast Ventriculography

Florence H. Sheehan, M.D.

VENTRICULOGRAPHIC TECHNIQUE _____ 164
QUALITATIVE ASSESSMENT OF THE CONTRAST
 LEFT VENTRICULOGRAM _____ 165
QUANTITATIVE ANALYSIS OF THE CONTRAST
 LEFT VENTRICULOGRAM: VOLUME
 DETERMINATION _____ 167
Volume Determination in Theory _____ 169
Volume Determination in Practice _____ 170
Parameters Derived From Volume
 Measurements _____ 175
 Volumes, Indices, and Output _____ 175
 Regurgitant Flow and Valve Areas _____ 175
 Left Ventricular Mass and Stress _____ 175
QUANTITATIVE ANALYSIS OF REGIONAL LEFT
 VENTRICULAR WALL MOTION _____ 176

Wall Motion Analysis in Theory _____ 176
Methods of Wall Motion Analysis _____ 177
 Assumptions in Methods of Wall Motion
 Analysis _____ 177
 Parameters of Regional Function _____ 180
 Definition of Normal Motion _____ 182
 Definition of Abnormal Motion _____ 182
 Variability _____ 182
 Measuring Wall Motion in the Region of
 Interest _____ 182
 Method Selection: Theoretical, Empirical, and
 Clinical Considerations _____ 182
SUMMARY _____ 187

Contrast angiography allows visualization of the left ventricle and other chambers as a projection image. Assessment can be made of chamber dimensions and function through the phases of the cardiac cycle. Angiograms can be evaluated subjectively or with the use of quantitative techniques to assess chamber volume, ejection fraction and wall motion, and valve orifice area and flow.

VENTRICULOGRAPHIC TECHNIQUE

The goal in cardiac angiography is to obtain images of the left ventricle contracting in normal sinus rhythm, with adequate con-

trast quality to allow confident identification of the endocardial contour throughout the cardiac cycle. Placing the catheter in the inflow tract or reducing the acceleration in the flow of contrast material from the injector minimizes ectopy.[1] The volume and rate of injection needed to adequately opacify the left ventricle depend on the size of the chamber, the heart rate, and the function of the heart and valves. Patients with hypercontractile hearts, tachycardia, or mitral or aortic regurgitation require a higher volume and rate of contrast injection. Good-quality ventriculograms can be obtained in patients unable to tolerate ordinary contrast volume by injection at low flow rates through a six-hole catheter in the apex.[1] The 30-degree right anterior oblique (RAO) projection allows visualization of the left ventricle at full length, without overlap of the heart with the spine, as occurs in the anteroposterior (AP) view. Orthogonal views provide additional information about regional function, which may be of use in evaluating patients with ischemic heart disease.

QUALITATIVE ASSESSMENT OF THE CONTRAST LEFT VENTRICULOGRAM

The shape of the normal left ventricle in diastole is elliptical (Fig. 19–1). Normally, some asynchrony is present, but it is barely perceptible. Normality in regional function is uniform inward motion of the walls in systole (Fig. 19–2) and uniform outward motion in diastole.

Abnormality in volume can be appreciated from the size and shape of the ventricle. With dilation the ventricle becomes more spherical as wall stresses redistribute (Fig. 19–3).[2] In patients with hyperkinesis due to hypertrophic cardiomyopathy, the end-systolic volume may be reduced nearly to the point of "cavity obliteration" at the apex (Fig. 19–4).

Abnormality in ventricular function may be either diffuse or regional. Depression of regional wall motion usually indicates the presence of coronary artery disease, although it has also been reported in valvular disease of rheumatic origin.[3] For purposes of qualitative assessment, the ventricular contour is commonly divided into segments whose motion is graded individually as normal, as hypokinetic when wall motion is reduced, as akinetic when the segment is motionless, or as dyskinetic when the segment displays paradoxical outward motion during systole. When numeric values

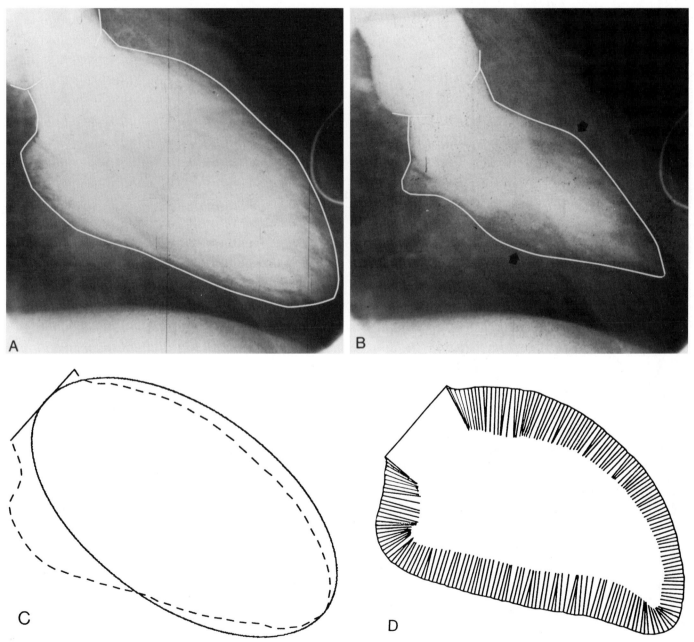

FIGURE 19–1. Contrast ventriculogram (30 degrees RAO) of a patient with normal cardiac function and anatomy at end-diastole (*A*) and end-systole (*B*). The papillary muscles, visible only at end-systole (*arrows*), are included in the chamber volume when one is tracing the endocardial contour. Chamber volume is calculated by comparing the contour to an ellipse of equivalent area and long-axis length (*C*, end-diastole only). Normal wall motion was calculated as the mean motion of 52 patients with normal cardiac anatomy and function (*D*).

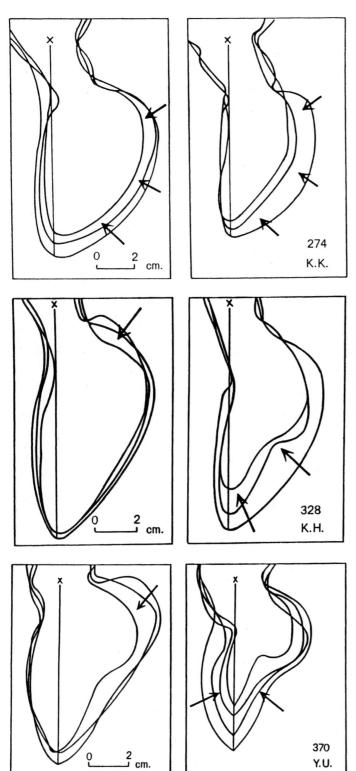

FIGURE 19–2. Left ventricular endocardial contours in the 60-degree LAO view in subjects with a normal heart *(top)*, mitral regurgitation *(middle)*, or hypertrophic cardiomyopathy *(bottom)*. Boxes on the left display the contours at end-diastole and 50 msec and 100 msec later. Boxes on the right display contours from the second 100 msec after end-diastole. The normal subject has uniform inward motion. In the two heart disease patients, motion begins at the base and apical contraction is delayed. (From Ueda, H., Ueda, K., Morooka, S., et al.: A cineangiocardiographic study of the regional contraction sequence of the normal and diseased left ventricle in man. Jpn. Heart J. 10:95–112, 1969, with permission.)

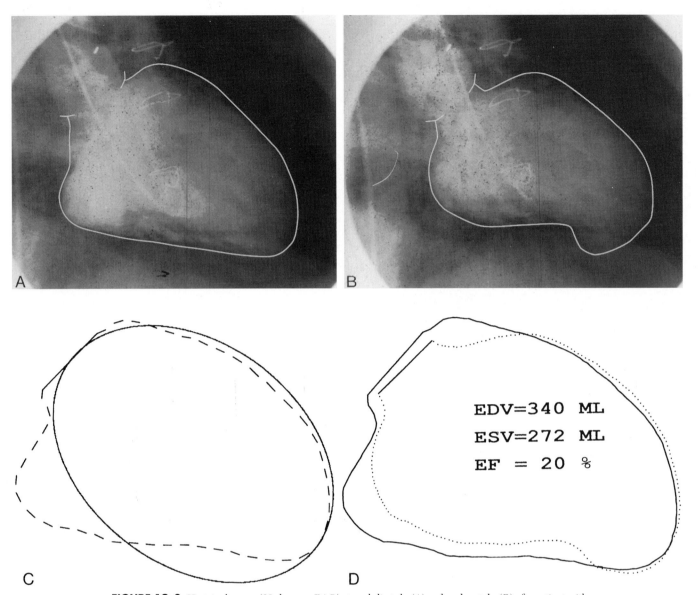

EDV=340 ML

ESV=272 ML

EF = 20 %

FIGURE 19–3. Ventriculogram (30 degrees RAO) at end-diastole (A) and end-systole (B) of a patient with left ventricular dilation and congestive heart failure due to acute myocardial infarction and three-vessel coronary artery disease. The ventricle is more spherical than normal (C), the ejection fraction is reduced, and there is anteroapical akinesis (D).

are assigned to each grade, their summed total over all the segments provides a wall motion score. Such visual assessment of the size and function of the left ventricle can be used to gauge surgical risk and prognosis in patients with coronary artery disease.[4] Asynchrony or abnormal timing of wall motion can also be appreciated from a visual inspection of the ventriculogram. In patients with ischemia or infarction, contraction of the affected region may be delayed into early diastole.[5]

The severity of mitral regurgitation can be estimated from the ventriculogram by comparing the relative opacification of the atrium and ventricle (Fig. 19–5). The artifactual appearance of mitral regurgitation may result from poor catheter placement near or even across the valve, or from arrhythmia. In mitral valve prolapse, one can see the valve ballooning into the atrium during systole (Fig. 19–6).

Other valve disease entities may also result in ventriculographic abnormalities, but of a less specific or diagnostic nature. Mitral stenosis is associated with a small but normally functioning ventricle. In patients with aortic stenosis, the severity of hypertrophy may be appreciable from the thickness of the anterior wall, where the epicardium is most visible.[6] Limitation of aortic valve motion

or calcification or thickening of the leaflets may also be appreciated. Aortic regurgitation results in left ventricular dilation and hypertrophy (Fig. 19–7).

On inspection of the ventriculogram, other pathology, such as aneurysms (Fig. 19–8), may be visible. Filling defects due to intraventricular thrombi are not uncommon in patients with myocardial infarction. In a patient suspected of having ventricular septal defect, ventriculography in the 45-degree left anterior oblique (LAO) view may show a systolic passage of contrast material into the right heart.

QUANTITATIVE ANALYSIS OF THE CONTRAST LEFT VENTRICULOGRAM: VOLUME DETERMINATION

Volume determination by contrast ventriculography is the "gold standard" by which other imaging modalities are judged, because of its demonstrated accuracy. The area-length method[7] was validated with the use of postmortem hearts filled with barium paste

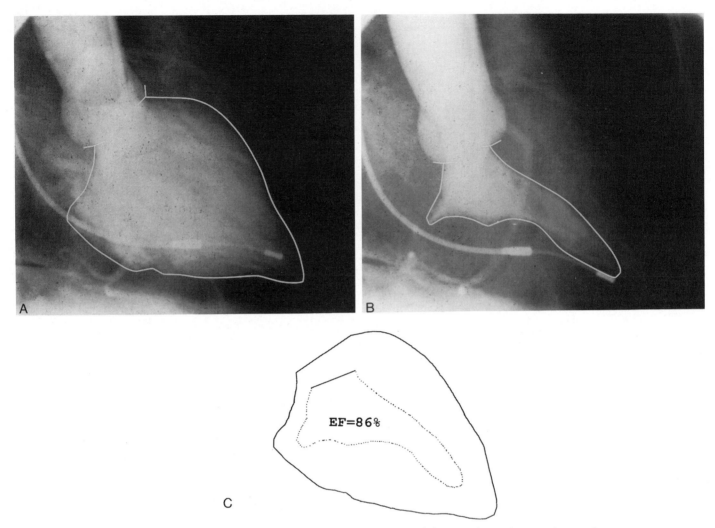

FIGURE 19–4. Ventriculogram (30 degrees RAO) of a patient with hypertrophic cardiomyopathy at end-diastole (A). At end-systole (B), there is "cavity obliteration." The ejection fraction is elevated (C).

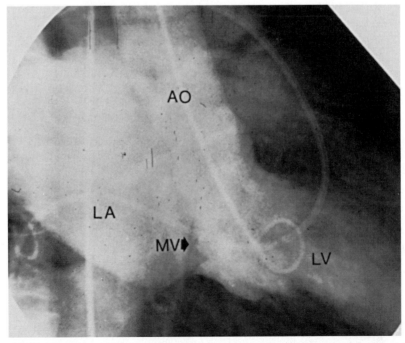

FIGURE 19–5. The backward flow of blood across the mitral valve (MV) has opacified the left atrium (LA) in this patient with grade 4+ mitral regurgitation. LV = left ventricle; AO = aorta.

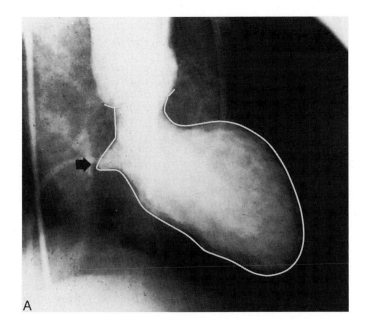

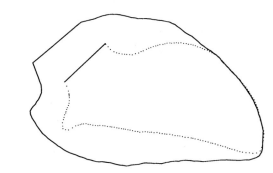

FIGURE 19–6. Mitral valve prolapse is evident at end-systole (*A, arrow*). The end-diastolic contour (*B*) is normal. The view is 30 degrees RAO.

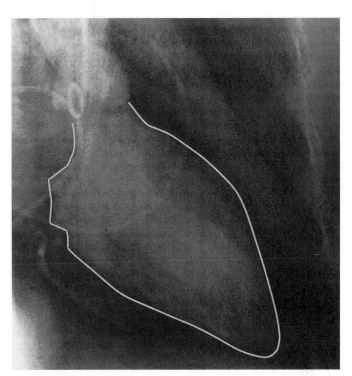

FIGURE 19–7. In aortic valvular regurgitation, contrast injected into the aortic root opacifies the left ventricle.

and has a standard error (SE) of only 8.2 mL (Fig. 19–9). The accuracy of angiographic stroke volume determination in vivo was demonstrated by comparison with volumes measured with the Fick or indicator dilution techniques (Fig. 19–10).

Volume Determination in Theory

The area-length method calculates volume by relating the left ventricle to an ellipsoid of revolution (see Fig. 19–1). The diameter of the contour is calculated from the area and long-axis length with the use of the formula for an ellipse. The method was originally validated for biplane ventriculograms in the AP and lateral views, but it is also accurate for the 30-degree RAO and 60-degree LAO projections.[8] Because the long axis is frequently foreshortened in the straight LAO view (Fig. 19–11), addition of 15 to 30 degrees of cranial angulation has been advocated.[9] The short-axis diameters are similar in orthogonal projections, so volume can be accurately determined from single-plane ventriculograms in the 30-degree RAO or AP projections.

Most of the other methods invented for determining left ventricular volume have proved to be less accurate.[7] The Simpson rule method has an accuracy that is comparable to that of the area-length method but requires more complex computation. The accuracy or validity of the area-length method may appear questionable for grossly abnormal ventricles, such as those with aneurysms. However, despite its inherent assumption of an ellipsoidal chamber, the area-length method has proved accurate for determining the volume of the right ventricle and atria.[10]

The papillary muscles, trabeculae carneae, and chordae tendineae occupy a volume that is not calculable. Instead, correction is made with the use of regression equations.[7, 8] Correction must also be made for magnification in the imaging chain, which includes magnification when the cine film is projected for tracing, and pincushion distortion. Previously, a grid of known dimension was placed at the level of the patient's heart and filmed with the imaging equipment positioned as it was during ventriculography (Fig. 19–12). It is easier to place an aluminum sphere in the axilla at the midchest level and film it immediately after the ventriculogram. From the projected image, the correction factor is calculated as the ratio of the true size of the calibration figure to its measured size. The correction factor can also be determined with the use of a pigtail catheter with metallic bands at known spacing.[11] This

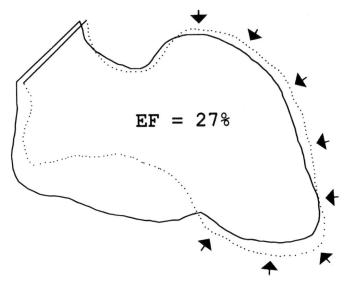

FIGURE 19–8. End-diastolic and end-systolic contours (30 degrees RAO) of a patient with aneurysm due to recent anterior myocardial infarction. There is dyskinesis around the anteroapical region (*arrows*).

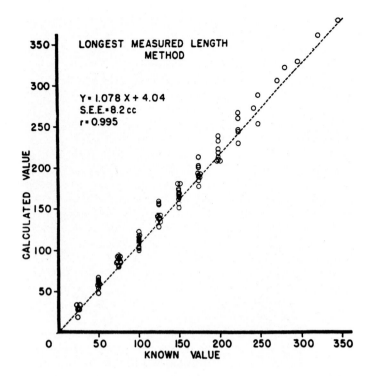

FIGURE 19–9. The area-length method of measuring left ventricular chamber volume was validated by comparing the volume calculated from angiograms of barium-filled heart casts with the true volume of these hearts. (From Dodge, H.T., Sandler, H., Ballew, D.W., et al.: The use of biplane angiocardiography for the measurement of left ventricular volume in man. Am. Heart J. 60:762–776, 1960, with permission.)

method requires simultaneous biplane ventriculography and does not correct for pincushion distortion. For accuracy in volume calculation, the calibration figure should be heart sized and imaged in midfield.[12]

Volume Determination in Practice

The accuracy of volume determination is also influenced by technical factors. Quantitative analysis requires higher quality images than qualitative assessment, simply because the projector must be stopped for tracing. Qualitative assessment is performed with the projector running and thus is aided by the visual integration of motion. It is helpful to record the electrocardiogram with the ventriculogram (Fig. 19–13), to check the regularity of the rhythm, select a normal sinus beat of representative cycle length, and determine the RR interval. Otherwise, cycle length and rhythm

regularity can be estimated by counting the number of frames from each end-diastole to the next. The first normal beat after ectopy is not analyzed, because it is subject to postextrasystolic potentiation.

Because of the cardiodepressive effect of contrast agents, analysis should be performed on the earliest normal sinus beat after chamber opacification. Using epicardial clips to track serial ventricular functional changes (Fig. 19–14), Vine and associates found that contrast material causes the end-systolic volume and ejection fraction to deviate significantly from their preinjection values after seven cardiac cycles.[13] The new nonionic contrast media cause less hypotension, arrhythmias, or fluctuation in ventricular function than Renografin.

For clinical studies, only the end-diastolic and end-systolic endocardial contours are traced. End-diastole is the frame at which ventricular volume appears to be largest or, when the electrocardiogram is recorded, at the peak of the R wave (see Fig. 19–13). In

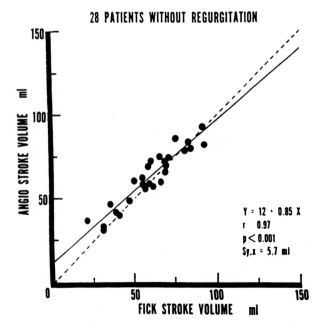

FIGURE 19–10. The area-length method of volume determination has been further validated in vivo by comparing the angiographic stroke volume against that measured by the Fick technique. (From Hunt, D., Baxley, W.A., Kennedy, J.W., et al.: Quantitative evaluation of cineaortography in the assessment of aortic regurgitation. Am. J. Cardiol. 31:696–700, 1973, with permission.)

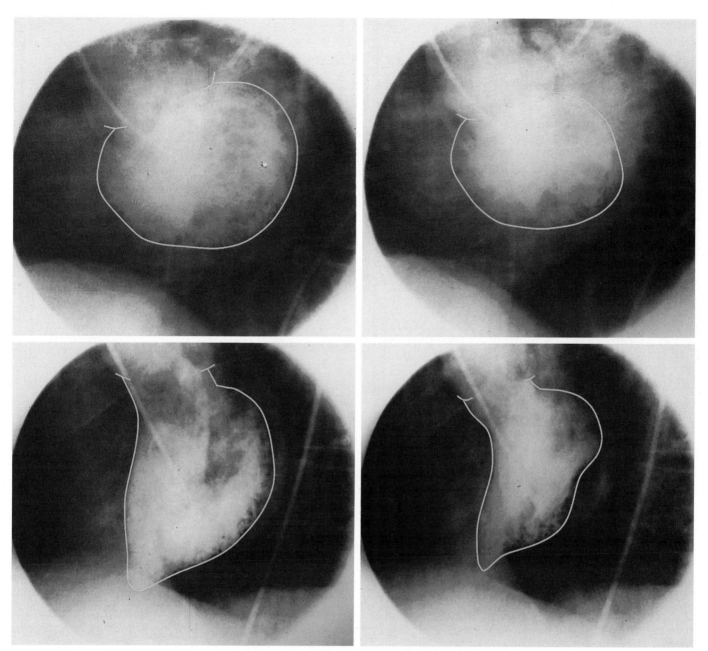

FIGURE 19–11. End-diastolic *(left)* and end-systolic *(right)* contours in the 60-degree LAO view of two patients. When the left ventricle is foreshortened *(top)*, the motion of the apex cannot be assessed. To visualize the full length of the ventricle *(bottom)*, some angiographers advocate addition of cranial angulation.

patients with sinus rhythm, end-diastole can be seen to follow immediately after the "kick" of atrial systole. End-systole is the frame of minimum chamber volume. In patients with asynchronous motion, it may be necessary to trace several frames to find the frame of minimum volume.

One of the most important factors influencing the accuracy of quantitative analysis is the care with which the endocardial contours are identified, traced, and digitized. Tracing is less fatiguing on a horizontal or upward-sloped table on which the cine images are displayed from an overhead mounted projector (Fig. 19–15). The tracing room should be darkened; otherwise, function is overestimated because the faintly opacified fingers of contrast material between trabeculae at end-systole are hard to see, and the contour is mistakenly traced at the tips of the trabeculae, rather than at their roots. By convention, the endocardial contours begin and end where they intersect with the aortic valve. The papillary muscles and trabeculae carneae are not traced (see Fig. 19–1). Correction

for their volume is made with the use of regression equations (see earlier). The projector should be played back and forth to track endocardial motion as an aid to tracing, error checking, and editing (Fig. 19–16). The x-y coordinates of the final endocardial contours are then entered into the computer with the use of a digitizing tablet (Fig. 19–17). For accurate analysis from digital images, the system should allow endocardial motion to be tracked by playing a "cine loop" of images under the traced border. Such systems are preferable to more primitive systems that require the user to trace the entire contour in a single sweep from the stopped frame, unaided by visual tracking of the motion of the walls.

Training is obviously a factor influencing the accuracy of volume determination. At the University of Washington, interobserver variability is minimized by requiring that new tracers pass a variability test after their training. Variability studies have shown that tracing is most difficult in the anterobasal region, where a faintly opacified left anterior descending artery may be mistaken for the ventricular

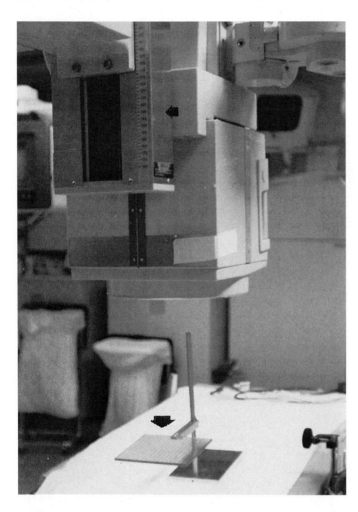

FIGURE 19-12. The calibration grid is filmed at the level of the patient's midchest *(large arrow)*. The height of the image intensifier is recorded at the time ventriculography was performed *(small arrow)* so that the equipment can be returned to this position to film the grid.

FIGURE 19-13. Continuous recording of the electrocardiogram (ECG) during contrast ventriculography. This tracing was recorded at 100 mm per second. The timing of angiographic (angio) frames is indicated by the vertical lines for comparison with the ECG. The RR interval preceding beat 4 is nearly normal and approaches the interval preceding beats 2 and 3. Nevertheless, beat 4 is a slightly premature ventricular contraction, with a wide QRS interval, and is associated with reduced pressure. If this angiogram was evaluated without the ECG, the slight prematurity of beat 4 might be overlooked; it could then be identified only by the lack of an atrial kick.

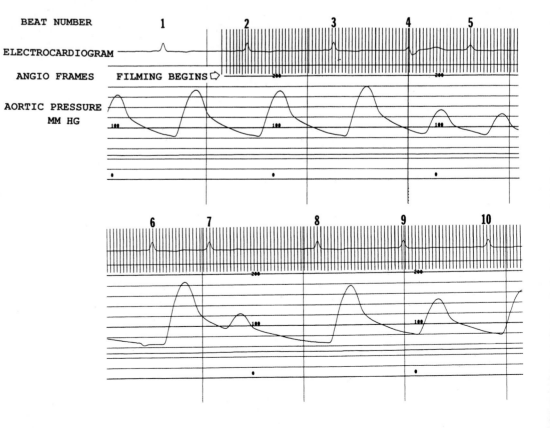

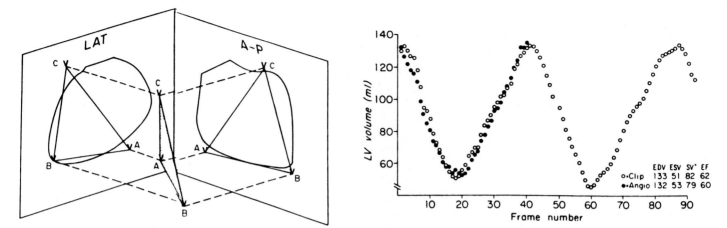

FIGURE 19–14. To measure the effect of contrast material on left ventricular volume and ejection fraction, volume was determined continuously, beginning before contrast injection from the motion of epicardial clips *(left)*. There was close agreement between clip-derived volume and angiographic volume *(right)*. (From Vine, D.L., Dodge, H.T., Frimer, M.J., et al.: Quantitative measurement of left ventricular volumes in man from radio-opaque epicardial markers. Circulation 54:391, 1976, with permission from the American Heart Association, Inc.)

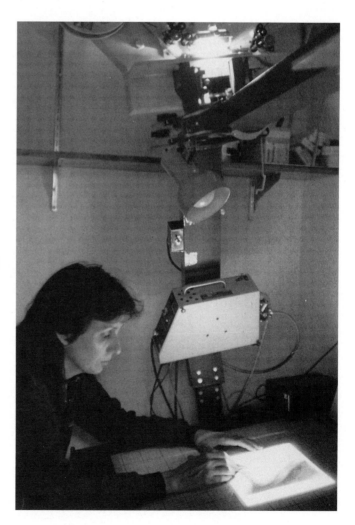

FIGURE 19–15. With an overhead mounted projector, the image is projected onto the table, where it can be traced more comfortably.

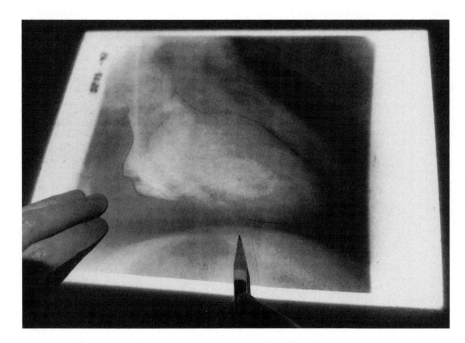

FIGURE 19–16. The endocardial contour of this end-diastolic frame has been traced. The operator covers the tracing with a blank sheet of paper, mentally retraces the endocardial contour, slides off the blank paper, and checks to see whether the new impression of the contour agrees with the pencilled tracing.

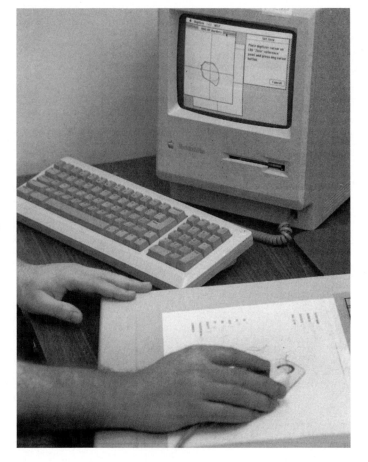

FIGURE 19–17. The endocardial contours are entered into the computer with the use of an x-y digitizing tablet.

contour, and at the apex, because it is often less well opacified.[14] In experienced laboratories, interobserver variability ranges from 6.6 to 20 mL for end-diastolic volume, from 5.7 to 10 mL for end-systolic volume (Fig. 19–18), and from 4 to 5 percent for ejection fraction.[15] Beat-to-beat variability and intraobserver variability are similarly low.[15] However, study-to-study variability is considerably greater, even when measured from serial ventriculograms in clinically stable patients. This variability is probably due to differences in hemodynamic state, in addition to variability in tracing the ventricular contours.

Parameters Derived From Volume Measurements

Volumes, Indices, and Output

The end-diastolic volume is that measured when the ventricle has reached peak dilation for a given cardiac cycle. The end-systolic volume is a measure of the residual volume of blood remaining in the ventricle at the end of contraction. The difference between them is the stroke volume. The product of stroke volume and heart rate yields the cardiac output, the volume of blood ejected from the ventricle per minute. These measurements are normalized for differences in patient size by dividing by the body-surface area to yield volume or cardiac index. The ratio of the stroke volume to the end-diastolic volume is the ejection fraction. It can be measured with a high degree of reproducibility and is useful as an index of prognosis (Fig. 19–19).

Regurgitant Flow and Valve Areas

Because the angiographic stroke volume is the volume output from the left ventricle, but the Fick or dilution stroke volume is the forward output, the difference between them is the regurgitant flow per beat. The severity of regurgitation may be expressed as a percentage of the angiographic stroke volume. Quantitative measurements correlate only roughly with the grades of aortic regurgitation assessed visually from the aortogram (r = 0.56, Fig. 19–20),[16] because the visual grade is affected by the size and function of the left ventricle and the presence of valvular stenosis. From the cardiac output and the pressure gradient across a stenotic valve, the cross-sectional area of the valve can be calculated with the use of a hydraulic formula. The accuracy of this approach has been established by comparing the calculated area with the valve area measured at surgery or autopsy.

Left Ventricular Mass and Stress

Myocardial wall thickness is measured from the distance between the epicardial and the endocardial contours along the anterior wall, where the epicardium is visible (Fig. 19–21). Myocardial mass is calculated by assuming the measured wall thickness to be homogeneous around the ventricle. Comparison of calculated mass with postmortem weight has revealed a close agreement (r = 0.97, standard error of the estimate [SEE] = 32.4 g) (Fig. 19–22),[17] except in patients with right ventricular hypertrophy or pericardial disease.

Left ventricular stress can be calculated from measurements of dimensions, wall thickness, and pressure. Because of trabecular thickening, the mass calculated from direct measurement of wall thickness at end-systole exceeds the mass at end-diastole. To avoid this artifactual increase in mass, wall thickness at end-systole is determined by measuring mass at end-diastole and homogeneously spreading it over the chamber volume at end-systole.[6]

The capability of measuring wall thickness and stress has led to increased understanding of the effect of pressure or volume overload on the left ventricle and of compensatory response (Fig.

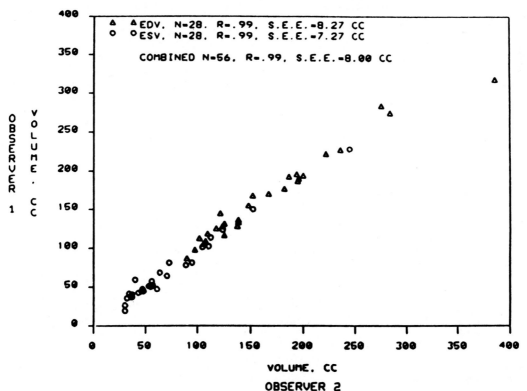

FIGURE 19–18. Variability in left ventricular volume between measurements made independently by different observers. (From Dodge, H.T., Sheehan, F.H., and Stewart, D.K.: Estimation of ventricular volume, fractional ejected volumes, stroke volume, and quantitation of regurgitant flow. *In* Just, H., and Heintzen, P.H. [eds.]: Angiocardiography: Current Status and Future Developments. Berlin, Springer-Verlag, 1986, p. 99, with permission.)

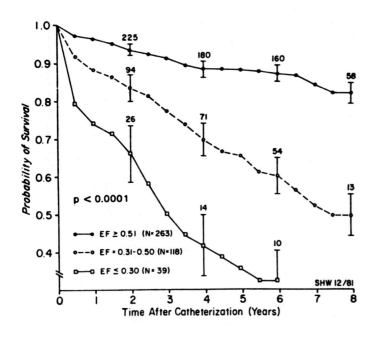

FIGURE 19-19. Left ventricular ejection fraction was found to be one of the strongest prognostic indicators in the Seattle Heart Watch Study. This figure displays survival in patients randomized to medical therapy, subgrouped according to initial ejection fraction. (From Hammermeister, K.E., DeRouen, T.A., Zia, M.S., et al.: Survival of medically treated coronary artery disease patients in the Seattle Heart Watch Angiography Registry. *In* Hammermeister, K.E. [ed.]: Coronary Bypass Surgery: The Late Results, p. 185. Reprinted with permission of Greenwood Publishing Group, Inc., Westport, CT. © 1983.)

19–23). In pressure overload, the myocardium thickens without dilating; in volume overload, on the other hand, wall thickness remains normal, but total mass increases with the increase in volume. The two types of load cause different patterns of hypertrophy,[18] but both act to reduce wall stress. In decompensated patients with impaired ventricular performance, the ventricle becomes more spherical and stresses redistribute.[2, 19] The adaptations to volume overload are analogous to normal cardiac growth.

QUANTITATIVE ANALYSIS OF REGIONAL LEFT VENTRICULAR WALL MOTION

The illustrative examples were prepared with the centerline method developed at the University of Washington, to allow a more uniform presentation (Fig. 19–24).

It has long been recognized that coronary artery occlusion causes dysfunction in the ischemic region. Wall motion abnormalities in

the nonischemic region in patients with chronic or acute ischemia have also been identified and their relationship to the ejection fraction measured.[20, 21] The ejection fraction reflects the net effect of abnormalities in the various regions of the left ventricle. The value of wall motion analysis derives from its greater sensitivity to the function of the region of interest and its usefulness for interpreting observed changes in the ejection fraction.

Wall Motion Analysis in Theory

The accuracy of volume determination by each proposed method was established by postmortem heart studies. However, no such gold standard exists for verifying the accuracy of wall motion measurements. Metallic markers have been implanted in the epicardium, midwall, or endocardium and have been tracked to validate one or another approach to wall motion analysis.[22–24] None of these marker methods has won universal acceptance. That wall thickening contributes half of the perceived endocardial wall mo-

$$\text{Valve orifice area} = \frac{\text{valve flow}}{K \sqrt{\text{pressure gradient}}}$$

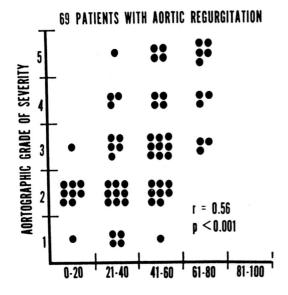

FIGURE 19-20. Correlation between visual assessment and quantitative measurement of aortic regurgitation expressed as a percentage of stroke volume. (From Hunt, D., Baxley, W.A., Kennedy, J.W., et al.: Quantitative evaluation of cineaortography in the assessment of aortic regurgitation. Am. J. Cardiol. 31:696, 1973, with permission.)

The problem is further complicated by the translational motion of the heart within the chest, which cannot be distinguished angiographically from the perceived inward motion of the projected endocardial contours. To correct for translational motion, a number of approaches have been proposed, which realign the end-systolic contour relative to the end-diastolic contour (Fig. 19–25). However the validity of performing realignment has been questioned on theoretical grounds, and more recent studies indicate that realignment worsens variability in wall motion measurement and may, in an artifactual fashion, give the appearance of motion to patients with akinesis.[14, 26, 27] For these reasons, it is more appropriate to consider the various methods as models rather than as measures of regional wall motion.

Methods of Wall Motion Analysis

In the absence of a gold standard by which to gauge the accuracy of wall motion analysis, it is necessary to consider other criteria in selecting a method. All the methods carry inherent assumptions concerning the directionality of wall motion. It is important to identify the assumption implied in each method under consideration and to evaluate its validity in the light of available experimental data. The selection of a method involves more than the definition of motion vectors. Additional considerations include the parameter used to express regional function and how abnormality will be defined and measured. Practically, performance is assessed by four empirical criteria. First, the measurements made should be reproducible; variability should be minimal to increase accuracy in detecting abnormalities and changes. Second, the motion of normal subjects should have a narrow standard deviation to enhance sensitivity for abnormality (Fig. 19–26). Third, the method used to measure wall motion should be able to focus on the region of interest. Fourth, it should demonstrate sensitivity and specificity in distinguishing the function of normal subjects from that of patients with hypokinesis or hyperkinesis.

Assumptions in Methods of Wall Motion Analysis

Most methods use either a rectangular or a radial coordinate system (Fig. 19–27). To adjust for patient-to-patient differences in

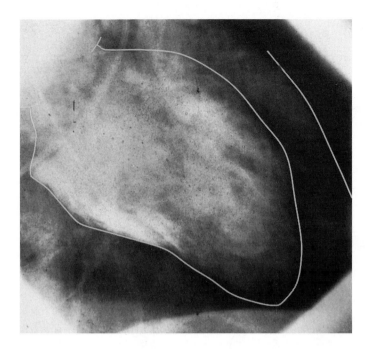

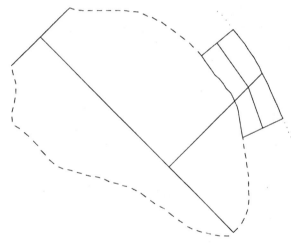

FIGURE 19–21. The thickness of the myocardium is measured along the anterior wall, in the neighborhood of the hemiaxis between the middle and the distal thirds of the long axis, where the epicardium is visible.

tion implies that epicardial or midwall marker motion underestimates the extent of endocardial motion. The methods defined with the use of midwall markers and endocardial markers measure motion along vectors that differ by nearly 90 degrees at the apex; this discrepancy weakens confidence in validation by marker tracking. Furthermore, endocardial marker motion may not correspond to the motion measured from a contrast ventriculogram, because the markers become embedded in the trabeculae as the latter thicken in systole. Thus, a one-to-one correspondence cannot be established between points on the end-diastolic contour and points on the end-systolic contour.[6]

The lack of a gold standard for wall motion has led to a proliferation of methods, promoted on the basis of empirical criteria, such as the accuracy with which the resulting wall motion measurements distinguished normal subjects from patients with ischemic heart disease or how homogeneous the motion in the normal group appeared. These criteria are influenced by the size and selection of the normal subjects and patient populations used for testing and by the statistical approach.[25]

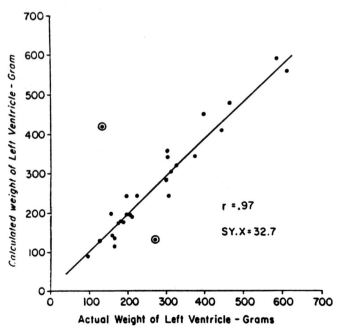

FIGURE 19–22. Validation of the method for measuring left ventricular mass. The two outliers had right ventricular hypertrophy and were excluded from statistical analysis. (From Kennedy, J.W., Reichenbach, D.D., Baxley, W.A., et al.: Left ventricular mass: A comparison of angiocardiographic measurements with autopsy weight. Am. J. Cardiol. 19:221, 1967, with permission.)

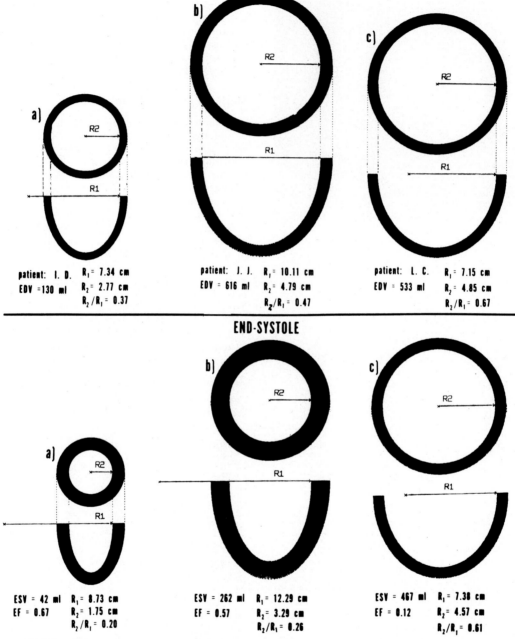

FIGURE 19–23. Schematic drawings for three subjects: (*a*) normal, (*b*) volume overload with hypertrophy and intact left ventricular function, and (*c*) dilated hypertrophied ventricle with depressed function. The ventricle of c is rounder, as is evident from the elevated ratio of the principal radii of curvature R2/R1, calculated by comparing the ventricle to an ellipsoid of revolution. In the more spherical ventricle, wall stress in the meridional direction increases relative to stress in the equatorial direction. (From Dodge, H.T., Frimer, M., and Stewart, D.K.: Functional evaluation of the hypertrophied heart in man. Circ. Res. 34–35 [Suppl. II]:122–127, 1974, with permission from the American Heart Association, Inc.)

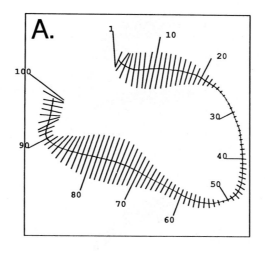

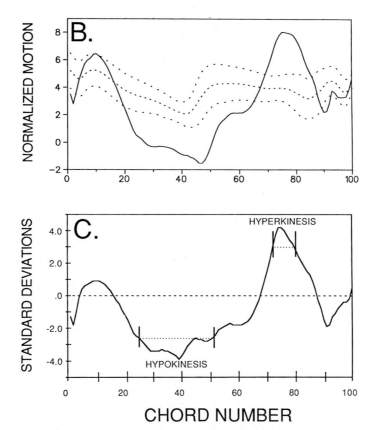

FIGURE 19–24. Wall motion measured by the centerline method. A centerline is constructed midway between the end-diastolic and the end-systolic endocardial contours. Motion is measured along 100 chords perpendicular to the centerline *(A)*. To adjust for heart size, the motion of each chord is normalized by the length of the end-diastolic perimeter. *B,* When one compares the patient's motion *(solid curve)* with the normal range (mean ± 1 SD; *dotted curves*), the regional variability of normal motion is apparent. *C,* Therefore, motion is converted to units of SDs from the normal mean, represented by the horizontal axis. Abnormality in a region of interest is calculated as the mean motion of chords lying in the most abnormally contracting part of the respective coronary artery territory.

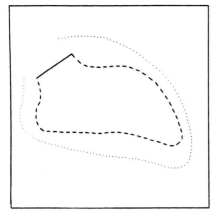

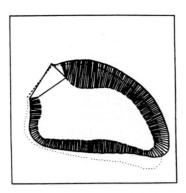

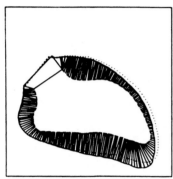

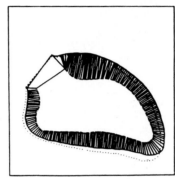

FIGURE 19–25. The displacement of the endocardial contour between end-diastole and end-systole measures the net effect of inward wall motion and translational motion of the heart in the chest. However, realignment to correct for translational motion can, in the fashion of an artifact, create anterior hypokinesis, normal motion, or inferior hypokinesis (proceeding clockwise). (Original contours traced under external reference are on *upper left*).

heart size, the measured motion is normalized by the end-diastolic length of the hemiaxis or radius to calculate a shortening fraction, a linear version of the ejection fraction. In addition, the coordinate system may be used to divide the ventricle into regions, whose area ejection fractions can be calculated.

Two of the methods developed on the basis of metallic marker studies use a coordinate system. The method of Ingels and associates measures motion along radii to an origin located 69 percent down the long axis. This approach yielded the closest agreement with the motion of midwall markers.[23] Slager and co-workers developed their method based on the motion of endocardial markers implanted in pigs. They subsequently extended their studies to include normal human ventriculograms, using an automated border-recognition system to identify and track the motion of individual irregularities on the endocardial contour. The mean motion of these irregularities was used to define 20 pathways in a rectangular coordinate system, along which wall motion can be measured.[24]

Several problems are associated with coordinate system methods. First, most methods rely on identification of the apex to define the coordinate system. However, the apex is not an anatomical landmark, is often poorly visualized, and is subject to the highest variability in tracing.[14] Second, many studies have challenged the assumption that wall motion proceeds toward the long axis or a central origin. The direction of wall motion is multicentric,[28] and the motion pattern depicted in the various marker studies consistently shows systolic descent of the base toward the apex.[22–24] This observation invalidates methods that use a rectangular coordinate system to measure motion at the base, because the vectors run perpendicular to the long axis. It has been suggested that the center of mass be used as the origin of a radial system, both for wall motion analysis and as a reference for realignment to correct for cardiac translation.[29] However, only the center of the chamber can be calculated from the endocardial contour; delineation of the epicardium is required to determine the center of mass. The so-called center of mass approach has proved to be less sensitive than other methods on empirical testing.[25] Third, coordinate system methods are not suitable for contours of varying shapes, such as

the LAO view of the left ventricle (see Fig. 19–11), or the right ventricle (Fig. 19–28).

A few methods do not rely on construction of a coordinate system. One approach is to divide the end-diastolic and end-systolic contours evenly into the same number of points, then measure motion between the two contours at corresponding points. The problem with this approach is that the ventricular contour does not shorten homogeneously around its circumference in patients with ischemic heart disease. Local hypokinesis may cause the end-systolic borders of an akinetic region to be related to normally contracting sections of the end-diastolic contour, giving the artifactual appearance of motion. Gibson and co-workers connected points on the end-diastolic contour to the nearest point on the end-systolic contour.[30] This method is free from serious theoretical drawbacks, although it occasionally creates undesirable motion vectors in tightly curved sections of the contour. The centerline method (see Fig. 19–24) measures wall motion along chords perpendicular to a centerline drawn midway between the end-diastolic and the end-systolic contours.[31] The measured motion is normalized by the end-diastolic perimeter length to generate a shortening fraction.

Parameters of Regional Function

The results of wall motion analysis may be expressed in terms of the magnitude of inward motion or of the circumferential extent of wall motion abnormality (Fig. 19–29). The latter, usually referred to as the hypokinetic segment length, is determined as the percentage of the contour with motion depressed below a specified threshold. Measurements of hypokinetic or akinetic segment length indicate the length of the dysfunctional segment but are uninformative concerning the magnitude of dysfunction beyond the threshold. Measurements of inward motion express the level of function of a point or region on the ventricular contour but indicate nothing about the function of surrounding regions. Which parameter is preferable depends on the question being addressed. For example, the effect of thrombolytic therapy in salvaging myocardium is most sensitively detected by measuring inward motion in the infarct

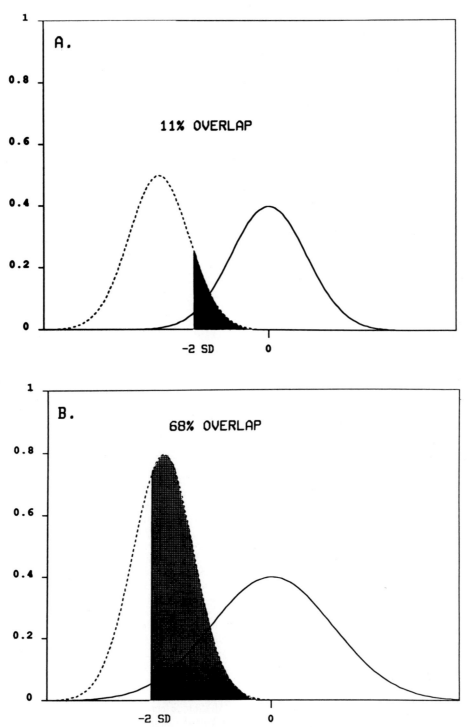

FIGURE 19–26. Distribution of wall motion in normal subjects and in patients with recent myocardial infarction by different imaging modalities. In method "A," there is relatively little variability in the normal group's motion, and the SD is low. Consequently, separation of normals from diseased patients is much greater than that for method "B," indicating that method "A" can more accurately distinguish between these two populations. (Reprinted from Sheehan, F.H.: Measurement of left ventricular function from contrast angiograms in patients with coronary artery disease. *In* Brundage, B. H. [ed.]: Comparative Cardiac Imaging, p. 107, with permission of Aspen Publishers, Inc., © 1990.)

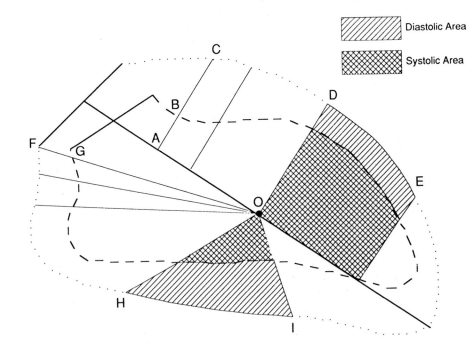

Diastolic Area

Systolic Area

FIGURE 19–27. Most wall motion analysis methods use a rectangular or radial coordinate system. In a rectangular system, motion is measured along a hemi-axis, such as AC; fractional shortening is calculated as BC/AC. Similarly, a fractional shortening can be determined from motion along radius FO as FG/FO. Alternatively, the area ejection fraction may be determined from the areas spanned by two hemiaxes or two radii. For the border segments DE or HI, the calculation is (diastolic area − systolic area)/diastolic area.

region.[21] Measuring hypokinetic segment length introduces variability because of dysfunction in regions outside the acute infarct, such as in the site of previous infarction. On the other hand, a comparison of function in patients with stenosis of the left anterior descending versus the right coronary artery would be more appropriately done with a parameter of hypokinetic segment length, to demonstrate that the former affects a larger segment of the ventricle.

Definition of Normal Motion

Most investigators calculate the mean and standard deviation for normal motion with the use of the data from patients with normal findings on diagnostic cardiac catheterization. Such "cath normals" are closer in age to the patients with ischemic heart disease, who are the most likely subjects of a wall motion analysis, than to Bayesian normals, asymptomatic subjects who by age, sex, or other criteria have a low probability of cardiac disease.

Definition of Abnormal Motion

Abnormality should be assessed in reference to the normal range. The threshold value of 55 percent for the ejection fraction represents two standard deviations below the mean of a normal population. The normal extent of inward motion varies by region around the ventricle (see Fig. 19–24),[32] because of the local architecture of the ventricle.[33] Consequently, there is no single threshold for abnormal wall motion. For example, in the anterior or inferior walls, akinesis represents a grave dysfunction, but at the apex it lies within 2 standard deviations (SDs) of the normal mean for motion (see Fig. 19–24).

Gelberg and colleagues have suggested that motion be expressed in terms of the number of standard deviations by which it differs from the normal mean.[32] By means of this simple conversion, the motion of all regions is expressed in equivalent units, allowing the function of different regions to be summed, averaged, or compared (see Fig. 19–24). The standard deviation units indicate not only the magnitude but also the clinical significance of the abnormality. Positive values indicate hyperkinesis, and negative values hypokinesis.

Variability

The greatest variability arises from differences between repeated studies, but there is also beat-to-beat, intraobserver, and interobserver variability.[14] Variability affects the measurement of volume less than that of wall motion, because wall motion measurements are subject to point-to-point variability, which is "averaged out" when motion is measured over regions rather than at discrete points on the contour (Fig. 19–30).[31, 32]

Measuring Wall Motion in the Region of Interest

The American Heart Association guidelines divide the contour seen in the 30-degree RAO view into five regions. However, in a study of patients with acute myocardial infarction due to isolated stenosis of the left anterior descending artery, the dysfunctional segment spanned two adjacent regions in about one half of the patients (Fig. 19–31). In such cases, the severity of dysfunction is underestimated by both regions because each contains only part of the infarction and partly normal myocardium (see Fig. 19–31).

To address this problem, the centerline method measures wall motion in the region of interest, which in coronary disease is the perfusion territory of the stenosed artery (Fig. 19–32). The most abnormally contracting 50 percent of the artery territory is sought, and the motion of its chords is averaged. This approach yields a greater correlation between wall motion and coronary stenosis severity than the mean motion of larger or smaller proportions of the artery territory. Each artery's territory is defined simply as the set of chords whose motion is significantly depressed, compared with that normal hearts, when measured in patients with isolated stenosis of that artery.[21] The centerline method thus yields a single parameter that expresses the severity of wall motion abnormality within a region of interest. Either hypokinesis or hyperkinesis can be measured with this approach.

Method Selection: Theoretical, Empirical, and Clinical Considerations

Several comparisons have been made, testing the diagnostic accuracy of 2 to 19 methods against the same patient population. These studies have had somewhat variable results, but, in general, radial methods and the centerline method perform better than methods based on a rectangular coordinate system.[23, 25] The methods of Gibson and co-workers and Slager and associates have never been compared to others.[24, 30] A final test of a method's usefulness may be more practical criteria, such as which method is flexible enough to answer all analysis needs and which method produces results that are easy to interpret or to correlate with the results of other diagnostic tests.

Text continued on page 187

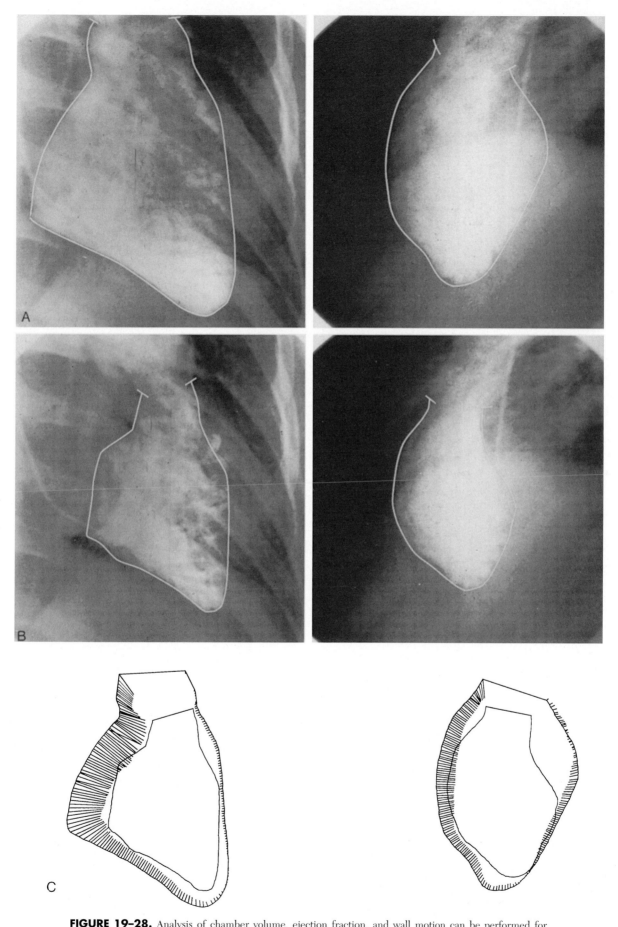

FIGURE 19–28. Analysis of chamber volume, ejection fraction, and wall motion can be performed for the right ventricle as well as for the left. The end-diastolic (A) and end-systolic (B) images, contours, and wall motion analysis (C) are displayed in the 30-degree RAO *(left column)* and 60-degree LAO *(right column)* projections. This patient, a sudden cardiac death survivor, has normal left ventricular function and normal cardiac anatomy. The right ventricular ejection fraction (by the Simpson rule) is 61 percent, and wall motion is hyperkinetic (contours) compared with that of a normal reference population (chords).

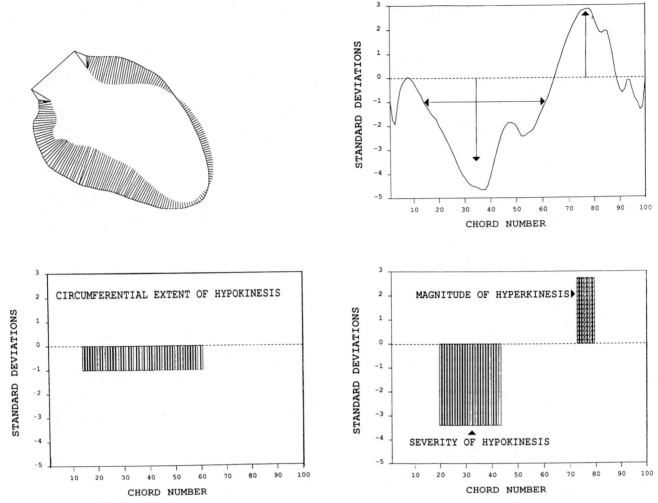

FIGURE 19–29. Wall motion abnormality is commonly expressed in terms of its severity within a region of interest *(lower right)* or its circumferential extent *(lower left)*. The two parameters give quite different impressions of the heart's function. The original contours and full wall motion analysis are shown above.

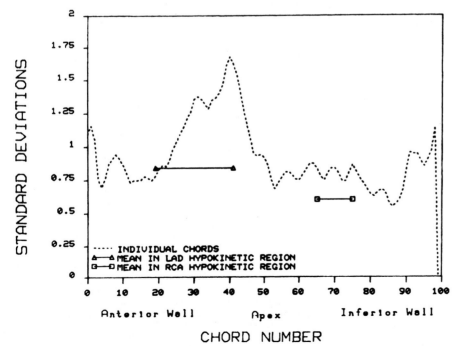

FIGURE 19–30. Variability in the motion of individual chords between repeated angiographic studies is relatively high, even in stable patients. This variability is reduced by averaging the motion of chords lying in the region of interest. (From Sheehan, F.H., Stewart, D.K., Dodge, H.T., et al.: Variability in the measurement of regional ventricular wall motion from contrast angiograms. Circulation 68:550, 1983, with permission from the American Heart Association, Inc.)

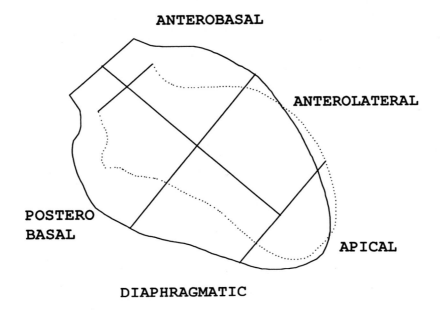

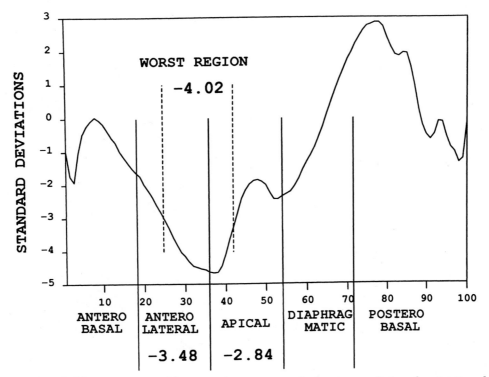

FIGURE 19–31. Segmentation of the ventricular contour into fixed regions results in underestimation of the severity of wall motion because the location of the hypokinetic segment often spans adjacent segments.

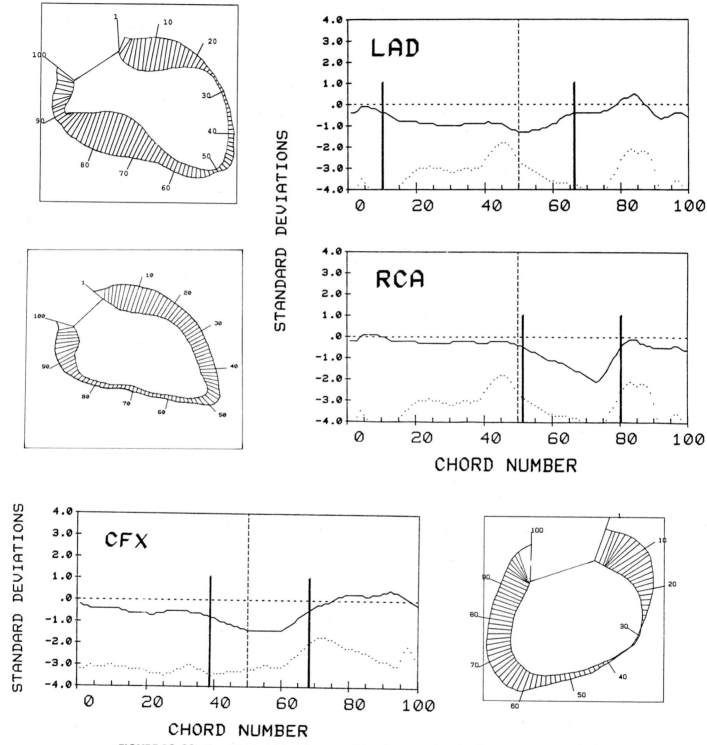

FIGURE 19–32. The territories of the left anterior descending artery (LAD), right coronary artery (RCA), and circumflex artery (CFX) were defined as the sequence of contiguous chords having significantly depressed wall motion in patients with isolated stenosis of the respective artery. The LAD and RCA territories are well visualized in the 30-degree RAO projection, and the CFX in the 60-degree LAO projection.

SUMMARY

In summary, methods for quantitative assessment of the size and function of the atria and ventricles from angiograms have been extensively validated. Because of the accuracy of these methods, and owing to the inherent high spatial and temporal resolution of this imaging modality, angiography continues to serve as the gold standard by which other methods are evaluated.

References

1. Hildner, F.J., Furst, A., Krieger, R., et al.: New principles for optimum left ventriculography. Cathet. Cardiovasc. Diagn. 12:266, 1986.
2. Dodge, H.T., Frimer, M., and Stewart, D.K.: Functional evaluation of the hypertrophied heart in man. Circ. Res. 34–35 (Suppl. II):II-122, 1974.
3. Thompson, R., Ahmed, M., Seabra-Gomes, R., et al.: Influence of preoperative left ventricular function on results of homograft replacement of the aortic valve for aortic regurgitation. J. Thorac. Cardiovasc. Surg. 77:411, 1979.
4. Kennedy, J.W., Kaiser, G.C., Fisher, L.D., et al.: Clinical and angiographic predictors of operative mortality from the Collaborative Study in Coronary Artery Stenosis (CASS). Circulation 63:793, 1981.
5. Holman, B.L., Wynne, J., Idoine, J., et al.: Disruption in the temporal sequence of regional ventricular contraction. Circulation 61:1075, 1980.
6. Hugenholtz, P.G., Kaplan, E., and Hull, E.: Determination of left ventricular wall thickness by angiocardiography. Am. Heart J. 78:513, 1969.
7. Dodge, H.T., Sandler, H., Ballew, D.W., et al.: The use of biplane angiocardiography for the measurement of left ventricular volume in man. Am. Heart J. 60:762, 1960.
8. Wynne, J., Green, L.H., Mann, T., et al.: Estimation of left ventricular volumes in man from biplane cineangiograms filmed in oblique projections. Am. J. Cardiol. 41:726, 1978.
9. Rogers, W.J., Smith, L.R., Bream, P.R., et al.: Quantitative axial oblique contrast left ventriculography: Validation of the method by demonstrating improved visualization of regional wall motion and mitral valve function with accurate volume determinations. Am. Heart J. 103:185, 1982.
10. Lange, P.E., Onnasch, D., Farr, F.L., et al.: Angiocardiographic right ventricular volume determination. Accuracy, as determined from human casts, and clinical application. Eur. J. Cardiol. 8:477, 1978.
11. Cha, S.D., Incarvito, J., and Maranhao, V.: Calculation of magnification factor from an intracardiac marker. Cathet. Cardiovasc. Diagn. 9:79, 1983.
12. Sheehan, F.H., and Mitten-Lewis, S.: Factors influencing accuracy in left ventricular volume determination. Am. J. Cardiol. 64:661, 1989.
13. Vine, D.L., Hegg, T.D., Dodge, H.T., et al.: Immediate effect of contrast medium injection on left ventricular volumes and ejection fraction: a study using metallic epicardial markers. Circulation 56:379, 1977.
14. Sheehan, F.H., Stewart, D.K., Dodge, H.T., et al.: Variability in the measurement of regional ventricular wall motion from contrast angiograms. Circulation 68:550, 1983.
15. Dodge, H.T., Sheehan, F.H., and Stewart, D.K.: Estimation of ventricular volume, fractional ejected volumes, stroke volume, and quantitation of regurgitant flow. *In*
16. Just, H., and Heintzen, P.H. (eds.): Angiocardiography: Current Status and Future Developments. Berlin, Springer-Verlag, 1986, pp. 99–108.
16. Hunt, D., Baxley, W.A., Kennedy, J.W., et al.: Quantitative evaluation of cineaortography in the assessment of aortic regurgitation. Am. J. Cardiol. 31:696, 1973.
17. Kennedy, J.W., Reichenbach, D.D., Baxley, W.A., et al.: Left ventricular mass: A comparison of angiocardiographic measurements with autopsy weight. Am. J. Cardiol. 19:221, 1967.
18. Grossman, W., Jones, D., and McLaurin, L.P.: Wall stress and patterns of hypertrophy in the human left ventricle. J. Clin. Invest. 56:56, 1975.
19. Gould, K.L., Lipscomb, K., Hamilton, G.W., et al.: Relation of left ventricular shape, function and wall stress in man. Am. J. Cardiol. 34:627, 1974.
20. Stack, R.S., Phillips, H.R., III, Grierson, D.S., et al.: Functional improvement of jeopardized myocardium following intracoronary streptokinase infusion in acute myocardial infarction. J. Clin. Invest. 72:34, 1983.
21. Sheehan, F.H., Mathey, D.G., Schofer, J., et al.: Effect of interventions in salvaging left ventricular function in acute myocardial infarction: A study of intracoronary streptokinase. Am. J. Cardiol. 52:431, 1983.
22. McDonald, I.G.: The shape and movements of the human left ventricle during systole. Am. J. Cardiol. 26:221, 1970.
23. Ingels, N.B., Jr., Daughters, G.T., II, Stinson, E.B., et al.: Evaluation of methods for quantitating left ventricular segmental wall motion in man using myocardial markers as a standard. Circulation 61:966, 1980.
24. Slager, C.J., Hooghoudt, T.E.H., Serruys, P.W., et al.: Quantitative assessment of regional left ventricular motion using endocardial landmarks. J. Am. Coll. Cardiol. 7:317, 1986.
25. Karsch, K.R., Lamm, U., Blanke, H., et al.: Comparison of nineteen quantitative models for assessment of localized left ventricular wall motion abnormalities. Clin. Cardiol. 3:123, 1980.
26. Clayton, P.D., Jeppson, G.M., and Klausner, S.C.: Should a fixed external reference system be used to analyze left ventricular wall motion? Circulation 65:1518, 1982.
27. Leighton, R.F., Drobinski, G., Fontaine, G.H., et al.: Effects of correcting apical displacement on regional wall motion in severely damaged ventricles. *In* Computers in Cardiology. Long Beach, CA, IEEE Computer Society, 1983, pp. 173–176.
28. Goodyer, A.V.N., and Langou, R.A.: The multicentric character of normal left ventricular wall motion: Implications for the evaluation of regional wall motion abnormalities by contrast angiography. Cathet. Cardiovasc. Diagn. 8:225, 1982.
29. Papapietro, S.E., Smith, L.R., Hood, W.P., Jr, et al.: An optimal method for angiographic definition and quantification of regional left ventricular contraction. *In* Computers in Cardiology. Long Beach, CA, IEEE Computer Society, 1978, pp. 293–296.
30. Gibson, D.G., Doran, J.H., Traill, T.A., et al.: Abnormal left ventricular wall movement during early systole in patients with angina pectoris. Br. Heart J. 40:758, 1978.
31. Sheehan, F.H., Bolson, E.L., Dodge, H.T., et al.: Advantages and applications of the centerline method for characterizing regional ventricular function. Circulation 74:293, 1986.
32. Gelberg, H.J., Brundage, B.H., Glantz, S., et al.: Quantitative left ventricular wall motion analysis: A comparison of area, chord and radial methods. Circulation 59:991, 1979.
33. Brutsaert, D.L.: Nonuniformity: A physiologic modulator of contraction and relaxation of the normal heart. J. Am. Coll. Cardiol. 9

CHAPTER

20 Applications of Contrast Ventriculography

Florence H. Sheehan, M.D.

APPLICATIONS OF QUANTITATIVE ANALYSIS ____ 188
Normal Values ____ 188
Ventricular Function in Coronary Artery Disease ____ 188
Relationship Between Coronary Artery Stenosis Severity and Function ____ 188
Stress Ventriculography: Assessment of Cardiac Reserve and Viability ____ 188
Wall Motion at the Site of Acute Myocardial Infarction ____ 188

Wall Motion Remote From an Infarction ____ 188
Evaluating the Response to Therapeutic Intervention ____ 188
Theoretical Considerations ____ 188
Timing of Measurements ____ 192
Evaluating the Response to Therapy ____ 192
Ventricular Function Analysis to Assess Prognosis ____ 192
FURTHER APPLICATIONS OF ANGIOGRAPHIC ANALYSIS ____ 192

Right Ventriculography _____ 192
Atrial Angiography _____ 192
Analysis of Left Ventricular Function Throughout
   the Cardiac Cycle _____ 193

Volume Curve _____ 193
Pressure-Volume Relationship _____ 194
Regional Function _____ 194

The accuracy and reproducibility of measurements from contrast ventriculograms have made these techniques useful for a number of research and clinical applications. Quantitative ventriculography is used to define the range of normality, evaluate the effect of disease processes on the heart, and compare the efficacy of therapeutic interventions in salvaging function and improving prognosis.

APPLICATIONS OF QUANTITATIVE ANALYSIS

Normal Values

Normal ranges for end-diastolic volume, end-systolic volume, stroke volume, and the ejection fraction have been determined for both adults and children (Table 20–1). Normal ranges for wall motion have also been published; values vary from study to study with the method used to measure wall motion and to realign to correct for translational motion.

Ventricular Function in Coronary Artery Disease

Relationship Between Coronary Artery Stenosis Severity and Function

In experimental studies and in patients, ventricular function is preserved during progressive coronary artery stenosis until a critical stenosis is reached at which resting coronary flow falls below normal.[1] In humans, function is preserved until unstable angina or infarction occurs. The finding of mild to moderate hypokinesis is not specific for ischemic heart disease, because hypokinesis has also been reported in valvular regurgitation and cardiomyopathy.[2, 3] However, severe regional hypokinesis generally indicates infarction.

Stress Ventriculography: Assessment of Cardiac Reserve and Viability

The purpose of stress ventriculography is to determine cardiac reserve in those with normal resting function or viability in patients with resting hypokinesis or akinesis. The stress may be supine bicycling, handgrip, arm ergometry, cold pressor testing, or atrial pacing. Pharmacologic and metabolic stresses have also been tested. Viability testing is performed clinically to determine whether hypokinetic myocardium might benefit from revascularization. Studies have shown that patients responding to an infusion of epinephrine or nitroglycerin, or to postextrasystolic potentiation, are more likely to recover ventricular function after coronary artery bypass graft surgery. The response to postextrasystolic potentiation during acute myocardial infarction has also been found to predict later functional recovery with or without thrombolytic therapy.[4]

TABLE 20–1. NORMAL VALUES FOR LEFT VENTRICULAR VOLUME AND MASS IN ADULTS

End-diastolic volume	70 ± 20 mL/m^2
End-systolic volume	24 ± 10 mL/m^2
Ejection fraction	0.67 ± 0.08
Mass	92 ± 16 g/m^2
Wall thickness	10.9 ± 2.0 mm

Modified from Dodge, H.T., and Sheehan, F.H.: Quantitative contrast angiography for assessment of ventricular performance in heart disease. J. Am. Coll. Cardiol. 1:73–81, 1983. Reprinted with permission from the American College of Cardiology.

Currently, viability testing is usually performed noninvasively from perfusion or metabolism studies.

Wall Motion at the Site of Acute Myocardial Infarction

Hypokinesis due to occlusion of the left anterior descending and right coronary arteries is similar in severity, averaging -2.7 SD. The circumferential extent of hypokinesis is greater after occlusion of the left anterior descending artery, resulting in a lower ejection fraction. Dysfunction due to circumflex artery occlusion usually resembles that of right coronary artery occlusion but may vary in location, depending on the location of the occlusion. It is slightly better appreciated in the LAO view (Fig. 20–1), which allows visualization of the posterior wall, although the RAO view gives an adequate measure of the severity of hypokinesis.[5, 6]

Infarct size is overestimated by measurement of hypokinetic segment length, because dysfunction extends beyond the ischemic zone. This phenomenon has been attributed to several mechanisms. First, hypofunction in the normally perfused "border zone" may be due to tethering of normal muscle fibers to adjacent infarcted akinetic fibers. Alternatively, the border region may be a zone in which infarction is restricted to a thin layer of the subendocardium, because regional hypokinesis occurs after fibrosis of as little as 6 percent of the wall, and akinesis occurs with fibrosis of only 14 percent of the wall.[7] The dysfunction of the border zone has also been attributed to amplification of local stress in the border zone.[8] The error from including the border zone with the infarct can be reduced by measuring the length of the severely hypokinetic region, rather than the region with mild to moderate hypokinesis.[9] In patients with acute infarction, the hypokinetic region may include myocardium that is ischemic but salvageable; measurements of hypokinetic segment length made at least 48 hours later correlate better with pathologic infarct size, because the risk region has either infarcted or recovered. Another factor is asynchronous motion. Determination of the full extent of akinesis or dyskinesis from frame-by-frame analysis of function throughout the cardiac cycle yields a closer estimate of infarct size than assessment of hypokinetic segment length at end-systole alone.[10]

Infarct size correlates significantly with measurements of either the severity of hypokinesis or the length of the hypokinetic segment measured by the centerline method. The strength of the correlation varies with the method used to measure infarct size: $r = 0.69$ for thallium scintigraphy, $r = 0.78$ for creatine phosphokinase release, $r = 0.79$ for antimyosin antibody scintigraphy or technetium pyrophosphate imaging, and $r = 0.85$ for nuclear magnetic resonance imaging[11, 12] (Fig. 20–2).

Wall Motion Remote From an Infarction

Motion in the wall opposite the site of acute infarction may be increased (Fig. 20–3), normal, or reduced. The incidence of hyperkinesis ranges from 16 to 67 percent in different studies[13, 14] and is independent of the severity of hypokinesis in the infarct site.[15] Hyperkinesis is more common in patients with single-vessel disease than with multivessel disease.[14, 16] It is not surprising, therefore, that patients with hyperkinesis have a higher, even normal ejection fraction and a better prognosis: they also have less severe hypokinesis.[13, 14, 16] Conversely, patients with hypokinesis in the noninfarct region may have an ejection fraction lower than expected from the severity of hypokinesis in the infarct region.[15]

Evaluating the Response to Therapeutic Intervention

Theoretical Considerations

Ventricular function is often measured as an end point in clinical trials of interventions to reduce ischemia or salvage myocardium,

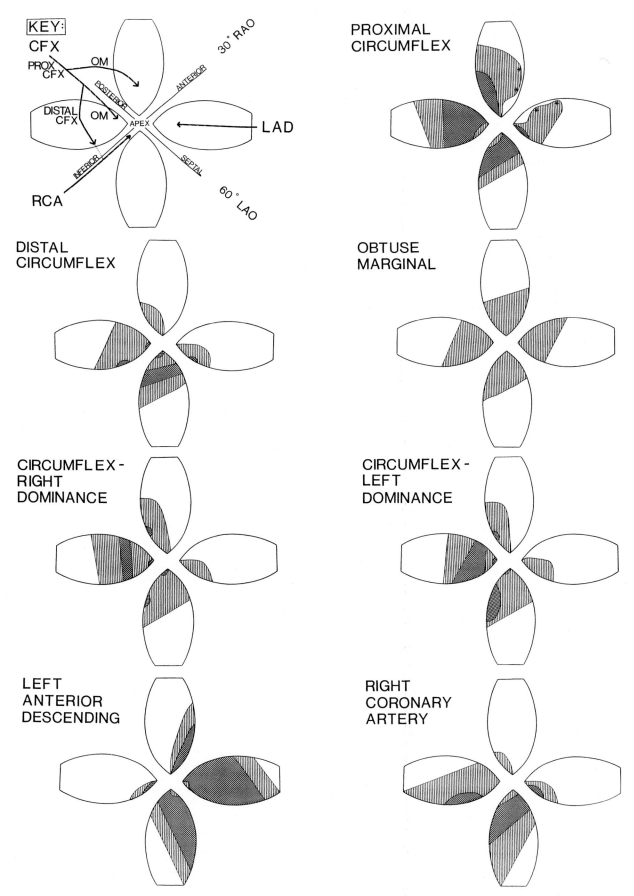

FIGURE 20–1. Biplane analysis of regional wall motion. The display presents the location, extent, and severity of regional dysfunction. This example shows the patterns of dysfunction observed in acute myocardial infarction resulting from isolated stenosis of the left anterior descending (LAD) coronary artery, the right coronary artery (RCA), and the circumflex (CFX). The key is at the upper left. OM = obtuse marginal branch. (From Sheehan, F.H.: Left ventricular dysfunction in acute myocardial infarction due to isolated left circumflex coronary artery stenosis. Am. J. Cardiol. 64:440, 1989, with permission.)

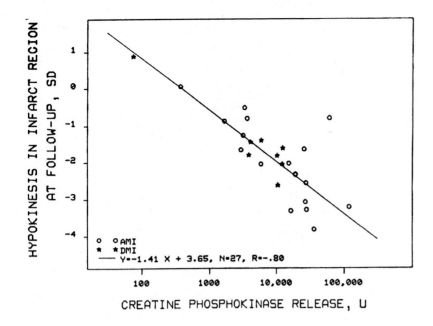

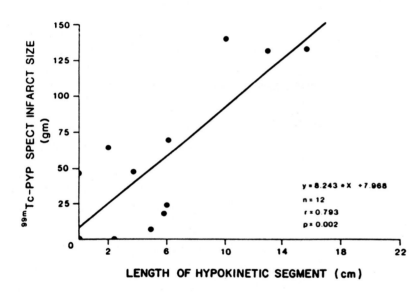

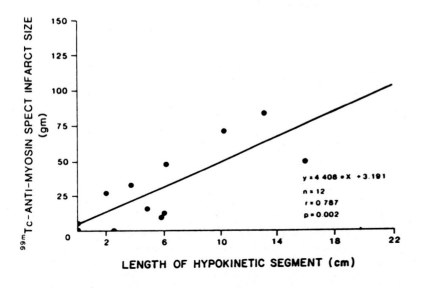

FIGURE 20–2. The severity of hypokinesis in left ventricular wall motion correlates significantly with infarct size estimated from release of creatine phosphokinase *(top)*, technetium pyrophosphate imaging *(center)*, or antimyosin antibody scintigraphy *(bottom)*. (*Top* from Sheehan, F.H., Bolson, E.L., Dodge, H.T., et al.: Advantages and applications of the centerline method for characterizing regional ventricular function. Circulation 74:293, 1986. *Middle and bottom* from Ban An Khaw, Gold, H.K., Yasuda, T., et al.: Scintigraphic quantification of myocardial necrosis in patients after intravenous injection of myosin-specific antibody. Circulation 74:501, 1986, with the permission of the American Heart Association, Inc.)

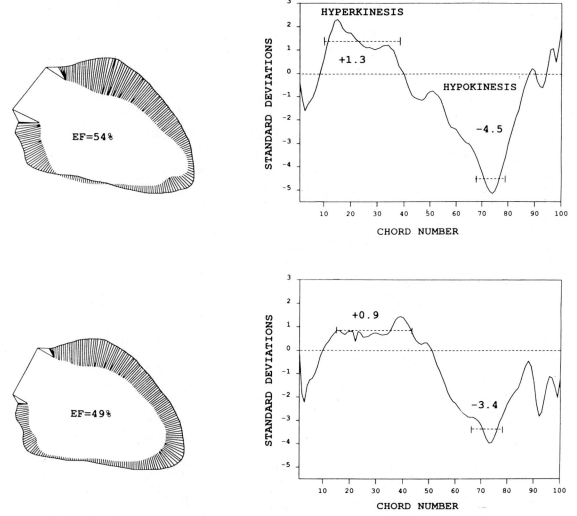

FIGURE 20–3. The development of compensatory hyperkinesis during acute myocardial infarction improves global function *(top)*. However, the effect of thrombolytic therapy on functional recovery in the infarct region may be underestimated by measurement of the ejection fraction because of concomitant regression of hyperkinesis following infarction *(bottom)*.

or both. Ventricular function reflects not only infarct size and adequacy of myocardial perfusion but also prognosis. In general, quantitative end points are more accurate, less variable, and more powerful, requiring fewer study patients to detect a treatment effect.

Timing of Measurements

The effect of therapy on function may be assessed either from the change observed between the baseline and follow-up studies or from the level of function achieved by the time of follow-up. Measurement of function prior to treatment allows (1) comparison of treatment groups to be sure that they were similar at baseline, (2) measurement of the change in function after the intervention, and (3) adjustment for the influence of patient-to-patient variability in baseline function. On the other hand, it is the absolute level of function achieved, not the change in function, which correlates with survival. Thus, the measurement of function at follow-up, and of the severity of residual dysfunction, may be more pertinent to outcome.

In studies of acute myocardial infarction, the time at which ventricular function is measured has critical importance, because of the time course of changes. For example, recovery may be underestimated when measured too soon, because there is a delay before function recovers after reperfusion, even in viable myocardium. This delay ranges from 15 minutes after a 5-minute occlusion to 4 weeks after a permanent occlusion.[17, 18] Both the magnitude and the rate of recovery are related to the severity of the ischemic result. Thus, recovery is more rapid in the peripheral than in the central infarct region.[18-20] In humans, function begins to recover 3 to 5 days after thrombolysis.[21, 22] This phenomenon of the "stunned" myocardium has been attributed to the need to repair damaged metabolic processes. In the noninfarcted region, compensatory hyperkinesis regresses within 3 days after infarction, before function in the infarcted region recovers, causing a transient fall in ejection fraction.

Evaluating the Response to Therapy

The ejection fraction is usually measured as the principal functional end point. However, for studies of thrombolytic therapy for acute myocardial infarction, wall motion in the infarcted region has proved to be more sensitive to the effect of reperfusion, because the ejection fraction is influenced by the sometimes-opposing changes in the infarcted and noninfarcted regions.[15, 23] Wall motion analysis is useful not only in measuring functional recovery after treatment but also in pinpointing the factors that influence recovery.[24] Analysis of wall motion also aids in the interpretation of trial results.

Measurement of left ventricular function can also be used to identify subsets of patients who are likely to benefit from a therapeutic intervention. For example, survival is better after coronary artery bypass graft surgery than with medical therapy for angina in patients with three-vessel disease and an ejection fraction less than 50 percent,[25] despite their higher operative mortality.[26] In contrast, patients with three-vessel disease and an ejection fraction of 50 percent or more did not clearly benefit from surgery.[27] Another example is the preoperative evaluation of patients with aneurysms. Studies agree that the ejection fraction of the nonaneurysmal part of the ventricle correlates with survival.[28]

Ventricular Function Analysis to Assess Prognosis

The ejection fraction is the most powerful predictor of survival in patients with coronary artery disease. In the Seattle Heart Watch Study, which surveyed more than 2000 patients with angina, the ejection fraction was one of the best correlates of survival in both medically and surgically treated groups[29] (see Fig. 19–19). In patients with myocardial infarction, the ejection fraction predicts survival, whether it is measured acutely, after 3 days, before hospital discharge, or later.[21, 30, 31]

Measurements of regional function correlate closely with the ejection fraction and, therefore, closely parallel it as a prognostic indicator. In the Western Washington Intracoronary Streptokinase Study, the hypokinetic segment length was slightly more predictive of the 6-month survival rate than the ejection fraction, but the opposite was true for the 1-year survival rate.[31] The end-systolic volume also correlates strongly with survival, in a manner independent from that of the ejection fraction.[32] In the recent GUSTO trial, the ejection fraction, end-systolic volume, severity of hypokinesis in the infarct region, and circumferential extent of hypokinesis all correlated closely with survival (Fig. 20–4).[33] The question is not "Which parameter is best?" but "What information does each provide?" For assessment of treatment efficacy, wall motion analysis provides accurate information specific to the coronary artery being revascularized. For assessment of left ventricular function as a surrogate end point for mortality, the global ejection fraction should be measured.

FURTHER APPLICATIONS OF ANGIOGRAPHIC ANALYSIS

Right Ventriculography

Until recently, interest in evaluating right ventricular function was restricted to pediatric cardiologists for management of congenital heart disease patients. Experimental studies had suggested that the right ventricle was a superfluous structure. It was not until after the clinical consequences of right ventricular infarction were recognized that methods for measurement of right ventricular volume and ejection fraction were developed.

Even though the right ventricle bears no resemblance to an ellipsoid of revolution, its volume can be calculated with the area-length method from biplane angiograms with an accuracy comparable to that of the left ventricle and of the multiple-slice method.[34] The right ventricle has also been compared to other geometric structures, such as a parallelogram or a prism. In a recent analysis of 21 methods, the pyramid method yielded the greatest accuracy.[35] Measurement of right ventricular volume from single-plane angiograms increases the SEE by 2.7 mL and results in a systematic underestimation of stroke volume and ejection fraction: the error can be reduced by applying phase-specific correction factors at end-diastole and end-systole.[34]

Studies in normal subjects indicate that right ventricular ejection fraction is lower than for the left ventricle.[36] Because the stroke volumes of the two ventricles are equal in the absence of a shunt, normal volumes are greater in the right ventricle than in the left ventricle. This has been demonstrated indirectly by Lange and associates, who showed that the relationship between right ventricular volume and body-surface area has a higher coefficient than the relationship between left ventricular volume and body-surface area.[34] A direct comparison of right and left ventricular volumes is difficult in vivo because biventricular angiograms are not performed on patients with normal hearts. The normal extent of inward wall motion is lower in the right ventricle (see Fig. 19–28).[36] Consequently, it is more difficult to identify abnormalities in wall motion, unless the disease process results in frank dyskinesis.

Reports on right ventricular function in coronary artery disease have been recent and few. Right ventricular infarction occurs much less frequently than, and is virtually always associated with, left ventricular infarction.[37] Occlusion of the right or left anterior descending coronary arteries causes hypokinesis in the free wall or septum, respectively,[38] but the circumferential extent of hypokinesis is small.

Atrial Angiography

As for the ventricles, methods for left and right atrial volume determination have been developed and validated by casts. Al-

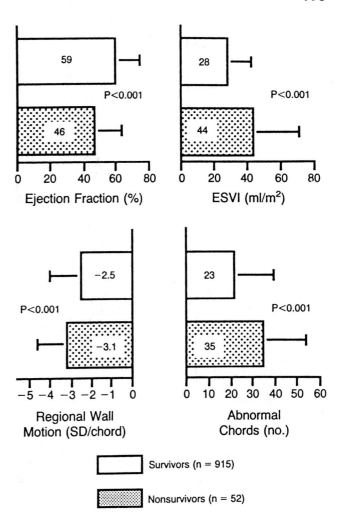

FIGURE 20–4. Left ventricular function 90 minutes after the start of thrombolytic therapy in patients who survived for 30 days after infarction and patients who died before 30 days. Values are means; horizontal T bars indicate the standard deviation. ESVI = end-systolic volume index. Regional wall motion is expressed as the severity of hypokinesis in the infarct zone, in units of standard deviations from the normal mean. Chords in the infarct zone were considered abnormal when their motion was more depressed than 2 SDs below the normal mean. (From The GUSTO Angiographic Investigators: The effects of tissue plasminogen activator, streptokinase, or both on coronary artery patency, ventricular function, and survival after acute myocardial infarction. N. Engl. J. Med. 329:1620, 1993. Reprinted by permission of the New England Journal of Medicine.)

though the Simpson rule approach yielded slightly but not significantly better results for the right atrium, left atrial volume was most accurately determined by the area-length method. Studies of atrial volumes have provided information on the normal range in children and adults and the effect of congenital and valvular heart disease. Analysis of the left atrial pressure-volume relationship has provided information on the function of the left atrium and on the mechanism of left atrial enlargement.

Analysis of Left Ventricular Function Throughout the Cardiac Cycle

Volume Curve

From calculations of volume at each frame through a cardiac cycle, a volume-time curve can be constructed (Fig. 20–5). Rapid filming at 30 to 60 frames per second allows accurate determination of the rate of ejection or filling from the slopes of the systolic or

FIGURE 20–5. From frame-by-frame analysis of left ventricular chamber volume, the volume-time curve can be plotted. At slow heart rates (heart rate = 46 in this study), the diastasis period is prolonged.

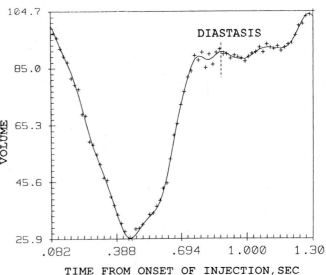

diastolic portions of the volume-time curve. The peak ejection rate is a parameter of ventricular performance but offers no advantage over the ejection fraction.[39]

Because the ejection fraction is normal in patients with coronary disease without infarction, there has been a search for a functional parameter that is more sensitive to ischemia. The partial ejection fraction, or volume ejected in early systole, was not consistently found to be reduced in patients with a normal end-systolic ejection fraction.[40] On the other hand, diastolic filling rates are reduced in patients with coronary artery disease and normal systolic function.[41] These findings have been confirmed with the radionuclide techniques.

Pressure-Volume Relationship

Integration of volume and ventricular pressure data allows measurement of stroke work.[42, 43] Systolic stroke work is calculated from the area under the systolic portion of the pressure-volume curve and the work of filling from the diastolic portion. Systolic stroke work increases when the ventricle dilates or afterload increases, as with aortic stenosis. The work of filling the ventricle in diastole is related to its distensibility. In patients with increased wall thickness, compliance is chronically reduced. This is manifested by an elevation in end-diastolic pressure, shifting the diastolic portion of the pressure-volume upward. Acute myocardial ischemia can also decrease compliance, by increasing muscle stiffness without changing the volume:mass ratio, which has been attributed to impaired relaxation or to sustained contraction. Even without performing further quantitative analysis, the effect of heart disease on stroke work can be appreciated from the shape and location of the pressure-volume loop (Fig. 20–6).

The elastance of the left ventricle can be determined from repeated measurements of the pressure-volume relationship under varying loading conditions.[44] The maximum elastance (Emax) has been used as a load-independent measure of contractility. In clinical studies, Emax is generally approximated by calculating the elastance at end-systole. More recent studies report that the end-systolic pressure-volume relationship is curvilinear under conditions of regional myocardial ischemia and is not adequately described by a simple slope and intercept.[45] The preload recruitable stroke work is another parameter of contractility that is load independent. It can be determined from the same set of pressure-volume loops as that for elastance.[46]

Regional Function

Assessment of regional wall motion throughout the cardiac cycle provides information on the synchrony of contraction (Figs. 20–7 to 20–9). A method is needed to adjust for heart rate and to express the wall motion results so that they are clearly understandable (Fig. 20–10). The duration of systole is fairly constant, varying within narrow limits of 0.36 ± 0.04 second over the clinical spectrum of heart rates.[41] Consequently, the extent of motion can be measured at each fraction of systole and compared between patients (see Fig. 20–9). Alternatively, the linearity of the correlation between wall motion and time through systole can be used as an index of function.[47] The strength of the correlation indicates the linearity of motion with time; the slope of the regression and its direction indicate whether motion is hyperkinetic or hypokinetic. The situation is more difficult for diastole. The duration of diastasis correlates highly with the length of the cardiac cycle ($r = 0.87$) in normal subjects[41] and thus adjusts the duration of diastole for changes in heart rate. When the duration of diastole is fractionated, measurements of function made at a given fraction correspond to different parts of diastole in patients with different heart rates (see Fig. 20–10).

In normal patients there is regional variability in the timing of the phases of diastole, in the timing of the onset of systolic inward motion,[48] in the extent and velocity of outward motion during isovolumic relaxation,[49] and in the peak velocity of systolic inward motion,[50] as well as in the extent of motion at end-systole.[51] This regional, temporal variability has been related to the sequence of activation[52] and to loading conditions.[53]

In patients with coronary artery disease, the extent of wall motion in the ischemic region is not accurately reflected by the measurement at end-systole.[54] The onset of contraction may be delayed, or there may be paradoxical outward motion during isovolumic contraction.[55] These abnormalities are associated with abnormal inward motion during isovolumic relaxation.[49] Asynchrony can be defined as the difference between the time of end-systole and the time at which each region around the ventricular contour

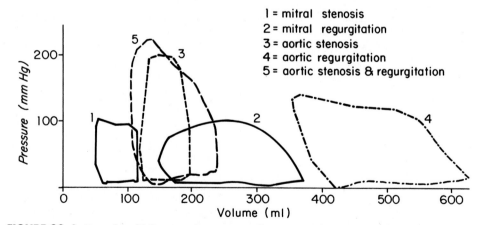

1 = mitral stenosis
2 = mitral regurgitation
3 = aortic stenosis
4 = aortic regurgitation
5 = aortic stenosis & regurgitation

FIGURE 20–6. Examples of left ventricular pressure-volume curves from patients with different types of heart diseases. The curve from the patient with mitral stenosis (1) shows well-defined isovolumic contraction and relaxation periods, a normal stroke volume, and relatively normal stroke work. The other patients have large stroke work values, as estimated by the areas under the systolic limb of the curves. The patients with aortic (4) or mitral (2) regurgitation and aortic stenosis and regurgitation (5) have elevated stroke work values with large stroke volumes, as is shown by excursion of the curves along the horizontal or volume axis. Patients with valvular insufficiency have shortening or absence of isovolumic contraction and relaxation periods. Patients with aortic valve stenosis (3) have elevated systolic pressures. Patients with large stroke volumes have elevated end-diastolic volumes. (From Dodge, H.T., and Kennedy, J.W.: Cardiac output, cardiac performance, hypertrophy, dilation, valvular disease, ischemic heart disease, and pericardial disease. *In* Sodeman, W.A., Jr., and Sodeman, W.A. (eds.): Pathologic Physiology: Mechanisms of Disease. 7th ed. Philadelphia, W.B. Saunders, 1985, pp. 292–331.)

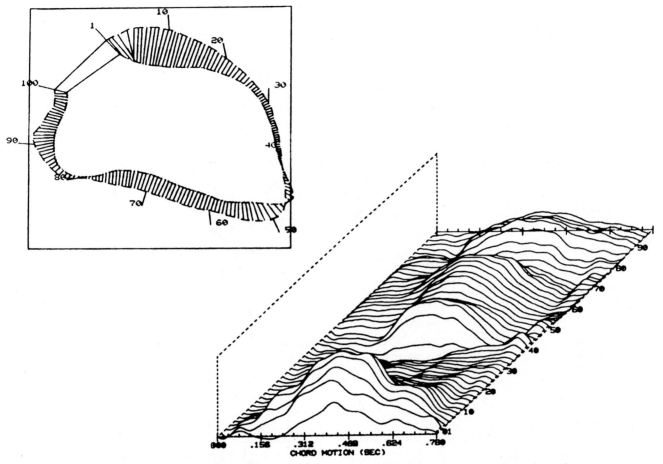

FIGURE 20–7. Wall motion throughout the cardiac cycle can be plotted as a three-dimensional plot, with chord number, time, and motion on the x, y, and z axes. Normal motion is a "mountain range" extending the length of the y axis. Akinesis is depicted as a flat "plain." The patient was studied during acute anterior myocardial infarction.

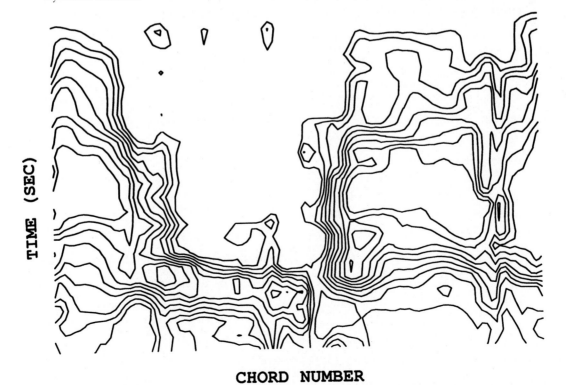

CHORD NUMBER

FIGURE 20–8. The timing of motion depicted with the use of a contour plot.[55] All data can be seen; none is hidden behind the "mountain range." Same patient as in Figure 20–7.

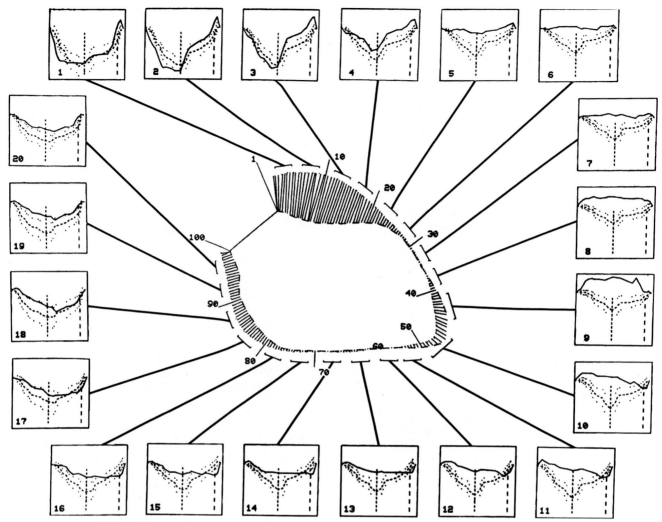

FIGURE 20–9. Wall motion *(vertical axis)* in 20 regions around the left ventricle plotted versus time *(horizontal axis)* through the cardiac cycle from end-diastole to end-diastole. End-systole is marked by the finely dashed vertical line. The time in diastole at which inward motion ceases is marked by the coarsely dashed vertical line. The solid curve is the patient's motion. The dotted curves indicate the mean ± 1 SD for motion in 31 normal patients. Motion is akinetic along the anterior wall (regions 6–8) in this patient with acute thrombosis of the left anterior descending artery. There is apical dyskinesis. Along the inferior wall, postsystolic shortening can be seen. In segments with normal synchronous motion (segment 3) or akinesis (segment 6 or 7), the correlation of motion with time is linear, differing only in slope. In some regions, motion is asynchronous. For example, segment 14 displays slight paradoxical motion at the onset of systole, contraction at a normal rate in early systole, then near akinesis through mid-diastole.

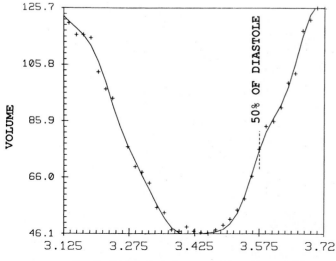

FIGURE 20–10. Differences in heart rate primarily affect the duration of diastole by prolonging diastasis. Consequently, when function is measured at fractions of the duration of diastole, different parts of the cardiac cycle are compared in patients with different heart rates. In this study, the heart rate is 96, and mid-diastole occurs near midfilling. In contrast, mid-diastole occurs after the rapid filling period has ended, at the beginning of diastasis, at a heart rate of 46 as seen in Figure 20–5.

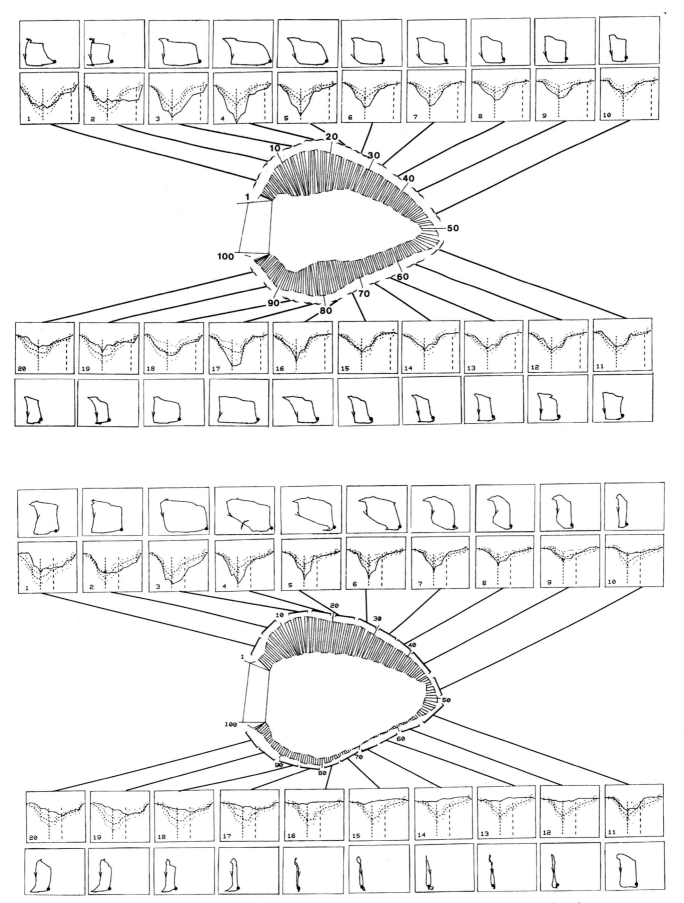

FIGURE 20–11. Pressure-motion loops relate the motion measured throughout the cardiac cycle with changes in intraventricular pressure. These studies were performed before *(top)* and during *(bottom)* occlusion of the right coronary artery in a patient undergoing angioplasty. The motion-time curves of the same regions are presented for comparison.

reaches maximum contraction, or it can be defined as the difference between the systole and the time each region reaches peak rate of contraction or peak rate of relaxation and can be measured from the first derivative of the motion-time curve.[56] It has been suggested that inward motion occurring in diastole represents residual contractile activity in patients with acute myocardial infarction.[57] These patterns of asynchrony can be classified into a progression of abnormality with increasing severity of coronary artery disease.[58]

Examination of asynchrony has not proved useful in studies attempting to correlate function with infarct size, the clinical status of the patient, or the presence of surgical aneurysm.[59, 60] On the other hand, analysis of regional diastolic function has been helpful in elucidating observed abnormalities in global diastolic function. For example, prolongation of the time constant of pressure decay and decrease in the diastolic filling rate at rest and during acute ischemia have been related to reduced regional outward wall motion in the ischemic region.[61, 62]

Measurements of the displacement of the ventricular wall with time can be combined with intraventricular pressure data in a manner analogous to that of pressure-volume curves (Fig. 20–11). The area enclosed within the loop provides an index of regional stroke work, and the shape of the loop graphically displays the effect of disease processes on regional contraction. Sasayama and associates have demonstrated the differing effects of pacing-induced ischemia on diastolic pressure-length relationships in normal and ischemic regions, and their contribution to the global pressure-volume relation.[63] In pressure-dimension analyses, as in two-frame wall motion studies, it must be remembered that the translational motion of the heart within the chest cannot be distinguished from endocardial motion.

References

1. Schwarz, F., Flameng, W., Thiedemann, K.-U., et al.: Effect of coronary stenosis on myocardial function, ultrastructure and aortocoronary bypass graft hemodynamics. Am. J. Cardiol. 42:193, 1978.
2. Osbakken, M.D., Bove, A.A., and Spann, J.F.: Left ventricular regional wall motion and velocity of shortening in chronic mitral and aortic regurgitation. Am. J. Cardiol. 47:1005, 1981.
3. Wallis, D.E., O'Connell, J.B., Henkin, R.E., et al.: Segmental wall motion abnormalities in dilated cardiomyopathy: A common finding and good prognostic sign. J. Am. Coll. Cardiol. 4:674, 1984.
4. Azancot, I., Beaufils, P., Masquet, C., et al.: Detection of residual myocardial function in acute transmural infarction using postextrasystolic potentiation. Circulation 64:46, 1981.
5. Sheehan, F.H., Schofer, J., Mathey, D.G., et al.: Measurement of regional wall motion from biplane contrast ventriculograms: A comparison of the 30-degree RAO and 60-degree LAO projections in patients with acute myocardial infarction. Circulation 74:796, 1986.
6. Sheehan, F.H.: Left ventricular dysfunction in acute myocardial infarction due to isolated left circumflex coronary artery stenosis. Am. J. Cardiol. 64:440, 1989.
7. Ideker, R.E., Behar, V.S., Wagner, G.S., et al.: Evaluation of asynergy as an indicator of myocardial fibrosis. Circulation 57:715, 1978.
8. Bogen, D.K., Rabinowitz, S.A., Needleman, A., et al.: An analysis of the mechanical disadvantage of myocardial infarction in the canine left ventricle. Circ. Res. 47:728, 1980.
9. Gallagher, K.P., Gerren, R.A., Stirling, M.C., et al.: The distribution of functional impairment across the lateral border of acutely ischemic myocardium. Circ. Res. 58:570, 1986.
10. Kaul, S., Pandian, N.G., Gillam, L.D., et al.: Contrast echocardiography in acute myocardial ischemia: III. An in vivo comparison of the extent of abnormal wall motion with the area at risk for necrosis. J. Am. Coll. Cardiol. 7:383, 1986.
11. Sheehan, F.H., Bolson, E.L., Dodge, H.T., et al.: Advantages and applications of the centerline method for characterizing regional ventricular function. Circulation 74:293, 1986.
12. Khaw, B.A., Gold, H.K., Yasuda, T., et al.: Scintigraphic quantification of myocardial necrosis in patients after intravenous injection of myosin-specific antibody. Circulation 74:501, 1986.
13. Stadius, M.L., Maynard, C., Fritz, J.K., et al.: Coronary anatomy and left ventricular function in the first 12 hours of acute myocardial infarction: The Western Washington Randomized Intracoronary Streptokinase Trial. Circulation 72:292, 1985.
14. Jaarsma, W., Visser, C.A., Van, M.J.E., et al.: Prognostic implications of regional hyperkinesia and remote asynergy of noninfarcted myocardium. Am. J. Cardiol. 58:394, 1986.
15. Sheehan, F.H., Mathey, D.G., Schofer, J., et al.: Effect of interventions in salvaging left ventricular function in acute myocardial infarction: A study of intracoronary streptokinase. Am. J. Cardiol. 52:431, 1983.
16. Grines, C.L., Topol, E.J., Califf, R.M., et al.: Prognostic implications and pre-

17. Heyndrickx, G.R., Millard, R.W., McRitchie, R.J., et al.: Regional myocardial functional and electrophysiological alterations after brief coronary artery occlusion in conscious dogs. J. Clin. Invest. 56:978, 1975.
18. Lavallee, M., Cox, D., Patrick, T.A., et al.: Salvage of myocardial function by coronary artery reperfusion 1, 2, and 3 hours after occlusion in conscious dogs. Circ. Res. 53:235, 1983.
19. Ellis, S.G., Henschke, C.I., Sandor, T., et al.: Time course of functional and biochemical recovery of myocardium salvaged by reperfusion. J. Am. Coll. Cardiol. 1:1047, 1983.
20. Roan, P.G., Buja, M., Izquierdo, C., et al.: Interrelationships between regional left ventricular function, coronary blood flow, and myocellular necrosis during the initial 24 hours and 1 week after experimental coronary occlusion in awake, unsedated dogs. Circ. Res. 49:31, 1981.
21. Sheehan, F.H., Doerr, R., Schmidt, W.G., et al.: Early recovery of left ventricular function after thrombolytic therapy for acute myocardial infarction: An important determinant of survival. J. Am. Coll. Cardiol. 12:289, 1988.
22. Widimsky, P., Cervenka, V., Gregor, P., et al.: First month course of left ventricular asynergy after intracoronary thrombolysis in acute myocardial infarction: A longitudinal echocardiographic study. Eur. Heart J. 6:759, 1985.
23. Stack, R.S., Phillips, H.R., III, Grierson, D.S., et al.: Functional improvement of jeopardized myocardium following intracoronary streptokinase infusion in acute myocardial infarction.
24. Sheehan, F.H., Mathey, D.G., Schofer, J., et al.: Factors determining recovery of left ventricular function following thrombolysis in acute myocardial infarction. Circulation 71:1121, 1985.
25. CASS Principal Investigators and Their Associates: Myocardial infarction and mortality in the coronary artery surgery study (CASS randomized trial). N. Engl. J. Med. 310:750, 1984.
26. Kennedy, J.W., Kaiser, G.C., Fisher, L.D., et al.: Clinical and angiographic predictors of operative mortality from the Collaborative Study in Coronary Artery Stenosis (CASS). Circulation 63:793, 1981.
27. European Coronary Surgery Study Group: Long-term results of prospective randomized study of coronary artery bypass surgery in stable angina pectoris. Lancet 2:1172, 1982.
28. Kiefer, S.K., Flaker, G.C., Martin, R.H., et al.: Clinical improvement after ventricular aneurysm repair: Prediction by angiographic and hemodynamic variables. J. Am. Coll. Cardiol. 2:30, 1983.
29. Hammermeister, K.E., DeRouen, T.A., and Dodge, H.T.: Variables predictive of survival in patients with coronary disease. Circulation 59:421, 1979.
30. Multicenter Postinfarction Research Group: Risk stratification and survival after myocardial infarction. N. Engl. J. Med. 309:331, 1983.
31. Stadius, M.L., Davis, K., Maynard, C., et al.: Risk stratification for 1 year survival based on characteristics identified in the early hours of acute myocardial infarction: The Western Washington Intracoronary Streptokinase Trial. Circulation 74:703, 1986.
32. White, H.D., Norris, R.M., Brown, M.A., et al.: Left ventricular end-systolic volume as the major determinant of survival after recovery from myocardial infarction. Circulation 76:44, 1987.
33. The GUSTO Angiographic Investigators: The effects of tissue plasminogen activator, streptokinase, or both on coronary artery patency, ventricular function, and survival after acute myocardial infarction. N. Engl. J. Med. 329:1615, 1993.
34. Lange, P.E., Onnasch, D., Farr, F.L., et al.: Angiocardiographic right ventricular volume determination: Accuracy, as determined from human casts, and clinical application. Eur. J. Cardiol. 8:477, 1978.
35. Dubel, H.P., Romaniuk, P., and Tschapek, A.: Investigation of human right ventricular cast specimens. Cardiovasc. Intervent. Radiol. 5:296, 1982.
36. Sheehan, F.H., Mathey, D.G., Wygant, J., et al.: Measurement of regional right ventricular wall motion from biplane contrast angiograms using the centerline method. *In* Computers in Cardiology. Long Beach, CA, IEEE Computer Society, 1985, pp. 149–152.
37. Rackley, C.E., Russell, R.O., Jr., Mantle, J.A., et al.: Right ventricular infarction and function. Am. Heart J. 101:215, 1981.
38. Morrison, D.A., Hartnett, S.D., and Adcock, K.: Radionuclide and angiographic assessment of the right heart. Cardiovasc. Clin. 17:19, 1987.
39. Hammermeister, K.E., Brooks, R.C., and Warbasse, J.R.: Rate of change of left ventricular volume in man: I. Validation and peak systolic ejection rate in health and disease. Circulation 49:729, 1974.
40. Sheehan, F.H., Dodge, H.T., Bolson, E.L., et al.: Value of partial ejection fraction and volume increment in distinguishing patients with and without clinically significant coronary artery disease. Circulation 68:756, 1983.
41. Hammermeister, K.E., and Warbasse, J.R.: The rate of change of left ventricular volume in man: II. Diastolic events in health and disease. Circulation 49:739, 1974.
42. Dodge, H.T., Sandler, H., Baxley, W.A., et al.: Usefulness and limitations of radiographic methods for determining left ventricular volume. Am. J. Cardiol. 18:10, 1966.
43. Rackley C.E., Behar, V.S., Whalen, R.E., et al.: Biplane cineangiographic determinations of left ventricular function: Pressure-volume relationships. Am. Heart J. 74:766, 1967.
44. Sagawa, K.: Editorial: The end-systolic pressure-volume relationship of the ventricle: Definition, modifications and clinical use. Circulation 63:1223, 1981.
45. Kass, D.A., and Maughan, W.L.: From "Emax" to pressure-volume relations: A broader view. Circulation 77:1203, 1988.
46. Glower, D.D., Spratt, J.A., Snow, N.D., et al.: Linearity of the Frank-Starling

relationship in the intact heart: The concept of preload recruitable stroke work. Circulation 71:994, 1985.

47. Chen, C., Bonzel, T., Just, H., et al.: Quantitative assessment of temporal and spatial ventricular wall motion in normal and infarcted human left ventricles. Am. Heart J. 112:712, 1986.

48. Clayton, P.D., Bulawa, W.F., Klausner, S.C., et al.: The characteristic sequence for the onset of contraction in the normal human left ventricle. Circulation 59:671, 1979.

49. Gibson, D.G., Prewitt, T.A., and Brown, D.J.: Analysis of left ventricular wall movement during isovolumic relaxation and its relation to coronary artery disease. Br. Heart J. 38:1010, 1976.

50. Gibson, D.G., Sanderson, J.E., Traill, T.A., et al.: Regional left ventricular wall movement in hypertrophic cardiomyopathy. Br. Heart J. 40:1327, 1978.

51. Gelberg, H.J., Brundage, B.H., Glantz, S., et al.: Quantitative left ventricular wall motion analysis: A comparison of area, chord and radial methods. Circulation 59:991, 1979.

52. Klausner, S.C., Blair, T.J., Bulawa, W.F., et al.: Quantitative analysis of segmental wall motion throughout systole and diastole in the normal human left ventricle. Circulation 65:580, 1982.

53. Gaasch, W.H., Blaustein, A.S., and Bing, O.H.L.: Asynchronous (segmental early) relaxation of the left ventricle. J. Am. Coll. Cardiol. 5:891, 1985.

54. Weyman, A.E., Hogan, T.D., Jr., Gillam, L.D., et al.: Importance of temporal heterogeneity in assessing the contraction abnormalities associated with acute myocardial ischemia. Circulation 70:102, 1984.

55. Gibson, D.G., Doran, J.H., Traill, T.A., et al.: Abnormal left ventricular wall

56. Melchior, J.P., Doriot, P.A., Chatelain, P., et al.: Improvement of left ventricular contraction and relaxation synchronism after recanalization of chronic total coronary occlusion by angioplasty. J. Am. Coll. Cardiol. 9:763, 1987.

57. Takayama, M., Norris, R.M., Brown, M.A., et al.: Post-systolic shortening of acutely ischemic canine myocardium predicts early and late recovery of function following coronary artery reperfusion. Circulation 78:994, 1988.

58. Holman, B.L., Wynne, J., Idoine, J., et al.: Disruption in the temporal sequence of regional ventricular contraction. Circulation 61:1075, 1980.

59. Dawson, J.R., and Sutton, G.C.: Incoordinate left ventricular wall motion after acute myocardial infarction. Br. Heart J. 51:545, 1984.

60. Leighton, R.F., Drobinski, G., Eugene, M., et al.: The timing of paradoxical wall motion in ventricular aneurysms and in asynergic ventricles. Int. J. Cardiol. 12:321, 1986.

61. Takeuchi, M., Fujitani, K., and Fukuzaki, H.: The relation between left ventricular asynchrony, relaxation, outward wall motion and filling characteristics during control period and pacing-induced myocardial ischemia in coronary artery disease. Int. J. Cardiol. 9:45, 1985.

62. Serruys, P.W., Wijns, W., Van denBrand, M., et al.: Left ventricular performance, regional blood flow, wall motion, and lactate metabolism during transluminal angioplasty. Circulation 70:25, 1984.

63. Sasayama, S., Nonogi, H., Miyazaki, S., et al.: Changes in diastolic properties of the regional myocardium during pacing-induced ischemia in human subjects. J. Am. Coll. Cardiol. 5:599, 1985.

movement during early systole in patients with angina pectoris. Br. Heart J. 40:758, 1978.

CHAPTER

21 Role of Aortography in the Age of Imaging

Colleen Sanders, M.D.

TECHNICAL ASPECTS _____ 199
Aortographic Technique _____ 199
  Catheterization Technique _____ 199
  Choice of Contrast Agent _____ 200
  Risks of Aortography _____ 200
Filming Techniques _____ 200
  Screen-Film Methods _____ 200
  Digital Techniques _____ 200
  Advantages of Digital Imaging _____ 200
  Disadvantages of Digital Imaging _____ 200
  Screen-Film Versus Digital Methods _____ 201
  Cineangiography _____ 202
CLINICAL ASPECTS _____ 202

Aortic Aneurysm _____ 202
  Imaging of Aortic Aneurysm _____ 202
  Angiographic Diagnosis of Aortic Aneurysm _____ 202
Aortic Dissection _____ 202
  Imaging of Aortic Dissection _____ 202
  Angiographic Diagnosis of Aortic Dissection _____ 203
Aortic Trauma _____ 204
  Angiographic Diagnosis of Aortic Injury _____ 204
  Role of Computed Tomography in Aortic Trauma _____ 205

Aortography was established as the diagnostic standard in aortic disease in the 1960s[1, 2] and remains an extremely useful and important tool. It offers greater than 95 percent diagnostic accuracy, and its superb delineation of smaller arterial branches is unmatched by any other examination. The newer techniques of computed tomography (CT) and magnetic resonance imaging (MRI) are less invasive and have fewer complications with little, if any, loss of accuracy. The advent of these alternatives requires reexamination of the uses of and indications for angiography.

TECHNICAL ASPECTS

Aortographic Technique

Catheterization Technique

Except in intravenous digital subtraction angiography (DSA), a femoral artery puncture is usually used. Catheter sizes range from 4 to 7 Fr., with the smaller catheters being used in intraarterial digital studies. For the thoracic aortogram, the end of the catheter is positioned approximately 2 to 3 cm above the aortic valve. For abdominal aortograms, the catheter is placed with its tip at the level of the celiac axis.

In cases of severe distal aortic or ileofemoral disease, an axillary artery puncture may be performed. However, this procedure has a higher complication rate than femoral artery puncture, and hematomas requiring surgical evacuation to alleviate neural compression occur in 1 to 2 percent of cases.[2] Axillary puncture is contraindicated in patients with abnormal coagulation, hypertension, or obesity because these conditions increase the likelihood of hematoma.

If a femoral Dacron graft is present, puncture of the graft is preferable to the axillary approach if the graft is more than 6 months old and the puncture site is proximal to the femoral anastomosis. Careful attention to sterile technique is required, and the catheter must be removed over a guidewire to avoid shearing of catheter fragments. In rare instances, a translumbar approach may be used.[3]

Choice of Contrast Agent

Pain, heat, and transient hypotension are the common side effects of angiography with ionic contrast agents such as metrizoate (Renografin). These effects result from dilatation of the vascular bed, which causes a decrease in systemic vascular resistance and a drop in arterial pressure. A reflex rise in cardiac output and pulse then occurs, typically lasting 2 to 3 minutes. In a study comparing subjective and hemodynamic reactions to aortic injections of iohexol (a nonionic agent), metrizamide (a low-osmolality ionic agent), and metrizoate, the high-ionic agent caused more pain and heat sensation and had more pronounced systemic hemodynamic effects than the other agents.[4] Because of their high cost, however, the newer contrast agents are not routinely used in angiography unless there is a history of allergy to contrast media (see also Chapter 18).

Risks of Aortography

Aortography is a very safe procedure. It has a mortality rate of 0.032 percent and a complication rate for the transfemoral approach of 1.73 percent.[5] Adverse effects may be related to the catheterization itself (e.g., hematomas, arterial thromboses, cholesterol emboli[2]) or to the administration of the contrast agent. Renal dysfunction, usually transient, develops in up to 30 percent of patients after angiography.[6] Development of renal dysfunction is not reduced by the use of nonionic media, but serious allergic reactions are decreased significantly with use of the newer agents (see also Chapter 18).

Filming Techniques

Screen-Film Methods

Conventional aortography uses screen-film combinations to display full-sized images on film (Fig. 21–1). Whether conventional or digital imaging is used, filming rates should not be less than 3 films per second, with an optimum filming rate of 4 or more

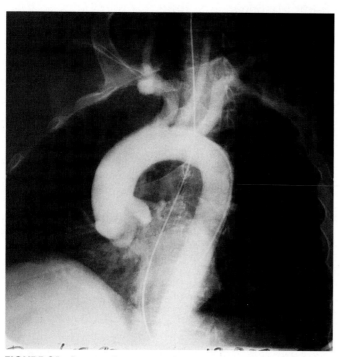

FIGURE 21–1. Normal conventional screen-film thoracic aortogram. The right posterior oblique (RPO) projection displays the long axis of the thoracic aorta.

films per second.[2] Filming is performed initially at an angle of approximately 40 degrees right posterior oblique to display the long axis of the thoracic aorta. Other projections are obtained as necessary. For congenital aortic abnormalities, anteroposterior and lateral views are the most informative. The field of view should include the entire thoracic aorta and the origins of the brachiocephalic vessels. For thoracic aortograms, 60 mL of diatrizoate meglumine (Renografin-76) is injected at a rate of 30 mL per second. Abdominal aortograms usually require less contrast material, 40 to 50 mL over seconds. In the abdomen, a single anteroposterior projection is usually sufficient. Lateral views provide additional needed information in cases of abdominal aortic aneurysms or if stenoses of the origins of the visceral arteries are suspected.

Digital Techniques

In digital radiography, the information from the x-rays is recorded in digital format from the photodiode tube, rather than in analog format on film. Because the information is in digital form, image processing and transmission are easily performed. The most common method of image processing is subtraction. In this procedure, a mask (an initial image of the area taken before injection of the contrast agent) is subtracted from the digital image, leaving only the vessels that contain contrast material in view.

In intravenous DSA, the contrast medium is injected in an antecubital vein or, less commonly, into the superior vena cava or the right atrium.[7] Images of the area in question are then obtained as the bolus of contrast material passes through the systemic circulation. The site of injection is an important aspect of image quality, particularly with the prolonged circulation times common in left ventricular failure; in general, right atrial and central venous injections produce better images than injections in peripheral veins.[8, 9] Subtraction artifacts are a problem[10, 11] because of the long time gap between the taking of the mask and the appearance of contrast material in the vessels, and because of the diffuse nature of the bolus. In view of its relatively poor image quality and the continued improvements in noninvasive vascular imaging methods such as MRI,[12, 13] intravenous DSA has not found general acceptance.

Angiographic images may also be obtained with injection into the arterial system. Intraarterial DSA is essentially identical in performance to conventional aortography except that smaller catheters may be used. DSA has become widely used, particularly in neuroangiography. Images can be obtained with or without subtraction of the background anatomy and in either positive or negative phase. For the rest of this discussion, the term "digital study" refers to intraarterial DSA unless otherwise specified.

Advantages of Digital Imaging

In general, digital methods are more convenient, more cost-effective, and faster than traditional screen-film methods of angiography.[14] Digital images have greater contrast resolution than film images. This increase in the contrast resolution, a result of both digitization and subtraction, allows marked reduction in contrast dose with subsequent reduction in toxicity and discomfort. Digital studies typically require about 30 to 50 percent of the contrast dose used for screen-film methods.[15, 16] Reduction in contrast dose compared with that used in conventional angiography is an important factor in examinations of children and of patients who are predisposed to renal dysfunction. Because only the images of interest are recorded on film for archiving, rather than the dozen or more images obtained during a typical conventional study, there are significant film savings. Manipulation of digital data also allows instant availability of the images, without waiting for development of the film, and compatibility with teleradiology systems. Because less contrast material is used and because images are available immediately, multiple projections of the area in question are easily obtained.

Disadvantages of Digital Imaging

The major disadvantages of DSA are decreased spatial resolution compared with screen-film methods, "bright spots" on the image caused by variability in x-ray transmission through different types of tissues in the field, and subtraction artifacts caused by patient motion, either voluntary or involuntary. The best spatial resolution with DSA is 2 to 2.5 line pairs per millimeter, compared with 7 to 10 line pairs per millimeter for conventional film methods.[1] Although the improved contrast resolution of digital images offsets the decrease in spatial resolution somewhat, there is an intrinsic problem with identification of fine detail in digital images.

Bright spots are more of a problem in the thorax than in other areas of the body because there is a hundred-fold greater transmission of x-rays through the lung compared with the mediastinum. This difference in exposure cannot adequately be captured with either film or the photodiode tube. Tight coning of the x-ray field and use of filters diminish but do not abolish this problem.

Motion or misregistration artifacts are caused by movement that occurs between the time the mask is taken and the time the bolus of contrast material appears in the artery of interest. Motion is minimal in the cerebral vessels and in the peripheral arteries of the legs because these areas can be immobilized, and DSA is frequently used to image these areas. However, in the thorax, and to a lesser degree in the abdomen, reprocessing techniques are often necessary to reduce artifacts caused by cardiac and respiratory motion. These techniques may include remasking, integration, pixel-shifting, matched filtering, and edge enhancement.

One way to minimize motion artifacts is to display the digital images without subtraction of the background, so that the resulting images resemble a minified conventional angiogram. Image quality improvement with DSA may come with development of newer image processing techniques[1] and of more refined video cameras with higher signal-to-noise ratios. Electrocardiographic gating has also been shown to improve image quality,[17, 18] as it does in MRI of the thorax, but it is not commonly available in conventional angiographic suites at this time.

Screen-Film Versus Digital Methods

Aortography performed with current digital imaging methods (i.e., arterial injections) provides significant savings in contrast load, examination time, film cost, and film storage. However, because of the decrease in spatial resolution compared with screen-film systems, the possibility exists of missing subtle abnormalities. For medium-sized and large vessels, there is no difference in diagnostic accuracy. Multiple studies have shown equivalent diagnostic value or even superior performance of DSA in the arteries of the lower extremity,[19, 20] hepatic arterial supply,[21] and brain.[22] Controlled studies comparing the two methods in the thorax, however, are difficult to find. In a large series of 61 patients with blunt chest trauma, Mirvis and co-workers[14] compared DSA to conventional angiography in 10 patients and to clinical follow-up or surgery in the remaining patients. There were 10 patients whose diagnosis was confirmed by surgery, and there was 100 percent correlation between the diagnosis by DSA and follow-up in the remaining patients. Still, close examination of digital and conventional screen-film images for the same patient indicated that conventional aortography was inherently superior for imaging of subtle abnormalities (Fig. 21–2).

Care should be used in relying solely on DSA in cases requiring high spatial resolution, such as aortic dissection and transection. Further controlled studies are needed before substitution of DSA

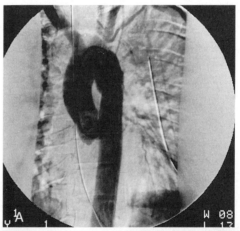

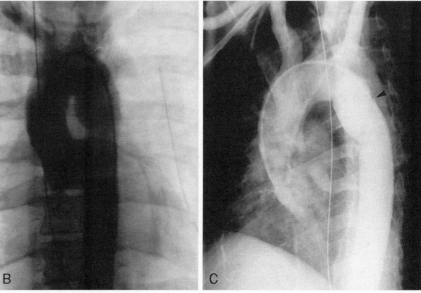

FIGURE 21–2. A 30-year-old man involved in a motorcycle accident. Intra-arterial digital aortograms, with (A) and without (B) background subtraction, and the screen-film aortogram (C) all demonstrate widening of the aorta at the level of the ligamentum arteriosum resulting from pseudoaneurysm formation. However, the intimal irregularity along the outer aortic wall (*arrowhead*) is best demonstrated on the conventional angiogram.

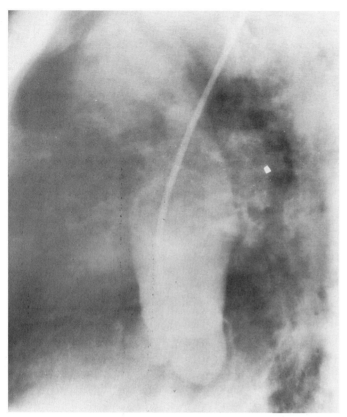

FIGURE 21–3. Cineangiogram of the thoracic aorta in the left anterior oblique projection (equivalent to the right posterior oblique projection). The entire aorta cannot be imaged with the 9-inch diameter image intensifier.

for conventional aortography in these situations is warranted. For maximal flexibility, most new angiographic rooms are equipped with both digital and conventional capability.

Cineangiography

Cineangiography of the thoracic aorta can be performed in conjunction with coronary angiography[23, 24] (Fig. 21–3) with injection of 40 mL Renografin-76 at 20 mL per second. The bolus of contrast material is followed by panning, or moving the image intensifier tube manually along the length of the aorta, and acquiring images at 30 frames per second. The largest image intensifier tube in common use in cardiac catheterization laboratories is 9 inches in diameter; therefore, the entire aorta cannot be encompassed in a single view. Larger image intensifiers are available, but there is considerable decrease in spatial resolution compared with the smaller diameter tubes unless the resolution of the television camera is increased.

Few studies have directly compared cineangiography and conventional screen-film methods for image quality and diagnostic accuracy. Arcinegas and colleagues,[24] in a study comparing these two methods in different patients with aortic dissection, reported 100 percent accuracy with both techniques. Although cineangiography has increased temporal resolution (30 frames per second, compared to 4 films per second available with most screen-film methods), image quality suffers from the poorer spatial resolution and higher levels of noise compared with conventional methods. In most centers, aortography is performed by either conventional or digital methods.

CLINICAL ASPECTS

The last 15 years have witnessed an explosion of new methods for evaluation of thoracic vascular disease, including CT,[25–27] MRI,[28, 29]

and transesophageal echocardiography.[30] All are safer and better tolerated by the patient than angiography. The risk of CT is mainly limited to reactions to contrast materials, and MRI and ultrasound have few, if any, hazards in the thorax. These imaging modalities differ widely in their physical principles, but they share the ability to evaluate both the aortic lumen and the aortic wall and perivascular soft tissues. Angiography, on the other hand, is limited to examination of the vascular lumen only. CT and MRI have some disadvantages, particularly for imaging of the brachiocephalic vessels and in demonstration of small intimal abnormalities. Echocardiography is limited to views of the aortic root and the descending aorta; the aortic arch cannot reliably be visualized. The greatest advantage of angiography is that its spatial resolution is superior to that of CT, MRI, or ultrasound and that vascular anatomy and pathology are displayed in exquisite detail not yet matched by other methods. In general, aortography is now used after other imaging techniques have yielded negative or incomplete results[29] or if vasculitis[31] or aortic trauma[32] is suspected.

Aortic Aneurysm

Imaging of Aortic Aneurysm

Computed tomography[25, 33] and MRI[28] have been shown to be highly accurate in detection of thoracic and abdominal aneurysms and in most cases are sufficient for surgical planning. CT is more commonly used because it is cheaper and more readily available. Angiography with either digital or screen-film technique should be reserved for those cases in which more accurate determination of brachiocephalic, mesenteric, or renal artery involvement is thought to be necessary.[34]

Angiographic Diagnosis of Aortic Aneurysm

The angiographic diagnosis of aneurysm is straightforward: the lesion produces dilatation of the aortic lumen, either localized or generalized.[35, 36] The extent of the aneurysm and branch involvement is well shown. If the aneurysm is largely thrombosed, the luminal wall shows irregularity, and the nonopacified wall of the aorta is seen as an extraluminal shadow. Most thoracic aneurysms are fusiform and are caused by atherosclerosis, although the differential for aneurysms of the ascending aorta also includes cystic medial necrosis, tertiary syphilis, and Marfan syndrome. Unlike atherosclerotic aneurysms of the ascending aorta, the aneurysms seen in Marfan syndrome and annuloaortic ectasia extend inferiorly to involve the sinuses of Valsalva (Fig. 21–4). Differentiation of Marfan syndrome from the more common atherosclerotic aneurysm of the ascending aorta is important because of the high prevalence of aortic insufficiency and aortic dissection in this condition.

Focal aneurysms may be true aneurysms or pseudoaneurysms. A pseudoaneurysm is basically a contained rupture. Most true aneurysms have a neck that is as broad or broader than the base; pseudoaneurysms typically have a smaller neck than base. Any focal aneurysm in the area of the ligamentum arteriosum should arouse suspicion of a post-traumatic pseudoaneurysm.

Aortic Dissection

Imaging of Aortic Dissection

CT has acquired a dominant role in the diagnosis of dissection and is highly accurate in demonstrating the presence and extent of dissection.[25, 37–39] MRI has become more widely available and may eventually replace CT as the method of choice in the diagnosis and evaluation of subacute and chronic aortic dissection. In many large institutions, there is growing use of transesophageal echocardiography in the acute situation.[30] CT and MRI are often diagnostic in cases of completely thrombosed dissections, and they complement angiography in this situation. However, the diagnosis of branch involvement is difficult, and the coronary arteries cannot be evalu-

of the catheter from the outer aortic wall. During angiography, it is necessary to determine whether the catheter is in the true or false lumen before power injection of the contrast agent. The true lumen is characterized by the presence of systemic blood pressure, normal blood flow, and visualization of anatomic landmarks, especially the sinuses of Valsalva, coronary arteries, and aortic valve[45] (Fig. 21–6). The false lumen, as shown on a test or hand injection, typically has few or no aortic branches, has slow flow, and has a lower arterial blood pressure (Fig. 21–7). The aortic valve and the sinuses of Valsalva never arise from the false lumen.

Determining whether the catheter is in the true or false lumen is difficult if branch vessels are supplied by the false lumen. In this situation, the false lumen usually has both an entrance and an exit, thus allowing a large amount of flow. Power injections of the false lumen are safe if there is a large amount of flow through the false channel,[36, 46] but most angiographers agree that limiting injections to the true lumen is the safest procedure. As a practical matter, angiography should show the extent of dissection, particularly with regard to the entry site in the ascending or proximal descending aorta, the presence of aortic regurgitation, and the involvement of proximal coronary arteries or brachiocephalic vessels. If the dissection extends into the abdomen, the true lumen is often anterior in position and perfuses the visceral arteries, whereas the false lumen is posterior. However, this relation is variable, and the renal arteries, in particular, may be occluded or supplied on either side by the false lumen (Fig. 21–8).

Falsely negative angiographic studies occur in 2 to 3 percent of cases[47] and are caused predominantly by a completely thrombosed false lumen; in these cases, no false lumen or intimal flap can be seen, but the true lumen remains compressed in the characteristic

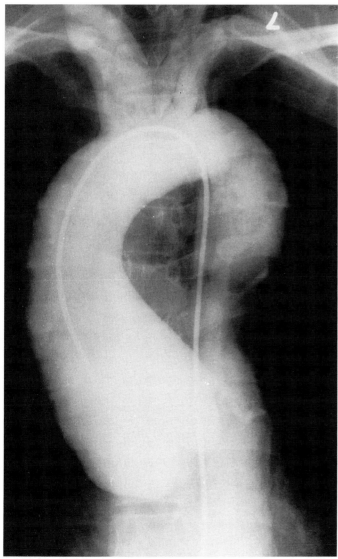

FIGURE 21–4. Aortogram in anteroposterior (AP) projection in a patient with Marfan syndrome, demonstrating an aneurysm of the ascending aorta that involves the sinuses of Valsalva. No dissection is present.

ated. The exact choice and sequence of imaging methods remains somewhat controversial and varies from institution to institution, depending on local experience and expertise. Angiography is usually reserved for complicated cases in which knowledge of brachiocephalic, mesenteric, or renal involvement is necessary, or for cases in which initial imaging studies are negative. Because of its low risk and its ability to visualize periaortic tissues, CT is currently the method of choice for follow-up of patients treated medically or surgically for aortic dissection.[40–42] There is growing evidence that MRI provides the same information.[43]

Angiographic Diagnosis of Aortic Dissection

Angiography has an extremely high accuracy (greater than 95 percent) in the diagnosis of aortic dissection. The angiographic diagnosis of aortic dissection, as with CT, MRI, or echocardiography, depends on demonstration of the intimal flap or the false lumen, or both.[36, 39, 44] The true lumen is typically compressed in a spiral fashion, with slow opacification of the false lumen (Fig. 21–5). Visualization of the intimal flap depends on the entrance of sufficient contrast material into the false channel. If the false lumen fills very slowly, the intimal flap is seen as an undulating edge rather than a line.

Additional angiographic signs of dissection include displacement

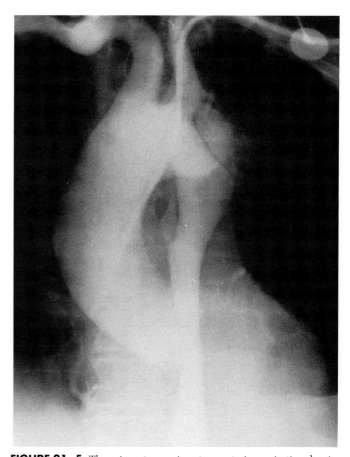

FIGURE 21–5. Thoracic aortogram in anteroposterior projection showing a type III dissection. An intimal flap is present, with faint filling of the false lumen distal to the left subclavian artery. There is marked compression of the true lumen distal to this point, owing to the presence of the false channel, which has not yet filled with contrast.

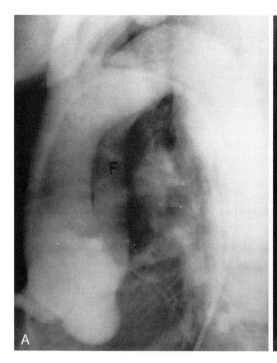

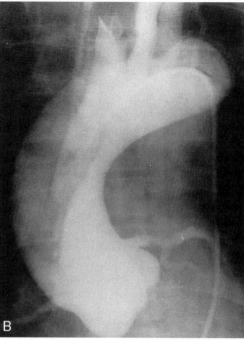

FIGURE 21-6. Anteroposterior *(A)* and lateral *(B)* thoracic aortograms in type I dissection. The true lumen has been injected, and contrast material fills the coronary arteries and sinuses of Valsalva. The dissection involves the innominate artery. F = false lumen.

fashion. Another, less common cause of a false-negative study is simultaneous and equal opacification of true and false channels; orthogonal views are then necessary to show the intimal flap (Fig. 21–9).

Aortic Trauma

Traumatic pseudoaneurysms of the aorta and aortic transections are increasing in frequency and currently account for 15 to 20 percent of fatalities from high-speed motor vehicle accidents. They are almost always caused by blunt chest trauma, usually associated with sudden deceleration. Because the injury is caused by a shearing force, regions fixed in position suffer the most stress and are most prone to damage. The isthmus of the aorta, located immediately distal to the left subclavian artery and tethered by the ligamentum arteriosum and the origin of the great vessels, is the most common location of rupture, accounting for 95 percent of injuries seen angiographically.[48, 49] At angiography, 1 percent of aortic lacerations are located in the distal descending aorta and 5 percent in the ascending aorta.[49, 50] As motor vehicle accidents become more common, and as CT and MRI have become the methods of choice in the diagnosis and staging of most nontraumatic aortic disease, evaluation of aortic trauma has become an increasingly important use of aortography. In the author's institution, almost 50 percent of thoracic aortograms are performed for either blunt or penetrating trauma.

Angiographic Diagnosis of Aortic Injury

Pathologic examination of the aorta in blunt trauma demonstrates either a complete transection of the aortic wall or a laceration limited to a small intimal tear.[51] Intimal and medial lacerations may progress to pseudoaneurysm formation and rupture, with at least 50 percent mortality within 24 hours among those patients lucky enough to reach the hospital. Angiographic findings mirror the pathologic ones. The diagnosis rests on demonstration of either a pseudoaneurysm or intimal irregularity.

Because the area of laceration is extremely fragile, the utmost care should be taken during angiography. Patients may be extremely unstable hemodynamically. Complete transection and exsanguination have been reported after angiography, possibly related to the pressure of the injection or to guidewire manipulation.[52] The pigtail catheter should be formed in the distal thoracic aorta and gently advanced under fluoroscopy. If resistance is met to the advance of the catheter, a hand injection should be performed. If extravasation is seen, the diagnosis of aortic transection has been made, and a power injection study should not be performed. If there is no resistance to advancement of the catheter, then the usual aortic study should be performed. Because the intimal tears are often small and subtle, more than one view is often necessary to completely exclude injury. Angiography should image the entire thoracic aorta as well as the intrathoracic portions of the brachiocephalic vessels, because injury to brachiocephalic vessels occurs in approximately 5 percent of cases.[53]

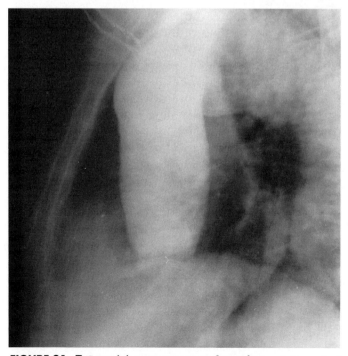

FIGURE 21-7. Lateral thoracic aortogram of ascending aorta in a patient with type I dissection. The false lumen has been injected. Notice the featureless appearance and absence of the aortic valve.

has become more common in the past decade. Because many patients who survive the initial event proceed directly to surgery, angiography is often unnecessary. Indications for angiography include proximity of injury to the great vessel, mediastinal hematoma on chest films, and absent peripheral pulse.[56] Falsely negative angiographic studies are more common with penetrating trauma than with deceleration injuries, probably because the abnormalities are more subtle and often are seen in one view only. Two views are always recommended in these cases to detect subtle intimal punctures that may be clinically silent until rupture.[56]

There is disagreement among angiographers as to the role of digital angiography in aortic trauma. Mirvis[14, 57] has been a proponent of digital imaging for these patients, citing the decrease in examination time that results from immediate availability of images and the overall high image quality. Others have raised concerns about the decreased spatial resolution of digital imaging compared with screen-film studies and the often subtle findings in aortic trauma. In a study of 61 patients with potential aortic injury studied with DSA, only 10 also had conventional angiograms as well.[14] Many angiographers prefer to perform an initial digital imaging analysis in the left posterior oblique projection and follow this with a screen-film study in another projection if the initial views are negative; others prefer to perform only conventional angiography.

Role of Computed Tomography in Aortic Trauma

The role of CT in the evaluation of aortic trauma remains controversial. Mirvis and colleagues[57] compared CT and angiography in 20 patients with abnormal or equivocal chest radiographs after blunt chest trauma. All patients with normal CT scans also had normal angiograms. Positive CT findings such as focal aortic wall irregularity or mediastinal hematoma, or both, were less reliable as an indicator of aortic damage. Most studies have found that abnormal findings have only 10 to 30 percent predictive value for aortic injury.[32, 58] Although the number of positive angiograms in patients with CT evidence of mediastinal hematoma is small, it is still higher than the number found with the use of chest radiography as a screening examination. The low incidence of aortic injury

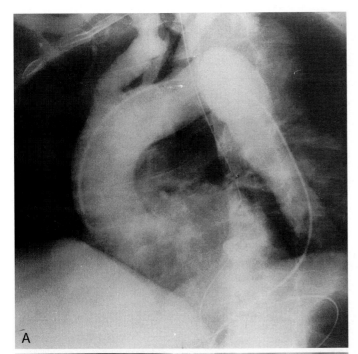

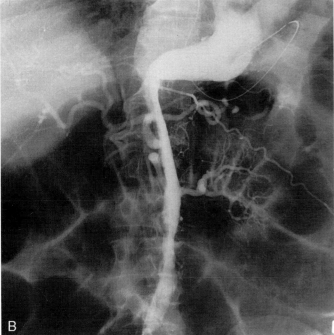

FIGURE 21–8. Extensive type III dissection extending into the abdomen in a patient with worsening abdominal pain. *A,* Thoracic aortogram in right posterior oblique (RPO) projection shows an intimal flap with filling of the true and false channels. *B,* The abdominal aortogram in anteroposterior (AP) view shows abrupt narrowing and compression of the aorta with nonfilling of the right renal artery and superior mesenteric artery. The distention and thickening of the small bowel is consistent with ischemia.

Rare false-positive studies may occur, probably in less than 1 percent of cases, as a result of the presence of either atherosclerotic ulcers or a prominent aortic diverticulum.[54] This remnant of closure of the ductus diverticulum is seen in 9 to 26 percent of normal aortograms as a small focal bulge with oblique borders in the area of the ligamentum arteriosum. Goodman and colleagues state that aortic diverticula are differentiated from pseudoaneurysms by absence of an intimal flap and lack of retention of the contrast medium, features usually seen in pseudoaneurysms.[55]

Penetrating thoracic trauma caused by gunshot or stab wounds

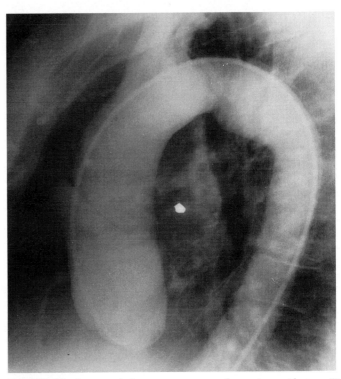

FIGURE 21–9. Lateral thoracic aortogram of a patient with type II dissection limited to the ascending aorta. The small intimal flap was seen only in this projection.

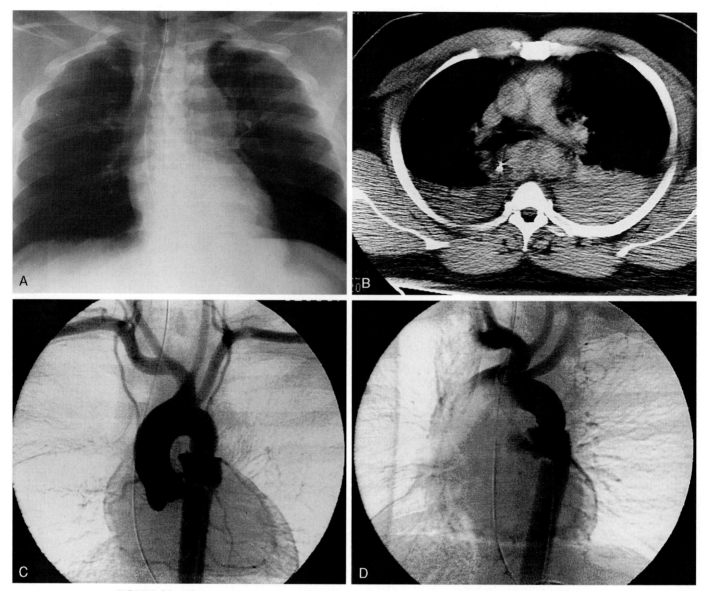

FIGURE 21–10. A young man involved in a high-speed car accident. *A*, Initial chest film taken in the emergency department shows mediastinal widening with deviation of the nasogastric tube to the right side. *B*, Chest computed tomography (CT) with contrast performed concurrently with abdominal CT shows bilateral hemothoraces and increased density of the mediastinum caused by hematoma. The aortic contour is poorly defined, suggesting aortic injury. Intra-arterial digital aortograms in anteroposterior (AP) *(C)* and right posterior oblique (RPO) *(D)* projections show a large pseudoaneurysm with active extravasation.

in known mediastinal hematoma is not surprising because bleeding may be caused by arterial, venous, or vertebral injury. The size of the hematoma visualized by CT does not predict the likelihood of aortic injury[51, 59] and does not confirm or deny the existence of aortic transection.

In many series, the predictive value of a normal CT has been 100 percent.[57–59] Because of the high reliability of a normal CT study (i.e., no evidence of mediastinal hematoma with a good quality contrast-enhanced CT image), some researchers have proposed using CT as a screening technique in patients with low to moderate risk of aortic rupture.[32] Protocols such as those proposed by Madayag,[32] Morgan,[60] and Richardson[61] begin with the chest films obtained in the emergency room. If the chest films show a definite mediastinal hematoma, angiography is performed immediately. Patients with equivocal mediastinal contours or normal chest films with clinical evidence of blunt chest trauma (e.g., high-speed deceleration accident such as a motor vehicle crash or a fall from a significant height, anterior chest wall contusion, broken steering wheel) are referred for initial chest CT, particularly if their injuries

also require assessment with abdominal CT.[32] If the mediastinum is within normal limits and without hematoma, patients may be observed clinically and with repeated chest films. If there is evidence of mediastinal hematoma or focal aortic irregularity or enlargement, or if the examination is suboptimal owing to motion artifact or other difficulty, angiography is performed (Fig. 21–10). With this protocol, Madayag observed a 73 percent decrease in the number of angiograms performed for trauma, with no false-negative CT studies. Several studies have reported a 50 to 70 percent reduction in angiography with this approach, compared with performing angiography in all patients with blunt chest trauma, with significant savings in time and money and no loss of diagnostic accuracy.[32, 58]

Rare false-negative CT examinations have been reported in patients with aortic transection.[27, 60, 62] In the five cases of aortic injury with negative CTs reported by Miller,[63] two occurred in patients with vertebral artery injury and one in a patient with injury to the subclavian artery—injuries that rarely cause mediastinal hematomas. One of their five cases was interpreted as showing a mediastinal hematoma in retrospect and therefore did not represent a false-negative study; in the last case, the CT was performed without the use of an intravenous contrast agent and cannot be regarded as an optimal study. In the case reported by Kubota,[62] the CT image that is presented is degraded by significant artifact, and it is not clear whether this image is representative of the study in general. However, Morgan[60] described a single case of negative CT and positive angiogram in a patient who was found to have a small, contained aortic rupture at the time of surgery. For this reason, serial chest films are recommended in patients after negative CT examination, with angiography performed for any change in clinical status or mediastinal contour on follow-up films.

Although MRI is better capable of imaging the aortic isthmus, MRI is unsuitable for unstable patients, who are often intubated and require an immediate definitive diagnosis.

CONCLUSIONS

Angiography is a highly accurate examination in aortic disease and is unmatched in demonstration of anatomic detail. Because CT and MRI also have extremely high accuracy with less cost and risk to the patient, these imaging methods have replaced angiography as the initial examination in aortic aneurysm and dissection, with angiography usually reserved for difficult or ambiguous cases. Angiography remains the gold standard in the diagnosis of aortic trauma and should be the initial examination in clinically unstable patients or those with obvious mediastinal hematoma on chest radiography. CT has a valuable role to play as a screening examination after equivocal chest film findings in more stable patients, but all patients with mediastinal hematoma still require aortography for definitive diagnosis.

References

1. Crummy, A.B.: Digital subtraction angiography. *In* Taveras, J.M., and Ferruci, J.T. (eds.): Radiology: Diagnosis—Imaging—Intervention. Philadelphia, J.B. Lippincott, 1983.
2. Abrams, M.L.: Thoracic aortography: Technique, indications and hazards. *In* Abrams, H.L. (ed.): Angiography. 3rd ed. Boston, Little, Brown, 1983.
3. Bakal, C.W., Friedland, R.J., Sprayregen, S., et al.: Translumbar arch aortography: A retrospective controlled study of usefulness, technique, and safety. Radiology 178:225, 1991.
4. Nyman, U., Nilsson, P., and Westergren, A.: Pain and hemodynamic effects in aortofemoral angiography. Acta Radiol. Diagn. 23:389, 1982.
5. Hessels, J., Adams, D.F., and Abrams, H.L.: Complications of angiography. Radiology 138:273, 1981.
6. Lang, E.K., Foreman, J., Schlegel, J.U., et al.: Incidence of contrast medium-induced acute tubular necrosis following angiography. Radiology 138:203, 1981.
7. Grossman, L.B., Buonocore, E., Modic, M.T., et al.: Digital subtraction angiography of the thoracic aorta. Radiology 150:323, 1984.
8. Saddekni, S., Sos, T.A., Sniderman, K.W., et al.: Optimal injection for intravenous digital subtraction angiography. Radiology 150:655, 1984.
9. Rubin, D.L., Burbank, F.H., Bradley, B.R., et al.: An experimental evaluation of central versus peripheral injection for intravenous digital subtraction angiography. Invest. Radiol., 19:30, 1984.
10. Guthaner, D.F., Brody, W.R., and Miller, D.C.: Intravenous aortography after aortic dissection repair. AJR 137:1019, 1981.
11. Buonocore, E., Meaney, T.F., Borkowski, G.P., et al.: Digital subtraction angiography of the abdominal aorta and renal arteries. Radiology 139:281, 1981.
12. Bissett, G.S., III, Strife, J.L., Kirks, D.R., et al.: Vascular rings: MR imaging. AJR 149:251, 1987.
13. Kersting-Sommerhoff, B.A., Sechtem, U.P., Fisher, M.R., et al.: MR imaging of congenital anomalies of the aortic arch. AJR 149:9, 1987.
14. Mirvis, S.E., Pais, S.O., and Gens, D.R.: Thoracic aortic rupture: Advantages of intraarterial digital subtraction angiography. AJR 146:987, 1986.
15. Kaufman, S.L., Chang, R., Kadir, S., et al.: Intraarterial digital subtraction angiography in diagnostic arteriography. Radiology 151:323, 1984.
16. Levin, D.C., Schapiro, R.M., Boxt, L.M., et al.: Digital subtraction angiography: Principles and pitfalls of image improvement techniques. AJR 143:447, 1984.
17. Foley, W.D., Lipchik, E.O., Larson, P.A., et al.: Evaluation of ECG gating and hybrid subtraction for intraarterial digital subtraction thoracic aortography. AJR 149:1269, 1987.
18. Kelly, W.M., Gould, R., Norman, D., et al.: EKG-synchronized DSA exposure control: Improved cervicothoracic image quality. AJR 143:857, 1984.
19. Smith, T.P., Cragg, A.H., Berbaum, K.S., et al.: Comparison of the efficacy of digital subtraction and film-screen angiography of the lower limb. AJR 158:431, 1992.
20. Sibbitt, R.R., Palmaz, J.C., Garcia, F., et al.: Trauma of the extremities: Prospective comparison of digital and conventional angiography. Radiology 158:255, 1986.
21. Flannigan, B.D., Gomes, A.S., Stambuk, E.C., et al.: Intra-arterial digital subtraction angiography: Comparison with conventional hepatic arteriography. Radiology 148:17, 1983.
22. Brant-Zawadski, M., Gould, R., Norman, D., et al.: Digital subtraction cerebral angiography by intra-arterial injection: Comparison with conventional angiography. AJR 140:347, 1983.
23. Gutierrez, F.R., Gowda, S., Ludbrook, P.A., et al.: Cineangiography in the diagnosis and evaluation of aortic dissection. Radiology 135:759, 1980.
24. Arcincgas, J.C., Soto, B., Little, W.C., et al.: Cineangiography in the diagnosis of aortic dissection. Am. J. Cardiol. 47:890, 1981.
25. Godwin, J.D., Herfkens, R.L., Skioldebrand, C.G., et al.: Evaluation of dissections and aneurysms of the thoracic aorta by conventional and dynamic CT scanning. Radiology 136:125, 1980.
26. Egan, T.J., Neiman, H.L., Herman, R.J., et al.: Computed tomography in the diagnosis of aortic aneurysm, dissection, or traumatic injury. Radiology 136:141, 1980.
27. White, R.D., Lipton, M.J., and Higgins, C.B., et al.: Noninvasive evaluation of suspected thoracic aortic disease by contrast-enhanced computed tomography. Am. J. Cardiol. 57:282, 1986.
28. Dinsmore, R.E., Liberthson, R.R., Wisner, G.L., et al.: Magnetic resonance imaging of thoracic aortic aneurysms: Comparison with other imaging methods. AJR 146:309, 1986.
29. Link, K.M., and Lesko, N.M.: The role of MR imaging in the evaluation of acquired diseases of the thoracic aorta. AJR 158:1115, 1992.
30. Hashimoto, S., Kumada, T., Osakada, G., et al.: Assessment of transesophageal Doppler echography in dissecting aortic aneurysm. J. Am. Coll. Cardiol. 14:1253, 1989.
31. Miller, D.L., Reinig, J.W., and Volkman, D.J.: Vascular imaging with MRI: Inadequacy in Takayasu's arteritis compared with angiography. AJR 146:949, 1986.
32. Madayag, M.A., Kirshenbaum, K.J., Suryaprakasharao, R.N., et al.: Thoracic aortic trauma: Role of dynamic CT. Radiology 179:853, 1991.
33. Guthaner, D.F.: The use of computed tomography in assessing aneurysms and dissecting hematomas of the thoracic aorta. *In* Taveras, J.M., and Ferruci, J.T. (eds.): Radiology: Diagnosis—Imaging—Intervention. Philadelphia, J.B. Lippincott, 1983.
34. Todd, G.J., Nowygrod, R., Benvensity, A., et al.: The accuracy of CT scanning in the diagnosis of abdominal and thoracoabdominal aortic aneurysms. J. Vasc. Surg. 13:302, 1991.
35. Randall, P.A., and Jarmolowski, C.R.: Aneurysms of the thoracic aorta. *In* Abrams, H.L. (ed.): Angiography. 3rd ed. Boston, Little, Brown, 1983.
36. Guthaner, D.F.: Angiography in assessing aneurysms and dissecting hematomas of the thoracic aorta. *In* Taveras, J.H., and Ferruci, J.T. (eds.): Radiology: Diagnosis—Imaging—Intervention. Philadelphia, J.B. Lippincott, 1983.
37. DeSanctis, R.W., Doroghazi, R.M., Austen, W.G., et al.: Aortic dissection. N. Engl. J. Med. 317:1060, 1987.
38. Parienty, R.A., Couffinhal, J-C., Wellers, M., et al.: Computed tomography versus aortography in diagnosis of aortic dissection. Cardiovasc. Intervent. Radiol. 5:285, 1982.
39. Petasnick, J.P.: Radiologic evaluation of aortic dissection. Radiology 180:297, 1991.
40. Jacobs, N.M., Godwin, J.D., Wolfe, W.G., et al.: Evaluation of the grafted ascending aorta with computed tomography. Radiology 145:749, 1982.
41. Godwin, J.D., Turley, K., Herfkens, R.J., et al.: Computed tomography for follow-up of chronic aortic dissections. Radiology 139:655, 1981.
42. Landtman, M., Kivisaari, L., Standertskjold-Nordenstam, C-G., et al.: Computed tomography in pre- and post-operative evaluation of aortic dissection. Acta Radiol., 27:273, 1986.
43. White, R.D., Ullyot, D.J., and Higgins, C.B.: MR imaging of the aorta after surgery for aortic dissection. AJR 150:87, 1988.
44. Abrams, H.L.: Dissecting aortic aneurysm. *In* Abrams, H.L. (ed.): Angiography. 3rd ed. Boston, Little, Brown, 1983.
45. Soto, B., Harman, M.A., Ceballos, R., et al.: Angiographic diagnosis of dissecting aneurysm of the aorta. Am. J. Roentgenol. Radium Ther. Nucl. Med. 116:146, 1972.
46. Kirschner, L.P., Twigg, H.L., Conrad, P.W., et al.: Retrograde catheter aortography in dissecting aortic aneurysms. AJR 102:349, 1968.
47. Shuford, W.H., Sybers, R.G., and Weens, H.S.: Problems in the aortographic diagnosis of dissecting aneurysm of the aorta. N. Engl. J. Med. 280:225, 1969.
48. Sanborn, J.C., Heitzman, E.R., and Markarian, B.: Traumatic rupture of the thoracic aorta: Roentgen-pathological correlation. Radiology 95:293, 1970.
49. Daniels, D.I., and Maddison, F.E.: Ascending aortic injury: An angiographic diagnosis. AJR 136:812, 1981.
50. Lundell, C.J., Quinn, M.F., and Finck, E.J.: Traumatic laceration of the ascending aorta: Angiographic assessment. AJR 145:715, 1985.
51. Brooks, A.P., Olson, L.K., and Shackford, S.R.: Computed tomography in the diagnosis of traumatic rupture of the thoracic aorta. Clin. Radiol. 40:133, 1989.
52. LaBerge, J.M., and Jeffrey, R.B.: Aortic lacerations: Fatal complications in thoracic aortography. Radiology 165:367, 1987.
53. Fishbone, G., Robbins, D.L., Osborn, D.J., et al.: Trauma to the thoracic aorta and great vessels. Radiol. Clin. North Am. 11:543, 1973.
54. Morse, S.S., Glickman, M.G., Greenwood, L.H., et al.: Traumatic aortic rupture: False-positive aortographic diagnosis due to atypical ductus diverticulum. AJR 150:793, 1988.
55. Goodman, P.C., Jeffrey, R.B., Minagi, H., et al.: Angiographic evaluation of the ductus diverticulum. Cardiovasc. Intervent. Radiol. 5:1, 1982.

56. Fisher, R.G., and Ben-Menachem, Y.: Penetrating injuries of the thoracic aorta and brachiocephalic arteries: Angiographic findings in 18 cases. AJR 149:607, 1987.
57. Mirvis, S.E., Kostrubiak, I., Whitley, N.O., et al.: Role of CT in excluding major arterial injury after blunt aortic trauma. AJR 149:601, 1987.
58. Raptopoulos, V., Sheiman, R.G., Phillips, D.A., et al.: Traumatic aortic tear: Screening with chest CT. Radiology 182:667, 1992.
59. Heiberg, E., Wolverson, M.K., Sudaram, M., et al.: CT in aortic trauma. AJR 140:1119, 1983.
60. Morgan, P.W., Goodman, L.R., Aprahamian, C., et al.: Evaluation of traumatic

aortic injury: Does dynamic contrast-enhanced CT play a role? Radiology 182:661, 1992.
61. Richardson, P., Mirvis, S.E., Scorpio, R., et al.: Value of CT in determining the need for angiography when finding of mediastinal hemorrhage on chest radiographs are equivocal. AJR 156:273, 1991.
62. Kubota, R.T., Tripp, M.O., Tisnado, J., et al.: Evaluation of traumatic rupture of descending aorta by aortography and computed tomography: Case report with follow-up. J. Comput. Tomogr. 9:237, 1985.
63. Miller, F.B., Richardson, J.D., Hollis, A.T., et al.: Role of CT in the diagnosis of major arterial injury after blunt thoracic trauma. Surgery 106:596, 1989.

CHAPTER

22 Pulmonary Angiography

Antoinette S. Gomes, M.D.

INDICATIONS ____ 208
CONTRAINDICATIONS ____ 208
TECHNIQUE ____ 208
NORMAL ANATOMY OF PULMONARY
    VASCULATURE ____ 210
PULMONARY ANGIOGRAPHY IN PULMONARY
    EMBOLISM ____ 210
Timing ____ 211
Interpretation ____ 211
Complications ____ 212
Therapeutic Maneuvers at the Time of
    Angiography ____ 212

PULMONARY ANGIOGRAPHY FOR OTHER
    PULMONARY VASCULAR LESIONS ____ 214
Pulmonary Arteriovenous Fistula ____ 214
Pulmonary Artery Stenosis ____ 215
Pulmonary Artery Aneurysm ____ 215
Pulmonary Varix ____ 215
Neoplasm ____ 216
Pulmonary Sequestration ____ 216
Congenital Dysplasia of the Lung ____ 216
Anomalous Pulmonary Venous
    Connection ____ 217
NEWER VASCULAR IMAGING
    TECHNIQUES ____ 218

INDICATIONS

Pulmonary arteriography is the most reliable technique for evaluation of the status of the pulmonary vessels. It is indicated in the diagnosis of suspected pulmonary embolism and in the evaluation of other vascular abnormalities of the pulmonary arteries. Other vascular lesions diagnosed with angiography include pulmonary arteriovenous fistulas; pulmonary artery stenoses, aneurysms, neoplasms, and sequestration; and congenital lesions of pulmonary arteries and veins. By far the most frequent clinical indication is in the diagnosis of suspected pulmonary embolism.

CONTRAINDICATIONS

In the past, the only absolute contraindication to pulmonary angiography was the presence of a known allergy to contrast media.[1] Because medication before angiography has been shown to be effective, a history of allergy to contrast media is a relative contraindication. Other relative contraindications to angiography are severe pulmonary hypertension, recent myocardial infarction, ventricular irritability, left bundle branch block, and a severe bleeding diathesis. In patients with a previous documented reaction to contrast material, premedication with corticosteroids is necessary. Several regimens have been employed. Prednisone given orally, 50 mg for three doses (150 mg total) beginning 18 hours before the study, with the intramuscular administration of 50 mg of Benadryl just before angiography, has been found to be an effective means of blocking allergic reactions to contrast agents.[2] Use of the new nonionic contrast agents is also recommended because these agents have been suggested to reduce the overall incidence of reactions to contrast agents.

Pulmonary hypertension and right ventricular dysfunction have been found to be associated with a higher incidence of sudden death at angiography. In a large series, Mills and associates noted a similar incidence of major nonfatal complications in patients who had pulmonary hypertension compared with those who had normal right ventricular and pulmonary artery pressures.[3] Mortality, however, was higher in patients with severe pulmonary hypertension (pulmonary artery pressure greater than 70 mm Hg systolic) and moderate right ventricular dysfunction (right ventricular end-diastolic pressure greater than 20 mm Hg). The degree to which pulmonary angiography contributed to the death of these patients was not completely clarified, because they were all gravely ill. Nonetheless, others have observed that patients with pulmonary artery pressures tolerate large injections of contrast material poorly,[1] and, in these patients, low-volume subselective injection of contrast agents into high probability areas is recommended. Use of the new, low-osmolar contrast agents is recommended in this patient subgroup.

Patients with a left bundle branch block are at risk for developing complete heart block as the pulmonary angiography catheter is passed along the right ventricular wall into the pulmonary artery. Complete heart block can result in acute decompensation with hypotension. Patients with left bundle branch block who require pulmonary angiography should have a temporary pacemaker placed before angiography.

TECHNIQUE

Pulmonary angiography should be performed in a well-functioning angiographic fluoroscopic radiographic suite with, at minimum, single-plane rapid serial filming capability. The focal spot of the x-ray tube should be adequate for obtaining magnification films. Often, spot-filming capability may be of value. The availability of biplane filming capability, U or C arms, and cineangiography may in certain cases allow use of reduced volumes of contrast medium and facilitate the study. Because pulmonary embolism does not require a dynamic display, the use of cineangiography, with its attendant higher radiation dosage, is not recommended.

Digital angiography is not routinely employed in pulmonary angiography in the adult patient. Newer digital x-ray imaging systems equipped with a large field of view image intensifier (12 to 16 inches) permit visualization of the entire right or left pulmonary artery. High-resolution imaging (1024 gray levels) with rapid image acquisition is possible, and the images obtained may be viewed in the subtracted or unsubtracted mode. The images may be further processed to permit magnification and filtering. Dilute contrast may be employed. However, there have been no studies to date comparing the accuracy of high-resolution unsubtracted digital images with those obtained with conventional film-screen techniques in the diagnosis of pulmonary embolism.

Digital subtraction angiography is of value in the diagnosis of large congenital lesions in children. In the older patient, although the main pulmonary artery may be well visualized, misrepresentation caused by motion artifact may make digital subtraction angiography unreliable for the diagnosis of pulmonary embolism or evaluation of abnormalities of the smaller pulmonary artery branches. The angiography suite must be equipped with an electrocardiographic monitor, a blood pressure monitor, and a physiologic monitor for measurement of right heart and pulmonary artery pressures. The physiologic monitor should allow collection of a printed record of these pressures. Pulse oximetry should be used. A life support cart should be readily available, and the angiographers should be knowledgeable in its use.

If a pulmonary angiogram is requested, the indications for the study and the patient's overall condition should be discussed with the referring physician. All of the patient's pertinent studies should be reviewed, in particular the chest films and, in patients being studied for pulmonary embolism, the lung scan. A radionuclide lung scan before arteriography is strongly recommended because it may obviate the need for the angiographic study, and, if angiography is indicated, the lung scan directs the angiographer to the most suspicious areas of the lung. Baseline serum creatinine and coagulation studies should be obtained. Severe bleeding abnormalities should be corrected, if possible, before the study. If the patient is receiving heparin therapy, however, such therapy needs to be stopped 1 to 2 hours before the study. The ECG should be examined to rule out acute myocardial infarction, a conduction defect, or a cardiac arrhythmia.

As before any type of arteriography, informed consent should be obtained. Patients with renal insufficiency should be well hydrated, and patients on dialysis should have provisions made for dialysis after arteriography. The patient should be sedated beforehand, with the drug selected and the dosage adjusted appropriately for the patient's degree of hypoxia.

Pulmonary angiography can be performed with an approach through the arm, through the groin, or through a jugular vein. The femoral vein approach is the one most frequently used. If such access is not possible because of occlusion of the femoral vein or inferior vena cava, an antecubital vein approach via the basilic vein may be performed. Percutaneous puncture with the modified Seldinger technique is used at both sites. Infrequently, a cutdown may be required if the study is being performed through an arm vein.

If a Swan-Ganz catheter has been passed through a sheath positioned in the internal jugular vein, it may be exchanged for the angiographic catheter if the sheath size is at least 6 Fr. After the study had been completed, a new Swan-Ganz catheter is passed through the sheath. The catheter most frequently used for pulmonary angiography is the 7- to 8-Fr. Grollman pigtail catheter with multiple side holes.[4] A patient with a dilated heart may more easily be catheterized with a pigtail catheter.[5] Stiff, straight 8-Fr. catheters

with multiple side holes, such as the NIH catheter, are not recommended because of the increased risk of myocardial perforation attendant with their use.[6]

After administration of local anesthetic, the femoral vein is punctured below the inguinal ligament, using a single-wall or double-wall puncture needle. The position of the vein is medial to the femoral artery, and the femoral artery passes diagonally across the medial one third of the femoral head. After the vein has been entered and the needle stylet has been removed, a syringe or connecting tubing is attached to the needle, and suction is applied as the needle is slowly withdrawn. After freely aspirated venous blood is obtained, the tubing is removed from the needle hub, and a guidewire is passed into the vein and advanced up the vena cava to the right side of the heart under fluoroscopic guidance. Failure to pass the guidewire freely is a result of either passage of the wire up into the ipsilateral ascending lumbar vein, in which case the wire tip should be reoriented, or occlusion of the vein or of the inferior vena cava, in which case the procedure should be performed from the arm.

After the guidewire has entered the inferior vena cava, the catheter is passed over the guidewire and advanced into the inferior vena cava. Often, a test injection of contrast agent into the inferior vena cava is made to document free flow within it. A theoretical possibility is that a catheter could dislodge a caval thrombus; however, the likelihood of this occurrence is low, and for complete evaluation of the cava, a separate cavogram is necessary. In most instances, the catheter is passed directly up into the right side of the heart.

The guidewire is then exchanged for a Cook deflecting wire (Cook Inc., Bloomington, Ind.), and the deflecting wire is used to facilitate passage of the Grollman catheter across the tricuspid valve and into the right ventricle. With the use of clockwise torque, the catheter is pushed across the pulmonic valve. The catheter is then manipulated into the right or left pulmonary artery. The left pulmonary artery is entered most frequently. Fluoroscopically, if the tip of the catheter lies above the left mainstem bronchus, the catheter is committed to the left pulmonary artery. Deflection of the catheter when it is just below the left mainstem bronchus results in its passage into the right pulmonary artery. The deflecting wire is usually removed at this point and exchanged for a J guidewire or a soft-tip guidewire to assist in passage of the catheter out into the distal right or left pulmonary artery for injection. Pulmonary artery pressures are then recorded.

To reduce overall study time, and particularly in cases in which difficulty was encountered in reaching the pulmonary artery, pull-back pressures of the right side of the heart are not usually recorded before the angiogram is taken. Pulmonary artery pressures however, are always recorded, and if pulmonary artery pressures are markedly elevated, it may be useful to pull the catheter back and record right ventricular pressures, because patients with high right ventricular end-diastolic pressures may not tolerate the injection of large volumes of contrast material well.

If pulmonary artery pressures are elevated, subselective angiography is preferred. In patients with normal or near-normal pressures, the catheter is positioned in the proximal portion of the descending pulmonary artery on the selected side. In patients with suspected pulmonary embolism, the area of highest probability on the lung scan should be the site of the first injection. In selected instances, main pulmonary artery injections may be performed.

A test injection is made to determine catheter position and to assess the pulmonary flow rate. A standard injection is 40 mL of contrast medium injected at a flow rate of 20 to 25 mL per second, depending on the rate of pulmonary blood flow and the patient's heart rate. In general, patients with a higher heart rate require a higher injection rate. Rapid serial filming is performed at a rate of 3 films per second for 3 seconds and 1 film per second for 3 seconds. The initial position for filming is the anteroposterior projection. If thrombi are suspected in the lower lobes, oblique filming is performed in the ipsilateral posterior oblique position. If the suspected thrombus is in the upper lobe, the ipsilateral anterior oblique position is used.[7] The lateral view may be helpful in difficult cases. Each lung should be visualized in two projections. Magnification is recommended, although full two-to-one magnification is not necessary.

After filming is complete, the patient is allowed to stabilize after the final injection, and pullback pressures of the right side of the heart are performed with recording of pulmonary artery, right ventricular, and right atrial pressures. After the study, the patient is given bedrest for 2 to 4 hours with frequent monitoring of vital signs.

The antecubital approach is performed by puncture of a basilic vein or through a cutdown. Entry through the cephalic vein is not desirable, because it may be difficult to pass a catheter from the cephalic vein into the subclavian vein. A short 2-inch, 18-gauge needle may be used for the venous puncture, after which a guidewire is passed. If an 18-gauge needle is too large for the size of the vein, a smaller-gauge needle and guidewire may be used for entry and exchanged for a small dilator, through which a guidewire of larger bore may then be passed. After a guidewire of suitable size has been passed into the right atrium, a pigtail catheter is advanced over the wire. A straight pigtail catheter may be used; alternatively, a gentle, 6-cm curve is steamed into the distal portion of the catheter at a site that is proximal to that of the pigtail. This procedure facilitates passage of the catheter out into the right ventricular outflow tract. A Cook deflecting wire is used to manipulate the catheter out into the pulmonary artery. The pulmonary angiogram is then performed with the same technique used for the femoral vein approach.

In certain instances, balloon occlusion pulmonary arteriography may be performed. This technique is occasionally used for patients with severe pulmonary hypertension and suspected pulmonary embolism in whom standard arteriography is precluded, or in cases of suspected small pulmonary emboli and equivocal cut-film arteriography.[8] Under fluoroscopic guidance, a 7-Fr. pulmonary wedge balloon catheter is passed into the pulmonary artery, and the appropriate branch is subselectively catheterized. The balloon is inflated to obstruct flow, and 5 to 10 mL of contrast material is then injected slowly until the entire vessel is opacified. Three to four films are obtained (preferably 105-mm spot films). The balloon is deflated immediately after filming. Overinflation of the balloon should be avoided because it can cause vessel injury or rupture.

Another angiographic technique used in pulmonary arteriography is the pulmonary vein wedge arteriogram. This technique is used for evaluation of the patency and drainage pattern of pulmonary arteries, and it is used frequently in patients with congenital heart disease with pulmonary artery obstruction.[9] An end-hole catheter is wedged into a pulmonary vein branch, and 7 to 10 mL of contrast medium is hand injected over a period of 2 to 4 seconds. Cine film, spot film, or cut film recording is then done.

Pulmonary angiography can be performed with the use of either the new low-osmolar ionic or nonionic agents or the conventional ionic agents. The nonionic agents have been shown to be associated with less patient discomfort, diminished incidence of coughing, and consequently less motion artifact.[10] Similar findings were observed in a comparison study of ioxaglate 320 (a low-osmolar ionic agent), diatrizoate meglumine, and diatrizoate sodium.[11] The incidence of adverse reactions has been found to be significantly lower with the newer, lower-osmolar nonionic contrast media,[12] and there is some evidence that these low-osmolar agents are less nephrotoxic, particularly in patients with preexisting renal dysfunction.[13, 14] The use of low-osmolar contrast agents is therefore recommended in pulmonary arteriography.

NORMAL ANATOMY OF PULMONARY VASCULATURE

The main pulmonary artery arises from the right ventricle, anterior to the aorta, and lies within the pericardium. It passes to the left of the aorta and divides into the right and left pulmonary arteries. The left pulmonary artery is shorter than the right, courses higher and more posteriorly than the right, and is foreshortened in the frontal angiogram. In the left hilus, the left pulmonary artery divides into ascending and descending branches, which supply the left upper and left lower lobe, respectively. The right pulmonary artery passes behind the ascending aorta, superior vena cava, and right upper lobe pulmonary vein. Its position is anterior to the esophagus and the right upper lobe bronchus. At the level of the hilus of the right lung, it divides into superior and inferior branches. The ascending branch supplies the right upper lobe, and the descending branch supplies the right middle and right lower segments of the right lobe. The pulmonary artery branches to both lungs usually follow the segmental bronchi; however, variations occur frequently, usually in the upper lobes.

The pulmonary veins drain into the left atrium. On the right side, the middle lobe vein joins the upper lobe vein to form the right superior pulmonary vein. The inferior pulmonary vein drains the lower lobe. On the left, the three segmental upper lobe veins form the superior pulmonary vein. The two lower lobe veins join to form the inferior pulmonary vein. In general, filming during pulmonary angiography should be carried out to the levophase so that previously unsuspected venous disease is not missed.

PULMONARY ANGIOGRAPHY IN PULMONARY EMBOLISM

The clinical diagnosis of pulmonary embolism can be difficult because the signs and symptoms of pulmonary embolism are nonspecific and can mimic a variety of other disease processes. Because of difficulties in diagnosis, the precise incidence of pulmonary embolism is unknown. In 1975, Dalen and Alpert estimated that a total of 630,000 symptomatic cases of pulmonary embolism occur each year in the United States.[15] Pulmonary embolism is the direct cause of death or a major contributor to death in approximately 200,000 cases. Eleven percent of patients with pulmonary embolism died within the first hour. The correct diagnosis was not made in 71 percent of the 563,000 patients who survived beyond the first hour, and 30 percent of these patients died. In the 163,000 patients in whom the diagnosis was made and therapy was instituted, however, only 8 percent died. The diagnosis and treatment of pulmonary embolism are therefore imperative. Similarly, Barker observed that postoperative patients who suffered an episode of pulmonary embolism and were not treated with anticoagulants had a 33 percent chance of recurrence and an 18 percent chance of fatal recurrence.[16]

An autopsy study by Smith and associates demonstrated that most pulmonary emboli (46 percent) arise from thrombosis in veins of the leg.[17] Other sites of origin in that study were the right atrium (23 percent), the inferior vena cava (19 percent), and the pelvic veins (16 percent). Clinical studies indicate that 35 to 71 percent of patients with documented pulmonary emboli have deep vein thrombosis.[18, 19]

Usually, the symptoms of pulmonary embolism are misinterpreted as those of primary respiratory disease or ischemic heart disease. Pulmonary embolism can mimic myocardial infarction, arrhythmia, pneumonia, pneumothorax, and other systemic diseases. These disease processes should be excluded before pulmonary angiography is performed. The typical clinical workup of a patient with suspected pulmonary embolism should include an ECG, chest radiograph, complete blood count, arterial blood gases, and ventilation perfusion ($\dot{V}/\dot{Q}$) scan. This initial workup helps to exclude other causes of the patient's symptoms. It also provides valuable information regarding the patient's ability to tolerate angiography. $\dot{V}/\dot{Q}$ scanning is recommended in the initial evaluation of suspected pulmonary embolism because it helps to establish the relative probability of a pulmonary embolus and serves as a useful guide if the patient undergoes angiography.

As with clinical findings, the laboratory findings in pulmonary embolism are nonspecific. Although a chest radiograph should be obtained in all patients with suspected pulmonary embolus, the lack of specific findings with chest radiography make it unreliable for diagnosis.[20] The chest radiograph is often most helpful for exclusion of other conditions that can mimic pulmonary embolism, and it is essential for interpretation of the radionuclide lung scan. The radionuclide lung scan is the only currently available noninvasive imaging modality with documented sensitivity and specificity in the diagnosis of pulmonary embolism.[6, 21, 22]

$\dot{V}/\dot{Q}$ imaging has its limitations. The most reliable criterion for pulmonary embolus in $\dot{V}/\dot{Q}$ imaging is lack of perfusion with persistent ventilation. Although the $\dot{V}/\dot{Q}$ scan is sensitive to changes in pulmonary perfusion, perfusion abnormalities can occur from causes other than pulmonary embolus. In addition, the technique for performing $\dot{V}/\dot{Q}$ imaging, as well as the sensitivity and specificity of the various criteria used in interpretation of the scan, have been the subject of controversy.[23–26]

Pulmonary angiography is indicated in those instances in which the diagnosis of pulmonary embolism must be made with certainty. The most frequent indication is an indeterminate $\dot{V}/\dot{Q}$ scan. This situation often occurs in the presence of pulmonary parenchymal disease and congestive heart failure. Pulmonary angiography is indicated after a $\dot{V}/\dot{Q}$ study suggesting high probability of pulmonary embolism if anticoagulation is contraindicated, and in patients with $\dot{V}/\dot{Q}$ scan results showing a low probability of embolism if the clinical suspicion of pulmonary embolism is strong. It is also indicated if the patient has an underlying disease process that may cause a perfusion defect. Angiography should be performed before caval filter placement and before treatment with thrombolytic therapy.

Timing

Both clinical and experimental evidence indicate considerable variability in the resolution rate of pulmonary emboli.[27–30] The rate of resolution may be adversely affected by the presence of concomitant cardiac or lung disease.[28] Angiographic evidence of complete resolution has been reported at 25 and 128 days[31] and at 6 weeks after embolism.[32] Dalen and colleagues reported the results of follow-up arteriography in 15 patients with previous angiographically documented bilateral pulmonary emboli.[33] The follow-up arteriograms were performed 1 to 7 days after the initial study in 7 patients, 10 to 21 days afterward in 10 patients, and at 34 days in 2 patients. Only minimal angiographic and hemodynamic signs of resolution were present at 7 days. By 10 to 21 days, pressures in the right side of the heart had returned to almost normal levels and unmistakable angiographic evidence of resolution was visible. Complete resolution of emboli with normal arteriography and hemodynamics was observed in three patients at 14, 15, and 34 days, respectively. In other patients, hemodynamic abnormalities persisted for weeks. In another series of nine patients with major pulmonary embolism who were free from cardiopulmonary disease, follow-up angiography performed an average of 26.5 hours after initiation of heparin therapy showed that little resolution of major pulmonary embolism occurs during the first 24 to 48 hours of heparin therapy.[34]

The rate of early resolution of pulmonary embolus was also assessed in the Urokinase Pulmonary Embolism Trial (UPET).[35] Lung scans and pulmonary angiograms were repeated 18 hours after a 12-hour heparin infusion in 78 patients with documented emboli. The follow-up angiograms documented slight improvement at 24 hours, with a 20 percent decrease in the degree of embolic obstruction. Repeat lung scans demonstrated an 8 percent resolution at 24 hours. These studies indicate that pulmonary embolism is not likely to be missed if arteriography is performed within 24 to 48 hours of the event. Studies performed within 7 days of the embolic event also should not result in a significant incidence of misdiagnosis.

The overall condition of the patient should be taken into consideration in the determination of the optimal time for performance of the arteriogram. In acutely ill patients who are in shock and under consideration for emergency embolectomy or thrombolytic therapy, the study may have to be performed on an emergency basis. In other patients, delay of the arteriography until heparin therapy has been instituted and the patient's condition has stabilized may be more appropriate. Many patients, shortly after embolism, are acutely ill and dyspneic and are unable to lie flat or cooperate for angiography. These same patients, if brought to arteriography 12 to 14 hours after institution of heparin, are typically more stable and tolerate angiography better. This improved tolerance may be a reflection of several hemodynamic factors. Early improvement may result from in vivo fibrinolysis or decrease in pulmonary vascular obstruction owing to subtle changes in the locations of the pulmonary emboli.[15]

Miller and associates evaluated right atrial, right ventricular, and pulmonary artery hemodynamics in two groups of patients with massive pulmonary embolism.[36] Hemodynamics were measured within 24 hours of embolism in one group, and 24 to 48 hours after the clinical event in the other group. All but two of the 23 patients studied were free from preexisting cardiorespiratory disease. Right atrial, right ventricular, and pulmonary artery hemodynamics were found to be significantly more abnormal in those patients studied within 24 hours. Patients studied more than 24 hours after the event no longer showed evidence of right ventricular failure. Because massive pulmonary embolism was still present, this finding suggests an adaptation of the right ventricle to the stress.

The hypotension sometimes seen after pulmonary angiography may be caused by the vasodilator effects of contrast medium in patients with right ventricular failure and a fixed cardiac output. This finding suggests that the acutely stressed right ventricle is unable to increase right ventricular pressure to a degree adequate to maintain pulmonary artery pressure and systemic output. Adaptation of the right ventricle is the most likely explanation for the improved ability of patients to tolerate angiography after a delay of some hours.

Other important considerations are the vasoconstriction and bronchoconstriction that frequently accompany pulmonary embolism.[37] If an embolus is examined within a few minutes of the event, degranulation of platelets is evident, with release of serotonin, adenine nucleotides, histamine, catecholamines, prostaglandins, thromboxanes, and other substances, which result in smooth muscle constriction of the pulmonary arteries and bronchi.[38] Acute bronchoconstriction, which occurs with pulmonary embolism, involves the small peripheral airways (terminal bronchioles and alveolar ducts) that are perfused by the pulmonary artery. Thrombin stimulates the degranulation of platelets. Heparin, by its inhibitory effect on thrombin, blocks this vasoconstrictive response.

Given that angiographic studies indicate only minimal resolution of pulmonary emboli within 24 hours of the embolic event and hemodynamic responses in most patients improve with therapy during this period, the indications for emergency pulmonary arteriography would appear to be limited to extreme situations.

Interpretation

The two most reliable signs of pulmonary embolism are an intraluminal filling defect and a vessel cutoff, which may occur singly or in combination.[39] Intraluminal filling defects appear as negative defects outlined by surrounding radiopaque contrast medium (Figs. 22–1 through 22–3). Oligemia and asymmetry of blood flow are frequently observed in pulmonary embolism but are not specific findings. These abnormalities may occur in chronic lung disease or congestive heart failure without pulmonary embolism.[39] If strict criteria (i.e., presence of intraluminal filling defect or vessel cutoff) are used for the diagnosis of pulmonary embolism, interobserver variation is low (less than 3 percent).[35]

Novelline and co-workers followed the clinical course of 180 patients with clinically suspected pulmonary embolism and a negative pulmonary arteriogram.[40] The arteriography was performed

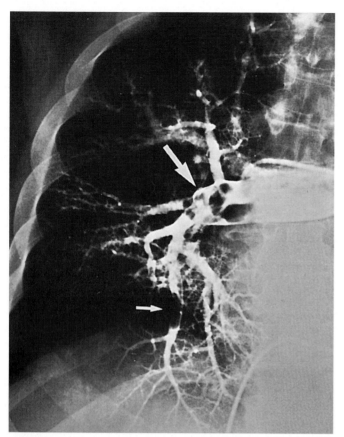

FIGURE 22–1. Selective right pulmonary artery injection angiogram shows the typical appearance of multiple pulmonary emboli involving the right main pulmonary artery and multiple right lower lobe segmental pulmonary arteries. Pulmonary emboli appear as radiolucent filling defects surrounded by contrast medium *(arrows)*.

with selective injections and subselective magnification views of areas of lung scan abnormality within 24 to 48 hours after the onset of symptoms. None of the untreated 167 patients died as a result of thromboembolic disease during their acute illness. During a follow-up period of 6 months or more, 20 patients died from unrelated causes, and none of the 147 patients who survived suffered from "recurrent" pulmonary embolism. These findings indicate that a negative pulmonary arteriogram of good quality can effectively exclude the presence of clinically significant pulmonary embolism.

In cases of chronic pulmonary embolism, organization of the thrombus occurs if the emboli do not lyse and fragment. Organization may result in little or no persistent recognizable abnormality, total occlusion of the vessel, transverse webs, eccentric plaques, or longitudinal strands. Multiple small recurrent peripheral pulmonary emboli may occur over time, causing pulmonary hypertension and right ventricular failure. Angiographically, these tend to appear as a lacy network of vessels, and they may be associated with bronchial arterial dilatation and pleural collateral flow, especially if infarction has occurred.[41] These changes are not specific, and neoplastic, postinflammatory, and other fibrotic obliterations may have a similar appearance.

A variety of nonembolic pathologies may be seen on pulmonary angiography during evaluation for pulmonary embolus. These disorders include arteritis, primary and metastatic pulmonary artery neoplasms, extrinsic compression of the pulmonary arteries by granulomatous or neoplastic hilar lymph nodes, and pulmonary arteriovenous malformations.[42]

Complications

The complications of pulmonary arteriography fall into three broad categories: those related to the angiographic technique, those

resulting from altered hemodynamics caused by contrast injections, and those arising from adverse reactions to contrast material. Two large series, one involving 367[39] and the other 298 patients,[43] reported a total of three deaths as a consequence of pulmonary arteriography. Two of these patients had more than 90 percent occlusion of the pulmonary vascular bed, and one had severe pulmonary hypertension. Dalen and colleagues reported an overall 3 percent incidence of complications.[39] In the UPET, five cases of ventricular tachycardia and one cardiac perforation occurred, all of which were treated successfully.[35]

Mills and associates evaluated the incidence of complications in 1350 pulmonary arteriograms.[3] He reported an overall 4 percent incidence of complications. Three deaths (0.2 percent) were directly attributable to the procedure. All three patients had severe pulmonary hypertension with systolic pulmonary artery pressures greater than 75 mm Hg and diastolic right ventricular pressures greater than 20 mm Hg. The precipitating event was the injection of contrast medium, which produced a sudden drop in systemic pressure. In the same series, cardiac perforation occurred in 1 percent of patients, and endocardial stain in 0.04 percent. These latter complications occurred exclusively in catheterizations performed with either the NIH or the Gensini catheter. No perforations occurred with the pigtail configuration catheter. Other complications included cardiac arrhythmias (0.08 percent of patients), cardiac arrest (0.03 percent), and contrast reaction (0.08 percent). This study confirmed the general experience regarding the safety of pulmonary arteriography when it is performed by experienced personnel using appropriate techniques and precautions.

Therapeutic Maneuvers at the Time of Angiography

Traditional therapy for pulmonary embolism consists of anticoagulant therapy with intravenous heparin followed by anticoagulation with oral sodium warfarin (Coumadin). Heparin limits the propagation of existing thrombi while the body's endogenous fibrinolytic system lyses the clot. Heparin interferes with the activation of factor IX by activated factor XI (intrinsic pathway) and acts as a potent antithrombin (common pathway) to inhibit the conversion of fibrinogen to fibrin. Its effectiveness is measured by the activated partial thromboplastin time (APTT) test. Heparin is not a benign drug. Its administration is the most common cause of drug-related complications in hospitalized patients. Serious bleeding complications have been reported in 10 to 15 percent of patients who were being treated with appropriately adjusted doses.[44, 45]

Systemic heparinization is accomplished through administration of an intravenous loading dose of 5000 units, followed by 800 to 1000 intravenous units per hour with the dose adjusted to maintain the APTT at 1.5 to 2.5 times the control value. Oral anticoagulation with sodium warfarin is usually started several days after institution of heparin therapy. Sodium warfarin inhibits hepatic synthesis of vitamin K–dependent factors and interferes with fibrin formation and growth of thrombi. Warfarin is administered orally, and its effectiveness is monitored by the prothrombin time.

Another form of treatment is thrombolytic therapy. Suitable candidates for thrombolytic therapy are patients with large pulmonary emboli that produce an obstruction of two or more segmental arteries or of one lobar artery and patients with multiple smaller pulmonary emboli that produce hemodynamic compromise in the presence of severe left ventricular dysfunction (Fig. 22–4). Patients should be screened to exclude those with a contraindication to thrombolytic therapy. Contraindications include active or recent internal bleeding, recent cerebrovascular accident, recent major surgery, serious trauma, and severe arterial hypertension.[46]

Both the UPET[44] and the Urokinase/Streptokinase Pulmonary Embolism Trial (USPET)[47] documented the value of thrombolytic therapy. The phase I study established that urokinase increased the resolution rate of pulmonary emboli, especially massive emboli, as judged by arteriography, hemodynamics, and lung scanning. The

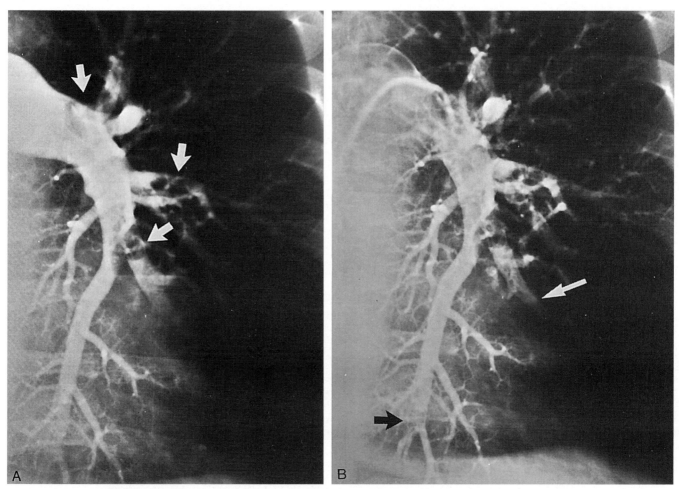

FIGURE 22–2. *A,* Left pulmonary artery injection angiogram shows multiple filling defects consistent with multiple pulmonary emboli in the distal left pulmonary artery and in the lobar branches to the left upper lobe and lower lobe *(arrows). B,* Next film from the angiographic series shows a vessel cutoff *(white arrow)* and an additional embolus in the segmental pulmonary artery to the left lower lobe *(black arrow).* Intravascular filling defects and vessel cutoffs are the two most reliable angiographic signs of pulmonary embolism.

trial was not designed to demonstrate a difference in mortality, and none was found. Patients selected at random for lytic therapy had the best hemodynamic response, with a significantly greater reduction in their pulmonary artery and right atrial pressures compared with patients treated with heparin.

The phase II trial was organized to determine whether 24 hours of urokinase therapy further increased clot resolution compared with 12 hours of urokinase therapy. Another goal was to compare 24 hours of streptokinase therapy with 24 hours of urokinase therapy. All three phase II dosage regimens were found to be superior to heparin alone in accelerating the rate of resolution of acute pulmonary embolism. Patients treated with urokinase achieved the best angiographic and hemodynamic response, although the difference between the response to urokinase and the response to streptokinase was not statistically significant. Mortality did not differ significantly. Two-week follow-up of participants in the UPET and USPET showed significant improvement in both diffusing capacity and pulmonary capillary blood flow for patients treated with lytic agents compared with those receiving heparin therapy. Long-term studies showed that patients who receive lytic therapy for massive pulmonary embolism have improved capillary blood volume at 2 weeks and at 1 year, compared with heparin-treated patients, who demonstrated decreased capillary blood volume at 1 year.[48] In these studies, however, no difference among the drug treatments was shown in recurrence rate of pulmonary embolism, and the use of thrombolytic agents was associated with a significantly higher rate of bleeding complications.

Forty-five percent of patients who received urokinase had bleeding complications, compared with 27 percent of those given heparin alone. Both of these bleeding rates were considered unacceptable for clinical practice, and this issue has been readdressed on several occasions.[46, 49] The 45 percent incidence of bleeding with the use of urokinase included both moderate and severe bleeding, and superficial oozing from a venous cutdown site was considered in the same manner as a retroperitoneal or other major hemorrhage. The incidence of clinically meaningful bleeding episodes (i.e., those that occurred during the infusion and required transfusion or discontinuation of therapy, as opposed to those that could easily be prevented or managed) was 9 percent for patients treated with urokinase and 4 percent for patients treated with heparin.[44] In these trials, both the heparin and the thrombolytic agent were administered through a peripheral intravenous line. Systemic doses of lytic therapy were used.

More recently, a newer thrombolytic agent, recombinant human tissue plasminogen activator (human rt-PA), has undergone evaluation in the treatment of acute pulmonary embolism. This agent has greater affinity for fibrin-bound plasminogen than for circulating unbound plasminogen and therefore should allow effective lysis of fibrin clots with minimal systemic fibrinogenolysis, which in turn should reduce the risk of hemorrhagic complications.

The effectiveness of this agent was tested against that of urokinase in a randomized controlled trial.[50] The principal end points of the study were clot lysis at 2 hours, as assessed by angiography, and pulmonary reperfusion at 24 hours, as assessed by lung scan-

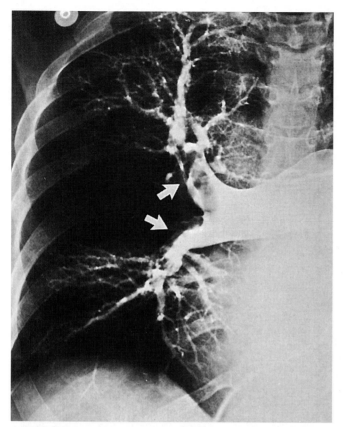

FIGURE 22–3. Acute and chronic pulmonary embolism. A right pulmonary artery injection angiogram shows a large acute saddle embolus involving the right upper lobe artery, right middle lobe artery, and right lower lobe pulmonary artery *(arrows)*. Note the severe oligemia in the right middle lobe distribution. Although observed with pulmonary embolism, oligemia can occur with other pulmonary disorders. The paucity of vessels and the stringy appearance in the right lower lobe segmental arteries suggest chronic recurrent emboli.

ning. By 2 hours, a significantly greater number of patients treated with rt-PA demonstrated clot lysis, compared with the patients treated with urokinase (82 percent versus 48 percent, respectively). A significantly lower incidence of hemorrhagic complications occurred among patients treated with rt-PA. The results indicated that, in the dosage regimens employed (rt-PA, 100 mg delivered at 50 mg per hour; or urokinase, 2000 units per pound of body weight as a bolus, followed by 2000 U/lb per hour for 24 hours), rt-PA acted more rapidly and was safer than urokinase in the treatment of acute pulmonary embolism.[50]

In a small series of patients, Verstraete and associates were unable to show that intrapulmonary infusion of rt-PA offered significant benefit over the intravenous route.[51] Their results suggested that a prolonged infusion of 100 mg of rt-PA over 7 hours was superior to a single infusion of 50 mg delivered over 2 hours. Nonetheless, administration of rt-PA or other thrombolytic agent through the pulmonary angiographic catheter has the advantages of obviating the need for repeat venipuncture when follow-up arteriogram is performed and of permitting a higher concentration of the agent to be delivered to the thrombus. This is the preferred approach at the University of California at Los Angeles Medical Center.

Other therapeutic maneuvers that can be performed at angiography are percutaneous embolectomy and percutaneous placement of an inferior vena cava filter. Transvenous percutaneous embolectomy was first proposed by Greenfield in the early 1970s.[52] This technique involves aspiration of the clots after passage of a specially designed catheter with a suction tip through the right ventricle and out into the pulmonary artery. The technique has never gained widespread popularity.

The placement of an inferior vena cava filter, however, is an often-used and effective therapy. Placement of a filter is indicated in patients with an absolute contraindication to anticoagulant therapy, acute bleeding in the presence of anticoagulant therapy, or recurrent emboli occurring in the presence of appropriately managed full anticoagulation. The first caval filter was the Mobin-Uddin filter.[53] It was placed by means of a jugular vein cutdown. Its use was limited by its tendency to generate caval thrombosis and to migrate to the right ventricle. It was followed by the Kimray-Greenfield filter, which was associated with a lower incidence of complications.[54] Initially, these filters were placed through a jugular or femoral vein cutdown. Currently, a variety of inferior vena cava filters are commercially available for percutaneous transfemoral or transjugular placement through sheath sizes ranging from 9 to 12 Fr. Among the filters frequently used are the Gianturco-Roehm Bird's Nest Filter (Cook, Inc., Bloomington, IN), the Titanium Greenfield Vena Cava Filter (Medi-Tech Boston Scientific Corp., Watertown, MA), the LGM Filter (Braun Vena Tech, Evanston, IL), and the Simon Nitinol Filter (Nitinol Medical Technologies, Woburn, MA).[55, 56]

A follow-up study of 320 patients by Ferris and colleagues in which a variety of filters were evaluated reported a 4 percent incidence of documented pulmonary embolism after filter placement.[57] The prevalence of caval thrombosis was 19 percent, and the incidence of new or increased deep venous thrombosis was found to be 22 percent. Placement of a caval filter is typically performed in the angiographic suite after an inferior vena cavogram to identify the location of the renal veins (Fig. 22–5). The filter is usually placed below the renal veins. Neuerburg and associates have described early experience with a filter that may be placed prophylactically and removed after the risk of embolism has been resolved.[58]

PULMONARY ANGIOGRAPHY FOR OTHER PULMONARY VASCULAR LESIONS

Pulmonary arteriography is essential for accurate diagnosis of other pulmonary vascular lesions. Among these are pulmonary artery stenosis, pulmonary arteriovenous fistula, arteritis, and pulmonary artery aneurysm. The technique of pulmonary angiography applied in cases of these suspected lesions is the same as that employed in the evaluation of suspected pulmonary embolism. A different pulmonary vascular abnormality is often found in a patient initially suspected of having a pulmonary embolus. The preangiographic workup should include routine laboratory admission studies, chest radiograph, and ECG, and it should be tailored to the patient's suspected underlying disease process. The risks of pulmonary arteriography are similar to those previously described.

Pulmonary Arteriovenous Fistula

Pulmonary arteriovenous fistulas are abnormal communications between pulmonary arteries and veins; most of them are congenital. They may occur as an isolated anomaly, but they occur most frequently in cases of hereditary hemorrhagic telangiectasia, in which 30 to 40 percent of the patient's family members may be affected.[59] Acquired fistulas are rare and are often secondary to pulmonary arterial hypertension resulting from mitral stenosis or to hepatic cirrhosis with portal hypertension. Other acquired causes include schistosomiasis, trauma, and metastatic disease to the lung, especially thyroid carcinoma. Pulmonary arteriovenous fistulas may often be suspected from the chest radiograph. At angiography, selective injections into the area of corresponding radiographic abnormality disclose the typical angiographic findings of a fistula.

Fistulas may be simple or complex.[60, 61] The simple type are characterized by a single feeding artery draining into a bulbous, nonseptated aneurysmal part with two or more draining veins. Complex fistulas have two or more pulmonary artery branches communicating with a bulbous, septated, cirsoid, aneurysmal part with two or more draining veins. In both types, the feeding artery may also give rise to branches to the uninvolved adjacent lung.

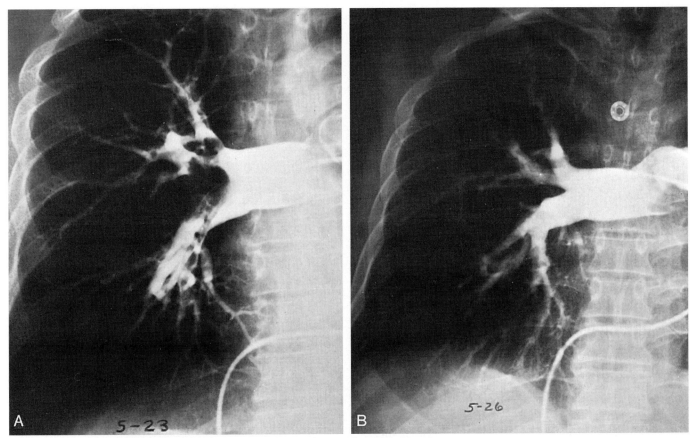

FIGURE 22–4. *A,* Patient with a large saddle embolus to the right upper and lower lobe pulmonary artery. This patient was treated with systemic doses of a thrombolytic agent infused into the right pulmonary artery. *B,* Repeat pulmonary arteriogram at 72 hours shows lysis of the thrombus, with improved pulmonary perfusion.

Both types can occur in the same patient, and diffuse involvement can occur with evidence of multiple large or small lesions (Fig. 22–6). Fistulas vary in size from microscopic to large bulbous structures.

In the past, surgical excision of single or several of the largest pulmonary arteriovenous malformations was the therapy of choice. With time, however, symptoms recurred as smaller malformations grew. Currently, the preferred treatment of these fistulas involves transcatheter embolization therapy. Particular skill is required in the transcatheter embolization of these lesions, because faulty technique can result in inadvertent passage of the embolic agent to the pulmonary veins and subsequent systemic embolization.[61]

Pulmonary Artery Stenosis

Pulmonary artery stenosis is characterized by narrowing of the pulmonary artery or of its branches. The stenoses may be central, peripheral, or combined. The condition exists as an isolated anomaly in approximately 40 percent of cases, and in the remaining 60 percent it is associated with valvular pulmonic stenosis or other congenital heart disease, usually tetralogy of Fallot or ventricular septal defect.[62] Acquired stenosis of a main branch pulmonary artery can occur secondary to a hilar mass, such as an aortic aneurysm, thymoma, or bronchogenic carcinoma. Peripheral branch pulmonary artery stenosis may occur as part of the congenital rubella syndrome, the supravalvular aortic stenosis syndrome, or Takayasu arteritis.

Takayasu arteritis primarily involves the aortic arch and great vessels but may involve the pulmonary arteries in as many as 50 percent of patients.[63, 64] Usually, the main pulmonary arterial branches are involved. Segmental stenosis, vessel irregularity, and occlusion are usually seen on the angiography (Fig. 22–7). Pulmonary hypertension is common, and most patients have exertional dyspnea. If pulmonary hypertension is severe, subselective injections should be performed during arteriography. Because the disease often occurs in young patients, the disease process should be considered so that early angiography may be obtained.

Pulmonary Artery Aneurysm

Almost 90 percent of pulmonary artery aneurysms involve the main pulmonary artery and are asymptomatic.[65] They may occur in Marfan syndrome. Most peripheral pulmonary artery aneurysms are multiple, are of mycotic origin, and are associated with a high incidence of rupture (Fig. 22–8). They may also occur after trauma. Solitary peripheral aneurysms are usually tuberculous in origin. Rasmussen aneurysms, as they are called, are false aneurysms of the pulmonary arteries that result from arterial erosion in chronic cavitary tuberculosis. They are most often found in the upper lobe, usually with hemoptysis, and are associated with a high incidence of fatal rupture.[66]

Pulmonary Varix

On the chest radiograph, pulmonary varices appear as cylindrical or oval-shaped densities that are centrally located. They may be unilateral or bilateral, and they may congenital or acquired in origin. The acquired lesions are usually secondary to venous hypertension or mitral insufficiency. They may bleed, but such bleeding is rare. They are usually asymptomatic, and their diagnosis is important to prevent unnecessary operation. They are identified on the venous phase of pulmonary arteriography.

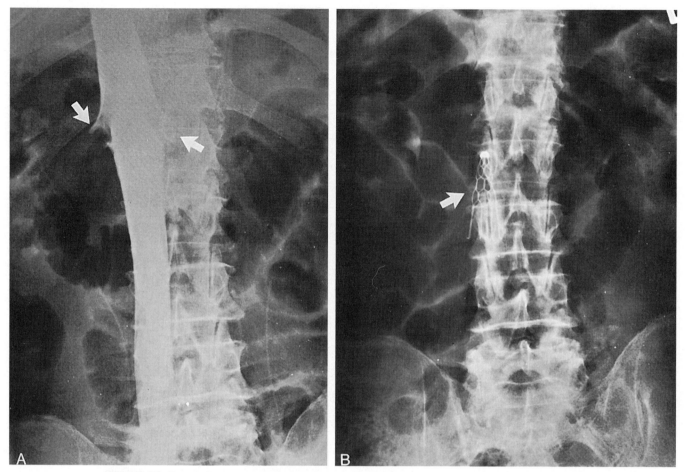

FIGURE 22–5. *A,* Inferior venacavogram. Radiolucent defects in the upper vena cava indicate the site of drainage of the right and left renal veins *(arrows).* The location of the renal veins should be determined before filter placement because the filter should be placed below their site of entrance into the vena cava. *B,* A Kimray-Greenfield filter has been percutaneously placed in the inferior vena cava. Note the upright position of the filter. If the filters are placed incorrectly and tilted, they are less effective in trapping thrombi.

Neoplasm

Malignant lesions involving the pulmonary arteries can also be identified at arteriography (Fig. 22–9). Arterial narrowing and occlusion have been documented in patients with bronchogenic carcinoma and large mass lesions.[67] Primary pulmonary artery sarcoma can mimic pulmonary embolism. It is rare and typically arises from the main pulmonary artery. Pulmonary infarcts caused by tumor emboli or by small thrombi that arise on the mass may produce symptoms similar to those of pulmonary emboli. The clinical symptoms of this tumor more typically simulate those of chronic or recurrent embolism.

Pulmonary carcinosarcoma is an uncommon pulmonary neoplasm. Two varieties occur. The central type is a pedunculated endobronchial lesion that produces bronchial obstruction. The peripheral type grows rapidly and has a propensity to invade the chest wall, mediastinum, and vascular structures. Symptoms may be indistinguishable from those of pulmonary embolism, and neoplasia should be included in the differential diagnosis of acute pulmonary embolism in patients in whom perfusion scan defects do not change with appropriate anticoagulation or who show a progression of perfusion defects on lung scanning despite adequate anticoagulation.[68]

Pulmonary Sequestration

Pulmonary sequestration is a condition in which a portion of a lung tissue is detached from the remainder of the lung, is not connected with the pulmonary artery, and sometimes is not connected with the bronchial tree. The abnormal lung tissue receives its blood supply from an artery that arises from the thoracic or abdominal aorta. In intralobar sequestration, the nonfunctional segment of lung is enclosed within the visceral pleura of a pulmonary lobe. The posterior-basilar segment is usually involved, and the majority of cases occur on the left side.[69] In intralobar sequestration, venous drainage to pulmonary veins occurs. In extralobar sequestration, the abnormal lung segment is contained within its own visceral pleura and may be located in or outside the pleural space, either above or below the diaphragm. The blood is supplied from a systemic source, typically the thoracic aorta, but venous drainage involves a systemic vein such as the inferior vena cava, the azygous vein, or the hemiazygos system. These abnormalities usually occur on the left side.

Congenital Dysplasia of the Lung

Embryologically, the aorta and the main pulmonary artery arise from a common trunk that septates to form the ascending aorta and the main pulmonary artery. The main right and left pulmonary arteries arise from the ventral portions of the sixth primitive arches; the dorsal portions form the ductus on the side, which retains its fourth arch, the forerunner of the descending aorta. The lung buds develop as a ventral outgrowth from the foregut and transiently receive blood from small systemic vessels that arise from the paired dorsal aortas. Pulmonary parenchymal vessels then develop and join on each side with the corresponding sixth arch.

Abnormalities of the pulmonary arteries are seen in conjunction with congenital dysplasia of the lung. Hypoplasia, interruption, agenesis, or anomalous origin of the pulmonary vessels may be

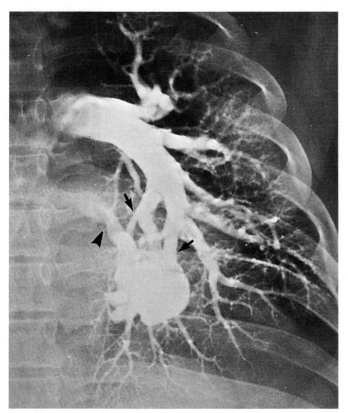

FIGURE 22–6. Left pulmonary arterial injection angiogram shows a large pulmonary arteriovenous fistula involving the left lower lobe in a patient with hereditary hemorrhagic telangiectasia. This complex fistula is supplied by two lower lobe segmental pulmonary arteries (*arrows*) that communicate with a bulbous aneurysm. The draining pulmonary vein opacifies (*arrowhead*).

evident. Chest radiographs may show a unilaterally small hemithorax, decreased or absent pulmonary vascular markings, a small or absent hilus, or a mediastinal shift to the affected side. Hypogenetic lung syndrome causes lobar or segmental absence of pulmonary tissue, bronchi, and vessels. Occasionally, it involves anomalous systemic arterial supply and partially or totally anomalous venous drainage from the right lung into systemic veins, usually the inferior vena cava or the right atrium ("scimitar syndrome").[70]

Interruption of the right or left pulmonary artery occurs when the ventral portion of the sixth arch does not communicate with its corresponding pulmonary parenchymal plexus. Usually, a left-sided arch is present when the right pulmonary artery is interrupted, and a right-sided arch when the left pulmonary artery is interrupted. In agenesis of the lung, no pulmonary vessels or parenchymal tissue is present.

The pulmonary artery can also arise anomalously from the aorta. This phenomenon is explained embryologically by persistence of the dorsal portion of the sixth arch (ductus) with agenesis of its ventral portion. Typically, anomalous origin of the right pulmonary artery is associated with a left aortic arch, and that of the left pulmonary artery with a right aortic arch. The left pulmonary artery may also arise anomalously from the right pulmonary artery, pulmonary artery "sling" or, rarely, the abdominal aorta. The pulmonary artery sling can produce obstruction of the distal trachea or the right bronchus, or both.[71]

Anomalous Pulmonary Venous Connection

Anomalous pulmonary venous return can be diagnosed on the venous phase or levophase of a pulmonary arteriogram. The anomalous drainage may be partial or complete. If partial, it most frequently consists of drainage of the right upper lobe pulmonary vein

to the right superior vena cava. In total anomalous pulmonary venous connection, the anomalous return, in order of frequency, is to the left superior vena cava, the coronary sinus, the right atrium, the right superior vena cava, or below the diaphragm. Less frequently, the connection may be mixed, with one or more veins draining into a different site. These anomalies are typically associated with an atrial septal defect that allows oxygenated blood to reach the systemic circulation. These anomalies are best identified with selective pulmonary arterial injections and delayed filming.

Summary

Pulmonary arteriography is currently the most reliable test for the diagnosis of abnormalities of the pulmonary vessels. The most frequent indication is for diagnosis of pulmonary embolism. Pulmonary angiography can be performed by experienced physicians with little morbidity. The procedure should be performed in a well-equipped angiographic suite with ECG and pressure monitoring. Selective right and left pulmonary arterial injections should be performed. Particular care should be taken in examination of patients with pulmonary hypertension. In these patients, subselective injections of contrast material should be made into the area of highest probability. In patients with pulmonary embolism, heparin therapy followed by oral anticoagulation is usually sufficient to prevent recurrence. Patients with massive pulmonary embolism should be considered for treatment with thrombolytic therapy if no contraindications exist. If heparin therapy fails or the patient's medical condition precludes anticoagulation, vena caval filter placement can be performed. Filter placement should not be undertaken in the absence of angiographically documented pulmonary

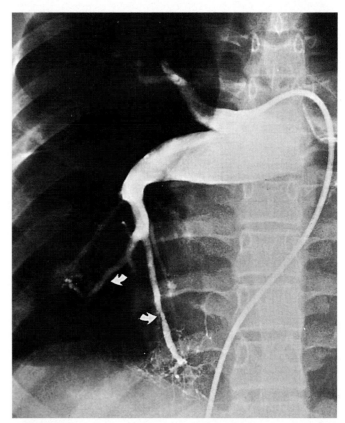

FIGURE 22–7. Takayasu arteritis involving the pulmonary artery. A right pulmonary arterial injection angiogram shows rapid tapering of distal vessels, with occlusion of several segmental branches and areas of irregular stenosis typical of vasculitis (*arrows*). This patient had severe pulmonary hypertension. (From Cassling, R.J., Lois, J.F., and Gomes, A.S.: Unusual pulmonary angiographic findings in suspected pulmonary embolism. AJR 145:995, 1985, with permission. © American Roentgen Ray Society.)

embolism. These filters can now be placed percutaneously, avoiding the need for operative placement. Pulmonary angiography is also indicated in the diagnosis of other pulmonary vascular lesions, such as pulmonary arteriovenous fistulas, vasculitis, and pulmonary artery stenosis.

NEWER VASCULAR IMAGING TECHNIQUES

Both magnetic resonance imaging (MRI) and computed tomography (CT) allow the noninvasive imaging of the vascular system. ECG-triggered spin-echo MRI techniques provide high-resolution images of the central pulmonary arteries in multiple projections. Gradient echo techniques allow functional assessment. The size and configuration of the central pulmonary vessels can readily be determined without the use of intravascular contrast agents. MRI techniques have been shown to be useful in the evaluation and follow-up of congenital abnormalities of the pulmonary vessels.[72] Central pulmonary emboli can be detected, but evaluation of the segmental and subsegmental vessels is unreliable. The application

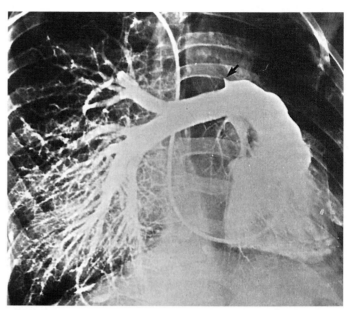

FIGURE 22–9. Metastatic rectal carcinoma to the lung. A main pulmonary artery injection angiogram shows an oblique view of left upper lobe lung infiltrate. The left upper lobe pulmonary artery is occluded by tumor encasement (*arrow*).

of MRI techniques in the evaluation of the pulmonary vessels is currently investigational.

Pulmonary emboli have been detected using conventional, non-dynamic CT techniques.[73, 74] The recently developed spiral (helical) volumetric and fast CT scanning techniques allow denser and more consistent opacification of the central pulmonary artery and its proximal subdivisions, and the role of these techniques in the diagnosis of pulmonary embolism has also been assessed.[75, 76] Pulmonary emboli in lobar and segmental arteries have been diagnosed by the use of these newer CT techniques with contrast media injection.[76] Subsegmental pulmonary vessels, however, cannot be reliably evaluated. Consequently, the use of these newer CT techniques in the diagnosis of pulmonary emboli is limited, and these techniques cannot currently be relied on to exclude the presence of small distal pulmonary emboli.

References

 1. Dalen, J.E.: Pulmonary angiography in pulmonary embolism. Bull. Physiopathol. Respir. 6:45, 1970.
 2. Kelly, J.F., Patterson, R., Lieberman, P., et al.: Radiographic contrast media studies in high-risk patients. J. Allergy Clin. Immunol. 62:181, 1978.
 3. Mills, S.R., Jackson, D.C., Older, R.A., et al.: The incidence, etiologies, and avoidance of complications of pulmonary angiography in a large series. Radiology 136:295, 1980.
 4. Grollman, J.H., Jr., Gypes, M.T., and Helmer, E.: Transfemoral selective bilateral pulmonary arteriography with a pulmonary-artery–seeking catheter. Radiology 96:202, 1970.
 5. Green, G.S.: Use of the pigtail catheter for pulmonary angiography. Radiology 138:744, 1981.
 6. Alderson, P.O., and Martin, E.C. Pulmonary embolism: Diagnosis with multiple imaging modalities. Radiology 164:297, 1987.
 7. Gomes, A.S., Grollman, J.H., Jr., and Mink, J.: Pulmonary angiography for pulmonary emboli: Rational selection of oblique views. AJR 129:1019, 1977.
 8. Bynum, L.J., Wilson, J.E., III, Christenson, E.E., et al.: Radiographic techniques for balloon occlusion pulmonary angiography. Radiology 133:518, 1979.
 9. Nihill, M.R., Mullins, C.E., and McNamara, D.G.: Visualization of the pulmonary arteries in pseudotruncus by pulmonary vein wedge angiography. Circulation 58:140, 1978.
10. Saeed, M., Braun, S.D., Cohan, R.H., et al.: Pulmonary angiography with iopamidol: Patient comfort, image quality, and hemodynamics. Radiology 165:345, 1987.
11. Smith, D.C., Lois, J.F., Gomes, A.S., et al.: Pulmonary arteriography: Comparison of cough stimulation effects of diatrizoate and ioxaglate. Radiology 162:617, 1987.
12. Katayama, H., Yamaguchi, K., Kozuka, T., et al.: Adverse reactions to ionic and nonionic contrast media: A report from the Japanese Committee on the safety of contrast media. Radiology 175:621, 1990.
13. Katholi, R.E., Taylor, G.J., Woods, W.T., et al.: Nephrotoxicity of nonionic low-osmolality contrast media: Prospective double-blind randomized comparison in human beings. Radiology 186:183, 1993.

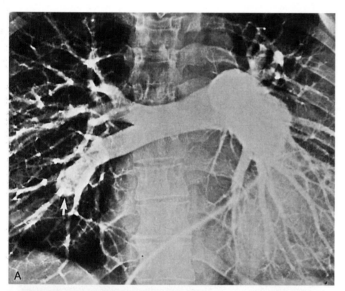

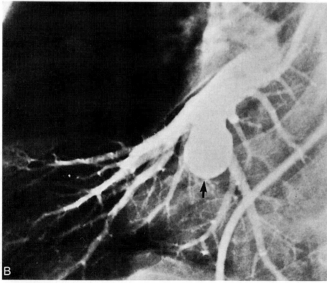

FIGURE 22–8. *A*, Peripheral pulmonary artery aneurysm. A pulmonary arteriogram in a patient with a history of intravenous drug abuse shows an aneurysm of the right lower lobe pulmonary artery (*arrow*). *B*, A selective pulmonary artery injection angiogram shows a mycotic aneurysm arising from the anterior basal segmental artery (*arrow*).

14. Barrett, B.J., and Carlisle, E.J.: Metaanalysis of the relative nephrotoxicity of high and low-osmolality iodinated contrast media. Radiology 188:171, 1993.
15. Dalen, J.E., and Alpert, J.S.: Natural history of pulmonary embolism. Prog. Cardiovasc. Dis. 17:259, 1975.
16. Barker, N.W.: The diagnosis and treatment of pulmonary embolism. Med. Clin. North Am. 42:1053, 1958.
17. Smith, G.T., Dexter, L., and Dammin, G.J.: Postmortem quantitative studies in pulmonary embolism. In Sasahara, A.A., and Stein, M. (eds.): Pulmonary Embolic Disease. New York, Grune & Stratton, 1965, p. 120.
18. Sasahara, A.: Clinical studies in pulmonary thromboembolism. In Sasahara, A.A., and Stein, M. (eds.): Pulmonary Embolic Disease. New York, Grune & Stratton, 1965, p. 256.
19. Hull, R.D., Hirsh, J., Carter, C.J., et al.: Pulmonary angiography, ventilation lung scanning and venography for clinically suspected pulmonary embolism with abnormal perfusion scan. Ann. Intern. Med. 98:891, 1983.
20. Greenspan, R.H., Ravin, C.E., Polansky, S.M., et al.: Accuracy of the chest radiograph in diagnosis of pulmonary embolism. Invest. Radiol. 17:539, 1982.
21. Wellman, H.N.: Pulmonary thromboembolism: Current status report on the role of nuclear medicine. Semin. Nucl. Med. 6:236, 1986.
22. Sostman, H.D., Rapoport, S., Gottschalk, A., et al.: Imaging of pulmonary embolism. Invest. Radiol. 21:443, 1986.
23. McNeil, B.J.: A diagnostic strategy using ventilation perfusion studies in patients suspected for pulmonary embolism. J. Nucl. Med. 17:613, 1976.
24. Biello, D.R., Mattar, A.G., McKnight, R.C., et al.: Ventilation-perfusion studies in suspected pulmonary embolism. AJR 133:1033, 1979.
25. Sostman, H.D., Ravin, C.E., and Sullivan, D.C.: Use of pulmonary angiography for suspected pulmonary embolism: Influence of scintigraphic diagnosis. AJR 139:673, 1982.
26. Sullivan, D.C., Coleman, R.E., and Mills, S.R.: Lung scan interpretation: Effect of of different observers and different criteria. Radiology 149:803, 1983.
27. Bjork, L., and Ansusinha, T.: Angiographic diagnosis of acute pulmonary embolism. Acta Radiol. Diagn. 3:129, 1965.
28. Fred, H.L., Axelrad, M.A., Lewis, J.M., et al.: Rapid resolution of pulmonary thromboemboli in man: An angiographic study. J.A.M.A. 196:1137, 1966.
29. Chait, A., Summers, D., Krasnow, N., et al.: Observations on the fate of large pulmonary emboli. AJR 100:364, 1967.
30. Murphy, M.L., and Bulloch, R.T.: Factors influencing the restoration of blood flow following pulmonary embolization as determined by angiography and scanning. Circulation 38:1116, 1968.
31. Sautter, R.D., Fletcher, F.W., Emanuel, D.A., et al.: Clinical notes: Complete resolution of massive pulmonary thromboembolism. J.A.M.A. 189:948, 1964.
32. Simon, M., and Sasahara, A.A.: Observations on the angiographic changes in pulmonary thrombolism. In Sasahara, A.A., and Stein, M. (eds.): Pulmonary Embolic Disease. New York: Grune & Stratton, 1965, p. 214.
33. Dalen, J.E., Banas, J.S., Brooks, H.L., et al.: Resolution rate of acute pulmonary embolism in man. N. Engl. J. Med. 280:1194, 1969.
34. McDonald, I.G., Hirsh, J., and Hale, G.S.: Early rate of resolution of major pulmonary embolism: A study of angiographic and hemodynamic changes occurring in the first 24–48 hours. Br. Heart J. 33:432, 1971.
35. Urokinase Pulmonary Embolism Trial. A national cooperative study. Circulation 47 & 48(Suppl. 2):1, 1973.
36. Miller, G.A.H., and Sutton, G.C.: Acute massive pulmonary embolism: Clinical and hemodynamic findings in 23 patients studied by cardiac catheterization and pulmonary arteriography. Br. Heart J. 32:518, 1970.
37. Sasahara, A.A., Sidd, J.J., Tremblay, G., et al.: Cardiopulmonary consequences of acute pulmonary embolic disease. Prog. Cardiovasc. Dis. 9:259, 1966.
38. Stein, M., Hirose, T., Yasutake, T., et al.: Airway responses to pulmonary embolism: Pharmacologic aspects. In Moser, K.M., and Stein, M. (eds.): Pulmonary Thromboembolism. Chicago, Yearbook Medical Publishers, 1973, p. 166.
39. Dalen, J.E., Brooks, H.L., Johnson, L.W., et al.: Pulmonary angiography in acute pulmonary embolism: Indications, techniques, and results in 367 patients. Am. Heart J. 81:175, 1971.
40. Novelline, R.A., Baltarowich, O.H., Athanasoulis, C.A., et al.: The clinical course of patients with suspected pulmonary embolism and a negative pulmonary arteriogram. Radiology 126:561, 1978.
41. Bookstein, J.J., and Silver, T.M.: The angiographic differential diagnosis of acute pulmonary embolism. Radiology 110:25, 1974.
42. Cassling, R.J., Lois, J.F., and Gomes, A.S.: Unusual pulmonary angiographic findings in suspected pulmonary embolism. AJR 145:995, 1985.
43. Moses, D.L., Silver, T.M., and Bookstein, J.J.: The complementary roles of chest radiography lung scanning and selective pulmonary arteriography in the diagnosis of pulmonary embolism. Circulation 49:179, 1974.
44. Urokinase Pulmonary Embolism Trial. Phase I results: A cooperative study. J.A.M.A. 214:2163, 1970.
45. Mant, M.J., Thong, K.L., Kirtwhistle, R.V., et al.: Fibrinolytic therapy. Radiology 159:619, 1986.
46. Consensus Developmental Panel: Thrombolytic therapy in thrombosis: A National Institutes of Health Consensus Development Conference. Ann. Intern. Med. 93:141, 1980.
47. Urokinase-Streptokinase Pulmonary Embolism Trial Phase II results: A cooperative study. J.A.M.A. 229;1606, 1974.
48. Sharma, G.V.R.K., Burleson, V.A., and Sasahara, A.A.: Effect of thrombolytic therapy on pulmonary capillary blood volume in patients with pulmonary embolism. N. Engl. J. Med. 303:842, 1980.
49. Marder, V.J.: Are we using fibrinolytic agents often enough? (Editorial.] Ann. Intern. Med. 93:136, 1980.
50. Goldhaber, S.Z., Kessler, C.M., Heit, J., et al.: Randomised controlled trial of recombinant tissue plasminogen activator versus urokinase in the reatment of acute pulmonary embolism. Lancet 2:293, 1988.
51. Verstraete, M., Miller, G.A.H., Bounameaux, H., et al.: Intravenous and intrapulmonary recombinant tissue type plasminogen activator in the treatment of acute massive pulmonary embolism. Circulation 77:353, 1988.
52. Greenfield, L.J.: Pulmonary embolism: Diagnosis and management. Curr. Probl. Cardiol. 13:1, 1976.
53. Mobin-Uddin, K., McLean, R., and Jude, J.R.: A new catheter technique of interruption of inferior vena cava for prevention of pulmonary embolism. Am. J. Surg. 35:889, 1969.
54. Greenfield, L.J., Peyton, R., Crute, S., et al.: Greenfield vena caval filter experience: Late results in 156 patients. Arch. Surg. 116:1451, 1981.
55. Dorfman, G.S.: Percutaneous inferior vena caval filters. Radiology 174:987, 1990.
56. Grassi, C.J.: Inferior vena caval filters: Analysis of five currently available devices. AJR 156:813, 1991.
57. Ferris, E.J., McCowan, T.C., Carver, D.K., et al.: Percutaneous inferior vena caval filters: Follow-up of several designs in 320 patients. Radiology 188:851, 1993.
58. Neuerburg, J.M., Gunther, R.W., Rasmussen, E., et al.: New retrievable percutaneous vena cava filter: Experimental in vitro and in vivo evaluation. Cardiovasc. Intervent. Radiol. 16:224, 1993.
59. Dines, D.E., Arms, R.A., Bernatz, P., et al.: Pulmonary arteriovenous fistulas. Mayo Clin. Proc. 49:460, 1974.
60. Moyer, J.H., Glentz, G., and Brest, A.N.: Pulmonary arteriovenous fistulas. Am. J. Med. 32:417, 1962.
61. White, R.I., Jr., Mitchell, S.E., Barth, K.H., et al.: Angioarchitecture of pulmonary arteriovenous malformations: An important consideration before embolotherapy. AJR 140:681, 1983.
62. Gay, B., French, R.H., Shuford, W.H., et al.: The roentgenologic features of single and multiple coarctations of the pulmonary artery and branches. AJR 90:599, 1963.
63. Lupi-Herrera, E., Sanchez-Torres, G., Marcushamer, J., et al.: Takayasu's arteritis: Clinical study of 107 cases. Am. Heart J. 93:94, 1977.
64. Kawai, C., Ishikawa, K., Kato, M., et al.: Pulmonary pulseless disease: Clinical Conference in Cardiology from the Third Medical Division, Kyoto University Hospital, Kyoto, Japan. Chest 73:651, 1978.
65. Trell, E.: Pulmonary arterial aneurysm. Thorax 28:644, 1973.
66. Auerbach, O.: Pathology and pathogenesis of pulmonary arterial aneurysms in tuberculous cavities. Am. Rev. Tuber. 39:99, 1939.
67. Ballantyne, A.J., Clagett, O.T., and McDonald, J.R.: Vascular involvement in bronchogenic carcinoma. Thorax 12:294, 1957.
68. Olsson, H.E., Spitzer, R.M., and Erston, W.F.: Primary and secondary pulmonary artery neoplasia mimicking acute pulmonary embolus. Radiology 118:49, 1976.
69. Turk, L. Newton, III, and Lindskog, G.E.: The importance of angiographic diagnosis in intralobar pulmonary sequestration. J. Thorac. Cardiovasc. Surg. 41:299, 1961.
70. Roehm, J., Jue, K., and Amplatz, K.: Radiographic features of the scimitar syndrome. Radiology 86:856, 1966.
71. Ellis, K., Seamen, W.B., Griffiths, S.P., et al.: Some congenital anomalies of the pulmonary arteries. Semin. Roentgenol. 2:325, 1967.
72. Gomes, A.S., Lois, J.F., and Williams, R.G.: MR imaging of the pulmonary arteries in patients with congenital right ventricular outflow tract obstruction. Radiology 174:51, 1990.
73. Chintapalli, K., Thorsen, K., Olson, D.L., et al.: Computed tomography of pulmonary thromboembolism and infarction. J. Comput. Assist. Tomogr. 12:553, 1988.
74. Verschakelen, J.A., Vanwijck, E., Bogaert, J., et al.: Detection of unsuspected central pulmonary embolism with conventional contrast-enhanced CT. Radiology 188:847, 1993.
75. Geraghty, J.J., Stanford, W., Landas, S.K., et al.: Ultrafast computed tomography in experimental pulmonary embolism. Invest. Radiol. 27:60, 1992.
76. Remy-Jardin, M., Wattinne, L., and Giraud, F.: Central pulmonary thromboembolism: Diagnosis with spiral volumetric CT with single-breath-hold technique—comparison with pulmonary angiography. Radiology 185:381, 1992.

23 Principles and Practice of Coronary Angiography

Maryl R. Johnson, M.D.

HISTORIC EVENTS IN THE DEVELOPMENT OF
CORONARY ANGIOGRAPHY ____ 220
INDICATIONS ____ 221
CONTRAINDICATIONS ____ 223
COMPLICATIONS ____ 223
PATIENT PREPARATION AND
MANAGEMENT ____ 226
CORONARY ANGIOGRAPHIC
TECHNIQUES ____ 227
Sones Technique ____ 227
Judkins Technique ____ 227
Amplatz Technique ____ 228
Schoonmaker Technique ____ 229
Alternative Arterial Access Techniques ____ 229
General Principles of Safe and Optimal
Coronary Angiography ____ 229
Bypass Graft and Internal Mammary Artery
Angiography ____ 230
OUTPATIENT CORONARY
ANGIOGRAPHY ____ 230
Studies of Small-Diameter Catheters ____ 231
IMPORTANCE OF ADEQUATE ANGIOGRAPHIC
VIEWS ____ 232
NORMAL CORONARY ANATOMY ____ 233
CONGENITAL ANOMALIES OF THE CORONARY
ARTERIES ____ 235

Coronary Anomalies That Alter Myocardial
Perfusion ____ 235
Coronary Anomalies That Do Not Alter
Myocardial Perfusion ____ 237
CORONARY COLLATERALS ____ 238
CORONARY BRIDGING ____ 239
VALIDITY OF CORONARY
ANGIOGRAMS ____ 239
Comparison of Postmortem and Angiographic
Findings ____ 239
Intraobserver and Interobserver
Variability ____ 240
EVALUATION, INTERPRETATION, AND
IMPLICATIONS OF THE CORONARY
ANGIOGRAM ____ 241
Physiologic Significance of Coronary
Stenoses ____ 241
Prognostic Significance of Coronary
Stenoses ____ 241
Implications of Coronary Stenosis
Morphology ____ 244
TRAPS TO AVOID IN THE PERFORMANCE AND
INTERPRETATION OF CORONARY
ANGIOGRAMS ____ 247
GENERAL RECOMMENDATIONS ____ 248

Coronary artery disease remains the major cause of morbidity and mortality in the United States, and symptomatic coronary artery disease is present in more than 6 million individuals.[1] It is estimated that nearly 1.5 million myocardial infarctions occur each year, and coronary heart disease caused almost 500,000 deaths in 1990.[2] Coronary angiography has been used increasingly to define the coronary arterial lesions responsible for the morbidity and mortality caused by ischemic heart disease, and it is estimated that more than 1 million diagnostic cardiac catheterizations are performed in the United States each year.[3] In contrast with the early years of cardiac catheterization, during which coronary angiography was performed only when coronary bypass or valvular surgery was clearly indicated, coronary angiography is currently used to define coronary anatomy whenever the information obtained will be beneficial to patient management. Despite numerous attempts with other imaging modalities to define the presence, extent, and functional significance of coronary artery disease, coronary angiography remains the only method of defining the anatomy of the coronary tree, and coronary angiography remains the "gold standard" for determining the presence, extent, localization, and severity of coronary artery disease. Coronary angiography also allows visualization of lesion morphology, intracoronary thrombus, coronary collaterals, coronary artery spasm, and congenital anomalies of the coronary arteries. If coronary stenoses are present, coronary angiography permits analysis of the distal coronary vessels and also provides a rough index of the area "at risk" distal to a coronary stenosis.

Because of the prevalence of coronary artery disease and the more than 1 million diagnostic catheterizations performed each year in the United States, it is important to review the techniques of coronary angiography and the implications of the information found on coronary angiograms. This chapter reviews previously reported data, stressing aspects of clinical performance and interpretation of coronary angiograms that should be useful to the clinical cardiologist, to scientists working to improve the safety and validity of coronary angiography, and to clinicians interested in using angiographic information to define the prognostic significance of coronary artery stenoses and appropriate means of therapy. The references provided allow the interested reader to more fully explore selected areas.

HISTORIC EVENTS IN THE DEVELOPMENT OF CORONARY ANGIOGRAPHY

The history of coronary angiography began more than a century ago when catheters were placed into the arteries and veins of horses by Claude Bernard.[4] Subsequently, Chauveau and Marey were able to record pressures from such catheters.[4] Vascular catheterization in humans began in 1929 when Werner Forssman, a 25-year-old surgical resident, inserted a ureteral catheter into his left antecubital vein, advanced it to the right atrium, and climbed several flights of stairs to the radiology unit to document the intracardiac position of the catheter.[4] In 1937, Castellanos injected iodine into the antecubital vein to better define the anatomy of patients with congenital heart disease. In 1938, investigators placed catheters into the right atrium and injected contrast material.[5]

Although these reports served as the background for the development of coronary angiography, it was not until 1945 that Radner first saw human coronary arteries in vivo at the time of retrograde aortography (performed after direct needle puncture through the sternum into the aorta).[6] Similar observations were reported by Jönsson in 1948.[7] The development of angiography in general, and the pursuit of adequate coronary visualization in particular, was facilitated in 1952 when Seldinger reported his technique of obtaining vascular access.[8] In 1952, DiGuglielmo and Guttadauro published diagrams of the radiographic appearance of the coronary arteries based on thoracic aortograms. However, visualization was adequate in only 112 of 159 cases.[7] Attempts were subsequently made to increase opacification of the coronary arteries during thoracic aortography by balloon occlusion, as reported by Dotter in a dog model,[9] or by acetylcholine-induced circulatory arrest, as reported by Lehman.[7] Injections were also attempted in late systole or early diastole or with the Valsalva maneuver to decrease contrast dilution.[10] In 1960, Williams reported the injection of contrast material into the aortic root with a loop catheter containing side holes so that a larger volume of contrast agent was injected into the region of the coronary ostia.[11] He also suggested that carotid compression during injection of the contrast agent would slow the heart rate and decrease the cerebral flow of contrast material. In 27 of 32 males, the coronary arteries were seen with the use of the loop catheter and carotid compression.[11] Despite all of these advances, however, visualization of the coronary arteries was still inadequate in most cases.

In 1959, Sones reported a brachial approach in which better coronary opacification was produced by injection of 20 to 30 mL of contrast material directly into the coronary sinuses.[12] With this technique, coronary collaterals were seen angiographically for the first time. In April 1959, Sones began the era of selective coronary angiography with selective catheter entry of the right and left coronary arteries.[13] He entered both coronary arteries in 954 of 1020 cases, and entered at least one artery in every patient. Selective coronary injection decreased the interference arising from contrast medium in the aortic root, decreased the volume of contrast material needed for each injection, and made possible the use of additional projections to better define coronary anatomy. Ricketts and Abrams reported the use of selective catheterization from the femoral approach in 1962.[14] Judkins reported the use of preformed catheters from the femoral approach in 1967,[15] and Amplatz, in the same year, pioneered the use of selective catheters from the femoral approach with catheter tips designed to point perpendicular to the wall of the aorta and thus more easily enter the coronary ostia, which are funnel shaped and arise perpendicular to the sinuses.[16]

Coronary angiography has come a long way from the time when Werner Forssman showed that intravascular placement of catheters in humans was possible. Although many of these developmental techniques seem far-fetched, archaic, and dangerous today, they serve as the basis of our current techniques, and they still provide lessons concerning selective coronary angiography.

INDICATIONS

The primary purpose of coronary angiography is to delineate the presence or absence of significant narrowings of the coronary arteries. This information is then used to define patient prognosis and determine appropriate therapy. Although complications occur during coronary angiography, the risk of the procedure may be small compared with the risk of undertaking therapy with incomplete or inaccurate diagnostic information.

In the past, angiography was performed only in patients with symptoms significant enough to warrant surgical therapy. Improved angiographic techniques, advances in cardiac surgery, and new methods of therapy (particularly catheter-based interventional techniques, including balloon angioplasty, stenting, laser angioplasty, atherectomy, transluminal extraction techniques, and intracoronary ultrasound ablation) have expanded the list of indications for cardiac catheterization. Although general guidelines concerning patients in whom coronary angiography should be considered can be presented, it is impossible to provide absolute indications or contraindications, because the appropriateness of coronary angiography depends not only on the patient's cardiac status but also on his or her age (in particular, the physiologic age), overall health, occupation, and desired level of activity. Factors such as the availability of experienced angiographers, the physician's philosophy concerning appropriate therapy for coronary disease, and local results from interventional techniques and surgery also play a role. Although coronary angiography requires specialized technical skills for safe and adequate studies to be performed, it is essential that angiographers retain the clinical acumen necessary to individualize the use of angiography in each patient in whom it is considered.

An excellent review of the indications for coronary angiography was presented by Ross and colleagues for the American College of Cardiology/American Heart Association Task Force on Assessment of Diagnostic and Therapeutic Cardiovascular Procedures (ACC/AHA Task Force).[17] The following description of indications for coronary angiography has been compiled from proposals by several authors.[17–23]

History of Angina

ANGINA UNRESPONSIVE TO MEDICAL MANAGEMENT. The presence of angina that is unresponsive to medical management (or in a patient who is unable to tolerate accepted medical therapy) is perhaps the most uniformly agreed on indication for coronary angiography, as long as the patient is otherwise healthy enough to potentially undergo anatomical correction by coronary artery bypass grafting, angioplasty, or other catheter-based interventional techniques.

UNSTABLE ANGINA. The term unstable angina refers to anginal chest pain that is new in onset, is crescendo in character (i.e., increasing in frequency or duration or occurring with lesser degrees of exertion), or occurs at rest.

STABLE ANGINA WITH "HIGH-RISK" NONINVASIVE TESTS. If noninvasive tests indicate the probability of high-risk coronary artery disease, coronary angiography may be indicated in the patient with stable angina. High-risk treadmill results include those that are positive at a heart rate of less than 120 or a work load of less than 6.5 METS, those with greater than 2.0 mm or greater than 6 minutes of ST depression, and those with electrocardiographic changes in multiple leads or a decrease in blood pressure with exercise. A thallium scan with multiple areas of abnormal thallium uptake or an exercise decrease in ejection fraction of greater than 10 percent on radionuclide ventriculography are also considered indicative of high risk. Although it has been reported that the development of a wall motion abnormality on a stress echocardiogram at a heart rate of less than 125 beats per minute suggests the likelihood of multivessel coronary artery disease,[24] the prognostic significance of a positive stress echocardiogram at a low heart rate has not been strictly defined.

ANGINA AFTER MYOCARDIAL INFARCTION

RECURRENT ANGINA AFTER BYPASS SURGERY OR ANGIOPLASTY. The evaluation of recurrent angina after coronary artery bypass surgery or angioplasty, particularly if it is not readily responsive to medical management, should include coronary angiography.

ANGINA AND PLANNED MAJOR VASCULAR SURGERY

History of Myocardial Infarction

During evolving myocardial infarction, coronary angiography is considered if it can be performed within 6 hours in patients who are potential candidates for primary angioplasty. Coronary angiography is considered later in the course if thrombolytics have been given and the patient is being considered for angioplasty or coronary artery bypass graft surgery. Patients with completed myocardial infarction are considered for coronary angiography in the following circumstances.

RECURRENT ANGINA AFTER MYOCARDIAL INFARCTION. Coronary angiography is indicated, particularly if the angina occurs close to the time of the infarction.

NON–Q WAVE MYOCARDIAL INFARCTION

MYOCARDIAL INFARCTION AT A "YOUNG" AGE

SEVERE HEART FAILURE AFTER MYOCARDIAL INFARCTION THAT MAY BE DUE TO INFARCT COMPLICATIONS. Coronary angiography is indicated if heart failure has resulted from infarct complications (mitral regurgitation, ventricular septal defect, or ventricular aneurysm).

LEFT VENTRICULAR EJECTION FRACTION OF LESS THAN 45 PERCENT

INDICATION OF HIGH RISK ON NONINVASIVE STUDIES

RECURRENT VENTRICULAR TACHYCARDIA OR VENTRICULAR FIBRILLATION

Suspected Coronary Artery Disease in Asymptomatic Patients

A high degree of suspicion of significant coronary artery disease in an asymptomatic patient may be an indication for coronary angiography. The following conditions may contribute to the decision for coronary angiography in such a patient.

ABNORMAL ELECTROCARDIOGRAPHIC OR POSITIVE TREADMILL TEST RESULTS. Abnormal results on these tests indicate a need for coronary angiography, particularly if the patient's occupation affects the public safety (e.g., airline pilot, bus driver, truck driver, firefighter, air traffic controller).

NUMEROUS CORONARY RISK FACTORS

HISTORY OF MYOCARDIAL INFARCTION. A history of a myocardial infarction is an indication for coronary angiography, particularly if the patient is young.

SUSPECTED SILENT ISCHEMIA. Coronary angiography is indicated if a high likelihood of significant silent ischemia is suggested by results of noninvasive tests.

HISTORY OF CARDIAC ARREST. Coronary angiography is indicated if the patient has a history of a cardiac arrest, particularly if the cardiac arrest is thought to have resulted from ischemia.

Chest Pain of Uncertain Origin

This indication is one of the more controversial. However, in patients with atypical chest pain, subsequent therapy may be significantly aided if the coronary arteries are found to be normal. In patients in whom the coronary arteries are normal and the suspicion of a cardiac origin for chest pain remains high, ergonovine testing to diagnose coronary artery spasm[25] or testing to evaluate for "microvascular angina"[26] should be considered.

Planned Surgery for Valvular Heart Disease

If a patient undergoing surgery for valvular heart disease has significant coronary disease, the long-term prognosis may be better if coronary lesions are bypassed.[27] Preoperative coronary angiography is therefore indicated in a patient in whom valvular surgery is planned if the patient's age or risk factor profile suggests a significant likelihood of coronary disease. Noninvasive tests may be used to define those patients at the highest risk of having associated coronary disease; however, in many of these patients, left ventricular hypertrophy is present, making an exercise test difficult to interpret. It has been said that if patients with isolated aortic stenosis do not have angina, coronary angiography is not necessary; however, in a study of 103 patients with isolated aortic stenosis, Green and colleagues found that 25 percent of patients with no history of angina had significant coronary disease that would have been missed had coronary angiograms not been performed.[28]

Left Ventricular Dysfunction of Uncertain Origin

Coronary angiography in this setting determines whether ischemia is the cause of left ventricular dysfunction. This indication for coronary angiography has become more important as improved surgical techniques have allowed coronary bypass grafting to be performed more safely in patients with ventricular dysfunction, and in face of data from the Coronary Artery Surgery Study (CASS) revealing prolongation of life in patients with three-vessel coronary disease and left ventricular dysfunction who are treated surgically.[29]

Possible Coronary Anomaly

Coronary angiography may be performed to identify coronary anomalies. Coronary anomalies can be of functional significance, and they can complicate surgical repair in patients with congenital heart disease.

Intractable Ventricular Arrhythmias

Intractable ventricular arrhythmias provide another indication for coronary angiography, particularly if they occur after cardiac arrest.

Planned Interventional Therapy

If interventional therapy is being considered, such as angioplasty or other catheter-based interventional techniques, preprocedure coronary angiography is indicated.

Thrombolytic Therapy

Coronary angiography may be indicated after intravenous thrombolytic therapy, particularly if the results of noninvasive tests suggest the presence of high-risk coronary artery disease (as described in the section on stable high-risk angina with "high-risk" noninvasive tests).

Evaluation of a Potential Donor for Cardiac Transplantation

Coronary angiography may be used to evaluate a potential heart donor if donor age or history suggests a possibility of coronary disease. This indication will probably become more common with continued attempts to expand the cardiac donor pool.

Evaluation of Cardiac Transplant Recipients

Yearly surveillance catheterizations may also be required to evaluate the heart transplant recipient for graft atherosclerosis, which frequently does not result in angina because the heart is denervated.[30] This disease tends to be diffuse and is thought to be caused, at least in part, by an immune mechanism (Fig. 23–1).

Lack of Noninvasive Test Results

If conventional noninvasive tests cannot be performed (i.e., in amputees or patients with peripheral vascular disease) and coronary risk needs to be defined. This indication probably has become less common with the development of pharmacologic stress thallium[31] and echocardiographic[32] techniques.

A somewhat controversial study involving 168 medically stable patients referred by their physicians or insurance carriers (24 percent) or self-referred (76 percent) for a second opinion as to the need for coronary angiography was reported by Graboys and associates in 1992.[33] By the application of strict indications, only 4 percent of the patients were deemed to require angiography and 80 percent were not; in 16 percent, the decision was deferred pending further studies. During a follow-up period of almost 4 years, only 7 cardiac deaths (1.1 percent per year) and 19 new myocardial infarctions (2.7 percent per year) occurred. Unstable angina developed in 27 patients (4.3 percent), and 26 patients

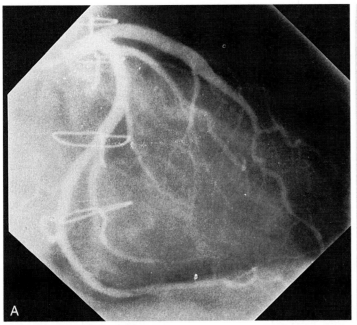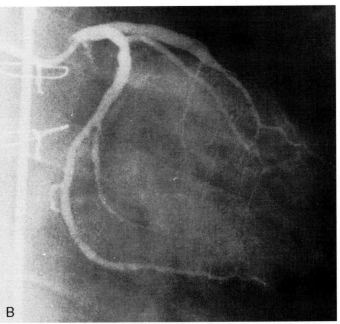

FIGURE 23-1. Serial coronary angiograms of a patient after cardiac transplantation, demonstrating the diffuse coronary disease that can develop in the transplanted coronary arteries. A, Left coronary angiogram (right anterior oblique projection) taken 2 years after transplantation. Only minimal irregularities are noted. B, The same vessel 3 years after transplantation reveals severe diffuse disease with pruning of the distal vessels. The patient was asymptomatic at the time the second angiogram was taken but died suddenly 2 months later, before a suitable donor heart for retransplantation was obtained.

(15.4 percent) ultimately underwent coronary angioplasty or bypass surgery. The authors concluded that up to 50 percent of coronary angiograms being done in the United States were unnecessary, and stated that because angiography did not alter medical management it should be performed only in patients being considered for angioplasty or bypass surgery. Controversy arose concerning these claims because of the small percentage of patients in the study with New York Heart Association functional class III or class IV angina (12 percent), because patients in whom a second opinion is sought are those in whom the need for angiography is already in doubt, because clinical events did occur in patients who did not undergo angiography, and because it was uncertain whether coronary artery disease even existed in the many patients who did not undergo angiography.

CONTRAINDICATIONS

Just as the indications for coronary angiography must be individualized, most of the contraindications are also relative, and the risks and benefits of proceeding to coronary angiography in a specific patient must be considered carefully. There are situations in which angiography is of enough clinical benefit to override the presence of factors that in general would be strong contraindications. Perhaps the only absolute contraindication to coronary angiography is the lack of an experienced angiographer and suitable laboratory facilities. However, in patients with any of the following conditions, the risk-benefit ratio of proceeding to coronary angiography, particularly before stabilization of the clinical condition, should be evaluated thoroughly.[17, 19, 20, 23]

1. Bleeding diatheses, whether caused by underlying illness or anticoagulation therapy
2. Advanced physiologic age
3. Uncontrolled hypertension
4. Significant electrolyte abnormalities or digitalis toxicity
5. Fever, particularly with documented infection
6. Decompensated congestive heart failure (which may prevent

the patient from assuming a posture that is supine enough to allow a complete study)
7. Uncontrolled ventricular irritability
8. Severe anemia
9. Active gastrointestinal bleeding
10. A mental or physical condition that precludes patient cooperation
11. A significant cerebrovascular accident within the previous few months
12. The presence of noncardiac disease that precludes long-term survival
13. Previous history of a reaction to contrast medium (although pretreatment may decrease the incidence of recurrence)
14. Significant renal insufficiency or anuria
15. Patient refusal to undergo any interventional therapy regardless of the outcome of the coronary angiogram

COMPLICATIONS

In evaluating the risk-benefit ratio of coronary angiography, the physician must be aware of the risk of complications from the procedure. Because coronary angiography is invasive and is usually performed in patients with cardiovascular disease, it is associated with complications. These complications may be cardiovascular in origin (e.g., myocardial infarction, cerebrovascular accident, arrhythmia, death), or they may be related to the vascular access site (e.g., local arterial damage, clot formation, embolism, infection). Although the early angiographers each reported complication rates, Adams and colleagues reported the first large series in which complications occurring during or within 24 hours after cardiac catheterization and coronary angiography were tabulated.[34] His survey concerned 46,904 patients studied in 173 centers during 1970 and 1971. The mortality rate was 0.45 percent. Cardiovascular complications were significantly higher for studies performed from the femoral than from the brachial approach, with death rates of 0.78 percent and 0.13 percent, respectively. The overall cardiovascular complication rate (including death, myocardial infarction, and cerebrovascular accident) was 2.22 percent for the femoral approach and 0.38 percent for the brachial approach. However, arterial clot formation was higher with the brachial approach (1.67 percent) than with the femoral approach (1.19 percent). A significant contributor to the cardiovascular complication rate for angiograms from the femoral approach was the high rate of cardiovascular complications for femoral cases in laboratories performing fewer than 100 cardiac catheterizations per year. The complication rate was higher in these laboratories than in laboratories performing more than 400 angiograms per year. The risk of complications also increased with longer procedures and with sicker patients.

In 1976, Bourassa and Noble reported complication rates in 5250 patients studied by the femoral approach (without heparin) between 1970 and 1974.[35] In patients with normal coronary arteries, no serious complications resulted. The mortality rate was 0.23 percent, and all 12 patients who died had left main coronary artery disease. The five patients who experienced myocardial infarction (0.09 percent) also had severe coronary artery disease. There was a 0.80 percent incidence of significant arrhythmias (i.e., ventricular fibrillation, ventricular tachycardia, or transient asystole). Cerebral ischemia occurred in 0.13 percent, femoral site complications in 0.85 percent (with a higher incidence in females), and impending pulmonary edema in 0.1 percent. The study concluded that complications were related mainly to disease severity.

In 1979, Davis and colleagues presented the complications of coronary angiography that occurred in the CASS.[36] In this study, 7553 patients were prospectively evaluated at 13 centers during 1975 and 1976. Eighty-four percent of the studies were performed by the femoral approach. The death rate was 0.20 percent, and the myocardial infarction rate was 0.25 percent. As with the results of Bourassa and Noble, the complications all occurred in patients with left main coronary artery disease or three-vessel disease. In 657 patients with significant left main coronary artery disease, there were 5 deaths and 3 myocardial infarctions, a complication rate 6.8 times that of the remainder of the group. In contrast with the earlier study of Adams and co-workers,[34] cardiovascular complications were increased in patients undergoing the procedure from the brachial approach. However, this was not true in centers that performed more than 80 percent of procedures by the brachial route. Therefore, complications appeared to be related to the familiarity of the operators with the technique used. In the CASS survey, there was an increased mortality rate in patients with congestive heart failure, hypertension, significant premature ventricular contractions, greater than 50 percent left main coronary artery disease, three-vessel disease, or a left ventricular ejection fraction of less than 30 percent. There was also an increased risk of myocardial infarction in patients with unstable angina. There were 48 episodes of ventricular fibrillation without myocardial infarction (0.63 percent), 2 cerebrovascular accidents (0.03 percent), 7 arterial emboli, and 56 vascular injuries. The authors found that heparin did not significantly alter any of the risks. As in the study of Adams and co-workers,[34] local complications were higher in patients catheterized by the brachial approach.

Kennedy reported complications compiled in the Registry of the Society for Cardiac Angiography.[37] In this report, data were included in 53,581 patients from 66 laboratories over a 14-month period in 1979 and 1980. Forty-three percent of procedures were brachial and 54 percent femoral, with the arterial access site not reported in 3 percent. Heparin was used in 71 percent of patients. The overall complication rate was 1.82 percent, and the mortality rate was 0.14 percent. The mortality rate was equal for males and females and for patients catheterized from the brachial or the femoral approach. However, it was increased for patients who were younger than 1 year of age or older than 60 years of age, for patients who were functional class IV versus those who were functional class I and II, for patients with left ventricular dysfunction, and for patients with left main coronary artery disease. Nonfatal myocardial infarctions occurred in 0.07 percent and significant arrhythmias in 0.56 percent (including ventricular fibrillation, ventricular tachycardia, and bradycardias). Vascular complications occurred in 0.57 percent, with local complications significantly higher for procedures performed by the brachial approach.

More recent data from the Registry of the Society for Cardiac Angiography, including 222,553 diagnostic procedures (68 percent femoral, 31 percent brachial, fewer than 1 percent both) performed between July 1984 and December 1987, reveal a mortality rate of 0.10 percent, with myocardial infarctions in 0.06 percent, arrhythmias in 0.47 percent, cerebrovascular accidents in 0.07 percent, vascular complications in 0.46 percent, hemorrhage in 0.07 percent, and an overall complication rate of 1.74 percent.[38] Total complications were similar for brachial and femoral approaches, although vascular complications occurred more frequently in brachial and hemorrhage more frequently in femoral cases. Significant cardiovascular complications were increased in patients who were older than 60 years of age, who had left main coronary artery disease, who had a decreased left ventricular ejection fraction, or who were functional class IV; however, there was a 1.5 percent incidence of complications (mainly arrhythmias and vascular complications) in patients with normal coronary arteries.

Wyman and colleagues reported complication data for 1609 diagnostic cardiac catheterizations performed between July 1986 and December 1987 at Beth Israel Hospital.[39] In these diagnostic studies (performed primarily by the femoral approach), the rates for mortality (0.12 percent), myocardial infarction (0 percent), and significant arrhythmias (0.31 percent) were the same as or decreased from those of previous studies, despite the fact that the patients included in this study were older and had more severe coronary disease. The incidence of cerebrovascular events was 0.25 percent. Vascular complications occurred in 1.62 percent of the procedures, but approximately one third of the vascular problems arose in patients who required intra-aortic balloon counterpulsation.

A more recent report from the Registry of the Society for Cardiac Angiography was published in 1991.[40] Among 59,792 patients undergoing diagnostic catheterization in 63 laboratories during 1990, 15 percent of the catheterizations were brachial and 83 percent were femoral; 19 percent of the catheterizations were performed on outpatients. Major complications occurred in 1.71 percent of cases, including death in 0.11 percent, myocardial infarction in 0.05 percent, arrhythmias in 0.38 percent, cerebrovascular events in 0.07 percent, vascular injuries in 0.43 percent, contrast reactions in 0.37 percent, hemodynamic instability in 0.26 percent, perforation in 0.03 percent, and other complications in 0.28 percent. The complications were similar to those reported from this registry for patients catheterized in previous years.

Table 23-1 summarizes the complications of coronary angiography reported in the series described. Overall, there has been a gradually decreasing risk of complications since 1970, despite the fact that patients being catheterized today are generally older and frequently have more severe cardiac disease.

In 1984, Nishimura and colleagues reported the arrhythmic complications occurring in 7915 patients who underwent coronary angiography between 1978 and 1983.[41] Thirty-nine significant ventricular arrhythmias occurred (0.5 percent), with 12 patients developing ventricular tachycardia, 23 ventricular fibrillation, and 4 ventricular tachycardia that degenerated into ventricular fibrillation. All of the patients were successfully cardioverted. Sixty-seven percent of the arrhythmias occurred with injections to normal or minimally diseased coronary arteries. In these patients, the arrhythmias were usually preceded by bradycardia and widening of the QRS complex and QT interval. On the other hand, arrhythmias occurring with injection into diseased coronary arteries began with a premature ventricular contraction on the T wave. Twenty-four of the arrhythmias occurred with injection of the right coronary artery (RCA). Seven arrhythmias were preceded by ventricularization of the pressure wave form monitored at the tip of the coronary catheter. The authors concluded that ventricular arrhythmias could be decreased by allowing time between injections, because many of the arrhythmias occurred late in the study (77 percent occurred with the last or next to the last coronary injection). They also emphasized paying

TABLE 23–1. COMPLICATIONS OF CORONARY ANGIOGRAPHY

	Adams et al.[34]	Bourassa et al.[35]	Davis et al.[36]	Kennedy et al.[37]	Johnson et al.[38]	Wyman et al.[39]	Noto et al.[40]
Number of angiograms	46,904	5250	7553	53,581	222,553	1609	59,792
Years of study	1970–1971	1970–1974	1975–1976	1979–1980	1984–1987	1986–1987	1990
Vascular approach (% femoral/% brachial)	49/51	100/0	84/16	54/43†	68/31‡	95/5	83/15
Deaths (%)	0.45	0.23	0.20	0.14	0.10	0.12	0.11
Myocardial infarctions (%)	0.61	0.09	0.25	0.07	0.06	0.00	0.05
Arrhythmias (%)°	1.28	0.80	0.63	0.56	0.47	0.31	0.38
Cerebrovascular events (%)	0.23	0.13	0.03	0.07	0.07	0.25	0.07
Vascular complications (%)	1.62	0.85	0.74	0.57	0.46	1.62	0.43

°Generally includes ventricular fibrillation or prolonged ventricular tachycardia requiring countershock or bradyarrhythmias significant enough to require medical or pacemaker therapy; the Davis series reported only ventricular fibrillation data.

†Site of vascular access was not reported in 3%

‡Both techniques were used in fewer than 1%.

close attention to the arterial pressure wave form. They hypothesized that atropine may prevent some arrhythmias, particularly those that occur after bradycardia.

In 1987, Gordon and associates reported on angiographic complications in 107 patients with left main coronary artery disease.[42] There were 3 deaths, 3 myocardial infarctions, 3 patients with angina requiring intra-aortic balloon pumping or coronary artery bypass grafting, 2 episodes of ventricular fibrillation, and 1 episode of hypotension requiring intra-aortic balloon pump support. The risk of complications was increased if angina occurred within the 24 hours before catheterization and if there was a short distance from the catheter tip to the left main coronary artery lesion. No significant differences in complication rates occurred related to functional class, femoral versus brachial artery approach, the number of coronary injections, the amount of contrast material used, the severity of left main coronary artery disease, the number of diseased vessels, or the patient's blood pressure, left ventricular end-diastolic pressure, or ejection fraction.

Recent reports have suggested that one of the local vascular complications that occurs with cardiac catheterization, the development of a pseudoaneurysm, may be treatable by ultrasound-guided compression rather than surgery.[43, 44] Success rates of 79 to 94 percent have been reported; however, the success rate is lower and the risk of recurrence higher in patients on chronic anticoagulation. It makes intuitive sense, and has been reported in at least one series,[45] that local vascular complications are increased in obese patients. Cohen and associates reported that 22 out of 7796 catheterization patients required surgical intervention for local vascular complications, and 18 of these 22 (82 percent) were 20 percent or more above their ideal body weight. Complication rates for outpatient catheterization have also been reported (see section on outpatient coronary angiography).

The question may arise as to whether complications related to catheterization result from the procedure itself or from the underlying coronary disease. In 1973, Hildner and colleagues reported on "pseudocomplications" occurring within the 48 hours before or longer than 24 hours after scheduled but unperformed catheterizations.[46] The pseudocomplication rate was 2.3 percent, with a 1.2 percent mortality rate during this time period. In the 24 hours immediately after catheterization, there was a 2.6 percent complication rate and a 0.56 percent mortality rate. Therefore, many complications probably resulted from the coronary disease itself rather than the catheterization. Hildner and colleagues followed up on this data in 1982 and reported a 0.81 percent incidence of complications with no catheterization-related deaths, compared with a 0.81 percent incidence of pseudocomplications including 4 deaths (0.24 percent).[47] Seven of the 13 pseudocomplications occurred within 2 hours before the scheduled procedure, suggesting that patient anxiety may have contributed to their occurrence.

Vagal responses, characterized by nausea, hypotension, and bradycardia also occur during and after angiography. Particularly in elderly patients, a vasodepressor response can occur without

bradycardia; it usually responds to discontinuation of catheter maneuvers, intravenous atropine, elevation of the legs, intravenous fluids, or combinations of these treatments. Pyrogenic reactions can also occur as a result of catheter contamination by foreign proteins; these problems usually respond to administration of morphine sulphate, antihistamines, or antipyretics. The radiation exposure occurring during coronary angiography varies from 0.2 to 0.45 Gy and presents little risk to the patient unless multiple procedures are performed.[48]

In summary, complications can and do occur during and after coronary angiography. The incidence is related to the patient's disease and to the experience of the angiographer and the laboratory. Therefore, Judkins has suggested that each angiographer select a particular approach (brachial or femoral) and become proficient at it.[49] It has been suggested that if a laboratory has a mortality rate of greater than 0.1 percent, patient selection and the skills of the angiographers should be re-evaluated; if the mortality rate is greater than 0.3 percent, procedures should be terminated.[50]

Although randomized studies have not defined specific means of decreasing angiographic complications, several precautions can be taken to minimize complication rates. The angiographer must carefully examine and evaluate each patient before the angiographic study. Any electrolyte or hemodynamic instability should be corrected, unless the catheterization is required on an emergency basis without further stabilization of the patient. Dehydration should be avoided, and premedication should be used to decrease patient anxiety. A temporary pacemaker should be available, and in some cases it should be inserted before the procedure begins.

Because use of more than 3 mL/kg of contrast medium has been said to increase complication rates, the amount used should be minimized; in high-risk patients, the use of low-osmolar or nonionic contrast agents should be considered. If patients are unstable, filling pressures should be monitored with a Swan-Ganz catheter, and if abnormalities are found they should be treated before coronary angiography is undertaken. If the patient is extremely unstable, an intra-aortic balloon pump can be used to stabilize the patient during catheterization.[51, 52] In techniques that use exchange wires, anticoagulation may be of benefit, but of even more importance is careful aspiration and flushing of the catheters, wiping of the wires, and restriction of the time that the wire remains in the vascular system to 3 minutes. During the procedure, the electrocardiogram (ECG) should be constantly monitored and careful attention should be paid to the catheter tip pressure. Minimal time should be spent in the coronary arteries (no longer than 2.5 to 4 minutes), and contrast material should not be injected during episodes of electrocardiographic changes or significant chest pain until therapy has been given. For patients with small or diseased arteries, the use of 5- to 7-Fr. rather than 8-Fr. catheters may decrease local complications (see discussion of small-diameter catheters). However, the most important factors in reducing complication rates are the skill of the operator (particularly for the technique chosen), meticulous attention to details, and expediency in obtaining the necessary information in the least possible amount of time.

PATIENT PREPARATION AND MANAGEMENT

Although each laboratory develops its own protocols for precatheterization management, use of medications during catheterization, and postcatheterization care, several guidelines have been proposed.[19, 20, 22, 23, 48, 50, 53] Some recommendations are summarized here.

One of the most important factors in determining the safety and usefulness of coronary angiography is the precatheterization evaluation of the patient by the angiographer. Complete review of the patient's history and physical examination, laboratory data, chest radiograph, ECG, past angiograms, and operative reports of any previous cardiac operations is essential for defining the questions that need to be answered during the procedure and for evaluating the risk of the procedure to the patient. A baseline ECG taken within 24 hours before catheterization is essential. After careful evaluation of the patient, the angiographer should define the catheterization protocol for the patient, including access site, sequence of studies, and contrast medium to be used. Contrast medium affects hemodynamic measurements and can depress left ventricular function; however, rather than always performing left ventricular angiography before coronary angiography, a better guideline is to obtain the most critical pieces of information first. For example, if it has been decided on the basis of noninvasive testing that the patient's left ventricular function is adequate to undergo coronary bypass surgery, perhaps the coronary angiogram should be performed before the left ventricular angiogram, because if any untoward events should occur that require emergency surgical intervention, the essential pieces of information would more likely have already been obtained. On the other hand, if there is a question as to the patient's ventricular function, performing the left ventricular angiogram first is prudent because this sequence allows the most accurate assessment of left ventricular function. In cases in which hemodynamic measurements are important (e.g., valvular heart disease), measurement of intracardiac pressures and cardiac output should usually be completed before any injection of contrast medium. A potential exception would be in cases of aortic stenosis in which the critical nature of the stenosis has been defined by noninvasive testing (e.g., Doppler echocardiography) and the most important information to be acquired is whether the patient has concomitant coronary artery disease. In this case, perhaps coronary angiography should be performed first, followed by hemodynamic measurements and the other required angiograms.

In addition to allowing for careful evaluation of the patient and planning of the catheterization protocol, the precatheterization meeting should also be the occasion of informing the patient about the procedure, the reasons for the procedure, the potential risks of the procedure, and the reasons why the risk-benefit ratio is in favor of proceeding. It is important that a family member also be present for this discussion. Educating the patient as to what to expect during the procedure and what will be expected of him or her afterward can decrease patient anxiety. The patient should be educated about the potential need to cough on request and to take deep breaths and hold them during coronary injections. It is particularly important that the patient not perform the Valsalva maneuver, because that maneuver elevates the diaphragm and makes coronary visualization more difficult.

After the precatheterization meeting, precatheterization orders should be written. In the past, there was concern about continuing antianginal drugs, particularly β-blockers, until the time of catheterization. However, experience has shown that all antianginal medications usually should be continued to prevent the development of increased angina caused by medication withdrawal. The patient should take nothing by mouth for 6 to 8 hours before the catheterization; however, if the study is to be performed in the afternoon, a light breakfast should be ordered. To prevent dehydration before the procedure, intravenous hydration should be considered during the time the patient is receiving nothing by mouth; this may decrease the incidence of vasovagal reactions and of renal insufficiency induced by the contrast agent. Antibiotics are not required. Prophylactic antiarrhythmic therapy, unless otherwise clinically indicated, is not necessary.

Premedication regimens vary, but a sedative is usually used to decrease patient anxiety. The sedative may be diazepam (5 to 10 mg by mouth or intravenously) or secobarbital (50 to 100 mg by mouth). An antihistamine is often included by mouth or intravenously, either diphenhydramine (25 to 50 mg) or promethazine (25 to 50 mg). The use of atropine is variable, but unless the patient is unstable, is tachycardiac, is to undergo an ergonovine study, or is in atrial fibrillation, atropine (0.4 to 0.6 mg subcutaneously) can decrease vasovagal reactions and the sinus bradycardia that follows injection of contrast agents. It has also been reported that atropine may reduce the frequency of ventricular arrhythmias during coronary angiography.[54] However, atropine can also increase the heart rate and thus myocardial oxygen consumption; the resultant increased coronary flow may decrease coronary opacification. Many physicians avoid intramuscular injections because they cause elevations of skeletal muscle creatine phosphokinase, which can complicate interpretation of creatine phosphokinase levels after catheterization. However, the group at Emory University reports using a premedication regimen of 6.25 mg of promethazine, 6.25 mg of chlorpromazine, and 25 mg of meperidine intramuscularly.[48] They use additional intravenous diazepam or midazolam as needed.

Medication protocols during angiography also vary. Many laboratories use intravenous heparin (2000 to 5000 U) at the beginning of the procedure, after the catheters have been inserted, in an attempt to decrease thromboembolic phenomena; this was not shown to be beneficial in data collected at 13 CASS clinics.[36] (If heparin is used and the catheterization is performed by the femoral approach, protamine is often given to reverse the anticoagulation at the end of the procedure.)

Nitroglycerin is commonly given (by either sublingual or intracoronary administration) to decrease coronary artery spasm, decrease coronary vascular tone, and allow better visualization of coronary lesions and collaterals. The author prefers to perform the first left coronary angiogram before giving nitroglycerin. In the absence of left main coronary artery disease or hemodynamic instability, the author routinely gives sublingual or intracoronary nitroglycerin after the first left coronary angiogram. If a significant left main coronary artery lesion is present or the patient is at all hemodynamically unstable, nitroglycerin should perhaps be withheld because it could result in hypotension and decreased coronary perfusion, which may lead to complications. In cases of left main coronary artery stenosis or hemodynamic instability in which nitroglycerin is thought to be essential to better visualize distal coronary vessels, a Swan-Ganz catheter should be placed before nitroglycerin therapy is instituted so that filling pressures can be monitored and treated appropriately.

Several additional medications should be available for emergency use. These include atropine, lidocaine, furosemide (or a similar diuretic), steroids, antihistamines, epinephrine, pressor agents (i.e., dopamine and norepinephrine), morphine, and nifedipine.

Angiographers also must be cognizant of the effects of intracoronary injection of contrast medium on the ECG and hemodynamics, adverse reactions that can occur, and the methods for prevention and treatment of such reactions. The potential benefits of using conventional versus nonionic or low-osmolar contrast agents must be evaluated in each patient, particularly in light of the fact that nonionic and low-osmolar agents are significantly more costly than conventional contrast agents. A knowledge of contrast agents and their effects is important to the angiographer for defining the risk-benefit ratio of coronary angiography in each patient and planning the study protocol to minimize the potential adverse effects. Chapter 18 contains a more complete discussion of contrast agents.

During catheterization, the ECG and arterial pressure should be continuously monitored. Time should be allowed for the ECG and arterial pressure to return to the baseline state before the next injection of contrast material. In cases of prolonged bradycardia or asystole with hypotension, having the patient cough can speed resolution of the hemodynamic and electrocardiographic changes by clearing contrast from the coronary vessels and by providing a mechanical stimulus to the heart. It also may be helpful to remove the catheter from the coronary ostium to allow more rapid return of blood to the coronary circulation. The ability to place a temporary transvenous pacemaker or an intra-aortic balloon pump, if indicated, is also important.[51, 52] Multiple projections of each coronary artery should be imaged with a 6 inch or higher magnification image intensifier. The angiographic study should be recorded on videotape or digitally for immediate review.

Patient care after cardiac catheterization depends on the approach used. If the brachial approach is used, the patient can sit up and, if stable, be out of bed almost immediately. If the procedure is performed by the femoral route, at least 4 to 8 hours of bedrest is required to achieve adequate hemostasis. The patient should have vital signs monitored frequently (for example, every 15 minutes for the first hour, every 30 minutes for the next 2 hours, every hour for the next 4 hours, and then every 4 hours until the following day). The arterial entry site and pulses distal to the site should be examined with each check of vital signs. Unless the patient has had nausea and vomiting with the procedure, resumption of fluid intake and gradual resumption of full diet can occur very soon after catheterization. It is essential that the patient remain well hydrated, so if the patient is not taking sufficient oral fluids (1 to 2 L within 8 hours after catheterization), intravenous hydration should be continued. Maintenance of good hydration appears to decrease the incidence of vasovagal episodes after catheterization. If such episodes still occur, they can be treated with atropine (1 to 3 mg intravenously) and additional intravenous fluids. Because patients may be uncomfortable after the procedure, particularly with the femoral approach, sedatives and analgesics should be given as needed. Postcatheterization care should also include palpation of the vascular site for an aneurysm and listening for a bruit, which could indicate the presence of an arteriovenous fistula. Previously ordered medications should be resumed as soon as possible.

If complications occur in the angiography laboratory, there are established techniques that can be used to stabilize the patient. If congestive heart failure is aggravated, it can be treated with intravenous nitroglycerin and diuretics and placement of a Swan-Ganz catheter for monitoring of right heart pressures if necessary. Angina can be treated with nitroglycerin (by sublingual, intravenous, or intracoronary administration) or with nifedipine. Elevation of left ventricular end-diastolic pressure frequently responds to administration of nitrates or oxygen. Hypertension and sinus tachycardia respond to intravenous β-blockers; hypertension can also be treated with nifedipine.

CORONARY ANGIOGRAPHIC TECHNIQUES

Before coronary angiography is performed, the arterial access site must be determined: brachial, femoral, or, less commonly, axillary,[55] translumbar,[56–58] transradial,[59, 60] or transseptal.[61] The access technique (cutdown and arteriotomy, or the Seldinger technique using either wire exchanges or a vascular sheath) and the specific catheters to be used must also be determined.

Brachial access may be advantageous in patients with peripheral vascular disease, abdominal aortic aneurysms, or ileofemoral clots. It may also be advantageous in patients with coarctation of the aorta and in obese patients, in whom hemostasis after femoral puncture may be difficult. The major disadvantages of the brachial approach are an increased incidence of local arterial complications and the fact that tortuous subclavian vessels may make coronary catheterization difficult.

The femoral technique is advantageous in patients with subcla-

vian arterial disease. The preformed catheters available for use with the femoral approach also make direct catheter entry into the coronary artery easier. However, this facilitation may be a disadvantage if less skilled operators perform the procedure and subject the patients to higher complication rates. Disadvantages of the femoral approach are that access may be difficult in the presence of aortoiliac disease and that the use of multiple catheters may increase the embolic risk.

The transaxillary approach, as reported by Weidner and colleagues,[55] has been less commonly used than either the brachial or the femoral approach. Its advantage is that it allows vascular access closer to the coronary arteries and in an artery that is large enough to allow re-examination by means of the same artery. A cutdown procedure on the brachial artery may be the least risky approach in patients who are anticoagulated, who have defective hemostasis, who are hypertensive, or who have significant aortic regurgitation (in whom bleeding complications after percutaneous access, particularly from the femoral approach, may be increased).

Thorough reviews of the techniques of arterial entry and coronary angiography are provided elsewhere,[18, 20–23, 48, 62–67] and four of the most commonly used techniques are summarized in the following sections. Some general points deserve emphasis, however. First, if arterial spasm develops during cutdown or percutaneous entry of the brachial artery, it can be treated with morphine sulfate or decreased by use of a smaller catheter. If a clot produces loss of distal pulses in either the brachial or femoral approach, a Fogarty catheter can be used to remove the clot and restore distal perfusion. During brachial approaches, particularly cutdowns, injection of heparin both proximal and distal to the cutdown site is recommended. For femoral approaches, the use of heparin is more variable. If femoral access is used, the level of arterial puncture is important. To decrease bleeding complications, the arterial entry site must be below the inguinal ligament; however, if vascular access is attempted too far distally, the separation of the artery and vein may cause difficulty. Almost all techniques of coronary angiography involve the use of a coronary manifold, in which three different ports are used for contrast medium, waste, and monitoring of arterial pressure. Such a setup allows rapid return after contrast injection to monitoring of intracoronary pressure through the coronary catheter.

Sones Technique

The Sones technique of brachial artery cutdown and use of a single catheter (with an endhole and four side holes) for left coronary angiography, right coronary angiography, and left ventriculography has the advantage of requiring only a single catheter. However, because of the presence of side holes as well as an end hole, obstruction at the distal tip may not dampen catheter pressure. The Sones technique requires that the angiographer learn the catheter manipulations involved to engage the coronary arteries, but because the catheter tip is closer to the manipulating hand, the operator has a "better feel" for the catheter than in many of the femoral techniques. Selective coronary entry is performed in a left anterior oblique (LAO) projection. Although several maneuvers can be used to perform selective coronary cannulation with the Sones catheter (as described in detail elsewhere[22, 64]), the catheter tip is usually placed in the left coronary sinus and a shallow loop is formed. With gradual rotation and advancement of the catheter tip, the left coronary ostium is entered (Fig. 23–2). For RCA entry, a shallow loop toward the left coronary artery is rotated clockwise, with slight withdrawal, and the catheter is manipulated toward the right sinus of Valsalva until the coronary artery is engaged. If ostial engagement is difficult, having the patient take a deep breath may allow easier catheter entry into the coronary artery.[18, 20]

Judkins Technique

Judkins catheters are preformed catheters; they are available in different designs for the right and left coronary arteries and with a

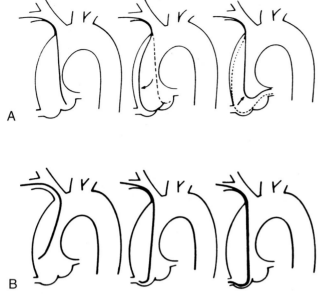

FIGURE 23–2. Illustration of the Sones technique for selective catheterization of the left (*A*) and right (*B*) coronary arteries. (From Conti, C.R.: Coronary arteriography. Circulation 55:228, 1977, with permission of the American Heart Association, Inc.)

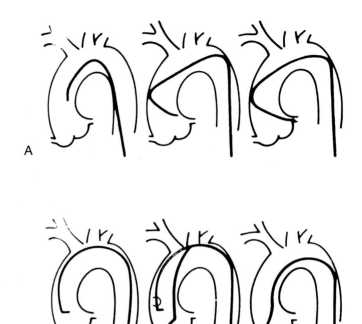

FIGURE 23–3. Selective catheterization of the left (*A*) and right (*B*) coronary arteries by the Judkins technique. (From Conti, C.R.: Coronary arteriography. Circulation 55:229, 1977, with permission of the American Heart Association, Inc.)

range of sizes appropriate for differently sized aortic arches. The key to the success of the Judkins technique is proper catheter selection. Judkins catheters come in sizes 3.5, 4, 5, and 6, with the size referring to the distance between the primary and secondary curvatures of the catheter. A size 4 catheter is for standard aortas; size 5 for older patients or those with unfolded aortas, hypertension, or medial disease; and size 6 for patients with aortic dilatation. If a Judkins left coronary catheter is too small, it will double back on itself as it reaches the coronary ostium; if it is too long, it will be positioned vertically and rest on the tip of the sinus rather than in the coronary ostium.[15]

The Judkins technique of selective coronary catheterization is illustrated in Figure 23–3. The left coronary artery is entered in a shallow LAO projection. In this orientation, the left coronary catheter is placed "en face" (i.e., in profile) and slowly advanced with continuous tip pressure monitoring. After the catheter has apparently entered the coronary ostium, contrast material is gently injected. If ventricularization or damping of the pressure occurs, the catheter is pulled back. If damping recurs after repositioning of the catheter in the artery, nonselective injections may be used to rule out ostial disease. For RCA entry, a shallow LAO projection is again used. The right coronary catheter is positioned between one half and one rib interspace cephalad to the aortic valve and rotated clockwise until the catheter enters the right coronary ostium. If damping occurs, it could imply stenosis, subselective entry into the conus branch, or spasm around the catheter (which is much more common in the RCA than in the left coronary artery). A question about whether spasm or a significant lesion exists can be resolved in many cases by repeating the angiograms after administration of nitroglycerin or by performing sinus injections of contrast material. The Judkins technique of coronary angiography has been reviewed in detail by Judkins and Judkins[65] and by Levin and Gardner.[67]

Amplatz Technique

Amplatz coronary catheters can also be used. These preformed catheters have the advantage that they can be used from either the brachial or the femoral approach. The disadvantage is that, from the femoral approach and on many occasions from the brachial approach, multiple catheter changes may be necessary, and if the angle of takeoff of the coronary artery from the aorta is unusual, selective coronary entry may be difficult.

To position the left Amplatz catheter in the left coronary ostium, the curve of the catheter is stabilized in the noncoronary cusp; to position the right Amplatz catheter, the curve of the catheter is placed in the left coronary cusp. The left catheter is advanced until its tip points upward and enters the coronary ostium; then, with gradual slight withdrawal, the catheter is locked in place (Fig. 23–4). Maneuvering of the right Amplatz catheter is similar to that previously described for the right Judkins catheter. If the catheters are too small, they may slip through the valve, recoil from the ostium with injection or valve motion, or be unable to reach the coronary ostium. Use of too large an Amplatz catheter may result in buckling of the catheter so that the tip does not ascend to the level of the ostium, or, alternatively, the tip may extend beyond the ostium itself.

Zir and colleagues reported on 500 catheterizations performed by the brachial approach using preformed catheters (Amplatz catheters modified for the brachial approach in that they had a smaller curve and less of a hook on the end).[68] In many cases, the RCA was difficult to cannulate because of its sharp angle of origin. The use of the preformed catheters rather than Sones catheters was thought to be advantageous, however, because it allowed easier

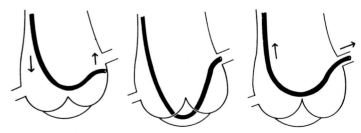

FIGURE 23–4. The technique of selective catheterization of the left coronary artery with an Amplatz catheter. (From Baim, D.S., and Grossman, W.: Coronary angiography. *In* Grossman, W., and Baim, D.S. [eds.]: Cardiac Catheterization, Angiography, and Intervention. 4th ed. Philadelphia, Lea & Febiger, 1991, p. 191, with permission.)

arterial entry, resulted in excellent opacification, allowed stable catheter position during contrast injection, and required minimal manipulation of the catheters.

Schoonmaker Technique

An additional catheter technique, reported by Schoonmaker in 1974, is illustrated in Figure 23–5. It uses a single catheter from the femoral approach.[69] This technique requires a bit more training than the use of preformed catheters from the femoral route, but, with experience, angiography can be performed in approximately 15 minutes by most operators. The catheter is an 8-Fr., 100-cm catheter with a 45-degree curve at its tip.

To position the Schoonmaker catheter in the left coronary artery, a 30-degree right anterior oblique (RAO) projection is used, and the catheter tip is placed in the noncoronary cusp. A loop of the tip of the catheter is then formed, and clockwise rotation results in the positioning of the tip at the mouth of the coronary orifice. To enter the RCA, a 45- to 60-degree LAO projection is used. The catheter body is placed in the left coronary cusp, and, with withdrawal and clockwise rotation, the tip of the catheter is rotated into the right coronary ostium. The maneuvers of these catheters are very much like those described by Sones for his brachial technique. Details of the technique of performing coronary angiography with the use of the Schoonmaker multipurpose technique are provided by King and Douglas[66] and by Schoonmaker and King.[69]

In 6800 procedures performed over a period of 7 years, only 10

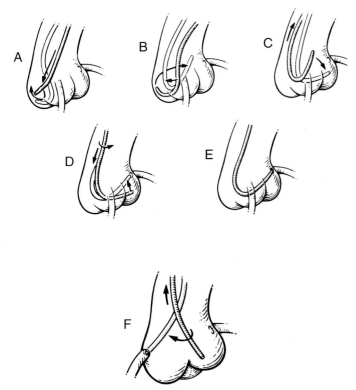

FIGURE 23–5. The Schoonmaker technique of selective catheterization of the left coronary artery in the right anterior oblique projection (*A through E*) and of the right coronary artery in the left anterior oblique projection (*F*). For entry into the left coronary artery, the catheter tip is positioned in the noncoronary cusp, and clockwise rotation and slight withdrawal followed by gradual catheter advancement result in selective entry into the artery. For selective catheterization of the right coronary artery, the catheter body is placed in the left coronary cusp. Withdrawal and clockwise rotation of the catheter are required to accomplish selective entry into the artery. (From King, S.B., III, and Douglas, J.S., Jr.: Coronary arteriography and left ventriculography: Multipurpose technique. *In* King, S.B., III, and Douglas, J.S., Jr. [eds.]: Coronary Arteriography and Angioplasty. New York, McGraw-Hill, 1985, pp. 252 & 256, with permission.)

percent of patients required use of a second catheter for selective coronary angiography. Because embolic complications occurred in this series only if catheter exchanges were necessary, proponents of this technique suggest that use of a single catheter decreases embolic complications.[69]

Alternative Arterial Access Techniques

Many authors have proposed changes in the methods used to obtain arterial access. In 1979, Barry and associates reported the use of a sheath with a side arm and a hemostasis valve.[70] The sheath made catheter changes easier and decreased patient discomfort during catheter changes. Side arm pressure could be monitored during coronary injection, and, because a wire was not essential for catheter insertion, catheters without an endhole could be placed. The investigators reported that if the arterial puncture did not occur at an angle of 45 degrees or less, the sheath would become kinked. Heparin was routinely used. Among 562 patients, 2 local complications required surgical repair, and 10 percent of patients required groin compression for longer than 10 minutes to achieve hemostasis. It was proposed that the sheath may decrease the occurrence of thromboemboli by decreasing the arterial trauma associated with catheter changes, by allowing aspiration and flushing between catheters, by reducing intravascular guidewire time, and by decreasing the length of the procedure.

In 1981, Fergusson and Kamada described percutaneous access through the brachial artery by use of a sheath without a hemostasis valve or side port.[71] In 1986, results of this technique with 1783 patients were reported.[72] Ninety-six percent of attempts were successful, with a 1.3 percent incidence of brachial occlusion, which in general was easily repaired. Three arteriovenous fistulas occurred. During catheter changes, a blood pressure cuff and not a hemostasis valve was used for hemostasis, because it was believed that the catheter was easier to maneuver without a hemostasis valve. In the 62 cases in which percutaneous brachial entry was unsuccessful, studies were completed with either brachial cutdown or the femoral technique. The authors recommended their technique for outpatient cardiac catheterization because of easier achievement of hemostasis.

In 1984, Pepine and colleagues reported a slightly different percutaneous brachial technique in which a 7-Fr. side arm sheath with a hemostasis valve was used.[73] One hundred patients underwent the procedure without failure or serious complications, including 12 patients who had had at least one previous brachial cutdown. There was one loss of a radial pulse, which was treated with cutdown and thrombectomy. The only other significant complications were 11 ecchymoses and 4 small hematomas. The authors suggested that the sheaths protected the artery from the trauma of catheter motion. Cohen and co-workers reported on a series of brachial catheterizations performed by two angiographers at Mount Sinai Hospital, New York, between 1982 and 1984.[74] Two hundred fifty-four brachial studies were done percutaneously and 184 by cutdown. The complication rates were 3.1 and 2.1 percent, respectively. In 4 patients in whom the percutaneous route failed, successful cutdown was performed. The average duration of the procedure was 39 ± 10 minutes for the percutaneous route and 44 ± 13 minutes for cutdown. Campeau reported on 400 consecutive patients in whom a percutaneous brachial approach was used.[75] In 3 percent, cannulation was not possible. The complication rate was low, with a 4 percent incidence of hematomas, 2 percent loss of radial pulse, and less than 1 percent late rebleeding (in a patient on Coumadin).

General Principles of Safe and Optimal Coronary Angiography

In addition to the specific observations made concerning each technique above, there are some pointers applicable to all techniques of coronary angiography. These are described as follows:

1. Damping or ventricularization of the pressure recorded at the catheter tip is indicative of restriction of inflow to the coronary artery. This can be caused by proximal stenosis, adverse catheter position, catheter-induced spasm, or subselective entry into a branch vessel. Although catheters with side holes near the tip have been developed to eliminate damping and still allow coronary blood flow and injection, they must be used cautiously because injection into a plaque may result in dissection.[76] It is also important to remember that, with the use of catheters with side holes, it is aortic and not coronary pressure that is being monitored.

2. A vessel needs to be imaged perpendicular to its course and in orthogonal views to allow adequate evaluation (see the later discussion concerning the importance of angulated views in coronary angiography).

3. If resistance is met or the catheter tip pressure damps, do not advance the catheter.

4. Do not wait for electrocardiographic changes to identify possible catheter obstruction of the coronary artery.

5. Perform cineangiography during deep inspiration to clear the liver from the field of view.

6. Inject contrast material in such a manner as to replace blood in the coronary artery for a period of 3 to 4 seconds (usually 3 to 9 mL in the left coronary artery and 2 to 4 mL in the RCA).

7. If contrast material does not clear after coronary injection, this may be an indication of catheter obstruction of the coronary ostium; the catheter should be withdrawn.

8. Tortuous peripheral and central arteries can interfere with torque control and may necessitate the use of coronary catheters requiring less manipulation.

9. Be cautious if the catheter tip does not rotate when the catheter is being rotated outside the body. Evaluate the entire course of the catheter by fluoroscopy to rule out "kink" formation in tortuous iliac or abdominal vessels.

10. If no lesions are seen on the angiograms and the patient's history strongly suggests coronary disease, take additional views to be certain no lesions have been missed.

11. When the angiographer lines up views for cineangiography, the left coronary artery should be positioned with the catheter tip near the top of the screen. The RCA should be positioned with the catheter tip in the upper quadrant and not at the top of the screen, because the conus and sinus node branches frequently course cephalad.

12. Allow hemodynamic and electrocardiographic changes to normalize before the next injection of contrast agent.

Although instability of the patient was formerly considered a contraindication to cardiac catheterization, the possibility of acute interventions for patients with unstable angina or acute myocardial infarction has resulted in clinical circumstances in which angiography is indicated despite patient instability. In addition to maximizing medical therapy in these patients to stabilize them as much as possible before catheterization, it has been suggested that an intra-aortic balloon pump can produce resolution of ischemia and stabilization of the patient.[51, 52] In the study by Gold and colleagues,[51] all 11 patients with rest angina had significant angina relief after intra-aortic balloon pumping, with angina recurring in 5 patients when balloon pumping was interrupted. Weintraub and co-workers studied 16 similar patients and found that balloon counterpulsation produced significant resolution of chest pain and electrocardiographic changes in 15.[52] The mechanism of stabilization with balloon pumping is unclear, although theories include decreased oxygen demand because of decreased afterload, increased coronary perfusion pressure and thus increased coronary blood flow, augmentation of collateral blood flow, and redistribution of coronary blood flow.

Bypass Graft and Internal Mammary Artery Angiography

The location of coronary artery bypass grafts is less predictable than that of native coronary arteries. In general, right coronary grafts are placed on the right anterolateral aorta and left anterior descending (LAD) and circumflex artery grafts are placed anteriorly. If the bypass graft itself or the stump of a graft is not defined by use of selective bypass graft catheters or right coronary catheters, an aortogram may define a graft stump or a patent graft that was unable to be selectively cannulated.

Internal mammary arteries are frequently studied in patients with previous vein bypass graft surgery (to confirm the integrity of these arteries should subsequent surgery be indicated) and in patients with recurrent angina after internal mammary artery grafting. One study suggests that internal mammary artery angiography should routinely be performed whenever internal mammary grafting is being considered because, in 15 percent of patients who had not undergone previous bypass surgery, significant findings were present that would alter the operative approach.[77]

For internal mammary artery angiography, an internal mammary artery catheter is guided into the subclavian artery over a wire and the catheter is then gradually withdrawn, with rotation anteriorly, until the internal mammary artery is selectively entered (Fig. 23–6). Because conventional high-osmolar contrast agents produce significant chest pain if they are injected undiluted into the internal mammary arteries, low-osmolar contrast agents or dilution with sterile saline should be used. Evaluation of bypass graft or internal mammary artery graft angiograms should include analysis not only of graft patency but also of the anastomosis to the native vessel and of the native vessel beyond the site of anastomosis.[67]

The right gastroepiploic artery has also been used as a coronary bypass conduit. To visualize this artery, a catheter is positioned in the celiac axis and advanced into the hepatic artery and then subselectively into the gastroduodenal branch.[67] Until cardiac angiographers gain additional experience in angiography of the gastroepiploic artery, collaboration with peripheral angiographers experienced in this technique is recommended.

OUTPATIENT CORONARY ANGIOGRAPHY

Although outpatient cardiac catheterization is considered relatively new, Fierens reported that 12,719 outpatient angiograms were performed between 1968 and 1982 at Butterworth Hospital in Detroit by use of the Sones technique.[78] Fierens reviewed the most recent 5107 cases, in which there were no deaths or myocardial infarctions and a 2.2 percent incidence of complications. Specific protocols were followed in these patients. Each patient was seen 1 to 2 weeks before the planned procedure. At that time, the procedure was explained and the patient was given a brochure to review. Chest radiograph, ECG, hematocrit and hemoglobin, leukocyte count, blood chemistries, electrolytes, and prothrombin time were obtained, and treadmill tests, thallium scans, or radionuclide ventriculograms were performed as indicated. On the day of the procedure, the patient fasted for 4 hours and reported to the catheterization facility 30 minutes before the scheduled procedure. Coronary angiography was performed by the Sones technique. After the procedure, the patient was allowed to leave the area but remained in the hospital and returned after 30 to 60 minutes for evaluation of the radial pulse, the catheterization site, blood pressure, and any evidence of complications. The following day, the patient again was seen and the angiograms were reviewed.

Ventricular fibrillation occurred in 0.14 percent of the patients in this series; most were discharged without hospital admission. Cerebrovascular complications occurred in 0.02 percent, anaphylactic complications in 0.02 percent, brachial artery lacerations in 0.04 percent, and loss of radial pulses in 2 percent. Twenty-four patients (0.5 percent) were hospitalized because of chest pain, angiographic findings, hypotension, malaise, nausea, or oozing at the catheterization site. No deaths occurred in this series.

Mahrer and Eshoo reported on 288 patients who underwent outpatient coronary angiography, 95 percent by the percutaneous Judkins technique and 5 percent by the Sones technique.[79] There

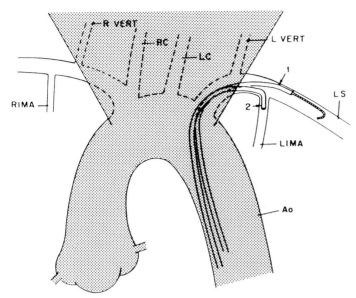

FIGURE 23–6. Schematic diagram showing the origin of the internal mammary artery from the subclavian artery and the technique of selective cannulation of the left internal mammary artery. After an internal mammary artery catheter is placed in the subclavian artery over a guidewire, selective internal mammary cannulation is achieved by withdrawal of the catheter with slight anterior rotation. Ao = aorta; LC = left carotid artery; LIMA = left internal mammary artery; L VERT = left vertebral artery; LS = left subclavian artery; RC = right carotid artery; RIMA = right internal mammary artery; R VERT = right vertebral artery. (From Baim, D.S., and Grossman, W.: Coronary angiography. *In* Grossman, W., and Baim, D.S. [eds.]: Cardiac Catheterization, Angiography, and Intervention. 4th ed. Philadelphia, Lea & Febiger, 1991, p. 193, with permission.)

were six complications (1 death, 2 myocardial infarctions, 1 air embolism, and 2 hematomas). Three of the six complications occurred in patients with left main coronary artery disease, and only two of the complications were thought to be related to the outpatient nature of the procedure. However, the authors emphasized careful patient selection and excluded patients with unstable angina, recent heart failure, severe arrhythmias, severe valvular heart disease, or concomitant insulin-dependent diabetes mellitus, chronic obstructive pulmonary disease, or steroid dependency. In those patients studied with the Judkins technique, the arterial site was treated with pressure for 6 to 10 minutes after catheter removal and with a pressure dressing for 4 hours. If there was no bleeding at that time, ambulation and discharge were allowed. The patients were to rest at home for 1 day and then resume normal activity. Ninety-one percent of patients were discharged at 4 hours. Eleven (3.6 percent) were hospitalized, predominantly for chest pain or hypotension, but were subsequently discharged without complications. Ten patients (3.2 percent) were hospitalized for emergency coronary artery bypass surgery, mainly for left main coronary artery disease.

Klinke and colleagues summarized the results of 3071 outpatient catheterizations performed from the femoral approach, reporting mortality in 0.13 percent, myocardial infarction in 0.07 percent, arrhythmias in 0.42 percent, cerebrovascular complications in 0.14 percent, and local vascular complications in 0.35 percent.[80] Mahrer, Young, and Magnusson reported a series of 2207 elective outpatient catheterizations performed from November 1983 to June 1986, in which the only exclusion was if the patient required hospitalization for symptoms.[81] Only 1 death (0.05 percent) occurred, and that was in a patient with left main coronary artery disease. Other complications included myocardial infarction in 0.05 percent, ventricular fibrillation in 0.6 percent, cerebrovascular accident in 0.05 percent, and vascular complications in 0.15 percent. Despite the less restricted patient population, outcomes were still quite good. However, the authors stressed the importance of staffing the pa-

tient observation area with nurses experienced in critical care of the cardiac patient to achieve these results. No patient required admission for late bleeding.

Block and associates reported a prospective randomized trial of outpatient versus inpatient cardiac catheterization.[82] Because of careful patient selection, only 20 percent of patients were eligible for study. There were no deaths and no cerebrovascular accidents, but hematoma, vascular insufficiency, and myocardial infarction were slightly more common among the outpatients. Twelve percent of outpatients were admitted as a result of disease severity or complications. As expected, costs were lower for the outpatients, and it was estimated that if 15 percent of the catheterizations performed in the United States were done on an outpatient basis, the savings would amount to approximately 51 million dollars per year.

During a 3-month period in 1987, 986 consecutive patients undergoing cardiac catheterization at Duke University Medical Center were prospectively classified as to their eligibility for outpatient catheterization. Of these patients, 24 percent underwent outpatient catheterization, 28 percent were inpatients but had no exclusion criteria for outpatient catheterization, and 47 percent were inpatients who had one or more exclusions for outpatient catheterization.[83] Those catheterized as outpatients averaged a 1-Fr. smaller catheter size. Overall, there was a 6 percent incidence of minor complications with no differences noted among the three groups. Of those catheterized as outpatients, 43 (18 percent) were admitted: 4 for observation, 31 for revascularization, and 8 as previously scheduled. The difference in charges between the outpatient and the inpatient procedures was $580 per case, whereas the difference in costs was only $218 per case.

Clements and Gatlin reported on 3000 outpatient catheterizations performed at Emory University from October 1986 through May 1990.[84] Despite careful screening to eliminate potentially high-risk patients, 2 percent of the patients had left main coronary artery disease. Seven patients had ventricular fibrillation, 2 had cerebral emboli, 2 had pulmonary edema, and 2 had allergic reactions. Three patients had late bleeding at home, and 3 developed pseudoaneurysms of the femoral artery. The overall complication rate was 0.8 percent, and no deaths occurred. Of the 3000 patients, 18.2 percent were admitted after the procedure, but in 17.7 percent admission was for revascularization.

In conclusion, coronary angiography, whether by the Judkins or the Sones technique, can be performed in a safe and cost-effective manner in selected cases on an outpatient basis. However, patient selection and meticulous postcatheterization care and follow-up (including ready access to catheter-based interventions and coronary bypass graft surgery) are critical, and the status of the patient as well as suspected pathology must be evaluated to determine whether inpatient or outpatient catheterization is appropriate. Patients who are not generally considered good candidates for outpatient cardiac catheterization because of increased risk for adverse outcomes include those who are at high risk for vascular complications (i.e., because of morbid obesity or significant peripheral vascular disease) and those who have a mechanical prosthetic valve, general debility or cachexia, an ejection fraction of 35 percent or less, anticoagulation or a bleeding diathesis, uncontrolled systemic hypertension, diabetes mellitus that is difficult to control, chronic steroid use, history of allergy to contrast medium, severe chronic obstructive lung disease, age younger than 21 years, complex congenital heart disease, a recent stroke, noninvasive test results indicating high risk, pulmonary hypertension, or arterial desaturation (Table 23–2).[85] Patients who live a significant distance from the laboratory should be encouraged to spend the night after the study close to the catheterization laboratory. Interventional procedures usually should not be done on an ambulatory basis.[85]

Studies of Small-Diameter Catheters

In an attempt to decrease entry site complications, and thereby further increase the feasibility of outpatient catheterization, while

TABLE 23–2. RISK FACTORS FOR ADVERSE OUTCOME THAT MAY MAKE PATIENTS UNSUITABLE FOR OUTPATIENT CATHETERIZATION

High risk for vascular complications
   Morbid obesity
   Severe peripheral vascular disease
Mechanical prosthetic valve
General debility or cachexia
Low ejection fraction (35% or less)
Anticoagulation or bleeding diathesis
Uncontrolled systemic hypertension
Patient's home a significant distance from catheterization laboratory
Diabetes mellitus that is difficult to control
Chronic use of corticosteroids
History of allergy to radiographic contrast material
Severe chronic obstructive lung disease
Age less than 21 years or complex congenital heart disease regardless
   of age
Recent stroke (within 1 month)
Severe ischemia during stress testing
Pulmonary hypertension
Arterial desaturation

From Pepine, C.J., Allen, H.D., Bashore, T.M., et al.: ACC/AHA guidelines for cardiac catheterization and cardiac catheterization laboratories. American College of Cardiology/American Heart Association Ad Hoc Task Force on Cardiac Catheterization. J. Am. Coll. Cardiol. 18:1156, 1991. Reprinted with permission from the American College of Cardiology.

preserving angiographic quality, smaller catheters have been developed that have the same flow characteristics as the larger ones. Brown and MacDonald reported on 100 angiograms performed with 5-Fr. catheters from July 1985 through February 1986. All angiograms were diagnostic, but 9 percent were of only fair quality.[86] Problems noticed with the smaller catheters included catheter instability, high degree of torque, and contrast streaming. The main difficulty was in engagement of the RCA, which was less problematic if a modified Amplatz rather than a right Judkins catheter was used. It was suggested that use of a sheath may decrease the "drag" on the catheter and make maneuverability easier. The only complications noted were two small groin hematomas.

Kern and colleagues reported the results of a five-center pilot trial in which 5-Fr. catheters were used and patients were ambulated a mean of 2.6 hours after the procedure.[3] In 92 percent of the patients, the catheterization could be completed with the large-lumen 5-Fr. catheter, and only 3 patients required switching to 7- or 8-Fr. catheters. Small site hematomas occurred in 5 percent of patients early and in an additional 3 percent later. The incidence of hematoma was increased in patients who received both heparin and aspirin and in whom compression time was shorter than 10 minutes. No other significant vascular complications were seen.

Talley and co-workers reported that, of 50 patients undergoing coronary angiography, 72 percent were successfully studied with 4.1-Fr. catheters through a percutaneous brachial approach,[87] and diagnostic-quality studies were obtained in all patients. A learning curve was noted in that arterial time (the total time during which the catheter was in the arterial system) decreased as experience with the technique increased. In a study of 200 patients who were randomized to 4- or 6-Fr. catheters for coronary angiography, no site complications occurred in either group, and adequate angiograms were obtained in 97 percent of patients.[88] There were no differences between the two groups with regard to procedure time, fluoroscopy time, quantity of contrast medium used, number of catheters used, cine length (length of cine film), or percent of adequate angiograms. The 4-Fr. catheters were more likely to dislodge, but they were also thought to have slightly better torque control. Streaming was not thought to be a significant problem as long as catheter position was good.

Whether 5-Fr. catheters are of any advantage compared with 6- or 8-Fr. catheters is called into question by the results of Brown

and co-workers.[89] In a randomized series, they found that 5-Fr. catheters were less maneuverable, were more difficult to place, and had poorer injection characteristics, but resulted in no obvious improvements in time to hemostasis or entry site complications. In addition, at least one study has reported an increased risk of coronary dissection with 6-Fr. compared with 8-Fr. catheters (0.67 percent versus 0.04 percent, respectively), particularly for inexperienced operators.[90] It was suggested that this complication was a result of poorer torque control and less stability of the 6-Fr. catheters and the development of increased tip pressure at similar contrast agent flow rates.

Although catheterization with smaller catheters that have high-flow characteristics is feasible, whether it is of significant advantage remains unclear.

IMPORTANCE OF ADEQUATE ANGIOGRAPHIC VIEWS

Despite the best efforts of the angiographer to obtain safe and correct catheter position and optimum opacification of the coronary vessels, unless angiographic views are selected properly, lesions will be missed. To completely evaluate a vessel for lesions, the entire vessel must be visualized in orthogonal projections, perpendicular to the x-ray beam, and without foreshortening or overlap. LAO and RAO views are routinely used. However, because of the oblique orientation of the heart in the thorax and the fact that the vessels curve around the epicardial surface of the heart, angles in the cranial-to-caudal plane are also required to adequately visualize all portions of the coronary tree. The widespread use of C-arm angiographic systems has greatly facilitated the acquisition of such cranial and caudal angulated views.

Because of confusion about the terminology of angulated views, Paulin proposed in 1981 that projections should be described as if the observer were seeing the object transilluminated by the x-ray source on the opposite side.[91] The projections referred to as caudocranial and craniocaudal are illustrated in Figure 23–7. The view is considered caudocranial (hereafter referred to as cranial) if the observer seems to be looking down from the patient's head, and craniocaudal (caudal) if the observer's view is upward from the patient's feet.

Although angulated views increase the demand on the x-ray generator and also increase radiation scatter, they are essential in some cases to adequately visualize the coronary arteries. Because of the increased demand and scatter, however, it is recommended that screening LAO and RAO views be done initially, followed by angulated projections to bring out areas in question.[22] For the left coronary artery, standard LAO and RAO views result in foreshortening and overlap of the proximal vessels; for the RCA, the LAO projection foreshortens the posterior descending and right ventricular branches, and the RAO projection foreshortens the proximal and distal portions of the RCA. The major problem areas that may require specific evaluation are therefore the left main coronary artery, the proximal circumflex and LAD coronary arteries, the diagonal branches of the LAD artery, and the distal RCA, as well as the proximal portions of the posterior descending and posterolateral branches.[50]

Numerous investigators have extolled the benefits of angulated projections.[92–100] In up to 50 percent of cases, angulated views result in improved visualization of lesions, if not the uncovering of lesions not previously seen. Bunnell and associates suggested that the angle most helpful for bringing out the proximal left coronary artery and its branches is a shallow LAO projection with cranial angulation.[92] Diagnosis was improved in 33 of 72 cases with this view. In 1974, using cut film technique, Sos and colleagues showed that lordotic views assisted in the evaluation of left main coronary artery disease, of proximal LAD and circumflex disease, and of LAD and diagonal disease.[93] Also in 1974, Eldh and Silverman proposed the elevation of the patient on a wedge to obtain cranial

Although it is hard to predict which angiographic view may be helpful in an individual patient because of variability in the position of the heart and in each patient's coronary anatomy, there are views that are considered helpful to bring out specific problem areas. The left main coronary artery can usually be visualized best in a shallow LAO or RAO projection (such that the vessel is just off the spine) with 20 to 25 degrees of caudal angulation; the proximal LAD artery can be brought out at 45 to 60 degrees LAO with 25 to 45 degrees of cranial angulation; and the proximal circumflex is often best seen in a 60- to 75-degree LAO projection with 20 to 45 degrees of caudal angulation. An RAO angle of 30 to 45 degrees with caudal angulation can also be used to bring out the proximal circumflex artery. To better evaluate the portion of the RCA adjacent to the crux or the posterior descending and posterolateral coronary arteries, a shallow LAO or RAO view with a small amount of either cranial or caudal angulation, variable from patient to patient, can be useful. The important thing is for the angiographer to be experienced enough to determine which areas are not adequately seen on routine views and then, beginning with these general guidelines, obtain the additional views that are necessary. Some of the more commonly used angulated angiographic projections are shown in Figure 23–8. Angiographic views that are beneficial for defining specific locations in the native coronary tree, coronary bypass grafts, and internal mammary artery grafts are reviewed elsewhere.[101, 102]

NORMAL CORONARY ANATOMY

The major coronary arteries run in the atrioventricular and interventricular grooves along the epicardial surface (Fig. 23–9). Although this description is straightforward, analysis is made somewhat difficult and angulated views are necessary for adequate visualization because the planes of the atrioventricular groove and the interventricular septum are set at 45-degree angles to the major planes of the body. The interventricular septum runs from right posterior to left anterior at an angle of 45 degrees from the frontal and sagittal planes. The atrioventricular groove runs from right anterior to left posterior and is also tilted 45 degrees to the horizontal and sagittal planes, running from right inferior to left superior. In addition, it is tilted 45 degrees to the horizontal and frontal planes, running from anteroinferior to posterosuperior. Although the coronary arteries follow the atrioventricular and interventricular grooves, the oblique positioning of the heart makes description and analysis of their course more difficult. The anterior descending and posterior descending arteries course along the anterior and posterior aspects, respectively, of the interventricular septum. The right and circumflex coronary arteries course in the atrioventricular groove.

Terms that describe certain borders of the heart can assist understanding of the descriptions of the coronary arteries. The obtuse margin of the heart is the superior (i.e., left) border of the heart, and the acute margin is the inferior (i.e., right) border of the heart. Other authors have described the course of the coronary arteries,[21, 22, 48, 50, 67] and the following description of coronary anatomy is based on a compilation of previous descriptions supplemented by the author's experience. The important thing to remember is that coronary anatomy is variable from person to person. This variability contributes to the challenge of correct interpretation of coronary angiograms, whether the coronary arteries are normal or abnormal.

The RCA arises from the right or anterior sinus of Valsalva; the left coronary artery arises from the left sinus of Valsalva, which is to the left and posterior; and the noncoronary cusp, which is slightly larger than either of the two coronary cusps, lies to the right and posterior, between the two coronary cusps. The left coronary ostium tends to arise higher in the aorta than the right coronary ostium.

The concept of coronary dominance was described by Schlesinger in 1940.[103] The classification refers to the relative dominance

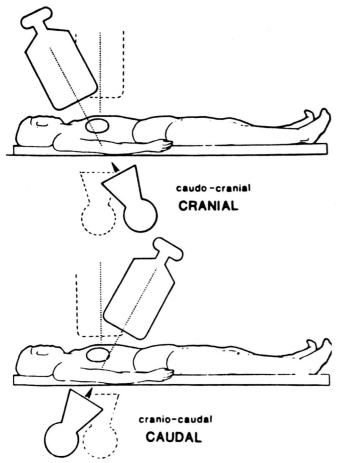

FIGURE 23–7. Illustration of the terminology used for describing angulations in the cranial-caudal plane. The arrowheads indicate the direction of travel of x-ray photons. The view is described as caudocranial, or simply cranial *(top)*, if the view is taken as if the observer were looking down from the patient's head; the craniocaudal, or caudal, view *(bottom)* is the projection as if the observer were looking upward from the patient's feet. (From Paulin, S.: Terminology for radiographic projections in cardiac angiography. [Letter.] Cathet. Cardiovasc. Diagn. 7:343, 1981, with permission. Copyright © 1981 John Wiley & Sons, Inc.)

angulation.[94] In 1975, Arani and co-workers reported that LAO angulation with cranial projection was helpful in 47 percent of cases.[95] Aldridge and colleagues found that additional views unmasked lesions in 20 percent of 100 consecutive coronary angiograms and that analysis was improved in an additional 34 percent.[96] In 4 of 12 cases in which the coronary arteries had been considered normal, angulated views unmasked lesions.

Gomes and associates reported that shallow LAO projections of the RCA with 15 to 25 degrees of cranial angulation allowed avoidance of errors in the interpretation of the takeoff of the posterior descending coronary artery in 6 of 20 cases.[98] RAO projections with 15 degrees of either cranial or caudal angulation also improved separation of the distal RCA and the posterior descending branch. In 1981, Elliott reported on 300 patients and found that cranial angulation in the RAO projection improved visualization of 80 percent of middle LAD lesions and that lesions were uncovered in 7 percent.[99] Similar projections improved the diagnosis of diagonal lesions in 75 percent. Among 50 RCA studies, a cranial RAO projection improved separation of the posterior descending and posterolateral coronary arteries in more 80 percent. Aldridge reported that angled projections improved lesion visualization in 54 to 93 percent of patients.[100] However, such angulation was problematic if patients were obese or if the diaphragms were interposed, because adequate x-ray penetration was not always possible.

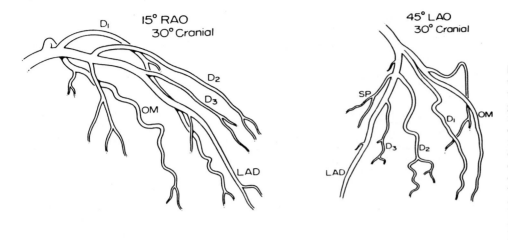

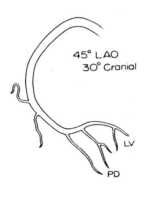

FIGURE 23–8. Specially angulated views of the coronary arteries designed to show areas that are frequently masked in conventional angiographic projections. *(Upper left)* A shallow right anterior oblique (RAO) view of the left coronary artery with cranial angulation is helpful for evaluation of the proximal left anterior descending coronary artery (LAD) and its diagonal branches. *(Upper right)* A left anterior oblique (LAO) view of the left coronary artery with cranial angulation is useful for evaluation of the proximal LAD and circumflex arteries because it decreases the foreshortening of the proximal left coronary artery. *(Bottom)* A cranially angulated LAO projection of the right coronary artery better defines the takeoff of the posterior descending coronary artery (PD) from the distal right coronary artery. OM = obtuse marginal coronary artery; D1, D2, D3 = diagonal branches of the LAD; SP = septal artery; LV = left ventricular branch. (From King, S.B., III, Douglas, J.S., Jr., and Morris, D.C.: New angiographic views for coronary arteriography. *In* Hurst, J.W. [ed.]: Update IV: The Heart. New York, McGraw-Hill, 1981, pp. 206, 208, & 210, with permission.)

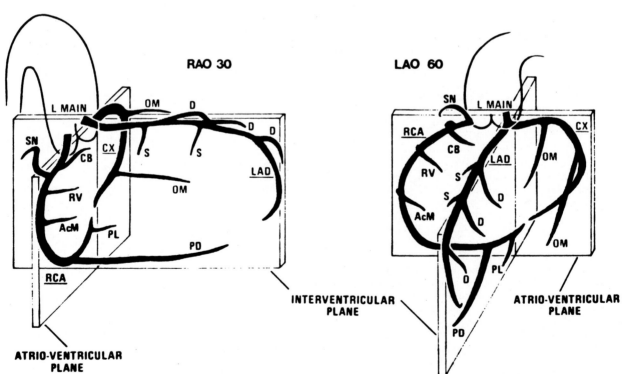

FIGURE 23–9. Relation of the right and left coronary arteries to the interventricular and atrioventricular planes of the heart. RAO = right anterior oblique; LAO = left anterior oblique; L Main = left main; LAD = left anterior descending; D = diagonal; S = septal; CX = circumflex; OM = obtuse marginal; RCA = right coronary artery; CB = conus branch; SN = sinus node artery; RV = right ventricular branch; AcM = acute marginal artery; PD = posterior descending; PL = posterolateral left ventricular branch. (From Baim, D.S., and Grossman, W.: Coronary angiography. *In* Grossman, W., and Baim, D.S. [eds.]: Cardiac Catheterization, Angiography, and Intervention. 4th ed. Philadelphia, Lea & Febiger, 1991, p. 200, with permission.)

of the right or the left circumflex coronary arteries; in humans, the left coronary artery always supplies the greatest portion of the left ventricular myocardium. The dominant coronary artery was described by Schlesinger as that which supplies the inferior portion of the septum and the diaphragmatic wall of the left ventricle. In Schlesinger's original series, coronary circulations were right dominant in 48 percent, balanced in 34 percent, and left dominant in 18 percent. However, subsequent series have shown the dominant artery to be the RCA in 77 to 90 percent of cases. Of the remaining patients, one half to two thirds have left-dominant coronary systems—that is, the inferior wall of the left ventricle and the atrioventricular nodal artery arise from the circumflex coronary artery and the entire septum is supplied by the left coronary system—and one third to one half have codominant coronary artery systems, in which both the right and circumflex coronary arteries provide blood to the inferior septum and the diaphragmatic wall of the left ventricle.

The left coronary artery arises from the left sinus of Valsalva, has an initial diameter of approximately 4.5 mm, and courses behind the right ventricular outflow tract for 0 to 10 mm before dividing into the LAD and circumflex coronary arteries. To differentiate these two branches, it is helpful to recall that they move in opposite directions, with the LAD artery showing less motion than the circumflex. In 20 to 37 percent of patients, the division of the left main coronary artery is actually a trifurcation, with a ramus medianus (ramus intermedius) branch arising between the LAD and the circumflex coronary arteries.

The LAD artery continues along the anterior interventricular groove and, in 70 to 80 percent of patients, courses around the apex to supply a portion of the apical inferior septum. In the RAO projection, the LAD coronary artery follows the anterior border of the heart, whereas in the LAO projection it is located in the midline of the heart. The LAD artery gives off septal branches and a variable number of diagonal branches that course to the anterolateral wall of the heart. In 90 percent of patients, one to three diagonal branches are present. The LAD coronary artery and its branches supply the anterior left ventricle, the anterior interventricular septum, and the anterolateral wall (the left ventricular free wall). Although variability in terminology exists, the proximal LAD artery usually includes that portion of the vessel proximal to the origin of the first septal perforator, and the middle LAD artery includes that portion of the vessel between the first septal and second diagonal branches.

The circumflex coronary artery runs in the left atrioventricular groove, with its more distal course paralleling that of the coronary sinus. The circumflex artery supplies the lateral and posterior left ventricle, giving off one to three obtuse marginal branches. These marginal branches are variable, and the terminology concerning these branches is among the most variable in coronary angiography. In some centers, the largest branch that courses to the actual obtuse margin of the heart is called the obtuse marginal, and all of the other branches are called lateral branches. In other centers, the marginals are simply numbered in order of takeoff from the circumflex artery (e.g., first marginal, second marginal), like the diagonal branches of the LAD coronary artery. Others refer to the branches of the circumflex coronary artery that go to the posterolateral wall as lateral branches and number them sequentially. The terminology used to describe coronary anatomy to other angiographers must therefore be clarified in each case.

The circumflex also gives off atrial branches. In 40 to 50 percent of patients the sinus node artery arises from the circumflex, and in 8 to 10 percent the atrioventricular nodal artery and the posterior descending artery arise from the circumflex coronary artery, making the circumflex the "dominant" coronary artery.

The RCA has an initial diameter of approximately 2.5 mm. It follows the right atrioventricular groove to the crux of the heart (the portion of the heart at which the right atrioventricular groove, the left atrioventricular groove, and the posterior interventricular groove join). In 50 percent of patients, the conus branch is the first branch of the RCA; otherwise, it arises from a separate ostium

in the right coronary sinus. This is an important anatomical variation, for the conus branch frequently supplies collaterals to the LAD artery system. The sinus node artery arises from the RCA in 50 to 60 percent of cases. (The fact that the conus and the sinus node arteries initially course in opposite directions can be helpful in distinguishing them.)

The RCA provides right ventricular branches and, in those patients with a right-dominant coronary circulation, it gives off the posterior descending coronary artery, which provides branches to the inferior portion of the ventricular septum. After the takeoff of the posterior descending artery, the dominant RCA continues in the atrioventricular groove to give off posterolateral left ventricular branches. The distal portion of the RCA is extremely variable; two posterior descending arteries can be present or, in some cases, one of the right ventricular branches provides a portion of the blood supply to the inferior ventricular wall. The acute marginal branches of the RCA arise below the right atrium and just before or at the acute margin of the heart. These branches run toward the apex of the heart and, in some cases, also reach the inferior ventricular wall and provide a portion of the blood supply to the interventricular septum.

In coronary angiograms, only large to medium coronary arteries (at least 100 to 200 μm in size) are seen. Only a small part of the entire coronary tree (the epicardial coronary arteries and some second-, third-, and fourth-order branches) can be visualized.

CONGENITAL ANOMALIES OF THE CORONARY ARTERIES

Congenital anomalies of the coronary arteries occur in 1 to 2 percent of patients. They frequently occur in association with other forms of congenital heart disease, but in many cases they are of no clinical significance. In angiographic series, the incidence of anomalous origin of the coronary arteries has been reported as 0.83 percent in 3750 patients at the Montreal Heart Institute,[104] 1.20 percent in 4250 patients at St. Thomas Hospital in Nashville,[105] 0.64 percent in 7000 angiograms performed at Hahnemann Hospital in Philadelphia,[106] and 1.33 percent among 126,595 patients undergoing coronary angiography at the Cleveland Clinic between 1960 and 1988 (Table 23–3).[107] In the Hahnemann series,[106] associated valvular heart disease was present in 31 percent of patients. The Cleveland Clinic series reported that the anomalies were equal in both sexes and that the prevalence of atherosclerosis was not increased in the anomalous vessels.[107] Variations in origin from the right coronary sinus are greater than those from the left, and origin of the coronary arteries from the noncoronary sinus is rare.

There are three reasons why knowledge of coronary anomalies is important for coronary angiographers. First, if an anomalous coronary origin is not realized, a totally occluded coronary artery may be mistakenly diagnosed. Second, some coronary anomalies can cause myocardial ischemia. And third, surgeons should be made aware of anomalous coronary arteries in order to avoid damaging them during cardiac surgery. For convenience, coronary artery anomalies can be divided into those that affect perfusion and those that do not.[50, 67, 108, 109]

Coronary Anomalies That Alter Myocardial Perfusion

CORONARY ARTERY FISTULA. These are the most common anomalies that can affect coronary perfusion. In half of patients, coronary fistulas are completely asymptomatic; in the other half, they may be detected because of a heart murmur or they may be associated with complications such as congestive heart failure, myocardial ischemia or infarction (resulting from a coronary steal phenomenon), endocarditis, or rupture of the aneurysmal segments of the coronary arteries. About fifty percent of fistulas arise from the RCA, 42 percent from the left coronary artery, and 5 percent

TABLE 23–3. ANOMALOUS AORTIC ORIGINS OF THE CORONARY ARTERIES

	Chaitman et al.[104]	Engel et al.[105°]	Kimbiris et al.[106†]	Yamanaka & Hobbs[107‡]
Number of patients	3750	4250	7000	126,595
Incidence of anomalous coronary arteries (%)				
Total	0.83	1.20	0.64	1.33
Origin of Cx from right sinus of Valsalva	0.45	0.71	0.37	0.37
Origin of both coronary arteries from left sinus of Valsalva	0.19	0.07	0.17	0.11
Origin of both coronary arteries from right sinus of Valsalva	0.19	0.11	0.06	0.02
Origin of LAD from right sinus of Valsalva	NR	0.07	0.03	0.03
Origin of first septal artery from right sinus of Valsalva	NR	0.09	0.04	NR

Cx = circumflex coronary artery; LAD = left anterior descending coronary artery; NR = not reported.

°The series reported by Engel et al. also included 1 case of left main coronary artery origin from the pulmonary artery, 1 case of LAD origin from the pulmonary artery and Cx origin from the right coronary sinus, and 8 cases of separate ostia for LAD and Cx in the left coronary sinus.

†In the series of Kimbiris et al., 2 patients had a combination of the listed coronary anomalies.

‡Separate origin LAD and Cx in the left sinus of Valsalva was considered an anomaly and occurred in 0.41%.

from both.[108] Coronary fistulas drain into the right side of the heart more commonly than into the left; in one series, the right ventricle was the site of drainage in 41 percent, the right atrium in 26 percent, the pulmonary artery in 17 percent, the coronary sinus in 7 percent, the left atrium in 5 percent, the left ventricle in 3 percent, and the superior vena cava in 1 percent.[108] An example of a fistula from the RCA that drains into the coronary sinus is shown in Figure 23–10. If patients are symptomatic because of a coronary artery fistula, the goal of treatment aims to obliterate the fistula but preserve forward coronary flow, usually by means of coronary artery bypass grafting.

Coronary fistulas can be acquired or congenital. Coronary fistulas can occur after myocardial infarction,[110] and recently an increased incidence of coronary artery fistulas has been described after car-

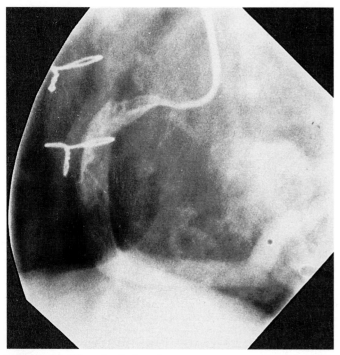

FIGURE 23–10. A fistula from the right coronary artery to the coronary sinus (left anterior oblique projection). The right coronary artery is markedly dilated because of the increased right coronary flow caused by the fistula.

diac transplantation.[111] An 8 percent incidence of coronary fistulas was found in 176 heart transplant patients, compared with a 0.2 percent incidence in 1000 control patients. In the transplant population, the fistulas were single in 9 patients and multiple in 5. Fifty-two percent arose from the RCA, 43 percent from the LAD, and 5 percent from the circumflex. All drained into the right ventricle, none was symptomatic, and no shunts were detected by oxymetry. However, the transplant patients with coronary fistulas had a slightly higher cardiac index and pulmonary arterial oxygen saturation than those without coronary fistulas. On follow-up angiograms, 3 fistulas had increased in size, 3 had remained the same, 2 had decreased in size, and 3 had disappeared. Fitchett and colleagues reported coronary arterial–right ventricular fistulas in five post-transplant patients.[112] Two of these fistulas were not seen on the first yearly angiogram, documenting that they were not congenital anomalies present in the donor heart. Although the cause of the increased incidence of coronary fistulas in the cardiac transplant population is uncertain, one hypothesis is that they are related to the right ventricular endomyocardial biopsies that are performed for the diagnosis of rejection.

ORIGIN OF THE LEFT CORONARY ARTERY FROM THE PULMONARY ARTERY. Origin of the left coronary artery from the pulmonary artery[108, 113, 114] usually produces myocardial ischemia early in life, resulting in an infant syndrome of failure to thrive, tachypnea, wheezing, and angina. Seventy-five to 90 percent of reported patients die as infants or children. Those who survive to adulthood present with mitral regurgitation, angina, and congestive heart failure. There is also a high incidence of sudden death in adults with this syndrome. Origin of the left coronary artery from the pulmonary artery results in low coronary perfusion pressure and low oxygen saturation in the blood perfusing the left coronary artery. Survival depends on the development of collaterals from the RCA. However, a steal syndrome can develop in which flow proceeds from the right coronary system to the left coronary artery and on into the pulmonary artery. In patients in whom the anomaly is diagnosed, treatment consists of ligation of the left coronary artery at its origin from the pulmonary artery, either alone or with coronary artery bypass grafting or reimplantation of the left coronary artery into the aorta.

CONGENITAL STENOSIS OR ATRESIA OF THE CORONARY ARTERIES. This rare anomaly usually occurs in association with other congenital heart diseases, including calcific coronary sclerosis, supravalvular aortic stenosis, homocystinuria, Hurler syndrome, progeria, or the congenital rubella syndrome.[108]

ORIGIN OF THE LEFT CORONARY ARTERY OR THE RCA FROM THE OPPOSITE CORONARY SINUS WITH

PASSAGE OF THE VESSEL BETWEEN THE AORTA AND THE RIGHT VENTRICULAR OUTFLOW TRACT. These anomalies[104, 106, 115] are shown in Figure 23–11. Origin of the left coronary artery from the right coronary sinus or the RCA with passage of the left main coronary trunk between the aorta and pulmonary artery occurred in 33 of 475,000 autopsies.[115] It has been associated with sudden death in 27 to 33 percent of patients. The mechanism of sudden death is not known, but it may be related to "squeezing" of the left main coronary artery between the two vessels (although this is unlikely because of the low pulmonary artery pressure involved), to the presence of a congenitally small left coronary artery, to kinking or spasm of the artery as it passes between the other vascular structures, or to the slit-like orifice of the left main coronary artery or the acute angle of its takeoff when it arises in this position.

Origin of the RCA from the left coronary sinus with passage of this vessel between the aorta and the right ventricular outflow tract was initially thought to be benign. However, angina, myocardial infarction, syncope, and sudden death (associated with left ventricular scarring in the absence of coronary artery disease) have been reported. Brandt, Martins, and Marcus described a patient in whom the RCA arose from the left coronary sinus and passed between the great vessels. They found that coronary flow reserve (evaluated with an epicardial Doppler probe in the operating room) was decreased by 50 percent in the RCA. The abnormality in flow reserve was corrected by coronary artery bypass grafting.[116] Thus, origins of the RCA from the left sinus of the left coronary artery can have pathophysiologic significance. The reason for the pathophysiologic significance of this anomaly is unclear, but it may be related to the slit-like origin of the RCA or to compression of the vessel between the aorta and pulmonary outflow tract. Kragel and Roberts have suggested that the dominance of the coronary system may be the most important factor in determining whether anomalous vessels coursing between the aorta and the pulmonary outflow tract are of clinical significance.[117]

Coronary Anomalies That Do Not Alter Myocardial Perfusion

ORIGIN OF THE LEFT MAIN CORONARY ARTERY FROM THE RIGHT CORONARY SINUS OR RCA WITH PASSAGE OF THE VESSEL ANTERIOR TO THE RIGHT VENTRICULAR OUTFLOW TRACT, WITHIN THE CRISTA SUPRAVENTRICULARIS, OR POSTERIOR TO THE AORTA. An anomalous origin to the left main coronary artery in which the vessel passes in these locations is not believed to cause symptoms or cardiac dysfunction.[118]

ORIGIN OF THE CIRCUMFLEX CORONARY ARTERY FROM THE RIGHT CORONARY SINUS OR THE RCA. This anomaly occurs in 0.45 percent of cases[104] and is the most common of all congenital coronary anomalies.[119] In one half of patients, it is found in association with other cardiac anomalies. The vessel courses posterior to the aortic root and the noncoronary sinus to enter the left atrioventricular groove and supply its usual territory of the posterolateral left ventricle. Two angiographic signs have been suggested for anticipating origin of the circumflex coronary artery from the right coronary sinus.[120] These are the aortic root sign, which is a profiling of the vessel across the aortic root during RAO left ventricular angiography, and, in the case of a separate origin of the circumflex coronary artery from the right coronary sinus, the presence of a nonperfused region of the heart in the left circumflex territory after completion of left and right coronary angiography. Although this coronary anomaly is generally thought to be benign, it has been associated with myocardial infarction and angina.[121]

ORIGIN OF THE LAD ARTERY FROM THE RCA OR RIGHT CORONARY SINUS. This anomalous vessel usually courses anterior to the pulmonary artery, and the anomaly is thought to be of no physiologic significance. If difficulty is noted in determining the course of the LAD coronary artery (i.e., whether it passes anterior or posterior to the pulmonary artery), positioning of a catheter in the pulmonary artery during coronary angiography may be helpful.

SINGLE CORONARY ARTERY. A single coronary artery has been reported in 0.024 percent[106] to 0.04 percent[122] of cases reviewed; in the former series, 40 percent of the cases were associated with other congenital cardiac anomalies. A single coronary artery is of potential importance only if the artery passes between the aorta and the pulmonary artery. Three types of single coronary artery have been described. In the first, the origin of the single artery follows the course of one of the normal coronary arteries

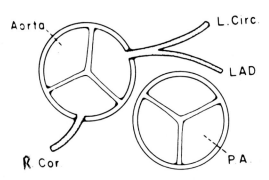

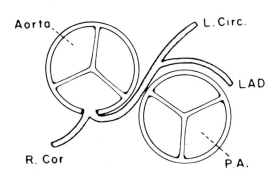

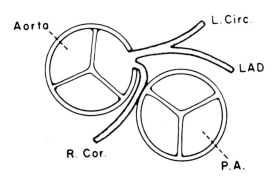

FIGURE 23–11. (*Top*) Normal positions of the aorta, the pulmonary artery (P.A.), and the origins of the right (R. Cor.), left circumflex (L. Circ.), and left anterior descending (LAD) coronary arteries. (*Middle*) Anomalous origin of the left main coronary artery from the right sinus of Valsalva. (*Bottom*) Anomalous origin of the right coronary artery from the left sinus of Valsalva. For the anomalous coronary origins illustrated here, the anomalous coronary artery passes between the aorta and the pulmonary artery; such anomalies may be of physiologic significance. (From Cheitlin, M.D., DeCastro, C.M., and McAllister, H.A.: Sudden death as a complication of anomalous left coronary origin from the anterior sinus of Valsalva: A not-so-minor congenital anomaly. Circulation 50:781, 1974, with permission of the American Heart Association, Inc.)

and then swings around the heart to supply the distribution of the second coronary artery. In the second, the ostium is located in the position of one of the normal coronary ostia, but branches come off proximally to supply the other coronary territory. In the third type, totally irregular coronary perfusion is seen. Because the corrected cross-sectional area of a single coronary artery is usually less than the total of the two normal arteries would be, it has been suggested that the anomaly may be of clinical significance. Accelerated atherosclerosis may also occur because of the irregular course and bending of the artery. Congestive heart failure and sudden death have been reported[122]; however, in the absence of coronary disease, only 15 percent of patients have evidence of myocardial ischemia.[123]

MULTIPLE OSTIA OF THE CORONARY ARTERIES. In a pathologic series, 50 percent of patients had a separate origin for the conus artery in the right coronary sinus. This is important because the conus artery can be a major source of collaterals in cases of LAD stenosis or occlusion. Separate origin of the LAD and circumflex coronary arteries was observed in 1 percent of 2000 autopsy cases.[119]

HIGH ORIGIN OF THE CORONARY ARTERIES. In a pathologic series, Vlodaver and colleagues found that in 30 percent of patients the left coronary ostium arose above the junction of the coronary sinuses and the tubular aorta, in 8 percent the RCA arose above this junction, and in 6 percent both coronary arteries arose from the tubular aorta.[119]

HORSESHOE CORONARY ARTERY WITH TWO OSTIA FROM THE AORTA

ORIGIN OF THE FIRST SEPTAL PERFORATOR FROM THE RCA OR RIGHT CORONARY SINUS

CONGENITAL CORONARY ANEURYSM. Congenital coronary aneurysms are rare. They most commonly affect the RCA, followed by the circumflex and the LAD coronary arteries.[124] They are usually asymptomatic but can be complicated by thrombus formation and distal embolization.

DOUBLE RCA. This anomaly has been discussed by Barthe and colleagues.[125]

FOUR CORONARY OSTIA ORIGINATING FROM THE RIGHT SINUS OF VALSALVA. This anomaly was described by Virmani and colleagues.[126]

In summary, although coronary anomalies are uncommon, they can be of clinical significance, and the presence of an anomalous coronary artery should be considered in a young person who presents with chest pain or sudden death.

CORONARY COLLATERALS

Coronary collaterals are said to be present when a coronary artery is seen beyond the site of an occlusion or a stenosis so severe that it prevents significant antegrade flow. In normal hearts at postmortem examination, small anastomotic vessels are seen, and it is suggested that these vessels actually increase in size to form collaterals in the presence of coronary artery disease, probably as a result of the pressure gradients that develop between normally perfused portions of the heart and small, nonfunctioning collaterals distal to sites of coronary occlusion. Collateral vessels usually are not seen until the stenosis reaches 75 to 90 percent severity. One hundred angiograms were reviewed by Gensini and DaCosta.[127] Fifty-three angiograms with no significant coronary artery disease showed no collateral vessels. Of 47 angiograms with significant coronary disease, 37 had collateral vessels, and all but 1 of 67 vessels with collaterals contained stenoses of greater than 90 percent severity.

Since collaterals were first seen, there has been controversy concerning their clinical importance. Initially, it was believed that collaterals indicated severe disease but were of no functional significance. Helfant and colleagues reported in 1970 on 111 patients with coronary artery disease; there was no difference in wall motion

abnormalities, left ventricular end-diastolic pressure, or cardiac index in patients with collaterals compared with those without collaterals.[128] Helfant and Gorlin reported in 1972 that coronary flow distal to the obstruction was not changed in the presence of collateral vessels, that ECGs were not different, and that treadmill tests were more commonly positive in patients with collaterals than in patients without them.[129] In 1976, Hamby and associates reported that collaterals appeared to be of benefit in patients with LAD coronary artery occlusions but of no benefit in patients with RCA occlusions.[130] In 1981, Tubau and co-workers reported on 37 patients with one-vessel coronary artery disease, 16 of whom had collaterals.[131] Some protective effect of collaterals was suggested, because only 40 percent of patients with collaterals had defects on exercise thallium perfusion scans, compared with 100 percent of patients without collaterals. However, ST segment depression and work capacity on the treadmill were not affected by the presence of collaterals.

The most convincing evidence of the functional significance of collaterals in humans is that angiographic total occlusions may be seen in patients in the absence of pathologic evidence of myocardial infarction. Furthermore, several studies suggest that coronary collateral vessels are functionally important. In 1975, Hecht and colleagues reported that, in 43 patients with coronary artery disease, normal wall motion was more common if good collateral filling was present than if there was no collateral filling.[132] They suggested that it was the size rather than the presence or absence of collaterals that was important in determining their functional significance. In 1976, Williams and co-workers reported on 20 patients with acute myocardial infarction, 6 of whom were believed to have "adequate" collateral vessels.[133] In this series, patients with adequate collaterals had lower left ventricular end-diastolic pressures, less dyssynergy, increased cardiac index, increased stroke work index, increased ejection fraction, and increased survival rate compared with patients without collaterals. In 1978, Schwarz and associates reported that ejection fraction and wall motion were better in patients with coronary collaterals, and that patients with collaterals had fewer myocardial infarctions.[134] However, rapid pacing resulted in wall motion abnormalities in 12 patients with LAD coronary occlusions and collaterals. This study suggested that although collateral vessels may preserve myocardial viability at rest, they are not adequate to prevent myocardial ischemia during stress. In 1982, it was reported that patients with collateral-dependent beds could have normal exercise thallium scans.[135] Patients who, on angiographic studies, had shorter times to appearance of contrast medium in the collaterals were more likely to have normal thallium perfusion scans.

Studies performed in patients undergoing coronary angioplasty also speak to the clinical significance of coronary collateral flow. In a study reported by Probst, Zangl, and Pachinger involving 63 patients with single-vessel coronary artery disease who underwent angioplasty, there was a significant positive relation between distal coronary occlusion pressure and the extent of collaterals seen on angiography.[136] There was also less of a difference in the distal coronary pressure before and during balloon occlusion in the presence of collaterals. In another study, of 24 patients observed during four sequential balloon dilations of the LAD coronary artery, 14 had angiographic collaterals and 10 did not; RCA flow and cross-sectional area increased during balloon inflation in patients with collaterals but did not change in those without collaterals.[137] Elevation of the anterior ST segment and chest pain were also more common in the patients without collaterals.

The pathways most commonly taken by coronary collaterals have been described in detail by other authors.[21, 138] Collaterals can arise either from the same artery in which the occlusive stenosis is seen (homocoronary or intracoronary collaterals) or from other coronary vessels (intercoronary collaterals). Some of the common coronary collateral pathways to the LAD artery are as follows:

1. From the posterior descending artery through septal branches
2. From the posterior descending artery around the apex

3. From the acute marginal branch of the RCA
4. From the conus branch of the RCA through Vieussen's circle
5. From the obtuse marginal branch of the circumflex artery
6. From diagonal branches of the LAD artery
7. From LAD septal-to-septal collaterals

The most common coronary collateral pathways to the RCA are as follows:

1. From the LAD through septal branches
2. From the LAD around the apex
3. From the distal circumflex to the RCA or the atrioventricular nodal artery
4. From the obtuse marginal artery through posterior left ventricular branches
5. From the right ventricular branch of the LAD artery to the marginal branch of the RCA
6. From Kugel's artery along the anterior atrial septum to the atrioventricular nodal artery
7. From the sinus node artery to the left atrial circumflex artery and subsequently to the RCA
8. From the conus branch or the acute marginal branch of the RCA to more distal branches
9. From the distal or left atrial circumflex artery to the atrioventricular nodal artery

The most common collateral pathways to the circumflex coronary artery are as follows:

1. From the left atrial circumflex to the more distal circumflex
2. From a proximal marginal branch to a more distal marginal branch
3. From a diagonal branch of the LAD artery to a marginal branch
4. From the distal RCA to the distal circumflex artery
5. From a posterior left ventricular branch of the RCA to the obtuse marginal branch

CORONARY BRIDGING

Bridging of myocardial vessels was first described by Block in 1796. Bridging refers to the intramural location of a coronary artery, which on angiogram appears as systolic narrowing. Although autopsy reports show a widely variable incidence of bridging (5 to 86 percent), angiographic studies report an incidence of 0.5 to 12 percent. The functional significance of coronary bridging remains controversial. Generally, bridging is not believed to result in symptoms, because the coronary narrowing occurs during systole and most coronary flow occurs during diastole. This was confirmed by Kramer and co-workers, who reported a 12 percent incidence of bridging in 658 otherwise normal cineangiograms.[139] In their series, all of the bridges occurred in the LAD distribution. The 5-year survival rate was 98 percent, and no myocardial infarctions occurred in the survivors.[139] Marcus reported that the coronary flow reserve of a human coronary artery with a prominent myocardial bridge studied intraoperatively was almost normal and that diastolic inflow to the vessel was not delayed.[140]

In 1976, Noble and colleagues reported a 0.51 percent incidence of intramyocardial LAD coronary arteries in 5250 coronary angiograms.[141] In a more extensive study of 11 of these patients, it was found that if the systolic narrowing resulted in greater than 75 percent obstruction of the vessel, ST segment depression and lactate production occurred with pacing. At 50 to 75 percent systolic narrowing, 2 of 4 patients developed angina and electrocardiographic changes but no changes in lactate metabolism; less than 50 percent systolic narrowing resulted in no angina, electrocardiographic changes, or metabolic changes. It has also been suggested that the duration of coronary obstruction caused by myocardial bridging (i.e., whether obstruction is purely systolic or extends into diastole) is a determinant of the physiologic consequences of

bridging. Krawczyk and associates found in a dog model of coronary bridging that the duration of occlusion did influence myocardial flow.[142] For systolic occlusion alone, mean flow decreased by 8 ± 5 percent, whereas occlusions extending into diastole reduced mean flow by 20 ± 14 percent. However, the delay in diastolic opening required to produce significant ischemia was equal to one quarter to one half of the diastolic interval at heart rates of 60 to 120 beats per minute, and the frequency with which this duration of occlusion occurs in humans in vivo is unknown. Faruqui and associates reported two symptomatic cases of coronary arterial bridging that responded to therapy with debridging and coronary artery bypass surgery.[143]

In summary, although coronary bridging is usually not of physiologic or pathologic significance, cases of documented abnormalities have been reported. Bridges may be important if they are prominent, if vascular occlusion extends into diastole, or if concomitant left ventricular hypertrophy or a hypercontractile state exists. One of the major questions concerning bridges is why patients develop symptoms later in life if bridges are present from birth. Possibilities include changes in vascular beds and flow that occur with aging, changes in oxygen requirements, or increases in systolic wall tension that occur with the development of hypertrophy.

VALIDITY OF CORONARY ANGIOGRAMS

Comparison of Postmortem and Angiographic Findings

In evaluating studies of angiographic-pathologic correlation, it must be remembered that a 50 percent diameter stenosis on angiography is equivalent to a histologic stenosis of 75 percent of the cross-sectional area; likewise, an angiographic 75 percent diameter stenosis correlates with a histologic 90 percent cross-sectional area stenosis. Keeping these facts in mind, it is important to consider how well the coronary angiogram defines the disease present in the coronary arteries. One of the first studies to address this point was published by Eusterman and colleagues in 1962.[144] At postmortem examination, 75 percent of adults had significant coronary disease. Of 479 coronary segments from 50 hearts, 19 percent contained focal as well as nonfocal disease. For areas with nonfocal disease, postmortem angiograms agreed with the pathologic diagnosis in 61 percent of cases, underestimated disease in 22 percent of cases, and overestimated disease in 17 percent of cases. For focally diseased areas, however, agreement was present in only 11 percent of cases, with angiographic underestimation occurring in 86 percent and overestimation in 3 percent.[144]

In 1967, Kemp and co-workers compared the postmortem diagnosis of disease to premortem angiographic findings in 145 coronary segments in 29 patients.[145] Twenty-three mismatches, only three of which were thought to be functionally significant, were noted. The greatest errors involved angiographic underestimations of disease severity. Problems were particularly noted in segments with crescentic lumens or in areas of vessel overlap on angiography. Errors were also common when the diagonal and circumflex branches were small but were erroneously interpreted as being diffusely diseased. The authors stressed the importance of quality angiograms and expert observers for obtaining accurate angiographic diagnoses.[145]

In 1972, Vlodaver and associates reported the pathologic distribution of disease in 50 adult hearts.[119] Coronary disease was most common in the RCA between the acute margin and the posterior descending branch; the next most common areas of disease were the proximal LAD artery and the proximal RCA. In the LAD and circumflex systems, proximal disease was more common than distal disease. There was a strong tendency for disease to be present in more than one artery. Pathologically, most atherosclerotic plaques were distributed in an arc around the periphery of the lumen, with few lesions showing circumferential distribution. The angiographic significance of diseased segments with a slit-like lumen was frequently misinterpreted. In patients with a false-negative angiogram, 68 percent of the lesions whose significance was underestimated had slit-like lumens.

In a follow-up study, Vlodaver and co-workers compared premortem angiograms with necropsy findings in 10 cases.[146] Of 135 coronary segments, the angiograms were falsely negative in 44 (33 percent). Many of the angiographic false-negative segments were diffusely diseased pathologically and contained slit-like lumens. Only 5 (4 percent) of coronary segments had false-positive angiograms. For only 5 of 10 left main coronary artery segments was agreement noted between angiographic and postmortem diagnoses. Angiographic underestimation of disease was especially common in the middle RCA, the left main coronary artery, and the proximal circumflex artery.[146]

Grondin and colleagues evaluated the hearts of 23 patients who died after coronary bypass grafting and in whom angiograms were available within 30 days of postmortem evaluation.[147] In 9 cases, there was an appreciable difference in the severity of coronary disease defined angiographically and at postmortem examination, and in 4 of these cases incomplete revascularization had occurred because of angiographic underestimation of disease. Eleven (8 percent) of 145 lesions were underestimated angiographically. Hutchins and co-workers compared clinical angiograms and pathologic findings in 28 patients who died within 3 months of angiography.[148] Of 315 segments with greater than 50 percent diameter narrowing on the angiogram, discrepancies were noted between angiographic and postmortem findings in 21 (7 percent). In 6 segments, the angiogram overestimated the disease, but in 3 of these spasm was clearly present. In 15 segments, the angiogram underestimated the coronary disease, and in 12 of these the discrepancy was caused by overlap of the LAD and diagonal coronary arteries.

Several subsequent studies also evaluated the correlation between angiographic and histologic diagnoses of coronary disease. Isner and associates studied 29 patients post mortem who had undergone angiography less than 6 weeks before death.[149] In 15 patients with a greater than 75 percent histologic decrease in luminal cross-sectional area, 7 (47 percent) had normal angiographic findings; in 14 patients with less than 75 percent histologic narrowing, 6 (or 43 percent) were thought to have severe narrowing on the angiogram. In almost 50 percent of cases, therefore, angiographic underestimation or overestimation of disease occurred. Arnett and colleagues compared premortem angiograms and postmortem findings in 10 patients.[150] In 61 coronary segments, there was no angiographic overestimation of disease. In 11 segments with 0 to 50 percent narrowing, there was perfect angiographic and pathologic correlation. For 8 segments with 51 to 75 percent cross-sectional narrowing, 7 were underestimated angiographically, and of 42 segments with 76 to 100 percent pathologic narrowing, 17 were underestimated on angiogram. Diffuse plaquing rather than focal disease was noted pathologically in 90 percent of 467 5-mm segments. Seventeen of 24 arteries with eccentric lumens were underestimated angiographically.

Murphy and colleagues compared pathologic and angiographic findings in 20 patients.[151] They evaluated 313 coronary segments on LAO and 311 on RAO angiograms. For single plane views, angiographic sensitivity was 72 to 78 percent and specificity 85 to 87 percent. For those segments in which both angiographic views were evaluated, the stenosis was seen in both views in only 61 percent; however, if narrowing was seen in both views, a 93 percent specificity was noted. Left main coronary artery disease was overestimated in 10 percent of cases. The most common area of false-positive diagnosis was the proximal RCA, possibly as a result of catheter-induced spasm.[151]

In summary, comparative studies of angiographic and postmortem definitions of coronary artery disease suggest that angiograms frequently underestimate coronary disease severity. However, this interpretation must be made with some caution, because many of the pathologic studies were not performed on arteries fixed by pressure-perfusion. Although pathologic studies report a significant incidence of crescentic or slit-like residual coronary lumens, such lumens are rarely seen in vivo.

Intraobserver and Interobserver Variability

An additional problem concerning the clinical validity of the coronary angiogram is the high degree of intraobserver and interobserver variability that occurs with interpretation of the degree and significance of coronary stenosis. In 1975, Detre and co-workers reported on a subset of 13 angiograms from the Veterans Administration Cooperative Study that had been reviewed by 22 physicians on two different occasions.[152] Those reviewers who showed the highest intraobserver variability also had the highest interobserver variability, and the more experienced angiographers tended to show less variability in angiographic interpretation. Highest agreement was noted for lesions in the RCA and the left main coronary arteries, and the most disagreement occurred with distal LAD and circumflex lesions.

In a more quantitative study, Zir and colleagues reported on the variability observed when four experienced angiographers (two radiologists and two cardiologists) independently assessed 20 coronary angiograms.[153] In only 65 percent of cases did all angiographers agree about the significance of stenoses in the proximal or middle LAD coronary artery. Agreement on the presence or absence of significant disease in the left main coronary artery existed in 85 percent of cases, in the circumflex coronary artery in 75 percent of cases, and in the proximal RCA in 65 percent of cases.[153] DeRouen and associates reported on 11 readers who evaluated 10 angiograms.[154] The standard deviation for diagnosis of coronary disease per segment was 18 percent. Disagreement as to which vessels contained 70 percent or greater stenosis occurred in 31 percent of cases, especially in distal vessels, in nonopacified segments, in diffusely diseased segments, and in angiograms of poor technical quality. Best agreement was found in the proximal RCA, the proximal LAD artery, and the left main coronary artery. Least agreement was seen for diagonal lesions, distal RCA lesions, and distal LAD lesions.[154]

Galbraith, Murphy, and deSoyza reported a study in which interpretation of premortem coronary angiograms was compared with postmortem histology.[155] Of 624 angiographic segments evaluated by three cardiologists, there was a higher incidence of false-positive than false-negative angiograms. In slightly more than 50 percent of the misinterpreted segments, at least two of three interpreters made the same misdiagnosis. Use of a consensus opinion may therefore not improve the validity of angiographic interpretation. In 82 to 84 percent of cases, the angiographic definition correlated with pathologic findings.

In 1982, Fisher and colleagues reported on the reproducibility between two readers who analyzed 870 coronary angiograms from participants in the CASS study.[156] Interpretation of left main coronary artery lesions was the least reproducible, and that of proximal RCA lesions was most reproducible. If one reader diagnosed a stenosis of 50 percent or more in the left main coronary artery, the second reader found no left main coronary artery disease 18.6 percent of the time (Fig. 23–12). However, in only 5.3 percent of cases did the number of vessels considered diseased differ between researchers by more than one vessel. It was found that good quality and complete studies resulted in less interobserver variability.

In summary, the standard method for interpretation of coronary angiograms, that of visually estimating percent diameter stenosis, frequently underestimates the severity of coronary artery disease[150] and also results in substantial intraobserver and interobserver variability.[152–156] Underestimation of the severity of coronary stenoses may be related to the presence of eccentric lesions, which cannot adequately be evaluated unless several perpendicular views of the lesion are seen, and of diffuse disease, such that the "normal" segment used as a denominator in defining percent diameter stenosis frequently is not normal.[150, 157]

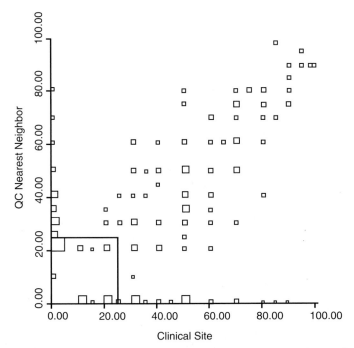

FIGURE 23–12. Variability between the quality control (QC) site (*vertical axis*) and the clinical site (*horizontal axis*) for readings of percent stenosis of the left main coronary artery in the Coronary Artery Surgery Study. The area of each square is proportional to the number of cases with that reading. The large square at the lower left represents cases in which both readers considered the segment nonstenotic. The marked variability in interpretation of the degree of disease in the left main coronary artery is readily apparent. (From Fisher, L.D., Judkins, M.P., Lesperance, J., et al.: Reproducibility of coronary arteriographic reading in the Coronary Artery Surgery Study (CASS). Cathet. Cardiovasc. Diagn. 8:569, 1982, with permission. Copyright © 1982 John Wiley & Sons, Inc.)

EVALUATION, INTERPRETATION, AND IMPLICATIONS OF THE CORONARY ANGIOGRAM

Eighty-one percent of patients referred for catheterization with the diagnosis of coronary artery disease are found to have coronary disease, and in 77 percent the disease is significant (defined as greater than 50 percent diameter narrowing of the left main coronary artery or greater than 75 percent narrowing of the other vessels).[50] One-vessel disease is found in 24 percent of cases, two-vessel disease in 27 percent, three-vessel disease in 49 percent, and left main coronary artery disease in 10 percent. Seventy-five percent of patients have complete or nearly complete occlusions, usually in association with disease elsewhere.

It is important to systematically evaluate the coronary angiogram to define the extent and severity of disease that is present. The course and caliber of each vessel should be carefully traced. The number of diseased vessels, the number of lesions in each vessel, and the severity of the lesions also must be evaluated. It is important to consider the area of myocardium supplied by each diseased vessel and whether the diseased vessel supplies viable or necrotic myocardium. The status of the distal vessel should also be considered. Lesion length and proximal versus distal location of the stenosis are also clinically important. The coronary angiogram should be evaluated not in isolation but in conjunction with information regarding the function of each left ventricular region. Collateral vessels should be looked for, time to filling of collaterals should be evaluated, and the presence of coronary artery spasm or bridging should be considered. Assessment of collaterally filled vessels is unreliable in determining the status of the vessel, and slow distal filling of vessels may imply proximal disease.

Physiologic Significance of Coronary Stenoses

Definitions of the significance of coronary stenoses are based mainly on the studies of Gould and his colleagues, in which the effects of varying degrees of stenosis on resting and hyperemic coronary blood flow were evaluated in a dog model.[158–160] These studies are illustrated in Figure 23–13. Resting coronary blood flow was found to be an insensitive indicator of the significance of coronary disease, because resting flow was unaffected until 85 percent stenosis was reached. However, hyperemic flow began to decrease at 30 to 45 percent diameter stenosis, and no hyperemia was noted when stenoses reached 88 to 93 percent in diameter.[158] Gould also found that the resistance to flow produced by stenoses in series was additive, so that each stenosis in the vessel was important, not only the most severe one.[159] In a follow-up study, Gould, Lipscomb, and Calvert reported that distal vasodilatation could be used to maintain almost normal resting flow with stenoses of up to 60 to 85 percent, but that resting flow decreased beyond this point.[160] Based on such reports, clinical studies have usually used 50 percent or 75 percent diameter narrowing to signify significant coronary artery disease.

That stenosis length as well as the number and severity of stenoses must be considered was confirmed in a dog study by Feldman and associates.[161] They reported that if the area of stenosis was short, a pressure gradient and change in resting coronary flow occurred only with a stenosis greater than 80 percent; however, if stenosis length was increased to 10 to 15 mm, a 40 to 60 percent stenosis resulted in a pressure gradient and a decrease in resting flow.

Subsequent studies have suggested that these indicators of coronary disease significance may not apply in humans, in whom diffuse coronary disease is often present. Diffuse disease was originally seen on pathologic studies[150] and more recently has been confirmed in vivo by high-frequency epicardial echocardiography[157] (Fig. 23–14) and intravascular ultrasound.[162] Ganz and colleagues found that, of 15 stenoses graded as 25 to 75 percent severity on angiograms, 7 had significant gradients at rest, with an increase in the gradient occurring after injection of contrast medium.[163] The problem with using percent diameter stenosis to reflect the significance of coronary lesions in the face of diffuse coronary artery disease is graphically shown in Figure 23–15.

Atherosclerosis is a disease of the vessel wall and not of the lumen (which is the part seen on the coronary angiogram), a fact that has been shown with intracoronary ultrasound.[164] Therefore, minor changes in the lumen may represent important, and frequently diffuse, changes in the vessel wall. This is particularly true in patients with multivessel coronary artery disease, in whom percent stenosis does not correlate with coronary flow reserve (Fig. 23–16).[165] It has been shown that minimum lesion luminal area is one of the major determinants of coronary lesion physiologic significance.[166] The minimum luminal area defined by quantitative coronary arteriography[167] (Fig. 23–17) or by videodensitometry[168] (Fig. 23–18) does predict coronary lesion physiologic significance. Coronary lesion minimal diameter defined by other geometric methods has also been shown to correlate with coronary lesion physiologic significance.[169] Quantitation of absolute luminal dimensions may also substantially decrease intraobserver and interobserver variability in angiographic interpretation. Physicians who use angiographic data for clinical decision-making need to be aware of the problems that exist with conventional use of percent diameter stenosis to define the clinical importance of coronary stenoses as well as potential approaches for improving the clinical significance of the information obtained with coronary angiography.

Prognostic Significance of Coronary Stenoses

In spite of the controversy concerning the use of percent diameter stenosis to define the significance of coronary artery disease,[170, 171] the classic definition of significant coronary artery disease—50 percent or 75 percent diameter stenosis—does predict coronary

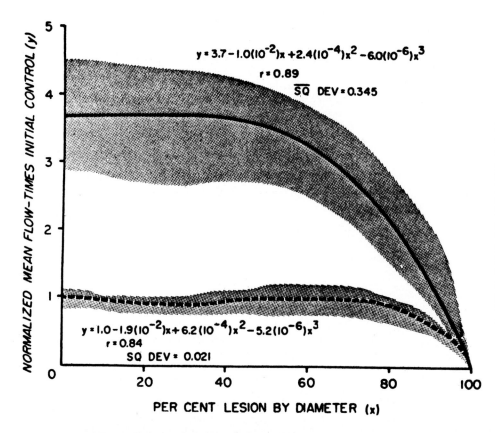

$$y = 3.7 - 1.0(10^{-2})x + 2.4(10^{-4})x^2 - 6.0(10^{-6})x^3$$

$$r = 0.89$$

$$\overline{SQ}\ DEV = 0.345$$

$$y = 1.0 - 1.9(10^{-2})x + 6.2(10^{-4})x^2 - 5.2(10^{-6})x^3$$

$$r = 0.84$$

$$SQ\ DEV = 0.021$$

FIGURE 23–13. These data from a study by Gould and his colleagues illustrate the effects of varying degrees of coronary stenosis on resting and hyperemic coronary blood flow as evaluated in a dog model. Resting mean flow is shown by the dashed line and hyperemic flow after intracoronary injection of Hypaque by the solid line. Flows are compared with control flow and expressed as ratios. The shaded area indicates the limits of the data when plotted for the individual dogs. SQ DEV = mean square of deviations. (From Gould, K.L., Lipscomb, K., and Hamilton, G.W.: Physiologic basis for assessing critical coronary stenosis: Instantaneous flow response and regional distribution during coronary hyperemia as measures of coronary flow reserve. Am. J. Cardiol. 33:91, 1974, with permission.)

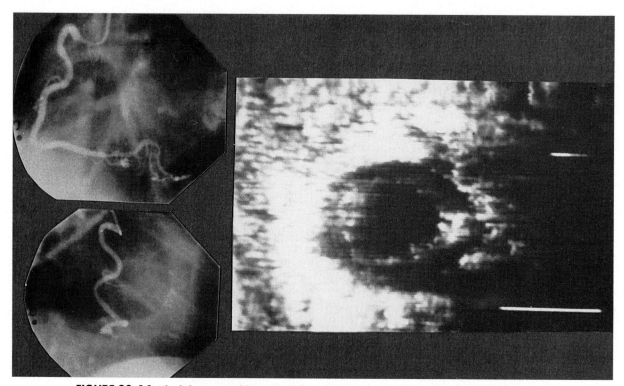

FIGURE 23–14. The left anterior oblique (*top left*) and right anterior oblique (*bottom left*) angiograms of this right coronary artery show only mild irregularities. However, the high-frequency echocardiographic image of the middle right coronary artery (*right*) shows diffuse thickening of the arterial wall. This confirms that vessels that are almost normal in angiographic appearance may be diffusely diseased. (From McPherson, D.D., Hiratzka, L.F., Lamberth, W.C., et al.: Delineation of the extent of coronary atherosclerosis by high-frequency epicardial echocardiography. N. Engl. J. Med. 316:306, 1987, with permission.)

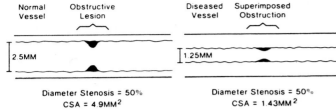

FIGURE 23–15. The markedly different effects of a 50 percent diameter stenosis in a vessel that is normal (*left*) and one that is diffusely diseased (*right*). In a normal vessel of 2.5 mm diameter, a 50 percent diameter lesion results in a luminal cross-sectional area (CSA) of 4.9 mm². If the same vessel is diffusely diseased with a luminal diameter of 1.25 mm, a 50 percent stenosis results in a markedly decreased luminal area of 1.43 mm². Because coronary disease often is a diffuse process, percent stenosis alone is an inadequate means of assessing the severity of coronary artery disease. (Adapted from Harrison, D.G., White, C.W., Hiratzka, L.F., et al.: The value of lesion cross-sectional area determined by quantitative coronary angiography in assessing the physiologic significance of proximal left anterior descending coronary arterial stenoses. Circulation 69:1117, 1984, with permission of the American Heart Association, Inc.)

risk. In 1970, Friesinger, Page, and Ross reported on 244 patients with chest pain who were followed for a mean of 53 months.[172] The 5-year survival rate was 97 percent in patients with normal coronary arteries and 73 percent in patients with coronary artery disease. Survival rate decreased with increasing coronary disease severity as defined by a coronary artery disease score. Bruschke and associates confirmed the importance of the presence or absence of coronary artery disease in relation to the risk of cardiac events.[173] In 342 patients with normal coronary arteries, there was a 0.6 percent 5-year cardiac mortality rate and a 0.9 percent incidence of myocardial infarction, compared with a 5.3 percent incidence of cardiac mortality and a 3.5 percent incidence of myocardial infarction in patients with minimal (30 to 50 percent) coronary narrowings.

In 1974, Webster reported on 469 patients with 80 to 100 percent proximal coronary lesions.[174] Yearly attrition was 4 percent with LAD coronary artery disease, 2.3 percent with RCA disease,

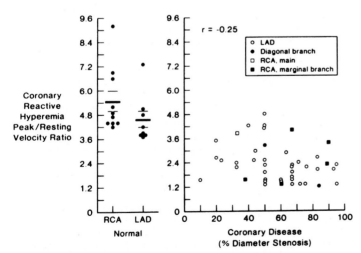

FIGURE 23–16. Relation between the coronary hyperemic response obtained during intraoperative Doppler studies (*vertical axis*) and percent diameter stenosis (*horizontal axis*) for normal coronary vessels (*left*) and for diseased coronary arteries (*right*). The normal ratio of peak to resting velocity is greater than 3.6:1. The right panel clearly shows that percent diameter stenosis does not adequately predict the coronary reactive hyperemic response and therefore does not accurately reflect the physiologic significance of coronary lesions. RCA = right coronary artery; LAD = left anterior descending coronary artery. (From White, C.W., Wright, C.B., Doty, D.B., et al.: Does visual interpretation of the coronary arteriogram predict the physiologic importance of a coronary stenosis? N. Engl. J. Med. 310:821, 1984, with permission.)

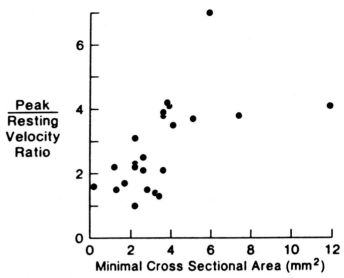

FIGURE 23–17. Relation between the ratio of peak to resting velocity (*vertical axis*) and coronary luminal minimal cross-sectional area defined by the Brown-Dodge method of quantitative coronary arteriography (*horizontal axis*). (From Harrison, D.G., White, C.W., Hiratzka, L.F., et al.: The value of lesion cross-sectional area determined by quantitative coronary angiography in assessing the physiologic significance of proximal left anterior descending coronary arterial stenoses. Circulation 69:1116, 1984, with permission of the American Heart Association, Inc.)

6.6 percent with two-vessel disease and 10 percent with three-vessel disease. The 6-year mortality rates were 25.5 percent, 14 percent, 41.5 percent, and 63 percent, respectively, in these patient groups, confirming the impact of coronary artery disease on mortality. In 1974, Humphries and colleagues also reported that the severity of coronary atherosclerotic disease, as expressed by a coronary score based on the number of vessels diseased and the severity of the disease, was an important predictor of survival for 244 patients at 5 to 12 years after coronary arteriography.[175]

Harris and colleagues reported that the 5-year survival rate of patients with coronary disease who were treated medically was inversely related to the number of vessels with 75 percent or greater stenosis, but that survival was also related to left ventricular function.[176] Burggraf and Parker, in a review of 259 patients, found that survival was inversely related to the number of vessels having greater than 50 percent or greater than 75 percent stenosis,[177] but survival was also affected by hypertension, congestive heart failure, abnormal hemodynamics, or left ventricular asynergy.

The CASS registry data for patients treated medically also show that the 4-year survival rate is inversely related to the number of vessels with greater than 70 percent stenosis; the 4-year survival rates were 92 percent for patients with one-vessel disease, 84 percent for those with two-vessel disease, and 68 percent for those with three-vessel disease (Fig. 23–19).[178] The survival rate was further decreased in patients who also had left main coronary artery stenosis.

Others have looked more specifically at the effect of left main coronary artery stenosis. Conley and associates reported that the 3-year survival rate was only 50 percent in patients with 50 percent or greater left main coronary artery stenosis and that this rate decreased to 41 percent in patients with 70 percent or greater stenosis.[179] Congestive heart failure, resting chest pain, cardiomegaly on chest radiography, ST-T segment changes, abnormal left ventricular function, and elevated left ventricular end-diastolic pressure also predicted mortality. Campeau and co-workers reported in 1978 that the 7-year survival rate of patients with greater than 50 percent left main coronary artery stenosis who were treated medically was 48.5 percent.[180]

In summary, although problems exist in interpretation of coronary angiograms in relation to pathologic specimens, in variability

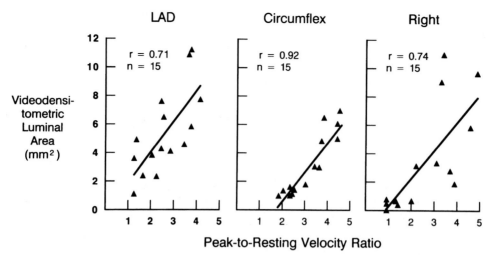

FIGURE 23–18. Absolute coronary luminal areas defined by videodensitometric techniques (*vertical axis*) also correlate with the coronary reactive hyperemic response as defined by studies of the ratio of peak to resting velocity (*horizontal axis*) in the left anterior descending (LAD, *left panel*), circumflex (*center panel*), and right (*right panel*) coronary arteries. (From Johnson, M.R., Skorton, D.J., Ericksen, E.E., et al.: Videodensitometric analysis of coronary stenoses: In vivo geometric and physiologic validation in humans. Invest. Radiol. 23:896, 1988, with permission.)

of angiographic interpretation, and in the definition of a significant coronary stenosis, the presence of coronary disease on coronary angiograms does have major prognostic significance.

Implications of Coronary Stenosis Morphology

It has been suggested that the morphologic characteristics of stenoses seen on coronary angiograms may also predict the clinical state. The classic paper of DeWood and colleagues concerning the high incidence of total thrombotic arterial occlusion in the early hours after myocardial infarction reported that in 59 patients with angiographic features suggestive of clot, a Fogarty catheter retrieved clot in 88 percent, suggesting that clot could be defined angiographically.[181] In only 5 patients was clot found intraoperatively that was not seen angiographically. Figure 23–20 shows an intravascular filling defect seen on a coronary angiogram that was confirmed to be thrombus because it disappeared after lytic therapy with urokinase. Others have determined the angiographic presence of coronary thrombi and correlated this with a patient's clinical status.

Capone and associates evaluated the angiograms of 119 patients with unstable and 35 with stable angina.[182] Intracoronary thrombi, defined as intravascular filling defects, were present in 37 percent of the patients with unstable angina but in no patients with stable angina. If the unstable angina patients had rest pain within 24 hours of catheterization, the incidence of intracoronary thrombus was 52 percent, compared with 28 percent in patients whose rest pain occurred 1 to 14 days before angiography. In a similar study, Bresnahan and co-workers evaluated 286 angiograms and in 29 of these found intracoronary thrombus, defined as contrast staining or an intravascular filling defect without associated calcification.[183] Eighty-three percent of patients with intracoronary thrombi had unstable angina. Likewise, thrombus was found in 36 percent of patients with unstable angina, compared with 2.5 percent of patients with stable angina. No clot was found in patients with stable angina unless they had a prior history of myocardial infarction.

It therefore appears that thrombus is commonly seen on the angiograms of patients with unstable angina, but whether this thrombus progresses to cause total occlusion and myocardial infarction requires further study.

Others have evaluated stenosis morphology and related it to the patient's clinical status. Levin evaluated 73 coronary stenoses by postmortem angiography and histology.[184] If a stenosis had a smooth

or hourglass angiographic appearance without associated intracoronary lucency, only 11.4 percent were histologically complicated by plaque rupture, hemorrhage, or clot. On the other hand, if angiographically the stenosis was irregular or there was intracoronary lucency, 78.9 percent were found to be histologically complicated plaques. The angiogram was 88 percent sensitive and 79 percent specific for defining histologically complicated plaques. Ambrose and colleagues reported that eccentric stenoses with a narrow neck or totally irregular stenoses were seen in 71 percent of patients with unstable angina but in only 16 percent of patients with stable angina.[185] They found no difference in the number of vessels diseased or the degree of coronary obstruction between the patient groups. In 41 patients with recent myocardial infarction and subtotal occlusions, 66 percent of infarct vessel stenoses were eccentric with a narrow neck or were irregular; this type of stenosis was found in only 11 percent of noninfarcted vessels.[186] There was also a high incidence (61 percent) of eccentric stenoses with narrow necks or irregular stenoses in infarct vessels after streptokinase therapy.

Wilson, Holida, and White described a quantitative definition of luminal irregularity, the ulceration index, and found that luminal irregularity was significantly greater in patients with unstable angina and after myocardial infarction than in patients with stable angina and in the noninfarct vessels of patients after myocardial infarction.[187] By quantitative angiography, the lesions in the patients with unstable angina were somewhat more severe than those in the other clinical syndromes.

Rehr and associates reviewed a series of patients, 50 with rest angina within the previous week and 42 with stable angina.[188] Patients with rest angina were significantly more likely to have angiographically defined thrombus or lesion complexity than were patients with stable angina, although there was no difference in the severity of coronary disease or frequency of collaterals in the two groups. Although few women (n = 29) were included in the study, it is of potential therapeutic importance that there were no significant differences in angiographic morphology between females with rest angina and those with stable angina. Kapashi and colleagues found a 43 percent incidence of type II eccentric lesions (asymmetric narrowing with a narrow neck and overhanging irregular edges) in 110 lesions of 100 patients with unstable angina; in contrast, this angiographic morphology was seen in only 11 percent of 51 lesions in 50 patients with stable angina.[189]

A more recent study has confirmed a relation between the

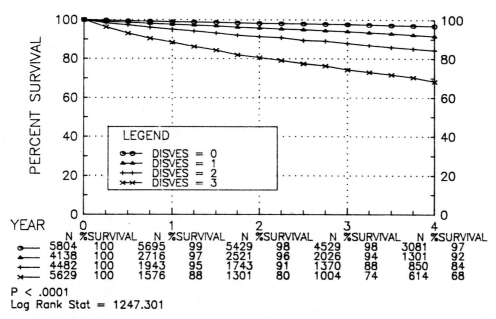

DISEASED VESSELS

FIGURE 23-19. Despite difficulties in interpretation of the data on coronary angiograms, survival is related to the number of coronary arteries containing significant disease (here defined as greater than 70 percent stenosis). DISVES = diseased vessels. (From Mock, M.B., Ringquist, I., Fisher, L.D., et al.: Survival of medically treated patients in the Coronary Artery Surgery Study (CASS) registry. Circulation 66:564, 1982, with permission of the American Heart Association, Inc.)

clinical syndrome with which the patient presents and angiographic lesion morphology, a relation that may shed additional light on the pathophysiology of acute coronary syndromes.[190] Of 160 patients with coronary disease who underwent angiography, 60 had stable angina, 78 had unstable angina, and 22 had a recent myocardial infarction that had been treated with thrombolytic therapy. Lesions were classified as complex on the basis of eccentricity, irregular borders, presence of ulceration, calcification, presence of thrombi, or presence of total occlusion. Although the number of diseased vessels and the location of disease were similar in the stable and unstable angina patient groups, significantly more patients with unstable angina or with recent myocardial infarction had complex

lesions (59 percent and 54 percent, respectively) than did patients with stable angina (25 percent). Angiographic signs of thrombus were seen in 34 percent of unstable angina patients and in 27 percent of postmyocardial infarction patients but in only 1.5 percent of stable angina patients. Thrombi were more commonly seen if angiographic evaluation was performed within 48 hours of pain in the patients with unstable angina.

In an attempt to decrease the subjectivity of qualitative analyses of lesion morphology, Kalbfleisch and colleagues have proposed an automated approach to quantitation of lesion morphology that involves automatic edge detection and sequential edge linking.[191] The method has been shown to be reproducible, and patients with

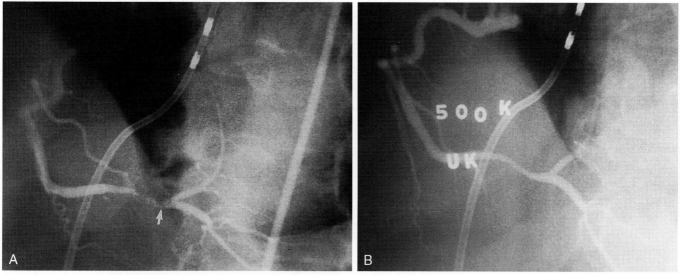

FIGURE 23-20. An intravascular filling defect has been said to represent intracoronary thrombus. In this case, an intravascular filling defect in the distal right coronary artery (*A, arrow*) disappeared after thrombolytic therapy with urokinase (*B*).

unstable angina had significant morphometric differences from patients with stable angina. Taken together, the studies of the association between coronary lesion morphologic characteristics and specific clinical syndromes imply that intimal disruption and clot formation are important in the pathophysiology of unstable ischemic syndromes.

Lesion morphology has also been suggested to be important in predicting the success, risk, and ultimate outcome after percutaneous transluminal coronary angioplasty. As reported by the Subcommittee on Percutaneous Transluminal Coronary Angioplasty of the ACC/AHA Task Force, lesions can be classified by the characteristics shown in Table 23–4 into type A, type B, or type C.[1] Examples of each lesion type are shown in Figure 23–21. Type A lesions have an anticipated success rate of greater than 85 percent and a low

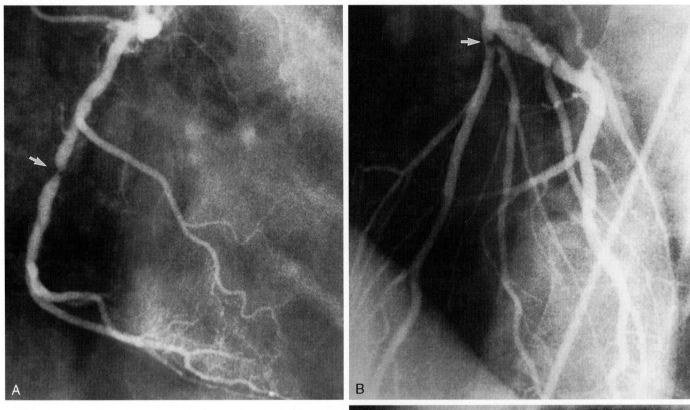

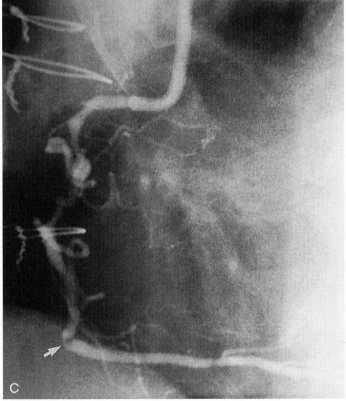

FIGURE 23–21. Panel *A*, shows a type A lesion *(arrow)* of the right coronary artery that is discrete and concentric and does not involve any major side branches. Panel B shows an example of a type B lesion *(arrow)* of the proximal left anterior descending coronary artery (left anterior oblique, cranial projection) that is eccentric and involves the origin of a large diagonal branch. Panel C shows a lesion *(arrow)* at the junction of the middle and distal right coronary artery that is classified as type C because of an extremely tortuous proximal segment and because of the location of the lesion in an extremely angulated segment (a bend of greater than 90 degrees).

TABLE 23–4. CHARACTERISTICS OF TYPE A, B, AND C LESIONS (Lesion-Specific Characteristics)

Type A Lesions (high success, >85%; low risk)
Discrete (<10 mm length)
Concentric
Readily accessible
Nonangulated segment, <45°
Smooth contour
Little or no calcification
Less than totally occlusive
Not ostial in location
No major branch involvement
Absence of thrombus

Type B Lesions (moderate success, 60 to 85%; moderate risk)
Tubular (10–20 mm length)
Eccentric
Moderate tortuosity of proximal segment
Moderately angulated segment, 45–90°
Irregular contour
Moderate to heavy calcification
Total occlusions <3 months old
Ostial in location
Bifurcation lesions requiring double guidewires
Some thrombus present

Type C Lesions (low success, <60%; high risk)
Diffuse (>2 cm length)
Excessive tortuosity of proximal segment
Extremely angulated segments >90°
Total occlusion >3 months old
Inability to protect major side branches
Degenerated vein grafts with friable lesions

From Ryan, T.J., Faxon, D.P., Gunnar, R.M., et al.: Guidelines for percutaneous transluminal coronary angioplasty: A report of the American College of Cardiology/American Heart Association Task Force on Assessment of Diagnostic and Therapeutic Cardiovascular Procedures (Subcommittee on Percutaneous Transluminal Coronary Angioplasty). J. Am. Coll. Cardiol. 12:538, 1988. Reprinted with permission from the American College of Cardiology.

risk of abrupt closure; type B lesions have a predicted success rate of 60 to 85 percent or a moderate risk of abrupt closure, or both; and type C lesions have a low success rate (less than 60 percent) or a high risk of abrupt closure, or both.

That clinical characteristics and lesion morphology predict occurrence of adverse events (i.e., death, myocardial infarction, bypass surgery, and reintervention) in patients during and immediately after angioplasty is confirmed by a review of data from the CARPORT and MERCATOR studies.[192] In these studies, although no quantitative angiographic variable was associated with adverse cardiac events, univariate analysis showed that major adverse cardiac events were associated with unstable angina, a type C lesion, a lesion located at a bend of greater than 45 degrees, a stenosis in the middle segment of the artery, and angiographically visible dissection. Multivariate predictors of adverse events included unstable angina, a lesion located at a bend of greater than 45 degrees, and angiographically visible dissection. Unfortunately, interobserver discordance in the definition of qualitative lesion morphology can be high, up to 39 percent for classification of lesions as type A, type B, or type C.[193]

Ellis and colleagues reported that both angiographic morphology and clinical factors are important in predicting acute closure after native vessel angioplasty.[194] Multivariate analysis revealed seven preprocedural and four procedural variables related to acute closure, including a long stenosis, female gender, stenosis at a bend point of greater than 45 degrees, stenosis at a branch point, stenosis-associated thrombus, other stenoses in the vessel, multivessel disease, postangioplasty percent stenosis, intimal tear or dissection, use of prolonged heparin infusion, and postangioplasty gradient of 20 mm Hg or more. A multivariate analysis including both preprocedural and procedural variables revealed that acute closure was related, in decreasing order, to postangioplasty percent stenosis, dissection, prolonged postangioplasty heparin use, branch point location, fixed bend point stenosis, and other stenoses in the vessel dilated. Therefore, although an estimation of risk can be made before angioplasty, the most powerful predictors of closure become apparent only during the procedure.

Ellis and colleagues confirmed the ability of the ACC/AHA classification scheme to predict relative angioplasty success and risk in patients with multivessel disease; however, they suggested that type B lesions be subdivided to better differentiate success and risk, with B1 lesions having one type B characteristic and B2 lesions having two or more type B characteristics.[195] With the use of this schema, success was achieved in 92 percent of type A, 84 percent of type B1, 76 percent type of B2, and 61 percent of type C lesions, with complications occurring in 2, 4, 10, and 21 percent of these same patient groups, respectively.

Moushmoush and co-workers analyzed stenosis morphology prospectively before angioplasty in 328 stenoses in 97 patients.[196] They found no difference in success rate between type A and type B lesions but did find a significantly decreased success rate for type C lesions. Although the ACC/AHA classification scheme did predict lesions with a higher likelihood of an adverse outcome, failed angioplasty was best predicted by a total occlusion for longer than 3 months, a total occlusion for less than 3 months, and a stenosis at a bend point of greater than 90 degrees in the vessel. Owing to the subjectiveness of many of the characteristics used to classify lesions as type A, B, or C (a 25 percent interobserver variability was noted in this study), the authors suggested that a simplified grading system based on fewer and more objective criteria was just as helpful.

A series by Myler and associates[197] has suggested that newer angioplasty catheters and techniques may have increased the success rate and decreased the adverse event rate for angioplasty of even complicated (i.e., type B or type C) lesions. In a series of 1000 lesions in 533 patients, success rates for the three lesion classes were 99 percent for type A (8 percent of lesions), 92 percent for type B (48 percent of lesions), and 90 percent for type C (44 percent of lesions). Untoward events (myocardial infarction or emergency bypass surgery; there were no in-hospital deaths) occurred in 1.2 percent of type A, 1.9 percent of type B, and 2 percent of type C lesions. The authors found that subdividing B and C lesions into B1, B2, C1 (one type C characteristic), and C2 (two or more type C characteristics) provided further prognostic information as to the probable success and risks of angioplasty. The only factor found to be associated with untoward events was the presence of thrombus.

These studies suggest that more precise characterization of the angiographic appearance of coronary stenoses is of clinical importance and that morphologic characteristics of the stenosis should be considered in deciding the best therapy to offer patients with coronary artery disease.

TRAPS TO AVOID IN THE PERFORMANCE AND INTERPRETATION OF CORONARY ANGIOGRAMS

Accurate diagnosis of coronary artery disease depends on performance of a complete angiographic study and on correct interpretation of the study. Several authors have described problems that commonly arise in coronary angiography.[18, 22, 50, 67, 198, 199] Potential errors that can be made in the performance or interpretation of the coronary angiogram and that can result in an incomplete or misinterpreted study include the following:

1. The use of a fixed number of projections or only specific projections, particularly without cranially or caudally angulated projections, results in an incomplete study. Unless each vascular segment is viewed perpendicular to the plane of the x-ray beam

(i.e., without foreshortening), it cannot be adequately analyzed. In addition, adequate views and angles are needed so that no superimposition of vessels masks lesions. To evaluate eccentric stenoses, angiograms in two views at least 90 degrees apart are essential.

2. Inadequate force of injection or pulsatile injection of contrast media may result in a misinterpreted study. Unless contrast is injected to produce almost complete opacification of the vessel (with some contrast reflux into the coronary sinus), pockets of unopacified blood may be interpreted as stenoses or ostial lesions may be missed.

3. Iatrogenically induced coronary artery spasm can be misinterpreted as a proximal coronary lesion. It is much more common in the RCA than in the left coronary artery. If a proximal lesion must be differentiated from spasm, repeating the angiogram after administration of nitroglycerin or nifedipine or performing sinus flush shots may help resolve the question. Spasm is also suggested if the narrowing occurs at or within a few millimeters of the catheter tip without any alteration in coronary flow, chest pain, or ST-T segment changes.

4. Superselective coronary injections can result not only in misinterpretation of a branch vessel as being totally occluded but also, in the case of injection into a RCA beyond the conal branch, in failure to identify collaterals to the LAD circulation. Superselective injection can also produce ventricular fibrillation. Reflux of contrast into the sinus of Vasalva should be seen, and the proximal segment of the vessel should be carefully analyzed.

5. Angiographic projections in which the vessels overlie dense structures such as the spine or the diaphragm make adequate visualization of the coronary arteries difficult. To get good opacification of the distal RCA, the patient must inspire during injections to move the diaphragm out of the way. Similarly, views in which the segment of interest is not obscured by the spine are critical.

6. To avoid missing left main coronary artery lesions, the artery should be filmed in the frontal projection and with the vessel off the spine. Catheter damping and absence of reflux into the coronary sinus suggest an ostial lesion.

7. Absent blood supply to a portion of the heart may be produced by a flush coronary occlusion or by an anomalous coronary vessel that has not yet been visualized. Collaterals suggest an occlusion or severe disease in a vessel proximal to the collateral dependent bed.

8. Recanalized vessels may be present. In one third of cases, vessels that have been totally occluded subsequently recanalize.

9. Coronary bridging must be differentiated from a coronary lesion because the implications of bridging are different from those of atherosclerotic coronary disease.

10. Coronary veins can be mistaken for arteries.

11. "Artifactual" collaterals may appear if contrast is injected too vigorously.

GENERAL RECOMMENDATIONS

The safest and most complete coronary angiographic study requires an expert and skilled angiographer, a competent and dedicated catheterization laboratory team, a good imaging system, and the briefest possible complete study. A catheterization laboratory should usually be operated only in conjunction with surgical facilities. Performance of safe and adequate coronary angiography requires not only technical skills but also good clinical judgment and attention to detail. Fewer than 25 percent of angiograms performed for chest pain in a catheterization laboratory should show no significant coronary artery disease.[17]

The Intersociety Commission on Heart Disease Resources recommended in 1983 that no fewer than 150 angiographic studies per year should be done by each physician to obtain the best quality studies at the least risk to the patient.[53] A laboratory minimum of 300 cases per year was also suggested. Additional performance

standards were that no more than 1 percent of studies should be considered inadequate or require a repeat procedure for diagnosis, unless the initial study had become prolonged for some reason, and that the mortality rate in stable patients undergoing elective angiography should be less than 0.1 percent.

References

1. Ryan, T.J., Faxon, D.P., Gunnar, R.M., et al.: Guidelines for percutaneous transluminal coronary angioplasty: A report of the American College of Cardiology/American Heart Association Task Force on Assessment of Diagnostic and Therapeutic Cardiovascular Procedures (Subcommittee on Percutaneous Transluminal Coronary Angioplasty). J. Am. Coll. Cardiol. 12:529, 1988.
2. American Heart Association: 1993 Heart and Stroke Facts Statistics. Dallas, American Heart Association, 1992, p. 8.
3. Kern, M.J., Cohen, M., Talley, J.D., et al.: Early ambulation after 5 French diagnostic cardiac catheterization: Results of a multicenter trial. J. Am. Coll. Cardiol. 15:1475, 1990.
4. Steckelberg, J.M., Vlietstra, R.E., Ludwig, J., et al.: Werner Forssman (1904–1979) and his unusual success story. Mayo Clin. Proc. 54:746, 1979.
5. Chavez, I., Dorbecker, N., and Celis, A.: Direct intracardiac angiography: Its diagnostic value. Am. Heart J. 33:560, 1947.
6. Radner, S.: An attempt at the roentgenologic visualization of coronary blood vessels in man. Acta Radiol. 26:497, 1945.
7. Lehman, J.S., Boyer, R.A., and Winter, F.S.: Coronary arteriography. Am. J. Roentgenol. 81:749, 1959.
8. Seldinger, S.I.: Catheter replacement of the needle in percutaneous arteriography: A new technique. Acta Radiol. 39:368, 1953.
9. Dotter, C.T., and Frische, L.H.: Visualization of the coronary circulation by occlusion aortography: A practical method. Radiology 71:502, 1958.
10. Amplatz, K.: Technics of coronary arteriography. Circulation 27:101, 1963.
11. Williams, J.A., Littmann, D., Hall, J.H., et al.: Coronary arteriography: II. Clinical experiences with the loop-end catheter. N. Engl. J. Med. 262:328, 1960.
12. Sones, F.M., Shirey, E.K., Proudfit, W.L., et al.: Cine-coronary arteriography. (Abstract.) Circulation 20:773, 1959.
13. Sones, F.M., Jr., and Shirey, E.K.: Cine coronary arteriography. Mod. Concepts Cardiovasc. Dis. 31:735-738, 1962.
14. Ricketts, H.J., and Abrams, H.L.: Percutaneous selective coronary cine arteriography. J.A.M.A. 181:620, 1962.
15. Judkins, M.P.: Selective coronary arteriography: Part 1. A percutaneous transfemoral technic. Radiology 89:815, 1967.
16. Amplatz, K., Formanek, G., Stanger, P., et al.: Mechanics of selective coronary artery catheterization via femoral approach. Radiology 89:1040, 1967.
17. Ross, J.R., Jr., Brandenburg, R.O., Dinsmore, R.E., et al.: Guidelines for coronary angiography: A report of the American College of Cardiology/American Heart Association Task Force on Assessment of Diagnostic and Therapeutic Cardiovascular Procedures (Subcommittee on Coronary Angiography). Circulation 76:963A, 1987.
18. Conti, C.R.: Coronary arteriography. Circulation 55:227, 1977.
19. Carabello, B.A., and Grossman, W.: Bedside hemodynamic monitoring, cardiac catheterization, and pulmonary angiography. In Cohn, P.F., and Wynne, J. (eds.): Diagnostic Methods in Clinical Cardiology. Boston, Little, Brown, 1982, p. 235.
20. Cohn, P.F., and Goldberg, S.: Cardiac catheterization and coronary arteriography. In Cohn, P.F. (ed.): Diagnosis and Therapy of Coronary Artery Disease. Boston, Martinus Nijhoff, 1985, p. 219.
21. Assessment of coronary artery disease. In Yang, S.S., Bentivoglio, L.G., Maranhao, V., et al. (eds.): From Cardiac Catheterization Data to Hemodynamic Parameters. 3rd ed. Philadelphia, F.A. Davis, 1988, p. 256.
22. Baim, D.S., and Grossman, W.: Coronary angiography. In Grossman, W., and Baim, D.S. (eds.): Cardiac Catheterization, Angiography, and Intervention. 4th ed. Philadelphia, Lea & Febiger, 1991, p. 185.
23. Grossman, W.: Cardiac Catheterization. In Braunwald, E. (ed.): Heart Disease: A Textbook of Cardiovascular Medicine. 4th ed. Philadelphia, W.B. Saunders, 1992, p. 180.
24. Segar, D.S., Brown, S.E., Sawada, S.G., et al.: Dobutamine stress echocardiography: Correlation with coronary lesion severity as determined by quantitative angiography. J. Am. Coll. Cardiol. 19:1197, 1992.
25. Heupler, F.A., Proudfit, S.L., and Razavi, M.: Ergonovine maleate provocative test for coronary arterial spasm. Am. J. Cardiol. 41:631, 1978.
26. Cannon, R.O., III, Watson, R.M., Rosing, D.R., et al.: Angina caused by reduced vasodilator reserve of the small coronary arteries. J. Am. Coll. Cardiol. 1:1359, 1983.
27. Richardson, J.V., Kouchoukos, N.T., Wright, J.O., III, et al.: Combined aortic valve replacement and myocardial revascularization: Results in 220 patients. Circulation 59:75, 1979.
28. Green, S.J., Pizzarello, R.A., Padmanabhan, V.T., et al.: Relation of angina pectoris to coronary artery disease in aortic valve stenosis. Am. J. Cardiol. 55:1063, 1985.
29. Passamani, E., Davis, K.B., Gillespie, M.J., et al.: A randomized trial of coronary artery bypass surgery: Survival of patients with a low ejection fraction. N. Engl. J. Med. 312:1665, 1985.
30. Gao, S.Z., Schroeder, J.S., Hunt, S., et al.: Retransplantation for severe accelerated coronary artery disease in heart transplant recipients. Am. J. Cardiol. 62:876, 1988.
31. Hays, J.T., Mahmarian, J.J., Cochran, A.J., et al.: Dobutamine thallium-201 tomography for evaluating patients with suspected coronary artery disease unable

to undergo exercise or vasodilator pharmacologic stress testing. J. Am. Coll. Cardiol. 21:1583, 1993.

32. Lane, R.T., Sawada, S.G., Segar, D.S., et al.: Dobutamine stress echocardiography for assessment of cardiac risk before noncardiac surgery. Am. J. Cardiol. 68:976, 1991.

33. Graboys, T.B., Biegelsen, B., Lampert, S., et al.: Results of a second-opinion trial among patients recommended for coronary angiography. J.A.M.A. 268:2537, 1992.

34. Adams, D.F., Fraser, D.B., and Abrams, H.L.: The complications of coronary arteriography. Circulation 48:609, 1973.

35. Bourassa, M.C., and Noble, J.: Complication rate of coronary arteriography: A review of 5250 cases studied by a percutaneous femoral technique. Circulation 53:106, 1976.

36. Davis, K., Kennedy, J.W., Kemp, H.G., Jr., et al.: Complications of coronary arteriography from the collaborative study of coronary artery surgery (CASS). Circulation 59:1105, 1979.

37. Kennedy, J.W., and the Registry Committee of the Society for Cardiac Angiography: Complications associated with cardiac catheterization and angiography. Cathet. Cardiovasc. Diagn. 8:5, 1982.

38. Johnson, L.W., Lozner, E.C., Johnson, S., et al.: Coronary arteriography 1984–1987: A report of the Registry of the Society for Cardiac Angiography and Interventions. I: Results and complications. Cathet. Cardiovasc. Diagn. 17:5, 1989.

39. Wyman, R.M., Safian, R.D., Portway, V., et al.: Current complications of diagnostic and therapeutic cardiac catheterization. J. Am. Coll. Cardiol. 12:1400, 1988.

40. Noto, T.J., Jr., Johnson, L.W., Krone, R., et al.: Cardiac catheterization 1990: A report of the Registry of the Society for Cardiac Angiography and Interventions (SCA&I). Cathet. Cardiovasc. Diagn. 24:75, 1991.

41. Nishimura, R.A., Holmes, D.R., Jr., McFarland, T.M., et al.: Ventricular arrhythmias during coronary angiography in patients with angina pectoris or chest pain syndromes. Am. J. Cardiol. 53:1496, 1984.

42. Gordon, P.R., Abrams, C., Gash, A.K., et al.: Pericatheterization risk factors in left main coronary artery stenosis. Am. J. Cardiol. 59:1080, 1987.

43. Rocha-Singh, K.J., Schwend, R.B., Otis, S.M., et al.: Frequency and nonsurgical therapy of femoral artery pseudoaneurysm complicating interventional cardiology procedures. Am. J. Cardiol. 73:1012, 1994.

44. Cox, G.S., Young, J.R., Gray, B.R., et al.: Ultrasound-guided compression repair of postcatheterization pseudoaneurysms: Results of treatment in one hundred cases. J. Vasc. Surg. 19:683, 1994.

45. Cohen, J.R., Sardari, F., Glener, L., et al.: Complications of diagnostic cardiac catheterization requiring surgical intervention. Am. J. Cardiol. 67:787, 1991.

46. Hildner, F.J., Javier, R.P., Ramaswamy, K., et al.: Pseudo complications of cardiac catheterization. Chest 63:15, 1973.

47. Hildner, F.J., Javier, R.P., Tolentino, A., et al.: Pseudo complications of cardiac catheterization: Update. Cathet. Cardiovasc. Diagn., 8:43, 1982.

48. Franch, R.H., King, S.B., III, and Douglas, J.S., Jr.: Techniques of cardiac catheterization including coronary arteriography. In Schlant, R.C., and Alexander, R.W. (eds.): The Heart: Arteries and Veins. 8th ed. New York, McGraw-Hill, 1994, p. 2381.

49. Judkins, M.P., and Gander, M.P.: Prevention of complications of coronary arteriography. (Editorial.) Circulation 49:599, 1974.

50. Gensini, G.G.: Coronary arteriography. In Braunwald, E. (ed.): Heart Disease: A Textbook of Cardiovascular Medicine. 2nd ed. Philadelphia, W.B. Saunders, 1984, p. 304.

51. Gold, H.K., Leinbach, R.C., Sanders, C.A., et al.: Intraaortic balloon pumping for control of recurrent myocardial ischemia. Circulation 47:1197, 1973.

52. Weintraub, R.M., Voukydis, P.C., Aroesty, J.M., et al.: Treatment of preinfarction angina with intraaortic balloon counterpulsation and surgery. Am. J. Cardiol. 34:809, 1974.

53. Friesinger, G.C., Adams, D.F., Bourassa, M.G., et al.: Optimal resources for examination of the heart and lungs: Cardiac catheterization and radiographic facilities. Examination of the Chest and Cardiovascular System Study Group. Circulation 68:893A, 1983.

54. Lehmann, K.G., and Chen, Y-C.J.: Reduction of ventricular arrhythmias by atropine during coronary arteriography. Am. J. Cardiol. 63:447, 1989.

55. Weidner, W., MacAlpin, R., Hanafee, W., et al.: Percutaneous transaxillary selective coronary angiography. Radiology 85:652, 1965.

56. Nath, P.H., Soto, B., Holt, J.H., et al.: Selective coronary angiography by translumbar aortic puncture. Am. J. Cardiol. 52:425, 1983.

57. Marcus, R., and Grollman, J.H., Jr.: Translumbar coronary and brachiocephalic arteriography using a modified Desilets-Hoffman sheath. Cathet. Cardiovasc. Diagn. 13:288, 1987.

58. Argenal, A.J., and Baker, M.S.: Selective coronary arteriography via translumbar catheterization. Am. Heart J. 121:198, 1991.

59. Campeau, L.: Percutaneous radial artery approach for coronary angiography. Cathet. Cardiovasc. Diagn. 16:3, 1989.

60. Otaki, M.: Percutaneous transradial approach for coronary angiography. Cardiology 81:330, 1992.

61. Pearce, A.C., Schwengel, R.H., Simione, L.M., et al.: Antegrade selective coronary angiography via the transseptal approach in a patient with severe vascular disease. Cathet. Cardiovasc. Diagn. 26:300, 1992.

62. Coronary arteriography. In Verel, D., and Grainger, R.G. (eds.): Cardiac Catheterization and Angiocardiography. 3rd ed. Edinburgh, Churchill Livingstone, 1978, p. 107.

63. King, S.B., III, and Douglas, J.S., Jr.: Indications, limitations, and risks of coronary arteriography and left ventriculography. In King, S.B., III, and Douglas,

64. Heupler, F., Jr.: Coronary arteriography and left ventriculography: Sones technique. In King, S.B., III, and Douglas, J.S., Jr. (eds.): Coronary Arteriography and Angioplasty. New York, McGraw-Hill, 1985, p. 137.

65. Judkins, M.P., and Judkins, E.: Coronary arteriography and left ventriculography: Judkins technique. Part I: The Judkins technique. In King, S.B., III, and Douglas, J.S., Jr. (eds.): Coronary Arteriography and Angioplasty. New York, McGraw-Hill, 1985, p. 182.

66. King, S.B., III, and Douglas, J.S., Jr.: Coronary arteriography and left ventriculography: Multipurpose technique. In King, S.B., III, and Douglas, J.S., Jr. (eds.): Coronary Arteriography and Angioplasty. New York, McGraw-Hill, 1985, p. 239.

67. Levin, D.C., and Gardner, G.A., Jr.: Coronary arteriography. In Braunwald, E. (ed.): Heart Disease: A Textbook of Cardiovascular Medicine. 4th ed. Philadelphia, W.B. Saunders, 1992, p. 235.

68. Zir, L.M., Dinsmore, R.E., Goss, C., et al.: Experience with preformed catheters for coronary angiography by the brachial approach. Cathet. Cardiovasc. Diagn. 1:303, 1975.

69. Schoonmaker, F.W., and King, S.B., III: Coronary arteriography by the single catheter percutaneous femoral technique: Experience in 6800 cases. Circulation 50:735, 1974.

70. Barry, W.H., Levin, D.C., Green, L.H., et al.: Left heart catheterization and angiography via the percutaneous femoral approach using an arterial sheath. Cathet. Cardiovasc. Diagn. 5:401, 1979.

71. Fergusson, D.J.G., and Kamada, R.O.: Percutaneous entry of the brachial artery for left heart catheterization using a sheath. Cathet. Cardiovasc. Diagn. 7:111, 1981.

72. Fergusson, D.J.G., and Kamada, R.O.: Percutaneous entry of the brachial artery for left heart catheterization using a sheath: Further experience. Cathet. Cardiovasc. Diagn. 12:209, 1986.

73. Pepine, C.J., VonGunten, C., Hill, J.A., et al.: Percutaneous brachial catheterization using a modified sheath and new catheter system. Cathet. Cardiovasc. Diagn. 10:637, 1984.

74. Cohen, M., Rentrop, K.P., Cohen, B.M., et al.: Safety and efficacy of percutaneous entry of the brachial artery versus cutdown and arteriotomy for left-sided cardiac catheterization. Am. J. Cardiol. 57:682, 1986.

75. Campeau, L.: Percutaneous brachial catheterization. (Letter.) Cathet. Cardiovasc. Diagn. 11:443, 1985.

76. Bourdillon, P.D.V.: Use of sideholes for diagnostic coronary arteriography by Judkins technique in patients with ostial coronary stenosis. Cathet. Cardiovasc. Diagn. 27:259, 1992.

77. Feit, A., Reddy, C.V., Cowley, C., et al.: Internal mammary artery angiography should be a routine component of diagnostic coronary angiography. Cathet. Cardiovasc. Diagn. 25:85, 1992.

78. Fierens, E.: Outpatient coronary arteriography. Cathet. Cardiovasc. Diagn. 10:27, 1984.

79. Mahrer, P.R., and Eshoo, N.: Outpatient cardiac catheterization and coronary angiography. Cathet. Cardiovasc. Diagn. 7:355, 1981.

80. Klinke, W.P., Kubac, G., Talibi, T., et al.: Safety of outpatient catheterizations. Am. J. Cardiol. 56:639, 1985.

81. Mahrer, P.R., Young, C., and Magnusson, P.T.: Efficacy and safety of outpatient cardiac catheterization. Cathet. Cardiovasc. Diagn. 13:304, 1987.

82. Block, P.C., Ockene, I., Goldberg, R.J., et al.: A prospective randomized trial of outpatient versus inpatient cardiac catheterization. N. Engl. J. Med. 319:1251, 1988.

83. Lee, J.C., Bengtson, J.R., Lipscomb, J., et al.: Feasibility and cost-saving potential of outpatient cardiac catheterization. J. Am. Coll. Cardiol. 15:378, 1990.

84. Clements, S.D., Jr., and Gatlin, S.: Outpatient cardiac catheterization: A report of 3000 cases. Clin. Cardiol. 14:477, 1991.

85. Pepine, C.J., Allen, H.D., Bashore, T.M., et al.: ACC/AHA Guidelines for cardiac catheterization and cardiac catheterization laboratories. American College of Cardiology/American Heart Association Ad Hoc Task Force on Cardiac Catheterization. J. Am. Coll. Cardiol. 18:1149, 1991.

86. Brown, R.I.G., and MacDonald, A.C.: Use of 5 French catheters for cardiac catheterization and coronary angiography: A critical review. Cathet. Cardiovasc. Diagn. 13:214, 1987.

87. Talley, J.D., Smith, S.M., Walton-Shirley, M., et al.: A prospective randomized study of 4.1 French catheters utilizing the percutaneous right brachial approach for the diagnosis of coronary artery disease. Cathet. Cardiovasc. Diagn. 26:55, 1992.

88. Pande, A.K., Meier, B., Urban, P., et al.: Coronary angiography with four French catheters. Am. J. Cardiol. 70:1085, 1992.

89. Brown, E.F., Hartnell, G.G., Morris, K., et al.: Limitations in the use of five French coronary catheters. Intl. J. Card. Imaging 7:43, 1991.

90. Prewitt, K.C., Zen, B., Worthham, D.C., et al.: Increased risk of coronary artery dissection during coronary angiography with 6F catheters. Angiology 44:107, 1993.

91. Paulin, S.: Terminology for radiographic projections in cardiac angiography. (Letter.) Cathet. Cardiovasc. Diagn. 7:341, 1981.

92. Bunnell, I.L., Greene, D.G., Tandon, R.N., et al.: The half-axial projection: A new look at the proximal left coronary artery. Circulation 48:1151, 1973.

93. Sos, T.A., Lee, T.G., Levin, D.C., et al.: New lordotic projection for improved visualization of the left coronary artery and its branches. Am. J. Radiol. 121:575, 1974.

94. Eldh, P., and Silverman, J.F.: Methods of studying the proximal left anterior descending coronary artery. Radiology 113:738, 1974.

95. Arani, D.T., Bunnell, I.L., and Greene, D.G.: Lordotic right posterior oblique

projection of the left coronary artery: A special view for special anatomy. Circulation 52:504, 1975.

96. Aldridge, H.E., McLoughlin, M.J., and Taylor, K.W.: Improved diagnosis in coronary cinearteriography with routine use of 110° oblique views and cranial and caudal angulations: Comparison with standard transverse oblique views in 100 patients. Am. J. Cardiol. 36:468, 1975.

97. Aldridge, H.E.: Better visualization of the asymmetric lesion in coronary arteriography utilizing cranial and caudal angulated projections. Chest 71:502, 1977.

98. Gomes, A.S., Esposito, V.A., Grollman, J.H., Jr., et al.: Angled views in the evaluation of the right coronary artery. (Abstract.) Circulation 59 & 60:II-161, 1979.

99. Elliott, L.P., Green, C.E., Rogers, W.J., et al.: Advantage of the cranial-right anterior oblique view in diagnosing mid left anterior descending and distal right coronary artery disease. Am. J. Cardiol. 48:754, 1981.

100. Aldridge, H.E.: A decade or more of cranial and caudal angled projections in coronary arteriography: Another look. (Editorial.) Cathet. Cardiovasc. Diagn. 10:539, 1984.

101. Native coronary angiography. In Vetrovec, G.W., and Goudreau, E. (eds.): Coronary Angiography for the Interventionalist. New York, Chapman & Hall, 1994, p. 7.

102. Bypass grafts. In Vetrovec, G.W., and Goudreau, E. (eds.): Coronary Angiography for the Interventionalist. New York, Chapman & Hall, 1994, p. 29.

103. Schlesinger, M.J.: Relation of anatomic pattern to pathologic conditions of the coronary arteries. Arch. Pathol. 30:403, 1940.

104. Chaitman, B.R., Lesperance, J., Saltiel, J., et al.: Clinical, angiographic, and hemodynamic findings in patients with anomalous origin of the coronary arteries. Circulation 53:122, 1976.

105. Engel, H.J., Torres, C., and Page, H.L.: Major variations in anatomical origin of the coronary arteries: Angiographic observations in 4250 patients without associated congenital heart disease. Cathet. Cardiovasc. Diagn. 1:157, 1975.

106. Kimbiris, D., Iskandrian, A.S., Segal, B.L., et al.: Anomalous aortic origin of coronary arteries. Circulation 58:606, 1978.

107. Yamanaka, O., and Hobbs, R.E.: Coronary artery anomalies in 126,595 patients undergoing coronary arteriography. Cathet. Cardiovasc. Diagn. 21:28, 1990.

108. Levin, D.C., Fellow, K.E., and Abrams, H.L.: Hemodynamically significant primary anomalies of the coronary arteries: Angiographic aspects. Circulation 58:25, 1978.

109. Taylor, A.J., Rogan, K.M., and Virmani, R.: Sudden cardiac death associated with isolated congenital coronary artery anomalies. J. Am. Coll. Cardiol. 20:640, 1992.

110. Rose, A.G.: Multiple coronary arterioventricular fistulae. Circulation 58:178, 1978.

111. Sandhu, J.S., Uretsky, B.F., Zerbe, T.R., et al.: Coronary artery fistula in the heart transplant patient: A potential complication of endomyocardial biopsy. Circulation 79:350, 1989.

112. Fitchett, D.H., Forbes, C., and Guerraty, A.J.: Repeated endomyocardial biopsy causing coronary arterial-right ventricular fistula after cardiac transplantation. Am. J. Cardiol. 62:829, 1988.

113. Wesselhoeft, H., Fawcett, J.S., and Johnson, A.L.: Anomalous origin of the left coronary artery from the pulmonary trunk: Its clinical spectrum, pathology, and pathophysiology, based on a review of 140 cases with seven further cases. Circulation 38:403, 1968.

114. Wilson, C.L., Dlabal, P.W., Holeyfield, R.W., et al.: Anomalous origin of left coronary artery from pulmonary artery: Case report and review of literature concerning teen-agers and adults. J. Thorac. Cardiovasc. Surg. 73:887, 1977.

115. Cheitlin, M.D., DeCastro, C.M., and McAllister, H.A.: Sudden death as a complication of anomalous left coronary origin from the anterior sinus of Valsalva: A not-so-minor congenital anomaly. Circulation 50:780, 1974.

116. Brandt, B., III, Martins, J.B., and Marcus, M.L.: Anomalous origin of the right coronary artery from the left sinus of Valsalva. N. Engl. J. Med. 10:596, 1983.

117. Kragel, A.H., and Roberts, W.C.: Anomalous origin of either the right or left main coronary artery from the aorta with subsequent coursing between aorta and pulmonary trunk: Analysis of 32 necropsy cases. Am. J. Cardiol. 62:771, 1988.

118. Roberts, W.C., and Shirani, J.: The four subtypes of anomalous origin of the left main coronary artery from the right aortic sinus (or from the right coronary artery). Am. J. Cardiol. 70:119, 1992.

119. Vlodaver, Z., Neufeld, H.N., and Edwards, J.E.: Pathology of coronary disease. Semin. Roentgenol. 7:376, 1972.

120. Page, H.L., Jr., Engel, H.J., Campbell, W.B., et al.: Anomalous origin of the left circumflex coronary artery: Recognition, angiographic demonstration and clinical significance. Circulation 50:768, 1974.

121. Piovesana, P., Corrado, D., Verlato, R., et al.: Morbidity associated with anomalous origin of the left circumflex coronary artery from the right aortic sinus. Am. J. Cardiol. 63:762, 1989.

122. Lipton, M.J., Barry, W.H., Obrez, I., et al.: Isolated single coronary artery: Diagnosis, angiographic classification, and clinical significance. Radiology 130:39, 1979.

123. Shirani, J., and Roberts, W.C.: Solitary coronary ostium in the aorta in the absence of other major congenital cardiovascular anomalies. J. Am. Coll. Cardiol. 21:137, 1993.

124. Chen, Y-T., Hwang, C-L., and Kan, M-N.: Large, isolated, congenital aneurysm of the anterior descending coronary artery. Br. Heart J. 70:274, 1993.

125. Barthe, J-E., Benito, M., Sala, J., et al.: Double right coronary artery. Am. J. Cardiol. 73:622, 1994.

126. Virmani, R., Chun, P.K.C., Rogan, K., et al.: Anomalous origin of four coronary ostia from the right sinus of Valsalva. Am. J. Cardiol. 63:760, 1989.

127. Gensini, G.G., and DaCosta, B.C.B.: The coronary collateral circulation in living man. Am. J. Cardiol. 24:393, 1969.

128. Helfant, R.H., Kemp, H.G., and Gorlin, R.: Coronary atherosclerosis, coronary collaterals, and their relation to cardiac function. Ann. Intern. Med. 73:189, 1970.

129. Helfant, R.H., and Gorlin, R.: The coronary collateral circulation. (Editorial.) Ann. Intern. Med. 77:995, 1972.

130. Hamby, R.I., Aintablian, A., and Schwartz, A.: Appraisal of the functional significance of the coronary collateral circulation. Am. J. Cardiol. 38:305, 1976.

131. Tubau, J.F., Chaitman, B.R., Bourassa, M.G., et al.: Importance of coronary collateral circulation in interpreting exercise test results. Am. J. Cardiol. 47:27, 1981.

132. Hecht, H.S., Aroesty, J.M., Morkin, E., et al.: Role of the coronary collateral circulation in the preservation of left ventricular function. Radiology 114:305, 1975.

133. Williams, D.O., Amsterdam, E.A., Miller, R.R., et al.: Functional significance of coronary collateral vessels in patients with acute myocardial infarction: Relation to pump performance, cardiogenic shock, and survival. Am. J. Cardiol. 37:345, 1976.

134. Schwarz, F., Flameng, W., Ensslen, R., et al.: Effect of coronary collaterals on left ventricular function at rest and during stress. Am. Heart J. 95:570, 1978.

135. Eng, C., Patterson, R.E., Horowitz, S.F., et al.: Coronary collateral function during exercise. Circulation 66:309, 1982.

136. Probst, P., Zangl, W., and Pachinger, O.: Relation of coronary arterial occlusion pressure during percutaneous transluminal coronary angioplasty to presence of collaterals. Am. J. Cardiol. 55:1264, 1985.

137. Kyriakidis, M.K., Petropoulakis, P.N., Tentolouris, C.A., et al.: Relation between changes in blood flow of the contralateral coronary artery and the angiographic extent and function of recruitable collateral vessels arising from this artery during balloon coronary occlusion. J. Am. Coll. Cardiol. 23:869, 1994.

138. Levin, D.C.: Pathways and functional significance of the coronary collateral circulation. Circulation 50:831, 1974.

139. Kramer, J.R., Kitazume, H., Proudfit, W.L., et al.: Clinical significance of isolated coronary bridges: Benign and frequent condition involving the left anterior descending artery. Am. Heart J. 103:283, 1982.

140. Rare diseases of the coronary vasculature which can impair myocardial perfusion. In Marcus, M.L. (ed.): The Coronary Circulation in Health and Disease. New York, McGraw-Hill, 1983, p. 320.

141. Noble, J., Bourassa, M.G., Petitclerc, R., et al.: Myocardial bridging and milking effect of the left anterior descending coronary artery: Normal variant or obstruction? Am. J. Cardiol. 37:993, 1976.

142. Krawczyk, J.A., Dashkoff, N., Mays, A., et al.: Reduced coronary flow in a canine model of "muscle bridge" with inflow occlusion extending into diastole: Possible role of downstream vascular closure. Trans. Assoc. Am. Physicians 93:100, 1980.

143. Faruqui, A.M.A., Maloy, W.C., Felner, J.M., et al.: Symptomatic myocardial bridging of coronary artery. Am. J. Cardiol. 41:1305, 1978.

144. Eusterman, J.H., Achor, R.W.P., Kincaid, O.W., et al.: Atherosclerotic disease of the coronary arteries: A pathologic-radiologic correlative study. Circulation 26:1288, 1962.

145. Kemp, H.G., Evans, H., Elliott, W.C., et al.: Diagnostic accuracy of selective coronary cinearteriography. Circulation 36:526, 1967.

146. Vlodaver, Z., Frech, R., VanTassel, R.A., et al.: Correlation of the antemortem coronary arteriogram and the postmortem specimen. Circulation 47:162, 1973.

147. Grondin, C.M., Dyrda, I., Pasternac, A., et al.: Discrepancies between cineangiographic and postmortem findings in patients with coronary artery disease and recent myocardial revascularization. Circulation 49:703, 1974.

148. Hutchins, G.M., Bulkley, B.H., Ridolfi, R.L., et al.: Correlation of coronary arteriograms and left ventriculograms with postmortem studies. Circulation 56:32, 1977.

149. Isner, J.M., Kishel, J., Kent, K.M., et al.: Inaccuracy of angiographic determination of left main coronary arterial narrowing. (Abstract.) Circulation 59 & 60:II–161, 1979.

150. Arnett, E.N., Isner, J.M., Redwood, D.R., et al.: Coronary artery narrowing in coronary heart disease: Comparison of cineangiographic and necropsy findings. Ann. Intern. Med. 91:350, 1979.

151. Murphy, M.L., Galbraith, J.E., and deSoyza, N.: The reliability of coronary angiogram interpretation: An angiographic-pathologic correlation with a comparison of radiographic views. Am. Heart J. 97:578, 1979.

152. Detre, K.M., Wright, E., Murphy, M.L., et al.: Observer agreement in evaluating coronary angiograms. Circulation 52:979, 1975.

153. Zir, L.M., Miller, S.W., Dinsmore, R.E., et al.: Interobserver variability in coronary angiography. Circulation 53:627, 1976.

154. DeRouen, T.A., Murray, J.A., and Owen, W.: Variability in the analysis of coronary arteriograms. Circulation 55:324, 1977.

155. Galbraith, J.E., Murphy, M.L., and deSoyza, N.: Coronary angiogram interpretation. Interobserver variability. J.A.M.A. 240:2053, 1978.

156. Fisher, L.D., Judkins, M.P., Lesperance, J., et al.: Reproducibility of coronary arteriographic reading in the Coronary Artery Surgery Study (CASS). Cathet. Cardiovasc. Diagn. 8:565, 1982.

157. McPherson, D.D., Hiratzka, L.F., Lamberth, W.C., et al.: Delineation of the extent of coronary atherosclerosis by high-frequency epicardial echocardiography. N. Engl. J. Med. 316:304, 1987.

158. Gould, K.L., Lipscomb, K., and Hamilton, G.W.: Physiologic basis for assessing critical coronary stenosis: Instantaneous flow response and regional distribution during coronary hyperemia as measures of coronary flow reserve. Am. J. Cardiol. 33:87, 1974.

159. Gould, K.L., and Lipscomb, K.: Effects of coronary stenoses on coronary flow reserve and resistance. Am. J. Cardiol. 34:48, 1974.

160. Gould, K.L., Lipscomb, K., and Calvert, C.: Compensatory changes of the

distal coronary vascular bed during progressive coronary constriction. Circulation 51:1085, 1975.

161. Feldman, R.L., Nichols, W.W., Pepine, C.J., et al.: Hemodynamic significance of the length of a coronary arterial narrowing. Am. J. Cardiol. 41:865, 1978.
162. Hermiller, J.B., Buller, C.E., Tenaglia, A.N., et al.: Unrecognized left main coronary artery disease in patients undergoing interventional procedures. Am. J. Cardiol. 71:173, 1993.
163. Ganz, P., Abben, R., Friedman, P.L., et al.: Usefulness of transstenotic coronary pressure gradient measurements during diagnostic catheterization. Am. J. Cardiol. 55:910, 1985.
164. Hermiller, J.B., Tenaglia, A.N., Kisslo, K.B., et al.: In vivo validation of compensatory enlargement of atherosclerotic coronary arteries. Am. J. Cardiol. 71:665, 1993.
165. White, C.W., Wright, C.B., Doty, D.B., et al.: Does visual interpretation of the coronary arteriogram predict the physiologic importance of a coronary stenosis? N. Engl. J. Med. 310:819, 1984.
166. Mates, R.E., Gupta, R.L., Bell, A.C., et al.: Fluid dynamics of coronary artery stenosis. Circ. Res. 42:152, 1978.
167. Harrison, D.G., White, C.W., Hiratzka, L.F., et al.: The value of lesion cross-sectional area determined by quantitative coronary angiography in assessing the physiologic significance of proximal left anterior descending coronary arterial stenoses. Circulation 69:1111, 1984.
168. Johnson, M.R., Skorton, D.J., Ericksen, E.E., et al.: Videodensitometric analysis of coronary stenoses: In vivo geometric and physiologic validation in humans. Invest. Radiol. 23:891, 1988.
169. Fleagle, S.R., Johnson, M.R., Wilbricht, C.J., et al.: Automated analysis of coronary arterial morphology in cineangiograms: Geometric and physiologic validation in humans. IEEE Trans. Med. Imaging 8:387, 1989.
170. Marcus, M.L., Skorton, D.J., Johnson, M.R., et al.: Visual estimates of percent diameter coronary stenosis: "A battered gold standard." (Editorial.) J. Am. Coll. Cardiol. 11:882, 1988.
171. Gould, K.L.: Percent coronary stenosis: Battered gold standard, pernicious relic, or clinical practicality? (Editorial.) J. Am. Coll. Cardiol. 11:886, 1988.
172. Friesinger, G.C., Page, E.E., and Ross, R.S.: Prognostic significance of coronary arteriography. Trans. Assoc. Am. Physicians 83:78, 1970.
173. Bruschke, A.V.G., Proudfit, W.L., and Sones, F.M., Jr.: Clinical course of patients with normal and slightly or moderately abnormal coronary arteriograms: A follow-up study on 500 patients. Circulation 47:936, 1973.
174. Webster, J.S., Moberg, C., and Rincon, G.: Natural history of severe proximal coronary artery disease as documented by coronary cineangiography. Am. J. Cardiol. 33:195, 1974.
175. Humphries, J.O., Kuller, L., Ross, R.S., et al.: Natural history of ischemic heart disease in relation to arteriographic findings: A twelve year study of 224 patients. Circulation 49:489, 1974.
176. Harris, P.J., Harrell, F.E., Jr., Lee, K.L., et al.: Survival in medically treated coronary artery disease. Circulation 60:1259, 1979.
177. Burggraf, G.W., and Parker, J.O.: Prognosis in coronary artery disease: Angiographic, hemodynamic, and clinical factors. Circulation 51:146, 1975.
178. Mock, M.B., Ringquist, I., Fisher, L.D., et al.: Survival of medically treated patients in the Coronary Artery Surgery Study (CASS) registry. Circulation 66:562, 1982.
179. Conley, M.J., Ely, R.L., Kisslo, J., et al.: The prognostic spectrum of left main stenosis. Circulation 57:947, 1978.
180. Campeau, L., Corbara, F., Crochet, D., et al.: Left main coronary artery stenosis: The influence of aortocoronary bypass surgery on survival. Circulation 57:1111, 1978.
181. DeWood, M.A., Spores, J., Notske, R., et al.: Prevalence of total coronary occlusion during the early hours of transmural myocardial infarction. N. Engl. J. Med. 303:897, 1980.
182. Capone, G., Wolf, N.M., Meyer, B., et al.: Frequency of intracoronary filling defects by angiography in angina pectoris at rest. Am. J. Cardiol. 56:403, 1985.
183. Bresnahan, D.R., Davis, J.L., Holmes, D.R., Jr., et al.: Angiographic occurence and clinical correlates of intraluminal coronary artery thrombus: Role of unstable angina. J. Am. Coll. Cardiol. 6:285, 1985.
184. Levin, D.C., and Fallon, J.T.: Significance of the angiographic morphology of localized coronary stenoses: Histopathologic correlations. Circulation 66:316, 1982.
185. Ambrose, J.A., Winters, S.L., Stern, A., et al.: Angiographic morphology and the pathogenesis of unstable angina pectoris. J. Am. Coll. Cardiol. 5:609, 1985.
186. Ambrose, J.A., Winters, S.L., Arora, R.R., et al.: Coronary angiographic morphology in myocardial infarction: A link between the pathogenesis of unstable angina and myocardial infarction. J. Am. Coll. Cardiol. 6:1223, 1985.
187. Wilson, R.F., Holida, M.D., and White, C.W.: Quantitative angiographic morphology of coronary stenoses leading to myocardial infarction or unstable angina. Circulation 73:286, 1986.
188. Rehr, R., DiSciascio, G., Vetrovec, G., et al.: Angiographic morphology of coronary artery stenoses in prolonged rest angina: Evidence of intracoronary thrombosis. J. Am. Coll. Cardiol. 14:1429, 1989.
189. Kapashi, K.A., Singh, S., Raju, R., et al.: Morphometric analysis of coronary lesions in patients with unstable angina: An arteriographic study. Indian Heart J. 43:165, 1991.
190. Cools, F.J., Vrints, C.J., and Snoeck, J.P.: Angiographic coronary artery lesion morphology and pathogenetic mechanisms of myocardial ischemia in stable and unstable coronary artery disease syndromes. Acta Cardiol. 47:13, 1992.
191. Kalbfleisch, S.J., McGillem, M.J., Simon, S.B., et al.: Automated quantitation of indexes of coronary lesion complexity: Comparison between patients with stable and unstable angina. Circulation 82:439, 1990.
192. Hermans, W.R.M., Foley, D.P., Rensing, B.J., et al.: Usefulness of quantitative and qualitative angiographic lesion morphology, and clinical characteristics in predicting major adverse cardiac events during and after native coronary balloon angioplasty. Am. J. Cardiol. 72:14, 1993.
193. Kleiman, N.S., Rodriquez, A.R., and Raizner, A.E.: Interobserver variability in grading of coronary arterial narrowings using the American College of Cardiology/American Heart Association grading criteria. Am. J. Cardiol. 69:413, 1992.
194. Ellis, S.G., Roubin, G.S., King, S.B., III, et al.: Angiographic and clinical predictors of acute closure after native vessel coronary angioplasty. Circulation 77:372, 1988.
195. Ellis, S.G., Vandormael, M.G., Cowley, M.J., et al.: Coronary morphologic and clinical determinants of procedural outcome with angioplasty for multivessel coronary disease: Implications for patient selection. Circulation 82:1193, 1990.
196. Moushmoush, B., Kramer, B., Hsieh, A-M., et al.: Does the AHA/ACC Task Force grading system predict outcome in multivessel coronary angioplasty? Cathet. Cardiovasc. Diagn. 27:97, 1992.
197. Myler, R.K., Shaw, R.E., Stertzer, S.H., et al.: Lesion morphology and coronary angioplasty: Current experience and analysis. J. Am. Coll. Cardiol. 19:1641, 1992.
198. Levin, D.C., Baltaxe, H.A., Lee, J.G., et al.: Potential sources of error in coronary arteriography: I. In performance of the study. Am. J. Radiol. 124:378, 1975.
199. Levin, D.C., Baltaxe, H.A., and Sos, T.A.: Potential sources of error in coronary arteriography: II. In interpretation of the study. Am. J. Radiol. 124:386, 1975.

CHAPTER

24 Digital Angiography

G. B. John Mancini, M.D.

ASSESSMENT OF VENTRICULAR FUNCTION ___ 252
Left Ventricle ___ 252
Intravenous Studies ___ 252
Direct Studies ___ 252
Videodensitometry ___ 253
Regional Function and Muscle Mass ___ 253
Assessment of Physiologic Interventions ___ 253
Assessment of End-Systolic Pressure-Volume Relations ___ 253
Right Ventricle ___ 255

ASSESSMENT OF THE CORONARY CIRCULATION ___ 255
Anatomic Assessment of the Coronary Arteries ___ 255
Digital Fluoroscopy ___ 255
Intravenous Angiography ___ 256
Aortic Root Angiography ___ 256
Direct Angiography ___ 256
Anatomic Assessment of Bypass Grafts ___ 256
Intravenous Angiography ___ 256
Aortic Root Angiography ___ 257
Direct Angiography ___ 257

**Functional Assessment of the Coronary
Circulation _____ 257**
Methodology _____ 257
  Transit Time Analysis _____ 257
  Indicator Dilution Analysis _____ 258
  Contrast Washout Analysis _____ 259
  Impulse Response (Transfer Function)
    Analysis _____ 261

Appearance Time and Density
  Analysis _____ 262
  General Comparative Summary _____ 264
Clinical Applications _____ 264
  Coronary Disease _____ 264
  Bypass Grafts _____ 267
CONCLUSIONS _____ 267

ASSESSMENT OF VENTRICULAR FUNCTION

Left Ventricle

Intravenous Studies

The assessment of left ventricular function by means of intravenous contrast injections was one of the first applications to be tested with digital angiography. Table 24–1 summarizes many of the available studies and demonstrates the considerable degree of accuracy that can be obtained by this approach.[1–17] Despite the less invasive nature of this approach compared with direct left ventriculography, it is not very popular because of numerous difficulties in implementation. It requires the use of volumes and rates of injection of contrast agent that are comparable to those used in traditional left ventriculographic studies and that have very similar adverse effects.[18] The poor contrast resolution of the levophase ventriculogram mandates some type of image enhancement, usually mask-mode subtraction. Yet, this type of image processing is commonly marred by misregistration artifact caused by the prolonged breath holding that is required between venous injection and arrival of contrast into the left ventricle. In addition, opacification may be inadequate despite image enhancement in patients with very poor ejection fractions or tricuspid regurgitation. One advantage of the digital angiographic approach over direct left ventriculography is the virtual absence of ventricular arrhythmias during left ventricular imaging. This advantage, however, does not offset the imminently greater ease with which echocardiography, radionuclide studies, and even magnetic resonance studies[19] can provide assessments of ventricular function noninvasively.

One notable exception to the problem of misregistration with intravenous studies is the use of dual energy subtraction instead of mask-mode subtraction, as proposed by Van Lysel and colleagues.[17]

Direct Studies

The use of low-dose, direct left ventriculography is a much more practical and beneficial application of digital image processing and contrast enhancement through mask-mode subtraction. The main benefit is that the procedure allows for a much-reduced contrast dose, thereby minimizing costs and side effects. This is of particular importance for patients with preexisting renal disease, diabetes, multiple myeloma, aortic stenosis, unstable angina, or poor ventricular function. Table 24–2 summarizes many studies that demonstrate the comparability of low-dose to standard-dose left ventriculography.[1, 4, 10, 20–26] In patients with extremely large ventricles or

TABLE 24–1. SUMMARY OF STUDIES COMPARING INTRAVENOUS DIGITAL LEFT VENTRICULOGRAPHY TO CONVENTIONAL LEFT VENTRICULOGRAPHY

Center	No. of Patients	Contrast Dose (mL)	Injection Rate (mL/sec)	Correlation Coefficients* ED	ES	EF	Comments
University of California, Los Angeles[2]	12	20	5	—	—	0.75–0.85	
University of California, Irvine[3]	30	30–40	10–14	0.82	0.93	0.96	Hand injected in <3 seconds
Vanderbilt University[4]	9	40	12–15	0.91		0.89	ED & ES volumes combined for regression analysis
Cornell[5]	31	30	20	0.96	0.97	0.98	
University of California, San Diego[6]	20	20	10	0.88	0.89	0.81	
Free University of Berlin[7]	46	30	18	0.98	0.93	0.94	
University of Kentucky[8]	40	30	30	0.88	0.92	0.93	
Royal Free Hospital, London[9]	20	0.5–0.6 mL/kg	16–18	—	—	0.90	
Dublin, Ireland[10]	12–23	40	20	—	—	0.88–0.95	Improved results by excluding studies with any ectopic beats
Kyoto University[11]	11	40	12	0.95	0.98	0.96	
Kumamoto University[12]	15	30–40	12–25	0.85	0.98	0.90	
Cleveland Clinic[13]	40	0.5 mL/kg	10–15	—	—	0.88	
Utrecht, Netherlands[14]	20	40	—	—	—	0.81	TID images
Zurich, Switzerland[15]	20	45	15	0.92 0.90	0.98 0.95	0.92 0.89	Mask mode TID
University of Milan[16]	32	40	15	0.95	0.98	0.98	
University of Wisconsin[17]	13	40	20	0.99			ED & ES volumes combined for regression analysis. Pulmonary artery injection. Dual energy subtraction.

*ED = end-diastolic volume; ES = end-systolic volume; EF = ejection fraction; TID = time interval difference.

TABLE 24–2. SUMMARY OF STUDIES COMPARING LOW-DOSE DIRECT VENTRICULOGRAPHY WITH CONVENTIONAL LEFT VENTRICULOGRAPHY

Center	No. of Patients	Contrast Dose (mL)	Dilution (%)	Correlation Coefficients*			Comments
				ED	**ES**	**EF**	
Kyoto University[20]	16	5	0	0.95	0.98	—	
Vanderbilt University[4]	8	5–10	0	0.96		0.91	ED & ES volumes combined for regression analysis
Columbia University[21]	28	7	14	0.97	0.97	0.97	
Columbia University[22]	23	7	14	0.94	0.97	—	
University of California, Irvine[23]	24	10	0	0.77	0.95	—	
University of Michigan[24]	31	10	50	0.85	0.93	0.92	
Dublin, Ireland[10]	10–21	10–15	0	—	—	0.92–0.97	Improved results by excluding studies with any ectopic beats
University of California, San Francisco[25]	15	0.2 mL/kg	25	0.90	0.93	0.92	
Erasmus University[26]	9	0.5 mL/kg	0	—	—	0.97	Contrast dose is 75% of amount usually used

*ED = end-diastolic volume; ES = end-systolic volume; EF = ejection fraction.

with particularly severe wall motion abnormalities, incomplete mixing of contrast may occur with the most dilute or lowest-dose protocols listed in the table. Accordingly, the most generally applicable approach is to use between 50 and 75 percent of the dose usually used in a given laboratory, injected over 3 to 4 seconds and in a volume of 20 to 40 mL.

Videodensitometry

The pixel density that has been logarithmically converted in subtracted images represents the integral of the amount of contrast traversed by the x-ray beam as long as corrections can be implemented to overcome nonlinearity of the image intensifier and television transfer functions, beam scatter, geometric distortions and energy variations of the x-ray beam, and veiling glare. The necessary corrections vary according to the exact location within a given image and according to the variable attenuation caused by noncardiac structures. There is also variation in the degree of periventricular opacification that results from opacification of background structures. Finally, contrast medium must be distributed homogeneously in blood for densitometric analyses to be valid. When the majority of these factors are taken into account, numerous investigators have demonstrated the validity of videodensitometric analyses of ventricular function.[13, 27–31] This approach is of advantage over geometric approaches because it does not require precise edge definition, nor is it invalidated if ventricles are distorted by wall motion abnormalities. Extensive functional analyses, such as measurements of peak filling rates and timing intervals, are also facilitated by this approach.[32] Greater availability of the dual energy subtraction method, which is immune to misregistration artifacts that invalidate videodensitometric analyses, would probably provide the most robust method for application of videodensitometry in clinical practice.[33]

Regional Function and Muscle Mass

The ejection fraction and ventricular volumes may remain within the normal range despite subtle or obvious abnormalities of regional wall motion, regional wall thickening, or ventricular shape. Digital angiography is particularly well suited to analyses of the latter parameters because they require more extensive computational assistance. This is especially important in assessing responses to ischemic stress (e.g., in pacing studies). Moreover, innovative methods of regional function analysis can be devised to create a more comprehensive analysis of regional ventricular function. For example, by use of a combination of mask-mode subtraction and

time-interval difference image processing, wall thickening and muscle mass calculations can be undertaken (Fig. 24–1).[34–38] Similarly, algorithms can be applied to quantitatively measure the shape of various regions of the ventricle to determine whether the shape is abnormal and how the ventricle remodels over time (Fig. 24–2).[39–43]

Assessment of Physiologic Interventions

As noted, intravenous ventriculography with digital image enhancement was one of the earliest applications of digital angiography in cardiology. There was an intense interest at the time in applying this methodology to stress testing, with either atrial pacing[44–49] or exercise as the ischemic stimulus.[15, 50–56] These studies showed clearly that patients with functionally significant coronary stenoses could be identified if the ejection fraction failed to rise or fell significantly or if new wall motion abnormalities were induced. The main advantage over radionuclide stress testing was the markedly enhanced spatial resolution, which allowed for excellent detection of wall motion abnormalities. Nevertheless, these methods are seldom used because of the difficulties with intravenous digital ventriculography already outlined and the marked increase in misregistration that occurs with exercise studies. Dual energy subtraction methods, which are immune to misregistration artifacts, would be ideal for such applications except that the problem of intravenous contrast injections would remain. Atrial pacing in conjunction with direct, low-dose ventriculography is a convenient adjunct for selected patients undergoing diagnostic catheterization.[44–46] Figure 24–3 demonstrates an example of images obtained before and after successful angioplasty.[1] Kitazume and colleagues[57] have also applied digital left ventriculography (pulmonary artery injection of contrast) during angioplasty to assess the effects of balloon occlusion on regional ventricular function.

Assessment of End-Systolic Pressure-Volume Relations

The end-systolic pressure-volume relations and the calculation of Emax as a measure of contractility are the most sophisticated and yet most difficult parameters of ventricular function to measure accurately in patients. Low-dose digital angiography, especially in combination with validated videodensitometric volume measurements, is ideal for this purpose, which requires repeated ventriculography, frame-by-frame volume analyses, and concomitant high-fidelity pressure measurements. The image enhancement and computational attributes of digital angiography could be used to make this analysis safer and more practical.[58] Sophisticated analysis of

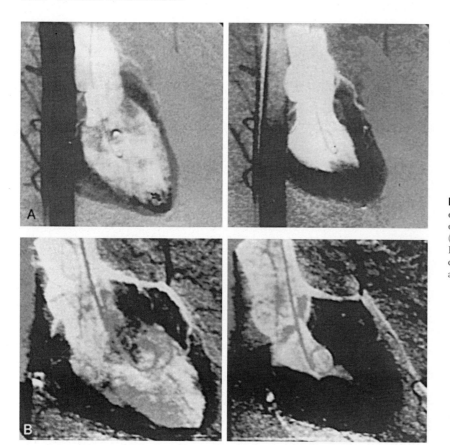

FIGURE 24–1. *A and B,* Left- and right-hand panels of each set show examples of wall thickness images at end-diastole and end-systole obtained in two different patients. (From McGillem, M.J., Pinto, I.M.F., and Mancini, G.B.J.: Determination of left ventricular wall thickness and myocardial mass by digital ventriculography. Am. J. Card. Imaging 3:244-252, 1989, with permission.)

FIGURE 24–2. Shape analysis of a patient with an inferior wall motion abnormality. The top left- and right-hand panels show the frame-by-frame outlines in systole and diastole, respectively. The bottom left-hand panel shows the color-coded shape analysis based on curvature calculations. The red streak indicates abnormalities of shape in the inferior wall throughout systole and diastole. The bottom right-hand panel conveys the same information in black and white. The dark streak in this image corresponds to the red streak in the bottom left-hand panel. (From Mancini, G.B.J., DeBoe, S.F., Gillon, J., et al.: Measurement of systolic and diastolic disorders of shape using frame-by-frame quantitative regional curvature analysis. Coron. Artery Dis. 2:179-187, 1991, with permission.)

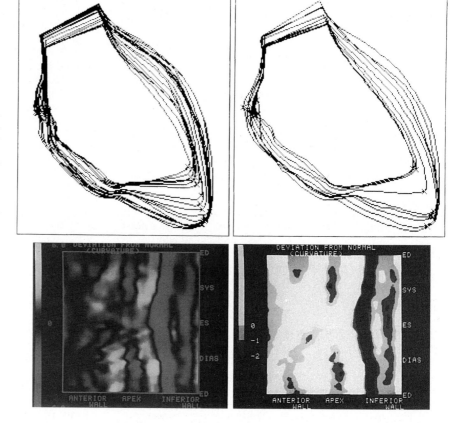

patients undergoing valve replacement or valvuloplasty have been performed with the use of these principles and methods.[59, 60]

Right Ventricle

Measurement of right ventricular function by geometric methods applied to radiographic images is problematic because of the complex shape of this chamber.[61, 62] Although most cardiologists rely on radionuclide assessments of right ventricular function, videodensitometric analysis of digital angiograms has been shown to be closely correlated with radionuclide measurements.[61–63] Moreover, the exquisite spatial resolution allows assessment of right ventricular wall motion disturbances as well as determination of hemodynamic deterioration in the setting of right ventricular infarction (Fig. 24–4).[64]

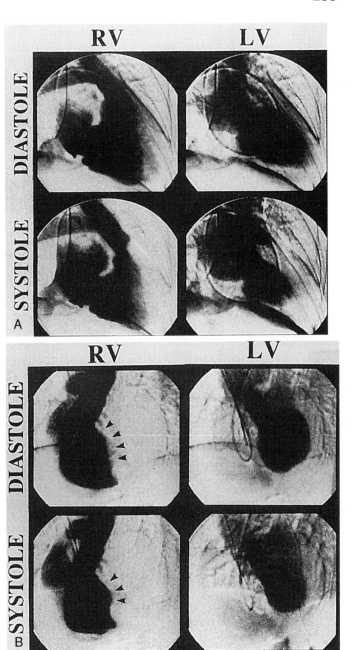

FIGURE 24–4. *A*, Thirty-degree right anterior oblique images at end-diastole and end-systole of the right and left ventricles in a patient with an inferior infarction involving the right ventricle. *B*, Right ventricular involvement is apparent only in 60-degree left anterior oblique views *(arrows)*. (From Honda, T., Hayasaki, K., Honda, T., et al.: Right ventricular wall motion disturbance and determinants of the appearance of hemodynamic right ventricular infarction. Jpn. Circ. J. 56:1106-1114, 1992, with permission.)

ASSESSMENT OF THE CORONARY CIRCULATION

Anatomic Assessment of the Coronary Arteries

Digital Fluoroscopy

An innovative application that does not require catheterization or contrast injection is digital subtraction fluoroscopy for detection of coronary calcifications as a screening test for the presence of significant underlying coronary disease. Detrano and co-workers[65] studied 191 subjects, who had no historical or electrocardiographic (ECG) evidence of previous myocardial infarction and had been

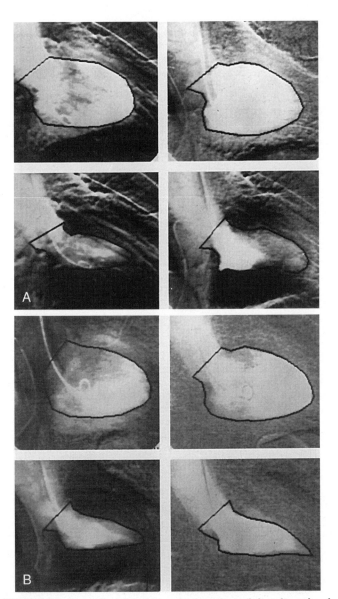

FIGURE 24–3. *A*, The left-hand panels show the end-diastolic and end-systolic images at baseline, and the right-hand panels show the same after atrial pacing. A new anterior wall motion abnormality is evident in the lower right-hand panel. *B*, These images were obtained in the same format after successful angioplasty of a lesion in the left anterior descending artery. Atrial pacing no longer induces an anterior wall motion abnormality. (From Mancini, G.B.J.: Assessment of left ventricular function by intravenous and direct low contrast dose digital ventriculography. *In* Mancini, G.B.J. [ed.]: Clinical Applications of Cardiac Digital Angiography. New York, Raven Press, 1988, p. 99-113, with permission.)

referred for coronary arteriography, with both conventional and digital subtraction fluoroscopy. Subtraction was used to enhance the visibility of coronary calcium. Higher overall accuracy was achieved with the digital fluoroscopy technique than with regular fluoroscopy for prediction of the presence of stenoses greater than 50 percent diameter, especially in younger patients.

This approach has been studied further[66] to assess the prognostic significance of cardiac cinefluoroscopy for coronary calcific deposits in asymptomatic high-risk subjects. A total of 1461 asymptomatic adults with an estimated 10 percent risk of having a coronary heart disease event within 8 years underwent this screening procedure. The prevalence of calcific deposits was 47 percent. The relative risk of having a coronary event within 1 year after detection of calcium was increased 2.7 times. The detection of calcium was found to be independent of other typical risk factors for coronary disease.

Intravenous Angiography

Much of the initial clinical enthusiasm for the technology of digital angiography was a result of the prospects of imaging the coronary arteries by intravenous contrast injection. But this very intriguing and important application of intravenous digital angiography has not yet successfully been achieved, for reasons elucidated by Mistretta and co-workers.[67-70] Overlying iodinated pulmonary and cardiac structures obscure the contrast material in the coronary arteries, which has undergone dilution by up to 20-fold. The large dynamic range of x-ray transmission between lung fields and cardiac structures leads to severe cross-scatter and image intensifier glare, increased television camera noise, and diminution in image contrast. Motion of vessels and of noniodinated structures also detracts from coronary visualization. Even high-pass temporal filtration techniques, dual energy subtraction, and hybrid subtraction have not provided practical solutions to these problems.[67, 71-75]

The largest clinical elucidation of the problems of intravenous digital angiography for coronary imaging has been provided by Haggman and Detrano and their colleagues.[76, 77] These investigators used a 30-degree right anterior oblique view and studied ideal, thin candidates. Even so, they were not uniformly successful in obtaining diagnostic images. The technique provided information primarily involving proximal coronary artery disease segments and did not adequately detect distally located disease. The method appeared to be better for assessment of the right coronary artery than the left anterior descending artery, even though the latter was also seen in most patients. The circumflex artery was extremely difficult to image, and only 84 percent of the studies demonstrated the left main trunk.

It is unlikely that intravenous digital coronary angiography using specialized processing of images generated by conventional x-rays will develop into a practical and widespread application, even for screening purposes. Synchrotron x-ray generation and dual energy subtraction techniques may rekindle this effort.[78] Whether the use of cine computed tomography or dynamic magnetic resonance imaging will provide images of sufficient anatomic detail and in a format useable by cardiologists and surgeons (i.e., longitudinal images of the coronaries and not just cross-sectional views) is also unknown, but much greater effort is being focused on these technologies for noninvasive coronary imaging than on digital angiography. Even so, intravenous angiography has been used successfully to assess aortitis and other vascular lesions outside the coronary tree in Takayasu disease.[79]

Aortic Root Angiography

Before the development of either selective angiography or digital angiography, several investigators examined the utility of aortic root angiography for visualization of the coronary arteries.[80-82] Impressive film images were demonstrable provided that several procedural details were followed. For example, the Valsalva maneuver was necessary to slow aortic root outflow and washout of contrast material, specially designed catheters with single or double

coils perpendicular to the catheter shaft enhanced delivery of contrast medium to the coronary ostia, and high flow rates of contrast material were needed. Digital enhancement techniques were expected to alleviate some of these technical demands with respect to specialized catheters and volume of contrast. Clinical applications, however, have not demonstrated sufficiently detailed images to warrant widespread use of this approach,[83-86] although assessment of vasculitis of the aorta and its branches can be achieved,[87] and preoperative screening of the status of internal mammary arteries can be achieved easily.[88]

Aortic root angiography has never been intended as a replacement for standard coronary arteriography. There may be a definite role for this technique if the patient is already undergoing other vascular angiography procedures such as carotid or aortic angiography. A simple and rapid screening test performed by the radiologist may provide compelling evidence for the cardiologist that would justify subsequent coronary angiography. The decision to perform coronary arteriography in patients being evaluated for carotid, aortic, or femoral disease is required frequently in a consultative practice, and it is often based on nonexercise stress test results such as dipyridamole-thallium imaging. The demonstration of high-grade lesions with digital aortic root angiography may diminish the need for other noninvasive testing.

Direct Angiography

Modern cardiac catheterization laboratories are usually equipped with digital imaging capabilities. Although a main thrust of digital coronary angiography is in the area of quantification, the most common use of the technique is actually for improvement of image quality to facilitate procedures such as angioplasty. Therefore, digital roadmapping, spatial filters, magnification, and other refinements are now used routinely. Although quantitative coronary angiography is not unique to digital angiography, it can be applied much more expeditiously to images acquired digitally than to images stored on a cineangiogram that must subsequently be digitized before quantitative analysis. This important topic is covered in detail in Chapter 23.

It is generally agreed that image enhancement of direct injection coronary arteriograms by the traditional mask-mode subtraction method is not desirable because of misregistration artifacts that are introduced into the image. These artifacts are often severe enough to degrade the qualitative aspects of the image and to cause problems with videodensitometry and with videodensitometrically-based edge detection methods. However, dual energy subtraction may overcome this problem and allow for image enhancement through background subtraction without the introduction of major misregistration artifacts. The benefit of this approach would be to create an opportunity for improved quantitation by videodensitometric techniques. These techniques cannot be applied well to unsubtracted images because of the occurrence of superimposed tissue signals that vary nonlinearly across the vessel profile and that cannot be removed adequately through standard background removal methods. A series of investigations have demonstrated the potential value of dual energy quantitative coronary arteriography.[89-91]

Anatomic Assessment of Bypass Grafts

Intravenous Angiography

The problems associated with the use of intravenous angiography for delineation of coronary arteries also apply to the imaging of coronary bypass grafts. Because grafts are larger, farther away from the left ventricular cavity, and subject to less motion, the problems encountered in imaging them are somewhat less severe. However, difficulties continue to arise, especially because the grafts are in close proximity to the aortic contrast pool. Clinical studies have focused on the detection of graft patency because the fine detail of graft stenoses and anastomoses cannot be assessed with this technique. In a comparison of graft patency assessment by intravenous and selective angiography, Myerowitz and colleagues found that 11 of 15 truly patent grafts could be visualized by the digital technique (sensitivity of 73 percent) and that all of 11 truly occluded grafts were correctly identified digitally (100 percent specificity).[70, 92, 93] Drury and co-workers[94] identified 9 of 13 patent grafts (sensitivity of 69 percent) with a specificity of 100 percent. Guthaner and colleagues[95] identified only 13 of 32 patent grafts. Although the technique appears to be highly specific, its low sensitivity in comparison to cine computed tomography has generally tempered the enthusiasm for this approach. More recently, however, Lupon-Roses and associates[96] studied 101 venous grafts and 7 internal mammary grafts and were able to positively identify 95 out of 97 patent grafts and all 11 occluded grafts (98 percent sensitivity and 100 percent specificity). These excellent results were attributed to the routine use of two views, a priori knowledge about the location of each graft, and the use of radiographic x-ray exposures instead of lower, fluoroscopic exposure levels. Similarly, Guiraudon and co-workers[97] demonstrated 100 percent specificity and 98 percent sensitivity in the detection of internal mammary grafts in 42 patients. These results are attributed, in part, to the fact that internal mammary grafts are farther from the heart and great vessels, and their position varies less from patient to patient. In addition, these researchers achieved good to excellent imaging without significant misregistration in almost 90 percent of cases.

Aortic Root Angiography

In keeping with the trend toward intra-arterial administration of contrast material, aortic root digital angiography has been shown to be highly accurate for detection of saphenous vein bypass grafts. Two groups have reported 100 percent specificity and sensitivity for detection of patent grafts with this technique, although graft detail cannot be analyzed.[94, 98] Guthaner and associates[95] reported a sensitivity of 98 percent (101 of 103 patent grafts). Steffenino and colleagues[99] demonstrated an overall sensitivity of 83 percent and a specificity of 100 percent, but performance varied considerably, depending on the site and type of graft. Greatest success was achieved with venous grafts to the left anterior descending artery, and the worst performance was in assessment of internal mammary grafts to this artery. Additional views were helpful to delineate the status of venous grafts to the right or circumflex arteries.

Improved evaluation of internal mammary grafts was obtained by Kuttler and associates,[100] who successfully and safely used ipsilateral brachial artery injections of contrast agent postoperatively to assess early patency. In this application, details of anastomotic adequacy and perfusion were evident. Marvasti and colleagues[101] safely used intra-arterial digital angiography to follow up composite graft replacement of the ascending aorta and aortic valve. They were able to detect pseudoaneurysm at anastomotic sites requiring repair as well as clinically inapparent persistent dissection beyond the distal aortic anastomosis. Boonstra and colleagues[102] used this technique as an outpatient screening method to assess bypass graft patency. In the majority of cases, they were able to assess the proximal anastomosis and the body of the graft, but assessment of the distal anastomosis was not adequate. They projected savings in time and cost relative to standard, selective angiographic assessment of bypass grafts. Using a retrograde brachial approach, Kawasuji and co-workers[103] were able to assess both internal mammary and saphenous vein bypass grafts expeditiously.

Anecdotal reports of digital detection of patent grafts that were not found by selective angiography suggest that aortic root angiography may be superior to standard catheterization methods if graft patency alone is to be assessed. But even this procedure does not routinely provide sufficient detail to allow accurate assessment of stenoses, distal anastomoses, and adequacy of distal run-off (Fig. 24–5). Moreover, because this procedure entails the same risk and preparation as selective catheterization, the method is recommended only as a quick screening test at the time of regular catheterization, especially in patients who do not have implanted graft markers. The use of this procedure early in the course of the catheterization helps to expedite the examination. In many instances, the amount of contrast agent used for the aortogram is

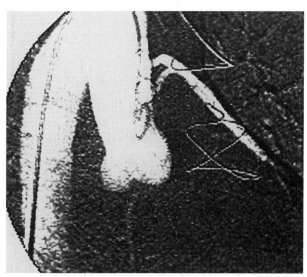

FIGURE 24–5. A direct digital aortogram obtained with 20 mL of a 50 percent solution of contrast material. This patient had aortocoronary bypass grafts to the left anterior descending artery and the first diagonal branches of the left coronary artery. Notice that, although the proximal segments are clearly seen, no definite anatomic information about the anastomoses or the distal vessels is available from this image. In addition, the main bodies of the grafts are overlapped in this projection. Despite these limitations, selective catheterization of grafts can be expedited by first screening for graft patency by this technique. (From Mancini, G.B.J., and Higgins, C.B.: Digital subtraction angiography: A review of cardiac applications. Prog. Cardiovasc. Dis. 18:111, 1985, with permission.)

offset by the time and amount of agent saved in the attempt to find unmarked grafts with selective catheters.

Direct Angiography

The specific use of digital angiography for assessment of graft anatomy by direct injection of contrast material is not different from that for assessment of the native coronary circulation. The major additional information that digital angiography has to offer with direct injection of contrast material is in the assessment of graft function and flow. These aspects are discussed in the next section.

Functional Assessment of the Coronary Circulation

Methodology

Transit Time Analysis

The concept of using transit time analysis to measure coronary velocity and flow is summarized in Figure 24–6. The transit time of a bolus of contrast material between two arterial regions of interest at a known distance apart can be used to calculate the velocity of the bolus. Measurement of the mean cross-sectional area of the arterial segment allows conversion of the velocity measurement to a flow measurement. The transit time can be measured from the peaks of the contrast density profile within each region of interest or from other portions of the curve (e.g., the point at which half of the maximal contrast density is achieved).

Rutishauser and co-workers[104–106] validated a method of measuring coronary flow based on transit time in a canine preparation and also demonstrated its application to measurement of right coronary artery flow in human patients. The densograms measured at two regions of interest in the arterial image were calibrated by filming a contrast wedge before image acquisition so that contrast depth and density could be linearized. The calculation of blood flow required geometric measurement of the distance between the two regions of interest and the volume of the coronary segment.

Smith and co-workers[107] used essentially the same technique as

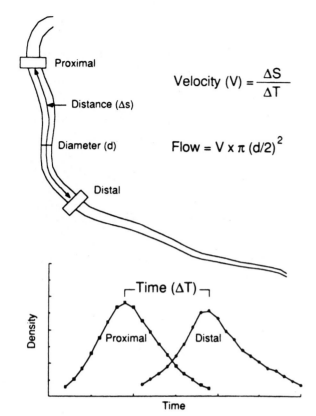

$$\text{Velocity (V)} = \frac{\Delta S}{\Delta T}$$

$$\text{Flow} = V \times \pi \, (d/2)^2$$

FIGURE 24–6. Schematic illustration of the scientific basis for calculation of coronary flow from transit time. The time (ΔT) for passage of a contrast bolus from a proximal to a distal coronary region of interest is measured. The velocity (V) and flow (F) can be calculated from the distance (ΔS) between the regions of interest and the diameter of the coronary segment. (From Nissen, S.E., Elion, J.L., and DeMaria, A.N.: Methods for calculation of coronary flow reserve by computer processing of digital angiograms. *In* Heintzen, P.H., and Bursch, J.H. [eds.]: Progress in Digital Angiocardiography. Dordrecht, Kluwer Academic Publishers, 1988, p. 237, with permission.)

Rutishauser and also demonstrated applications in humans.[108] These investigators emphasized the need for background subtraction to correct contrast densograms. The transit-time approach continues to be one of the most common fundamental applications in digital imaging for measurement of blood flow. Kruger and colleagues[109] described a method of temporal filtration of 30 frame-per-second fluoroscopic video sequences to establish a parametric image demonstrating the time to maximum opacification of arterial segments after injection of contrast material. Geometric length measurements were required to calculate flow velocity.

Spiller and colleagues[110] expanded on the combined transit-time and geometric measurement technique in two distinct ways. First, multiple contrast injections were used to enable calculations of *phasic* coronary flow, and second, the leading edge of the contrast bolus (appearance time) was tracked, instead of the peak of the contrast densograms (mean transit time). The leading edge of the contrast bolus was used to avoid the errors inherent in calculations of mean transit time in a pulsatile system and the alterations in densogram shape (and therefore in mean transit-time calculations) caused by layering and incomplete washout of contrast material. The appearance time was defined as the time at which the contrast density was half of the peak value in the regions of interest studied. The results of this method showed a strong linear correlation with saphenous vein bypass blood flow measurements made by electromagnetic probe at the time of surgery. A systematic overestimation of approximately 20 percent was noted. This technique was developed with high-frame-rate angiography (50 frames per second), and the calculations of phasic flow required repeated contrast injection at different phases of the cardiac cycle.

Swanson and co-workers[111] measured the linear distance that the contrast material waveform moved in each of 60 video fields per second and combined this with a densitometrically-based volume calculation[102] to establish phasic flow measurements. That is, instead of using two fixed regions of interest to calculate mean transit time, these investigators examined the changes in the distribution of contrast material along the arterial segment on a frame-by-frame basis. Excellent results for measures of phasic femoral flow in dogs were reported. A subsequent investigation[112] employed this technique to quantitate absolute phasic and mean flow in coronary artery bypass grafts. Correlations for mean and peak flows were high ($r = 0.91$ and 0.88, respectively). In contrast to the method of Spiller, this technique requires only a single injection of contrast material to measure phasic flow.

Shaw and Plewes[113] published a novel, pulsed-contrast injection method for measuring the velocity of blood flow. Contrast material is injected with a specially modified injector at a pulsing frequency as high as 15 Hz so that two or more boluses can be imaged simultaneously. Contrast injections are gated to an ECG signal. The velocity of flow is determined by measuring the spacing between the boluses and multiplying this distance by the pulsing frequency. In this application, the actual time measurement is not obtained from the contrast densogram, as it is in the usual transit-time applications; instead, it is obtained from the known injection frequency. The multiple contrast densograms are analyzed solely to determine the distance traveled by each bolus. In vivo, coronary applications have not yet been performed with this method.

These techniques are most suitable for assessments in relatively straight, long, and nonbranching arterial segments or bypass grafts that lie parallel to the image intensifier so that foreshortening does not affect arterial volume calculations and velocity changes at branch points do not alter transit-time measurements. Alternatively, biplane images, stereoscopic angiography, digital flashing tomosynthesis, or other geometric corrections for foreshortening can be employed.[114–116] The methods require high-frame-rate image acquisition to ensure adequate temporal resolution. The proposal of Shaw and Plewes requires both high-frame-rate angiography and high, pulsatile rates of injection of contrast agent. Because the contrast bolus must be compact, all of the methods are best applied with power injection of contrast material. More importantly, the mean transit time techniques assume constant flow even though flow is phasic. Consequently, mean transit times must be measured over at least one cardiac cycle, or precise gating of the contrast injections during a specified phase of the cardiac cycle is required.[117] Arrhythmias or contrast-induced heart rate changes also invalidate the transit-time calculations, so atrial pacing should be used with these techniques.

Indicator Dilution Analysis

The indicator dilution analysis method uses the theory embodied in the standard Stewart and Hamilton equations, which predict that the area under a curve of indicator density versus time is directly proportional to the quantity of indicator injected and inversely proportional to flow (Fig. 24–7). For angiographic applications, the indicator is contrast material itself, and the density is measured in an arterial region of interest. This method can be used to measure both absolute and relative flow. If cardiac output is known, then absolute flow can be calculated if indicator dilution curves are obtained from both a reference injection into the aorta and a separate injection of the same volume into the artery of interest. The technique requires precise knowledge of the amount of contrast material injected and full mixing of the indicator with blood. Alternatively, the measurement of absolute flow from single injections into an artery can be performed if complex corrections for the effects of radiographic scatter, veiling glare, and beam hardening are undertaken to optimize and linearize the effective mass absorption coefficient, the conversion factor of the image intensifier, the transfer function of the television system, the intensity of incident radiation, and the gains of the densitometry detectors. However, if the same quantity of contrast material can be

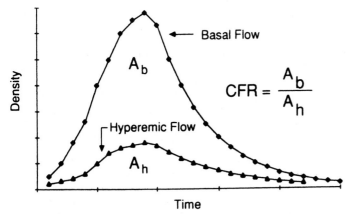

FIGURE 24–7. Calculation of coronary flow reserve from indicator-dilution curves. Coronary flow reserve is equal to the ratio of the area under a time-density curve for a coronary region of interest obtained under basal conditions (Ab) divided by the area of the curve of the same region of interest obtained under hyperemic flow conditions (Ah). CFR = coronary flow reserve. (From Nissen, S.E., Elion, J.L., and DeMaria, A.N.: Methods for calculation of coronary flow reserve by computer processing of digital angiograms. *In* Heintzen, P.H., and Bursch, J.H. [eds.]: Progress in Digital Angiocardiography. Dordrecht, Kluwer Academic Publishers, 1988, p. 237, with permission.)

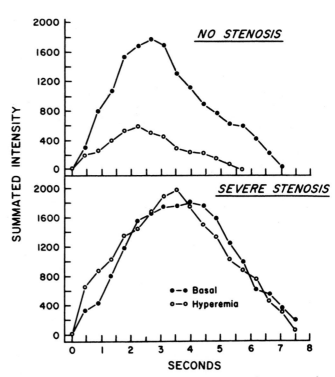

FIGURE 24–8. Representative intensity-time curves for a proximal circumflex coronary region of interest. The top panel illustrates the curves obtained in the absence of coronary stenosis and shows a marked decrease in the area under the curve for the hyperemic image *(open circles)* and the basal image *(closed circles)*. The bottom panel shows similar curves obtained under basal and hyperemic conditions in the presence of a severe coronary stenosis. (From Nissen, S.E., Elion, J.L., Booth, D.C., et al.: Value and limitations of computer analysis of digital subtraction angiography in the assessment of coronary flow reserve. Circulation 73:562, 1986, with permission. Copyright 1986, American Heart Association.)

administered under both basal and hyperemic conditions, and if the radiographic technique is relatively constant so that many effects are essentially canceled out, then a much less technically demanding measure of relative flow is possible.

A series of investigations from the University of California, Davis, extensively investigated the indicator-dilution technique for measures of blood flow.[118–121] Foerster and colleagues[120, 121] applied this method in animals and humans. Lois and colleagues[122] also demonstrated its validity in a phantom model and found it to be suitable for measurement of either absolute or relative coronary flow. Optimal results were achieved primarily with measurement of relative coronary flow. Nissen and associates[123, 124] and Gurley and co-workers[125] have reevaluated the method more recently, using digital angiography in a canine model. They demonstrated a correlation of 0.86 between electromagnetic measures of coronary flow reserve and ratios obtained from the integration of the time-density curves.

The most important technical prerequisite of this technique is that the administered dose of contrast agent must be known precisely and should be constant between injections. This mandates *subselective* cannulation of the coronary artery for the delivery of the contrast agent and avoidance of reflux. Complete mixing must also occur, so the sampling site must be sufficiently distal to the site of injection. This method is also best applied with power injection of contrast material and use of atrial pacing. The temporal resolution required for this application is not as great as with the methods based on transit time. For example, Nissen and colleagues[123] have used analysis of a single end-diastolic frame per cardiac cycle to produce the time versus density curves (Fig. 24–8).

Contrast Washout Analysis

Whereas the previously-described methods focus regions of interest over the arteries themselves, the contrast washout methods analyze the disappearance of contrast material from the myocardial bed. Digital subtraction enhances this technique because visualization of the myocardial blush phase is augmented. These analyses are predicated on use of an inert indicator and measurement of its monoexponential washout as embodied in the Kety-Schmidt relations (Fig. 24–9).

Ikeda and associates[126, 127] studied 53 patients with variable degrees of coronary stenosis isolated to the left anterior descending artery. One third of the patients had prior myocardial infarction. They manually injected 2 to 3 mL of contrast material into the left

main coronary artery and recorded an image run for 20 seconds at 30 frames per second. Mask-mode subtraction was used to provide background correction and enhancement of the myocardial phase of contrast. Eight 45-degree sectors emanating from the center of gravity of the diastolic left ventricular silhouette were analyzed to

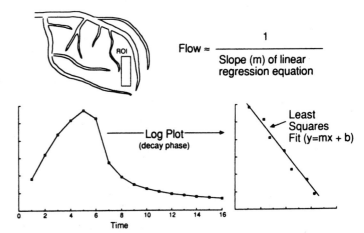

FIGURE 24–9. Measurement of coronary flow from the washout phase of myocardial contrast. The decay phase is assumed to be monoexponential and is plotted on a logarithmic scale. A linear regression least squares fit is determined for the decay phase. Flow is proportional to the inverse of the slope (m) of the regression equation. (From Nissen, S.E., Elion, J.L., and DeMaria, A.N.: Methods for calculation of coronary flow reserve by computer processing of digital angiograms. *In* Heintzen, P.H., and Bursch, J.H. [eds.]: Progress in Digital Angiocardiography. Dordrecht, Kluwer Academic Publishers, 1988, p. 237, with permission.)

produce sectorial time-density curves, and the sectors corresponding to the left anterior descending perfusion bed were evaluated. The disappearance half-life (T1/2) was calculated after the descending slope of the densograms was fitted to a monoexponential function. The T1/2 was given by the formula, T1/2 = ln(2/k), where ln is the natural logarithm and k is the exponential disappearance rate. Whenever the curves exhibited two components during the disappearance phase, T1/2 was calculated from the initial, fast portion of the curve. In a subset of patients, a strong inverse correlation was noted between the T1/2 value and great cardiac vein flow. The washout T1/2 was notably shortened by the presence of collateral vessels and lengthened by the presence of infarction, despite a comparable degree of stenosis of the left anterior descending coronary artery. A curvilinear relation was noted between the T1/2 and caliper-determined coronary stenosis (excluding patients with collaterals), such that prolonged T1/2 was associated with stenoses of greater than 75 percent. The number of instances in which the descending limb appeared to have two components was not provided, although this is generally recognized as a common problem. Moreover, because the T1/2 was calculated 3 to 10 seconds after injection of contrast material, the measures must have been obtained during some degree of hyperemia.[128, 129] This has two potential effects on the results. First, it may account for the outstanding separation of patients based on coronary stenosis, collateral status, and presence of wall motion abnormalities. Such separation based on coronary flow that is truly basal would not be anticipated until very severe stenoses are present. Second, and more problematic, the T1/2 measurements were very likely to have been made during a time when flow was not in a steady state.[128-130]

Takeda and associates[131] employed a similar technique in 10 control subjects and 8 patients with anterior myocardial infarction. Atrial pacing was used to avoid heart rate variability. In contrast to the study of Ikeda and colleagues, the washout time constants were calculated on a pixel-by-pixel basis and displayed as a parametric image. Washout time-constant images were almost homogeneous in the normal cases except at the basal region, where heterogeneity was thought to be a result of superimposed contrast material in the coronary sinus, right ventricle, and pulmonary arteries. In patients with myocardial infarction, regional heterogeneity was demonstrated, with prolonged washout times localized to the zones of contraction abnormality. The discrete areas with abnormal washout agreed more closely with discrete areas of wall thickening abnormalities than with the much broader areas of abnormal wall motion.[132]

Investigators at the University of California, Los Angeles, have provided an extensive evaluation of the role of washout analysis for measures of coronary flow and flow reserve. Whiting and colleagues[133] studied a dog model and developed algorithms for generating time-intensity curves from regions of interest over the proximal coronary artery (to accurately measure the time of contrast bolus onset and obviate ECG-gated power injection) and over the myocardium (to calculate time from injection to peak concentration and exponential washout rates), and from regions over a small lead blocker (to partially correct for scatter and veiling glare before logarithmic transformation of intensity data, thereby allowing assessment of absolute flow) (Fig. 24–10). Analyses were made on images acquired at 30 frames per second before and after hand injection of contrast material, and densograms were constructed from 10 sample-per-second data.

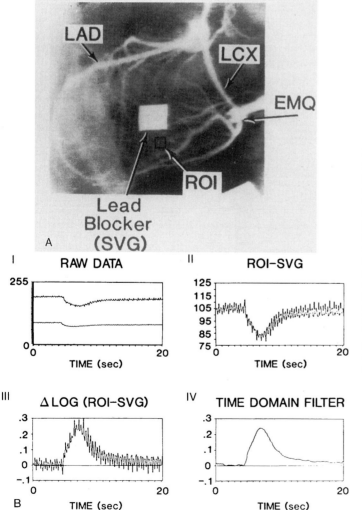

FIGURE 24–10. *A,* Digital angiogram illustrating the experimental configuration. Contrast material was injected into the left main coronary artery. The electromagnetic flowmeter probe (EMQ) was placed around the left circumflex coronary artery (LCX), and the snare occluder (not visualized) was placed just distal to the probe. The lateral projection was used to minimize overlap of the LCX and left anterior descending (LAD) perfusion beds. A 10 by 10 pixel region of interest (ROI) was placed over the myocardium served by the LCX. Scatter and veiling glare (SVG) was determined by measuring the intensity over a lead blocker placed adjacent to the myocardial region of interest. *B,* Processing steps used to obtain accurate time-concentration curves include (I) raw data over myocardium (region of interest, ROI) and lead blocker (scatter and veiling glare, SVG); (II) subtraction of SVG; (III) logarithmic subtraction of data from preinjection intensity; (IV) moving average (two cardiac cycles) applied to each point in (III) to filter high-frequency intensity variations. (From Whiting, J.S., Drury, J.K., Pfaff, J.M., et al.: Digital angiographic measurement of radiographic contrast material kinetics for estimation of myocardial perfusion. Circulation 73:789, 1986, with permission. Copyright 1986, American Heart Association.)

Some of the time-concentration curves displayed a secondary maximum 5 to 10 seconds after peak opacification, coincident with the arrival of contrast material in overlying pulmonary vessels. Therefore, the densogram analysis was limited to the arrival and initial washout portions of the curve. Analysis was considered possible only if three strict criteria were met: 1) the postinjection concentration had to remain above the preinjection baseline, 2) the curve had to exhibit a single smooth peak, and 3) the correlation coefficient of the logarithmic fit of the washout portion had to be greater than $r = .995$. Sixty-seven percent of all curves obtained were suitable for analysis, and the most common causes for exclusion resulted from respiratory motion or low myocardial iodine contrast detection. A linear correlation was found between absolute coronary arterial blood flow and both the washout rate ($r = 0.85$) and the inverse of the time to peak myocardial concentration ($r = 0.85$). Analyses during hyperemia significantly improved the ability of both indexes to distinguish between normal and ischemic re-

gions, and the effect was most marked for the washout rate analysis. This finding has been corroborated by Kusukawa and colleagues,[134] who found in patients that washout rate analysis was more sensitive than time-to-peak analysis. The authors argue that delayed contrast effects do not necessarily affect the diagnostic value of the washout portion of the densograms in these studies.

Impulse Response (Transfer Function) Analysis

Eigler and colleagues[135, 136] extended the work of Whiting and associates by introducing the concept of transfer function analysis and linear systems theory.[137-140] The approach is intended to address several unsolved problems, including lack of a validated physiologic model of contrast flow, systematic errors in densitometry, dependence on the technique of contrast agent injection, and the transient or variable effects of the contrast material itself and other hyperemic stimuli on flow. In the linear systems theory, the transfer function predicts the output of the system (obtained from a myocardial region of interest) to any input signal (obtained from a region of interest near the injection catheter tip) if the parameters describing the system have two essential characteristics. First, they must remain constant (principle of stationarity), and second, the output function in response to a combination of simultaneous inputs must equal the sum of the outputs in response to each input applied separately (principle of superposition). Unlike the washout method, this method uses the entire washin and washout curves, and these curves are obtained from both the input (proximal arterial) and output (myocardial) regions of interest (Fig. 24–11).

By investigating both phantom and animal models, these researchers were able to demonstrate that the transfer function analysis approach is insensitive to differences in hyperemic stimuli and contrast injection technique. Differences in the effects of hyperemic stimuli on vascular volume therefore do not affect the analysis, in contrast to techniques listed in the next section. In addition, gated, power injection of contrast becomes unnecessary. This research demonstrated that the mean transit time of the coronary system (the mean system transit time) obtained by this calculation is inversely proportional to actual flow per volume of contrast distribution, normalized for myocardial mass; that is, mean transit time is equal to the contrast vascular distribution volume times the myocardial mass, divided by the myocardial flow. In these experiments, the time to peak concentration and the washout time were found to be inferior to the system transit time as indices of flow. This method therefore uses the entire washin and washout curve, but an overall system transit time, not washout time, is calculated. However, because the relation between the mean system transit time calculation and myocardial flow is complicated by both the volume of distribution and the myocardial mass, analysis yielded higher flow per distribution volume in perfusion zones supplied by nonstenotic arteries than in zones supplied by stenotic arteries, even though actual flow per gram of myocardium was similar. This was interpreted to reflect the normal, autoregulatory vascular vasodilation that is expected to occur in the presence of a coronary stenosis. These investigators hypothesized that the observed flow-dependent changes in distribution volume were a consequence of the normal mechanism that regulates coronary flow.

As the myocardial microcirculation vasodilates to decrease vascular resistance and maintain flow in the presence of stenosis or to augment flow after a hyperemic stimulus, vascular capacitance simultaneously increases, as reflected by an increased distribution volume of the contrast material (see Fig. 24–11). This sensitivity of the mean transit time to autoregulatory vasodilatation, which in turn determines contrast vascular distribution, represents a new finding that may help differentiate normal from stenotic arteries at rest without requiring a prior hyperemic stimulus. The exquisite sensitivity of this approach to changes in vascular distribution volume was elegantly demonstrated in a canine model of contralateral occlusion that resulted in increased vascular distribution volumes through collateral recruitment.[141]

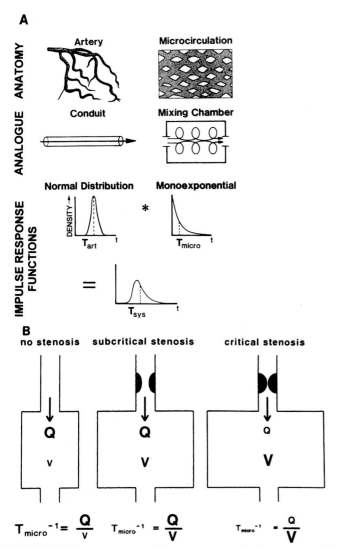

FIGURE 24–11. Derivation of the system transfer function. *A,* The coronary circulation is conceptualized as a conduit and a mixing chamber. The impulse response functions are shown below. T_{art} is the mean transit time from the arterial compartment. T_{micro} is the mean transit time from the microcirculatory compartment. After convolving these two curves, a lagged normal density function is produced from which the total system mean transit time (T_{sys}) can be determined. *B* indicates the sensitivity of the technique to the volume of distribution (V) even when flow (Q) is normal. (From Schuhlen, H., Eigler, N.L., and Whiting, J.S. Digital angiographic impulse response analysis of regional myocardial perfusion. Circulation 89:1004, 1994, with permission. Copyright 1994, American Heart Association.)

Appearance Time and Density Analysis

The appearance time and density analysis approach was developed empirically at the University of Michigan in two distinct stages. In the first phase of development, the concept that appearance of contrast agent in the myocardium was inversely proportional to flow was explored. This method was an outgrowth of the transit time analysis method, but it had the advantage of not requiring potentially inaccurate geometric calculations of arterial segments, it was geared toward measurement of relative, instead of absolute, flow, it did not require high temporal resolution or precise dosages of contrast medium, and it did not require subselective injection of contrast agent. Additionally, the early phase of contrast washin was analyzed to avoid the potential problems inherent in washout analyses that could coincide with the time when flow has been substantially perturbed by contrast material. The results with this early approach showed a good correlation with measures of coronary sinus and great cardiac vein flow in patients in whom variations in flow were induced with atrial pacing.[142, 143] Some degree of underestimation of flow ratios was noted in this early application, although the method was useful as a gauge of stenosis severity. Similarly, Rutishauser's group[144, 145] demonstrated that a variation of the appearance time technique based on pixel-by-pixel calculation of the time to maximal opacification or the time to mean ascending time[146] was effective in stratifying normal and ischemic myocardium. Haude and co-workers have recently suggested a modification of this approach that uses the myocardial contrast appearance curve to calculate the mean rise time from the time of onset of appearance to the time of peak myocardial opacification.[147]

Animal validation studies, however, demonstrated a substantial underestimation of flow reserve values by the appearance time method when flow was altered by papaverine or contrast material instead of atrial pacing.[148] Hodgson and co-workers[148] highlighted the potential importance of the density information in helping to rectify this problem (Fig. 24–12). In the absence of incorporation of the density information, appearance time can be considered to be inversely proportional to flow only if the contrast concentration remains constant and if the volume of dispersion remains constant. That is, $Q1 = RVV/t1$ and $Q2 = RVV/t2$, so that $Q1/Q2 = t2/t1$, where Q = flow, RVV = regional vascular volume, and t = transit time (appearance time in this application). Although this was apparently adequate with the relatively weak stimulus provided by atrial pacing,[146, 147] in the presence of papaverine or contrast material, or both, the effects on regional vascular volume were much more significant. Subjective analysis of the images revealed a distinctly brighter, more intense image after contrast medium or papaverine-induced hyperemia induction than after atrial pacing, and this suggested that the volume of distribution was not constant in the face of the profound, pharmacologically induced hyperemia.

FIGURE 24–13. See Color Plate 1.

Recruitment of capillaries,[149] capillary dilatation,[150, 151] fluid shifts into the vascular compartment,[152, 153] dilation of epicardial arteries,[154] and increases in the total myocardial vascular volume[155–159] have all been observed during pharmacologically induced hyperemia. Accordingly, an estimate of RVV for both the baseline and hyperemic images was obtained as follows: $RVV = (k/c)\int D$, where k is a radiographic constant, c is contrast medium concentration, and D is radiographic density. The radiographic constant (k) is a function of the attenuation coefficient of the iodine medium, the transfer function of the image intensifier and plumbicon, the radiographic parameters used, and the analog-to-digital conversion function. If sufficient contrast material is injected under both basal and hyperemic conditions, then c can be considered to be 100 percent under both conditions, and it cancels out. Similarly, if radiographic technique is maintained at a fixed value and if the same region of the image is analyzed in the basal and hyperemic states, then k also cancels out. Accordingly, an estimate of RVV is given by the accumulated radiographic density within a region. Thus, the relation between two flows can be given by $Q1/Q2 = (D1/t1)/\{D2/t2\}$. To compensate for uncertainties in timing caused by the limited temporal resolution of the images (one per cycle), ECG-gated contrast injections were used and appearance times were assigned as 0.5, 1.5, 2.5, and so on for each consecutive cardiac cycle after contrast injection. If heart rate stability cannot be maintained by atrial pacing, then cycle length appearance times are converted to absolute seconds. Using these empirical approaches, Hodgson and co-workers demonstrated a marked improvement over the previous method based solely on appearance times. A strong linear correlation with simultaneously-measured electromagnetic flow was demonstrated in the animal model.

The Hodgson method was subjected to a rigorous validation by Hess and associates,[160] who compared flow reserve measurements obtained by the parametric imaging technique to both electromagnetic and microsphere determinations of coronary flow reserve. This study was undertaken under conditions of unequivocal, maximal hyperemia induced by steady-state infusions of adenosine. The results demonstrated that the technique was associated with large variations that are greater than the variations inherent in the two reference techniques. The method was relatively accurate compared with the electromagnetic and microsphere methods (i.e., mean differences were small), but it lacked precision, as measured by the large standard deviation of mean differences. The low precision was thought to be caused by superposition of different cardiac structures in the two-dimensional display of a three-dimensional perfusion zone, potentially inhomogeneous contrast distribution, poor temporal resolution of the once-per-cycle imaging, inadequate displacement of blood by contrast material at high flow rates, and perturbations of microcirculatory flow caused by the contrast material itself. These problems caused underestimation of high flow reserves. Changes in coronary reserve of 40 percent or more could be detected by the technique, but more subtle differences would be difficult to measure. Graham and co-workers[161] noted similar findings in patients studied with both the digital technique and intravascular Doppler methods.

Cusma, Mistretta, and co-workers[162] investigated a refinement of

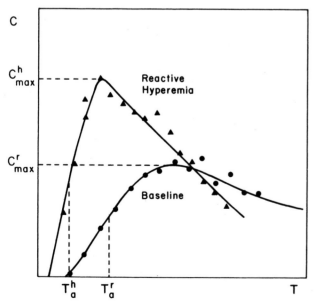

FIGURE 24–12. Contrast pass curve measured in a myocardial region of interest by videodensitometry for normal resting flow (r) and for flow during reactive hyperemia (h). The abscissa represents time (T), and the ordinate represents contrast density (C). (From Cusma, J.T., Taggart, E.J., Folts, J.D., et al.: Digital subtraction angiographic imaging of coronary flow reserve. Circulation 75:461, 1987, with permission.)

the Hodgson technique in an animal model that included single-vessel coronary stenoses. Several differences are noteworthy. The image acquisition was at a higher frame rate (15 frames per second), giving greater flexibility in selection of frames for analysis. The analyzed frames usually consisted of 8 to 10 end-diastolic images. Each pixel of the image was analyzed to create two separate data sets that encoded the time of peak opacification and the peak intensity (Fig. 24–14). The time of arrival of contrast material was determined on a pixel-by-pixel basis with a linear interpolation algorithm to estimate the time at which contrast density reached half of its maximal value. The time of arrival data set was mathematically divided into the peak opacification data set to obtain a composite parametric "flow" image, which was inversely proportional to flow and directly proportional to peak opacification. This process was repeated for a hyperemic image. The two resultant parametric images encoded the ratio of contrast density to arrival time, analogous to the method of Hodgson. The basal image encoded a pixel-by-pixel index of resting "flow," and the hyperemic image encoded the index of maximal flow. A final parametric image was produced by dividing the results from the basal analysis into those of the hyperemic analysis, thereby creating a single parametric image that encoded a "flow reserve" estimate for each pixel. Excellent image registration was mandatory to create this final image.

These investigators developed an explicit mathematical model that emphasized the importance of adequate administration of contrast agent to ensure that the concentration was virtually 100 percent during both basal and hyperemic conditions. That is, a sufficient bolus was required to prevent mixing between blood and contrast medium. Under such conditions, excellent correlations with measured flow reserves were demonstrated. Because mixing is more likely to occur during hyperemic flow, the result of insufficient contrast administration is an underestimation of the flow ratio at high values. With the use of this mathematical model, the investigators were also able to demonstrate the relative constancy of the effects of the radiographic parameters that have been discussed and the small effects of uncorrected scatter and veiling glare when measuring relative flow parameters.

The most significant modification of this approach was proposed by Pijls and colleagues.[163–165] It is based on the theory that at maximal vasodilation of the myocardial vascular bed, the maximally achievable blood flow through the myocardium is inversely proportional to mean transit time (T_{mn}) of contrast material. The T_{mn} is determined from ECG-triggered, digital coronary angiograms obtained during papaverine-induced, maximal coronary artery vasodilation. Contrast material is used as a perfusion agent, and videodensitometry is used to construct time-density curves that resemble dye-dilution curves. Pijls and colleagues argued that prior attempts to use this concept were limited by lack of a specific focus on T_{mn}, the only reliable and physiologically sound timing parameter. Moreover, because of the desire to make measurements analogous to coronary flow reserve—that is, the desire to compare hyperemic conditions to basal conditions—prior attempts were confounded by changes in vascular volume that occurred between basal and hyperemic states. Another problem to be dealt with was the changes in flow and volume induced by the contrast medium itself. Finally, the problem of videodensitometric calculations of contrast density, instead of contrast concentration, had to be overcome.

The conceptual leap taken by Pijls and colleagues was to recognize that these problems could be circumvented by performing all studies during maximal coronary hyperemia. This restriction provided assurance that the myocardial vascular bed would attain its maximal volume and that this volume would remain constant throughout the measurement period. Contrast material no longer was a factor in altering myocardial bed volume because the material could not induce any further increases once papaverine-induced maximal hyperemia had been achieved. Moreover, the videodensi-

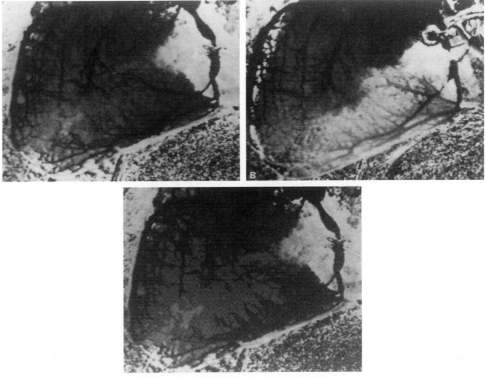

FIGURE 24–14. Parameteric flow ratio images. *A*, Flow ratio image for a normal dog heart. *B*, Image for the same heart with a severe stenosis placed on the circumflex branch, which reduced the coronary reserve in that vessel to unity. *C*, Image produced with temporal interpolation, that is, using one sample per cardiac cycle. (From Cusma, J.T., Taggart, E.J., Folts, J.D., et al.: Digital subtraction angiographic imaging of coronary flow reserve. Circulation 75:461, 1987, with permission. Copyright 1987, American Heart Association.)

tometric problem was circumvented because contrast concentration and contrast density are linearly proportional when vascular volume is constant and maximal.

The exercise then boiled down to one of paying meticulous attention to generation and measurement of time-density curves so that T_{mn} could be measured accurately and reliably. T_{mn} measurements were based on the assumption of a square-wave pulse injection of contrast material at the ostium of the coronary artery (time = 0 seconds) and then calculation of the mean time of onset of a time-density curve (after determining the best λ curve fit) detected in myocardial regions of interest.

The T_{mn} measurement, however, is of limited utility by itself. Its major value is as a means of assessing an intervention, such as angioplasty, in a given patient. Accordingly, these investigators developed the concept of the Maximal Flow Ratio (MFR), defined as follows:

$$MFR = \frac{T_{mn} \text{ at condition a}}{T_{mn} \text{ at condition b}}$$

For example, conditions "a" and "b" could be after angioplasty and before angioplasty, respectively. Alternatively, "a" and "b" could be totally normal vessel and diseased vessel, respectively.

General Comparative Summary

As is evident from the preceding discussion, the interest in the application of digital angiography to the measurement of coronary dynamics is intense and has led to a great variety of approaches. No consensus currently exists as to which method is most reliable or most applicable in a clinical setting.[166] Each method presents counterbalancing advantages and disadvantages, which can be summarized as follows. All methods designed to measure actual flow or flow per distribution volume must correct meticulously for the nonlinear relation between x-ray attenuation and iodine depth. All methods that do not employ atrial pacing and ECG-gated power injection must compensate by using high-frame-rate image acquisitions or mathematical corrections, or both. Methods based solely on transit time or appearance time are prone to errors caused by potential changes in vessel cross-sectional area or changes in regional vascular volume that are produced by coronary vasodilators. The method proposed by Pijls and associates, however, is a notable exception because all measurements are made during maximal hyperemia and, hence, constancy of vascular volume. These methods, in addition, must either be constrained to measures of mean transit time because of the phasic nature of coronary flow or applied after repeated boluses of contrast are injected at different phases of the cardiac cycle. These methods are even further compromised when they are coupled with geometric vessel volume measurements to calculate flow because of inaccuracies in quantification of the volume of arterial segments that may be tortuous or foreshortened. Methods based solely on the washout portion of contrast densograms must use high frame rate acquisitions and must invoke mathematical corrections to avoid errors caused by perturbations of the tail of the curves as a result of superimposition of contrast-laden structures, recirculation, and the delayed effects on flow of the contrast material itself. Strict indicator-dilution methods mandate subselective injection of precise volumes of contrast agent. Only additional research will determine which tradeoffs are appropriate for achieving an acceptable degree of accuracy in the clinical application of this important digital technique.

Clinical Applications

Coronary Disease

Several of the methods that have been outlined for measuring coronary flow or flow reserve have been applied in clinical settings. Most digital applications have been with the method described by Vogel and colleagues,[142, 143] its refinement proposed by Hodgson and colleagues,[148] and related methods.[144, 145, 167] The methods have also been applied in humans through postprocessing of cineangio-

grams[168] and found to correlate well with measurements obtained with intracoronary Doppler probes.

Legrand and co-workers[169] undertook a comparative study of flow reserve, quantitative percent stenosis, and exercise test measurements in patients with coronary disease. Two broad groups were investigated: those with and those without prior infarction or collateralized zones (or both). In patients without prior infarction or collateral vessels, a rough correlation between percent stenosis measurement and flow reserve values was found. This is in concordance with findings of several investigators (Figs. 24–15 through 24–22).[170–172] There was strong concordance among exercise-induced regional wall motion abnormalities or thallium defects, percent diameter stenosis greater than 50 percent in the artery serving that region, and flow reserve values of less than 2 measured by contrast-induced hyperemia and digital angiography. But the strongest concordances were noted with very severe (greater than 75 percent) and very mild (less than 25 percent) stenoses. The clinical, diagnostic value of the flow reserve and exercise test results was greatest for determination of the functional significance of the intermediate-grade lesions, especially if single-vessel disease was present. In the presence of multivessel disease, the exercise test results tended to reflect congruity only with the vascular bed showing the most severely depressed flow reserve or worst percent

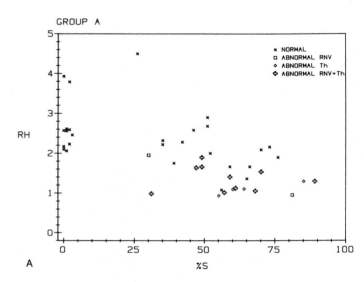

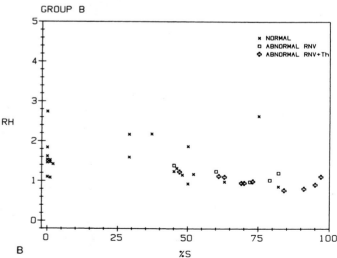

FIGURE 24–15. Relation between quantitative percent diameter stenosis (%S) and reactive hyperemia (RH) in Group A (without collaterals) and Group B (with collaterals). (From Legrand, V., Mancini, G.B.J., Bates, E.R., et al.: Comparative study of coronary flow reserve, coronary anatomy and results of radionuclide exercise test in patients with coronary artery disease. J. Am. Coll. Cardiol. 8:1022, 1986, with permission.)

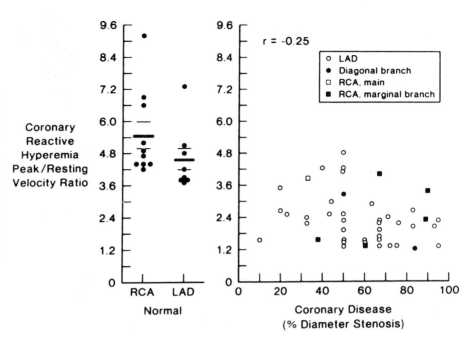

FIGURE 24–16. Relation between visually determined percent diameter stenosis and coronary reactive hyperemia (epicardial Doppler probe). Although the correlation is very poor within the stenotic segments, the overall relation is similar to the one shown in Figures 24–15, 24–17, and 24–18. If analyses are done with the inclusion of the results in normal segments, the *r* value is also similar to that shown in the other three figures. Notice that all stenoses greater than 70 percent are associated with low flow reserves. (From White, C.W., Wright, C.B., and Doty, D.B.: Does visual interpretation of the coronary arteriogram predict the physiologic importance of a coronary stenosis? N. Engl. J. Med. 310:819, 1984, with permission. Copyright 1984, Massachusetts Medical Society.)

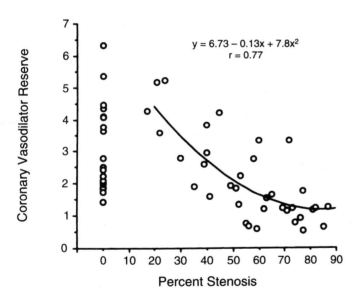

FIGURE 24–17. Relation between coronary vasodilator reserve (positron emission tomography) and percent stenosis (quantitative coronary arteriography). As in Figures 24–15, 24–16, and 24–18, a general relation is evident. In this assessment, low flow reserves are noted consistently only when stenoses are 80 percent or greater. (From Uren, N.G., Melin, J.A., de Bruyne, B., et al.: Relation between myocardial blood flow and the severity of coronary-artery stenosis. N. Engl. J. Med. 330:1782, 1994, with permission. Copyright 1994, Massachusetts Medical Society.)

FIGURE 24–18. Relation between the Doppler-derived distal coronary flow reserve and percent angiographic diameter stenosis. Open squares represent normal arteries, and solid squares represent stenotic arteries. The scatter and overall *r* values are similar to those shown by Legrand,[169] White,[170] and Uren.[171] All stenoses greater than 75 percent had flow reserves of less than 2.0, and all of them were associated with abnormal MIBI SPECT images. (From Miller, D.D., Donohue, T.J., Younis, L.T., et al.: Correlation of pharmacological ^{99m}Tc-Sestamibi myocardial perfusion imaging with poststenotic coronary flow reserve in patients with angiographically intermediate coronary artery stenoses. Circulation 89:2150, 1994, with permission. Copyright 1994, American Heart Association.)

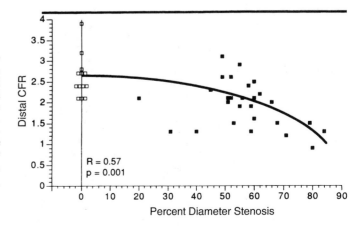

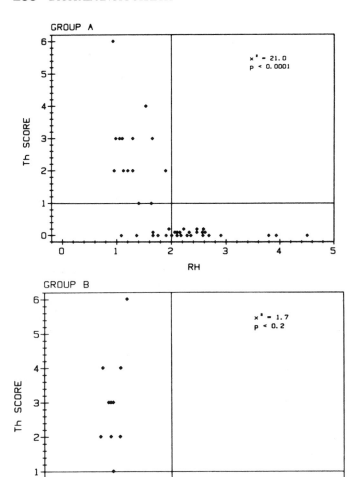

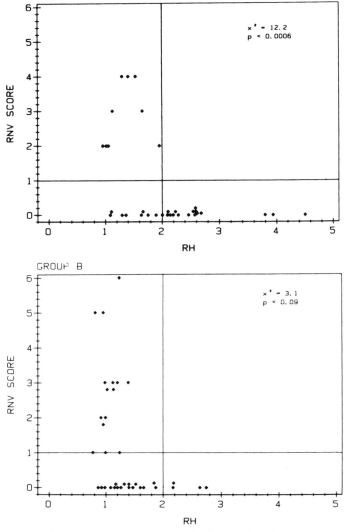

FIGURE 24–19. Relation between exercise thallium-201 tests and reactive hyperemia. Th score = the difference in regional thallium scores between exercise and redistribution images, with a score of 1 or greater signifying a positive test. (From Legrand, V., Mancini, G.B.J., Bates, E.R., et al.: Comparative study of coronary flow reserve, coronary anatomy and results of radionuclide exercise tests in patients with coronary artery disease. J. Am. Coll. Cardiol. 8:1022, 1986, with permission.) Group A = without collaterals; Group B = with collaterals.

stenosis. These conclusions were further extended by demonstration of a stronger relation between abnormal flow reserve and minimum lesion dimensions of less than 1.25 mm or 1.5 mm² than with percent diameter stenosis.[173]

In the setting of prior infarction or collateral flow, or both, there was a significant relation between abnormal exercise test results and stenoses greater than 50 percent. However, coronary flow reserve measurements tended to be extremely low and, therefore, were less well correlated with percent diameter stenosis. Moreover, the exercise-induced regional abnormalities were associated with lower flow reserve values (less than 1.3) than those for the group without infarction or collaterals (see Figs. 24–15 and 24–22). These results are similar to those of Uren and colleagues,[174, 175] who used positron emission tomography. They noted that after acute myocardial infarction, there was a severe vasodilator abnormality involving not only the infarcted region but also the regions perfused by normal coronary vessels. Although this improved over time, the flow reserve remote from the infarcted zone did not reattain normal values. Figure 24–22 shows a 30 percent reduction in the mean of the coronary vasodilator response in remote regions 6 months after infarction, compared with controls (i.e., mean flow reserves of 2.19 versus 3.17, respectively). This difference, measured by positron

emission tomography and dipyridamole, is similar to Legrand's suggested cutoff value of 1.3, which is reduced by 35 percent relative to the value of 2.0 in patients without prior infarctions.

These studies underscore the value of coronary flow reserve measurements for assessment of the true significance of moderate stenoses and the caution required when evaluating the meaning of isolated flow reserve measurements in the presence of prior infarction or collateralization.

Legrand and co-workers[176] also studied patients with atypical chest pain and normal coronary arteries and demonstrated that those individuals with exercise-induced radionuclide abnormalities also tended to have abnormal vasodilator reserve (see Fig. 24–21). These radionuclide abnormalities, sometimes considered to represent false-positive results, were actually true-positive results revealing underlying functional abnormalities of flow not attributable to epicardial stenoses.

Hodgson and co-workers[177] determined flow reserve before and after angioplasty in 20 patients with single-vessel disease. Using papaverine as the hyperemic stimulus, they demonstrated a doubling of the flow reserve value after the procedure that was of a similar magnitude in adjacent, nonstenotic, and nondilated arteries. The flow reserve in these arteries, however, was decidedly less than

FIGURE 24–20. Relation between reactive hyperemia and exercise radionuclide ventriculography demonstrated as in Figure 24–19. (From Legrand, V., Mancini, G.B.J., Bates, E.R., et al.: Comparative study of coronary flow reserve, coronary anatomy and results of radionuclide exercise tests in patients with coronary artery disease. J. Am. Coll. Cardiol. 8:1022, 1986, with permission.) Group A = without collaterals; Group B = with collaterals.

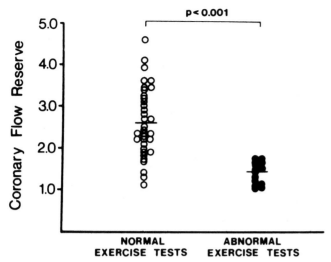

FIGURE 24–21. Coronary flow reserve for arterial distributions without *(open circles)* and with *(closed circles)* radionuclide abnormalities (exercise thallium-201 scintigraphy or radionuclide ventriculography, or both). (From Legrand, V., Hodgson, J. McB., Bates, E.R., et al.: Abnormal coronary flow reserve and abnormal radionuclide exercise tests in patients with normal coronary angiograms. J. Am. Coll. Cardiol. 6:1245, 1985, with permission.)

that measured by the same technique in totally normal individuals, thereby suggesting the presence of unrecognized coronary disease in angiographically normal coronary arteries.

Suryapranata and colleagues[178] evaluated coronary reserve in reperfused myocardium and its relation to regional myocardial function. They were able to show inducible vasodilator reserve in reperfused, ischemic myocardium after successful angioplasty in patients with acute myocardial infarction. The vasodilator reserve was improved at a 10-day follow-up study. The coronary flow reserve correlated well with regional myocardial function both during the acute phase and at follow-up angiography. Moreover, the coronary flow reserve measurement on reperfusion, immediately after acute angioplasty, was of value for prediction of regional myocardial function at follow-up angiography.

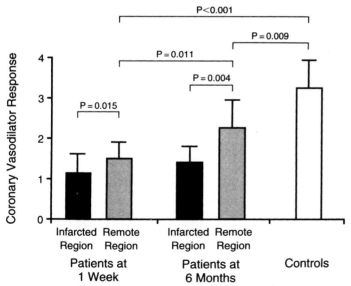

FIGURE 24–22. Mean (± standard deviation) of coronary vasodilator response in the infarcted region and the remote region in patients and controls. (From Uren, N.G., Crake, T., Lefroy, D.C., et al.: Reduced coronary vasodilator function in infarcted and normal myocardium after myocardial infarction. N. Engl. J. Med. 331:222, 1994, with permission. Copyright 1994, Massachusetts Medical Society.)

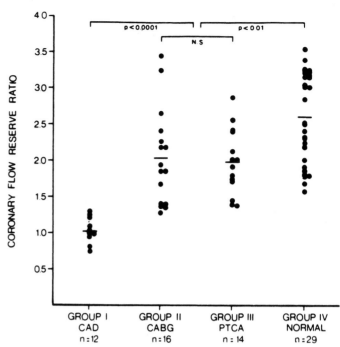

FIGURE 24–23. Long-term coronary flow reserve values for different patient groups. CAD = coronary artery disease; CABG = coronary artery bypass graft; PTCA = percutaneous transluminal coronary angioplasty. (From Bates, E.R., Aueron, F.M., LeGrand, V., et al.: Comparative long-term effects of coronary artery bypass graft surgery and percutaneous transluminal coronary angioplasty on regional coronary flow reserve. Circulation 72:833, 1985, with permission. Copyright 1985, American Heart Association.)

Bypass Grafts

Bates and associates[179–181] used digital angiography to assess the adequacy of bypass grafts soon and late after surgery. Immediate and sustained improvements were measured that were equivalent to results achieved by angioplasty, but flow reserve measurements were still depressed relative to normal values (Fig. 24–23). This latter finding remains controversial. It possibly reflects residual, diffuse atherosclerosis, alterations of adrenergic tone, arteriolar intimal thickening and fibrosis, or chronic microembolization of platelet aggregates. Others[181] have argued that methodological limitations may have precluded measurements of high flow reserves because the contrast material was used as the vasodilator.

Hodgson and colleagues[182] compared the flow reserve of sequential internal mammary bypass grafts to that of sequential and single saphenous vein grafts. All results were comparable but, overall, the values achieved were less than expected in totally normal patients, a finding similar to that of Bates and co-workers.

CONCLUSIONS

In the first edition of this textbook, digital angiography was considered a very new methodology and was discussed as a separate imaging modality. In this edition, the gradual integration of digital angiography in the traditional cardiac catheterization laboratory is evident. However, the applications described in this chapter and others have not yet reached their full potential in clinical practice. The ultimate role of cardiac digital angiography will rest on the demonstration that quantitative cineangiography and functional imaging provide diagnostically important information that may also be of prognostic benefit. Although there is increasing evidence that this is indeed the case, this information must be obtainable in an efficient and cost-effective manner. As industry standards are developed, the "all-digital" cardiac catheterization laboratory may become a reality. The acquisition, storage, and transfer of digital images will then be efficient and cost-effective and will promote greater use of the computational and image enhancement powers of digital angiography.

References

1. Mancini, G.B.J.: Assessment of left ventricular function by intravenous and direct low contrast dose digital ventriculography. *In* Mancini, G.B.J. (ed.): Clinical Applications of Cardiac Digital Angiography. New York, Raven Press, 1988, p. 99.
2. Vas, R., Diamond, G.A., Forrester, J.S., et al.: Computer-enhanced digital angiography: Correlation of clinical assessment of left ventricular ejection fraction and regional wall motion. Am. Heart J. 104:732, 1982.
3. Tobis, J.M., Nalcioglu, O., Johnston, W.D., et al.: Left ventricular imaging with digital subtraction angiography using intravenous contrast injection and fluoroscopic exposure levels. Am. Heart J. 104:20, 1982.
4. Kronenberg, M.W., Price, R.R., Smith, S.W., et al.: Evaluation of left ventricular performance using digital subtraction angiography. Am. J. Cardiol. 51:837, 1983.
5. Goldberg, H.L., Borer, J.S., Moses, J.W., et al.: Digital subtraction intravenous left ventricular angiography: Comparison with conventional intraventricular angiography. J. Am. Coll. Cardiol. 1:858, 1983.
6. Norris, S.L., Slutsky, R.A., Mancini, G.B.J., et al.: Comparison of digital intravenous ventriculography with direct left ventriculography for quantitation of left ventricular volumes and ejection fractions. Am. J. Cardiol. 51:1399, 1983.
7. Felix, R., Eichstadt, H., Kempter, H., et al.: A comparison of conventional contrast ventriculography and digital subtraction ventriculography. Clin. Cardiol. 6:265, 1983.
8. Nissen, S.E., Booth, D., Waters, J., et al.: Evaluation of left ventricular contractile pattern by intravenous digital subtraction ventriculography: Comparison with cineangiography and assessment of interobserver variability. Am. J. Cardiol. 52:1293, 1983.
9. Greenbaum, R.A., and Evans, T.R.: Investigation of left ventricular function by digital subtraction angiography. Br. Heart J. 51:163, 1984.
10. O'Connor, M.K., Quigley, P.J., and Gearty, G.F.: Digital subtraction angiography in the evaluation of left ventricular function and wall motion in man. Eur. Heart J. 5:652, 1984.
11. Nonogri, H., Sasayama, S., Sakurai, T., et al.: Intravenous left ventriculography utilizing digital subtraction technique. Jpn. Circ. J. 48:559, 1984.
12. Takahashi, M., Tsuchigame, T., Tomiguchi, S., et al.: Feasibility of ventricular function analysis by digital subtraction angiography. Comput. Radiol. 8:331, 1984.
13. Detrano, R., MacIntyre, W.J., Salcedo, E.E., et al.: Videodensitometric ejection fractions from intravenous digital subtraction left ventriculograms: Correlation with conventional direct contrast and radionuclide ventriculography. Radiology 155:19, 1985.
14. Engels, P.H.C., Ludwig, J.W., and Verhoeven, L.A.J.: Left ventricular evaluation by digital video subtraction angiography. Radiology 144:471, 1982.
15. Birchler, B., Hess, O.M., Murakami, T., et al.: Comparison of intravenous digital subtraction cineangiocardiography with conventional contrast ventriculography for the determination of the left ventricular volume at rest and during exercise. Eur. Heart J. 6:497, 1985.
16. Perondi, R., Gregorini, L., Pomidossi, G., et al.: Use of intravenous digital subtraction ventriculography in the evaluation of left ventricle volumes and ejection fraction. Eur. Heart J. 12:363, 1991.
17. Van Lysel, M.S., Miller, W.P., Senior, D.G., et al.: Left ventricular dual-energy digital subtraction angiography: A motion immune digital subtraction technique. Int. J. Card. Imaging 7:55, 1991.
18. Mancini, G.B.J., Ostrander, D.R., Slutsky, R.A., et al.: Comparative effects of ionic contrast agents injected intravenously or directly into the left ventricle: Implications for digital angiography. AJR 140:425, 1981.
19. Matsumura, K., Nakase, E., Haiyama, T., et al.: Determination of cardiac ejection fraction and left ventricular volume: Contrast-enhanced ultrafast cine MR imaging vs IV digital subtraction ventriculography. AJR, 160:979, 1993.
20. Sasayama, S., Nonogi, H., Kawai, C., et al.: Automated method for left ventricular volume measurement by cineventriculography with minimal doses of contrast medium. Am. J. Cardiol. 48:746, 1981.
21. Nicols, A.B., Martin, E.C., Fles, T.P., et al.: Validation of the angiographic accuracy of digital left ventriculography. Am. J. Cardiol. 51:224, 1983.
22. Seldin, D.W., Esser, P.D., Nichols, A.B., et al.: Left ventricular volume determined from scintigraphy and digital angiography by a semi-automated geometric method. Radiology 149:809, 1983.
23. Tobis, J.M., Nalcioglu, O., Johnston, W.D., et al.: Correlation of 10-millilitre digital subtraction ventriculograms compared with standard cineangiograms. Am. Heart J. 105:946, 1983.
24. Mancini, G.B.J., Hodgson J.McB., LeGrand, V., et al.: Quantitative assessment of global and regional ventricular function with low contrast dose digital subtraction ventriculography. Chest 87:598, 1985.
25. Denardo, S.J., Anderson, D.J., Gould, R.G., et al.: Feasibility, reliability and advantages of utilizing low contrast dose digital subtraction ventriculography in a conventional catheterization laboratory. Am. Heart J. 110:631, 1985.
26. Koning, G., van den Brand, M., Zorn, I., et al.: Usefulness of digital angiography in the assessment of left ventricular ejection fraction. Cathet. Cardiovasc. Diagn. 21:185, 1990.
27. Tobis, J., Nalcioglu, O., Seibert, J.A., et al.: Measurement of left ventricular ejection fraction by videodensitometric analysis of digital subtraction angiograms. Am J. Cardiol. 52:871, 1983.
28. Bursch, J., Heintzen, P.H., and Simon, R.: Videodensitometric studies by a new method of quantitating the amount of contrast medium. Eur. J. Cardiol. 1:437, 1974.
29. Takahashi, M., Tsuchigame, T., Tomiguchi, S., et al.: Feasibility of ventricular function analysis by digital subtraction angiography. Comput. Radiol. 8:331, 1984.
30. Trenholm, B.G., Winter, D.A., Reimer, G.D., et al.: Automated ventricular volume calculations from single plane images. Radiology 112:299, 1981.
31. Takahashi, M., Tsuchigame, T., Tomiguchi, S., et al.: Determination of left ventricular volumes with use of DSA density values. Comput. Radiol. 10:1, 1986.
32. Mustafa, A.A., Peregrin, J.H., Simo, M., et al.: A densitometric method for quantitative analysis of the left ventricle performance using I.V. digital subtraction angiography. Comput. Med. Imaging Graph. 15:293, 1991.
33. McCullough, C., Miller, W.P., Van Lysel, M.S., et al.: Densitometric assessment of regional left ventricular systolic function during graded ischemia in the dog by use of dual-energy digital subtraction ventriculography. Am. Heart J. 125:1667, 1983.
34. Bursch J, H.: Assessment of wall thickening, muscle mass and infarct size. *In* Mancini, G.B.J. (ed.): Clinical Application of Cardiac Digital Angiography. New York, Raven Press, 1988, p. 99.
35. Grob, D., Hess, O.M., Monrad, E., et al.: Determination of left ventricular wall thickness and muscle mass by intravenous digital subtraction angiocardiography: Validation of the method. Eur. Heart J. 9:73, 1988.
36. Jakob, M., Hess, O.M., Jenni, R., et al.: Determination of left ventricular systolic wall thickness by digital subtraction angiography. Eur. Heart J. 12:573, 1991.
37. McGillem, M.J., Pinto, I.M.F., and Mancini, G.B.J.: Determination of left ventricular wall thickness and myocardial mass by digital ventriculography. Am. J. Card. Imaging 3:244, 1989.
38. Haag, U.J., Hess, O.M., Maier, S.E., et al.: Left ventricular wall thickness measurements by magnetic resonance: A validation study. Int. J. Card. Imaging 7:31, 1991.
39. Mancini, G.B.J., DeBoe S.F., Anselmo, E., et al.: A comparison of traditional wall motion assessment and quantitative shape analysis: A new method for characterizing ventricular function in man. Am. Heart J. 114:1183, 1987.
40. Mancini, G.B.J., DeBoe, S.F., McGillem, M.J., et al.: Quantitative regional curvature analysis: A prospective evaluation of ventricular shape and wall motion measurements. Am. Heart J. 116:1616, 1988.
41. Mancini, G.B.J., DeBoe, S.F., Gillon, J., et al.: Measurement of systolic and diastolic disorders of shape using frame-by-frame quantitative regional curvature analysis. Coron. Artery Dis. 2:179, 1991.
42. Mancini, G.B.J., and McGillem, M.J.: Quantitative regional curvature analysis: Validation in animals of a method for assessing regional ventricular remodelling in ischemic heart disease. Int. J. Card. Imaging 7:73, 1991.
43. Sabbah, H.N., Kono, T., Stein, P.D., et al.: Left ventricular shape changes during the course of evolving heart failure. Am. J. Physiol. 163:H266, 1992.
44. Tobis, J., Nalcioglu, O., Johnson, W.D., et al.: Digital angiography in assessment of ventricular function and wall motion during pacing in patients with coronary artery disease. Am. J. Cardiol. 51:668, 1983.
45. Tobis, J., Iseri, L, Johnston, W.D., et al.: Determination of the optimal timing for performing digital ventriculography during atrial pacing stress tests in coronary heart disease. Am. J. Cardiol. 56:426, 1985.
46. Tobis, J., Sato, D., Nalcioglu, O., et al.: Correlation of minimum lumen diameter with left ventricular functional impairment induced by atrial pacing. Am. J. Cardiol. 61:697, 1988.
47. Mancini, G.B.J., Peterson, K.L., Gregoratos, G., et al.: Effects of atrial pacing in global and regional left ventricular function in coronary heart disease assessed by digital intravenous ventriculography. Am. J. Cardiol. 53:456, 1984.
48. Johnson, R.A., Wasserman, A.G., Leiboff, R.H., et al.: Intravenous digital left ventriculography at rest and with atrial pacing as a screening procedure for coronary artery disease. J. Am. Coll. Cardiol. 2:905, 1983.
49. Wasserman, A.G., Johnson, R.A., Katz, R.J., et al.: Detection of left ventricular wall motion abnormalities for the diagnosis of coronary artery disease: A comparison of exercise radionuclide and pacing intravenous ventriculography. Am. J. Cardiol. 54:497, 1984.
50. Goldberg, H.L., Moses, J.W., Borer, J.S., et al.: Exercise left ventriculography utilizing intravenous digital angiography. J. Am. Coll. Cardiol. 1:1092, 1983.
51. Detrano, R., Yiannikas, J., and Simpfendorfer, C.: Exercise digital subtraction angiography as a diagnostic test for coronary artery disease in patients without myocardial infarction. Br. Heart J. 56:131, 1986.
52. Yiannikas, and Detrano, R.: Exercise digital subtraction ventriculography. *In* Mancini, G.B.J. (ed.): Clinical Applications of Cardiac Digital Angiography. New York, Raven Press, 1988, p. 131.
53. Detrano, R., Simpfendorfer, C., Day, K., et al.: Comparison of stress digital fluoroscopy in the diagnosis of coronary artery disease in subjects without prior myocardial infarction. Am. J. Cardiol. 56:434.
54. Detrano, R., Yiannikas, J, Simpfendorfer, C., et al.: Prospective comparison of exercise digital subtraction and exercise first pass radionuclide ventriculography. Clin. Cardiol. 9:417, 1986.
55. Bellamy, G.R., Yiannikas, J., Detrano, R., et al.: Detection of multivessel disease after myocardial infarction using intravenous stress digital subtraction angiography. Radiology 161:685, 1986.
56. Lyons, J., Norell, M., Gardener, J., et al.: Phase and amplitude analysis of exercise digital left ventriculograms in patients with coronary disease. Br. Heart J. 62:102, 1989.
57. Kitazume, H., Kubo, I., Iwama, T., et al.: Left ventricular function during transient coronary occlusion: Digital subtraction left ventriculograms during coronary angioplasty. Clin. Cardiol. 14:665, 1991.
58. Starling, M.R., and Mancini, G.B.J.: The end-systolic pressure-volume relationship: Current concepts and the role of imaging in its calculation. *In* Mancini,

G.B.J. (ed.): Clinical Applications of Cardiac Digital Angiography. New York, Raven Press, 1988, p. 143.

59. Harpole, D.H., Skelton, T.N., Davidson, C.J., et al.: Validation of pressure-volume data obtained in patients by initial transit radionuclide angiocardiography. Am. Heart J. 118:983, 1989.

60. Harrison, J.K., Davidson, C.J., Leithe, M.E., et al.: Serial left ventricular performance evaluated by cardiac catheterization before, immediately after and at 6 months after balloon aortic valvuloplasty. J. Am. Coll. Cardiol. 16:1351, 1990.

61. Detrano, R., MacIntyre, W.J., Salcedo, E., et al.: Videodensitometric ejection fraction from intravenous digital subtraction right ventriculograms: Correlation with first pass radionuclide ejection fraction. J. Am. Coll. Cardiol. 5:1377, 1985.

62. Nissen S.E., Elion, J.L., and De Maria, A.M.: Value and limitations of densitometry in the calculation of right and left ventricular ejection fraction from digital angiography. In Mancini, G.B.J. (ed.): Clinical Applications of Cardiac Digital Angiography, New York, Raven Press, 1988, p. 115.

63. Nissen, S.E., Friedman, B.J., Waters, J., et al.: Right ventricular ejection fraction by videodensitometry of intravenous digital subtraction angiograms: Experimental validation and initial clinical results. J. Am. Coll. Cardiol. 3:589, 1987.

64. Honda, T., Hayasaki K., Honda, T., et al.: Right ventricular wall motion disturbance and determinants of the appearance of hemodynamic right ventricular infarction. Jpn. Circ. J. 56:1106, 1992.

65. Detrano, R., Markovic, D., Simpfendorfer, C., et al.: Digital subtraction fluoroscopy: A new method of detecting coronary calcifications with improved sensitivity for the prediction of coronary disease. Circulation 71:725, 1985.

66. Detrano, R.C., Wong, N.D., Tang, W., et al.: Prognostic significance of cardiac cinefluoroscopy for coronary calcific deposits in asymptomatic high risk subjects. Am. J. Coll. Cardiol. 24:354, 1994.

67. Taggart, E.J., and Mistretta, C.A.: Digital coronary angiography: Approaches using intravenous and direct methods. In Mancini, G.B.J. (ed.): Clinical Applications of Cardiac Digital Angiography. New York, Raven Press, 1988, p. 253.

68. Peppler, W.W., Van Lysel, M.S., Dobbins, J.T., et al.: Progress report on the University of Wisconsin Digital Video Image Processor (DVIP 11). In Heintzen, P.H., and Brennecke, R. (eds.): Digital Imaging in Cardiovascular Radiology. New York, George Thieme Verlag, 1983, p. 56.

69. Mistretta, C.A.: X-ray image intensifiers. In Haus, A.G. (ed.): The Physics of Medical Imaging: Recording System Measurements and Techniques. New York, American Institute of Physics, 1979, p. 11.

70. Myerowitz, P.D., Turnipseed, W.D., Shaw C-G., et al.: Computerized fluoroscopy: New technique for the non-invasive evaluation of the aorta, coronary artery bypass grafts, and left ventricular function. J. Thorac. Cardiovasc. Surg. 83:65, 1982.

71. Brody, W.R.: Hybrid subtraction for improved arteriography. Radiology 141:828, 1981.

72. Riederer, S.J., Brody, W.R., Enzmann, D.R., et al.: Work in progress: The application of temporal filtering techniques to hybrid subtraction in digital subtraction angiography. Radiology 147:859, 1983.

73. Riederer, S.J., Enzmann, D.R., Hall, A.L., et al.: The application of matched filtering to x-ray exposure reduction in digital subtraction angiography: Clinical results. Radiology 146:349, 1983.

74. Riederer, S.J., Hall, A.L., Maier, J.K., et al.: The technical characteristics of matched filtering in digital subtraction angiography. Med. Phys. 10:209, 1983.

75. Riederer, S.J., and Krager, R.A.: Intravenous digital subtraction: A summary of recent developments. Radiology 147:633, 1983.

76. Haggman, D., Detrano, R., and Simpfendorfer, C.: The value of coronary artery visualization during routine intravenous digital subtraction ventriculography. Cathet. Cardiovasc. Diagn. 12:5, 1986.

77. Detrano, R., Haggman, D.L., Simpfendorfer, C., et al.: Digital fluoroscopy and intravenous cardiac angiography for the detection of coronary artery disease in selected subjects. Cleve. Clin. J. Med. 55:129, 1988.

78. Akisada, M., Hyodo, K., Ando, M., et al.: Synchrotron radiation at the photon factory for non-invasive coronary angiography: Experimental studies. J. Cardiol. 16:527, 1986.

79. Yamamoto, S., Ogawa, S., Kitano, T., et al.: Complete evaluation of the cardiovascular lesions in 24 patients with Takayasu's aortitis using four-image, intravenous digital subtraction angiography. Am. Heart J. 114:1426, 1987.

80. Paulin, S.: Assessing the severity of coronary lesions with angiography. N. Engl. J. Med. 316:1405, 1987.

81. Paulin, S.: Nonselective coronary arteriography. Semin. Roentgenol. 7:369, 1972.

82. Bellman, S., Frank, H.A., Lambert, P.B., et al.: Coronary arteriography: I. Differential opacification of the aortic stream by catheters of special design. N. Engl. J. Med. 262:325, 1960.

83. Goldberg, H.L., Moses, J.W., Fisher, J., et al.: Diagnostic accuracy of coronary angiography utilizing computer-based digital subtraction methods: Comparison to conventional cineangiography. Chest 90:793, 1986.

84. Ross, A.M., Johnson, R.A., Katz, R.J., et al.: Diagnosis of coronary disease by aortic digital subtraction angiography. Circulation 63:III-43, 1983.

85. Lassar, T., Roden, R., Grenier, R., et al.: Nonselective coronary artery and bypass graft angiography utilizing density gated aortic root digital subtraction angiography. (Abstract.) Clin. Res. 34:318A, 1986.

86. Wholey, H.: Cardiovascular applications of digital subtraction angiography. Radiol. Clin. North Am. 23:627, 1985.

87. Talwar, K.K., Ramachandran, S.V., Sanjiv, S., et al.: Non-specific aortoarteritis: Long term follow-up on immunosuppressive therapy. Int. J. Cardiol. 39:79, 1993.

88. Finci, L., Meier, B., Steffenino, G., et al.: Nonselective preoperative digital subtraction angiography of internal mammary arteries. Cathet. Cardiol. Diagn. 19:13, 1990.

89. Molloi, S.Y., Weber, D.M., Peppler, W.W., et al.: Quantitative dual-energy coronary arteriography. Invest. Radiol. 25:908, 1990.

90. Molloi, S.Y., Ersahin, A., Roeck, W.W., et al.: Absolute cross-sectional area measurements in quantitative coronary arteriography by dual-energy DSA. Invest. Radiol. 26:119, 1990.

91. Weber, D.M., Sabee, Y.M., Folts, J.D., et al.: Geometric quantitative coronary arteriography. A comparison of unsubtracted and dual energy-subtracted images. Invest. Radiol. 26:649, 1991.

92. Myerowitz, P.D., Turnipseed, W.D., Swanson, D.K., et al.: Digital subtraction angiography as a method for screening for coronary artery disease during peripheral vascular angiography. Surgery 92:1042, 1982.

93. Myerowitz, P.D.: Digital subtraction angiography: Present and future uses in cardiovascular diagnosis. Clin. Cardiol. 5:623, 1982.

94. Drury J.K., Gray, R., Diamond, G.A., et al.: Computer enhanced digital angiography visualizes coronary bypass grafts without need for selective injection. (Abstract.) Circulation 66(Suppl.):229, 1982.

95. Guthaner, D.F., Wexler, L., and Bradley, B.: Digital subtraction angiography of coronary grafts: Optimization of technique. AJR 145:1185, 1985.

96. Lupon-Roses, J., Montana, J., Domingo, E., et al.: Venous digital angio-radiography: An accurate and useful technique for assessing coronary bypass graft patency. Eur. Heart J. 7:979, 1986.

97. Guiraudon, G.M., Rankin, R.N., Kostuk, W.J., et al.: Visualization of internal mammary artery bypass graft by digital intravenous angiography: Experience with 42 consecutive patients. (Abstract.) J. Am. Coll. Cardiol. 7:152A, 1986.

98. Goldberg, H.L., Moses, J.W., Borer, J.S., et al.: The role of digital subtraction angiography in coronary and bypass graft arteriography. (Abstract.) Circulation 66(Suppl. II):11, 1982.

99. Steffenino, G., Meier, B., Bopp, P., et al.: Non-selective intra-arterial digital subtraction angiography for the assessment of coronary artery bypass grafts. Int. J. Card. Imaging 1:209, 1985.

100. Kuttler, H., Hauestern, K.H., Kameda, T., et al.: Significance of early angiographic follow-up after internal thoracic artery anastomosis in coronary surgery. Thorac. Cardiovasc. Surg. 36:96, 1988.

101. Marvasti, M.A., Parker, F.B., Jr., Randall, P.A., et al.: Composite graft replacement of the ascending aorta and aortic valve. J. Thorac. Cardiovasc. Surg. 95:924, 1988.

102. Boonstra, P.W., Boeve, W.J., Mooyaart, E.L., et al.: Intra-arterial digital subtraction angiography as an outpatient screening method for the follow up of graft patency in coronary surgery. J. Cardiovasc. Surg. 30:764, 1989.

103. Kawasuji, M., Tsujiguchi, H., Sawa, S., et al.: Intraarterial digital subtraction angiography for evaluation of internal mammary artery graft in coronary bypass surgery. Jap. Circ. J. 53:773, 1989.

104. Rutishauser, W., Bussman, W-D., Noseda, G., et al.: Blood flow measurement through single coronary arteries by roentgen densitometry: Part I. A comparison of flow measured by radiologic techniques applicable in the intact organism and by electromagnetic flowmeter. AJR 109:12, 1970.

105. Rutishauser, W., Noseda, G., and Bussman, W.D.: Blood flow measurements through single coronary arteries by roentgen densitometry: Part II. Right coronary artery flow in conscious man. AJR 109:21, 1970.

106. Rutishauser, W.: Kreislanganalyse mettels montgendensitometrie. Stuttgart, Verlag Hans Huber Bern, 1969.

107. Smith, H.C., Frye, R.I., Donald, D.E., et al.: Roentgen videodensitometric measurement of coronary blood flow: Determination from simultaneous indicator-dilution curves to selected sites in the coronary circulation and in coronary artery saphenous vein grafts. Mayo Clin. Proc. 46:800, 1971.

108. Smith, H.C., Sturm, R.E., and Wood, E.H.: Videodensitometric system for measurement of vessel blood flow, particularly in the coronary arteries, in man. Am. J. Cardiol. 32:144, 1973.

109. Kruger, R.A., Bateman, W., Lin, P.Y., et al.: Blood flow determination using recursive processing: A digital radiographic method. Radiology 149:293, 1983.

110. Spiller, P., Schmeil, F.K., Politz, B., et al.: Measurement of systolic and diastolic flow rates in the coronary artery system by x-ray densitometry. Circulation 68:337, 1983.

111. Swanson, O.K., Myerwitz, P.D., Hegge, J.D., et al.: Arterial blood-flow waveform measurement in intact animals: New digital radiographic technique. Radiology 161:323, 1986.

112. Swanson, D.K., Kress, D.C., Pasaoglu, I., et al.: Quantitation of absolute flow in coronary artery bypass grafts using digital subtraction angiography. J. Surg. Res. 44:326, 1988.

113. Shaw, C.G., and Plewes, D.B.: Pulsed-injection method for blood flow velocity measurement in intra-arterial digital subtraction angiography. Radiology 160:556, 1986.

114. Fencil, L.E., Doi, K., Chua, K.G., et al.: Measurement of absolute flow rate in vessels using a stereoscopic DSA system. Phys. Med. Biol. 34:659, 1989.

115. Stiel, G.M., Stiel, L.S.G., Donath, K., et al.: Digital flashing tomosynthesis (DFTS): A technique for three-dimensional coronary angiography. Int. J. Card. Imaging 5:53, 1989.

116. Sitomer, J., LeFree, M.T., Anselmo, E.G., et al.: Computer image-guided gantry positioning for optimization of quantitative coronary arteriography. Am. J. Card. Imaging 117:1283, 1989.

117. Hoffman, K.R., Doi, K., and Fencil, L.: Determination of instantaneous and average blood flow rates from digital angiograms of vessel phantoms using distance-density curves. Invest. Radiol. 26:207, 1991.

118. Lantz, B.M.T., Foerster, J.M., Link, D.P., et al.: Determination of relative blood flow in single arteries: New video dilution technique. AJR 134:1161, 1980.

119. Link, D.P., Foerster, J.M., Lantz, B.M.T., et al.: Assessment of peripheral blood

flow in man by video dilution technique: A preliminary report. Invest. Radiol. 16:298, 1981.

120. Foerster, J., Lantz, B.M.T., Holcroft, J.W., et al.: Angiographic measurement of coronary blood flow by video dilution technique. Acta Radiol. Diagn. 22:121, 1981.

121. Foerster, J., Link, D.P., Lantz, B.M.T., et al.: Measurement of coronary reactive hyperemia during clinical angiography by video dilution technique. Acta. Radiol. Diagn. 22:209, 1981.

122. Lois, J.F., Mankovich, N.J., and Gomes, A.S.: Blood flow determinations utilizing digital densitometry. Acta Radiol. 28:635, 1987.

123. Nissen, S.E., Elion, J.L., Booth, D.C., et al.: Value and limitations of computer analysis of digital subtraction angiography in the assessment of coronary flow reserve. Circulation 73:562, 1986.

124. Nissen, S.E., Elion, J.L., and DeMaria, A.N.: Methods for calculation of coronary flow reserve by computer processing of digital angiograms. In Heintzen, P.H., and Bursch, J.H.(eds.): Progress in Digital Angiocardiography. Dordrecht, Kluwer Academic Publishers, 1988, p. 237.

125. Gurley, J.C., Nissen, S.E., Elion, J.L., et al.: Determination of coronary flow reserve by digital angiography: Validation of a practical method not requiring power injection or electrocardiographic gating. J. Am. Coll. Cardiol. 16:190, 1990.

126. Ikeda, H., Shibao, K., Okabe, K., et al.: Functional myocardial perfusion imaging by digital subtraction coronary arteriography: Comparison of contrast decay rates in normal and ischemic myocardium. Heart Vessels 2:45, 1986.

127. Ikeda, H., Koga, Y., Utsu, F., et al.: Quantitative evaluation of regional myocardial blood flow by videodensitometric analysis of digital subtraction coronary arteriography in humans. J. Am. Coll. Cardiol. 8:809, 1986.

128. Friedman, H.Z., DeBoe, S.F., McGillem, M., et al.: The immediate effects of iohexol on coronary blood flow and myocardial function. Circulation 74:1416, 1986.

129. Friedman, H.Z., DeBoe, S.F., McGillem, M.J., et al.: Immediate effects of graded ionic and nonionic contrast injections on coronary blood flow and myocardial function: Implications for digital coronary angiography. Invest. Radiol. 22:722, 1987.

130. Bookstein, J.J., and Higgins, C.B.: Comparative efficacy of coronary vasodilatory methods. Invest. Radiol. 12:121, 1977.

131. Takeda, T., Matsuda, M., Akatsuka, T., et al.: Clinical validity of wash-out time constant images obtained by digital subtraction angiography. J. Cardiol. 16:841, 1986.

132. McGillem, M.J., Mancini, G.B.J., DeBoe, S.F., et al.: Modification of the center-line method for assessment of echocardiographic wall thickening and motion: A comparison with areas of risk. J. Am. Coll. Cardiol. 11:861, 1988.

133. Whiting, J.S., Drury, J.K., Pfaff, J.M., et al.: Digital angiographic measurement of radiographic contrast material kinetics for estimation of myocardial perfusion. Circulation 73:789, 1986.

134. Kusukawa, R., Matsuzaki, M., Kohtoku, S., et al.: Analysis of digital subtraction coronary angiography for estimation of flow reserve in critical coronary stenosis. Am. J. Cardiol. 63:52E, 1989.

135. Eigler, N.L., Pfaff, J.M., Whiting, J.S., et al.: Digital angiographic transfer function analysis of regional myocardial perfusion: Measurement system and coronary contrast transit linearity. In Heintzen, P.H., and Bursch, J.H. (eds.): Progress in Digital Angiocardiography. Dordrecht, Kluwer Academic Publishers, 1988, p. 265.

136. Eigler, N.L., Schuchlen, H., Whiting, J.S., et al.: Digital angiographic impulse response analysis of regional myocardial perfusion. Circ. Res. 68:870, 1991.

137. Bassingthwaighte, J.B., Warner, H.R., and Wood, E.H.: A mathematical description of the dispersion in blood traversing an artery. Physiologist 4:8, 1961.

138. Bassingthwaighte, J.B., Ackerman, F.S., and Wood, E.H.: Applications of the lagged normal density curve as a model for arterial dilution curves. Circ. Res. 18:398, 1966.

139. Bassingthwaighte, J.B.: Plasma indicator dispersion in arteries of the human leg. Circ. Res. 19:332, 1966.

140. Nicholes, K.R.K., Warner, H.R., and Wood, E.H.: A study of dispersion of an indicator in the circulation. Ann. N.Y. Acad. Sci. 115:721, 1964.

141. Schuhlen, H., Eigler, N.L., and Whiting, J.S.: Digital angiographic impulse response analysis of regional myocardial perfusion. Circulation 89:1004, 1994.

142. Vogel, R., LeFree, M., Bates, E., et al.: Application of digital techniques to selective coronary arteriography: Use of myocardial contrast appearance time to measure coronary flow reserve. Am. Heart J. 107:153,1984.

143. Vogel, R.A., Bates, E.R., O'Neill, W.W., et al.: Coronary flow reserve measured during cardiac catheterization. Arch. Intern. Med. 144:1773, 1984.

144. Ratib, O., Chappuis, F., and Rutishauser, W.: Digital angiographic technique for the quantitative assessment of myocardial perfusion. AJR 28:193,1985.

145. DeBruyne, B., Dorsaz, P.A., Doriot, P.A., et al.: Assessment of regional coronary flow reserve by digital angiography in patients with coronary artery disease. Int. J. Card. Imaging 3:47, 1988.

146. Bursch, J.H., and Heintzen, P.H.: Parametric imaging. Radiol. Clin. North Am. 23:321, 1985.

147. Haude, M., Brennecke, R., Erbel, R., et al.: Parametric assessment of myocardial perfusion during interventional cardiac catheterization by means of X-ray densitometry: Short- and long-term results. Int. J. Card. Imaging 5:183, 1990.

148. Hodgson, J.McB., Legrand, V., Bates, E.R., et al.: Validation in dogs of a rapid digital angiographic technique to measure relative coronary blood flow during routine cardiac catheterization. Am. J. Cardiol. 55:188, 1985.

149. Tillmans, H., Steinhausen, M., Dart, A., et al.: New aspects of myocardial capillary recruitment during hypoxia and reactive hyperaemia. (Abstract.) Circulation 66(Suppl. II):11, 1982.

150. Branemark, P.L., Jacobsson, B., and Sorensen, S.E.: Microvascular effects of topically applied contrast media. Acta Radiol. Diagn. 8:547, 1969.

151. Read, R.C., Johnson, J.A., Vick, J.A., et al.: Vascular effects of hyperionic solutions. Circ. Res. 8:538, 1960.

152. Lehan, P.H., Harman, M.A., and Oldewurtel, H.A.: Myocardial water shifts induced by coronary arteriography. (Abstract.) J. Clin. Invest. 42:950, 1963.

153. Friesinger, G.C., Schaffer, J., Criley, J.M., et al.: Hemodynamic consequences of the injection of radiopaque material. Circulation 31:730, 1965.

154. Gould, K.L., and Kelley, K.O.: Physiologic significance of coronary flow velocity and changing stenosis geometry during coronary vasodilation in awake dogs. Circ. Res. 50:695, 1982.

155. Howe, B.B., and Winbury, M.M.: Effect of pentrinitrol, nitroglycerin and propranol on small vessel blood content of the canine myocardium. J. Pharmacol. Exp. Ther. 187:465, 1973.

156. Weiss, H.R., and Winbury, M.M.: Nitroglycerin and chromonar on small-vessel blood content of the ventricular walls. Am. J. Physiol. 228:838, 1974.

157. Corsini, G., Puri, P.B., Duran, P.V., et al.: Effect of nicotine on capillary flow and terminal vascular capacity of the heart in normal dogs and in animals with restricted coronary circulation. J. Pharmacol. Exp. Ther. 163:353, 1968.

158. Crystal, G.J., Downey, H.F., and Bashour, F.A.: Small vessel and total coronary blood volume during intracoronary adenosine. Am. J. Physiol. 241:H194, 1981.

159. Wueten, B., Busa, D.D., Deiet, H., et al.: Dilatory capacity of the coronary circulation and its correlation to the arterial vasculature in the canine left ventricle. Basic Res. Cardiol. 72:636, 1977.

160. Hess, O.M., McGillem, M.J., DeBoe, S.F., et al.: Determination of coronary flow reserve by parametric imaging. Circulation 82:1438, 1990.

161. Graham, S.P., Cohen, M.D., and Hodgson, J.McB.: Estimation of coronary flow reserve by intracoronary Doppler flow probes and digital angiography. Cathet. Card. Diagn. 19:214, 1990.

162. Cusma, J.T., Taggart, E.J., Folts, J.D., et al.: Digital subtraction angiographic imaging of coronary flow reserve. Circulation 75:461, 1987.

163. Pijls, N.H., Aengevaeren, W.R., Uijen, G.J., et al.: The concept of maximal flow ratio for immediate evaluation of percutaneous transluminal coronary angioplasty results by videodensitometry. Circulation 83:854, 1991.

164. Pijls, N.H., Uijen, G.J.H., Hoevelaken, A., et al.: Mean transit time for the assessment of myocardial perfusion by videodensitometry. Circulation 81:1331, 1990.

165. Pijls, N.H., den Arend, J., van Leeuwen, K., et al.: Maximal myocardial perfusion as a measure of the functional significance of coronary artery disease. In Reiber, J.H.C., and Serruys, P.W.: Advances in quantitative coronary arteriography. Dordrecht, Kluwer Academic Publishers, 1993, p. 213.

166. Simon, R., Herrmann, G., and Amende, I: Comparison of three different principles in the assessment of coronary flow reserve from digital angiograms. Int. J. Card. Imaging 5:203, 1990.

167. Ratib, O., and Rutishauser, W.: Parametric imaging in cardiovascular digital angiography. In Mancini, G.B.J. (ed.): Cardiac Applications of Digital Angiography. New York, Raven Press, 1988, p. 239.

168. Serruys, P.W., Zulstra, F., Laarman, G.J., et al.: A comparison of two methods to measure coronary flow reserve in the setting of coronary angioplasty: Intracoronary blood flow velocity measurements with a Doppler catheter, and digital subtraction cineangiography. Eur. Heart J. 10:725, 1989.

169. Legrand, V., Mancini, G.B.J., Bates, E.R., et al.: Comparative study of coronary flow reserve, coronary anatomy and results of radionuclide exercise tests in patients with coronary artery disease. J. Am. Coll. Cardiol. 8:1022, 1986.

170. White, C.W., Wright, C.B., and Doty, D.B.: Does visual interpretation of the coronary arteriogram predict the physiologic importance of a coronary stenosis? N. Engl. J. Med. 310:819, 1984.

171. Uren, N.G., Melin, J.A., de Bruyne, B., et al.: Relation between myocardial blood flow and the severity of coronary-artery stenosis. N. Engl. J. Med. 330:1782, 1994.

172. Miller, D.D., Donohue, T.J., Younis, L.T., et al.: Correlation of pharmacological ^{99m}Tc-Sestamibi myocardial perfusion imaging with poststenotic coronary flow reserve in patients with angiographically intermediate coronary artery stenoses. Circulation 89:2150, 1994.

173. Legrand, V., Mancini, G.B.J., LeFree, M.T., et al.: Clinical value of digital radiographic coronary quantification: Comparison with visual assessment and coronary flow reserve. Eur. Heart J. 13:95, 1992.

174. Uren, N.G., Crake, T., Lefroy, D.C., et al.: Reduced coronary vasodilator function in infarcted and normal myocardium after myocardial infarction. N. Engl. J. Med. 331:222, 1994.

175. Uren, N.G., Marraccini, P., Gistri, R., et al.: Altered coronary vasodilator reserve and metabolism in myocardium subtended by normal arteries in patients with coronary artery disease. J. Am. Coll. Cardiol. 22:650, 1993.

176. Legrand, V., Hodgson, J. McB., Bates, E.R., et al.: Abnormal coronary flow reserve and abnormal radionuclide exercise tests in patients with normal coronary angiograms. J. Am. Coll. Cardiol. 6:1245, 1985.

177. Hodgson, J.McB., Riley, R.S., Most, A.S., et al.: Assessment of coronary flow reserve using digital angiography before and after successful percutaneous transluminal coronary angioplasty. Am. J. Cardiol. 60:61, 1987.

178. Suryapranata, H., Zijlstra, F., MacLeod, D.C., et al.: Predictive value of reactive hyperemic response on reperfusion on recovery of regional myocardial function after coronary angioplasty in acute myocardial infarction. Circulation 89:1109, 1994.

179. Bates, E.R., Vogel, R.A., LeFree, M.T., et al.: The chronic coronary flow reserve provided by saphenous vein bypass grafts as determined by digital coronary radiography. Am. Heart J. 108:462, 1984.

180. Bates, E.R., Aueron, F.M., LeGrand, V., et al.: Comparative long-term effects of

coronary artery bypass graft surgery and percutaneous transluminal coronary angioplasty on regional coronary flow reserve. Circulation 72:833, 1985.

181. Bates, E.R., and Mancini G.B.J.: Digital radiographic assessment of coronary angioplasty and bypass graft revascularization results. *In* Mancini, G.B.J. (ed.): Cardiac Applications of Digital Angiography. New York, Raven Press, 1988, p. 291.

182. Wilson, R.F., and White, C.W.: Does coronary artery bypass surgery restore normal maximal coronary flow reserve? The effect of diffuse atherosclerosis and focal obstructive lesions. Circulation 76:563, 1987.

183. Hodgson, J.McB., Singh, A.K., Drew, T.M., et al.: Coronary flow reserve provided by sequential internal mammary artery grafts. J. Am. Coll. Cardiol. 7:32, 1986.

CHAPTER

25 Echocardiography: Physics and Instrumentation

Edward A. Geiser, M.D.

INTRODUCTION _____ 273
Historical Perspective _____ 273
WAVES AND PERIODIC MOTION _____ 274
PIEZOELECTRICITY AND THE GENERATION OF
    ULTRASOUND _____ 275
ULTRASOUND TRANSMISSION _____ 275
Measurement of Sound Amplitude _____ 275
Mechanical Wave Transmission in an Imperfect
    Medium _____ 276
    Reflection and Refraction _____ 276
    Scatter _____ 277
INSTRUMENTATION _____ 278
Pulse Transmission and Beam Insertion _____ 278
Other Determinants of Axial Resolution _____ 279
Beam Patterns and Determinants of Lateral
    Resolution _____ 279
Electronic Focusing: The Annular Array _____ 280
    Transmission _____ 280
    Dynamic Focusing During Reception _____ 280
DISPLAY FROM SINGLE-BEAM SYSTEMS _____ 281

MECHANISMS FOR FORMING REAL-TIME B-MODE
    IMAGES _____ 281
Electronic Beam Steering: Linear Array _____ 282
Electronic Beam Steering: Phased
    Array _____ 283
Electronic Beam Steering: The Orthogonal
    Phased Array and Three-Dimensional Beam
    Formation _____ 283
RECEPTION, AMPLIFICATION, AND IMAGE
    FORMATION _____ 284
DIGITAL SCAN CONVERSION _____ 286
PREPROCESSING AND
    POSTPROCESSING _____ 288
FREEZE-FRAME AND CONTINUOUS LOOP
    DISPLAY _____ 288
BIOEFFECTS _____ 289
Thermal Bioeffects _____ 289
Mechanical Bioeffects _____ 290
CONCLUSION _____ 290

INTRODUCTION

Ultrasonic imaging of the heart has become one of the mainstays of diagnosis, treatment evaluation, and research in cardiology. Part of the reason for this acceptance is the safety, portability, and versatility of the technique. However, the true reason for the growth and development of new applications of ultrasound is that ultrasound provides information that is helpful in understanding the mechanisms and evaluating the status and causes of cardiovascular disease in patients. It provides knowledge of a patient's cardiac anatomy in terms of chamber size, chamber function, valvular structure and motion, and pericardial structure, as well as knowledge of blood flow patterns and velocities. All of this is done in real time with immediate feedback to the physician.

The versatility of echocardiography continues to be demonstrated as further advances in material science, biomechanics, and computers impact on instrumentation. Transesophageal echocardiography has already been shown to improve diagnostic accuracy in special cases and to improve the early diagnosis of ischemia and volume status (see Chapter 38). Intravascular ultrasound imaging is now readily available (see Chapter 40).

Despite their great promise and great utility, these applications do have some limitations. It is the goal of this chapter that, through a better understanding of the physical principles and instrumentation used in ultrasound, those who utilize it for patient care will come to a better appreciation of both the strengths and weaknesses of the technique.

Historical Perspective

From the scientific perspective, research and understanding of the transmission of sound waves have paralleled those of light waves. For this reason, many of the names of people responsible for elucidation of these physical principles are frequently encountered in descriptions of ultrasound research, including those of Doppler, Rayleigh, Fresnel, Fraunhofer, and Huygen. More than a century of dedicated experimentation took place before Langvin was able to develop sonar in the early part of the 20th century. In its early form, sound was used mainly to map the ocean floor or to detect submerged objects. By the 1940s, other methods for production of sound waves had been explored and measurement of sound velocities in various media, including human tissues, had been carried out by Ludwig.[1] At about this same time, pulsed wave echocardiographic techniques were developed.[2] Finally, in 1954, Edler and Hertz[3] described the use of ultrasound for dynamic cardiac imaging. This was rapidly followed by A-mode and B-mode methods for displaying the information. Continuous wave Doppler ultrasound was applied to the cardiovascular system in the late 1950s by Yoshiba and colleagues in Japan,[4] and B-mode displays were developed by Wild and Reid[5] in the early 1950s. Further improvements in piezoelectric materials, computer materials, and electronic design made two-dimensional real-time B-mode imaging practical by the late 1960s. Some of these two-dimensional images were produced with either wobbling or rotating mechanical head scanners. Phased array radar technology was adapted to produce two-dimensional B-mode scans by Somer.[6] This technology was specifically applied to imaging of the heart in the mid-1970s by Kisslo, von Ramm, and Thurstone.[7]

In spite of the technological developments, ultrasound images remained relatively noisy because of poor penetration through the lung. Intravascular approaches were discussed in the early 1960s, and catheter-mounted transducers were developed and tested into the late 1970s. Also in the early 1970s, Frazin and co-workers[8] used the esophagus as a window to the heart. The 1980s were dominated by advances in computer technology and speed that allowed the development of color flow imaging and improved image processing and scan conversion. Further advances in computer processing speed and memory have come in the 1990s, allowing expansion of digital review capability, digital beam formation, and more advanced digital and image processing.

Other imaging techniques that have developed concurrently with echocardiography during the past 30 years include computed tomography, magnetic resonance imaging, and radionuclide techniques. All of these alternative techniques use electromagnetic energy to form the images. Echocardiography is unique among imaging techniques in that it uses a mechanical wave—that is, an energy that must be transmitted in a medium and cannot traverse a vacuum. Although sound waves can produce extremely high energy concentrations, as in lithotripsy, those used to create images are high-frequency, low-energy waves.

The techniques of ultrasound also differ from those of other imaging modalities in that the energy producing the image is reflected. Sound traveling into the body must be reflected from structures and returned along the same path before being received at the transducer. With x-ray techniques, the energy completely penetrates, but with magnetic resonance and nuclear methods, the energy source is within the tissue being imaged. Therefore, although x-ray, magnetic resonance, and nuclear images are usually formed with the use of a backprojection technique, ultrasound depends on line-of-sight and time-of-flight information. In addition, mechanical waves are much more susceptible to attenuation and, therefore, image quality differs greatly with ultrasound images. The attenuation correction, which is dependent on the distance traversed, becomes extremely important.

All of these features that are unique to ultrasound have provided challenges to the development of the imaging technique. Yet it is because of these challenges that ultrasound technology has acquired the unique features of safety, portability, and versatility that it now has. In the remainder of this chapter, the causes and magnitude of, and some of the solutions to, these basic problems are discussed.

WAVES AND PERIODIC MOTION

A wave is a cyclic disturbance that is nature's way of moving energy from one place to another. In the case of mechanical waves, the energy must be passed through matter or a medium and not through a vacuum. Waves are cyclic in nature. Each particle in the medium is displaced as the energy disturbance passes through. Subsequently, the displaced particle experiences a restoring force that is dependent on the properties of the medium and proportional to the displacement. This restoring force tends to return each particle to its previous position. In an ideal situation in which there are no frictional forces, each particle is again at its original position after the wave has passed, and there has been no net movement of particles or permanent changes in the medium. Such cyclic disturbances of particles are sinusoidal in nature. In its simplest form, the equation of a sinusoidal wave can be expressed as

$$A = A_0 \sin(kt) \tag{1}$$

where A is the amplitude of the displacement at any point in time, t; A_0 is the original amplitude of the wave; and k is a constant that depends on both the frequency of the disturbance and the properties of the medium through which it travels. Mechanical waves can be of two types. In the transverse type, the particle displacement is perpendicular to the direction of propagation of the wave. Waves of this type are usually on the surface of the medium. For example, a wave on the ocean displaces the water particles up and down as it travels slowly along the surface. Figure 25–1A shows a transverse displacement of particles around a zero resting position. The vertical or perpendicular restoring forces are represented by the vertical springs. The transverse energy is stored in the vertical springs but passed along by the horizontal springs tethering the particles together.

Figure 25–1B shows an example of the second type of mechanical wave, a longitudinal wave through the same particles. In this case, the energy propagation is parallel to the direction of motion of the particles. The restoring force exerted on the particles is now supplied by the tethering springs as the particles move back and forth in an oscillatory pattern.

Waves, whether transverse or longitudinal, are described by several parameters. Among these are the frequency, f; the period, T; the wavelength, λ; the amplitude, A; and the propagation velocity, v. The wavelength is defined as the distance between any

A

TRANSVERSE WAVE

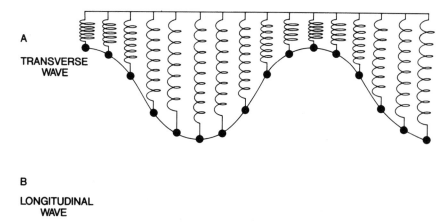

B

LONGITUDINAL WAVE

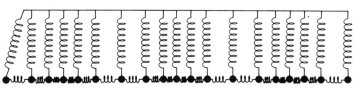

FIGURE 25–1. Diagrammatic representation of the two types of mechanical wave motion. *A,* A transverse wave moving from left to right. Particle motion is perpendicular to the direction of propagation of the wave. *B,* A longitudinal wave analogous to that of sound. Particle motion oscillates in a direction parallel to the propagation of energy in the wave. The time to complete one cycle is referred to as the period, T. The length of one complete cycle is referred to as the wavelength.

two particles simultaneously experiencing the same displacement amplitude. The wavelength is usually expressed in meters, but for the purpose of ultrasound it is often given in millimeters. The period is expressed in seconds and is defined as the time that it takes for a particle to undergo one complete cycle of oscillation. The number of complete cycles of oscillation that occur in 1 second is called the frequency. The frequency is expressed in Hertz, which is abbreviated Hz. One Hz is defined as one cycle per second. The propagation velocity can be measured or calculated from the relation $v = \lambda f$.

The human ear can hear mechanical waves in its environment, between the limits of 20 Hz and 20 KHz (1 KHz = 1000 Hz). Frequencies below 20 Hz are called subsonic; those greater than 20 KHz are out of the range of audible sound and are referred to as ultrasonic. Diagnostic ultrasound uses frequencies in the range of 1 to 20 MHz (1 MHz = 1,000,000 Hz). The velocity of sound in various materials depends on the properties of each material. Velocity differences are related to the forces between molecules in the materials, because these intermolecular forces are the basic restoring forces that attempt to return the disturbed particles to their equilibrium position. The velocity of sound in air is approximately 330 m per second; in soft tissue, the velocity is approximately 1540 m per second.[9] In general, the velocity of sound in a material can be expressed as $v = K/\rho$, where ρ is the density of the material and K is the elastic modulus. Although this relation seems simple, in practice it is somewhat more complex. Consider that the density of most materials changes with temperature (e.g., ice has a lower density than water). Therefore, the velocity of sound in a medium also depends on the temperature of the medium. Because the propagation velocity of sound is 1540 m per second at 40° C, normal saline solution at that temperature is used to test ultrasound equipment.

PIEZOELECTRICITY AND THE GENERATION OF ULTRASOUND

The longitudinal wave depicted in Figure 25–1B was initiated by pulling on the particle at the left-hand side of the figure. The displacement could have been initiated by compression or by pushing on this first particle with a piston. This would be analogous to the introduction of ultrasound into the body by use of a piezoelectric crystal. Piezoelectricity is the property of certain materials such that, if pressure is placed on them, a small electrical current is generated. One of the first substances in which this phenomenon was recognized was quartz. If pressure is applied to thin wafers of ground quartz crystal, a current is generated. One of the first uses of this property was in the microphone; voice waves supplied the pressure on the crystal and the small current generated from the quartz crystal was amplified.

The inverse is also true in piezoelectric materials. That is, if a high voltage is placed across the crystal, the crystal expands. The reason for this is that piezoelectric materials consist of microscopic, asymmetric, molecular structures that are highly polarized. If the material is subjected to a high electric potential, the molecules orient their long axes toward the surfaces of the wafer and the thickness of the wafer increases. This concept is shown diagrammatically in Figure 25–2. If the electrical charge is removed, the particles return to their resting position and the thickness of the wafer decreases. The wafer does not thin abruptly after the charge is removed but "rings down" in the manner of a damped oscillation. The frequency of this oscillation depends on many factors, but the most important are the nature of the material itself and the thickness of the wafer. Other ceramic materials displaying piezoelectricity, such as lead-zirconate-titanate and barium titanate, have now replaced the quartz crystal in ultrasound applications. However, the oscillation of thin quartz wafers is still important in the manufacture of watches.

Because the frequency of oscillation of the crystal is fixed by the

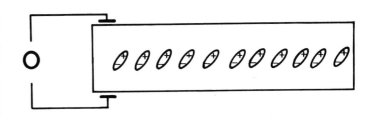

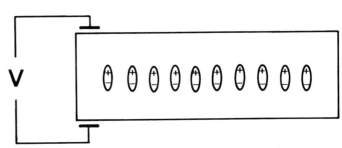

FIGURE 25–2. Diagrammatic representation of a piezoelectric crystal. In the resting state with no voltage applied, the crystal and particles may be aligned but they are not parallel to faces of the crystal. If a voltage, V, is applied to the surfaces of the crystal, the polarized particles align in the electric field, more perpendicular to the faces of the crystal, and cause it to expand.

material and its thickness, the wavelength of the sound traveling through a medium must vary directly with the propagation velocity of the medium in order to maintain the relationship of $v = \lambda f$, Table 25–1 shows the wavelengths of a distribution of frequencies commonly used in diagnostic ultrasound. The table assumes a propagation of 1540 m per second. These wavelengths in part determine the axial resolution of the ultrasound system. Many other factors come into play, however. Therefore, before considering the basic elements of transducer design, it is important to consider in more detail the factors that influence movement of these mechanical waves through the many complex media found in the human thorax.

ULTRASOUND TRANSMISSION

Measurement of Sound Amplitude

The basic unit of measurement of ultrasound amplitude (or intensity) is the decibel (dB). The decibel is not an absolute amplitude measurement. Rather, it is a unit that expresses the ratio between sound intensities (or amplitudes) at two different points. Because the difference in ultrasound energy varies over many orders of magnitude, the decibel scale is logarithmic rather than linear. The decibel is defined as being equal to $10 \log_{10}(I_2/I_1)$,

TABLE 25–1. WAVELENGTHS AT VARIOUS ULTRASOUND FREQUENCIES*

Frequency (MHz)	Wavelength (mm)
1.6	0.962
2.5	0.616
3.5	0.440
5.0	0.308
7.5	0.205
10.0	0.154
12.0	0.128

*In tissue with propagation velocity of 1540 m per second.

where I_1 and I_2 are the sound intensities to be compared. Because intensity is proportional to the square of the amplitude, A, the decibel can also be defined, in terms of the ratio of the amplitudes, as $20 \log_{10}(A_2/A_1)$.

Whether attenuation or amplification has occurred is indicated by the sign. For instance, if the amplitude of returning sound was measured at one half of the transmitted amplitude, then the decibel value is $20 \log_{10}(0.5)$; because the $\log_{10}$ of 0.5 is -0.3, the attenuation is said to be -6 dB. Similarly, if the amplitude of a sound wave is increased by a factor of 2 by an amplifier, this is expressed as $20 \log_{10}(2)$; because the $\log_{10}$ of 2 is 0.3, a doubling of the amplitude is expressed as a 6 dB gain. Table 25–2 shows the corresponding decibel values and amplitude ratios for both attenuation and amplification over a range that is commonly encountered in ultrasound images. As an example, the range of returning amplitudes encountered in a B-mode scan is approximately 100 dB. This means that the largest returning amplitude is 100,000 times greater than the smallest reflected amplitude.

Mechanical Wave Transmission in an Imperfect Medium

In the absence of frictional forces within the medium, the amplitude of a sinusoidal wave would remain the same regardless of the distance of propagation. Body tissues, however, are not perfect media. Muscle, lung, fat, cardiac muscle and blood all have internal friction and viscous forces between their molecules. Therefore, part of the energy of the propagating mechanical wave is lost because of these forces. The overall loss of wave amplitude is referred to as attenuation. The major factors contributing to the loss of amplitude are scatter by very small targets that disperse the wave in many directions; mode conversion, which is represented principally by conversion of the wavefronts into shear waves in large specular targets such as bone; and absorption, which refers to the conversion of wave energy into heat, primarily as a result of frictional forces.

The overall attenuation of ultrasound by a specific medium is characterized by the attenuation coefficient. The sound amplitude, A, along any path of propagation into the medium may be expressed as

$$A(x) = A_0 e^{-\alpha x} \qquad (2)$$

where A_0 is again the initial displacement amplitude, α is the amplitude attenuation coefficient, and x is the distance traversed in the medium. Because absorption is caused by frictional and viscous forces in the medium, it seems intuitive that the faster one tries to move particles in this medium, the more resistance will be encountered. Indeed, as the frequency is increased, more viscous

TABLE 25–3. ATTENUATION COEFFICIENTS (α) AND CHARACTERISTIC IMPEDANCES (Z) OF SELECTED TISSUES

Tissue	α (cm^{-1})°	Z
Water	0.0003	1.52
Blood	0.02	1.62
Heart	0.25–0.38	1.65–1.74
Liver	0.07–0.13	1.64–1.68
Lung	—	0.26
Fat	0.04–0.09	1.35
Bone	—	7.80

°At 1 MHz.

and inertial opposition to motion is present, and the attenuation is greater. Attenuation therefore depends on both the frequency of the transmitted wave and the properties of the medium. The values for attenuation are often given in units of decibels per centimeter per megahertz (dB/cm per MHz). Table 25–3 gives the attenuation coefficients for tissues of interest in echocardiography.

The foregoing discussion has been oriented toward the amplitude of displacement of the particles in the medium or tissue. Much of the ultrasound safety literature refers to the intensity. Intensity is the concentration of energy in a mechanical wavefront, that is, the power divided by the insonified cross-sectional area. Therefore, the units of intensity are watts per centimeter squared (W/cm^2). Written in terms of intensity, the equation for sound amplitude becomes

$$I(x) = I_0 e^{-2\alpha x} \qquad (3)$$

Because of attenuation, the intensity varies and is again dependent on the medium, the frequency of oscillation, and the distance traversed. With diagnostic ultrasound equipment, these intensities are quite low and are within defined safety limits.[10, 11] Studies of the bioeffects of ultrasound, however, have shown hemorrhage in lung tissue of mammalian species even at these low limits. This is discussed further in the section on bioeffects.

Reflection and Refraction

Thus far, only propagation of ultrasound in a single homogeneous medium has been considered. In biomedical imaging, however, ultrasound must encounter, and in part traverse, the boundaries between many types of tissues. Although the shapes of the interfaces between tissues in the body may be quite complex, the laws that determine reflection and refraction at any point on the surface are similar to those governing the reflection and refraction of light passing through prisms or lenses. Ultrasound images are formed by a process of reflection of a portion of the energy at an interface while the remainder of the energy propagates into the next tissue. The relative amount of reflected ultrasound depends on the difference in characteristic impedance, Z, between the two types of tissue. This type of interaction (reflection or refraction) occurs only at interfaces that are referred to as specular (coming from the Greek word for mirror). In light as well as sound, a specular reflector is described as an approximately planar surface that is greater in size than the wavelength of the incident energy; any irregularities in the surface must be much smaller than the wavelength of the incident energy. For this reason, light is not reflected from paper because the irregularities in the surface of paper are much larger than the wavelength of light. On the other hand, light is reflected from a mirror because the irregularities in the surface of the glass and the irregularities between silver molecules are much smaller than the wavelength of light. Because the wavelength of microwaves is measured in meters, a parabolic television dish that appears to be made out of wire screen is actually a perfect

TABLE 25–2. DECIBEL VALUES AND CORRESPONDING AMPLITUDE RATIOS FOR ATTENUATION AND AMPLIFICATION

Attenuation		Amplification	
dB	**Ratio**	**dB**	**Ratio**
0	1.000	0	1.000
-1	0.891	$+1$	1.122
-2	0.794	$+2$	1.259
-4	0.631	$+4$	1.585
-6	0.501	$+6$	1.995
-12	0.251	$+12$	3.981
-20	0.100	$+20$	10
-40	0.010	$+40$	100
-50	0.003	$+50$	316
-60	0.001	$+60$	10^3
-100	10^{-5}	$+100$	10^5
-120	10^{-6}	$+120$	10^6

parabolic mirror; the irregularities of the screen are much smaller than the wavelength of broadcast television.

When the specular surface conditions of size and smoothness are met, the intensity, I, of the reflected wave is given by

$$I_r = I_i \left(\frac{Z_2 - Z_1}{Z_2 + Z_1} \right)^2 \tag{4}$$

where r refers to the intensity of the reflected wave, i refers to the intensity of the incident wave, and 1 and 2 refer to the tissues on either side of the interface. The quantity by which I_i is multiplied is referred to as the reflection coefficient. Some characteristic impedances for biologic tissues are given in Table 25–3. For example, insertion of the appropriate values from the table into the equation shows that only 0.06 percent of the incident beam is reflected at a blood-muscle interface, but approximately 54 percent of the beam is reflected at the interface between heart and lung.

As with light, the angle of reflection is equal to the angle of incidence for ultrasound reflection from a specular interface. This is shown diagrammatically in Figure 25–3. The sound energy that continues on does not necessarily continue in the same direction. The change in direction of the energy that continues on is referred to as refraction. The relation between the angle of incidence, θ_i, and the angle of refraction, θ_t, depends on the propagation velocity in the two tissues:

$$\frac{\sin \theta_i}{\sin \theta_t} = \frac{v_1}{v_2} \tag{5}$$

where v_1 and v_2 are the velocity of sound in tissue 1 and tissue 2, respectively.

Ultrasound image formation occurs along lines of sight. Therefore, only sound that is incident on a specular target that is perpendicular to the line of sight contributes importantly to the image. Because the face of the transducer is large, approximately 1 cm², some ultrasound energy that undergoes only small angular change during reflection and refraction can still contribute to image formation. An example of image degradation from excessive reflection is frequently seen in parasternal short-axis views of the lateral left ventricular wall. In this region, not only is there increased attenuation from lung tissue but the epicardial and pericardial surfaces are oriented so that much of the beam energy is reflected out of the line of sight.

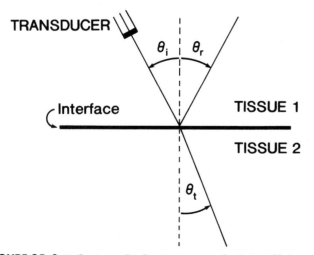

FIGURE 25–3. Reflection and refraction at a specular (mirror-like) acoustic interface. The ultrasound waves coming from the transducer encounter the interface at an incident angle, θ_i, and are reflected at the same angle, θ_r, with respect to the surface normal. Sound transmitted through the interface does not necessarily continue in a straight line. It is bent at an angle, θ_t, that depends on the acoustic impedance of the two tissues.

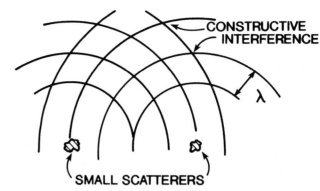

FIGURE 25–4. Diagrammatic representation of acoustic scatter. The two small scatterers serve as point sources of the reflected ultrasonic waves. Their interaction gives rise to a standing wave interference pattern with nodes of constructive interference.

Scatter

Reflection from specular targets accounts for only a portion of the interactions of the ultrasound beam with tissues in the body. The majority of time is spent interacting with various tissues during its propagation. Each of these tissues consists of cellular structures that are much smaller than the wavelength of incident ultrasound. The interaction of ultrasound with these much smaller targets is very different from the specular reflection that has been discussed.

Huygen's principle states that all points on a wavefront can be considered as point sources for the production of spherical secondary wavelets. Incident energy falling on a small spherical particle of radius r is scattered in all directions, such that the intensity, I, of the scattered wave is inversely proportional to the fourth power of the wavelength and directly proportional to the sixth power of the radius:

$$I \propto (2\pi/\theta)^4 r^6 \tag{6}$$

This is shown diagrammatically in Figure 25–4. Two small scatterers are shown a small distance apart. After the wave energy reaches the two particles, each serves as a secondary source, generating spherical wavefronts that radiate in all directions. As these spherical wavefronts propagate from the two particles, they eventually overlap. At points at which the maximum amplitudes of oscillation occur together (i.e., the oscillations are in phase), the wave amplitudes sum together. At points at which the overlapping waves are out of phase by 180 degrees, cancellation occurs. These phenomena of interaction are known as constructive and destructive interference. In the classic high school physics experiment, two point sources generate waves at the same frequency in a water tank; the positions of the points of constructive and destructive interaction between the waves do not change but form a standing wave pattern. In the case of an ultrasound image, thousands of point scatterers contribute, but the resulting standing wave pattern follows the same principle. The standing wave interference pattern is detected by the ultrasound transducer and displayed in the image; this portion of the image is referred to as acoustic speckle. Speckle is also referred to as noise, and it is a major contributor to the description of ultrasound images as being "noisy."

As can be seen from the last equation, the coarseness of the speckle is related to the wavelength and therefore to the frequency of the transducer. It is also related to the radius (r) of the scatterers and therefore to the microscopic structure of the tissue causing the scatter. This relation between the pattern of backscatter energy and the microscopic structure of the scattering particles forms the basis for research into ultrasonic tissue characterization (see Chapter 41).

INSTRUMENTATION

Pulse Transmission and Beam Insertion

In the section on historical perspective, special reference was made to the development of pulsed wave echocardiographic techniques. The importance of this development for modern ultrasound imaging cannot be overestimated. In order to understand this point, it is helpful to approach the problem of transducer design from an engineering perspective wherein the objective is to optimize both the introduction of energy into the body and the resolution capabilities of the system.

The piezoelectric materials act as a piston to inject or insert ultrasound into the body. In the ultrasound application, the current is applied to the element in what is called "shock excitation." This shock is normally on the order of several hundred volts, and its duration is roughly 1 µsec. After a short burst, the crystal resonates or "rings down." This ring-down time may be of the order of 10 µsec. If the speed of sound in the medium is 1540 m per second, this 10-µsec ring-down time would produce a pulse of 15.4 mm in length. This is shown diagrammatically in Figure 25–5A. Notice that the two targets have been placed in the line of sight of the generated pulse at 10 and 10.5 cm from the surface of the element. Figure 25–5B shows the returning pulse at some time after the incident pulse has encountered both targets. Because of the long pulse length, the echoes from the two targets are superimposed and the system would not be able to resolve the two targets in the image.

The axial resolution is defined as the minimum reflector separation along the sound path that is required to produce separate reflections. The primary determinants of axial resolution are the frequency of the transducer (the wavelength), the bandwidth, and the pulse length (also referred to as the "burst" length of the pulse). Although all of these factors contribute, a safe approximation of the axial resolution is a value equal to one half of the spatial pulse length. In order to shorten the pulse length and improve axial resolution, the ring-down time must be shortened. This is accomplished by applying a sound-absorbing backing to the piezoelectric element, a process referred to as damping. With the use of this technique, most ultrasound systems can cut the ring-down time to approximately 1 µsec. Using a common frequency such as 3 MHz as an example, only three waves of sound are injected into the body. Figures 25–5C and 25–5D diagrammatically show this short burst after transmission and the two separate wave packets returning after being reflected from the targets. The two packets now can be resolved into two separate reflecting structures.

Damping, however, is not without its limitations. Although damping decreases the pulse length, it also increases the bandwidth, which is the range of frequencies contained within the ultrasound pulse. Furthermore, more than 90 percent of the acoustic energy of the output of the piezoelectric material may be lost in the damping material and not transmitted into the body. Optimal damping therefore requires a tradeoff between transmitted energy, increased resolution caused by shortened pulse length, and decreased resolution caused by increased bandwidth. One of the descriptors of transducer design is the quality factor, which is expressed as $Q = f/BW$, where f again represents the center operating frequency of the transducer and BW is the bandwidth.

Yet another problem in injecting sound into the body is the acoustic mismatch between the piezoelectric material and the skin. For the piezoelectric ceramic, a typical acoustic impedance is approximately 30 rales. An average acoustic impedance for the skin and body tissues is close to 1.6 rales. The equation for intensity of the reflected wave shows that, under these conditions, more than 80 percent of the energy at the surface of the transducer will be reflected back into the transducer and not enter the body. One method of overcoming this mismatch is to place another layer of material, between the piezoelectric crystal and the skin, that has an intermediate impedance value. This concept of impedance matching is common in many types of electronic equipment.

The thickness of the impedance matching layer is very important. With the impedance matching layer in place, there is an interface between the piezoelectric material and the matching layer and another between the matching layer and the skin. Sound waves become trapped and reflected back and forth within this matching layer, a phenomenon referred to as reverberation. If the matching layer were left random in thickness, this reverberation would result in a loss of energy and increase in pulse length. Consider, however, that when a wave is reflected at an interface between a high-impedance medium and one of lower impedance, there is a 180-degree phase shift in the reflected portion of the wave. If the matching layer is made one-quarter wavelength in thickness, the reflected wave will undergo a shift of one-half wavelength as a result of round-trip propagation within the matching layer. Therefore, the reflected portion of the wave, when it returns to its point of origin on the surface of the piezoelectric material, will be exactly in phase with the motion of the surface at that point in time. The use of one-quarter wavelength impedance matching layers has been an important step in the improvement of image quality. More complete descriptions of the theory behind impedance matching can be found in the works of Wells[12] and of Kinsler and Fry.[13]

Impedance matching layers do not result in 100 percent insertion of the ultrasound energy into the body. Even with multiple matching layers, some portion of the wave is still reflected; and because there is a finite bandwidth, the one-quarter wavelength matching is not perfect. Impedance matching layers are now commonplace in all types of ultrasound systems. The principles are the same whether they are applied to single crystals, linear arrays, or phased arrays.

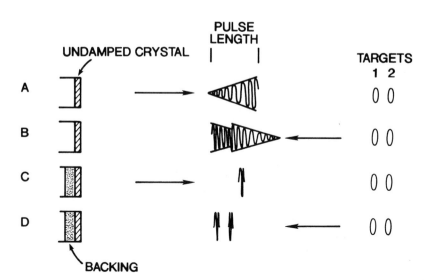

FIGURE 25–5. Effect of pulse length on axial resolution. In A, the undamped crystal gives rise to a burst of ultrasound with a pulse length greater than 15 mm. Targets 1 and 2 are separated by 5 mm. In B, the reflected pulses, after encountering targets 1 and 2, are indistinguishable because the reflected pulse from target 2 has merged with that from target 1. In C, a sound-absorbent backing has been applied to the transmitting crystal. Ring-down is markedly shortened, so that spatial pulse length is now approximately 1 mm. As a result (D), pulses reflected from targets 1 and 2 remain separate and easily distinguishable.

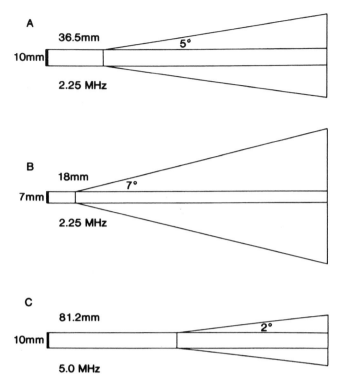

FIGURE 25–6. Effect of crystal diameter and crystal frequency on beam pattern. *A,* A 10-mm diameter crystal with a frequency of 2.25 MHz. The near field (Fresnel zone) is 36.5 mm in length, whereas the far field (Fraunhofer zone) diverges at an angle of approximately 5 degrees. *B,* The crystal diameter has been decreased to 7 mm but the frequency is kept constant. The near-field length is reduced by 50 percent, and the far-field divergence angle is increased. *C,* The crystal diameter remains at 10 mm but the crystal frequency has been increased to 5 MHz. The near field is now increased in length to 81 mm, and the far-field divergence angle has decreased to only 2 degrees.

Other Determinants of Axial Resolution

The transmitted ultrasound pulse injected into the body has both a center frequency and a bandwidth, as has been described. Because higher frequencies are attenuated to a higher degree as they pass through the tissues, there is an apparent decrease in the center frequency of the ultrasound pulse as it propagates through the tissues of the body. This frequency downshift is more pronounced in reflected pulses from deeper structures because it depends also on the distance of propagation. The axial resolution is in part, therefore, also dependent on the ability of the transducer to respond to a wider range of frequencies than its designed natural center frequency. In other words, a wider bandwidth can provide better axial resolution of deeper structures.

Beam Patterns and Determinants of Lateral Resolution

Lateral resolution is defined as the minimum reflector separation perpendicular to the direction of propagation that will produce separate representations in the image. Because the lateral resolution is defined perpendicular to each line of sight, the lateral resolution can be thought of as sweeping across the image in an arc; it is, therefore, frequently referred to as azimuthal resolution. Factors that determine the lateral resolution are the frequency of the transducer, focusing, aperture (width) of the transducer, bandwidth, and finally side lobe and grating lobe levels (described in a later section). The dominant factor of these is the focusing or beamwidth at any given depth.

In the single-element, circular-faced transducer, such as that used for M-mode echocardiography, the beam pattern is fairly

simple. In this situation, there is a near zone (called the Fresnel zone), where the beam remains columnar, and a far zone (called the Fraunhofer zone) where the beam starts to diverge. The length of the Fresnel zone, F1, is defined by $F1 = D^2/4\lambda$, where D is the transducer diameter. In the Fraunhofer zone, beam divergence occurs at an angle of divergence, θ, that is defined by $\sin \theta = 1.22$ λ/D. Notice that both of these equations show dependence on wavelength, and therefore frequency, and on the size of the transducer face.

In Figure 25–6, the dependency of the near- and far-field beam pattern on both frequency and diameter is shown. In Figure 25–6A, the piezoelectric crystal face is assumed to have the diameter of 10 mm and a frequency of 2.25 MHz. The near zone is 36.5 mm in length, and the far-field divergence angle is approximately 5 degrees. Figure 25–6B shows that, with a decrease in diameter to 7 mm, a transducer of the same frequency will have half the near-field depth and a wider divergence angle of approximately 7 degrees. The effect of increasing frequency to 5 MHz, without changing the 10-mm diameter, is to markedly increase the near-field length to 81.2 mm and to decrease the far-field divergence to only 2 degrees (see Fig. 25–6C). The influence of both aperture and transducer frequency on lateral resolution for targets at varying depths is apparent.

The discussion so far has assumed that the transducer is unfocused. One method of focusing, and thus of improving the lateral resolution, is to make the surface of the piezoelectric material concave (Fig. 25–7A). This forces the radiation at all points on the surface of the transducer to converge toward a point (the focal point). The beamwidth at that point may be quite narrow. This technique of accomplishing focusing by modification of the surface of the crystal is referred to as internal focusing.

A second method of focusing is to leave the surface of the piezoelectric material flat but apply an acoustic lens to the front surface of the crystal (Fig. 25–7B). The acoustic lens can be made from a material with refractive properties appropriate to force beam convergence. These lenses are analogous to optical lenses made for focusing light, and this method is referred to as external focusing. Again, the beam is much narrower at the focal point of the transducer.

No matter which method of focusing is used, the beamwidth at the focal point and the depth of the focal point can be controlled. Although this is an advantage in the near field and in the focal zone, the disadvantage of focusing is that far-field divergence occurs at a more rapid rate than with an unfocused transducer. Lateral resolution in the far field is therefore sacrificed.

Lateral resolution is also diminished by the presence of "secondary lobes," which, in the case of single-crystal transducers, are frequently referred to as "side lobes." These side lobes exist because not all the acoustic energy is propagated in the direction perpendicular to the face of the transducer (i.e., parallel to the

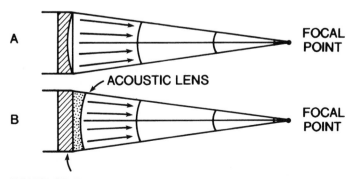

FIGURE 25–7. Focusing of the single-crystal transducer. *A,* Focusing is achieved by grinding the surface of the crystal. This method of forcing convergence of the transmitted sound pulse toward a focal point is referred to as internal focusing. *B,* The acoustic pulse is focused by an added epoxy lens. This is referred to as external focusing.

central axis of the beam). Figure 25–8 shows an unfocused single-crystal transducer. Acording to Huygen's principle, any point on the surface of the crystal can be considered as a point source for the transmitted ultrasound. At any point that the path lengths from the opposite ends of the transducer differ by exactly one wavelength, there will be a node of constructive interference or a secondary lobe. From Figure 25–8, it can be appreciated that the angle between the side lobes and the central axis of the beam is given by $\sin \theta = m\lambda/D$, where θ is the angle at which the side lobe occurs, m is an integer, and D is, again, the diameter of the transducer.

Transducers are frequently evaluated with the use of a beam intensity plot, as shown in the lower portion of Figure 25–8. In order to form this plot, which characterizes the beam quality of the transducer, the transducer is placed in a bath that contains a liquid with a conduction velocity of approximately 1540 m per second, similar to that of tissue. A device known as a hydrophone probe, which measures sound intensity, is swept in an arc at a constant distance near that of the focal length, F, from the surface of the transducer. A specific method of testing single-element transducers has been standardized by the American Institute of Ultrasound in Medicine (AIUM).[14] The resultant beam intensity plot shows the nominal beamwidth, which is defined as the width of the main lobe at the point at which the intensity has fallen to one half of the maximum intensity. Another way of expressing this is to define the beamwidth as the point at which the main lobe has decreased by 3 dB in intensity. The beam intensity plot also shows

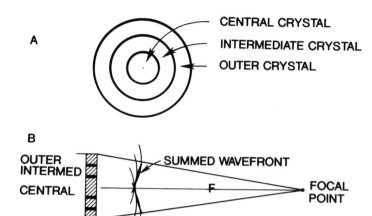

FIGURE 25–9. Focusing the annular array transducer. *A*, The face of a simple annular array transducer consisting of three independent crystals. *B*, A cross section of the crystal face. The outer crystal has been fired first, followed by the intermediate and central crystals, so that when the wavefronts sum, a single focused wavefront is formed. The focusing is electronic, in contrast to the mechanical internal and external focusing methods depicted in Figure 25–7.

the characteristics of the side lobes, which should be more than 50 dB below the main lobe.

Electronic Focusing: The Annular Array

Transmission

Thus far, only single-crystal transducers have been considered. One final method of focusing a single-beam, circular-faced transducer remains to be discussed. This method makes use of Huygen's principle to accomplish the focusing. Multiple circular elements are placed in the face of the transducer and fired at slightly different times. This technology is referred to as the annular array.

Such a transducer face is shown in Figure 25–9A. There is a small circular element with two concentric elements placed around it. In Figure 25–9B, a cross section of the set of circular crystal elements is depicted. If all three of the elements are fired simultaneously, the resultant beam characteristics are the same as those for an unfocused circular transducer. If the outer circular element is fired slightly ahead of the intermediate element and the central element is fired last, then the resultant summation of these wavefronts results in focusing of the beam at some distance (F) from the face of the transducer. Focusing is accomplished by purely electronic means, as opposed to the external and internal methods described previously. Although this may seem somewhat unimportant at first glance, the results are far-reaching. For instance, a laboratory performing both pediatric and adult echocardiography may require both a 4 cm and an 8 cm focal length in a 3.25 MHz transducer. Both needs could be satisfied simply by changing the time delay between the outer and the inner elements in a single annular array transducer. The focal point of the transmitted beam can be set to any depth by changing the timing of the shocks to the circular array elements. The previous discussions regarding the backing of the transducer elements to damp ring-down and the use of impedance matching layers also apply to the surfaces of the individual annular array elements. The result is that, after a focal point for the transmitted wave has been selected, a single pulse of approximately 1 μsec of sound can be injected into the body toward that single focal point.

Dynamic Focusing During Reception

The processes of point pulse generation, impedance matching, and focusing are involved with insertion of the ultrasound beam into the body. This entire process takes but a few microseconds. After generation of the pulse, the transducer's function is inverted

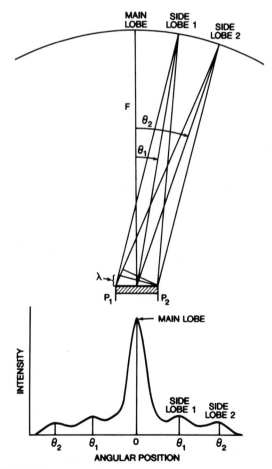

FIGURE 25–8. Diagram showing the positions at which side lobes will form. Side lobes occur at points at which the distances traversed by the ultrasound pulses from opposite edges of the crystal face differ by exactly one wavelength. Notice that the distance from the left edge of the crystal at point P1 to side lobe position 1 is exactly one wavelength longer than the distance from point P2 at the extreme right edge of the crystal to side lobe position 1. The lower portion of the figure shows the beam intensity plot formed by sweeping along an arc at the focal length, F.

and it essentially operates as a microphone to listen for returning pulses. Any reflecting target along the path of the beam serves as a point source of radiation of sound back toward the transducer. In the case of the single-crystal transducer, the external or internal focusing lens is still attached to the front of the transducer. If a reflector is very close to the transducer, the reflected wavefronts are quite curved; that is, they have a small radius. In this case, the excessive curvature of the wavefront means that the sound arrives at the center of the transducer crystal slightly before it arrives at the edges. This is shown diagrammatically in Figure 25–10A. On the other hand, the reflected wavefront from a target that is very distant has a large radius of curvature and is almost planar when it arrives back at the crystal (Fig. 25–10C). This radius of curvature is larger than that accommodated by the focusing lens; therefore, the reflected wavefront arrives at the edges of the transducer slightly before it arrives at the center. Thus, reflected waves from both very near and far targets are slightly "smeared" in time; it is only with waves reflected from targets in the focal zone of the transducer (Fig. 25–10B) that the whole wavefront arrives at the crystal face in phase and maximally vibrates the crystal.

In the annular array transducer, the returning sound activates the center, intermediate, and outer circular crystals. The small voltage outputs from the compression of all three of these elements must be added together to produce the single output analogous to the output of the single-crystal transducer. If the outputs of the three crystals are simply added together, the results are, in fact, the same as with a single, unfocused crystal. But the signals coming from each crystal can be delayed before they are added together, similar to the way the shock excitation voltages were delayed in order to produce focusing. In the case of a reflector close to the transducer, where the wavefront is quite curved, the sound arriving at the central crystal can be slightly delayed before being added to the sound arriving at the intermediate crystal, which in turn can be slightly delayed from that arriving to the outer crystal. These delays before summation assure that the voltages produced by the reflected wavefront from a nearby object are placed in phase; this allows them to sum together to form a maximum estimate of

the reflected wavefront amplitude from that depth. The reflected wavefront from a very distant target has a large radius of curvature; no time delays are necessary to ensure the highest possible sum, because the wavefront is, again, almost planar. This process of changing the focal point along the scan line during reception in order to assure optimal transducer response to the spherical wavefronts returning from each depth is referred to as dynamic focusing. The ability to change the focal point during both transmission and reception is a marked advantage of multiple-element transducers.

DISPLAY FROM SINGLE-BEAM SYSTEMS

From the preceding discussions it can be seen that echocardiography systems are phase-sensitive ultrasound systems designed to measure the distance from the transducer face to structures within and surrounding the heart. This distance measurement is accomplished by measuring the time between pulse generation and reception of a reflected signal while assuming the velocity of sound propagation through tissue.

This time-of-flight information, or distance, can be displayed in several ways. The first method is to display the depth on one axis and the relative amplitude of the returning sound on the other axis. This type of display is often placed on the side of the two-dimensional image and is referred to as the A-mode or amplitude-mode display. The second method is to display a peak in amplitude as a spot whose brightness is proportional to the amplitude of returning ultrasound from that depth. This type of display is referred to as the B-mode or brightness mode. If the B-mode display is routed through a fiberoptic cable onto photographic paper, while the paper is moved along at a constant speed, the M-mode or motion-mode display is obtained.

The A-, B-, and M-mode displays are all designed to provide graphic representation of the position of the reflecting sites along single-beam paths. Recall that the pulse generated along a single line can require as little as 1 μsec. After pulse generation, the transducer is switched into a receiving or listening mode for 999 μsec. This means that a single line of sight, such as an M-mode line, can be obtained in 0.001 second. This results in the very high temporal resolution of the M-mode tracing, which allows accurate representation of rapidly moving structures such as the mitral valve. In most cardiac applications, the display of anatomic structure and spatial relations is more important than this very high temporal resolution. Two-dimensional images are generated by display of multiple B-mode lines on the screen at the same time. The methods by which these multiple B-mode lines are generated and displayed at frame rates high enough to form moving images are described in the next section.

MECHANISMS FOR FORMING REAL-TIME B-MODE IMAGES

Three basic methods are used to form multiple scan line B-mode images. The first and simplest method is to move a single-element transducer back and forth through an arc of interest. The second is to rotate several single-element transducers and allow each to form a portion of the image as it rotates through the arc of interest. The third method is to form and move the beam electronically with the use of multiple phased elements. In the early wobbling transducer and the rotating head transducer, only single internally or externally focused elements were used. The limitations of single-crystal beam formation and single-crystal reception were seen in these scanners. For this reason, the annular array has replaced the single crystal in newer wobbling head mechanical scanners. The advantages of variable transmission focusing and dynamic focusing during reception can be implemented while the two-dimensional image itself is formed by mechanical means. Although this type of transducer overcomes some of the disadvan-

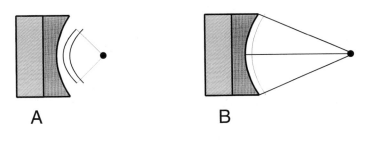

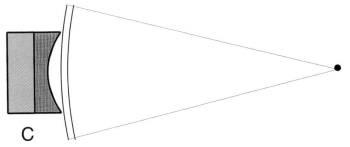

FIGURE 25–10. Schematic drawing showing the arrival of a wavefront from a near target (A), a target in the far field (C), and a target at the focal point B. The near- and far-field wavefronts contact only part of the transducer face to begin with and then progressively encounter the remainder. The encounter is "smeared" in time and therefore has a lower peak amplitude. Only the wavefronts returning from the target at the focal point encounter the entire face at the same time and thereby maximally compress the crystal.

tages inherent in fixed focal length, single-element transducers, the problems of impedance matching through the medium in which oscillation or rotation occurs and maintenance of the moving parts within the plastic housing that provides the contact with the skin continue to be obstacles to acceptance. Therefore, it is not surprising that the competing technology of electronic beam steering in stationary array transducers has developed.

Electronic Beam Steering: Linear Array

In addition to the annular array transducer, two other types of array technology are commonplace. These are the linear array and the phased array. The linear array finds its highest use in obstetrics and abdominal ultrasound, and phased array systems are most common in cardiac applications. The linear array transducer has a rectangular face with a width, W, and a height, H. Within the face of the transducer, there are many small rectangular crystals that are placed parallel to each other and parallel to the height dimension of the transducer (Fig. 25–11A). The linear array image is formed along multiple scan lines that are perpendicular to the face of the transducer. If the number of transducer elements activated is chosen such that the total active surface is approximately a square of dimensions H by H, then the same near- and far-field equations apply as if the beam were formed by a single circular element. Again, the beam travels in a line of sight perpendicular to the face of the transducer. Because the linear array image is formed by multiple parallel B-mode lines that are perpendicular to the face of the transducer, the first B-mode line in Figure 25–11 would be formed by firing elements 1, 2, 3, and 4. The next line would be formed by firing elements 2, 3, 4, and 5. Thus, each of the B-mode lines composing the image would be formed by sequential activation of the individual elements down the face of the array.

The individual beams formed for each line in this situation are unfocused. At this point, it becomes necessary to introduce the third dimension of resolution that becomes a factor in the formation of two-dimensional echocardiographic images. The axial and lateral resolution have already been discussed; the third dimension is the cross-plane resolution or beam thickness, which is the thickness of the beam perpendicular to the plane of the image. In other words, the plane of the scan is not thin like a sheet of paper, but may be 2 mm or more in thickness. The image is formed from the average reflection of all structures contained within this thickness. The larger the cross-plane beam thickness, the more blurred the image will be; the narrower the cross-plane beam thickness, the sharper the image will be. Because mechanical sector scans are formed by the use of either a single element or rotating circular elements with cylindrical beam shapes, the elevation resolution is usually the same as the lateral resolution at any specified depth.

Neither the fixed methods of focusing (external or internal) nor the variable technique of focusing described with the annular array will, by itself, solve the problems of focusing with the linear array transducer. Therefore, a combination of the techniques must be used. In the elevation dimension, the thickness of the beam must be focused with the use of one of the fixed methods. In Figure 25–11B, an external focusing lens has been applied to the surface of the array. Notice the narrowing of the cross-plane dimension and the more rectangular shape of the beam. The lateral or azimuthal focusing cannot be accomplished in the same way. Therefore, in a manner similar to that described for the annular array, elements 1 and 4 can be fired earlier than 2 and 3, forcing convergence toward a point (Fig. 25–11C). Again, the time interval between the firing of the lateral and central elements can be changed so that the azimuthal focal point is variable.

The linear array transducer accomplishes focused two-dimensional image generation by rapidly producing parallel B-mode scan lines with no moving parts. Side lobes still exist, but their positions become more complex. In the elevation dimension, side lobe positions are determined by the frequency of the transducer elements and by the height, H, of the transducer. In the lateral dimension, however, side lobe position is determined by the number of ele-

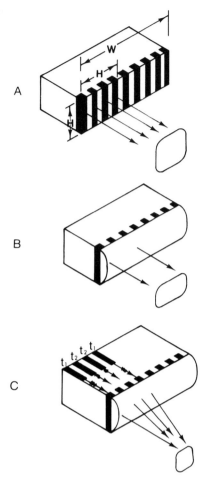

FIGURE 25–11. Diagrammatic representation of beam formation and focusing along each B-mode line generated by a linear array transducer. *A,* Four parallel crystal elements are fired simultaneously to form the beam. In this case, the beam would be unfocused and the cross-sectional beam shape is depicted as approximately square. *B,* Addition of an acoustical external focusing lens in the elevation dimension results in a rectangular beam cross-section. In this illustration, the assumption is made that the propagation velocity of sound through the lens is slower than through tissue, and therefore a convex lens is appropriate. *C,* Crystals 1 and 4 have been fired slightly earlier than crystals 2 and 3 in order to obtain the focusing in the lateral (azimuthal) direction. Although focusing in the elevation dimension is accomplished by a fixed external focusing means, focusing in the lateral dimension is accomplished electronically. (From Geiser, E.A., and Oliver, L.H.: Echocardiography: Physics and Instrumentation. *In* Collins, S.M., and Skorton, D.J. (eds.): Cardiac Imaging and Image Processing. New York, McGraw-Hill, 1986, with permission.)

ments fired to form an individual beam, because the number of elements determines the width of the active transducer face for each beam.

In addition to the side lobes, a new problem develops in the multiple-element-array transducers. One of these problems is a secondary lobe, which degrades the resolution of the images and is usually more serious than the side lobe. This secondary lobe is usually referred to as a grating lobe. Figure 25–12 shows the development of grating lobes in the same format as Figure 25–8 for side lobes. Each of the crystal elements in the face of the transducer is again considered a point source for sound, and the beam is formed by the summation of these wavefronts, again by Huygen's principle. However, at some angle θ to the side of the main beam, the first wavefront emitted from element 1, having traveled a longer distance, will arrive exactly in phase with the second wavefront emitted from element 4. At this point there will be constructive interference and the appearance of a grating lobe. The position of the grating lobes is given by the equation,

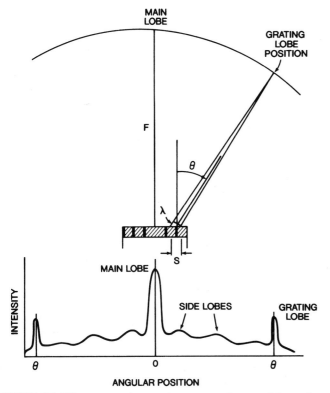

FIGURE 25–12. Diagram showing the position of grating lobes in linear array transducers. The position of grating lobes is determined by the spacing between the centers of independent crystal elements in the transducer. At any point where the path length between the two crystal elements differs by one wavelength, a grating lobe will be formed. The angular position of the grating lobe, θ, depends on the wavelength of the crystals, λ, and the spacing, S, between the crystal elements. The beam intensity plot formed at the focal length, F, is also shown.

$\sin \theta = m\lambda/S$, where θ is now the angle at which the grating lobe will appear, m is again an integer, and S is the center-to-center spacing between the individual transducer elements.

Because grating lobes can have a serious effect on image quality, the careful matching of transducer frequency to element spacing is one of the critical points in transducer design. Other critical points include electrical isolation, sealing of the transducer, and aspects of element isolation in order to suppress resonance modes.[15, 16]

Electronic Beam Steering: Phased Array

In the linear array transducer, the B-mode lines were formed parallel to each other and by firing a limited number of the transducer array elements. In the phased array transducer, each of the individual 100 to 130 B-mode lines in each image is formed as if from the same point source, through an arc of usually 90 degrees. Because each line is considered to have as its origin the center of the transducer face, each line is formed by firing all of the elements (usually 32 to 64) in the array.

Figure 25–13 depicts a simple, 9-element transducer array. If element 9 is first fired and each lower numbered element is fired at a slightly later time, the wavefronts summate into a single planar wavefront moving at an angle to the face of the transducer that is determined by the delay in time between the firing of the individual successive elements. This planar wavefront would form an unfocused beam at that angle, with similar characteristics to that from a single element aimed in the same direction. By compounding the time delay patterns, this beam can be focused in the lateral direction, as were both the linear array and the annular array beam. This is shown diagrammatically in Figure 25–14.

As with the linear array transducer, the elevation or cross-plane focusing is for the most part accomplished by a fixed external or internal acoustic lens. Therefore, the depth of field focus is again variable in the lateral or azimuthal direction but fixed in the cross-plane direction and the two focal points may not coincide (Fig. 25–15). Some manufacturers have developed means for changing the apparent lateral aperture of the transducer. This is referred to as dynamic elevation beam forming. Dynamic focusing during reception can also be accomplished, as was explained for the annular array. Side lobes and grating lobes continue to be present and are in general found at the locations predicted by the previously described equations.

Because there are no moving parts and both the transmission and receiving focal points can easily be adjusted, the phased array transducer has become the most widely used transducer for cardiology. The compact size of the element arrays not only accommodates beam insertion between the ribs but also allows adaptation to other windows. Although rotating head technology has been used for transesophageal imaging,[17] phased array transesophageal transducers are most commonly found.

Electronic Beam Steering: The Orthogonal Phased Array and Three-Dimensional Beam Formation

Within the past several years, development has proceeded on transducers that contain crystal arrays in two different directions. This new type of transducer facilitates display of two-dimensional orthogonal B-mode images and is referred to as "O-mode" scanning. One such crystal face design and the resultant orthogonal planes are shown in Figure 25–16A. This work was first reported and has continued to develop under the direction of Snyder, Kisslo and von Ramm.[18] In its original form, the cross-plane resolution was primarily dependent on fixed techniques. Simultaneous short- and long-axis images could be obtained at the same point in time. Although these two simultaneous views are helpful in assessing cardiac geometry, the methodology remained merely a modification or union of two phased array transducers.

More recently, investigators have succeeded in building transducers that provide true three-dimensional volumetric imaging.[19, 20]

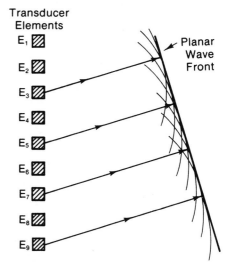

FIGURE 25–13. Diagrammatic representation of the formation of a planar wavefront moving away from a transducer array at an angle. In this situation, transducer element E9 would have been fired first and each successive crystal element at a slightly delayed time from its predecessor. The individual wavefronts have summed by Huygen's principle into a single planar wavefront. This formation of a single wavefront moving away from the transducer face at an angle is an example of electronic beam steering. (From Geiser, E.A., and Oliver, L.H.: Echocardiography: Physics and Instrumentation. *In* Collins, S.M., and Skorton, D.J. (eds.): Cardiac Imaging and Image Processing. New York, McGraw-Hill, 1986, with permission.)

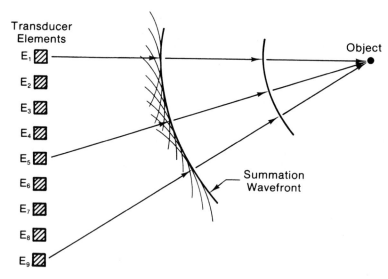

FIGURE 25-14. Diagrammatic representation of the formation of a curved wavefront. The time delay between elements is not constant. The delay is set so that the summation of the individual waves forms a circular or parabolic wavefront that converges at the focal point in addition to moving away from the transducer at an angle. This is an example of simultaneous electronic beam steering and electronic focusing. (From Geiser, E.A., and Oliver, L.H.: Echocardiography: Physics and Instrumentation. *In* Collins, S.M., and Skorton, D.J. (eds.): Cardiac Imaging and Image Processing. New York, McGraw-Hill, 1986, with permission.)

Within a transducer face of approximately 15 mm by 15 mm, multiple square crystal elements are positioned so that the scan lines can be directed, through two-dimensional phasing, in any direction within a pyramidal volume (Fig. 25–16*B*). This transducer appears to be the final step in which variable transmission focusing and dynamic focusing during reception along any desired line of sight can be accomplished.

Because the received signals can be gated so that only reflected structures at a predetermined depth from the transducer face are displayed, it is possible to display a plane that is parallel to the surface of the transducer. Furthermore, the thickness of this plane is now dependent on the axial resolution. Display of this plane that is parallel to the transducer face is referred to as C-scan imaging; because the cross-plane resolution is approximately that of the axial resolution, the scan thickness is on the order of 1 to 2 mm.

Display of an entire three-dimensional volumetric image is not a trivial task. In the present implementation, the on-screen display contains a single parasternal long axis and four C-scans of the heart at increasing depths. Image quality and frame rate have improved to the point that clinical utility will soon be tested. This area is extremely exciting. The advantages to echocardiography in terms of quantitation of surface area of infarction, volumes, and perfusion regions with contrast agents are hard to estimate. Reconstruction offers these advantages, but the two-dimensional images to be included in the reconstruction occur at different points in time. Therefore factors such as phase of respiration, preceding cardiac cycle length, and ectopy must be taken into account to produce an accurate synthesis of data. Three-dimensional volumetric scanning obviates these problems by obtaining all of the information at one point in time. Undoubtedly, this technology will impact the importance of echocardiography as an imaging tool in the future.

RECEPTION, AMPLIFICATION, AND IMAGE FORMATION

The process of converting the returning ultrasound into a visible image in television format is no less complicated than the process of beam formation. Figure 25–17 is a generalized flow diagram of the processes involved. The process of dynamic focusing during reception has been described. Notice that this process is carried out in the first five blocks of the flow diagram. The actual delay that forms the dynamically focused line occurs in the block labeled "Summing of Single Crystal Inputs." Before this, there are three other steps.

In the first, the reflected ultrasonic waves returning to the face of the transducer cross the impedance matching layers and cause oscillation of each piezoelectric element. This oscillation of the element (which has now been placed in reception mode) produces an electric voltage. These oscillations are slightly downshifted in frequency owing to the frequency dependence of attenuation, but they are still quite close to the nominal frequency of the transducer. The high-frequency signals coming from each transducer element, indicated as the "signal path" in Figure 25–17, are extremely weak, and before any further processing is performed, they must be linearly amplified.

Recall also that attenuation is expressed as dB/cm per MHz. Therefore, reflected sound from deeper structures is much weaker than that received from a shallower depth. Frequently, this difference is great enough that the amplitude of sound returning from the deeper portions of the image are one tenth to one thousandth of the amplitude of sound returning from the near field. Thus, more amplification of the signals must be performed on those signals returning to the transducer at a later time. This process of applying an increased gain to signals returning at a later time is referred to as time-gain compensation (TGC). TGC is usually accomplished by setting slide potentiometers on the control panel. This allows individual selection of amplification factors at varying depths during the performance of the study. Figure 25–17 shows

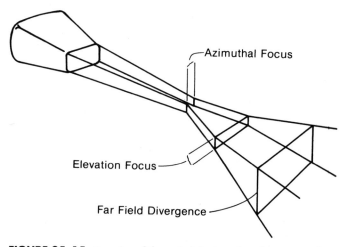

FIGURE 25-15. Focusing of the main lobe in a phased array transducer. The elevation focus is accomplished by an acoustic lens. The focus in the azimuthal direction is determined in the manner of electronic focusing shown in Figure 25–14. Notice that the azimuthal focal point and the elevation focal point are not necessarily the same. (From Geiser, E.A., and Oliver, L.H.: Echocardiography: Physics and Instrumentation. *In* Collins, S.M., and Skorton, D.J. (eds.): Cardiac Imaging and Image Processing. New York, McGraw-Hill, 1986, with permission.)

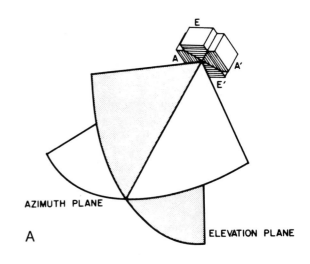

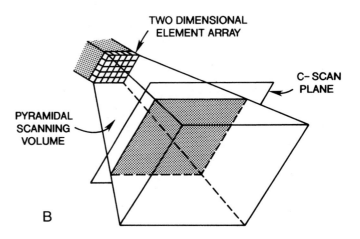

FIGURE 25–16. *A,* The "bow-tie" arrangement of transducer elements for simultaneous orthogonal-plane two-dimensional echocardiographic scanning. *B,* Diagram of a two-dimensional crystal array transducer whose transducer face consists of a 5 by 5 crystal array. Such a transducer is capable of three-dimensional pyramidal volumetric scanning. With this type of scanning, an image can be reconstructed that represents the echoes returning at a chosen distance from the transducer. This type of image, in which the plane is parallel to the face of the transducer, is referred to as C-scan imaging. (*A* from Snyder, J.E., Kisslo, J., and von Ramm, O.T.: Real-time orthogonal mode scanning of the heart. I. System design. J. Am. Coll. Cardiol. 7:1280, 1986, with permission.)

TGC being applied to the output of each individual crystal element. Whether TGC is applied to scan line formation or after the dynamic focusing time delay and summation depends on the manufacturer.

After linear amplification and TGC, the output of the individual crystal elements in the transducers is appropriately phased to accomplish dynamic focusing and summed together to form a single scan line. This scan line still contains the very-high-frequency information. The scan line formed at this point is therefore called the radio frequency (RF) scan line data.

Not all of the scan lines formed across the image are of equal quality. Many times, the lateral aspects of the short-axis view will have dropped out in either the epicardium or endocardium. In these cases, it is helpful to be able to increase the gain in a separate direction instead of only at a certain depth. This adjustment of the gain of a single scan line or a group of scan lines over their entire depth is referred to as lateral gain compensation (LGC). Many systems implement a fixed, angle-dependent gain adjustment.

The information contained in a scan line at this point is still too complex to be displayed. Part of the reason for this is that the difference between the lowest amplitude and highest amplitude signals along the scan line may be as much as 80 to 100 dB. On the other hand, video display devices and the human eye have the ability to display and perceive only 25 to 30 dB of information. Thus, the 80 to 100 dB must be compressed into 25 to 30 dB of dynamic range for the display device. Many of the low-amplitude signals in the scan line may represent background noise. It would be inappropriate to use part of the display capabilities unnecessarily for this portion of the signal. Therefore, the lower level background noise can be thresholded or rejected from the RF scan line. The remaining dynamic range is then compressed into the capabilities

of the display device. This can be done either linearly or logarithmically. In most situations, linear amplification results in failure of display of the majority of the very-low-level signals. Therefore, logarithmic amplification, which favors enhancement of the lower level signals in the RF data, is preferred.

After amplification, the polar scan line RF data still contains radio frequency sinusoidal waves with both positive and negative values. Individual echocardiographic specular targets consist of groups of these high-frequency spikes. To display these sets of spikes as single targets, the RF signal is next "envelope detected." Analog systems first rectify the RF signal, folding the negative portion into the positive portion of the signal. In digital systems, analytic detection is used to find the best curve outlining each set of high-frequency spikes (i.e., the envelope). This process consolidates the multiple spikes into single outlines that represent the targets. The targets are thus displayed as single bright spots on the scan line instead of a series of tiny bright spots.

After envelope detection, the signal undergoes a final low-pass filtration that removes much of the remaining high-frequency signal. The resulting detected and filtered signal is referred to as the *video signal* or the polar scan line data. Most of the processing required to form this line or beam of ultrasound is performed in analog signal-processing systems within the ultrasound machine. As computers become faster and processing of the signals for image improvement becomes more complex and requires more flexibility, the advantages of carrying out these steps in digital computer formats grow. The clear trend is for digital processing to move earlier into the processing chain. Figure 25–17 shows the point at which the signal for a line can be converted to digital format in systems that employ digital beam-forming technology.

After all of the individual polar lines have been obtained, the

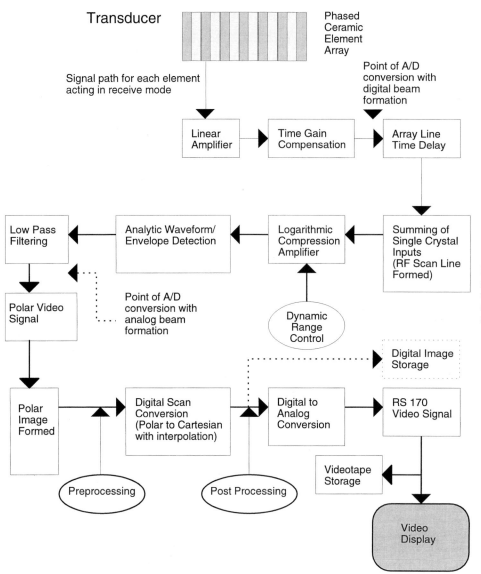

FIGURE 25–17. Block flow diagram of the steps involved in the reception of the reflected ultrasound and formation of a two-dimensional echocardiographic image. RF = radio frequency; A/D = analog-to-digital.

data necessary to form one two-dimensional echo image has been gathered. In this polar image data, each scan line has been obtained at a different angle and the data along each line is a radial distance, R, from the theoretical center point of the transducer. Figure 25–18 shows a polar video image. In this format, the data is not particularly useful and appears to be distorted. Only after the data have been redisplayed at the appropriate angles and depths can appropriate target positions be placed in their correct anatomic locations.

DIGITAL SCAN CONVERSION

The polar scan line data cannot be presented in standard video format without conversion. In early two-dimensional ultrasound machines, these data were presented on an oscilloscope that had independent steering of the beam in the x and y directions so that the lines could be displayed at the angles at which they had been obtained. However, display of this type of image cannot be placed on videotape because it is not a standard horizontal and vertical video signal. The only methods of storing the scanned image were by photography of the screen or by placing a television camera in front of the screen and recording the image on videotape. Furthermore, the overlap of the scan lines in the near field made this

portion of the picture extremely bright while there were wide gaps in the far field. The display was not visually optimal.

To circumvent these problems, digital scan conversion was developed. Scan conversion refers to the process of converting from analog polar scan line data to analog standard video by means of a digital, computerized process. If the ultrasound system employs analog beam formation, then each line must first go through analog-to-digital conversion. In most modern equipment, the voltage amplitude of the polar video signal is converted to a numeric (digital) value at 512 equally spaced points along each scan line. If the system employs digital beam formation, the polar lines will already be in the correct format. As each line enters the scan converter, each digital point along the line is mapped to the nearest Cartesian (x,y) location in a rectangular image that has 512×512 points. Because a picture is to be produced, each of these points is referred to as a picture element or pixel.

In the near field close to the apex of the scan, the polar lines overlap. Much of the information from the polar data must be deleted or averaged in order to fit the digitized data into the limited number of Cartesian matrix positions. Conversely, in the far field the polar scan lines are quite separated in the Cartesian space, and there will be only enough data to fill one half to one third of the available matrix positions. Figure 25–19 shows the result of this 1:1 mapping of the polar scan line points to the appropriate (x,y) pixel locations that correspond to their positions

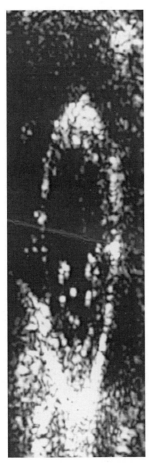

FIGURE 25–18. Display of the polar video data without scan conversion. Values along the ordinate represent axial distance from the face of the transducer. Values along the abscissa represent the angle along which the individual B-mode lines were obtained.

in the sector scan. Figure 25–19 can be thought of as the digital equivalent to the older analog x,y,z oscilloscope displays. In this figure, the polar scan line data presented in Figure 25–18 have, in part, been mapped into a 256 × 200 Cartesian array. This lower resolution was chosen so that the individual pixel elements in mapping were more easily illustrated. Notice that the process of mapping the polar data to the discrete locations in the Cartesian array produces a regular pattern of unfilled matrix elements between and through the scan lines. These curved lines sweeping upward and outward are referred to as a moiré pattern.

Clinicians find both the unfilled regions between scan lines and the moiré pattern distracting in evaluating clinical studies. Therefore, various schemes have been developed to fill in or interpolate the existing data in order to smooth the image.

The simplest method of filling blank matrix elements is to perform a linear interpolation in the horizontal or x direction. If there is only one pixel value to be filled, as in the case of matrix element M_{AB} in Figure 25–20, then the digital gray level value assigned to matrix element M_{AB} would be $(M_A + M_B)/2$. If two matrix elements were to be interpolated, then the values assigned to pixels M_{AB2} and M_{AB3} would be given by

$$M_{AB2} = M_B + \frac{(M_B - M_A)}{3}$$

$$M_{AB3} = M_B + \frac{2(M_B - M_A)}{3}$$

(7)

Notice that this linear interpolation assumes that the actual spacing

between the known gray levels along scan lines is equal in the x direction and that the nearest gray levels in the y direction are not considered. For this reason, simple linear interpolation in the horizontal direction produces a somewhat coarse quality in the image. Because this coarseness is also found objectionable by most observers, simple interpolation has been replaced by a more complex form of interpolation, referred to, in general, as R, θ scan conversion.[21] In this interpolation scheme, the gray level assignment for all matrix elements is derived by interpolation of the digital gray level values of the four nearest positions in the digital polar scan line data. Not only do all four contribute, but the contribution of each is also dependent on the relative distance to the new pixel in both radial and azimuthal directions. Thus, in Figure 25–20, the value of matrix element M_{AB} would now be filled by first interpolating new gray level values along scan line A and scan line B in the radial directions. The two new points corresponding to the radial length to the center of M_{AB} are labeled G_{AI} and G_{BI} and their values are given by

$$G_{AI} = \frac{1 - R}{\Delta R} G_{A1} + \frac{R}{\Delta R} G_{A2}$$

$$G_{BI} = \frac{1 - R}{\Delta R} G_{B1} + \frac{R}{\Delta R} G_{B2}$$

(8)

The value of M_{AB} is then calculated as

$$M_{AB} = \frac{1 - \theta}{\Delta \theta} G_{BI} + \frac{\theta}{\Delta \theta} G_{AI}$$

(9)

which shows that the relative contributions of G_{AI} and G_{BI} are again proportional to the distances to these respective points.

This method of filling the matrix and forming a final image in which the gray level of each picture element is proportional to the relative position of that pixel in relation to the original digital amplitudes from the polar video signal produces a very smooth image (Fig. 25–21). As computer power and speed progress, even higher-order interpolation is being implemented to enhance image quality.

The actual image content (in terms of real data) of the analog polar oscilloscope presentation, the digital interpolated image, and the R, θ scan–converted image are identical. The image quality,

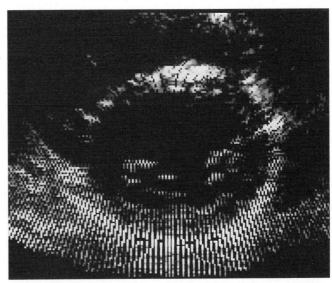

FIGURE 25–19. Simple digital scan conversion without interpolation. Here, the brightness values from Figure 25–18 have been placed in the nearest appropriate (x,y) location in Cartesian space. Notice the symmetrical, curved pattern of unfilled pixels around the central axis of the scan. This is referred to as a moiré pattern.

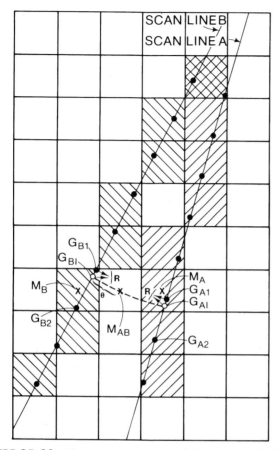

FIGURE 25–20. Schematic representation of the mapping of polar scan line data into Cartesian coordinates by the digital scan converter. The digitized gray levels or brightness at equally spaced positions along polar scan lines are represented by the letter G. The gray level assigned to a position in the scan converter Cartesian matrix is designated by the letter M. Position M_{AB} is an unfilled position in the matrix and must be interpolated. Two methods for determining the gray level of position M_{AB} are described in the text. (From Geiser, E.A., and Oliver, L.H.: Echocardiography: Physics and Instrumentation. *In* Collins, S.M., and Skorton, D.J. (eds.): Cardiac Imaging and Image Processing. New York, McGraw-Hill, 1986, with permission.)

however, varies greatly. Because the image content is the same, image quality is to a large extent cosmetic and a matter of preference.

PREPROCESSING AND POSTPROCESSING

The advent of the digital scan converter has made possible almost limitless variation in the display of the image to satisfy user preference. The polar video signal arriving at the scan converter is a logarithmically compressed, envelope detected, and low-pass filtered signal in which the amplitude at any point is proportional to the amplitude of the returning ultrasonic waves. (With a well-designed beam former, the phase of the returning wave should no longer contribute to the image.)

Part of the reason for logarithmic compression was to reduce the range of amplitudes in the polar video signal. Even after this compression, however, patient variation makes it desirable to manipulate the amplitudes and thereby enhance some low-level signals or decrease very-high-level signals that may saturate the display. This further manipulation of gray scale can be accomplished at one of two points. The first is the point at which the polar scan line data is placed into image memory; manipulation at this point means that the modified gray levels will be used in the

R, θ interpolation scheme and thus modify the image. The second point of modification is at the point of digital-to-analog conversion, when the digital scan converter matrix is read horizontally along each sequential line and converted into horizontal video signals. Modification at this level produces slightly different control such that all pixels having the same value after interpolation can be either suppressed or enhanced. The process of modifying the image entering the digital scan converter is referred to as preprocessing, and manipulation during digital-to-analog formation of the standard video signal is referred to as postprocessing (see Fig. 25–17).

Both preprocessing and postprocessing are usually accomplished through the use of a computerized "look-up table." During preprocessing, the polar video signal has an amplitude variation between 0 and a peak digital value of 255 units, the highest value an 8-bit gray scale resolution will allow. A target of intermediate amplitude in the polar video signal may have, for example, a value of 127. In a linear system this would be assigned a digital gray level in the scan converter of 127. However, if one wished to enhance the brightness of intermediate level targets by 10 percent, a value of 127 could simply be assigned a new value of 140 on entering the scan converter. This analog-to-digital conversion is handled by a table that specifies what output value should be given to any incoming value. Most manufacturers supply four to six such look-up tables, which are referred to as preprocessing curves.

Postprocessing is analogous, but in this case the digital value prompts assignment of an output voltage. One application of postprocessing is inversion of the image. In this situation, a value of 255 is assigned a voltage of 0, and a value of 0 a voltage of 5. This converts the image from a white-on-black digital image to a black-on-white television image.

FREEZE-FRAME AND CONTINUOUS LOOP DISPLAY

With previous analog and early digital scan conversion equipment, an image could not be saved on the screen and analyzed. The incorporation of analog-to-digital conversion and scan converter technology has substantially enhanced the ability to study and make measurements with the two-dimensional ultrasound equipment. In the previous section, the polar video signal was considered to be digitized, and the digital gray levels were mapped into the appropriate (x,y) location in the Cartesian coordinate image in the scan converter. If, instead of going directly into the scan converter, the digital gray levels at every point along each scan line are kept in

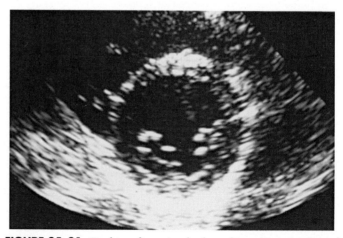

FIGURE 25–21. Final two-dimensional echocardiographic image formed from the data in Figure 25–18. Scan conversion has been accomplished in a larger matrix scan converter than in Figure 25–19, and all the matrix elements have been filled by an R, θ scan conversion similar to that described in the text.

random access memory (RAM), then at any point the digital polar data can be fed into the scan converter and displayed in video format for the operator. A single image displayed in this fashion is termed a "freeze frame." Because of freeze-frame technology, images can be stored during the examination and restored for comparison later.

This concept of storing images in RAM for later recall can be expanded by increasing the available RAM storage capabilities of the ultrasound machine. Sixteen, 32, or even 128 polar images in digital format can be stored. Any sequence or portion of a sequence of these stored images can then be read in real time into the scan converter and displayed. This capability is commonly referred to as continuous loop memory.

Finally, a polar digital image stored in RAM can be read into one half or even one quarter of the rectangular scan converter memory. Such manipulation allows side-by-side or four-quadrant simultaneous comparison of images.

After an image is in the rectangular scan converter and interpolated, various structures can be marked by use of a cursor. Because the depth of the scan is known from other machine settings, both the number of pixels per centimeter and the number of pixels per square centimeter can be calculated. Therefore, measurements of distance and area can be made with relative ease from the screen.

Because any output from the scan converter is in standard video format, whatever is seen on the screen can be recorded on videotape, which is the usual mode of storage for two-dimensional echocardiography. Many contemporary systems allow review of videotapes through the system. During this process of review, any video frame obtained from tape can be passed through a video analog-to-digital converter and passed to a section of memory that is similar to the scan converter. This allows postprocessing curves to be applied, so that even after a videotape is made, some changes in gray scale can be accomplished to enhance visual appreciation of structures. This digitization process also allows measurements to be made from the videotape images.

BIOEFFECTS

Bioeffects, as the name implies, is the study of changes, both temporary and permanent, in biological tissues that are placed in an ultrasonic field. For this discussion, an ultrasonic field is defined as any elastic medium containing ultrasonic waves. As discussed previously, mechanical waves are a means of transferring energy through a medium. That such energy can affect biological tissue is easily recognized because of such uses as shock-wave lithotripsy.

As ultrasonic waves pass through an imperfect medium, some energy is transferred to the surrounding medium; this is termed attenuation. With this loss of energy, mechanical work is performed in the tissues. The final common pathway for the loss of energy is the generation of heat, which is subsequently dissipated to the surroundings and contributes, ultimately, to the entropy of the universe.

An excellent review of the status of bioeffects research and regulatory issues concerning power output of diagnostic ultrasound machines was published by Skorton and associates in 1988.[22] In 1990, Child and colleagues[23] described lung hemorrhage resulting from exposure to pulsed ultrasound. Much work before this time had been done by placing tissues, cells, or intact organisms in ultrasound beams under free-field conditions. Essentially, "free field" means that the experiments were performed in a water bath with no obstructions to the target tissue. Although the experiments of Child and colleagues were performed in a water bath, young mice were exposed intact to ultrasound intensities that were comparable to those used in diagnostic equipment. The best explanation proposed was that the hemorrhage was caused by cavitation-related injury and not by thermal injury secondary to temperature rise of the tissue. This important finding of a measurable adverse effect caused by the mechanical interaction of ultrasound with

mammalian tissues has led to further research, discussion, and redirected interests regarding bioeffects. Although experimental work continues, knowledge concerning bioeffects and their importance to patients in clinical medicine is still sketchy. More and more work is being done on intact animals, and the previous free-field experiments are yielding to experiments with more relevance to the clinical situation.

When expressing ultrasound exposures at a depth into tissue, attenuation must be taken into account. A "derating factor" has now been agreed on. This derating factor is an attenuation of 0.3 dB/cm per MHz. If an estimate of an ultrasound field parameter has been made at the point of exposure, then the derated parameter usually has ".3" in the subscript of the notation. For example, peak rarefactional pressure, P_r, is an important parameter in the development of cavitation within a tissue or fluid. If the estimate is being made at a particular point in tissue, then the derated peak rarefactional pressure has the notation, $P_{r.3}$. An important descriptor of field intensity related to temperature is the spatial peak temporal average intensity, I_{spta}; if this is to be expressed at a depth in tissue, then the derated parameter is indicated by $I_{spta.3}$.

Thermal Bioeffects

The equation describing the intensity of an unfocused ultrasound beam at a particular depth in the tissues, as described in the section on ultrasound transmission, is given by

$$I(x) = I_0 e^{-2\alpha x}$$

where I_0 is the intensity at the surface, α is the amplitude attenuation coefficient, and x is the distance traversed in the tissue. The rate of rise in temperature for the tissue exposed to the ultrasound beam at the same depth is described by

$$\frac{dT}{dt} = 2\frac{\kappa I(x)}{\rho c_h} \tag{10}$$

where T is the temperature, t is time, κ is the absorption coefficient, ρ is the density of the tissue, and c_h is the specific heat of the tissue expressed in calories per gram per degree Celsius.

Both of these equations are for unfocused beams. If the beam is focused, the intensity is increased at the focal point, compared with the unfocused situation. Thermal effects are related to the peak intensity of ultrasound delivered over time, as shown by the use of the spatial peak temporal average intensity, or I_{spta}, to express part of the risk from thermal effect.

At the same time that heat is being generated in the tissues, heat loss occurs through conduction (heat flow to the surrounding tissue) and through convection (the removal of thermal energy by transfer to fluids such as blood moving through the area). Recall also that, in imaging mode, the pulsed ultrasound energy may be transmitted for as little as 1 μsec, with the transducer being placed in receiving mode for the remainder of the time that images are being formed. The time during which the transducer is actively transmitting sound, compared with the time during which it is off or in receiving mode, is referred to as the "duty cycle" of the transducer, and this parameter must also be taken into account in considerations of exposure. If the same transducer is placed in pulsed Doppler mode, the result is a considerably different ultrasound exposure. Within the tissues, there is also scatter, diffraction, absorption, reflection, and mode conversion, each of which can occur before the beam reaches the focal zone. All of these various interactions are lumped and considered in the derating factor.

The AIUM has developed a Thermal Index (TI) that has now been accepted by both the National Electronics Manufacturers Association and the Food and Drug Administration (FDA). The TI is defined as the ratio of total acoustic power to the acoustic power required to raise tissue temperature 1° C under defined assumptions. Separate assumptions are made for soft tissue and for bone. These are referred to as the "soft tissue model" and the "bone model." The AIUM[24] concludes that

> *Under most clinically relevant conditions, the soft tissue thermal index, TIS, and the bone thermal index, TIB, either overestimate or closely approximate the best available estimate of the maximum temperature increase (ΔT_{max}). . . . TIS and TIB track changes in the maximum temperature increase, ΔT_{max} thus allowing for implementation of the ALARA (As Low As Reasonably Achievable) principle, whereas $I_{spta.3}$ does not.*

There is good evidence that local elevations of 2° C are tolerated for prolonged periods without permanent tissue damage. It is unlikely that elevations of this magnitude can be reached in soft-tissue applications related to cardiac imaging. Technologists and physicians should keep in mind that exposure times should be considered, especially in patients who are febrile at the start of the examination.

Mechanical Bioeffects

The lung hemorrhage described by Child and co-workers[23] is clearly defined as a nonthermal effect of ultrasound. The damage seen has many of the characteristics of cavitation injury. With this in mind, the AIUM has also developed a Mechanical Index (MI), which is designed to be a worst-case scenario for mechanical tissue injury. The mechanical index is defined as "the derated peak rarefactional pressure (in MPa [megapascals]), at the point of the maximum pulse intensity integral, divided by the square root of the ultrasonic center frequency (in MHz)."[24] Expressed in the form of an equation, the MI is

$$MI = \frac{P_{r.3} x_{max\ sp}}{\sqrt{f_c}} \qquad (11)$$

The risk of cavitation increases with P_r and decreases with the frequency and depth (attenuation). In spite of the official look of this equation, there is still no consensus as to whether cavitation events are frequency dependent. However, this index has been accepted and is now part of the on-screen labeling in new diagnostic ultrasound equipment. The FDA-defined output limit of MI for two-dimensional scanning is 1.9.

Subsequent to the work of Child and colleagues, other investigators have pursued the possibility of mechanical bioeffects in mammalian tissue. Penney and associates[25] exposed intact mice to 10-µsec impulses at 1.6 MPa for 3 minutes. By both light and transmission electron microscopy, hemorrhagic areas were seen. These areas were sharply defined, with injury produced in both pneumocytes and capillary endothelial cells. These injuries caused direct continuities between vessel lumina and alveolar spaces. Raeman and colleagues[26] extended the murine observations and suggested that exposure modifies the tissue in a way that facilitates further, more extensive damage. The probability of damage from a scan across the lung, for example, is less than if the scan is directed at a single site in the lung for an extended period. More recently, Tarantal and Canfield[27] described lung hemorrhage in the primate. In their experiments, a clinical two-dimensional scanner was set for maximum output conditions, which included imaging with pulsed and color Doppler features being employed simultaneously. This resulted in a P_r of 3.7 MPa at 4 MHz, and an MI of approximately 1.8. Monkeys involved in the study ranged from 1 day to 16 years of age, and exposure times were approximately 5 minutes. Well-defined, circular hemorrhagic foci of 0.1 to 1.0 cm in diameter were seen.

All of these reports have noted hemorrhage in the lung. Similar searches for hemorrhage in solid tissues have not yielded similar results. The implication is that such injury occurs in tissue that contains microscopic gas bodies that can serve as cavitation nuclei.

It seems clear that the dominant physical factor in all of these cases is the temporal peak acoustic pressure and that there is a marked increase in the extent of tissue damage with increasing peak pressure once a threshold has been exceeded. Of interest is the fact that similar hemorrhage was not found in fetal lung tissue, also suggesting that microscopic bubbles of gas must be present to initiate the injury. The observations to date suggest that the mechanism of injury is related to mechanical bioeffects and probably to acoustic cavitation.

Acoustic cavitation is defined as the formation or activity of gas-filled or vapor-filled cavities (bubbles) in a medium exposed to an ultrasonic field.[28] Stable cavitation is the continuous oscillation of bubbles in response to the alternating positive and negative pressures in the acoustic field. If clinical ultrasound or microsecond pulses are employed, cavitation effects are most likely to be associated with bubble collapse rather than stable cavitation. However, pulse Doppler devices may have sufficiently high pulse pressure amplitudes, pulse lengths, and pulse repetition frequencies to support stable oscillations. Another factor that seems necessary is that the medium must constrain the growth of such bubbles within a biological structure such as a capillary or an alveolus.

A phenomenon that may relate to this injury is known as "rectified diffusion." This refers to inward diffusion of gas during rarefaction, with an unequal outward diffusion during the pressurization phase of the wave. This results in an increase in size of the bubble. Mechanisms of potential injury in the neighborhood of an oscillating bubble include microstreaming, high sheer stresses, and radiation forces that result in particle aggregation. Acoustic microstreaming refers to the streaming of fluids along the surface of an ultrasonically resonating cavitation. This phenomenon is especially seen in stable cavitation and can result in cell membrane breakage and hemolysis. An excellent review of these effects has recently been published.[29] Williams and colleagues[30] have demonstrated hemolysis of human red cells insonated in a rotating chamber into which a commercially available echocardiographic contrast agent had been introduced. This effect was decreased by increasing hematocrit; above a hematocrit of 5.5 percent, there was no detectable cell lysis.

In summary, it is clear that in the presence of microbubbles or cavitation nuclei, mechanical bioeffects may be seen with ultrasound exposures that can easily be produced by today's clinical scanners. This has prompted the AIUM to summarize[24] as follows:

> *Thresholds for adverse nonthermal effects depend upon tissue characteristics and ultrasound parameters such as pressure amplitude, pulse duration and frequency. Thus far, biologically significant adverse nonthermal effects have only been identified with certainty for diagnostically relevant exposures in tissues that have well-defined populations of stabilized gas bodies. For extravasation of blood cells in post-natal mouse lung, the threshold values of MI increase with decreasing pulse duration in the 1–100 µs range, increase with decreasing exposure time, and are weakly dependent upon pulse repetition frequency. The threshold value for MI for extravasation of blood cells in mouse lung is approximately 0.3. The implication of these observations for human exposure are yet to be determined.*

In other words, the threshold MI decreases (i.e., extravasation is more likely) with increasing pulse duration, increasing exposure time, and change in the pulse repetition frequency. In the near future, the TI and MI will be displayed as an on-screen reminder to practice the ALARA principle while further research regarding mechanical bioeffects and interactions between biological tissues, ultrasound, and microbubble contrast agents continues.

CONCLUSION

This chapter has been an attempt to explain basic principles of ultrasound and the methods that allow formation of diagnostic images. In brief, contemporary ultrasound machines are quite sophisticated and powerful computers that are designed specifically to provide real-time visualization of structure and motion in the heart. Although the specifics of implementation may differ somewhat among manufacturers, the individual components and methods remain fairly constant. Through increased knowledge of these principles, the reader may achieve a better understanding of the strengths and weaknesses of the technique.

References

1. Ludwig, G.D.: The velocity of sound through tissues and the acoustic impedances of tissues. J. Acoust. Soc. Am. 22:862, 1950.
2. Firestone, F.A.: The supersonic reflectoscope for interior inspection. Metal Progress 48:505, 1945.
3. Edler, I., and Hertz, C.H.: Use of ultrasonic reflectoscope for continuous recording of movement of heart walls. Kungl. Fysiogr. Sallsk. i Lund. Forhandl. 24:40, 1954.
4. Yoshiba, T., Mori, M., Nimura, Y., et al.: Study on examining the heart with ultrasonics. III: Kinds of Doppler beats. IV: Clinical applications. Jpn. Circ. J. 20:228, 1956.
5. Wild, J.J., and Reid, J.M.: Further pilot echographic studies on the histologic structure of tumors of the living intact human breast. Am. J. Pathol. 28:839, 1952.
6. Somer, J.C.: Electronic sector scanning for ultrasonic diagnosis. Ultrasonics 6:153, 1968.
7. Kisslo, J., von Ramm, O.T., and Thurstone, F.L.: Cardiac imaging using a phased array ultrasound system: II. Clinical technique and application. Circulation 53:262, 1976.
8. Frazin, L., Talano, J.V., Stephanides, L., et al.: Esophageal echocardiography. Circulation 54:102, 1976.
9. Wells, P.N.T.: Wave fundamentals. In Wells, P.N.T.: Biomedical Ultrasonics. New York, Academic Press, 1977, p. 1.
10. Carson, P.L., Fischella, P.R., and Oughton, T.V.: Ultrasonic power and intensities produced by diagnostic ultrasound equipment. Ultrasound Med. Biol. 3:341, 1978.
11. American Institute of Ultrasound in Medicine: Safety considerations for diagnostic ultrasound. J. Ultrasound Med. 3(Suppl.):S1, 1984.
12. Wells, P.N.T.: Biomedical Ultrasonics. New York, Academic Press, 1977. p. 20.
13. Kinsler, L.E., and Frey, A.R.: Fundamentals of Acoustics. 2d ed. New York, Wiley, 1962.
14. American Institute of Ultrasound in Medicine: Standard methods for testing single-element pulsed-echo ultrasonic transducers. J. Ultrasound Med. 1(Suppl.):S1, 1982.
15. Aero-Tech Reports: Linear Arrays: Theory of operation and performance. KB-Aerotech 2:(#1), 1981.
16. Larson, J.D., III: An acoustic transducer array for medical imaging: Part I. Hewlett-Packard J. 34:17, 1983.
17. Fearnot, N.E., Babbs, C.F., Bourland, J.D., et al.: Dynamic intraesophageal imaging of the heart with ultrasound. Ultrason. Imaging 2:78, 1980.
18. Snyder, J.E., Kisslo, J., and von Ramm, O.T.: Real-time orthogonal mode scanning of the heart: I. System design. J. Am. Coll. Cardiol. 7:1279, 1986.
19. Smith, S.W., Trahey, G.E., and von Ramm, O.T.: Two-dimensional arrays for medical ultrasound. Ultrason. Imaging 14:213, 1992.
20. von Ramm, O.T., and Smith, S.W.: Real time volumetric ultrasound imaging system. J. Digit. Imaging 3:261, 1990.
21. Leavitt, S.C., Hunt, B.F., and Larsen, H.G.: A scan conversion algorithm for displaying ultrasound images. Hewlett-Packard J. 34:32, 1983.
22. Skorton, D.J., Collins, S.M., Greenleaf, J.F., et al.: Ultrasound bioeffects and regulatory issues: An introduction for the echocardiographer. J. Am. Soc. Echocardiogr. 1:240, 1988.
23. Child, S.Z., Hartman, C.L., Schery, L.A., et al.: Lung damage from exposure to pulsed ultrasound. Ultrasound Med. Biol. 16:817, 1990.
24. AIUM updates bioeffects statements. AIUM Reporter 10:2, 1994.
25. Penney, D.P., Schenk, E.A., Maltby, K., et al.: Morphological effects of pulsed ultrasound in the lung. Ultrasound Med. Biol. 19:127, 1993.
26. Raeman, C.H., Child, S.Z., and Carstensen, E.L.: Timing of exposures in ultrasonic hemorrhage of murine lung. Ultrasound Med. Biol. 19:507, 1993.
27. Tarantal, A.F., and Canfield, D.R.: Ultrasound-induced lung hemorrhage in the monkey. Ultrasound Med. Biol. 20:62, 1994.
28. ten Haar, G.: Ultrasonic biophysics. In Hill, C.R. (ed.): Physical principles of medical ultrasound. Chichester, Eng., Ellis Horwood, 1986, p. 378.
29. Barnett, S.G., ter Haar G.R., Ziskin, M.C., et al.: Current status of research on biophysical effects of ultrasound. Ultrasound Med. Biol. 20:205, 1994.
30. Williams, A.R., Kubowicz, G., Cramer, E., et al.: The effects of the microbubble suspension SH U 454 on ultrasound-induced cell lysis in a rotating tube exposure system. Echocardiography 8:423, 1991.

CHAPTER

26 Principles and Instrumentation for Doppler

Edward G. Cape, Ph.D.
Ajit P. Yoganathan, Ph.D.

DOPPLER PRINCIPLE _____ 292
Angle of Incidence Concept _____ 292
VELOCIMETRIC IMPLEMENTATION _____ 292
Continuous-Wave Doppler _____ 292
 Limitations _____ 292
Pulsed-Wave Doppler _____ 293
 Limitations _____ 293
IMAGING IMPLEMENTATION _____ 293
Color Flow Doppler Mapping _____ 294
 Data Processing: Spectral Versus Autocorrelation _____ 294
 Limitations _____ 294
 Angle of Incidence Effects (Due to Beam Sweep) _____ 295

Angle of Incidence Effects (Due to Angulation) _____ 295
INSTRUMENT SETTINGS _____ 295
Gain _____ 295
Pulse Repetition Frequency _____ 295
Wall Filter Setting _____ 295
Carrier Frequency _____ 296
Frame Rate _____ 296
Tissue-Priority Algorithm _____ 296
TRANSDUCER CONFIGURATIONS _____ 296
Spectral Doppler _____ 296
Color Doppler _____ 296

Chapter 25 discussed principles and instrumentation for echocardiographic imaging, which allows tomographic images of the cardiac structures to be obtained in real time. Doppler ultrasound allows for measurement of blood flow velocities within the heart.

It is the purpose of this chapter to illustrate the capabilities and limitations of current Doppler echocardiographic techniques by constructing from basic principles the Doppler spectral display and the color flow Doppler image.

DOPPLER PRINCIPLE

Doppler ultrasound is commonly implemented in three different modalities in the clinical setting, depending on the desired information: spectral continuous-wave Doppler, spectral pulsed-wave Doppler, and color flow Doppler mapping. All of these techniques rely on the basic Doppler principle first described by the scientist whose name it bears. When a wave strikes a moving target, it will be reflected, and the reflected wave will show a frequency shift proportional to the component of target velocity that is parallel to the path of the wave. This general principle can be applied to patients with heart disease. First, the "wave" described in this general principle can be light, sound, or other entities capable of traveling through the medium between the wave source and the target. In Doppler echocardiography, sound is chosen as the entity, and beams capable of penetrating tissue exceed 1 million Hz, when expressed in terms of frequency. (The upper limit of audible sound is approximately 20,000 Hz, and anything above that is referred to as ultrasound, thus Doppler *ultrasound*.)

In humans, red blood cells follow flow patterns. Their size (a biconcave disc 3×8 μm) and concentration (40 to 45 percent by volume) allow them to reflect significant amounts of ultrasound energy. Thus, their velocities can be calculated with the Doppler principle, which is expressed mathematically as follows:

$$f_d = (cv)/2f_o\cos\theta \qquad (1)$$

where f_d is the shifted, or Doppler, frequency; c is the speed of sound in the medium (approximately 1560 m per second in blood and tissue); f_o is the emitted or carrier frequency, and θ is the angle of incidence between the ultrasound beam path and the blood-cell velocity vector. Rearranging this basic equation allows one to calculate blood-cell velocities as a function of the Doppler shift, since the speed of sound and emitted frequency are known.

$$v = (cf_d)/2f_o\cos\theta \qquad (2)$$

Angle of Incidence Concept

The angle of incidence is generally assumed to be zero in most cardiology instruments; thus, the user must keep in mind that velocities passing at an angle to the beam path will be underestimated, unless manually corrected. Because cardiac flows often have complex three-dimensional characteristics, the angle of incidence can vary significantly throughout a flow of interest for a given transducer position. This concept is important in all of the following modalities of Doppler: continuous-wave, pulsed-wave, and, especially, color flow mapping, in which the angle of incidence varies to different extents at different points throughout the imaging plane. As a rule, one should attempt to achieve angles of incidence of less than 20 degrees, because such angles produce an error of only 6 percent. Because of the curved nature of the cosine function, however, velocities calculated at angles larger than 20 degrees begin to produce considerable error. Additional complexities concerning the angle of incidence develop when one is considering velocity measurements displayed as an image. These complexities are discussed below.

VELOCIMETRIC IMPLEMENTATION

Blood flow velocities are useful for a number of clinical diagnostic methods that have been derived from fluid mechanical considerations, for example, estimation of pressure gradients with the Bernoulli equation. For quantitative derivation of blood flow velocities, one of two *spectral* modalities of Doppler is chosen, continuous-wave or spectral Doppler.

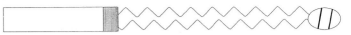

FIGURE 26–1. Schematic of ultrasound beam path. Sound is emitted from a transducer at a known frequency. A portion of the wave is reflected after striking the moving target. Returning sound has a frequency shift proportional to the velocity of the target.

Continuous-Wave Doppler

If ultrasound is continuously emitted from and received by a transducer, and velocities are calculated with equation 2, a spectrum of velocity values is obtained as the beams reflect and return from moving targets all along the line of interest, as shown in Figure 26–1. A spectral display consists of what may be thought of as a series of vertical strips, as diagrammed in Figure 26–2. Each vertical strip consists of a number of bins representing small velocity intervals. These bins are shaded with a brightness corresponding to the number of particles traveling at speeds within that interval. (It is sometimes useful to think of each vertical strip as a histogram, with *shading* of each bin replacing the bars seen in a traditional histogram.) Over time, a rapid updating of these strips produces a spectral signal, as diagrammed. By measuring the peak velocity at any given time, one obtains the maximum velocity along the line of the ultrasound beam. The advantage of this technique is that it allows quick and easy acquisition of a maximum velocity. For example, to characterize aortic valve stenosis one desires the maximum velocity distal to the valve for use in the Bernoulli equation. By aiming the ultrasound beam path down the centerline of the aorta, one can obtain the maximum velocity immediately. Signals other than the maximum are buried beneath the envelope of the spectrum when displayed on the instrument monitor (i.e., all of these velocities fall into lower velocity bins).

Limitations

The price of the ease in acquiring maximum velocities quickly is a lack of range-depth resolution. Although the maximum velocity along the ultrasound beam path is easily obtained, the depth from which the maximum velocity signal has returned is unknown without simultaneous consideration of cardiac anatomy and physiology. It is also an important limitation that low-velocity signals from other points along the beam path are buried beneath the maximum and are not recoverable.

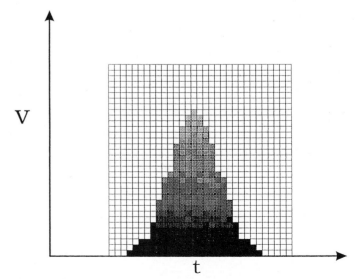

FIGURE 26–2. Spectral display of velocities. Particles traveling within specific velocity intervals are represented by shading of that interval within a vertical "strip." The strips are rapidly updated to produce a spectral display of velocity over time.

Pulsed-Wave Doppler

To acquire velocities at specific distances, or depths, from the transducer, pulsing of ultrasound is required. A burst of sound is emitted, the transducer waits a specific time (t), and then it opens a window for a very short time (W) to receive returning signals. Similar to continuous-wave Doppler, velocities are calculated with equation 2. However, for this limited burst of signal delivered in the pulsed-wave modality, we know the signal must have returned from a distance d, defined as

$$d = ct/2 \qquad (3)$$

where d is commonly referred to as the sample volume depth, c is the speed of sound in the medium, and t is time between emission and reception of the signal. The velocities are again displayed spectrally in a bin format, as described previously for continuous-wave Doppler. However, the spectrum for pulsed-wave data, compared with continuous-wave data, is usually much less broad because it contains only signals returning from a specific distance away from the transducer. Laminar flows with low temporal variation produce a narrow band, as shown in Figure 26–3A, whereas turbulent flows or those with significant temporal variation over the time of acquisition show some spectral broadening, which can be seen by comparing Figure 26–3A and B.

The axial and lateral dimensions of the sample volume are determined by two different factors. The axial length of the sample volume is determined by the length of time, W, during which the acquisition window stays open. As the window first opens at a time, t_1, the near boundary of the sample volume is established and can be calculated with equation 3, evaluated at the time $t = t_1$. The window closes at a time $t_1 + W$, and the far boundary of the sample volume is established and can be calculated with equation 3, evaluated at the time $t = t_1 + W$. It follows that the axial length of the sample volume can then be calculated with equation 3, evaluated with $t = W$.

The lateral dimension of the sample volume depends on transducer focusing considerations and is commonly referred to as the lateral resolution of the instrument. For a given transducer and choice of instrument settings, to be described later, an optimum focal point exists within the range of the transducer. Proximal and distal to this point, quality signals can still be obtained, but the beam and sample volume width gradually increase when one moves away from the focal point in either direction. (Newer transducers have multifocus capabilities, which partially overcome the problem of singular optimum acquisition points.)

Limitations

By switching from continuous- to pulsed-wave Doppler, one develops range resolution but must deal with two new limitations. First, a maximum detectable velocity limit is imposed (Fig. 26–4). Like any frequency-based sampling method, pulsed-wave Doppler is governed by the Nyquist criterion: the signal must be sampled at least twice as fast as the frequency of the measured phenomenon. In our case, this means that the pulse repetition frequency (PRF) must be at least twice that of the Doppler-shifted frequency produced by the blood-cell velocity for a given emitted frequency. If the true velocity produces a Doppler shift more than one half the PRF, then the signal will *alias*, meaning it will wrap to the opposite end of the full scale. For example, if the PRF and carrier frequency dictate that the maximum detectable velocity is 60 cm per second, and a region of flow is interrogated at which the maximum velocity is 80 cm per second, the spectrum will indicate that the velocity is −40 cm per second. If the signal is wrapped only once, baseline shifting can be applied to determine the correct velocity magnitude and direction. If more than one wrap is produced, the situation becomes quite complex. Although in principle such an erroneous signal could be "unwrapped," the sharp velocity decays found in many flow fields, such as turbulent mitral regurgitant jets, prohibit such algorithms, as they may be wrapped several times near the lesion but rapidly fall to levels below the Nyquist limit within a short distance.

The second limitation is range ambiguity. To overcome the Nyquist limit (i.e., to increase the maximum detectable velocity), the PRF can be increased. This must be done with caution. Equation 3 shows the desired distance from which pulsed-wave signals must have returned. In principle, signals could be received from any integer multiple of this distance. Increasing the PRF to overcome the Nyquist limit can shorten the time, t, in equation 3 and pulls in the distant sample volumes, such that they obscure the signals of interest when they exceed them. In practice, PRF values are chosen so that sample volumes beyond that calculated by equation 3 are too far away to return measurable signals, or so that the sample volumes not in the region of interest return lower velocity signals.

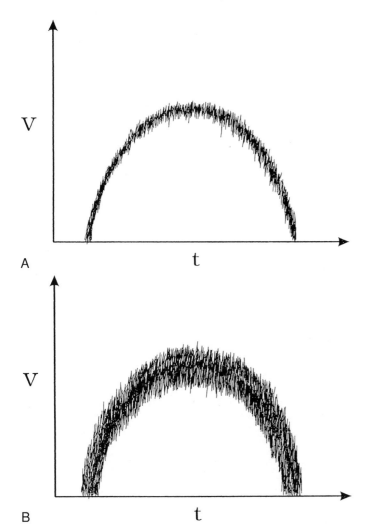

FIGURE 26–3. Spectral broadening. *A*, For uniform or laminar flows within a sample volume, a narrow band of frequencies-velocities is filled according to the principles noted in Figure 26–2. *B*, For turbulent flows, which are characterized by fluctuating velocities about a mean, the spectral signal broadens. Spectral broadening is commonly used to detect turbulent flow.

IMAGING IMPLEMENTATION

The imaging of anatomic structures provided by two-dimensional echocardiography led to the development of color flow Doppler imaging in the early 1980s. By extending the concept of pulsed-

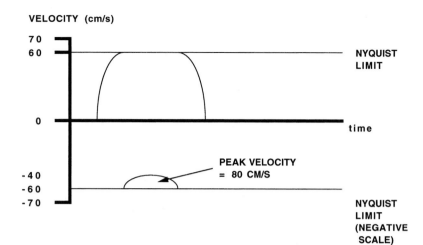

FIGURE 26–4. Aliasing. The pulse-repetition frequency of the instrument determines the maximum detectable velocity in pulsed-wave Doppler by the Nyquist principle. Velocities above this limit wrap around to the negative scale, as shown.

wave Doppler, with the use of multiple interrogation lines, each with multiple sample volumes, color-coded velocity patterns became available for superimposition on the echocardiographic anatomic images.

Color Flow Doppler Mapping

Figure 26–5 illustrates the principles involved in extending pulsed-wave Doppler to obtain a two-dimensional array of velocities. As in the spectral modality, a burst of ultrasound is emitted from the transducer. At a time t, a window opens and receives signals from a distance governed by equation 3, then closes. Then, it opens again, receiving signals at a slightly greater distance away, because the value of t in equation 3 has increased. This window is sequentially opened and closed until a string of sample volumes has been formed, as shown in Figure 26–5. This technique is called multigating. By mounting multiple piezoelectric crystals in the face of the transducer, or mechanically shifting the face of the transducer (see below), this string can be focused along many adjacent paths or lines, forming a two-dimensional matrix of velocity sample volumes in the same sector shape as that of the echocardiographic image. Because it is impossible to view spectra for many sample volumes in a given frame simultaneously, the samples for each are averaged to obtain a single value, and this value is color-coded, based on a predetermined color scale as shown in Figure 26–6. It is common practice to use shades of orange or red for flow toward the transducer and blue for flow away from the transducer. The set of velocities that are averaged within a single sample volume for a single frame is called a packet, or packet size.

FIGURE 26–6. See Color Plate 1.

Data Processing: Spectral Versus Autocorrelation

In the spectral modalities of pulsed-wave and continuous-wave Doppler, all returning signals are, at least in principle, displayed on the screen if not intentionally filtered. Individual particles contribute to the brightness of specific velocity intervals on the spectrum, as described previously. Magnitudes are calculated with the Doppler principle and distributed in the spectrum with the use of fast Fourier transformation techniques. Because of the large amount of data processing required in two-dimensional color flow mapping (in excess of 1 million calculations per second), it is common practice to use autocorrelation techniques instead of fast Fourier transformation methods. In this simpler calculation method, phases of subsequent signals are compared, to produce an estimate of their velocity, and multiple signals (which make up the packet size described earlier), are averaged to obtain one value of velocity. This value is then placed within a small interval of velocity and is represented by a color assigned to that interval. Although the variance of the average value (the square of the standard deviation, by statistical definition) may be added to the map as a shade of green, it is important to note that the visual display of velocity *distribution* within the sample volume is lost in this method, compared with spectral Doppler techniques.

Limitations

The major limitation of color flow Doppler mapping is related to its interpretation. Color flow Doppler images are constructed on the basis of Doppler velocity calculations. Unfortunately, the velocity magnitudes indicated by individual color pixels are approximate, and the technology is useful mainly for *detection* of abnormal flows

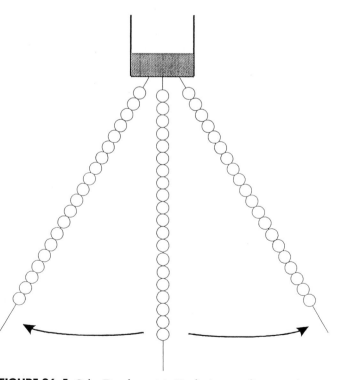

FIGURE 26–5. Color Doppler matrix. To obtain a two-dimensional matrix of velocities for subsequent color encoding, multigating and scan line sweeping are used. Multigating, sequential acquisition of returning signals, allows a string of sample volumes to be constructed along a line. Focusing of the scan line along angled paths produces a pie-shaped matrix of velocities for this transducer (see Fig. 26–7).

and delineation of flow direction and spatial extent. In conventional pulsed-wave Doppler imaging, many signals are acquired and displayed in spectral format. In color flow mapping, because the speed of sound is the limiting factor, the same amount of information must be spread throughout the two-dimensional image. In practice, this limitation produces packet sizes on the order of 8 to 16 samples per frame, a very small number to be averaged to obtain an accurate velocity for color encoding. For turbulent flows, such as that of mitral regurgitant jets, calling these pixels inaccurate would be an understatement. Indeed, not only do they fall short of representing an accurate average value, but also turbulent flows are often high-velocity flows, so they are also aliased. The display is most useful simply to show that flow is present. The use of these pixel velocities to calculate more complex quantities that are based on velocity measurements (pressure, flow rate, momentum) is very dangerous in high-velocity and disturbed-turbulent flow fields.

Packet sizes can be increased, but only by trading off other valuable factors. For example, decreasing imaging depth allows for increased packet sizes when all other factors are held constant. Packet sizes can also be increased by slowing the frame rate (see later), but slowing frame rate introduces the possibility of missing dynamic cardiac events, especially as heart rate goes up. Line density can be reduced, but such a reduction sacrifices lateral resolution to severe degrees for high-depth settings. Table 26–1 illustrates the interplay between depth, packet size, sector lines, and frame rate for a typical instrument.

To overcome spatial resolution difficulties in the axial and lateral directions, manufacturers generally use *smoothing algorithms* before final display of the color image. Although such steps make the images more pleasing to the eye and provide a picture of the flow field that is certainly continuous in physical reality, these algorithms make legitimate interpretation of data especially difficult, because the basic Doppler data has been altered by cosmetic factors. The smoothing algorithms, which are generally proprietary, are a major reason for significant intermachine variability, which can be readily observed for a single patient and flow condition.

In addition to these limitations specific to color flow Doppler mapping, it is important to note that the two primary limitations of pulsed-wave Doppler imaging discussed earlier must also be considered when one uses color Doppler, because each image is constructed of a matrix of pulsed-wave sample volumes. For example, aliasing occurs in color flow mapping and is represented by wrapping from red to blue, or vice versa. Range ambiguity cannot be tolerated in the setting of color flow Doppler mapping, because the essence of the modality is to place color-coded velocities in their correct spatial location. Thus, PRF values for color flow Doppler imaging are typically lower than those commonly used in spectral pulsed-wave Doppler. This important point is worth rephrasing. Although in principle the color and spectral modalities both make use of the pulsed-wave Doppler concept and should have the same velocity limitations, in practice, color Doppler aliasing velocities are lower for a given carrier frequency, because of limited PRFs in the color setting, which are chosen to prevent range ambiguity.

The angle of incidence effects, which apply to all Doppler calculations of velocity, express themselves in two ways with two-dimensional color flow imaging:

Angle of Incidence Effects (Due to Beam Sweep)

Sector and vector image geometries introduce complexities related to the angle of incidence. Consider a jet-type flow oriented parallel to the centerline of the imaging sector. Velocities along the centerline are correctly calculated with the use of the Doppler equation, with the angle of incidence assumed to be zero. For all points away from the centerline, however, velocities are underestimated as the scan line intersects velocity vectors at angles greater than 0 degrees. This angle varies throughout the imaging sector.

Angle of Incidence Effects (Due to Angulation)

When the transducer is angled with respect to the jet direction, further error is superimposed on the scan-line effects described above; that is, the net error will be due to a combination of scan line position and transducer orientation. Because color flow Doppler mapping represents, in principle, a two-dimensional matrix of velocities, these effects are very important in the development of quantitation techniques that rely on flow velocities, rather than on arbitrarily defined color images.

INSTRUMENT SETTINGS

Having described how Doppler data are obtained, we can now discuss the dependence of the signal on various instrument settings. Such factors as gain, pulse repetition frequency, wall filter, carrier frequency, and frame rate directly influence the appearance of data on the screen and therefore its qualitative and "quantitative" interpretation.

Gain

As sound waves propagate, their intensity (amplitude) decreases with distance, and it is common practice in most instruments to amplify waves received from distant structures. In the spectral modality, increasing the gain increases the intensity of the spectra and allows display of signals within velocity bins with only a few particles. The latter produces "feathering" of the envelope of the spectrum and, unless care is taken, can lead to an apparent increase in peak velocity at a particular instant. Similarly, in the color Doppler modality, increasing the gain of the color Doppler channels generally introduces noise, which can distort the color flow structure. Also, in contrast to the spectral artifacts, an increase in gain clearly affects the *low end* of the velocity scale in color flow imaging, reflected by additional color on the fringes of a jet, for example, making it appear larger.

Pulse Repetition Frequency

Pulse repetition frequency simply determines the maximum detectable velocity for a given carrier frequency, and this concept has clear relevance to both spectral and color flow modalities. Maximum PRF values are limited by the chosen depth setting in a given configuration. In addition, in the color flow modality, increases in PRF are generally accompanied by a preprogrammed increase in wall filter, which can trim the boundaries of jets (see next section).

Wall Filter Setting

High-pass filters have been installed in Doppler echocardiographic instruments to eliminate low-frequency, high-amplitude signals returning from moving cardiac structures. If not filtered,

TABLE 26–1. RELATIONSHIPS AMONG DEPTH, PACKET SIZE, NUMBER OF SECTOR LINES, AND FRAME RATE FOR COLOR FLOW DOPPLER IMAGING

Depth (cm)	Packet Size	Sector Lines	Frame Rate
6	4	30	30
8	8	45	20
10	8	30	30
12	4	45	30
14	8	30	20
16	8	45	15
18	4	30	30
18	4	45	20
18	8	45	12

these high-amplitude signals would saturate the Doppler processing circuitry and produce cluttered images. In the spectral modality, increasing the high-pass filter (or, low-velocity reject, as it is often called) tends to produce clearer spectra along the envelope. It is desirable to select the level of a high-pass wall filter low enough that the maximum dynamic range of the signal is spanned, but high enough to eliminate noise resulting from moving cardiac structures. Caution must be taken when one increases the wall filter setting, because these filters abolish any signals returning from low-velocity blood cells producing a Doppler shift less than the wall filter, and also because the wall filter reveals itself each time the signal passes through zero because of multiple aliasing. Removal of low-velocity signals can result in an overestimation of true mean velocities and frequencies. It is also important to recognize that the filter defines the boundary of color Doppler jets and other flows where spatial measurements are taken.

Carrier Frequency

Ultrasound transducers are available in a wide range of carrier frequencies. The carrier frequency affects the quality of the echocardiographic and color flow Doppler images. Varying the carrier frequency affects both the depth of penetration and the resolution of the cardiac image and color flow. In the spectral modality, lower frequency transducers allow higher velocities to be detected for a given PRF and depth, and the depth of penetration is higher for low-frequency transducers. This guideline holds in imaging implementations but must be balanced by the fact that higher frequencies produce better quality images of the cardiac structures.

Frame Rate

The frame rate, or sweep speed, is the number of frames of two-dimensional color Doppler data acquired per unit time. Slower frame rates generally produce better color flow images, because more time is allotted for data processing, and packet sizes can be increased. However, despite better quality, such images are often not accurate, because at higher heart rates some cardiac events may be missed, or single frames can represent events that occur *relatively* far apart in time (e.g., simultaneously opened mitral and aortic valves as the scan line sweeps from posterior to anterior at end-diastole). These adverse effects of lower frame rate can be counteracted by shortening imaging depths, if possible, or decreasing the scan line density at the expense of lateral resolution. Unfortunately, it is impossible to overcome the basic limitation of slow frame rates in the context of high heart rates without basic modification to the color Doppler system, for example, use of parallel processing methods whereby the amount of data acquired per unit time is increased to produce a proportionate increase in frame rate.

Tissue-Priority Algorithm

Conventional color Doppler instruments generally have tissue-priority algorithms that give B-mode tissue signals display priority over color flow data. When one looks at flow near a surface, for example, the color sample volume may encroach on a wall because of the sample volume's relatively large size. The resulting color pixels would then make it appear that flow is passing into the wall. Tissue-priority algorithms cancel color signals when solid structures are detected in the same location. It is important to note that the tissue-priority algorithm works in conjunction with instrument gain. With increasing B-mode gain, B-mode signals increase and begin to cancel legitimate color signals, as reverberations of the B-mode may appear within chambers. New imaging methods, such as Doppler tissue imaging (Acuson Corp., Mountain View, CA), which displays tissue velocities and not blood cell velocities, presumably require removal or modification of the

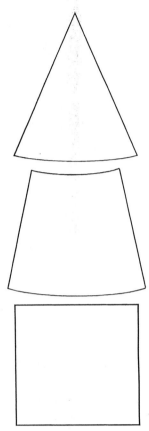

FIGURE 26–7. Image geometries. Sector (*top*), vector (*center*), and linear (*bottom*) image geometries are common.

tissue-priority algorithm because colors must be placed on the moving cardiac structures.

TRANSDUCER CONFIGURATIONS

Spectral Doppler

Transducers designed to implement the spectral Doppler modalities are relatively simple. Continuous-wave transducers consist of two crystals, with one emitting and one continuously receiving sound. Pulsed-wave transducers generally consist of a single crystal, alternately emitting and receiving sound. These transducers can stand alone or are embedded in the more complex imaging transducers described later, so that continuous- or pulsed-wave Doppler measurement locations can be steered into place on the two-dimensional image.

Color Doppler

Color Doppler images are obtained with the use of a phased array of crystals or a physically moving transducer head (mechanical transducer). Phased-array devices consist of multiple crystals arranged along a face, which allow focusing of the scan line along adjacent paths. These paths may fan out from a single point, forming a sector array, from an arc of points forming a vector array, or parallel to each other, forming a linear array. These various geometries are illustrated in Figure 26–7. In a mechanical transducer, a single line is swept from the transducer head as it physically oscillates.

Acknowledgment

We thank John Strobel for technical assistance in preparation of this chapter.

PLATE 1

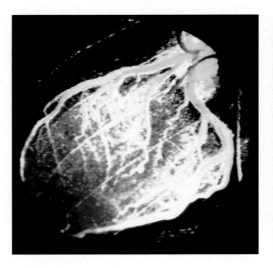 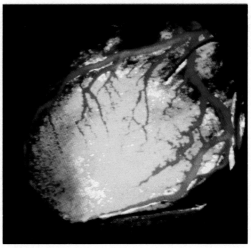

FIGURE 24–13. A set of contrast myocardial appearance pictures taken in the basal state *(left)* and after papaverine-induced hyperemia *(right)*. Color coding depicts the transit of contrast agent for each cycle (cycle 1 = red, cycle 2 = yellow, etc.). Density information is encoded in the intensity of each pixel. Analyses from regions of interest in both coronary beds showed normal flow reserve in this patient.

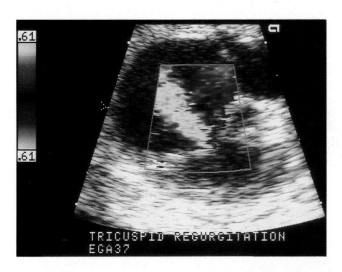

FIGURE 26–6. Color Doppler image from a patient with tricuspid regurgitation. The high-velocity turbulent jet is shown in the right atrium as a mosaic pattern of pixels, representing the chaotic flow patterns in the jet.

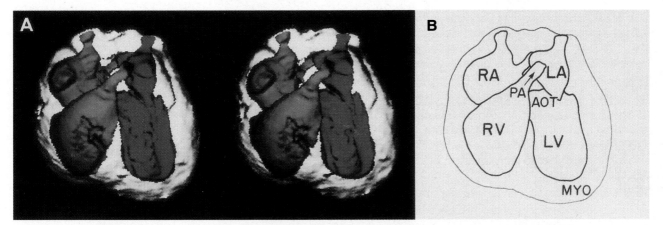

FIGURE 27–7. *A,* Three-dimensional volume-rendered canine heart with a translucent effect, generated from a set of data obtained from an excised heart scanned in a water tank. The left *(red)* and right *(blue)* chambers of the heart are depicted as solid objects in their natural relationship to each other within the myocardium. The images are a stereo pair to enhance the multidimensional effect. The image should be viewed with the figure held about 6 inches from the eyes. When the eyes relax, the two images merge into one. *B,* Corresponding diagram of cardiac structures. AOT = aortic outflow tract; LA = left atrium; LV = left ventricle; MYO = myocardium; PA = pulmonary artery; RA = right atrium; RV = right ventricle. (From Greenleaf, J.F., Belohlavek, M., Gerber, T.C., et al.: Multidimensional visualization in echocardiography: An introduction. Mayo Clin. Proc. 68:219, 1993, with permission.)

PLATE 2

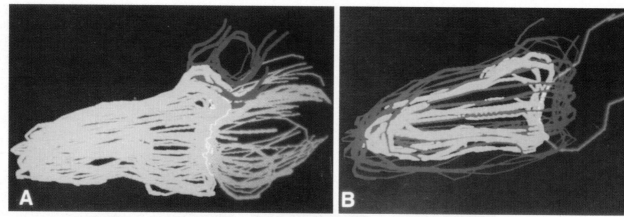

FIGURE 27-8. *A,* Normal human left ventricle reconstructed from apical views in vivo at peak systolic contraction. The endocardial border is shown in yellow with the apex to the left. The left atrium is traced in blue, and the aortic root in green. A papillary muscle indentation can be seen along the inferior surface of the ventricle, and the curvature of the mitral ring is evident at the atrioventricular junction. *B,* Superimposed endocardial borders in systole *(yellow)* and diastole in another subject. (The centers of the systolic and diastolic ventricular traces are superimposed.) (From Handschumacher, M.D., Lethor, J.P., Siu, S.C., et al.: A new integrated system for three-dimensional echocardiographic reconstruction: Development and validation for ventricular volume with application in human subjects. J. Am. Coll. Cardiol. 21:743, 1993. Reprinted with permission from the American College of Cardiology.)

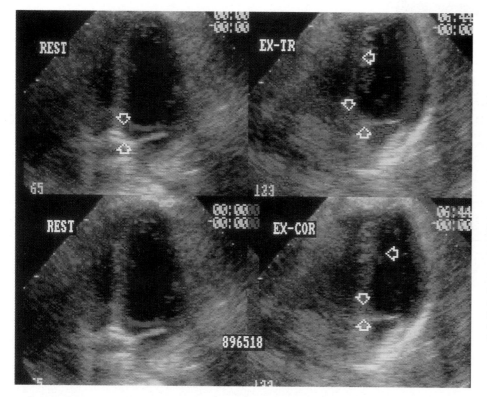

FIGURE 27-25. Color coding applied to digitized apical four-chamber view at rest (REST) and peak exercise. End-systolic images are displayed. Arrows mark position of mitral valve annulus in diastole *(upward arrow)* and systole *(downward arrow)* and ventricular septum *(horizontal arrow).* Rest images demonstrate normal basal-to-apical shortening without transverse displacement of mitral valve annulus. Peak exercise image (EX-TR) demonstrates translation with leftward displacement of mitral valve annulus during systole. As a result, the interventricular septum appears dyskinetic, and the lateral wall hyperkinetic. After correction for translation by realigning the mitral valve annulus to eliminate transverse displacement, peak exercise image (EX-COR) displays normal left ventricular wall motion. (From Bates, J.R., Ryan, T., Rimmerman, C.M., et al.: Color coding of digitized echocardiograms: Description of a new technique and application in detecting and correcting for cardiac transplantation. J. Am. Soc. Echocardiogr. 7:363, 1994, with permission.)

PLATE 3

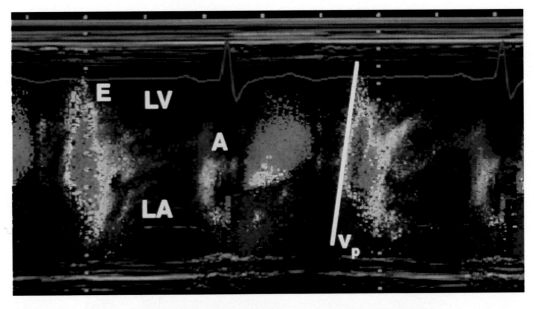

FIGURE 29–24. Color Doppler M-mode display of transmitral flow. This shows the spatiotemporal velocity distribution along a scan line from the middle left atrium (LA) to the middle left ventricle (LV), demonstrating the flow propagation occurring with early filling (E) and atrial contraction (A). A key derived parameter is the propagation velocity of the E wave, v_p, given by the slope of the leading edge of the E wave as it moves into the ventricle.

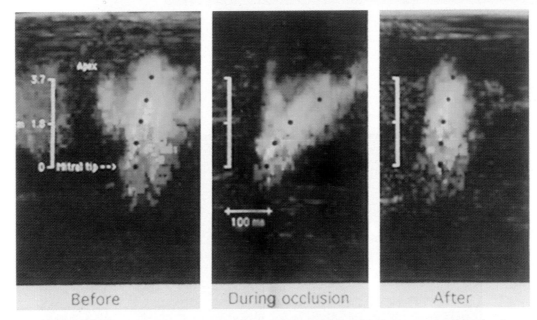

FIGURE 29–25. Delay in flow propagation caused by angioplasty-induced acute myocardial ischemia. (From Stuggard, M., et al.: Intraventricular early diastolic filling during acute myocardial ischemia: Assessment by multigated color M-mode Doppler echocardiography. Circulation 88:2705–2713, 1993, with permission from the American Heart Association.)

FIGURE 29–26. Doppler tissue imaging of left ventricular contraction (*left*) and relaxation (*right*) in amyloidosis, parasternal short-axis view. By eliminating the high-pass wall filter from the color Doppler processing chain and utilizing low-gain amplification to suppress the blood signal, intramyocardial velocity can be visualized.

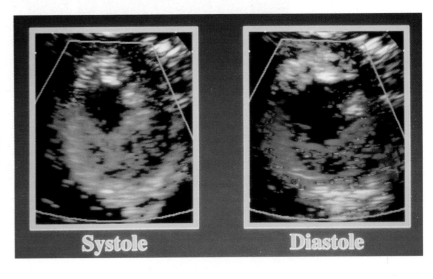

PLATE 4

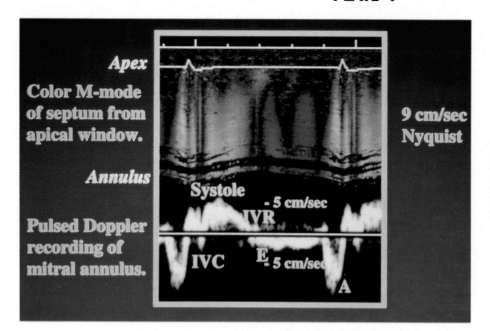

Apex

Color M-mode of septum from apical window.

Annulus

Pulsed Doppler recording of mitral annulus.

9 cm/sec Nyquist

Systole

- 5 cm/sec

IVR

IVC   E. 5 cm/sec

A

FIGURE 29–27. Color Doppler M-mode tissue imaging of longitudinal septal motion *(top)* in amyloidosis, with pulsed-wave display of annular velocity *(bottom)*. These data were obtained from the apical window with the scan line directed along the longitudinal extent of the interventricular septum.

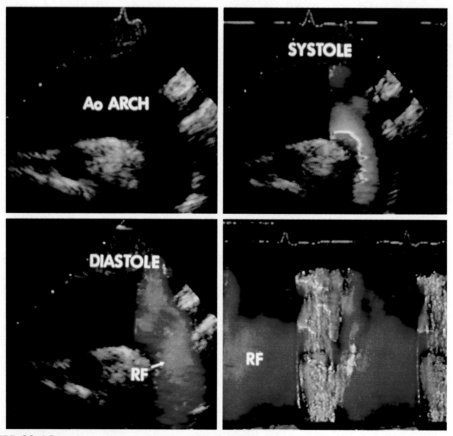

FIGURE 30–10. Flow reversal in the descending aorta in a patient with severe aortic regurgitation demonstrated from the suprasternal window. *Top Left,* Two-dimensional image of aortic arch and descending aorta. *Top Right,* Systolic frame demonstrates anterograde flow, which appears blue, in descending aorta. *Bottom Left,* Diastolic frame demonstrates retrograde flow, which appears red, in descending aorta. *Bottom Right,* Color M-mode demonstrates holodiastolic regurgitant flow. Ao arch = aortic arch; RF = regurgitant flow.

PLATE 5

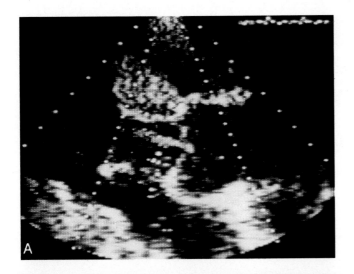

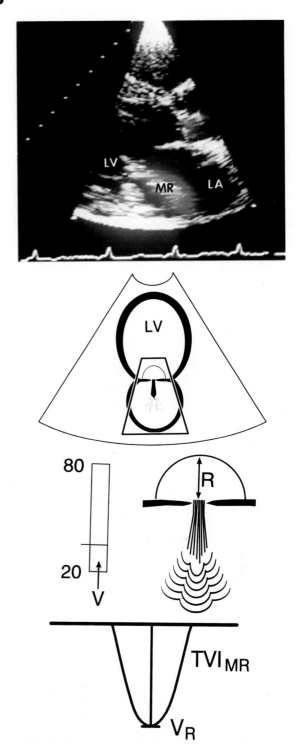

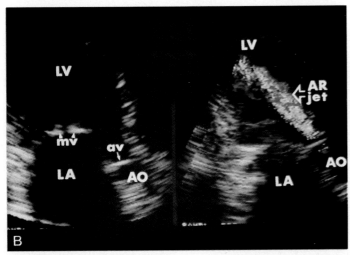

FIGURE 30–11. Assessment of severity of aortic regurgitation by color-flow imaging. *A,* Parasternal long-axis view. Proximal minimal width of regurgitant jet is less than 20 percent of width of left ventricular outflow tract, indicative of mild aortic regurgitation. *B,* Apical long-axis views, with and without color flow. Long, broad jet of aortic regurgitation in a patient with moderate aortic regurgitation. AO = aorta; AR = aortic regurgitation; av = aortic valve; LA = left atrium; LV = left ventricle; mv = mitral valve.

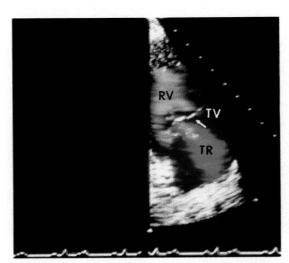

FIGURE 30–22. Moderate tricuspid regurgitation. Color flow imaging from an apical four-chamber view demonstrates systolic regurgitant flow through the tricuspid orifice into the right atrium. RA = right atrium; RV = right ventricle; TR = tricuspid regurgitation; TV = tricuspid valve.

FIGURE 30–19. *Top,* Moderate mitral regurgitation seen from parasternal long-axis view. High-velocity, turbulent flow (mosaic pattern) is characteristic because of the large systolic pressure gradient between left ventricle and left atrium. LA = left atrium; LV = left ventricle; MR = mitral regurgitation. *Bottom,* Schematic representation of the flow convergence method with instructions for calculation of regurgitant volume. (1) *Optimize two-dimensional image* of mitral regurgitant orifice (use zoom function). (2) *Optimize color flow detail* of the flow convergence region. (3) *Shift the color flow baseline downward* to decrease the color flow aliasing velocity. (4) Note the *alias velocity* (V). (5) Using online calipers, *measure "R" from aliased region to orifice.* (6) *Measure the time-velocity integral (TVI) and peak regurgitant velocity* (V$_R$) of the continuous-wave (CW) Doppler echocardiography jet.

PLATE 6

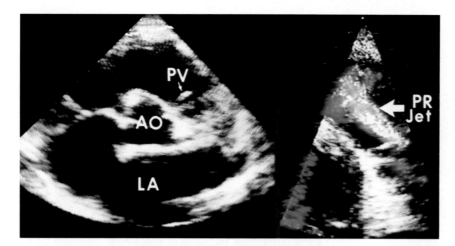

FIGURE 30–25. Pulmonary regurgitation (PR) by color flow imaging. Parasternal short-axis view demonstrates diastolic, red-encoded jet in the right ventricular outflow tract, representing a mild to moderate degree of pulmonary regurgitation. Ao = aorta; LA = left atrium; PV = pulmonary valve.

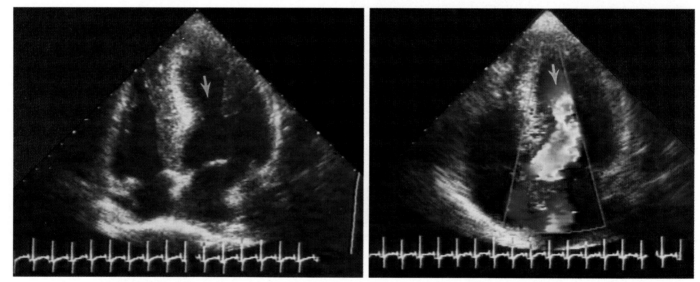

FIGURE 31–5. Two-dimensional echocardiographic image (left) with superimposed color flow Doppler (right), demonstrating midcavity ventricular hypertrophy, with flow acceleration occurring just proximal to the point of obstruction (arrow).

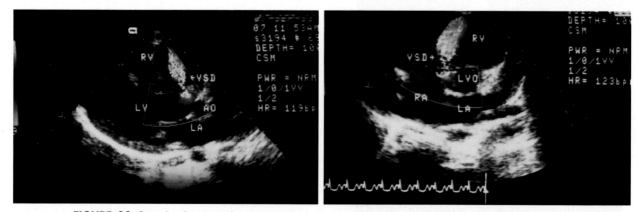

FIGURE 33–4. Color flow Doppler examination from a patient with a small membranous ventricular septal defect (VSD). The jet flow through the VSD is seen in the parasternal long-axis (left) and short-axis (right) views. The mosaic appearance of the jet is caused by the presence of high-velocity, disturbed flow. AO = aorta; LA = left atrium; LV = left ventricle; LVO = left ventricular outflow tract; RA = right atrium; RV = right ventricle.

PLATE 7

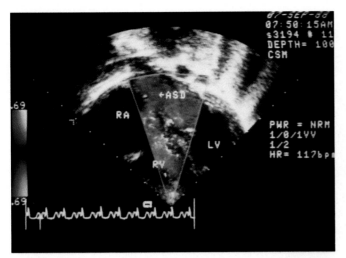

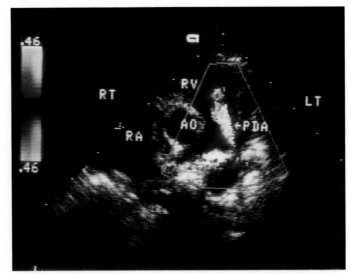

FIGURE 33–7. Color flow Doppler examination of a child with a large secundum atrial septal defect (ASD). In the four-chamber view, the jet flow through the ASD is seen. The red color of the jet indicates low-velocity flow directed toward the transducer. The yellow areas within the jet indicate variance or disturbed flow. LV = left ventricle; RA = right atrium; RV = right ventricle.

FIGURE 33–13. Color flow Doppler examination in the parasternal short-axis view of a child with a patent ductus arteriosus (PDA). The jet flow through the PDA appears as a mosaic of colors, which indicates disturbed high-velocity flow toward the transducer. AO = aorta; LA = left atrium; LT = left; RA = right atrium; RT = right; RV = right ventricle.

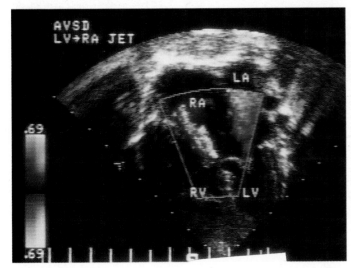

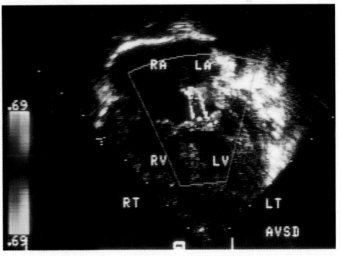

FIGURE 33–18. Color Doppler examination in the apical four-chamber view of a patient with an atrioventricular septal defect (AVSD) and left ventricular (LV)–to–right atrial (RA) shunting. LA = left atrium; RV = right ventricle.

FIGURE 33–19. Color Doppler examination in the apical four-chamber view of a patient with an atrioventricular septal defect (AVSD) and several small regurgitant jets (*blue*) arising from the left side of the common atrioventricular valve. LA = left atrium; LT = left; LV = left ventricle; RA = right atrium; RT = right; RV = right ventricle.

FIGURE 33–43. Color Doppler imaging in the subcostal long-axis view of the abdomen of an infant with infra-diaphragmatic total anomalous pulmonary venous connection. Doppler signals arising from blood flow in the common pulmonary vein are shown in red, indicating blood flow away from the heart and toward the abdomen. The common pulmonary vein drains into the portal vein. Note the area of aliasing in the common pulmonary vein due to obstruction of the vein as it passes through the diaphragm.

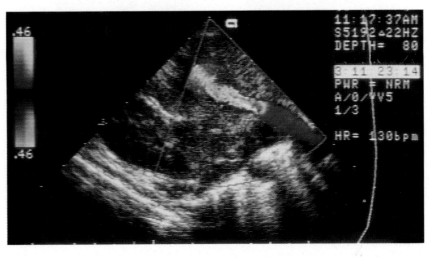

PLATE 8

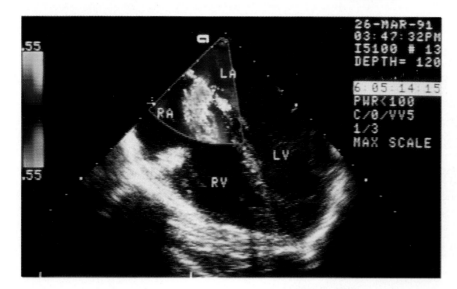

FIGURE 33–59. Transesophageal echocardiographic image of the apical four-chamber view of a child with a large secundum atrial septal defect. The left-to-right shunt across the atrial septal defect is seen on the color Doppler examination as a mosaic flow area. LA = left atrium; LV = left ventricle; RA = right atrium; RV = right ventricle.

FIGURE 33–60. Transesophageal imaging of the same patient as in Figure 33–59 after placement at interventional catheterization of a double-disk button device for closure of the atrial septal defect. Only a small residual shunt is seen on the color flow examination. Abbreviations are as in Figure 33–59.

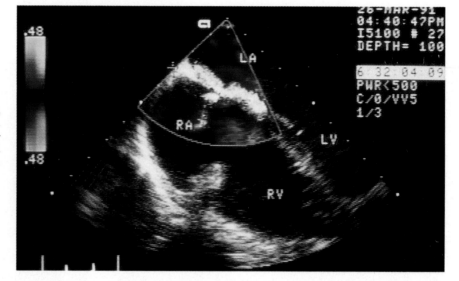

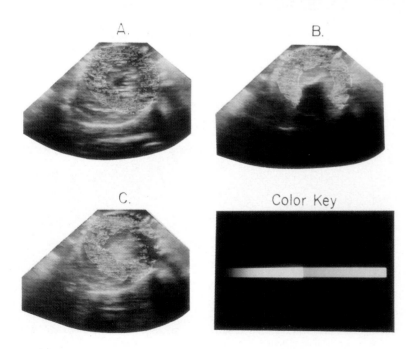

FIGURE 35–7. Color-coded data from an injection sequence similar to that noted in Figure 35–6. All regions except the myocardium have been "masked." The color code is shown in the bar, with red being minimal echo brightness and yellow being brighter. *A*, An image prior to contrast opacification of the myocardium. The red is homogeneously distributed. This image corresponds to *A* in Figure 35–6. *B*, An image taken during maximal myocardial opacification when the contrast present in the left ventricular cavity is producing posterior wall attenuation. Note the yellow. This image corresponds to *B* and *C* in Figure 35–6. *C*, An image obtained a few cycles later when posterior wall attenuation is no longer present. Although the myocardial contrast effect is not as great as in *B*, it is still present. This image corresponds to *D* in Figure 35–6. (From Villanueva, F.S., Glasheen, W.P., Sklenar, J., et al.: Successful and reproducible myocardial opacification during two-dimensional echocardiography from right heart injection of contrast. Circulation 85:1557, 1992, with permission.)

PLATE 9

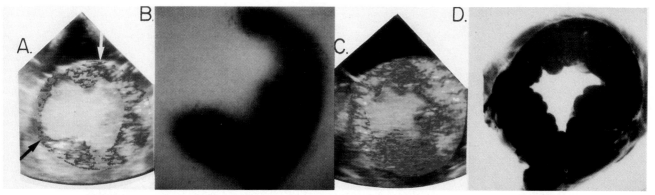

FIGURE 35–11. An example of successful reperfusion with no infarction and, hence, complete myocardial salvage. An anterior perfusion defect is noted on myocardial contrast echocardiography during left anterior descending artery occlusion (A), with a corresponding defect on technetium autoradiography (B). After reperfusion, there is no defect noted on myocardial contrast echocardiography (C), and no infarction is noted on postmortem triphenyltetrazolium chloride staining of the heart (D). (From Villanueva, F.S., Glasheen, W.D., Sklenar, J., et al.: Assessment of risk area during coronary occlusion and infarct size after reperfusion with myocardial contrast echocardiography using left and right atrial injections of contrast. Circulation 88:596, 1993, with permission.)

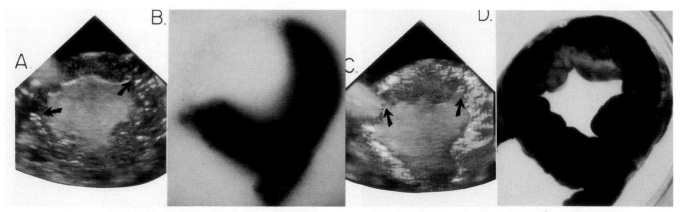

FIGURE 35–12. An example of successful reperfusion with partial myocardial salvage. An anterior perfusion defect is noted on myocardial contrast echocardiography during left anterior descending coronary artery occlusion (A), with a corresponding defect on technetium autoradiography (B). After reperfusion, an endocardial defect is noted on myocardial contrast echocardiography (C), and a subendocardial infarction is noted on postmortem triphenyltetrazolium chloride staining of the heart (D). (From Villanueva, F.S., Glasheen, W.D., Sklenar, J., and Kaul, S.: Assessment of risk area during coronary occlusion and infarct size after reperfusion with myocardial contrast echocardiography using left and right atrial injections of contrast. Circulation 88:596, 1993, with permission.)

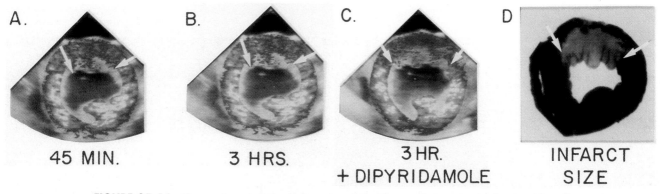

45 MIN. 3 HRS. 3 HR.
+ DIPYRIDAMOLE INFARCT SIZE

FIGURE 35–16. Changes in reperfusion patterns in a dog with a nearly transmural infarction. After 45 minutes of reperfusion, a small relative color defect localized to the endocardium in the anterior wall is noted, as shown by arrows in A. After 3 hours of reperfusion, this defect was slightly larger, as depicted by arrows in B. The addition of dipyridamole resulted in a much larger relative contrast defect, shown by arrows in C, which closely delineated the true size and shape of the infarct on tissue staining with triphenyltetrazolium chloride, which is indicated by arrows in D. (See text for details.) (From Villanueva, F.S., Glasheen, W.D., Sklenar, J., et al.: Characterization of spatial patterns of flow within the reperfused myocardium using myocardial contrast echocardiography: Implications for determining extent of myocardial salvage. Circulation 88:2596, 1993, with permission.)

PLATE 10

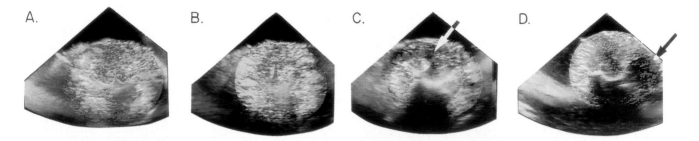

FIGURE 35–26. Color-coded end-systolic images at baseline (*A*) and during pharmacologically induced hyperemia (*B to D*), in the absence of any stenosis (*B*), in the presence of a left anterior descending artery stenosis (*C*), and during left circumflex artery stenosis (*D*). (See text for details.) (From Ismail, S., Jayaweera, A.R., Goodman, N.C., et al.: Detection of coronary artery stenoses and quantification of blood flow mismatch during coronary hyperemia with myocardial contrast echocardiography. Circulation 91:821, 1995, with permission.)

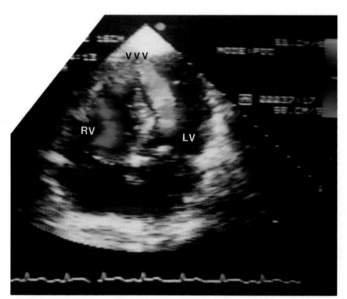

FIGURE 37–9. Color Doppler demonstration of ventricular septal defect secondary to myocardial infarction. Abnormal left ventricle–to–right ventricle flow across the defect is depicted by arrowheads. The orange color indicates blood flow toward the transducer; blue indicates flow away from the transducer. LV = left ventricle; RV = right ventricle.

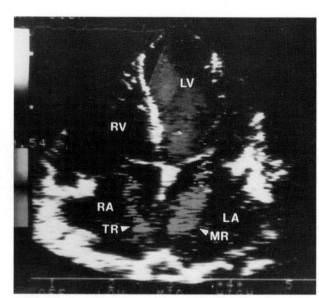

FIGURE 37–11. Color Doppler echocardiogram obtained from the apical four-chamber view. An eccentric turquoise mitral regurgitant jet (MR) and a tricuspid regurgitant jet (TR) are evident in this patient with ischemic myocardiopathy and papillary muscle dysfunction. LA = left atrium; LV = left ventricle; RA = right atrium; RV = right ventricle. (From Kotler, M.N., Goldman, A.P., and Parry, W.R.: Acute consequences and chronic complications of acute myocardial infarction. *In* Kerber, R.E. [ed.]: Echocardiography in Coronary Artery Disease. Mt. Kisco, NY, Futura Publishing Company, 1988, p. 17, with permission.)

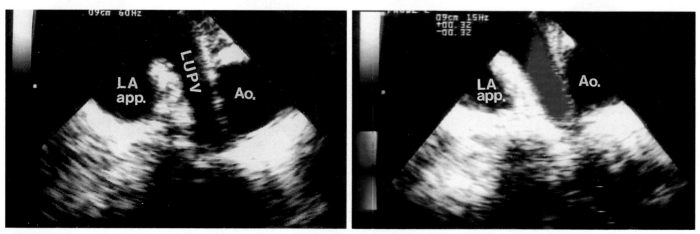

FIGURE 38–5. *Left,* Transverse view of left atrial appendage and left upper pulmonary vein (LUPV). *Right,* Color flow toward the transducer from the left upper pulmonary vein emptying into the left atrium. (From Schiller, N.B., and Himelman, R.B.: Echocardiography and Doppler in clinical cardiology. *In* Parmley, W.W., and Chatterjee, K. [eds.]: Cardiology. Vol. 1, Philadelphia, J.B. Lippincott, 1987, pp. 1–97, with permission.)

PLATE 11

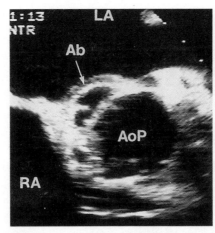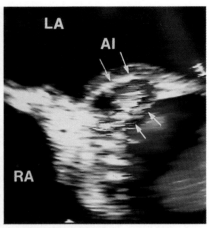

FIGURE 38-19. Transesophageal echocardiographic views of a posterior aortic prosthetic sewing ring abscess (AoPAb) in the region of the fibrous trigone (region of His bundle crossing) in a patient with prosthetic endocarditis and a new second-degree heart block. Color flow images demonstrate paravalvular aortic regurgitation (AI) *(arrows)* through the ring abscess. LA = left atrium; RA = right atrium.

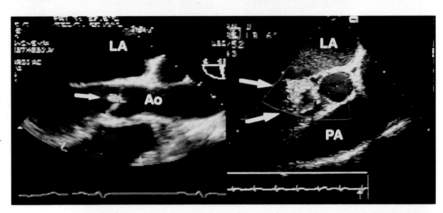

FIGURE 38-21. Trivial aortic insufficiency *(left panel, arrow)* compared with severe aortic insufficiency *(right panel, double arrows)*. *Left Panel,* The single arrow is within the left ventricular outflow tract. Compare its diameter with the diameter of the color flow regurgitant diastolic aortic jet to which the arrow points. Note that the jet occupies no more than 20 percent of the outflow tract diameter. *Right Panel,* The two solid arrows are in the left ventricular outflow tract and span the edges of the aortic insufficiency jet. Note that this jet occupies at least 80 percent of the diameter of the left ventricular outflow tract.

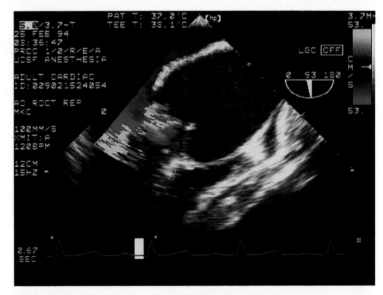

FIGURE 38-22. Transverse multiplane view (93 degrees) of the long axis of the aortic root in a patient whose aortic insufficiency is due to aortoannular ectasia. Note the enlargement of the aortic root relative to the right ventricular outflow tract that lies anteriorly at the bottom of the picture. Compare this relationship with that shown in Figure 38-21.

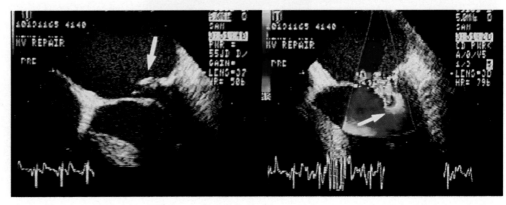

FIGURE 38-25. Flail mitral valve leaflet. *Left Panel,* The arrow points to thickened and displaced posterior mitral valve leaflet that has entered the left atrium during systole and is displaced from the coaptation plane, which is defined by the tip of the longer anterior leaflet. *Right Panel,* Color flow imaging *(arrow)* reveals concentric rings typical of a proximal acceleration phenomenon that accompanies mitral regurgitation. The size of this process and the broadness of its jet as it crosses the disrupted valve are two signs of the severity of the regurgitation.

PLATE 12

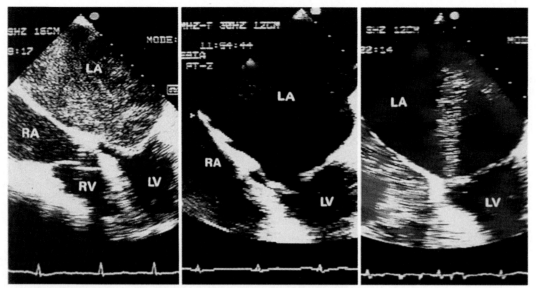

FIGURE 38–26. Mitral stenosis. *Left Panel,* Four-chamber view showing greatly enlarged left atrium, diastolic doming of the mitral valve, and dense spontaneous contrast within the left atrium (LA). *Middle Panel,* The limited orifice of the mitral valve is better appreciated with the gain lowered in the left atrium. Note how minor gain adjustments can prevent detection of spontaneous contrast. *Right Panel,* Tricuspid regurgitation (moderate) and mitral insufficiency (mild) are seen in systole and complicate the picture of rheumatic mitral and tricuspid valve disease. RA = right atrium; LV = left ventricle; LA = left atrium; RV = right ventricle. (From Schiller, N.B., and Himelman, R.B.: Echocardiography and Doppler in clinical cardiology. *In* Parmley, W.W., and Chatterjee, K. [eds.]: Cardiology. Vol. 1. Philadelphia, J.B. Lippincott, 1987, pp. 1–97, with permission.)

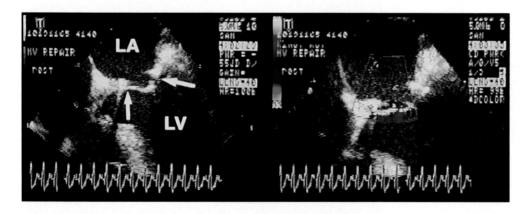

FIGURE 38–29. Mitral valve appearance after valve repair. The arrows denote the valvuloplasty ring, which has been placed to decrease the size of the mitral annulus and to improve coaptation. The right panel is a color flow study in systole showing that only trivial mitral regurgitation persists after this repair.

FIGURE 38–30. Paravalvular mitral regurgitation in a St. Jude prosthesis. *Left Panel,* A disastolic frame showing the twin discs in their open position parallel to one another *(double arrows).* *Right Panel,* The wall-hugging mitral regurgitation jet that arises outside the limits of the sewing ring of the prosthesis *(arrow).* LA = left atrium.

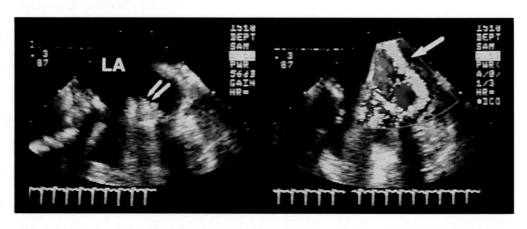

PLATE 13

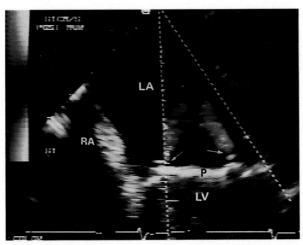

FIGURE 38-31. Transesophageal echocardiographic image of normal "physiologic" regurgitation (arrows) in a St. Jude mitral prosthesis. P = prosthesis; LA = left atrium; RA = right atrium; LV = left ventricle.

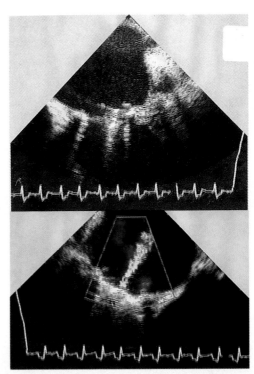

FIGURE 38-32. Top, Low-profile Medtronic-Hall prosthetic valve in the mitral position characterized by a single disc and prominent shadowing distal to the mitral valve ring. With color flow imaging (lower panel), this valve characteristically shows two jets of mitral regurgitation. The normal regurgitation pattern as shown here consists of a large central jet and a very small peripheral jet. Note that both jets lie within the sewing ring and do not extend deeply into the left atrium.

FIGURE 38-33. Transesophageal echocardiography of this patient with severe aortic regurgitation due to prosthetic valve endocarditis demonstrates a flail porcine cusp (arrow) prolapsing into the left ventricular outflow tract. The torn cusp was confirmed at surgery. Pathologic specimen at bottom. AoP = aortic prosthesis; LA = left atrium; RA = right atrium.

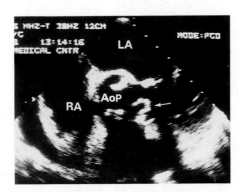

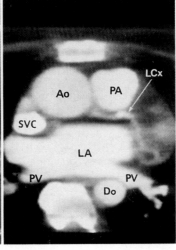

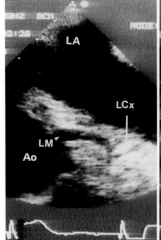
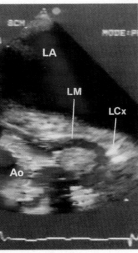
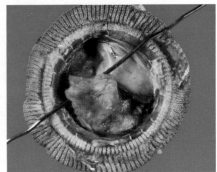

FIGURE 38-37. Left Panel, Transesophageal echo imaging of coronary vasculature. Middle Panel, Color detection of blood flow in the left main (LM) can be seen as well as a calcific plaque at the take-off of the left circumflex coronary artery (LCx). Cine-computed tomography scan of the thorax (right panel) in the same patient confirms a calcific plaque at the take-off of the left circumflex (arrow). Ao = ascending aorta; Do = descending aorta; PA = pulmonary artery; PV = pulmonary vein; SVC = superior vena cava; LA = left atrium.

PLATE 14

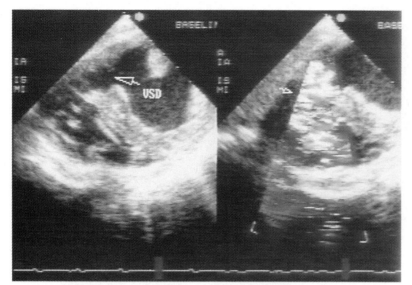

FIGURE 38–38. *Left Panel,* Short-axis transgastric view showing an enlarged ventricular septal defect (VSD) in the septum (posteroinferior portion) that appears to communicate directly with the right ventricle. *Right Panel,* The same view, centered over the right ventricle. Note that the flow crossing this defect during systole *(arrow)* is nearly laminar, indicating torrential left-to-right shunting.

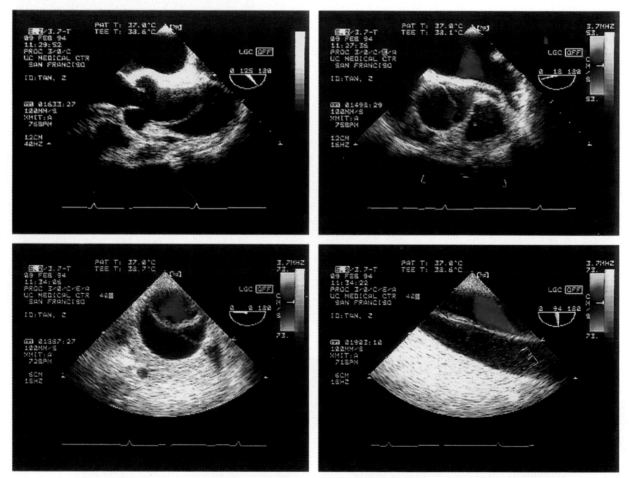

FIGURE 38–39. Proximal and distal aortic dissection. In this patient, the dissection involves both the aortic root and the distal descending thoracic aorta. *Upper Left Panel,* Longitudinal plane view of the long axis of the aorta at 125 degrees from the transverse. Note the intimal flap running from the superior aspect of the right coronary sinus (sinotubular junction) to the superior limits of the image. *Upper Right Panel,* In the short-axis view, the intimal flap can be seen and appears to partition the superior portion of the sinus. Note that in the right portion of the partition (patient's left) the left main coronary artery can be seen exiting from the true lumen. Inspecting the proximal aortic root reveals that the dissection begins at the sinotubular junction and thus comes very close to coronary involvement; it appears to spare the aortic valve, however. There is also no evidence of pericardial effusion. The lower panels show a short-axis *(left)* and a long-axis *(right)* view of the midthoracic descending aorta. Note that there is a true lumen (with color flow) and a false lumen (without color flow). Also note that there is no thrombus seen in the false lumen.

PLATE 15

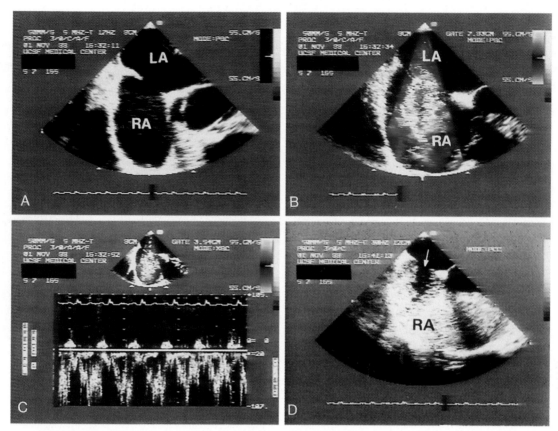

FIGURE 38–40. Secundum atrial septal defect. *A,* Direct visualization of a large secundum atrial septal defect with two-dimensional echocardiographic imaging. *B,* Prominent left-to-right shunting can be seen with color flow and pulsed Doppler interrogation *(C). D,* Saline contrast administration demonstrated a "negative contrast effect" *(arrow)* of left-to-right shunting. LA = left atrium; RA = right atrium.

FIGURE 38–41. *Upper Panel,* Unroofed atrial view in an anatomic specimen showing the relationship between the left atrial cavity and a St. Jude mitral prosthesis. *Lower Panel (Middle Image),* A patient with a St. Jude prosthesis has undergone three-dimensional transesophageal echocardiographic imaging. In this diastolic still-frame, the authors have re-created the unroofed atrial view seen in the anatomic image above. The landmarks that surround the prosthesis are identified in the diagram to the left. *Lower Panel (Right Image),* Another unroofed left atrial view of the same prosthesis. In this case, the cut extends more deeply into the free wall of the left atrium, and the prosthesis is viewed from a more lateral aspect. The overall orientation is the same, with the atrial appendage at the top of the image. *(Upper Panel* courtesy of Dr. Philip C. Ursell.)

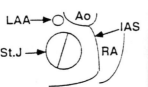

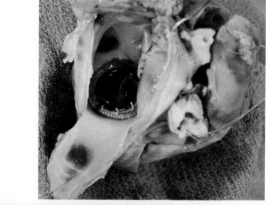

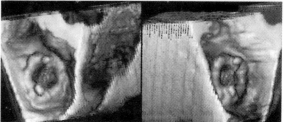

PLATE 16

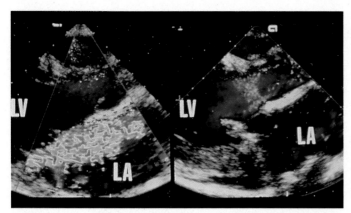

FIGURE 39–5. Epicardial color flow images before and after successful mitral valve repair. *Left,* Anteriorly directed jet of severe (3+ to 4+) mitral regurgitation resulting from a posterior leaflet prolapse. *Right,* Epicardial color flow image after successful repair showing no mitral regurgitation. LA = left atrium; LV = left ventricle.

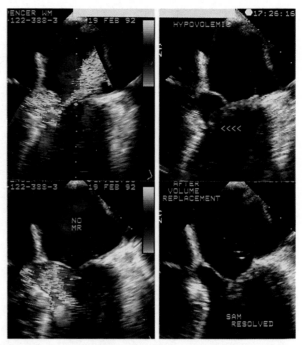

FIGURE 39–8. Transesophageal transverse views of dynamic left ventricular outflow tract obstruction occurring during postoperative hypovolemia immediately after mitral valve repair for mitral regurgitation (MR). *Upper Left,* Color flow image showing moderate, persistent mitral regurgitation, and high-velocity flow in the left ventricular outflow tract. *Upper Right,* Systolic anterior motion (SAM) of the mitral valve *(arrows). Lower Left,* After volume replacement and cessation of dobutamine administration, the mitral regurgitation has resolved. *Lower Right,* Two-dimensional image showing resolution of the SAM.

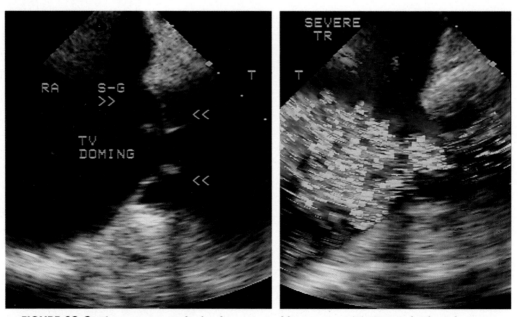

FIGURE 39–9. Rheumatic tricuspid valve disease imaged by transverse (T) TEE. *Left,* The right atrium (RA) is enlarged with doming of the tricuspid valve (TV) *(arrows).* A Swan-Ganz (S-G) catheter is shown *(arrows). Right,* Severe tricuspid regurgitation (TR) by color Doppler imaging.

PLATE 17

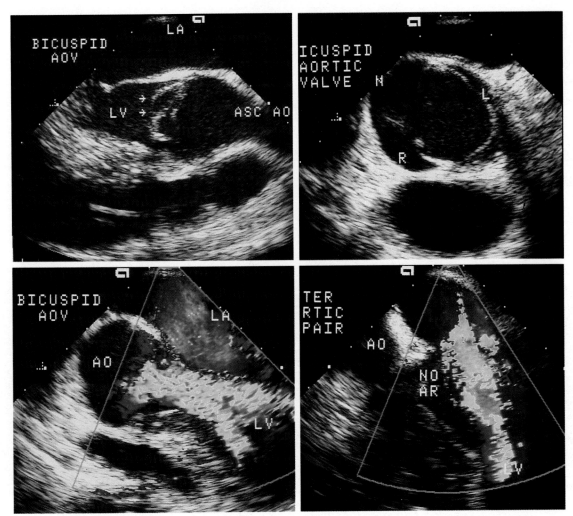

FIGURE 39–10. *Upper Left,* Longitudinal (L) TEE image of a bicuspid aortic valve (AOV) showing prolapse *(arrows)* into the left ventricle (LV). *Upper Right,* Transverse (T) TEE image showing what would be the non- (N) and right (R) cusps, which are fused, with a raphe in the middle of the large conjoined medial cusp, which is larger than the left (L) single cusp. *Lower Left,* Transverse (T) color image showing severe aortic regurgitation. *Lower Right,* Transverse TEE image after aortic repair, showing no aortic regurgitation (AR). The color represents mitral diastolic flow. ASC AO = ascending aorta; LA = left atrium.

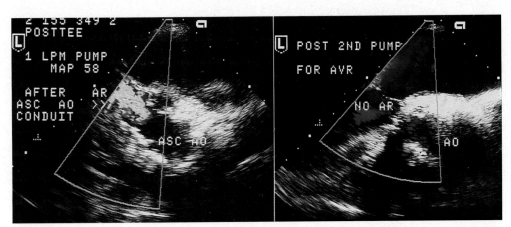

FIGURE 39–11. Longitudinal (L) color flow images in failed aortic valve repair. *Left,* After replacement of the ascending aorta (ASC AO) with a conduit and resuspension of the aortic valve, aortic regurgitation (AR) persists *(arrows)* as the patient was weaned down to 1 L per minute (LPM) of flow on the cardiopulmonary bypass pump, with the mean arterial pressure (MAP) at 58 mm Hg. *Right,* Repeat study after a second pump run for aortic valve replacement (AVR), showing no aortic regurgitation.

PLATE 18

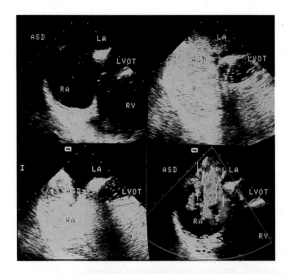

FIGURE 39–13. Intraoperative assessment of atrial septal defect (ASD) in the transverse (T) TEE view. *Upper Left,* Two-dimensional echocardiography showing the septal defect between the left atrium (LA) and the right atrium (RA), with enlargement of the right ventricle (RV). *Upper Right,* Intravenous contrast injection showing passage of contrast into the left atrium. *Lower Left,* Nonopacified left atrial blood is entering the right atrium. *Lower Right,* Color flow image showing left-to-right flow across the atrial septal defect. LVOT = left ventricular outflow tract.

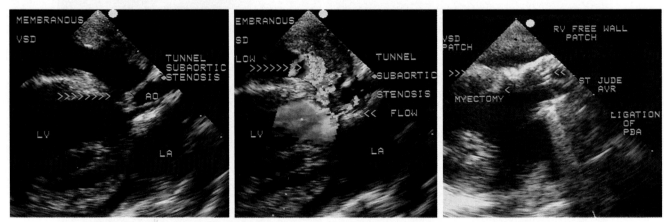

FIGURE 39–15. IOE in complex congenital heart disease. *Left,* Prepump epicardial parasternal long-axis equivalent image of complex congenital heart disease showing the opening *(arrows)* of a membranous ventricular septal defect (VSD), with a small aorta (AO) and tunnel subaortic stenosis, with left ventricular (LV) enlargement. *Middle,* Prepump epicardial color flow image showing flow *(arrows)* through the ventricular septal defect, and high-velocity flow *(arrows)* across the subaortic stenosis. LA = left atrium. *Right,* Postpump intraoperative epicardial image showing the heart after myectomy *(left, arrow),* patch repair of the ventricular septal defect *(arrows),* and St. Jude aortic valve replacement (AVR) *(arrows).* The patient also had ligation of a patent ductus arteriosus (PDA) and a patch of the right ventricular (RV) free wall (not shown in this figure).

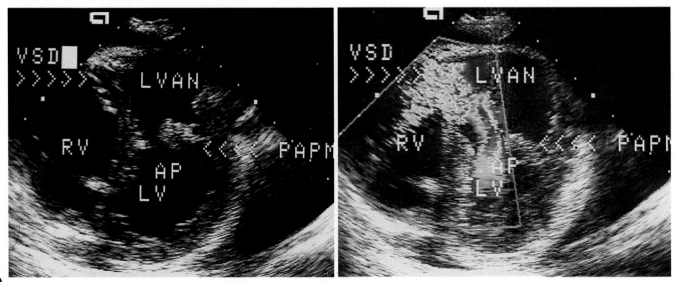

FIGURE 39–16. Transesophageal transverse images of an ischemic ventricular septal defect (VSD) and posterior left ventricular aneurysm (LVAN). *A,* Two-dimensional echocardiographic image at the papillary muscle (PAPM) level showing the dyskinetic aneurysm, with the apical and anterior left ventricle (AP LV) contracting normally. *B,* Color image showing flow *(arrows)* through the posteriorly positioned basilar ventricular septal defect. RV = right ventricle.

PLATE 19

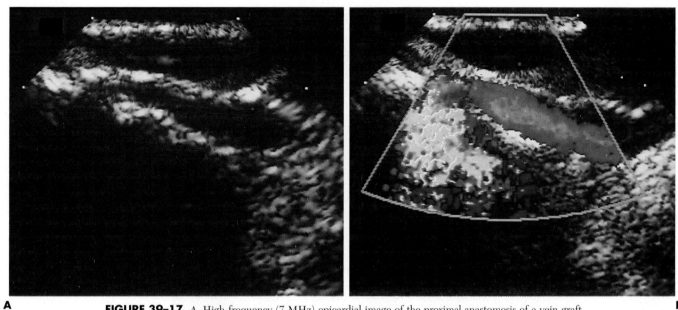

FIGURE 39–17. *A*, High-frequency (7 MHz) epicardial image of the proximal anastomosis of a vein graft with the aorta. *B*, Color flow image showing the multicolored flow in the aorta and the normal nonstenotic homogeneous red flow in the vein graft.

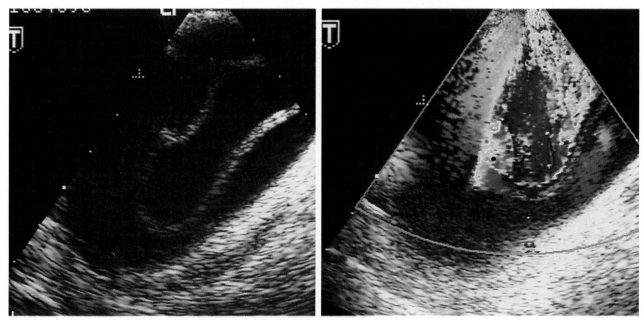

FIGURE 39–18. Transesophageal echocardiographic images of the upper ascending aorta in aortic dissection. *A*, Structural image showing the intimal flap spiraling across a 4-cm aneurysm of the ascending aorta and arch. *B*, Color flow image showing high-velocity flow in the true lumen and homogeneous (orange) lower velocity flow outside the intimal flap in the false lumen.

PLATE 20

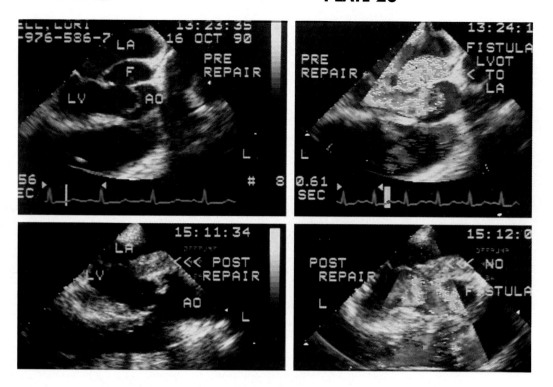

FIGURE 39-19. Longitudinal (L) transesophageal echocardiographic image in surgical correction of a periaortic fistula (F) originating in the left ventricular outflow tract (LVOT). The fistula dissected up the interatrial septum and emptied (not shown on this figure) into the left atrium (LA). *Upper Left,* Two-dimensional image before repair, showing the fistula (F) posterior to the aortic annulus. *Upper Right,* Color image showing flow into the fistula. *Lower Left,* Two-dimensional image after repair, showing closure of the mouth of the fistula (*arrows*). *Lower Right,* Color image after repair, showing no flow into the posterior annulus, where the fistula had been.

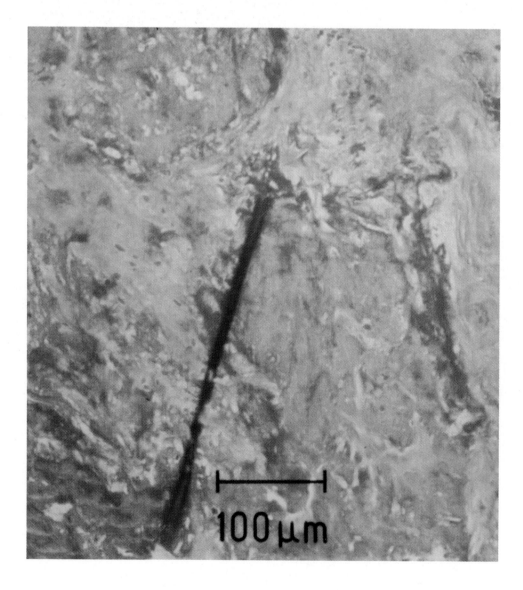

FIGURE 40-3. Histopathology findings implicating plaque rupture as the cause of crescendo claudication in patient from Figure 40–2. Atherectomy specimen from right external iliac artery shows foci of plaque hemorrhage within fibrous, hypocellular plaque.

PLATE 21

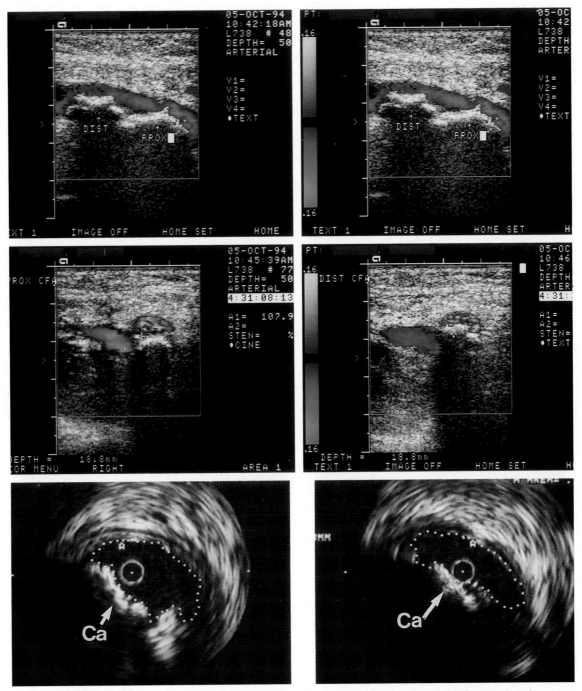

FIGURE 40-16. Color-flow Doppler and images of heavily calcified common femoral artery (CFA) recorded 1 day after IVUS for CFA angioplasty. *Top,* Two longitudinal views of CFA (red) each show eccentric calcific spur at site of minimum luminal diameter. Common femoral vein (CFV) is indicated in blue. *Middle,* Two cross-sectional views of CFA (color mosaic indicates turbulent flow at site of heavy calcific deposit). CFV appears blue. *Bottom,* Two cross-sectional views of CFA recorded immediately after angioplasty. Heavy calcific deposit attenuates image of subjacent arterial wall. Note correspondence of lumen geometry between IVUS and color-flow images (luminal boundaries in IVUS images have been planimetered to measure cross-sectional area). Patient remains asymptomatic at 1-year follow-up.

Suggested Reading

Bommer, W.J., and Miller, L.: Real-time two-dimensional color-flow Doppler: Enhanced Doppler flow imaging in the diagnosis of cardiovascular disease. (Abstract.) Am. J. Cardiol. 49:944, 1982.

Feigenbaum, H.: Two-Dimensional Echocardiography. Philadelphia, Lea & Febiger, 1986.

Goldberg, B., and Kimmelman, B.: Medical Diagnostic Ultrasound: A Retrospective on its 40th Anniversary. Washington, DC, and Rochester, American Institute of Ultrasound in Medicine and Eastman Kodak, 1988.

Goldberg, B.B. (ed.): Abdominal Ultrasonography. New York, Wiley, 1984.

Kremkau, F.W.: Diagnostic Ultrasound: Principles, Instruments, and Exercises. Philadelphia, W.B. Saunders, 1989.

Kremkau, F.W.: Doppler Ultrasound: Principles and Instruments. Philadelphia, W.B. Saunders, 1990.

Lee, R.: Physical principles of flow mapping in cardiology. In Nanda, N.C. (ed.): Textbook of Color Doppler Echocardiography. Philadelphia, Lea & Febiger, 1989.

Merritt, C.R.B.: Doppler color flow imaging. J. Clin. Ultrasound 15:591, 1987.

Miyatake, K., Okamoto, M., Kinoshita, N., et al.: Clinical applications of a new type of real-time two dimensional Doppler flow imaging system. Am. J. Cardiol. 54:857, 1984.

Switzer, D.F., and Nanda, N.C.: Doppler color flow mapping. Ultrasound Med. Biol. 11:403, 1985.

Taylor, K.J.W., Burns, P.N., and Wells, P.N.T. (eds.): Clinical Applications of Doppler Ultrasound. New York, Raven Press, 1988.

Vieli, A., Jenni, R., and Anliker, M.: Spatial velocity distributions in the ascending aorta of healthy humans and cardiac patients. I.E.E.E. Trans. Biomed. Eng. BME 33:28, 1986.

CHAPTER

27 Echocardiographic Assessment of Ventricular Systolic Function

Alan S. Katz, M.D.

Thomas L. Force, M.D.

Edward D. Folland, M.D.

Nicole Aebischer, M.D.

Satish Sharma, M.D.

Alfred F. Parisi, M.D.

GLOBAL LEFT VENTRICULAR SYSTOLIC FUNCTION _____ 297
Background Considerations _____ 298
Models for Estimation of Volume _____ 298
Echocardiographic Measurements of Left Ventricular Volume _____ 299
Left Ventricular Ejection Fraction _____ 303
Automatic Border Detection and Ejection Fraction _____ 304
End-Systolic Pressure-Volume Relationship _____ 306
Left Ventricular Mass _____ 306
REGIONAL LEFT VENTRICULAR FUNCTION _____ 307
Relation of Systolic Dysfunction to Ischemia and Infarction _____ 310
Analysis Algorithms _____ 310
Preliminary Considerations _____ 310
Endocardial Motion _____ 311
Reference Systems _____ 311
Types of Measurements _____ 313
Numbers of Measurements _____ 314
Sampling Frequency in the Cardiac Cycle _____ 314
Reference-Independent Systems _____ 314
Quantification of Infarct Size With Endocardial Motion _____ 314
Single-Plane Analyses _____ 314
Integrative Approaches to the Whole Ventricle _____ 315
Analysis of Apical Endocardial Motion _____ 315
Systolic Wall-Thickening Analysis _____ 316
RIGHT VENTRICULAR FUNCTION _____ 317
Echocardiographic Examination _____ 317
M-Mode Echocardiography _____ 317
Two-Dimensional Echocardiography _____ 317
Right Ventricular Dimension _____ 317
Global Right Ventricular Function: Volumes and Ejection Fraction _____ 317
Regional Right Ventricular Function _____ 318

Echocardiography has become widely accepted as an expeditious and practical means of assessing ventricular systolic function, particularly on the left side of the heart. Echocardiography can detect left ventricular endocardial and epicardial borders throughout the cardiac cycle in multiple well-defined anatomical planes. A visual assessment of global left ventricular function is usually possible in 90 percent of adults and nearly all children. As a result, evaluation of left ventricular function is probably the most frequent reason that echocardiography is used today. Using quantitative algorithms, one can not only measure volumes and ejection fraction (EF) but also determine other important aspects of left ventricular size and function, including myocardial mass, pressure-volume relationships, and regional performance.

GLOBAL LEFT VENTRICULAR SYSTOLIC FUNCTION

Over the past 5 years, widespread interest has developed in characterizing global left ventricular function by automated methods, and multiple studies have appeared that indicate the feasibility of this approach. In addition, more investigations have appeared that use three-dimensional reconstructions, the latter being facilitated by newer multiplane transducers and more sophisticated computer reconstruction techniques. Three-dimensional imaging can yield even more precise and accurate assessment of left ventricular volumes and topographic displays that have enormous potential in guiding reconstructive surgical techniques, particularly for congenital heart disease.

Background Considerations

Virtually all indices of left ventricular pump performance have been derived from measurements of volume and pressure. Historically, this development has required cardiac catheterization and contrast left ventricular angiography. Volume measurements and indices derived from them have proved to be of great clinical value.[1]

End-diastolic volume (EDV) is useful for evaluating and following the course of patients with left ventricular volume overloading lesions or myocardial disease. End-systolic volume (ESV) is determined by EDV, myocardial contractility, and afterload; thus, it is often ambiguous as an isolated measurement. When both EDV and ESV are measured, however, left ventricular stroke volume (SV) can be derived:

$$SV_{mL} = EDV_{mL} - ESV_{mL} \qquad (1)$$

In the absence of valvular regurgitation, cardiac output (CO) is the product of SV and heart rate (HR):

$$CO_{mL/min} = HR_{beats/min} \times SV_{mL/min} \qquad (2)$$

When EDV and ESV are known, EF can be calculated as the ratio of SV to EDV:

$$EF = \frac{SV}{EDV} \qquad (3)$$

Ejection fraction is the most widely used index of global left ventricular function and is generally considered the best single predictor of prognosis in both coronary and valvular heart disease, whether treated medically[2, 3] or surgically.[4, 5]

Models for Estimation of Volume

Angiographic estimates of left ventricular volume are usually based on the assumption that the left ventricle approximates the geometry of an ellipsoid, that is, a three-dimensional figure created by rotating an ellipse on its long axis (Fig. 27-1). The volume of such a figure can be calculated if the lengths of its three hemiaxes, a, b, and c, are known:

$$Volume = \frac{4}{3} \pi a \times b \times c \qquad (4)$$

In the earliest application of this model, the hemiaxes were measured directly from angiographic anteroposterior and lateral projections of the left ventricle. In comparing the angiographic volume with the true volume of barium-filled ventricles from fresh autopsy hearts, Dodge and associates[6] found that accuracy was enhanced when the minor axes were derived arithmetically from idealized ellipses of the same area and length as the two respective angiographic projections. The area of an ellipse is the product of π and its two hemiaxes. Thus, when c is the major hemiaxis, a the minor hemiaxis in the anteroposterior plane, b the minor hemiaxis in the lateral plane, and A_{AP} and A_{lat} the respective measured angiographic areas, the minor hemiaxes can be expressed as follows:

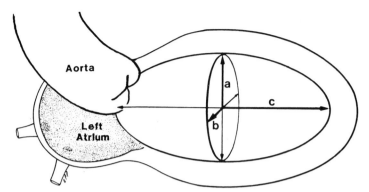

FIGURE 27-1. The ellipsoid model for left ventricular volume. This model is commonly used to estimate left ventricular volume for angiographic and echocardiographic images. The minor hemiaxes (a and b) and the major hemiaxis (c) are indicated by heavy arrows. The minor hemiaxes can be either directly measured from appropriate views or derived from the respective area and largest length of the appropriate views. (From Folland, E.D., and Parisi, A.F.: Ventricular volume and function. In Talano, J.V., and Gardin, J.M. [eds.]: Textbook of Two-Dimensional Echocardiography. New York, Grune & Stratton, 1983, p. 165, with permission.)

$$a = \frac{A_{AP}}{\pi c} \qquad (5)$$

$$b = \frac{A_{lat}}{\pi c} \qquad (6)$$

Then, by substitution in equation 4, volume is derived from the respective areas of the two projections and their common major hemiaxis:

$$Volume = \frac{4\pi}{3} \times \frac{A_{AP}}{\pi c} \times \frac{A_{lat}}{\pi c} \times c \qquad (7)$$

which simplifies to

$$Volume = \frac{4A_{AP}A_{lat}}{3\pi c} \qquad (8)$$

This formula is commonly referred to as a biplane area-length volume model. In applications in which angiography is performed only in a single plane, the formula is simplified by assuming that both minor hemiaxes (a and b) are equal. Thus, volume can be derived from the length and area of the single ventricular silhouette:

$$Volume = \frac{4A^2}{3\pi c} \qquad (9)$$

This formula is commonly referred to as the single-plane area-length volume model. Because half the length (L) of the left ventricle (L/2) is equivalent to c, the latter formula is practically simplified to the following:

$$Volume = \frac{0.85A^2}{L} \qquad (10)$$

An alternative model for measuring left ventricular volume uses the concept of the Simpson rule, whereby the volume of a solid may be estimated by subdividing it along one axis into a series of slices or discs, each with a finite thickness and measurable area. The volume of each disc is the product of its area and thickness. The volume of the complete solid is the sum of the volumes of all its discs. The greater the number of discs, the greater the accuracy of the volume estimation. According to the Simpson rule, the left ventricle can be envisioned as a series of discs from the base to the apex, analogous to a stack of coins with uniform thickness but variable area (Fig. 27-2).

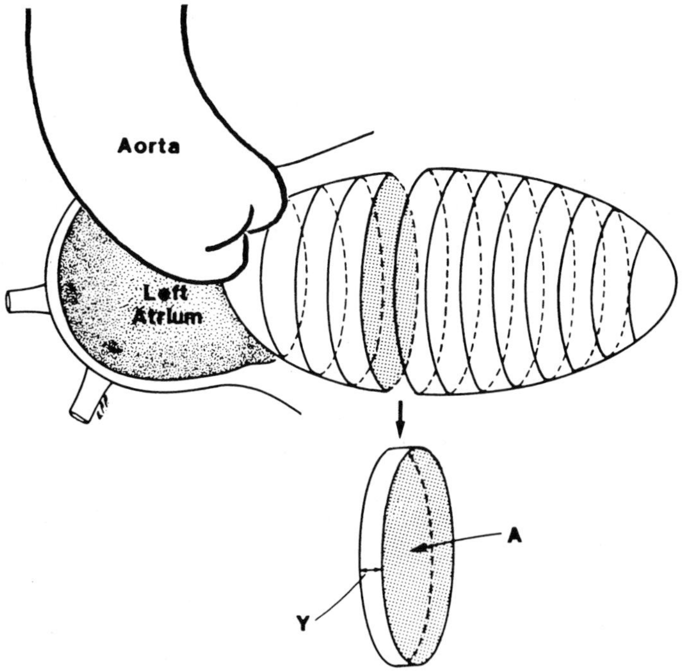

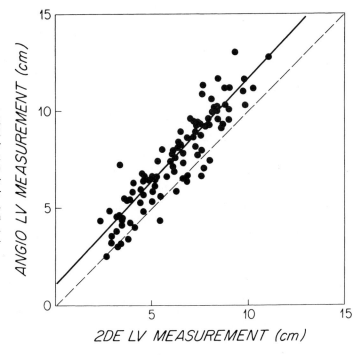

FIGURE 27-2. Simpson rule model for left ventricular volume, with the left ventricle sliced perpendicularly to the long axis. The total left ventricular volume is the sum of the volumes of individual slices, each with known thickness (Y) and area (A). (From Folland, E.D., and Parisi, A.F.: Ventricular volume and function. *In* Talano, J.V., and Gardin, J.M. [eds.]: Textbook of Two-Dimensional Echocardiography. New York, Grune & Stratton, 1983, p. 165, with permission.)

Echocardiographic Measurements of Left Ventricular Volume

Image formation is fundamentally different in angiography and ultrasound. Angiographic images are silhouettes or shadows, whereas ultrasound images are tomographic slices. Nevertheless, there is ample evidence that left ventricular dimensions measured with the two techniques correlate well, provided that the ultrasound section is properly oriented.

Figure 27–3 shows a plot of 100 corresponding linear measurements from right anterior oblique angiograms and two-dimensional echocardiograms performed in the laboratory of Moynihan and co-workers.[7] The echocardiographic long axis (in the apical four-chamber view) was measured from the midpoint of the mitral valve to the apex. The short axis (in a parasternal long-axis view at mitral

valve level) was measured at the tips of the mitral valve leaflets perpendicular to the long axis. Echocardiographic and angiographic measurements were made at end-diastole and end-systole, for a total of four measurements in each patient. The plot shows excellent agreement (r = .92; standard error of the estimate [SEE] = 0.97 cm); however, as evident from the relationship to the line of identity, the echocardiographic measurements consistently tended to underestimate the angiographic measurements, which is not surprising in view of the differences in projection in the respective techniques. An x-ray silhouette represents the largest area of the ventricle perpendicular to the x-ray beam. The analogous ultrasound slice is very likely to be smaller, unless it is perfectly oriented through the central axis to the true anatomical apex of the ventricle. In fact, it is usually impossible to locate the transducer precisely at the anatomical cardiac apex. When Barrett and associates per-

FIGURE 27-3. Correlation of 100 analogous measurements of left ventricular (LV) dimensions made from angiograms (ANGIO) and two-dimensional (2DE) echocardiograms in 25 patients. The short axis from the parasternal view at the mitral valve level and the long axis from apical four-chamber views were measured at end-diastole and end-systole and compared with analogous measurements from the right anterior oblique left ventricle (LV) angiogram, as shown by the solid regression line (r = .92, standard error of the estimate [SEE] = .97). The dashed line of identity is shown for reference. (Reprinted with permission of the publisher from Moynihan, P.F., Parisi, A.F., Folland, E.D., et al.: A system for quantitative evaluation of left ventricular function with two-dimensional ultrasonography. Med. Instrument. 14:113, 1980. Copyright 1980 by the Association for the Advancement of Medical Instrumentation, Arlington, Va.)

formed simultaneous x-ray contrast and two-dimensional echocardiographic imaging of a series of patients, they attributed uniform underestimation of x-ray contrast volumes by echocardiography to the finding that the apical ultrasound window was 33 degrees cephalad to the true cardiac apex.[8] In addition, angiographic images are ordinarily traced at the outermost boundary of contrast, which tends to include trabeculae within the cavity profile. Echocardiographic images are traced along the innermost edge of endocardial echoes, which would tend to exclude trabeculae from the cavity. Despite these differences, the correlation in measurement between the two techniques is good enough so that formulas for angiographic volume should apply equally well to echocardiographic volume determination, provided that systematic differences are corrected by regression formulas.

The earliest attempt to estimate left ventricular volumes from echocardiography used left ventricular short-axis dimensions from M-mode echocardiograms. This method employed the single-plane area-length volume formula, which required several assumptions: (1) that the left ventricular dimension in the standard position at the level of the chordae tendineae coincides with the minor axis of the left ventricle, (2) that both minor axes are equal in length, and (3) that the long axis is twice the length of the minor axis. This approach is commonly referred to as the "cube method" for left ventricular volume determination.[9] If D represents the short-axis dimension (at end-diastole or end-systole), then volume is estimated as follows:

$$\frac{4\pi}{3} \times \frac{D}{2} \times \frac{D}{2} \times D \tag{11}$$

which simplifies to

$$\text{Volume} = D^3 \tag{12}$$

Modifications of this formula have been proposed to compensate for systematic deviations from the foregoing assumptions in unusually large and unusually small ventricles.[10, 11] Formulas based on the cube assumption produced fair correlations with angiographic volume ($r = .64$ to $.74$)[9-11] but suffer from the inherent inaccuracy of making multiple geometric assumptions in an attempt to derive three-dimensional data from a single measurement. Furthermore, an important degree of correlation is expected only in the absence of asynergy.

Two-dimensional echocardiography offers a considerable advantage over the M-mode technique, because it enables direct measurement of left ventricular contours and dimensions in the planes of all three hemiaxes. It also allows application of other volume formulas, such as the Simpson rule. It has been well demonstrated that correlations between angiographic and echocardiographic volumes are improved when two-dimensional rather than M-mode methods are used.[12-15] Approaches that use the Simpson rule[13, 14, 16-20] and single-plane and biplane area-length methods[12-14, 21-23] have yielded such results. Furthermore, correlations between two-dimensional echocardiographic and angiographic volumes have been equally good ($r = .80$ to $.90$), regardless of the presence of left ventricular asynergy.[16, 22]

The American Society of Echocardiography charged a subcommittee to make recommendations for quantitation of the left ventricle, based on observations made with the use of two-dimensional echocardiography.[24] This group favored the use of apical views to determine left ventricular volumes, pointing out that methods that also required multiple short-axis images were time consuming and lowered the success rate of the procedure, because high-quality, short-axis images were less frequently obtained. They recommended that left ventricular volumes be determined from paired 90-degree orthogonal apical views, a biplane method of discs (Fig. 27-4, top). If only one apical view of adequate quality is available, it was deemed acceptable to use the single-plane area-length formula (see Fig. 27-4, bottom). With the widespread availability of computer support for quantifying echocardiographic measure-

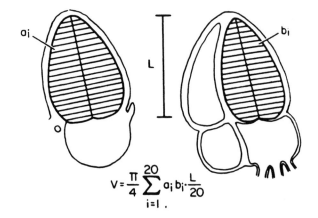

$$V = \frac{\pi}{4} \sum_{i=1}^{20} a_i b_i \cdot \frac{L}{20}$$

BY SINGLE PLANE AREA LENGTH

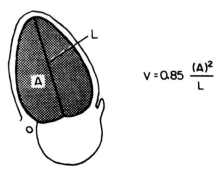

$$V = 0.85 \frac{(A)^2}{L}$$

FIGURE 27–4. Biplane and single-plane algorithms calculating chamber volume from two-dimensional echocardiograms. *Top Panel*, Biplane method of discs or disc summation method (modified Simpson's rule), based on nearly orthogonal planes from apical two- and four-chamber views. (Although the algorithm is also known as modified Simpson's rule, *method of discs* or *disc summations method* is a preferable term.) Calculation of volume (formula 1) results from summation of areas from diameters a_i and b_i of 20 cylinders or discs of equal height; these are apportioned by dividing the left ventricular longest length into 20 equal sections. This method is preferred because it is less sensitive to geometric distortions. Although 20 slices are commonly employed in many laboratories, there are no data about the ideal number. Weiss and colleagues (Circulation 67:889, 1983) suggest that the minimum number under experimental conditions is 4, whereas Erbel and associates (Clin. Cardiol. 3:377, 1980) have used as many as 256. The general formula for volume that does not designate the number of slices is as follows:

$$V = \frac{\pi}{4} \sum_{i=1}^{n} a_i b_i \cdot \frac{L}{n}$$

Bottom Panel, Single-plane area-length method (formula 2). This is the single-plane method developed for angiography and is applicable if only one apical view is obtainable. V = volume of left ventricular cavity; A = area of left ventricular cavity *(shaded area)*; L = length of left ventricular cavity. (From Schiller, N.B., Shah, P.M., Crawford, M., et al., Recommendations for quantitation of the left ventricle by two-dimensional echocardiography. J. Am. Soc. Echocardiogr. 2:358, 1989, with permission.)

ments, these algorithms should be incorporated into the operations of any laboratory that is systematically pursuing quantification of left ventricular volumes.

A summary of angiographic-echocardiographic correlations for various two-dimensional approaches to left ventricular volumes is presented in Table 27–1. Although the correlations are good, some of the estimating errors are rather large. Appropriate judgment should be exercised, therefore, in applying these echocardiographic estimates of left ventricular volume to individual patients.

Measurement of left ventricular volume has been simplified by inclusion of quantitative software programs in most commercially available two-dimensional echocardiography systems. Images must still be traced by hand, which is often tedious and time consuming.

TABLE 27–1. COMPARISON BETWEEN ECHOCARDIOGRAPHIC AND ANGIOGRAPHIC VOLUMES AND EJECTION FRACTIONS

Investigators	Method	No. of Patients	EDV		ESV		EF		Comments
			r	SEE	r	SEE	r	SEE	
Teichholz et al.°	B scan	25	—	—	—	—	.87		14 of 25 had asynergy
Folland et al.[13]	Modified Simpson rule	35	.76	43 mL	.86	32 mL	.78	0.10	10 of 35 had asynergy
Parisi et al.[14]	Modified Simpson rule	50	.82	39 mL	.90	29 mL	.80	0.09	25 of 50 had asynergy
Carr et al.[12]	Biplane area-length	22	.93	—	—	—	.93		23 of 24 volumes clustered: EDV r fell to .46 when 1 patient was excluded; 6 of 22 had asynergy
Schiller et al.[19]	Modified Simpson rule	30	.80	15 mL/m²	.90	8.5 mL/m²	.87	0.08	16 of 30 had asynergy
Ohuchi et al.[22]	Single-plane area-length	38	.84	(For all volumes)			.88		Patients with and without asynergy
		18	.86	(For all volumes)			.88		Only patients with asynergy
Erbel et al.†	Single-plane Simpson rule	50	.94	22 mL	.97	15 mL	.91	0.06	Same model and view (RAO equivalent) used for both echo and angiographic volumes
Kan et al.‡	Single-plane area-length	30	.84	—	.85	—	.91		RAO equivalent view
Quinones et al[43]	Multiple linear measurements in three planes	35	—	—	—	—	.91	0.07	See Figure 27–8

EDV = end-diastolic volume; ESV = end-systolic volume; EF = ejection fraction; r = correlation coefficient; SEE = standard error of the estimate; RAO = right anterior oblique.

°Teichholz, L.E., Cohen, M.V., et al. N. Engl. J. Med. 291:1220, 1974.
†Erbel, R., Schweizer, P., et al. Clin. Cardiol. 3:377, 1980.
‡Kan, G., Visser, C.A., et al. Eur. Heart J. 2:337, 1981.

Technically good images and painstaking care are required to achieve accurate results. Consequently, many laboratories, including our own, perform full quantitation only in selected cases and routinely report M-mode dimensions as indicators of volume. Laboratories may develop their own normal values for these dimensions or rely on comprehensive normal values developed by others,[25] keeping in mind that normal ranges vary with sex and body-surface area.[23]

The accuracy of volume estimation increases with the number of image planes sampled. Computer-generated three-dimensional reconstructions of left ventricular geometry can be derived from multiplane two-dimensional images. Three-dimensional reconstruction of the heart requires several steps: (1) data acquisition, (2) measurement of properties of the image (feature extraction), (3) identification of various elements of the image (classification), and (4) separation of elements from one another within the three-dimensional volume (segmentation), and display of selected elements in a comprehensible, information-dense format (image rendering).[26] Currently, most three-dimensional reconstruction is performed off-line, after image acquisition. When the image is displayed as a cine loop over time, it is often referred to as four-dimensional echocardiography.

Two basic techniques have been used for image acquisition. The first technique requires precisely locating the transducer in three-dimensional space, and the second involves obtaining sequential images of known relationship to each other. The first method allows for acquisition of images in a random order and for reconstructing images with the use of data acquired from multiple windows. The second method is particularly applicable to transesophageal imaging.

The exact position of the tomographic planes from a given transducer position has been determined with mechanical arms (Geiser, Skorton, Rachlen), or acoustic emitters (Moritz, Moritz, Weiss, Harrison).[27–33] Handschumacher and colleagues have employed a device that locates the transducer position using spark-gap emitters that send an audible sound toward an array of microphones (Fig. 27–5).[34] Using the time of arrival of the sound, the transducer location can be computed by triangulation. The location is encoded as a binary pattern on an unused portion of the video signal that comes directly from the ultrasound machine. The composite video signal is then recorded in real time on videotape. King and associates have also used an acoustic locator to acquire images.[35] Their system displays a reference image, for example, a parasternal long-axis image, with a line of intersection superimposed, displaying the relationship of the current image to the reference image. These techniques require a specialized examination room.

Devereux and co-workers have been using a transthoracic transducer that acquires sequential images.[36] The transducer rotates 180 degrees about a central axis at 3-degree increments, obtaining a fan of information. Thus, 63 equally spaced images are acquired, with the first and last images mirror rotations. The number of degrees from the starting image is displayed in the upper right-hand corner of the image (Fig. 27–6). Roelandt and colleagues[37] have reported on a transesophageal probe that acquires sequential images. The probe can be continuously rotated 180 degrees around

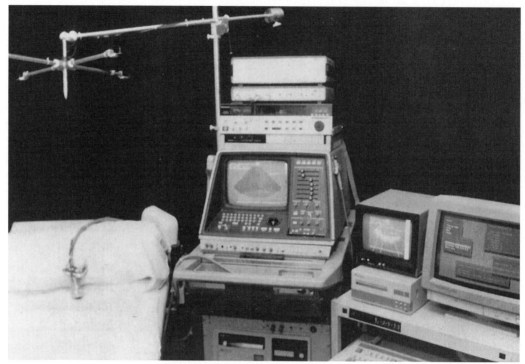

FIGURE 27–5. The three-dimensional echocardiography comprises a conventional two-dimensional real-time scanner *(center)*, a three-dimensional spatial locator system *(left)*, and a personal computer *(right)*. The line of intersection display appears on the computer video monitor. (From King, D.L., Harrison, M.R., King, D.L., Jr., et al.: Improved reproducibility of left atrial and left ventricular measurements by guided three-dimensional echocardiography. J. Am. Coll. Cardiol. 20:1238, 1992. Reprinted with permission from the American College of Cardiology.)

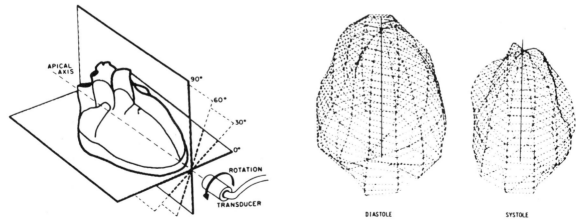

FIGURE 27–6. Three-dimensional reconstruction, apical axis rotation method. The transducer rotation and different planes intersecting the heart are shown on the left. Three-dimensional end-diastolic and end-systolic computer reconstructions of the left ventricle are shown on the right. These images represent a viewing angle of 45 degrees from the apical axis. (Reprinted with permission from Nanda, N.C., and Maurer, G.: Three-dimensional reconstruction of echocardiographic images using the rotation method. Ultrasound Med. Biol. 8:659, 1982. Copyright 1982, Pergamon Press, Inc.)

a central axis. A motorized stepwise pullback system controlled by an electrocardiogram and respiration-gated algorithm obtains parallel cross sections at equidistant intervals. Thus, their system obtains a cylinder of information. Sequential imaging requires holding the transducer in precisely the same position while acquiring multiple images and uses only a single window.

Von Ramm and associates[38] have described a novel system for acquiring three-dimensional data. They have modified a 32-channel, phased-array scanner to steer the ultrasound beam in two dimensions, acquiring a pyramidal scan of information from a single transducer position. To acquire high-resolution images with this method, a new generation of phased-array transducers capable of very small interelement spacing must be developed.

A comprehensive discussion of feature extraction and classification, as well as segmentation, is best left to textbooks and articles on image processing.[29] Briefly, feature extraction is used by the computer to distinguish one region from another within an image. Three pixel properties have been used: (1) texture (i.e., brightness), (2) spectral features (i.e., signal frequency), and (3) motion features (i.e., changes in position). Classification, or grouping of pixels into classes of objects, can be accomplished with the use of many different pattern recognition algorithms that compare pixel features to those of their nearest neighbors spatially. Segmentation refers to the process in which objects are separated into selected units (e.g., left ventricle from the entire heart), which is usually accomplished interactively because reliable automated methods are not available.

Displaying the three-dimensional image is the last stage in three-dimensional reconstruction. Two basic methods of image rendering have been used: surface rendering and volume rendering. Surface rendering reconstructs objects through surfaces visible to the computer at a particular point of view. Volume rendering produces a semitransparent object, allowing internal structures to be visible from the surface. Volume rendering is mathematically more difficult but can be more informative (Figs. 27–7 and 27–8).

FIGURES 27-7 and 27-8. See Color Plates 1 and 2.

Several studies have explored the usefulness of the methods of three-dimensional reconstruction. Working with a spark-gap locator to produce three-dimensional reconstructions, Handschumacher and associates[34] validated their method of determining ventricular volumes. Working with 11 ventricular phantoms and 11 excised canine ventricles, they produced estimates of ventricular volume that correlated closely with actual volumes. Furthermore, in 14 normal subjects, three-dimensional stroke volume estimates agreed well with those determined by means of an independent Doppler method. The group reported a correlation coefficient of .95 between the two methods, with an SEE of 3.2 mL. Similarly, Mensah and co-workers[39] reported comparable results on estimating volumes from ventricular phantoms, using a rotational transducer.

Using a spatial locator, Gopal and colleagues[40] found that volumes determined by three-dimensional reconstruction were comparable with those obtained by nuclear magnetic resonance imaging. For EDV the correlation coefficient was .92, with an SEE of 6.99 mL. For ESV the correlation coefficient was .81, with an SEE of 4.01 mL. The correlations between three-dimensional echocardiography and magnetic resonance imaging were superior to those obtained between two-dimensional echocardiographic apical biplane summation and magnetic resonance imaging. Their estimates were superior to those of the two-dimensional echocardiographic apical biplane summation method, because the technique eliminates geometric assumptions and image plane positioning error.

Using a rotating transducer, the authors were able to show that the assumption that the parasternal long-axis and short-axis images, and the apical four-chamber and two-chamber images, are orthogonal projections was not correct.[36] In rotations from the parasternal window, the best short-axis image was rotated an average of 100 ± 19 degrees from the best long-axis image. The rotation between the two views ranged from 64 to 156 degrees. From the apical window, the mean rotation between the best-appearing four- and two-chamber views was 95 ± 21 degrees, with ranges from 30 to 136 degrees. Similar results were reported by King and associates.[35] The assumption of orthogonality is important in the recommended biplane Simpson method for estimating ventricular volume and, thus itself, imposes errors in volume determination.[41]

Three-dimensional reconstruction of images obtained from the transesophageal window has also been reported. Working with the TomTec Corporation, Roelandt and associates[37] reported their experience with three-dimensional reconstruction using a multiplane transesophageal imaging transducer. The transducer has a 5-MHz, 64-element rotational-array transducer mounted at the distal end of a standard gastroscope. The scanning plane can be continuously rotated through 180 degrees, starting from a longitudinal image position. They were able to acquire data in 7 to 10 minutes and to reconstruct the image off-line in three-dimensions in 30 to 60 minutes.

Rendering three-dimensional images of the cardiac ventricles may not be an important phase of three-dimensional reconstruction. By merely assembling the three-dimensional data, we may gain important insights into ventricular dysfunction. Skorton and co-workers[28] used three-dimensional finite element reconstruction from two-dimensional echocardiograms for estimation of myocardial elastic properties. This technique, used in engineering applications for the evaluation of stress-strain relationships, requires accurate three-dimensional information and may provide important clues to ventricular diastolic dysfunction. Furthermore, an understanding of stress-strain relationships may be helpful in timing surgery for regurgitant valvular lesions or in deciding on revascularization.

It is apparent that one cannot understand complex three-dimensional structures solely by using two-dimensional projections. With advancements in parallel processing, image processing, and automated border definition, three-dimensional information and display should have important clinical applications in the near future. Early data indicate that three-dimensional echocardiography will yield more accurate estimations of ventricular volumes; it should also elucidate details of structural interrelationships in congenital malformations, has the promise of providing better topographic appreciation of regional contraction abnormalities, and can show features of adult hearts not previously appreciated. An example in this regard is the work of Levine and colleagues,[42] who reported an interesting insight into the geometry of the mitral valve. They confirmed that the mitral annulus is nonplanar and that the mitral valve is saddle-shaped, which explained the inconsistency in identifying mitral valve prolapse from the parasternal and apical windows.

Left Ventricular Ejection Fraction

The reliability of the echocardiographic estimate of EF depends on the accuracy of the method used to measure EDV and ESV. M-mode echocardiography is a particularly weak method, because of the adverse influence of left ventricular asynergy on its accuracy. Fair correlations with angiographic EF have been obtained for patients with symmetric contraction patterns (r = .64 to .74), but poor correlations have been found for ischemic heart disease patients with segmental contraction abnormalities.[9–11] Ejection fractions derived from two-dimensional echocardiography correlate well with those derived from angiography (r = .73 to .93; see Table 27–1). Furthermore, two-dimensional echocardiographic estimates are relatively accurate, even in the presence of asynergy, when either the Simpson rule or the area-length method is used. In a series of 50 patients, a modified Simpson rule algorithm provided good results (r = .80, SEE = 0.90), despite documentation that showed 25 patients with asynergy.[14] In 35 of the authors' patients whose EFs were also measured by radionuclide angiocardiography, the SEE (0.10) approached that of the radionuclide technique (0.07) when each method was compared to cineangiography.[13]

Quinones and associates[43] have developed a simplified method of measuring left ventricular EF from two-dimensional images, without planimetry and/or computer processing. The apical four-chamber, apical two-chamber, and parasternal long-axis views are used, and multiple diameters are measured by calipers in each of these views at end-diastole and end-systole. Diameters (D) are measured at the following locations: two in the parasternal long-axis view (at the tips of the mitral valve and halfway to the most distal point of the left ventricle) and three each in the two apical views (1 cm below the tips of the mitral valve, halfway from the mitral valve to the apex), and a more distal dimension at the same distance from the second dimension that the second is from the first. All these dimensions are averaged in diastole and in systole, and the fractional shortening is calculated (%ΔD). Finally, an arbitrary contraction factor (%ΔL) is assigned to the apex according to its visual grading (normal apical contraction, + 15 percent; hypokinetic, +5 percent; akinetic, 0 percent mild dyskinesis, −5 percent; and severe dyskinesis, − 10 percent). When these values are substituted into the formula

$$EF = (\%\Delta D^2) + [(1 - \%D^2)(\%\Delta L)] \qquad (13)$$

an estimate of EF results that agrees well with the EFs determined by both gated radionuclide and cineangiographic techniques for the same patients. By averaging fractional shortening at multiple locations, regional contraction defects are taken into account, and the shortcomings of the unidimensional M-mode fractional shortening measurement are avoided. Thus, good correlations were obtained, despite 42 of 55 patients who had coronary artery disease.

In the clinical setting, visual estimation of left ventricular EF has become a common practice.[44] Figure 27–9 displays the correlation between EFs visually estimated from echocardiography and measured radionuclide angiography in 48 patients studied in the authors' laboratory. The visual estimates were the averages of two independent observers who were blinded to the radionuclide re-

sults and were asked to estimate the left ventricular EF to the nearest 5 percent. The correlation between the EFs determined by the two methods is surprisingly good, especially for patients with impaired EF. The SEE (0.11), in this comparison, is similar to the SEE quoted earlier when quantitative echocardiographic and cineangiographic EFs were compared (0.10). Despite this, many prefer not to report a discrete number for EF, unless a quantitative or semiquantitative method has been used, because a numeric report conveys the impression of quantitative analysis, even when explicitly it is denoted as an estimate. Thus, some report left ventricular EF as mildly, moderately, or severely impaired.

Automatic Border Detection and Ejection Fraction

Automated quantification of left ventricular function has been a major goal in echocardiography, ever since quantification of left ventricular function was demonstrated and validated.[19] Although initial efforts were made with off-line edge-detection and tracking methods, more recently real-time quantitation of left ventricular function has been a major focus of research efforts.[45–51] A major obstacle had been the development of a reliable automated border tracking method. In 1992, two groups (those of Perez and Vandenberg) reported on an automatic border-detecting algorithm that grew from work on integrated ultrasonic backscatter for tissue differentiation.[52, 53] The system utilizes a computer-assisted algorithm to analyze unprocessed acoustic signals from blood-tissue interfaces in real time along every scan line and throughout every frame. A border is created between ventricular blood pools and myocardial tissue for any tomographic image plane. The area of the blood pool is outlined, superimposed on the real-time two-dimensional image (Fig. 27–10). Thus, area changes within the myocardial blood pool can be visually scrutinized on a beat-to-beat basis, allowing on-the-spot verification of accurate border detection. After the operator indicates a region of interest, the computer can report changes in area, percent fractional area change, and rates of change of area over time. Although area changes in any given tomographic plane are not equivalent to volume changes, from the apical four-chamber view instantaneous volume changes and EF can be estimated with the use of either a single-plane Simpson rule method or area-length calculation.

Using the canine heart, several groups have found a linear relationship between instantaneous backscatter calculated left ventricular area and left ventricular volume.[54, 55] In patient studies, backscatter-derived left ventricular volumes and EF were found to be comparable to those obtained by means of radionuclide ventriculography, when the single-plane rule of Simpson was applied off-line[56] and on-line[57] (Fig. 27–11). Similarly, left ventricular volumes obtained from ABD were found to be linearly related to those calculated from magnetic resonance imaging.[58] Using an in vivo canine model, in which left ventricular volumes were measured continuously from a balloon-lined, ejecting left ventricular cavity, Morrissey and co-workers[55] showed that, although automated boundary detection tended to underestimate volume, it correlated well with EF (Fig. 27–12). This underestimation likely emanates from the tomographic nature of the echocardiographic technique (see Fig. 27–3) and the inclusion of papillary muscles and other surface irregularities in the automated border boundary outlines.

This method of acoustic quantification (AQ) has some important limitations.[52, 53, 59–61] First, it is very gain dependent; hence, endocardial borders can be altered by incorrect settings of the gain controls. As in many aspects of ultrasound, the estimates are only as good as the ability and experience of the sonographer to set proper gain settings, so that borders can be precisely detected and tracked. Second, AQ is useful only for detecting blood-tissue borders, and so epicardial outlines cannot be obtained. Because blood-tissue interfaces are used for the estimates, the area of the mitral valve apparatus is subtracted when calculations are reported. Finally, although the heart translates in the thorax during the cardiac cycle and during respiration, the region of interest remains the same.

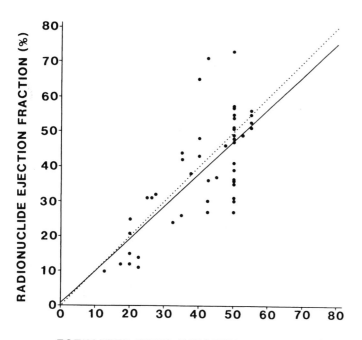

FIGURE 27–9. Comparison of left ventricular ejection fraction estimated visually from two-dimensional echocardiography and ejection fraction measured by radionuclide angiography. Each estimate was the average of two independent observers who were blinded to the radionuclide results. n = 48; r = .73; SEE = 10.8. The solid line is the linear regression (y = 0.94× + 0.61), and the dotted line is the line of identity.

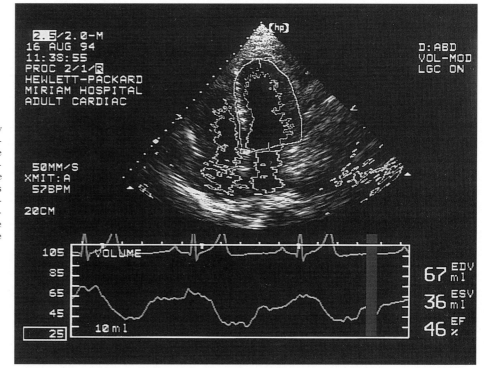

FIGURE 27-10. Four-chamber apical view showing instantaneous ejection fraction calculations using automatic border detection. The bell-shaped outline was traced by the echocardiographer to denote the region of interest. The waveform at the bottom shows instantaneous volumes in the region of interest, using the modified Simpson method. Digital readings of end-diastolic volume (EDV), end-systolic volume (ESV), and ejection fraction (EF) appear to the right of the waveform.

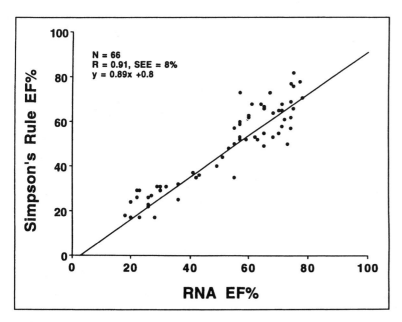

FIGURE 27-11. Relation of Simpson rule ejection fraction (EF%) using automated border detection short-axis area data to radionuclide (RNA) left ventricular ejection fraction. (From Gorcsan, J., III, Lazar, J.M., Schulman, D.S., et al.: Comparison of left ventricular function by echocardiographic automatic border detection and by radionuclide ejection fraction. Am. J. Cardiol. 72:810, 1993, with permission.)

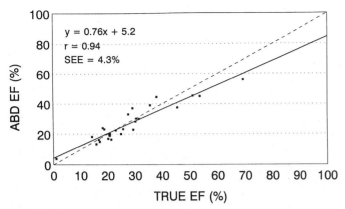

FIGURE 27–12. Correlation of ejection fraction by on-line automated border detection (ABD) and true ejection fraction (EF). The solid line is the line of identity; the dashed line is the regression line. (From Morrissey, R.L., Siu, S.C., Guerrero, J.L., et al.: Automated assessment of ventricular volume and function by echocardiography: Validation of automated border detection. J. Am. Soc. Echocardiogr. 7:112, 1994, with permission.)

The left atrium may move in and out of the selected area, reducing the accuracy of the method. Nevertheless, the method has been proved to be useful for clinical determinations in several laboratories.

Vandenberg and colleagues compared AQ-derived left ventricular area with that obtained by manual tracings off-line.[53] Thirty-seven normal subjects were imaged from the short-axis parasternal window during held expiration. Only 22 subjects (60 percent) had 75 percent or more of the endocardium visualized and were included in the study. Values of manually traced areas were obtained from serial frames (30 frames per second) from the electrocardiographic QRS onset until the end of systole (defined as the smallest apparent cavity area) and were compared with values obtained at the same time on-line. Manually drawn and real-time areas correlated for the group (r = .91), and correlation coefficients ranged from .94 to .99 in individual subjects.

Herregods and associates compared on-line area determinations with manual area tracings in 75 individuals, 25 of whom were normal subjects.[62] End-diastolic and end-systolic areas were analyzed from both the short-axis and apical four-chamber views. The correlation coefficient between the two methods from the short-axis view was .87 for end-diastole and .81 for end-systole. From the apical four-chamber view, the correlation coefficients for end-diastole and end-systole were .77 and .72, respectively.

Perez and co-workers found AQ area measurements to be reproducible over intervals of 2 to 3 weeks.[59] Furthermore, they found that there was a statistical difference in the average end-diastolic and end-systolic left ventricular area, as reported from AQ between normal subjects and subjects with visually dilated left ventricles. Marcus and colleagues compared AQ area measurements with those derived by ultrafast computer tomography.[63] They found an excellent correlation between the two methods but also found that real-time ultrasonic backscatter consistently underestimated end-diastolic area and overestimated end-systolic area. Martin and colleagues found the same results when AQ area estimation was compared with radionuclide ventriculography.[64]

Thus, the AQ method can accurately estimate manually drawn cavity areas. When compared with areas covered by ultrafast computed tomography, echo-derived left ventricular areas correlated but appeared to underestimate end-diastolic area and overestimate end-systolic area. The backscatter method is gain dependent, requires operator experience and judgment, and is applicable to only a subset of patients screened. In a small study, the method was noted to be reproducible and helpful in separating patients with dilated left ventricles from normal subjects.

Diastolic relaxation has been recognized as increasingly important in determining cardiac function. The cardinal problem in studying diastolic function has been the lack of a "gold standard." The Doppler signal of transmitral left ventricular filling has been cited as a marker of left ventricular diastolic function. Diastole is characterized by passive emptying of the left atrium (Doppler E wave), followed by atrial contraction (Doppler A wave). Presumably, when left ventricular end-diastolic pressure is high, atrial contraction contributes more to ventricular filling. AQ-derived percent atrial contribution to ventricular filling has been correlated with Doppler-derived measurements.[65]

Automated border detection provides a method of assessing left ventricular function in real time. With appropriate computer interfacing it allows multiple measurements of both systolic and diastolic performance to be made instantaneously. Thus, its use allows processing of large quantities of information that heretofore could be derived only by tedious off-line analyses, often with manual interaction by the observer. With improvements in the automated border detection algorithm and in processing of the measurements, it is likely that on-line readings of EF will come into more widespread use.

End-Systolic Pressure-Volume Relationship

The left ventricular pressure-volume relationship has received increasing interest as an index of left ventricular performance that takes into account loading conditions and, therefore, is thought to be more indicative of intrinsic muscle function than is EF. This phenomenon is particularly present under conditions in which augmented afterload may depress EF (aortic stenosis) or diminished afterload may enhance EF (mitral regurgitation). In either case, interpretation of EF in isolation from loading conditions may lead to an incorrect impression of the true state of left ventricular myocardial contractility.

This measurement of left ventricular function entails plotting end-systolic meridional wall stress against end-systolic volume (or short-axis dimension in M-mode applications) at various loading states. The slope of this plot is nearly linear and indicates the intrinsic contractile state: the steeper the slope, the greater the contractility.[66] Different loading states required for the plot are generated by administration of vasodilators or pure systemic pressors.

In its original form, this analysis was performed in the cardiac catheterization laboratory by obtaining ESVs and pressures from simultaneous left ventricular contrast cineangiography and pressure recording by high-fidelity catheter-tip manometry.[66] The noninvasive approach to systolic pressure-volume relations substitutes arm-cuff systolic pressure for left ventricular end-systolic pressure. The validity of this substitution is a subject of controversy, with some investigators finding that systolic cuff pressures do not alter the stress-volume slope[67] and others advising against such a substitution.[68] This technique has been used to demonstrate that afterload, rather than preload, reduction plays a more significant role in improving ventricular performance in patients with heart failure.[69]

The emergence of automated border determinations facilitates analysis of left ventricular pressure-volume relationships. In the operating room, left ventricular areas measured from automated boundary detection have been combined with simultaneous left ventricular pressures to construct pressure-area loops in real time.[70] Thus, this approach vastly facilitates data acquisition, which can be used to derive left ventricular volumes, holding considerable promise for more sophisticated assessment of left ventricular performance.

Left Ventricular Mass

Left ventricular mass is estimated most simply from the M-mode dimensions of interventricular septum and left ventricular posterior wall. A more quantitative approach to estimating mass from M-mode data uses these dimensions in a modification of the cube volume formula:

$$\text{Mass} = 1.05 \text{ g/mL} [(D + IVS + PW)^3 - D^3] \qquad (14)$$

In this formula, D is the left ventricular internal dimension, IVS the thickness of interventricular septum, and PW the thickness of the posterior wall; all these dimensions are measured at the level of chordae tendineae at end-diastole in units of centimeters. In this formula the difference between total left ventricular volume (including walls) and left ventricular chamber volume is multiplied by the specific gravity of heart muscle (1.05 g/mL).

This technique has been validated automatically by correlation of premortem echocardiographic measurements with postmortem left ventricular mass in 34 patients. The best agreement (r = .96) was obtained with a modified convention (Penn convention) for measuring left ventricular dimensions that *excluded* the thickness of endocardial echoes from wall thickness and included these echoes in the left ventricular internal dimension (D) (Fig. 27–13)[71] Corrected left ventricular mass calculated from measurements in which the Penn convention was used is as follows:

$$\text{Mass} = 1.04 \text{ g/cm} [(D + IVS + PW)^3 - D^3] - 14 \text{ g} \qquad (15)$$

Other investigators have had equally good results with standard convention (leading edge) measurements in this formula.[72] This technique has been shown to be a more accurate indicator of left ventricular hypertrophy than electrocardiography.[72, 73] Moreover, it has repeatedly been successfully related to adverse outcomes—both death and cardiovascular morbid events are more common in patients with left ventricular hypertrophy demonstrated with the Penn convention.[74]

Devereaux has defined left ventricular hypertrophy by means of

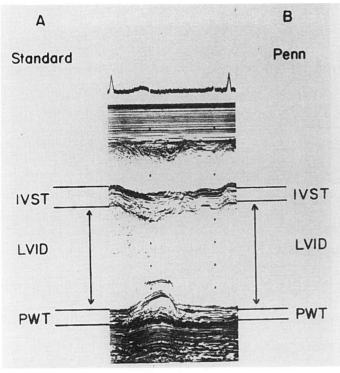

FIGURE 27–13. Methods of echocardiographic measurement of interventricular septal thickness (IVST), left ventricular internal dimension (LVID), and posterior wall thickness (PWT). *A,* Standard measurement convention includes the thickness of the right and left septal endocardial echoes in IVST and includes posterior wall endocardial echoes in PWT. *B,* The Penn convention excludes right and left septal endocardial echo thickness from IVST and excludes posterior wall endocardial echo thickness from PWT; thus, these structures are included in LVID by this method. (From Devereux, R.B., and Reichek, N.: Echocardiographic determination of left ventricular mass in man: Anatomic validation of the method. Circulation 66:613, 1977, with permission of the American Heart Association, Inc.)

this method as a mass index over 134 g/m² in men and 110 g/m² in women.[75] Woythaler and associates have developed a practical nomogram (Fig. 27–14) for determining the presence of left ventricular hypertrophy from standard M-mode measurements.[72] This nomogram was developed from a comparison of premortem echocardiographic data with postmortem left ventricular mass in 30 patients of both sexes.

The M-mode approach is theoretically limited by its unidimensional nature, which assumes that the walls measured are representative of the general thickness of the left ventricular wall. Consequently, this technique should be applied cautiously to hearts with regional left ventricular dysfunction or distorted geometry.

The limitations of M-mode data can be largely overcome by use of two-dimensional echocardiographic approaches to measurement of left ventricular mass.[76–78] Reichek and associates obtained better agreement between premortem echocardiographic measurements and postmortem left ventricular mass with two-dimensional formulation (area-length) than with their prior M-mode formulation.[78]

Both M-mode and two-dimensional echocardiographic approaches to measurements of left ventricular mass make geometric assumptions about the left ventricle. These assumptions are particularly inaccurate in the diseased ventricle. Gopal and co-workers have reported on a method of computing left ventricular mass, using three-dimensional echocardiography.[79] They determined left ventricular mass by subtracting endocardial volume from epicardial volume and multiplying the result by 1.05 g/mL, the density of myocardium. Endocardial and epicardial volumes were computed with the use of a polyhedral surface reconstruction algorithm.[40] Left ventricular mass, as determined by three-dimensional echocardiography, was superior to that determined by two-dimensional or M-mode echocardiography when 11 fixed animal hearts were studied. Furthermore, using 15 normal subjects, they reported that left ventricular mass, as determined by three-dimensional echocardiography, correlated more closely with mass, as determined by magnetic resonance imaging than with that determined by either two-dimensional echocardiography or M-mode techniques.

The formulation recommended by the American Society of Echocardiography is shown in Figure 27–15.[24] Both M-mode and two-dimensional echocardiography have been shown to be superior to electrocardiography in detecting left ventricular hypertrophy[72, 73] and have an accuracy rate similar to that of contrast angiography.[75, 78] Because of the ease of application of ultrasound, it plays an extremely important role in the determination of left ventricular mass for evaluation of therapy of patients with hypertension. Indeed, using M-mode measurements, both the Cornell group[80, 81] and the Framingham study[82, 83] have shown that left ventricular mass determined by the Penn convention has important predictive value regarding future cardiovascular morbid events.

REGIONAL LEFT VENTRICULAR FUNCTION

Abnormalities of regional systolic function occur very frequently as a consequence of important manifestations of coronary artery disease. These abnormalities may be acutely precipitated by ischemia ("stunning") and develop in chronic low-flow states ("hibernation") but are temporally limited when the ischemia resolves or the low-flow state is corrected without concomitant myocardial necrosis. When necrosis ensues, a permanent regional contraction abnormality results. The extent and severity of the latter abnormalities strongly predict subsequent clinical outcomes.[84–86]

Two-dimensional echocardiography is a very useful technique for assessing systolic function during and after acute myocardial infarction or thrombolytic therapy. Multiple studies have confirmed that qualitative analysis of two-dimensional echocardiograms can be used reliably to identify regional contraction abnormalities.[84–88] Furthermore, the reproducibility of qualitative review of echocardiograms used to identify regional wall motion abnormalities[86, 88, 89] generally compares favorably with that of qualitative angiogra-

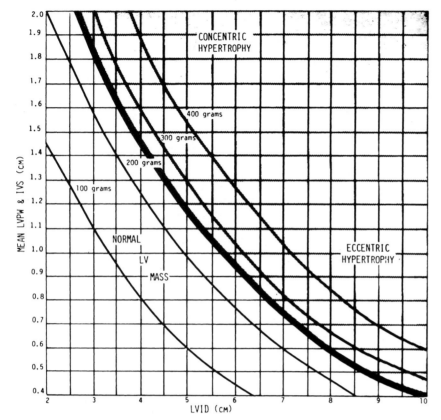

FIGURE 27–14. Nomogram for the clinical detection of left ventricular (LV) mass from M-mode echocardiographic measurements. After end-diastolic M-mode measurements are made, the mean of interventricular septal (IVS) and left ventricular posterior wall (LVPW) thickness is found on the vertical axis and followed to the place where it intersects the left ventricular internal chamber diameter (LVID) on the horizontal axis. Left ventricular mass is estimated from the relation of this point to the four plotted left ventricular mass meridians. All points above the 254-g mass meridian (*gray zone*) reflect an abnormally heavy left ventricle. Coordinates that lie in the upper left of the gray zone reflect concentric left ventricular hypertrophy with thickened left ventricular walls and no corresponding chamber dilation. Toward the middle and lower right of the gray zone lie regions where the chamber dilation is in proportion to the wall thickening in the situation of eccentric left ventricular hypertrophy. (From Woythaler, J.N., Singer, S.H., Kwan, O.H., et al.: Accuracy of echocardiography versus electrocardiography in detecting left ventricular hypertrophy: Comparison with postmortem mass measurements. J. Am. Coll. Cardiol. 2:310, 1983, with permission.)

FIGURE 27–15. *Upper Panel*, Diagram of left ventricular short axis at the level of papillary muscle tip, demonstrating epicardial and endocardial perimeters that are traced to calculate myocardial thickness (t), short-axis radius (b), and areas (A_1 and A_2). Note that papillary muscles are excluded (left within ventricular cavity) when measuring these perimeters. *Lower Panel*, Left ventricular mass by area length (AL) and truncated ellipsoid (TE). a = long or semimajor axis from the widest minor axis radius to apex; b = short-axis radius and is backcalculated from short-axis cavity area (A_2); t = myocardial thickness backcalculated from short-axis epicardial and cavity areas (A_1); d = truncated semimajor axis from widest short-axis diameter to mitral annulus plane. (From Schiller, N.B., Shah, P.M., Crawford, M., et al.: Recommendations for quantitation of the left ventricle by two-dimensional echocardiography. J. Am. Soc. Echocardiogr. 2:358, 1989, with permission.)

LV MASS BY AREA LENGTH (AL) AND TRUNCATED ELLIPSOID (TE)

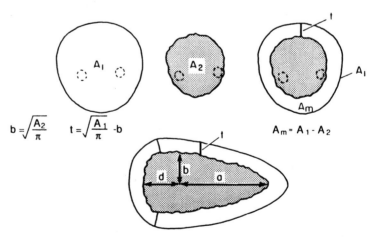

$$b = \sqrt{\frac{A_2}{\pi}} \qquad t = \sqrt{\frac{A_1}{\pi}} - b \qquad\qquad A_m = A_1 - A_2$$

$$\text{LV Mass (AL)} = 1.05 \left\{ \left[\tfrac{5}{6} A_1 \ (a + d + t) \right] - \left[\tfrac{5}{6} A_2 \ (a + d) \right] \right\}$$

$$\text{LV Mass (TE)} = 1.05 \, \pi \left\{ (b + t)^2 \left[\tfrac{2}{3}(a + t) + d - \frac{d^3}{3(a + t)^2} \right] - b^2 \left[\tfrac{2}{3} a + d - \frac{d^3}{3a^2} \right] \right\}$$

phy.[90, 91] When applied in a semiquantitative manner by experienced observers, the technique has provided important short-term prognostic information for patients with acute myocardial infarction.[84–86, 89, 92] For patients who survive the hospital phase of acute myocardial infarction, predischarge semiquantitative two-dimensional echocardiography predicts 1- to 2-year outcomes as well.[93–95]

Systematic division of the left ventricle into defined segments,[96] use of standard nomenclature for degree of asynergy,[97] and other conventions promote a unified approach and allow interstudy comparisons to be made. Based on the frequent use of semiquantitative evaluations of regional systolic function and their proven efficacy in relating to outcomes in patients with acute myocardial infarction, the American Society of Echocardiography has recommended a standardized approach to dividing the left ventricle into segments and grading the contractile function of each of these regions (Fig. 27–16). This model involves 16 segments, each of which is to be graded as follows: 1 = normal, 2 = mild hypokinesis, 3 = severe hypokinesis, 4 = akinesis, and 5 = dyskinesis. A global score index is obtained by dividing the sum of the segment scores by the number of scored segments; thus, the more the index deviates from a score of 1, the worse the regional contraction abnormality.

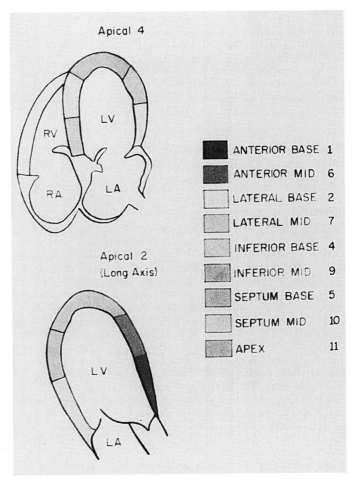

FIGURE 27–17. Schematic diagram showing the method used to visually identify myocardial segments from the apical four- and two-chamber echocardiographic views. RA = right atrium; LA = left atrium; LV = left ventricle; RV = right ventricle. (From Gibson, R.S., Bishop, H.L., Stamm, R.B., et al.: Value of early two-dimensional echocardiography in patients with acute myocardial infarction. Am. J. Cardiol. 49:1110, 1982, with permission.)

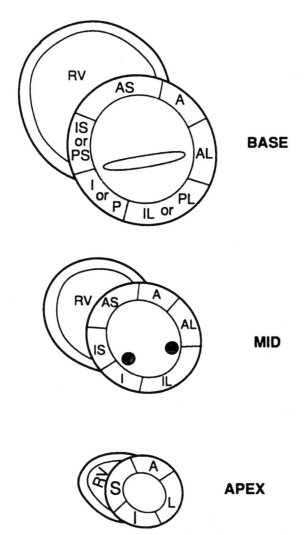

FIGURE 27–16. Sixteen-segment model for wall motion analysis, proposed by the American Society of Echocardiography. A = anterior; AL = anterolateral; IL = inferolateral; I = inferior; IS = inferior septum; AS = anterior septum; PL = posterior lateral; p = posterior; PS = posterior septum. (From Schiller, N.B., Shah, P.M., Crawford, M., et al.: Recommendations for quantitation of the left ventricle by two-dimensional echocardiography. J. Am. Soc. Echocardiogr. 2:358, 1989, with permission.)

A scheme for grading regional function in apical views is presented in Figure 27–17.

Qualitative analysis is also routinely used in the course of stress echocardiography (see Chapter 36). Herein, one looks for the stress (exercise or pharmacologic agent) to produce a new regional contraction abnormality. Most practitioners of stress echo rely primarily on apical two- and four-chamber views for diagnosis because these are easier to obtain and provide more comprehensive appreciation of the extent of a regional contraction abnormality.

Qualitative and semiquantitative wall motion analyses show poorer reproducibility than quantitative methods, even when trained observers are used.[90, 91] In nonquantitative methods, a ventricular region is identified as abnormal primarily by means of visual comparison of its systolic function to that of the remainder of the ventricle, rather than to a normally contracting ventricle or to segmental data averaged from a group of normal ventricles. The process of visually classifying subtle motion abnormalities is subjective and difficult.[98, 99] When interventions are made (e.g., to alter infarct size) and/or serial studies are performed to identify subtle changes in regional systolic function, more objective quantitative methods are desirable. Despite this phenomenon, no quantitative system for evaluating regional systolic function has been adopted by the consensus of an expert panel or the consistent reporting by a large number of users. This is the case because the quantitative analysis of regional left ventricular function is very difficult.

The left ventricle is a three-dimensional structure that moves and contracts simultaneously in three-dimensional space. Thus, the representation and analysis of this complex motion is fraught with limitations when an attempt is made to quantify regional contraction abnormalities with the use of two-dimensional methods. Nevertheless, extensive effort has been made to evaluate regional systolic function, using quantitative analytic algorithms applied to two-dimensional images.

Relation of Systolic Dysfunction to Ischemia and Infarction

Historically, the accuracy of most techniques used to examine regional systolic function has been evaluated by how closely they reflect the pathologic extent of ischemia or infarction. Several factors disrupt the linear relationship between size of the ischemic region and extent of regional systolic dysfunction, regardless of the method used to examine the latter.[100] Most of these factors cause the extent of systolic dysfunction to exceed the extent of ischemia.

The first of these factors is "tethering," that is, systolic dysfunction of nonischemic myocardium adjacent to ischemic or infarcted myocardium.[101, 102] On the basis of a spherical mathematical model of the ventricle, tethering has been explained as resulting from local increases in afterload.[103] Regardless of the mechanism involved, recent studies have indicated that the importance of tethering has been overstated by studies using two-dimensional echocardiography.[104] When tethering was examined by means of sonomicrometry, the extent of dysfunction caused by tethering was minimal (less than 8 mm or 30 degrees of endocardial circumference), and the degree of this dysfunction was modest.[105–109] However, the extent and severity of tethering can be expected to increase with increases in afterload and with increases in the severity of the wall motion abnormality of the ischemic zone (i.e., as the ischemic zone becomes increasingly dyskinetic).[110, 111]

A related factor involves the extent of transmural ischemia, as compared to the extent of transmural dysfunction. Gallagher and associates have shown that systolic wall thickening deteriorates significantly when blood flow to the subendocardium only is impaired.[112] A number of factors appear to account for this phenomenon. First, the epicardial third of the wall contributes minimally to overall wall thickening (approximately 17 percent).[113, 114] Therefore, even when the epicardium continued to function normally during periods of subendocardial ischemia, overall wall thickening would be significantly reduced. Second, there is some evidence that epicardial function is "tethered" to endocardial and midwall function, at least in the anterior wall of the heart.[115–117] Thus, not only does circumferential extent of dysfunction exceed circumferential extent of ischemia, but also transmural extent of dysfunction exceeds transmural extent of ischemia.

A third factor is the temporal relationship between resolution of ischemia and return of systolic function. The return of systolic function consistently lags behind the resolution of ischemia, often by prolonged periods (myocardial "stunning").[118–120] The time to complete return of systolic function is related to, but significantly greater than, the duration of ischemia. A transient 15-minute occlusion may produce changes in systolic function that persist for up to 6 hours[118] or more.[120] These data have obvious implications for examining return of function after reperfusion.[121–125]

Analysis Algorithms

Preliminary Considerations

The ideal system for analyzing regional ventricular function should be reproducible (i.e., intraobserver and interobserver, intersubject, and day-to-day variability should all be low) and accurate compared to some standard. Unfortunately, even the choice of an ideal reference standard is problematic. Pathologic data are suboptimal because of the factors (discussed above) that disrupt

the linear relationship between infarct size and extent of dysfunction and cause the latter to exceed the former. Therefore, the accuracy of two-dimensional echocardiography (or any method that examines systolic function) should not be determined solely by comparison to pathology.

One is left with in vivo methods of wall motion analysis that are, in reality, only historic standards (i.e., the "standard" technique predated two-dimensional echocardiography). Contrast ventriculography, one of the historic standards, also has problems with defining ideal analysis systems.[100, 126–132] In addition, contrast ventriculography is very difficult to equate one-to-one with two-dimensional echocardiography. Two-dimensional echocardiography images a tomographic cross section of the ventricle, whereas contrast ventriculography produces a silhouette of the ventricle. Thus, volume of the ventricle predicted by two-dimensional echocardiography is consistently less than that predicted by contrast ventriculography, even with model hearts.[133] Considerations such as these have led different investigators to choose widely differing reference standards—electrocardiography,[134] quantitative contrast ventriculography,[135–137] qualitative two-dimensional echocardiographic wall motion analysis,[138, 139] or some combination of these standards. These limitations should be kept in mind as various analytic algorithms for measuring regional function are considered. Observer variability is easy to define, but values for quantitative two-dimensional echocardiography rarely have been compared directly to values for other quantitative methods. However, with occasional exceptions,[140] most investigators have reported values for intraobserver and interobserver variability that compare favorably to values for quantitative contrast ventriculography.[90, 131, 136, 141] In general, 5 to 10 percent interobserver variability for regional fractional area change is an acceptable value.

The definition of the range of normal regional ventricular function (intersubject variability) from which to define abnormal regional function poses more difficult problems. The first problem is the wide range of normal or the large variability (defined here as standard deviation divided by the mean) reported for populations of normal subjects. Normal segmental cavity area shrinkage has been reported to vary from 0 percent (i.e., akinesis) to 100 percent and segmental wall thickening to vary from 0 to 150 percent.[142] Such extreme variability makes differentiation of normal and abnormal difficult in individual patients. If correct, these data suggest that quantitative wall-motion analysis may be of little value as a marker of ischemia in an individual and would be of value only for comparing groups of subjects.[140] Even in studies in which variability was not found to be so extreme,[135, 143, 144] the lower limit of normal for cavity-area shrinkage and systolic thickening, as defined by the mean minus two standard deviations (SDs), is near 0 percent for some regions. In reality, akinesis and failure of myocardium to thicken are rarely observed qualitatively in the hearts of normal humans or healthy animals.

It is this disagreement between mathematically derived quantitative ranges of normal for two-dimensional echocardiography and what one observes qualitatively that raises important concerns about the quantitative analysis algorithms currently being used. Further problems arise in technical execution of these algorithms (e.g., tracing of endocardial borders). Because of this extreme variability of regional performance, a conservative lower limit of normal is often chosen (arbitrarily) to be 0 percent thickening[142–145] and some minimal amount of endocardial motion (e.g., 0 to 10 percent radial shortening or cavity-area shrinkage).[145] However, there is no consensus about this arbitrary cutoff, and other values (10 to 20 percent shortening) have been used.[98, 146, 147] Sensitivity and specificity for detecting regional abnormalities thus will change significantly as different cutoffs for the normal range are chosen.

Several physiologic factors also compound the difficulties encountered with quantitative analysis. First, there is considerable heterogeneity of endocardial motion and thickening from level to level within the same ventricle. Left ventricular systolic thickening and endocardial motion increase from base to apex.[143, 144, 148–150] Intersegmental variation within the same level has also been shown with numerous techniques.[142, 149, 151, 152] Finally, temporal asynergy of contraction may contribute significantly to regional variability, especially in ventricles with regional wall motion abnormalities.[142, 153] Variability may be decreased by disregarding temporal asynergy and analyzing the maximum contraction of each segment, regardless of when it occurred in the cardiac cycle. The problems related to temporal asynergy can be solved by analyzing multiple frames within the cardiac cycle, but this approach creates new difficulties (see below).

Endocardial Motion

Analysis of endocardial motion antedated systolic thickening analysis for several reasons. First, endocardial borders were better imaged than epicardial borders because stop-frame tracing was used. Second, endocardial motion analysis is similar to the approach that had been used to evaluate regional motion with contrast ventriculography. The true course of endocardial motion in the 30-degree right anterior oblique plane has been elucidated, using endocardial markers implanted in experimental animals (Fig. 27–18).[154] This motion is a complex combination of inward transverse motion of the anterior and inferior wall and descent of the base toward the apex. It is clear from this study that none of the analysis algorithms currently in use track motion of individual endocardial points. Rather, they are simply a representation of endocardial motion.

As in contrast ventriculography, there are numerous choices in deciding on an analysis algorithm,[127] choices involving reference systems relating diastole to systole, the type of measurement to make, the number of such measurements to be made per ventricular section, and the frequency of such measurements.

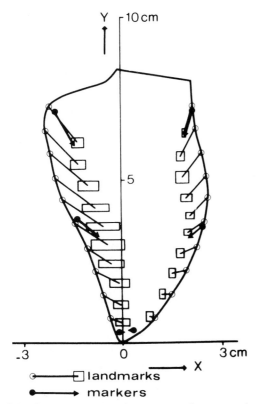

FIGURE 27–18. Mean end-diastolic contour and mean systolic pathways of implanted metal endocardial markers (*solid circles with arrows*) and of endocardial landmarks (*open circles*) in the right anterior oblique view in eight pigs. Boxes represent standard deviations of endocardial landmark motion. (From Slager, C.J., Hooghoudt, T.E.H., Serruys, P.W., et al.: Quantitative assessment of regional left ventricular motion using endocardial landmarks. J. Am. Coll. Cardiol. 77:317, 1986. Reprinted with permission from the American College of Cardiology.)

Reference Systems

Analysis of wall motion must account for the intrinsic centripetal motion ("contractile" motion) of the walls, as well as for the extrinsic or translational and rotational motion of the entire heart (Fig. 27–19). Systems with a fixed or external frame of reference ignore the heart's translational and rotational motion. Systems with a floating or internal frame of reference attempt to control for or correct for translation and rotation, so that only intrinsic motion is analyzed (Fig. 27–20). In general, as translational and rotational motion increases, fixed reference systems become less reliable and floating systems more reliable.[127] Hence, the need to choose one system in preference to another depends on the degree of translational and rotational motion occurring in a specific clinical or experimental setting.[127]

Fluoroscopic studies of myocardial markers implanted in the left ventricular midwall in the 30-degree right anterior oblique plane in humans indicate that there is very little rotational motion of the ventricular long axis in either the 30-degree right anterior oblique plane (roughly approximating the echocardiographic apical two-chamber view) (see Fig. 27–19C) or the 60-degree left anterior oblique plane (approximately the apical four-chamber view) (see Fig. 27–19D)[129, 155]; and for practical purposes can be ignored. Similarly, with two-dimensional echocardiography, the amount of rotational and translational motion of the ventricle (as measured by the amount of change in the position of the long axis in the apical four-chambers and two-chamber planes) in normal subjects and in preoperative coronary bypass patients is insignificant.[156, 157] In theory, because translation and rotation are minimal in these patients, one would expect a fixed-reference system to outperform a floating system, especially because the process of "floating" introduces unavoidable variability of its own.[129, 131, 132, 139] In practice, this has not always been the case for the apical views, and in some cases floating systems correcting for translation have performed better than fixed analysis. It is difficult to reconcile the theoretical advantage of fixed systems with the reported superiority of floating systems. The reason for this may be that the range of normal is smaller with floating systems in apical views. Even in normal individuals in whom translational motion is minimal, there is variability from individual to individual. Consequently, with a fixed external frame of reference, systems in the apical views have greater ranges of normal.[138, 139, 157] Thus, smaller intersubject variability of floating systems in the apical views probably accounts for their superior performance.[138, 139]

For patients who have undergone cardiac surgery in whom there is marked anteromedial translational motion of the ventricle, a floating reference system is clearly superior. The floating system has proved to be significantly better than a fixed system for differentiating patients with perioperative infarction from those without it and for localizing the area of infarction.[156–158] Thus, in the apical views, superiority of fixed versus floating-axis systems depends largely on the degree of translational motion of the ventricle in a particular clinical setting. Although the process of floating introduces a potential source of error, the smaller range of normal may allow more accurate identification of abnormal regions, especially where translational motion is great.

The choice of an analysis system is more difficult for the *parasternal short-axis view*, in which analysis systems must rely on a "centroid" as the internal reference to correct for translation. The centroid or center of mass (area) is a point in space that is defined by the endocardial or epicardial contour. Although a number of techniques exist for generating a centroid, all floating systems suffer from similar limitations. Figure 27–21 illustrates the problem. With normal, symmetric, and equal contractions and some anterior translation of the ventricle, the fixed-reference system leads to the conclusion that there is anterior hypokinesis. The floating endocardial center-of-mass system corrects for this situation and normalizes wall motion. Figure 27–21B is a schematic of a ventricle with an anterior wall motion abnormality and no translation. Here, the fixed-analysis system correctly localized the wall motion abnormal-

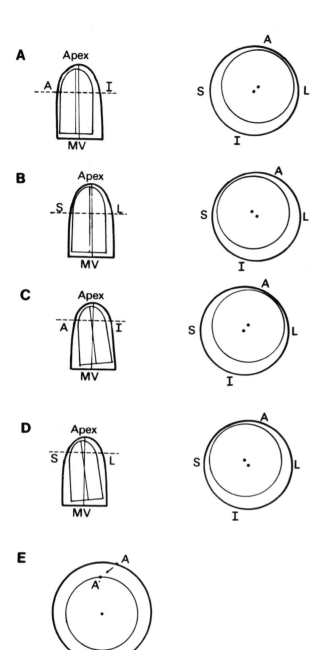

FIGURE 27–19. Schematic drawings of possible systolic translational and rotational motions of the ventricle, as described by movement of the ventricular long axis *(solid line)* in the apical four-chamber (A4C) or apical two-chamber (A2C) views *(left)* and parasternal short-axis (SAX) view *(right)*. The ventricular level of the short-axis section is identified by a dashed line on the A2C or A4C images. *A*, Anterior translation of the long axis of the ventricle seen in the A2C and SAX views. *B*, Medial translation of the long axis seen in the A4C *(left)* and SAX views. *C*, Rotation of the long axis in the A2C plane, as seen in A2C and SAX views. *D*, Rotation of the long axis in the A4C plane, as seen in the A4C and SAX views. *E*, Rotation of the ventricle about the long axis seen in the SAX view. S = septum; A = anterior wall; L = lateral wall; I = inferior wall; MV = mitral valve. (From Force, T.L., and Parisi, A.F.: Quantitative methods for analyzing regional systolic function with two-dimensional echocardiography. *In* Kerber, R.E. [ed.]: Echocardiography in Coronary Artery Disease. Mt. Kisco, NY, Futura, 1988, p. 193, with permission.)

FIGURE 27–20. Schematic of the fixed- and floating-axis systems used to analyze regional wall motion in the apical four-chamber view. For the fixed-axis system, radii are generated from the midpoint of the diastolic long axis. For the floating-axis system, the long axes of both diastolic and systolic images are defined, the midpoint is identified, the long axes are then superimposed, and radii are again generated from the midpoint. (From Force, T., Bloomfield, P., O'Boyle, J.E., et al.: Quantitative two-dimensional echocardiographic analysis of motion and thickening of the interventricular septum after cardiac surgery. Circulation 68:1013, 1983. By permission of the American Heart Association.)

AXIS RELATIONSHIPS

FIXED AXIS   FLOATING AXIS

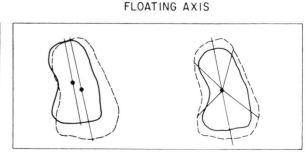

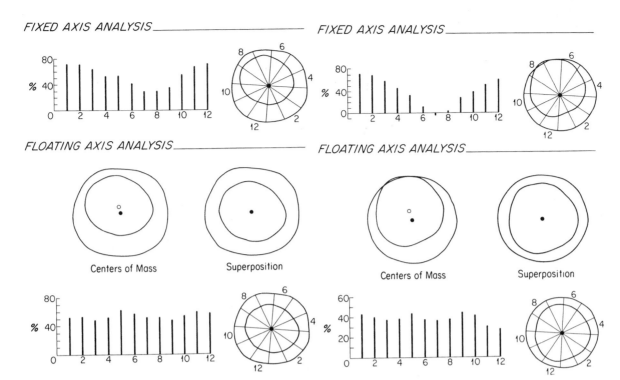

FIGURE 27–21. *A*, Fixed- and floating-axis wall motion analyses (area shrinkage) of a normally contracting ventricle with anterior translation of the ventricle. Fixed-axis analysis leads to the conclusion that anterior hypokinesis is present. Floating-axis analysis superimposes the diastolic *(solid circle)* and systolic *(open circle)* centroids and normalizes wall motion. *B*, Fixed- and floating-axis analyses of a ventricle with an anterior wall-motion abnormality and no translation of the ventricle. Fixed-axis analysis correctly localizes the abnormality. Because the centroid moves toward the wall motion abnormally in systole, superimposition of the diastolic and systolic centroids falsely normalizes anterior endocardial motion. (From Force, T.L., and Parisi, A.F.: Quantitative methods for analyzing regional systolic function with two-dimensional echocardiography. *In* Kerber, R.E. [ed.]: Echocardiography in Coronary Artery Disease. Mt. Kisco, NY, Futura, 1988, p. 193, with permission.)

ity. The floating endocardial center-of-mass system falsely normalizes anterior wall motion, because the centroid moves toward the abnormally contracting segment.

Not surprisingly, these theoretical concerns have been borne out repeatedly in experimental animal and human studies. Although fixed and floating systems may differ in their abilities to detect the presence of a regional abnormality or to separate patients with an abnormality from those without one, the floating system localizes the abnormality and quantifies it far less accurately than the fixed system.[135, 139, 143] Floating systems may incorrectly localize wall motion abnormalities more than 50 percent of the time.[139] These negative features of floating-axis analyses in the parasternal short-axis view more than outweigh the smaller range of normal, compared to that obtained with fixed analyses. However, an epicardial floating center-of-mass system may be a compromise that reduces the range of normal (albeit not to the extent that endocardial center systems do[147]) but does not falsely enhance motion of abnormal regions as much.[141, 159] With this system, the centroid still moves toward the wall motion abnormality, but less so than with an endocardial center-of-mass analysis (Fig. 27–22). With increasing degrees of dyskinesis, even the epicardial center of mass increasingly falsely improves apparent wall motion, although not to normal. Thus, identification of regional dysfunction remains good, but quantitation of the degree of asynergy is suspect.

In summary, the choice of a fixed or floating reference system and, if floating, the choice of what type of centroid to use are the most problematic decisions in quantitative two-dimensional echocardiography. Use of a fixed external frame of reference system is limited by a wider range of normal that is probably responsible for the suboptimal sensitivity for the apical four-chamber[138, 139] and apical chamber[138] views. In these views with more consistent internal landmarks to construct the long-axis of the left ventricle, a

floating analysis system may be superior. In the parasternal short-axis views, however, where a centroid must be used, endocardial center-of-mass floating-axis analysis leads to false normalization of regional wall motion abnormalities and poor localization. The use of an epicardial center-of-mass system leads to less movement of the centroid and less false normalization of wall motion. However, it produces inherent alterations that do not reflect true wall motion.

A related, though less problematic, issue is correction for systolic rotation of the ventricle about the long axis (see Fig. 27–19*E*). Normally, the ventricle "twists" slightly with ejection (i.e., more apical segments rotate relative to the base).[160] When the degree of systolic rotation is sufficient, analogous portions of the ventricle are not examined in diastole, compared to systole. The usual approach to this problem is to correct for such rotation by realigning the diastolic and systolic contours, based on the position of some internal landmarks (usually, the papillary muscles). In general, the basal two thirds of the heart rotates minimally (only 3 to 4 degrees),[104, 161] which suggests that correction for rotation about the long axis of the heart is unnecessary for short-axis views of the basal two thirds of the heart, unless precise alignment of papillary muscle contours is desired (i.e., when motion of the papillary muscles is being analyzed). This issue has not been examined adequately at the cardiac apex. It is the authors' impression that rotation here may be a more significant factor, just as it may be with inotropic stimulation.[160] When this is so, it poses a significant problem to quantitative analysis of short-axis apical images, because there are no internal landmarks with which to realign the diastolic and systolic contours.

Types of Measurements

The next choice to be made is between types of measurements—whether to use change in length of a chord or a

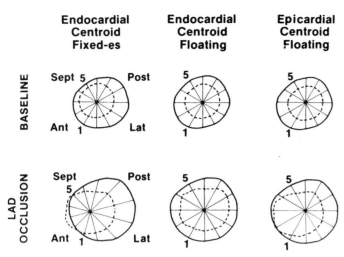

FIGURE 27–22. Reference systems used to determine radial shortening along 12 equidistant radii. Only one of the four fixed-reference systems (endocardial centroid fixed at end-systole [es]) and the two floating-reference systems are shown. The endocardial contours at end-diastole and end-systole are from before and after experimental coronary occlusion. Radius 1 is at the level of the anterolateral papillary muscle during end-diastole and end-systole. In this figure, the endocardial contours are already rotated, so that the respective radii are superimposed. In the case of floating references, the contours are further translated to superimpose the respective end-diastolic and end-systolic centroids. During baseline, with the use of either floating centroid system, radial shortening adequately reflects regional function, whereas the fixed reference delineates hypokinesia in the anteroseptal (Ant-Sept) area, secondary to cardiac translation. During left anterior descending (LAD) coronary occlusion, radial shortening in the involved region shows evidence of dyskinesia with the fixed reference, no abnormality with the floating endocardial centroid, and akinesia-hypokinesia with the floating epicardial centroid. Lat = lateral; Sept = septum; Ant = anterior; Post = posterior. (From Zoghbi, W.A., Charlat, M.L., Bolli, R., et al.: Quantitative assessment of left ventricular wall motion by two-dimensional echocardiography: Validation during reversible ischemia in the conscious dog. J. Am. Coll. Cardiol. 11:851, 1988. Reprinted with permission of the American College of Cardiology.)

radius emanating from a center point or change in a cavity area. In general, area methods are more reproducible, are more accurate, and have smaller ranges of normal than length-based methods.[128, 137, 138] However, as the number of areas into which the ventricle is subdivided increases, and the size of each such area decreases, the area methods increasingly resemble length methods, and any superiority of the former is lost.

An alternative to these coordinate systems is the "coordinateless" centerline method, developed for contrast ventriculography but applicable to two-dimensional echocardiography as well.[162, 163] In this system, radii are not generated from a predefined center point. Instead, a line is generated midway between the end-diastolic and the end-systolic contours, and then multiple chords are constructed perpendicular to this line (Fig. 27–23). Wall motion is assessed as the length of these chords, which avoids the problem, albeit of minor practical importance,[129] of where to place the center point for generation of radii. The use of this system also prevents tangential intersection of radii with endocardium, which may give a false impression of the extent of motion in a region. More important, motion is absolute and can be more reliably compared from region to region than when referenced to an end-diastolic radius or area and expressed as a percent change. However, this system does not solve the major problem of quantitative two-dimensional echocardiography: whether to correct for translation and rotation and, if so, how to accomplish it.

Numbers of Measurements

There are far fewer data regarding the optimum number of measurements in assessing regional ventricular function (i.e., the number of subdivisions of the left ventricle). Infarctions with small circumferential extent may be difficult to detect, even when they are transmural.[145] Theoretically, systems with more subdivisions would be more likely to detect small regional wall motion abnormalities. In practice, it is not clear whether more subdivisions increase detection of small infarctions significantly,[137] even when the ventricle is subdivided into 72 segments (at 5-degree intervals).[139] Balanced against any possible increase in sensitivity is the fact that reproducibility and variability deteriorate with greater subdivision of the left ventricle.[143] Hence, as the number of subdivisions decreases, so does the number of false-positive wall motion abnormalities.

Sampling Frequency in the Cardiac Cycle

Early attempts to quantify regional wall motion with radionuclide ventriculography or two-dimensional echocardiography examined only end-diastole and end-systole. This approach does not account for temporal heterogeneity of contraction. Dyskinesis is maximal in early systole in the vast majority of patients with previous infarction.[164–168] In one study, only 1 percent of regions were maximally dyskinetic at end-systole.[169] Thus, important regional wall motion abnormalities can be missed by sampling only end-diastole and end-systole.

Weyman and associates have extensively evaluated a system that samples endocardial motion every 16.7 msec and integrates the entire temporal course of systolic radial motion.[169] When digitized manually, this approach is extremely tedious and time consuming. Its reproducibility is surprisingly good when echocardiograms are of sufficiently high quality.[140, 146] However, a significantly greater amount of "noise" is inherent in such analyses. Such noise can be from irregularities of the endocardial surface, from the video image, or from errors in the digitization process (whether automated or manual). Fourier analysis is a logical approach to reducing the intraframe (spatial) and interframe (temporal) noise.[170] Unfiltered analyses show a large number of regional endocardial direction reversals for each systolic contraction sequence, which are largely caused by errors in tracing. Smoothing via Fourier transformation reduces the number of these endocardial direction reversals and produces an image that more closely resembles what the echocardiographer sees qualitatively that is, smooth, symmetric, centripetal contractions.

Reference-Independent Systems

Because all of the approaches to wall-motion analysis discussed above must address the issue of whether (and how) to correct for translation of the ventricle and what type of coordinate system to use, attempts have been made to develop systems that are truly independent of reference points. One such approach to identifying ischemic or infarcted segments is to analyze regional radius of curvature, rather than wall motion.[171] Curvature clearly changes when a region becomes ischemic or is infarcted.[172] However, it has still not been determined whether analysis of curvature is superior to any of the methods discussed above.

Quantification of Infarct Size With Endocardial Motion

Single-Plane Analyses

Although there are some limitations in comparing extent of regional wall motion abnormalities to observations of pathologic material, pathology at least offers an easily quantifiable and unequivocal standard. Numerous investigators have examined the accuracy of two-dimensional echocardiographic wall motion analyses for determining infarct size. In general, semiquantitative approaches,[173–176] that is, qualitative estimates of the percent circumference that is dysfunctional, reasonably predict pathologic infarct size,[173–176] even in humans.[175] Accuracy is, of course, critically dependent on the echocardiographer's experience, and all the inher-

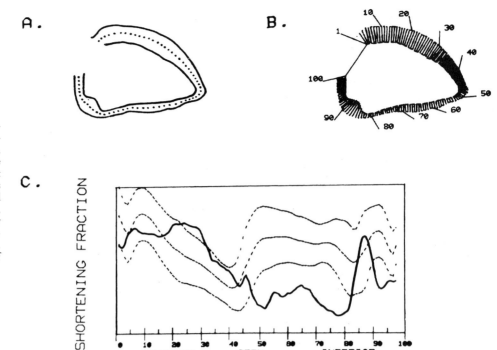

FIGURE 27–23. Centerline method of Bolson and associates. *A*, End-diastolic and end-systolic contours with dotted centerline. *B*, Chords constructed perpendicularly to the centerline. *C*, Wall motion in a patient *(heavy solid line)* with inferior hypokinesis and anterior hyperkinesis, plotted compared to the normal range. (From Sheehan, F.H., Stewart, A.K., Dodge, H.T., et al.: Variability in the measurement of regional left ventricular wall motion from contrast angiograms. Circulation 68:550, 1983. By permission of the American Heart Association, Inc.)

ent problems of qualitative analysis exist. Nevertheless, such approaches, as noted above, have been used successfully to stratify patients according to risk after myocardial infarction.

Although purely quantitative systems can identify normal and abnormal regional contraction reliably,[89, 177] they are less successful in quantifying the extent of an abnormality when they are related to another standard. Several studies that used quantitative analyses have consistently found the same problem: the size of an ischemic region is overestimated, and there is a large amount of "scatter," that is, the SEE is often 15 to 20 percent of the circumference of the left ventricle. One must realize that overestimation of ischemic region size is not necessarily a limitation, because the functional sequelae of myocardial infarction (i.e., the severity of left ventricular dysfunction) are excellent predictors of prognosis and are not necessarily inferior to other measures of ischemic region size.[178] However, although some of the overestimation occurs because extent of dysfunction truly exceeds pathologic extent of infarction, at least some of the overestimation is certainly due to limitations of analysis algorithms. Furthermore, the inaccuracy implicit in large SEEs is certainly a limitation.

It is not clear whether systems that examine for temporal heterogeneity of contraction by sampling multiple times in the cardiac cycle improve infarct size determinations. Initial reports have been encouraging.[98, 146] However, because the major advantage of the technique is that it increases the ability to detect abnormalities along individual radii by sampling throughout systole, it would seem that overestimation of infarct size might be a greater problem than with standard end-diastolic and end-systolic approaches.

Integrative Approaches to the Whole Ventricle

The problems of single-plane analyses are multiplied when one attempts to combine uniplanar images to reconstruct the entire ventricle. The most common approach is to use a Simpson rule algorithm for summating data from individual short-axis planes. However, to derive a percentage of the left ventricle that is infarcted, either one must know the "height" of the two-dimensional echocardiographic section (or, more accurately, the distance between sections) to calculate percent of myocardial mass infarcted (which is rarely possible clinically) or one must make assumptions concerning the height of the section or the relative proportion of

mass represented by each section (which is impossible clinically). Even in the experimental setting, such approaches have produced suboptimal correlations.[144]

A novel approach to this problem is the endocardial surface–mapping technique.[179, 180] Therein, the endocardial surface area of the ventricle is determined by computer algorithm with measured input from three short-axis views (circumference at each level) and two apical views (length of the long axis in the apical four-chamber and two-chamber views). The extent of dysfunction is determined qualitatively in each view, and then extent of dysfunction is calculated by the algorithm as a percentage of the total left ventricular surface area for the whole ventricle. Finally, for ease of viewing, the surface area of the ventricle is displayed as a planar map, in a manner similar to that of a Mercator projection of the globe (Fig. 27–24). Picard and associates[181] have used this approach to track the natural history of ventricular size and function in 57 patients with first acute myocardial infarctions. They showed that patients with anterior infarctions were considerably more prone to left ventricular dilation, based on measurements of their endocardial surface area index.

In the hands of trained operators, this approach accurately determines total endocardial surface area and extent of infarction in experimental animals and in autopsied human hearts.[179–182] This technique has some important advantages over approaches that combine data from multiple views to express global left ventricular dysfunction. First, it is free from major assumptions concerning the geometry of the ventricle (i.e., the ventricle does not have to be modeled as a geometric figure, its resemblance to which may be minimal, especially in the distorted ventricle). Second, regional aneurysmal dilations are handled easily when this system is used.[182] Although the initial reports used qualitative analysis of abnormal wall motion and no allowance was made for the severity of the wall motion abnormality, this algorithm can also easily be adapted to quantification.

Analysis of Apical Endocardial Motion

Apical regional wall motion abnormalities are extremely common with disease of the left anterior descending coronary artery. Unfortunately, the apex of the left ventricle is the most difficult area to evaluate, regardless of the technique used. With contrast ventricu-

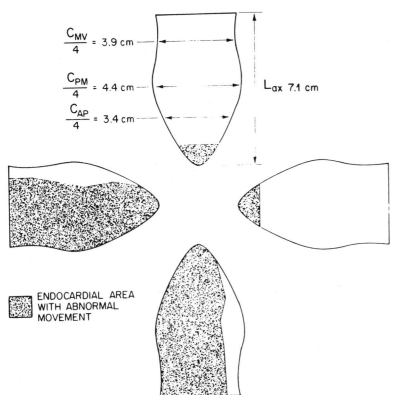

FIGURE 27–24. Planar map for an animal with a myocardial infarction from occlusion of the left circumflex coronary artery. C_{MV}, C_{PM}, and C_{AP} stand for short-axis circumference at the mitral valve level, papillary muscle level, and apex, respectively. Endocardial area with abnormal wall motion was 101.9 cm². (From Guyer, D.E., Foale, R.A., Gillam, L.D., et al.: An echocardiographic technique for quantifying and displaying the extent of regional ventricular dyssynergy. J. Am. Coll. Cardiol. 8:830, 1986. Reprinted with permission of the American College of Cardiology.)

lography, magnitude of motion is low and variability is high at the apex.[131] Therefore, reliability of motion measurement is worse there than in any other ventricular region, and motion must be nearly dyskinetic to be abnormal.[131]

Two-dimensional echocardiography has additional problems vis-à-vis the cardiac apex. In the short axis, lack of internal landmarks below the papillary muscles makes it difficult to define a reproducible section. In the apical views the true apex of the left ventricle is often truncated, because the operator-defined echocardiographic apex is often not identical to the anatomical apex. Because truncating the apex may falsely enhance wall motion, one would expect limited sensitivity to be a problem.[140] As with contrast ventriculography,[131] apical endocardial motion in the four-chamber view is minimal, making differentiation of abnormal and normal difficult.[157] Part of the reason for this may be difficulty in identifying endocardium.[50, 183, 184] Endocardial dropout is most prominent apicolaterally because of overlying lung. For this reason, one can expect false-positive wall motion abnormalities of the apex or apicolateral region when the criterion of hypokinesis is used.[139] Therefore, the authors consider isolated apical hypokinesis as normal.[158]

Systolic Wall-Thickening Analysis

Quantitative analysis of systolic wall thickening is the major alternative to analyzing the extent of endocardial motion. Thickening analysis has some important theoretical and practical advantages over motion analysis. Quantification of systolic thickening is relatively uninfluenced by translation of the ventricle, and correction for this situation with some sort of floating-axis system is unnecessary.[177, 185–187] Furthermore, thickening analyses are thought to be more independent of the particular center of mass chosen for the analysis. Endocardial motion may have passive components,[177] whereas systolic thickening does not. In addition, the analysis of systolic thickening has sounder experimental support: systolic wall thickening (determined with sonomicrometry) correlates closely with subendocardial shortening, subendocardial blood flow, and transmural blood flow.[107, 112, 188] In addition, it accurately separates infarcted and noninfarcted tissues.[188, 189] Finally, there is excellent qualitative agreement between systolic wall thickening determined

by means of two-dimensional echocardiography and that determined by sonomicrometry.[190, 191] Several studies have confirmed very good correlations between extent of abnormal systolic thickening and infarct size.[144, 191, 192]

In direct comparisons, however, systolic thickening analyses have not consistently outperformed endocardial motion analyses. Specifically, the sensitivity for detecting presence or absence of infarction is not significantly different,[134, 145, 192] and the sensitivity of both is limited when infarction is small.[145, 192] Furthermore, systolic thickening analyses are no more accurate at quantifying extent of infarction.[192] However, although both thickening and endocardial motion clearly separate infarcted from distant normal myocardium, systolic thickening is superior to wall motion analysis in distinguishing infarct zones from adjacent noninfarcted ones.[177, 192] Consequently, endocardial wall motion analyses systematically overpredict the circumferential extent of infarction more than thickening analyses do.

Systolic thickening analysis has some additional problems. It is often difficult to identify the epicardial borders sufficiently to trace them, even in experimental animals. This problem may produce large interobserver variability.[185] When the normal change from end-diastolic to end-systolic wall thickness can be only 1 to 2 mm, small errors in identifying epicardium can become important sources of variability. Definition of the range of normal systolic thickening has all the same problems as endocardial motion analyses. Intersubject, intersegment, and interlevel variability are just as high with systolic thickening, and temporal asynergy is also present.[142]

In addition, systolic thickening analyses may be subject to the "threshold phenomenon."[177] As the percentage of the transmural extent of ischemia or myocardial infarction exceeds some amount, systolic thickening deteriorates no further.[112, 116, 121, 177, 194, 195] Clarification is still needed on the transmural extent of infarction at which the threshold is reached; without this information precise sizing of transmural extent of infarction is prevented (although not necessarily circumferential extent of infarction). This phenomenon should not be viewed as a limitation of systolic thickening analyses but rather as another factor disrupting the linear relationship between extent of infarction and extent of dysfunction.

Finally, there are some problems with systolic thickening analysis algorithms. First, systolic thickening is often measured along radii generated from a center of mass. It is assumed that these radii will intersect the wall nearly perpendicularly to tangents to endocardium and epicardium, which may not be the case when contraction is asymmetric. Although this will introduce only small absolute errors in end-systolic thickness, it may be an important source of error when one is examining percent thickening. An adaptation of the centerline method of analysis (see Fig. 27–23)[116, 163, 177, 196] may be superior, because even with asymmetric contraction, the minimum thickness of the wall in both diastole and systole is measured, and the problem of tangential intersection of radii is avoided.

Of potential greater importance is that as with short-axis wall motion analyses, all systems reported to date use an analysis based on the percentage of circumference of the left ventricle that is dysfunctional in systole. Thus, overestimation of extent of dysfunction (compared to pathologic extent of infarction) is inherent in these systems. Systolic expansion of the dysfunctional segment would lead to larger estimates of dysfunctional region size, because the abnormal segment would then occupy an even larger percent of the systolic left ventricular circumference. The importance of tethering has been exaggerated by these flaws in analysis systems,[104, 197] because two-dimensional echocardiographic estimates of the amount of myocardium tethered significantly exceed estimates from sonomicrometry.[107, 109]

Automated methods of assessing regional performance are now possible. One such system tracks endocardial excursion in color, distinguishing the extent of endocardial motion by the thickness of a band of contrasting color within the ventricular end-diastolic contour.[198] This technique has particular promise for analysis of wall motion abnormalities unmasked by exercise echocardiography, provided that cardiac translation during exercise can be properly corrected (Fig. 27–25).

FIGURE 27–25. See Color Plate 2.

RIGHT VENTRICULAR FUNCTION

Just a few years ago, the right ventricle was regarded as a "passive conduit" not playing an important role in normal cardiac output. This notion was based on early canine experiments that demonstrated lack of hemodynamic compromise despite severe damage to the right ventricular wall by cauterization.[199, 200] Later clinical observations of right ventricular function in various disease states, especially right ventricular infarction, clearly demonstrated that severe hemodynamic compromise can occur without significant left ventricular involvement. These data have laid the passive-conduit theory to rest.[201]

Compared to the left ventricle, the right ventricle has a more complicated geometric shape that has defied full characterization by simple mathematical models. Consequently, quantitative evaluation of right ventricular function has been fraught with difficulty. As a result, despite the availability of several different geometric methods of evaluating left ventricular function, a historic standard or gold standard for quantifying right ventricular function has not emerged. The development and widespread availability of two-dimensional echocardiography provided a new opportunity to image the right ventricular chamber noninvasively and, hence, a new chance to study further its structure and function.

Echocardiographic Examination

The echocardiographic examination of the normal right ventricle has some limitations related to accessibility. A major portion of the

normal right ventricle is obscured by the sternum, which interferes with the transmission of ultrasound. An enlarged or dilated right ventricle is easier to image. This enlargement typically occurs in conditions that cause right ventricular volume overload, such as tricuspid regurgitation, atrial septal defect, and Ebstein's anomaly.[202] In addition, depending on the patient's position, there can be an important variation in the location of the right ventricle within the chest cavity in relationship to the chest wall,[203] which can lead to a significant variation in the measured dimension along a single axis, depending on the angle of the ultrasonic beam to the chamber.

M-Mode Echocardiography

M-mode echocardiography is commonly used to measure the internal right ventricular dimension. However, owing to the difficulty in obtaining clear images of the right ventricular endocardium anteriorly, accurate measurement of the true anteroposterior dimension of the right ventricle is quite difficult. Since the initial study of Popp and associates,[204] it had been estimated that the anterior wall of the right ventricle begins approximately 5 mm from the chest wall. However, the American Society of Echocardiography recommends that the dimensions of the right ventricle should be reported only when the endocardium of the anterior right ventricular wall and the right side of the septum are clearly imaged.[205] A second problem is that the right ventricular dimension is larger when the patient is in left lateral decubitus, rather than in a supine position. To standardize the dimensions, it is recommended that only the supine measurements be reported.

In summary, although M-mode echocardiography is not highly accurate for the measurement of right ventricular dimension in all patients, it can usually separate patients with a clearly dilated right ventricle from those with a normal one.

Two-Dimensional Echocardiography

Two-dimensional echocardiography, with its ability to image in multiple planes, offers a considerable advantage over M-mode echocardiography in qualitative and quantitative assessment of right ventricular size, shape, and function.

Right Ventricular Dimension

Qualitatively, with two-dimensional echocardiography the size of the right ventricle is usually assessed by visual comparison with the left ventricle. Normally, the transverse dimension of the right ventricle in the parasternal short-axis and apical four-chamber views is smaller than that of the left ventricle. In parasternal short-axis views of a normal heart, the body of the right ventricle has a crescent-like shape. Figure 27–26 shows the short-axis and four-chamber views of the heart in a patient with volume overload of the right ventricle. Note that the transverse right ventricular dimension appears equal to, or larger than, the left ventricular dimension. In addition, the left ventricle has lost its normal round shape in the parasternal short-axis view because of a change in the septal curvature at end-diastole.

Bommer and associates[206] were the first to attempt to determine right ventricular size by using two-dimensional echocardiography. In 50 subjects (25 patients with normal right ventricles and 25 patients with volume overload), they showed that the right ventricle short-axis dimensions and area better separated normal from overloaded right ventricles than did the long-axis or the standard M-mode study.

Global Right Ventricular Function: Volumes and Ejection Fraction

One approach to the complex geometric shape of the right ventricle is to consider it as comprising two chambers: a body

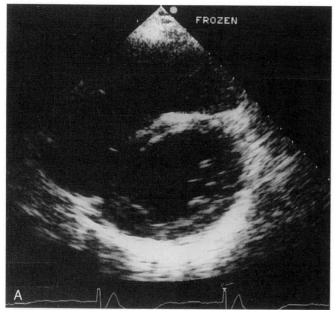

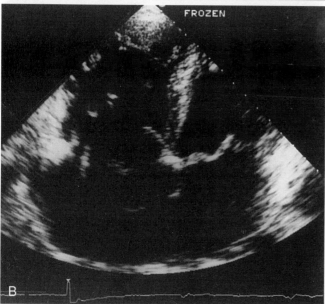

FIGURE 27–26. Volume-overloaded right ventricle. *A,* The parasternal short-axis view shows the increase in the width of the right ventricle, as well as the change in septal curvature. *B,* Apical four-chamber view with enlarged right ventricle and right atrium.

extending from the tricuspid annulus to the apex and an outflow tract, which is situated anteriorly and medially. The body of the right ventricle in short-axis section is shaped like a crescent, but its outflow tract is cylindrical. Because of this peculiar configuration, multiple different approaches have been used to quantify right ventricular function, including multiple geometric models,[187, 207-215] a tricuspid valve systolic excursion index,[208] contrast echocardiography,[216] and subtraction of left heart volume from total cardiac volume.[217]

Most of the early studies of right ventricular volumes used geometrical assumptions, modeling this chamber as an ellipsoid, a combination of half-cylinders and half-cones, or a combination of other tapering geometric solids. These models had fair correlations with end-diastolic volumes (r values from .65 to .85), with better and more consistent correlation with external measures of ejection fraction (r values .74 to .98). The details of each of these approaches have been presented in the first edition of this book.[218]

However, because none has gained widespread acceptance, they are not discussed further here.

It became apparent in the late 1980s that the body of the right ventricle might better be modeled as a tapering crescentic solid (Fig. 27–27). Using this model, Aebischer and Czegledy[207] found excellent correlations for the volume of the body of the right ventricle (r = .96), comparing two-dimensional echocardiographic measurements to actual volumes of casts of canine right ventricles (Fig. 27–28). Nevertheless, because of the limited views from two-dimensional echocardiography, no universally accepted approach to measuring the entire right ventricular volume has emerged.

The most promising estimates of right ventricular volume have come from recent studies that used three-dimensional echocardiography. Using a spark-gap device to locate three-dimensional positions of imaging planes. Jiang and colleagues[219] found excellent correlations of echocardiographic constructions of right ventricular volumes, as compared to those of gel casts of 12 excised human right ventricles (r = .99; SEE = 3.0 mL) (Fig. 27–29). In a further canine study of right ventricular volumes in vivo, using their three-dimensional approach, the same investigators[220] found superb correlations of actual right ventricular volumes measured by balloon displacements of right ventricular content (EDV: r = .99, SEE = 1.8 mL; ESV: r = .98, SEE = 2.5 mL). The mean difference between calculated and actual right ventricular volumes was 2.1 mL, which was only 4.9 percent of the mean volume measured. These studies indicate that the three-dimensional approach is the most promising of the methods so far attempted to measure right ventricular volume. They also serve to indicate the high level of accuracy in measuring cardiac chamber volumes with the use of three-dimensional techniques.

Regional Right Ventricular Function

Two-dimensional echocardiography can be used to confirm right ventricular involvement in patients with acute myocardial infarction. The three most common echocardiographic findings associated with right ventricular infarction are right ventricular dilation, regional wall motion abnormality, and paradoxic septal motion. Of these three conditions, regional wall motion abnormality is proba-

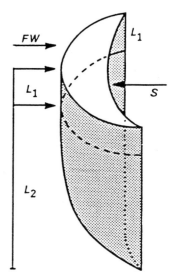

FIGURE 27–27. Schematic representation of the right ventricle, using a crescentic model. L_1 = length of the basal portion; L_2 = length of the apical portion; FW = right ventricular free wall; S = septum. The basal crescentic area is displayed in white. The dashed line separates a basal volume, where the midwidth of the crescent is constant, from the apical volume, where the crescentic width decreases progressively toward the apex. (From Aebischer, N.M., and Czegledy, F.: Determination of right ventricular volume by two-dimensional echocardiography with a crescentic model. J. Am. Soc. Echocardiogr. 2:110, 1989, with permission.)

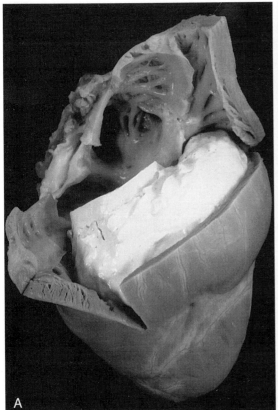

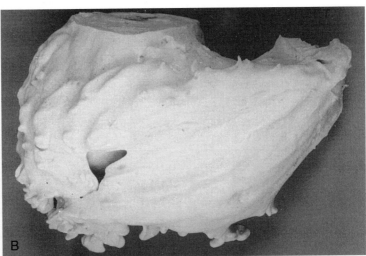

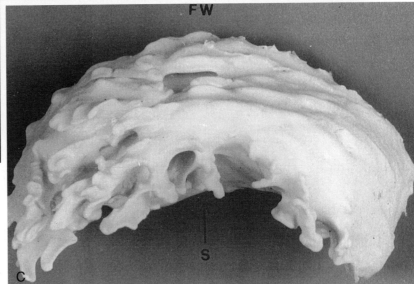

FIGURE 27–28. *A,* Right ventricle case in the right ventricular cavity. *B,* The anterior view of the right ventricle case illustrates the separate inflow and outflow regions of the right ventricle. *C,* The apical view shows the crescentic aspect of the right ventricle, delineated anteriorly by the right ventricular free wall (FW) and posteriorly by the interventricular septum (S).

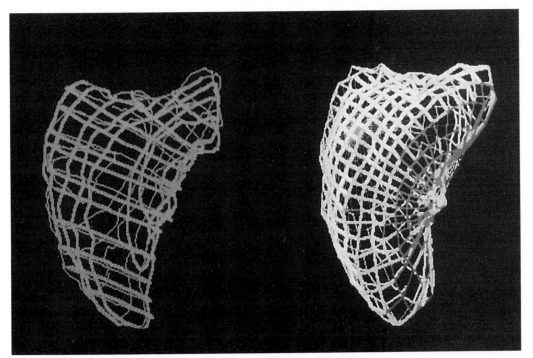

FIGURE 27–29. Reconstructed traced borders of human right ventricular cast *(left),* with inflow region at upper left, apex below, and outflow at upper right. (Curved septum lies behind anterior wall.) Corresponding surface used for volume calculation *(right).* (From Jiang, L., Handschumacher, M.D., Hibberd, M.G., et al.: Three-dimensional echocardiographic reconstruction of right ventricular volume: In vitro comparison with two-dimensional methods. J. Am. Soc. Echocardiogr. 7:153, 1994, with permission.)

bly the most useful. Although right ventricular enlargement has been reported commonly in the setting of acute right ventricular infarction,[221-224] Arditti and associates[225] did not find significant differences in the two-dimensional right ventricular end-diastolic dimension in patients with inferoposterior myocardial infarction and right ventricular dysfunction, compared to patients with inferoposterior myocardial infarction without right ventricular dysfunction and patients with normal hearts. However, the two-dimensional echocardiographic right ventricular end-systolic dimensions and the percent fractional shortening in the long and short axes of the right ventricle taken from the apical four-chamber view were significantly different in the group of patients with right ventricular dysfunction, as compared to the other two groups. The percent fractional shortening of the long-axis, maximal, and mid-short-axis dimensions were (mean ± standard deviation) 31.25 ± 9.60, 33.12 ± 7.80, and 30.68 ± 9.10 percent, respectively, in the normal group; 13.10 ± 8.20, 5.75 ± 13.80, and 5.80 ± 20.30 percent, respectively, in the group of patients with right ventricular dysfunction; and 20.42 ± 7.06, 35.30 ± 11.58, and 38.95 ± 16.70 percent, respectively, in patients with inferoposterior myocardial infarction but without right ventricular dysfunction.

Right ventricular infarction per se has been reported as a cause of paradoxic septal motion. In a closed-chest canine experiment, Sharkey and associates[226] showed that isolated infarction of the right ventricular free wall produced by right coronary artery embolization was associated with right ventricular dilation, right ventricular free-wall dyskinesis, and paradoxic septal motion with preserved systolic thickening. The paradoxic septal motion coincided with reversal of the transseptal end-diastolic pressure gradient because of an isolated increase in right ventricular end-diastolic pressure.

Regional wall motion abnormality has been repeatedly reported clinically in the setting of right ventricular infarction[221-223, 225, 227-229] and compared to bedside observations, electrocardiograms, hemodynamic data, and/or radionuclide studies. In a study of 50 patients with acute inferior myocardial infarction, in which an equilibrium-gated blood-pool study was used as a standard, Bellamy and associates[227] found that 20 of 50 patients had regional wall motion abnormalities according two-dimensional echocardiography, as compared to 22 patients by means of gated blood-pool study. The sensitivity and specificity for the detection of right ventricular infarction were 82 and 93 percent for two-dimensional echocardiography, compared to 50 and 71 percent for ST elevation in V_{4R}, 77 and 85 percent for elevation of venous pressure, and 59 and 89 percent for a positive Kussmaul sign.

In a study by Arditti and associates,[225] two-dimensional echocardiography and multigated acquisition radionuclide study revealed right ventricular dysfunction in 60 of 104 patients with acute inferoposterior myocardial infarction. Right ventricular dysfunction was diagnosed by means of two-dimensional echocardiography in the presence of regional wall motion abnormality and by multigated acquisition radionuclide study by a right ventricular EF lower than 2 SDs from the normal value. Eight patients presented with regional wall motion abnormality, as shown by means of two-dimensional echocardiography and normal EF on the radionuclide study, and five patients without regional wall motion abnormality showed a low right ventricular EF. Compared to the radionuclide study, two-dimensional echocardiography had a sensitivity of 92 percent and a specificity of 79 percent in the detection of right ventricular dysfunction. However, in this study a depressed EF, but not regional wall motion abnormality, was included in the diagnosis of right ventricular dysfunction by the radionuclide method. As the authors pointed out, the eight false-positive diagnoses of right ventricular dysfunction by two-dimensional echocardiography may, in fact, represent a higher sensitivity of this test.

In summary, two-dimensional echocardiography can provide valuable information about right ventricular global and regional function in a variety of clinical settings, such as coronary artery disease, congenital heart disease, valvular heart disease with secondary pulmonary hypertension, and chronic obstructive lung disease. In the future, further application of newer techniques, such as three-dimensional reconstruction, may provide the needed gold standard for right ventricular volume determination and for its full characterization as a geographic structure.

Acknowledgment

The authors acknowledge with gratitude the extraordinary help of Suzanne Bailey and Teresa Gadouas in preparation of this manuscript.

References

1. Kreulen, T.M., Bove, A.A., McDonough, M.T., et al.: The evaluation of left ventricular function in man. A comparison of methods. Circulation 51:677, 1975.
2. Murray, J.A., Chinn, N., and Peterson, D.R.: Influence of left ventricular function on early prognosis in atherosclerotic heart disease. (Abstract.) Am. J. Cardiol. 33:159, 1974.
3. Nelson, G.R., Cohn, P.F., and Gorlin, R.: Prognosis in medically treated coronary artery disease. Influence of ejection fraction compared to other parameters. Circulation 52:408, 1975.
4. Cohn, P.F., Gorlin, R., Cohn, L.H., et al.: Left ventricular ejection fraction as a prognostic guide in surgical treatment of coronary and valvular heart disease. Am. J. Cardiol. 34:136, 1974.
5. Hammermeister, K.E., and Kennedy, J.W.: Predictors of surgical mortality in patients undergoing direct myocardial revascularization. Circulation 50:II–112, 1974.
6. Dodge, H.T., Sandler, H., Ballew, D.W., et al.: Use of biplane angiocardiography for the measurement of left ventricular volume in man. Am. Heart J. 60:762, 1960.
7. Moynihan, P.F., Parisi, A.F., Folland, E.D., et al.: A system for quantitative evaluation of left ventricular function with two-dimensional ultrasonography. Med. Instrum. 14:111, 1980.
8. Barrett, M.J., Jacobs, L., Gomberg, J., et al.: Simultaneous contrast imaging of the left ventricle by two-dimensional echocardiography and standard ventriculography. Clin. Cardiol. 5:208, 1982.
9. Pombo, J.F., Troy, B.L., and Russell, R.O., Jr.: Left ventricular volumes and ejection fraction by echocardiography. Circulation 43:480, 1971.
10. Fortuin, N.J., Hood, W.P., Jr., Sherman, M.E., et al.: Determination of left ventricular volumes by ultrasound. Circulation 44:575, 1971.
11. Teichholz, L.E., Kreulen, T., Herman, M.V., et al.: Problems in echocardiographic volume determinations: Echocardiographic-angiographic correlations in the presence or absence of asynergy. Am. J. Cardiol. 37:7, 1976.
12. Carr, K.W., Engler, R.L., Forsythe, J.R., et al.: Measurement of left ventricular ejection fraction by mechanical cross-sectional echocardiography. Circulation 59:1196, 1979.
13. Folland, E.D., Parisi, A.F., Moynihan, P.F., et al.: Assessment of left ventricular ejection fraction and volumes by real-time, two dimensional echocardiography. A comparison of cineangiographic and radionuclide techniques. Circulation 60:760, 1979.
14. Parisi, A.F., Moynihan, P.F., Folland, E.D., et al.: Approaches to determination of left ventricular volumes and ejection fraction by real-time two-dimensional echocardiography. Clin. Cardiol. 2:257, 1979.
15. Silverman, N.H., Ports, T.A., Snider, A.R., et al.: Determination of left ventricular volume in children: Echocardiographic and angiographic comparisons. Circulation 62:548, 1980.
16. Gueret, P., Meerbaum, S., Wyatt, H.L., et al.: Two-dimensional echocardiographic quantitation of left ventricular volumes and ejection fraction: Importance of accounting for dyssynergy in short axis reconstruction mode. Circulation 62:1308, 1980.
17. Mercier, J.C., DiSessa, T.G., Jarmarani, J.M., et al.: Two-dimensional echocardiographic assessment of left ventricular volume and ejection fraction in children. Circulation 65:962, 1982.
18. Nixon, J.V., and Saffer, S.I.: Three-dimensional echoventriculography. (Abstract.) Circulation 58:II–157, 1978.
19. Schiller, N.B., Acquatella, H., Ports, T.A., et al.: Left ventricular volume from paired biplane two-dimensional echocardiography. Circulation 60:547, 1979.
20. Wyatt, H.L., Heng, M.K., Meerbaum, S., et al.: Cross-sectional echocardiography. II. Analysis of mathematical models for quantifying volume of the formalin-fixed left ventricle. Circulation 61:1119, 1980.
21. Gehrke, J., Leeman, S., Raphael, M., et al.: Non-invasive left ventricular volume determination by two-dimensional echocardiography. Br. Heart J. 37:911, 1975.
22. Ohuchi, Y., Kuwako, K., Umeda, T., et al.: Real-time, phased-array, cross-sectional echocardiographic evaluation of left ventricular asynergy and quantitation of left ventricular function: A comparison with left ventricular cineangiography. Jpn. Heart J. 21:1, 1980.
23. Devereux, R.B., Lutas, E.M., Casale, P.N., et al.: Standardization of M-mode echocardiographic left ventricular anatomic measurements. J. Am. Coll. Cardiol. 4:1222, 1984.
24. American Society of Echocardiography Committee on Standards, Subcommittee on Quantitation of Two-Dimensional Echocardiograms: Schiller, N.B., Shah, P.M., Crawford, M., et al.: Recommendations for quantitation of the left ventricle by two-dimensional echocardiography. J. Am. Soc. Echocardiogr. 2:358, 1989.
25. Pearlman, J.D., Triuizi, M.O., King, M.E., et al.: Limits of normal left ventricular dimensions in growth and development: Analysis of dimensions and variance in the two-dimensional echocardiograms of 268 normal healthy subjects. J. Am. Coll. Cardiol. 12:1432, 1988.

26. Greenleaf, J.F., Belohalavek, M., Gerber, T.C., et al.: Multidimensional visualization in echocardiography: An introduction. Mayo Clin. Proc. 68:213, 1993.

27. Geiser, E.A., Christie, L.G., Jr., Conetta, D.A., et al.: A mechanical arm for spatial registration of two-dimensional echocardiographic sections. Cathet. Cardiovasc. Diagn. 8:89, 1982.

28. Skorton, D.J., Chandran, K.B., Nikravesh, P.E., et al.: Three-dimensional finite element reconstruction from two-dimensional echocardiograms for estimation of myocardial elastic properties. *In* Computers in Cardiology. Long Beach, Calif, I.E.E.E. Computer Society, 1981, pp. 383–386.

29. Rachlen, J.S., Triveri, S.S., Herman, G.T., et al.: Dynamic three-dimensional reconstruction of the left ventricle from two-dimensional echocardiograms. J. Am. Coll. Cardiol. 8:364, 1986.

30. Moritz, W.E., and Shreve, P.L.: A microprocessor-based spatial locating system for use with diagnostic ultrasound. Proc. I.E.E.E. 64:966, 1974.

31. Moritz, W.E., Pearlman, A.S., McCabe, D.H., et al.: An ultrasonic technique for imaging the ventricle in three dimensions and calculating its volume. I.E.E.E. Trans. Biomed. Eng. 30:482, 1983.

32. Weiss, J.L., McGaughey, M., and Guier, W.H.: Geometric considerations in determination of left ventricular mass by two-dimensional echocardiography. Hypertension 9 (Suppl. 2):85, 1987.

33. Harrison, M.R., King, D.L., King, D.L., Jr., et al.: Influence of left ventricular dilatation upon reproducibility of diameter measurements: Evaluation by three-dimensional echo. (Abstract.) J. Am. Soc. Echocardiogr. 4:292, 1991.

34. Handschumacher, M.D., Lethor, J.P., Siu, S.C., et al.: A new integrated system for three-dimensional echocardiographic reconstruction: Development and validation for ventricular volume with application in human subjects. J. Am. Coll. Cardiol. 21:743, 1993.

35. King, D.L., Harrison, M.R., King, D.L., et al.: Ultrasound beam orientation during standard two-dimensional imaging: Assessment by three-dimensional echocardiography. J. Am. Soc. Echocardiogr. 5:569, 1992.

36. Katz, A.S., Wallerson, D.C., Pini, R., et al.: Visually determined long- and short-axis parasternal views and four- and two-chamber apical echocardiographic views do not consistently represent paired orthogonal projections. Am. J. Noninvasive Cardiol. 7:65, 1993.

37. Roelandt, J.R.T.C., ten Cate, F.J., Vletter, W.B., et al.: Ultrasonic dynamic three-dimensional visualization of the heart with a multiplane transesophageal imaging transducer. J. Am. Soc. Echocardiogr. 7:217, 1994.

38. von Ramm, O.T., Smith, S.W., and Pavy, H.G., Jr.: High-speed ultrasound volumetric imaging system. Part II: Parallel processing and imaging display. I.E.E.E. Trans. Ultrason. Ferroelec. Freq. Contr. 38:109, 1991.

39. Mensah, G.A., Pini, R., Monnini, E., et al.: Three-dimensional echocardiographic reconstruction: Experimental validation of volume measurement. (Abstract.) J. Am. Coll. Cardiol. 17:291, 1991.

40. Gopal, A.S., Keller, A.M., Rigling, R., et al.: Left ventricular volume and endocardial surface area by three-dimensional echocardiography: Comparison with two-dimensional echocardiography and nuclear magnetic resonance imaging in normal subjects. J. Am. Coll. Cardiol. 22:258, 1993.

41. Schröder, K.M., Sapin, P.M., King, D.L.: Three-dimensional echocardiographic volume computation: In vitro comparison to standard two-dimensional echocardiography. J. Am. Soc. Echocardiogr. 6:467, 1993.

42. Levine, R.A., Handschumacher, M.D., Sanfilippo, A.J., et al.: Three-dimensional echocardiographic reconstruction of the mitral valve with implications for the diagnosis of mitral valve prolapse. Circulation 80:589, 1989.

43. Quinones, M.A., Waggoner A.D., Reduto, L.A., et al.: A new, simplified and accurate method for determining ejection fraction with two-dimensional echocardiography. Circulation 64:744, 1981.

44. Rich, S., Sheikh, A., Gallastegui, J., et al.: Determination of left ventricular ejection fraction by visual estimation during real-time two-dimensional echocardiography. Am. Heart J. 104:603, 1982.

45. Cahalan, M.K., Ionescu, P., Melton, H.E.J., et al.: Automated real-time analysis of intraoperative transesophageal echocardiograms. Anesthesiology 78:447, 1993.

46. Garcia, E., Gueret, P., Bennett, M., et al.: Real time computerization of two-dimensional echocardiography. Am. Heart J. 101:783, 1981.

47. Geiser, E.A., Conetta, D.A., Limacher, M.C., et al.: A second generation computer-based edge detection algorithm for short axis, two-dimensional echocardiographic images: Accuracy and improvement in interobserver variability. J. Am. Soc. Echocardiogr. 3:79, 1990.

48. Jenkins, R.E., and Garrison, J.B.: Automatic contouring for two dimensional echocardiography. Johns Hopkins APL Tech. Digest: 1139, 1980.

49. Shah, P.M., Crawford, M., DeMaria, A., et al.: Recommendations for quantitation of the left ventricle by two-dimensional echocardiography. J. Am. Soc. Echocardiogr. 2:358, 1989.

50. Skorton, D.J., McNary, C.A., Child, J.S., et al.: Digital image processing of two-dimensional echocardiograms: Identification of endocardium. Am. J. Cardiol. 48:479, 1981.

51. Zhang, L.F., and Geiser, E.A.: An effective algorithm for extracting serial endocardial borders from two-dimensional echocardiograms. IEEE Trans. Biomed. Eng. 31:441, 1984.

52. Perez, J.E., Waggoner, A.D., Barzilai, B., et al.: On-line assessment of ventricular function by automatic boundary detection and ultrasonic backscatter imaging. J. Am. Coll. Cardiol. 19:313, 1992.

53. Vandenberg, B.F., Rath, L.S., Atuhlmuller, P., et al.: Estimation of left ventricular cavity area with an on-line, semiautomated echocardiographic edge detection system. Circulation 86:159, 1992.

54. Gorcsan, J., Morita, S., Mandarino, W.A., et al.: Two-dimensional echocardiographic automated border detection accurately reflects changes in left ventricular volume. J. Am. Soc. Echo Cardiogr. 6:482, 1993.

55. Morrissey, R.L., Siu, S.C., Guerrero, J.L., et al.: Automated assessment of ventricular volume and function by echocardiography: Validation of automated border detection. J. Am. Soc. Echocardiogr. 7:107, 1994.

56. Gorcsan, J., III Lazar, J.M., Schulman, D.S., et al.: Comparison of left ventricular function by echocardiographic automated border detection and by radionuclide ejection fraction. Am. J. Cardiol. 72:810, 1993.

57. Lindower, P.D., Rath, L., Preslar, J., et al.: Quantification of left ventricular function with an automated border detection system and comparison with radionuclide ventriculography. Am. J. Cardiol. 73:195, 1994.

58. Steward, W.J., Rodkey, S.M., Gunawardena, S., et al.: Left ventricular volume calculation with integrated backscatter from echocardiography. J. Am. Soc. Echocardiogr. 6:553, 1993.

59. Perez, J.E., Klein, S.C., Prater, D.M., et al.: Automated, on-line quantification of left ventricular dimensions and function by echocardiography with backscatter imaging and lateral gain compensation. Am. J. Cardiol. 70:1200, 1992.

60. Martin, R.P.: Real time ultrasound quantification of ventricular function: Has the eyeball been replaced or will the subjective become objective? J. Am. Coll. Cardiol. 19:321, 1992.

61. Foster, E., and Cahalan, M.K.: The search for intelligent quantitation in echocardiography: "Eyeball," "trackball," and beyond. J. Am. Coll. Cardiol. 22:848, 1993.

62. Herregods, M.C., Vermylen, J., Byness, B., et al.: On-line quantification of left ventricular function by automatic boundary detection and ultrasonic backscatter imaging. Am. J. Cardiol. 72(3):359, 1993.

63. Marcus, R.H., Bednarz, J., Coulden, R., et al.: Ultrasonic backscatter system for automated on-line endocardial boundary detection: Evaluation by ultrafast computed tomography. J. Am. Coll. Cardiol. 22:839, 1993.

64. Martin, G.R., Seibel, N.L., and Majd, M.: Real-time, automated echocardiographic measures of ventricular area and area change: Comparison with radionuclide technique. Echocardiography 11:111, 1994.

65. Stoddard, M.F., Keedy, D.L., and Longaker, R.A.: Two-dimensional transesophageal echocardiographic characterization of ventricular filling in real time by acoustic quantification: Comparison with pulsed Doppler echocardiography. J. Am. Soc. Echocardiogr. 7:116, 1994.

66. Grossman, W., Braunwald, E., Mann, T., et al.: Contractile state of the left ventricle in man as evaluated from end-systolic pressure-volume relations. Circulation 56:845, 1977.

67. Reichek, N., Wilson, J., St. John Sutton, M., et al.: Noninvasive determination of left ventricular end-systolic stress: Validation of the method and initial application. Circulation 65:99, 1982.

68. Borow, K.M., Neumann, A., and Wynne, J.: Sensitivity of end-systolic pressure-dimension and pressure-volume relations to the inotropic state in humans. Circulation 65:988, 1982.

69. Kameyama, T., Asanoi, H., Ishizaka, S., et al.: Ventricular load optimization by unloading therapy in patients with heart failure. J. Am. Coll. Cardiol. 17:199, 1991.

70. Gorcsan, J.J., III, Morita, S., Mandarino, W.A., et al.: Two-dimensional echocardiographic automated border detection accurately reflects changes in left ventricular volume. J. Am. Soc. Echocardiogr. 6:482, 1993.

71. Devereux, R.B., and Reichek, N.: Echocardiographic determination of left ventricular mass in man. Anatomic validation of the method. Circulation 55:613, 1977.

72. Woythaler, J.N., Singer, S.L., Kwan, O.L., et al.: Accuracy of echocardiography versus electrocardiography in detecting left ventricular hypertrophy: Comparison with post-mortem mass measurements. J. Am. Coll. Cardiol. 2:305, 1983.

73. Reichek, N., and Devereux, R.B.: Left ventricular hypertrophy: Relationship of anatomic, echocardiographic and electrocardiographic findings. Circulation 63:1391, 1981.

74. Bikkina, M., Levy, D., Evans, J.C., et al.: Left ventricular mass and risk of stroke in an elderly cohort. The Framingham Heart Study. JAMA 272:33, 1994.

75. Devereux, R.B.: Detection of left ventricular hypertrophy by M-mode echocardiography. Anatomic validation, standardization, and comparison to other methods. Hypertension 9:II–9, 1987.

76. Byrd, B.F., Wahr, D., Wang, Y.S., et al.: Left ventricular mass and volume/mass ratio determined by two-dimensional echocardiography in normal adults. J. Am. Coll. Cardiol. 6:1021, 1985.

77. Helak, J.W., and Reichek, N.: Quantitation of human left ventricular mass and volume by two-dimensional echocardiography: In vitro anatomic validation. Circulation 63:1398, 1981.

78. Reichek, N., Helak, J., Plappert, T., et al.: Anatomic validation of left ventricular mass estimates from clinical two-dimensional echocardiography: Initial results. Circulation 67:348, 1983.

79. Gopal, A.S., Keller, A.M., Shen, Z., et al.: Three-dimensional echocardiography: In vitro and in vivo validation of left ventricular mass and comparison with conventional echocardiographic methods. J. Am. Coll. Cardiol. 24:504, 1994.

80. Casale, P.N., Devereux, R.B., Milner, M., et al.: Value of echocardiographic measurement of left ventricular mass in predicting cardiovascular morbid events in hypertensive men. Ann. Intern. Med. 105:173, 1986.

81. Koren, M.J., Devereux, R.B., Casale, P.N., et al.: Relation of left ventricular mass and geometry to morbidity and mortality in uncomplicated essential hypertension. Ann. Intern. Med. 114:345, 1991.

82. Levy, D., Anderson, K.M., Savage, D.D., et al.: Echocardiographically detected left ventricular hypertrophy: Prevalence and risk factors (The Framingham Heart Study). Ann. Intern. Med. 108:7, 1988.

83. Levy, D., Garrison, R.J., Savage, D.D., et al.: Prognostic implications of echocardiographically determined left ventricular mass in the Framingham Heart Study. N. Engl. J. Med. 322:1561, 1990.

84. Gibson, R.S., Bishop, H.L., Stamm, R.B., et al.: Value of early two dimensional

echocardiography in patients with acute myocardial infarction. Am. J. Cardiol. 49:1110, 1982.

85. Heger, J.J., Weyman, A.E., Wann, L.S., et al.: Cross-sectional echocardiography in acute myocardial infarction: Detection and localization of regional ventricular asynergy. Circulation 60:531, 1979.

86. Nixon, J.V., Brown, C.N., and Smitherman, T.C.: Identification of transient and persistent segmental wall motion abnormalities in patients with unstable angina by two-dimensional echocardiography. Circulation 65:1497, 1982.

87. Kisslo, J.A., Robertson, D., Gilbert, B.W., et al.: A comparison of real-time, two-dimensional echocardiography and cineangiography in detecting left ventricular asynergy. Circulation 55:134, 1977.

88. Nixon, J.V., Narahara, K.A., and Smitherman, T.C.: Estimation of myocardial involvement in patients with acute myocardial infarction by two-dimensional echocardiography. Circulation 62:1248, 1980.

89. Horowitz, R.S., Morganroth, J., Parrotto, G., et al.: Immediate diagnosis of acute myocardial infarction by two-dimensional echocardiography. Circulation 65:323, 1982.

90. Chaitman, B.R., DeMots, H., Brislow, J.D., et al.: Objective and subjective analysis of left ventricular angiograms. Circulation 52:420, 1975.

91. Zir, L.M., Miller, S.W., Dinsmore, R.E., et al.: Interobserver variability in coronary angiography. Circulation 53:627, 1976.

92. Isaacsohn, J.L., Earle, M.G., Kemper, A.J., et al.: Postmyocardial infarction pain and infarct extension in the coronary care unit: Role of two-dimensional echocardiography. J. Am. Coll. Cardiol. 11:2, 246, 1988.

93. Bhatnagar, S.K., Moussa, M.A.A., and Al-Yusut, A.: The role of prehospital discharge two-dimensional echocardiography in determining the prognosis of survivors of first myocardial infarction. Am. Heart J. 109:472, 1985.

94. Nishimura, R.A., Reeder, G.S., Miller, F.A., Jr., et al.: Prognostic value of predischarge 2-dimensional echocardiogram after acute myocardial infarction. Am. J. Cardiol. 53:429, 1984.

95. Van Reet, R.E., Quinones, M.A., Poliner, L.R., et al.: Comparison of two-dimensional echocardiography with gated radionuclide ventriculography in the evaluation of global and regional left ventricular function in acute myocardial infarction. J. Am. Coll. Cardiol. 3:243, 1984.

96. Edwards, W.D., Tajik, A.J., and Seward, J.B.: Standardized nomenclature and anatomic basis for regional tomographic analysis of the heart. Mayo Clin. Proc. 56:479, 1981.

97. Herman, M.V., and Gorlin, R.: Implications of left ventricular asynergy. Am. J. Cardiol. 23:538, 1969.

98. Gillam, L.D., Hogan, R.D., Foale, R.A., et al.: A comparison of quantitative echocardiographic methods for delineating infarct-induced abnormal wall motion. Circulation 70:113, 1984.

99. Parisi, A.F.: Two-dimensional echocardiographic examination for quantitative detection of regional wall motion abnormalities. In Giuliani, E.R. (ed.): Two-Dimensional Real-Time Ultrasonic Imaging of the Heart. Boston, Martinus Nijhoff, 1985, p. 221.

100. Falsetti, H.L., Marcus, M.L., Kerber, R.E., et al.: Quantification of myocardial ischemia and infarction by left ventricular imaging. (Editorial.) Circulation 63:747, 1981.

101. Kerber, R.E., Marcus, M.L., Ehrhardt, J., et al.: Correlation between echocardiographically demonstrated segmental dyskinesis and regional myocardial perfusion. Circulation 52:1097, 1975.

102. Wyatt, H.L., Forrester, J.S., daLuz, P.L., et al.: Functional abnormalities in nonoccluded regions of myocardium after experimental coronary occlusion. Am. J. Cardiol. 37:366, 1976.

103. Bogen, D.K., Rabinowitz, S.A., Needleman, A., et al.: An analysis of the mechanical disadvantage of myocardial infarction in the canine left ventricle. Circ. Res. 47:728, 1980.

104. Force, T., Kemper, A.J., Perkins, L., et al.: Overestimation of infarct size by quantitative two-dimensional echocardiography—the role of tethering and of analytic procedures. Circulation 73:1360, 1986.

105. Cox, D., and Vatner, S.F.: Disparity between regional myocardial function and blood flow at the ischemic border. Circulation 66 (Suppl. II):II–1, 1982.

106. Cox D.A., and Vatner, S.F.: Myocardial function in areas of heterogenous perfusion after coronary artery occlusion in conscious dogs. Circulation 66:1154, 1982.

107. Gallagher, K.P., Gerren, R.A., Stirling, M.C., et al.: The distribution of functional impairment across the lateral border of acutely ischemic myocardium. Circ. Res. 58:570, 1986.

108. Gallagher, K.P., Gerren, R.A., Ning, X-H., et al.: The functional border zone in conscious dogs. Lab. Invest. 76:4, 1987.

109. Homans, D.C., Asinger, R., Elsperger, J., et al.: Regional function and perfusion at the lateral border of ischemic myocardium. Circulation 71:1038, 1985.

110. Gallagher, K.P., McClanahan, T.B., Lynch, M.J., et al.: Occlusion of the left anterior descending artery produces a larger functional border zone than circumflex occlusion. (Abstract.) Circulation 76(Suppl. IV):IV–373, 1987.

111. Weiss, R.M., and Marcus, M.L.: The extent of regional systolic dysfunction during acute ischemia is load-dependent. (Abstract.) Circulation 78 (Suppl. II)II–484, 1988.

112. Gallagher, K.P., Kumada, T., Koziol, J.A., et al.: Significance of regional wall thickening abnormalities relative to transmural myocardial perfusion in anesthetized dogs. Circulation 62:1266, 1980.

113. Myers, J.H., Stirling, M.C., Choy, M., et al.: Direct measurement of inner and outer wall thickening dynamics with epicardial echocardiography. Circulation 74:164, 1986.

114. Sabbah, H.N., Marzilli, M., and Stein, P.D.: The relative role of subendocardium and subepicardium in left ventricular mechanics. Am. J. Physiol. 240:4920, 1981.

115. Gallagher, K.P., Stirling, M.C., and Choy, M.: Dissociation between epicardial

and transmural function during acute myocardial ischemia. Circulation 71:1279, 1985.

116. Gallagher, K.P., Osakada, G., Hess, O.M., et al.: Subepicardial segmental function during coronary stenosis and the role of myocardial fiber orientation. Circ. Res. 50:352, 1982.

117. Weintraub, W.S., Hattori, S., Agarwal, J.B., et al.: The relationship between myocardial blood flow and contraction by myocardial layer in the canine left ventricle during ischemia. Circ. Res. 48:430, 1981.

118. Heyndrickx, G.R., Millard, R.W., McRitchie, R.J., et al.: Regional myocardial function and electrophysiologic alterations after brief coronary artery occlusion in conscious dogs. J. Clin. Invest. 56:978, 1975.

119. Kloner, R.A., DeBoer, L.W.V., Darsee, J.R., et al.: Recovery of cardiac function and adenosine triphosphate requiring 7 days of reperfusion following 15 minutes of ischemia. Clin. Res. 29:562A, 1981.

120. Theroux, P., Ross, J., Jr., Franklin, D., et al.: Regional myocardial function in the conscious dog during acute coronary occlusion and responses to morphine, propranolol, nitroglycerin, and lidocaine. Circulation 53:302, 1976.

121. Wyatt, H.L., Meerbaum, S., Heng, M.K., et al.: Experimental evaluation of the extent of myocardial dyssynergy and infarct size by two-dimensional echocardiography. Circulation 63:607, 1981.

122. Blumenthal, D.S., Becker, L.C., Bulkley, B.H., et al.: Impaired function of salvaged myocardium: Two-dimensional echocardiographic quantification of regional wall thickening in the open-chest dog. Circulation 67:225, 1983.

123. Ellis, S.G., Henschke, C.I., Sandor, T., et al.: Time course of functional and biochemical recovery of myocardium salvaged by reperfusion. J. Am. Coll. Cardiol. 1:1047, 1983.

124. Hammerman, H., O'Boyle, J.E., Cohen, C., et al.: Dissociation between two-dimensional echocardiographic left ventricular wall motion and myocardial salvage in early experimental acute myocardial infarction in dogs. Am. J. Cardiol. 54:875, 1964.

125. Taylor, A.L., Kieso, R.A., Melton, J., et al.: Echocardiographically detected dyskinesis, myocardial infarct size, and coronary risk region relationships in reperfused canine myocardium. Circulation 71:1292, 1985.

126. Chaitman, B.R., Bristow, J.D., and Rahimtoola, S.H.: Left ventricular wall motion assessed by using fixed external reference systems. Circulation 47:1043, 1973.

127. Clayton, P.D., Jeppson, G.M., and Klausner, S.C.: Should a fixed external reference system be used to analyze left ventricular wall motion? Circulation 65:1518, 1982.

128. Gelberg, H.J., Brundage, B.H., Glantz, S., et al.: Quantitative left ventricular wall motion analysis: A comparison of area, chord and radial methods. Circulation 59:991, 1979.

129. Ingels, N.B., Jr., Daughters, G.T., II, Stinson, E.B., et al.: Evaluation of methods for quantitating left ventricular wall motion in man using myocardial markers as a standard. Circulation 61:966, 1980.

130. Karsch, K.R., Lamm, U., Blanke, H., et al.: Comparison of nineteen quantitative models for assessment of localized left ventricular wall motion abnormalities. Clin. Cardiol. 3:123, 1980.

131. Sheehan, F.H., Stewart, A.K., Dodge, H.T., et al.: Variability in the measurement of regional left ventricular wall motion from contrast angiograms. Circulation 68:550, 1983.

132. Urie, P.M., Jensen, R.L., Clayton, P.D., et al.: Comparison of methods for quantifying segmental wall motion. (Abstract.) Circulation 56 (Suppl. III):III–238, 1977.

133. Erbel, R., Krebs, W., Henn, G., et al.: Comparison of single-plane and biplane volume determination by two-dimensional echocardiography. I. Asymmetric model hearts. Eur. Heart J. 3:469, 1982.

134. Henschke, C.I., Risser, T.A., Sandor, T., et al.: Quantitative computer assisted analysis of left ventricular wall thickening and motion by 2-dimensional echocardiography in acute myocardial infarction. Am. J. Cardiol. 52:960, 1983.

135. Fujii, J., Sawada, H., Aizawa, T., et al.: Computer analysis of cross sectional echocardiogram for quantitative evaluation of left ventricular asynergy in myocardial infarction. Br. Heart J. 51:139, 1984.

136. Loperfido, F., Mongiardo, R., Pennestri, F., et al.: Variability of normal regional wall motion and recognition of dyssynergy by angiography and two-dimensional echocardiography in myocardial infarction. J. Cardiovasc. Ultrasonogr. 4:175, 1985.

137. Parisi, A.F., Moynihan, P.F., Folland, E.D., et al.: Quantitative detection of regional left ventricular contraction abnormalities by two-dimensional echocardiography. II. Accuracy in coronary artery disease. Circulation 63:761, 1981.

138. Grube, E., Hanisch, H., Neumann, G., et al.: Quantitative evaluation of LV-wall motion by two-dimensional echocardiography (2-DE). (Abstract.) J. Am. Coll. Cardiol. 1:581, 1983.

139. Schnittger, I., Fitzgerald, P.J., Gordon, E.P., et al.: Computerized quantitative analysis of left ventricular wall motion by two-dimensional echocardiography. Circulation 70:242, 1984.

140. Zanolla, L., Marino, P., Golia, G., et al.: Intraobserver reproducibility of quantitative two-dimensional echocardiography. Analysis of left ventricular area-time curve and of regional wall motion with two-frame and frame-by-frame methods. J. Cardiovasc. Ultrasonogr. 4:211, 1980.

141. Zoghbi, W.A., Charlat, M.L., Bolli, R., et al.: Quantitative assessment of left ventricular wall motion by two-dimensional echocardiography: Validation during reversible ischemia in the conscious dog. J. Am. Coll. Cardiol. 11:4, 185, 1988.

142. Pandian, N.G., Skorton, D.J., Collins, S.M., et al.: Heterogeneity of left ventricular segmental wall thickening and excursion in 2-dimensional echocardiograms of normal human subjects. Am. J. Cardiol. 51:1667, 1983.

143. Moynihan, P.F., Parisi, A.F., and Feldman, C.L.: Quantitative detection of re-

gional left ventricular contraction abnormalities by two-dimensional echocardiography. I. Analysis of methods. Circulation 63:752, 1981.

144. Nieminen, M., Parisi, A.F., O'Boyle, J.E., et al.: Serial evaluation of myocardial thickening and thinning in acute experimental infarction: Identification and quantification using two-dimensional echocardiography. Circulation 66:174, 1982.

145. Pandian, N.G., Skorton, D.J., Collins, S.M., et al.: Myocardial infarct size threshold for two-dimensional echocardiographic detection: Sensitivity of systolic wall thickening and endocardial motion abnormalities in small versus large infarcts. Am. J. Cardiol. 55:551, 1985.

146. Kaul, S., Pandian, N.G., Gillam, L.D., et al.: Contrast echocardiography in acute myocardial ischemia. III. An in vivo comparison of the extent of abnormal wall motion with the area at risk for necrosis. J. Am. Coll. Cardiol. 7:383, 1986.

147. Mann, D.L., Foale, R.A., Ascah, K.J., et al.: Persistence of abnormal wall motion in the canine ventricle after subacute infarction: Implications for reperfusion therapy. (Abstract.) J. Am. Coll. Cardiol. 5:425, 1985.

148. Feiring, A.J., Rumberger, J.A., Reiter, S.J., et al.: Sectional and segmental variability of left ventricular function experimental and clinical studies using ultrafast computed tomography. J. Am. Coll. Cardiol. 12:2, 415, 1988.

149. Haendchen, R.V., Wyatt, H.L., Maurer, G., et al.: Quantitation of regional cardiac function by two-dimensional echocardiography. I. Patterns of contraction in the normal left ventricle. Circulation 67:1234, 1983.

150. LeWinter, M.M., Kent, R.S., Kroener, J.M., et al.: Regional differences in myocardial performance in the left ventricle of the dog. Circ. Res. 37:191, 1975.

151. Kong, Y., Morris, J.J., Jr., and McIntosh, H.D.: Assessment of regional myocardial performance from biplane cineangiograms. Am. J. Cardiol. 27:529, 1971.

152. Klausner, S.C., Blair, T.J., Bulawa, W.F., et al.: Quantitative analysis of segmental wall motion throughout systole and diastole in the normal human left ventricle. Circulation 65:580, 1982.

153. Marier, D.L., and Gibson, D.G.: Limitations of two frame method for displaying regional left ventricular wall motion in man. Br. Heart J. 44:555, 1980.

154. Slager, C.J., Hooghoudt, T.E.H., Serruys, P.W., et al.: Quantitative assessment of regional left ventricular motion using endocardial landmarks. J. Am. Coll. Cardiol. 7:317, 1986.

155. Ingels, N.B., Daughters, G.T., II, Stinson, E.B., et al.: Measurement of mid-wall myocardial dynamics in intact man by radiography of surgically implanted markers. Circulation 52:859, 1975.

156. Force, T., Bloomfield, P., O'Boyle, J.E., et al.: Quantitative two-dimensional echocardiographic analysis of motion and thickening of the interventricular septum after cardiac surgery. Circulation 68:1013, 1983.

157. Force, T., Bloomfield, P., O'Boyle, J.E., et al.: Quantitative two-dimensional echocardiographic analysis of regional wall motion in patients with perioperative myocardial infarction. Circulation 70:233, 1984.

158. Force, T., Kemper, A.J., Bloomfield, P., et al.: Non-Q wave perioperative myocardial infarction: Assessment of the incidence and severity of regional dysfunction with quantitative two-dimensional echocardiography. Circulation 72:781, 1985.

159. Sakamaki, T., Lang, D., Wong, O.Y., et al.: Comparative validation of two-dimensional echocardiographic segmental wall motion analysis methods. (Abstract.) J. Am. Coll. Cardiol. 1:581, 1983.

160. Shapiro, E.P., Buchalter, M.B., Rogers, W.J., et al.: LV twist is greater with inotropic stimulation and less with regional ischemia. (Abstract.) Circulation (Suppl. II):II–466, 1988.

161. Mirro, M.J., Rogers, E.W., Weyman, A.E., et al.: Angular displacement of the papillary muscles during the cardiac cycle. Circulation 60:327, 1979.

162. Bolson, E.L., Kliman, S., Sheehan, F., et al.: Left ventricular segmental wall motion—a new method using local direction information. IEEE Comput. Cardiol. 1980, p. 245.

163. McGillem, M.J., Mancini, G.B.J., DeBoe, S.F., et al.: Modification of the centerline method for assessment of echocardiographic wall thickening and motion: A comparison with areas of risk. J. Am. Coll. Cardiol. II:4, 861, 1988.

164. Gibson, D.G., Doran, J.H., Traill, T.A., et al.: Abnormal left ventricular wall movement during early systole in patients with angina pectoris. Br. Heart J. 40:758, 1978.

165. Johnson, L.L., Ellis, K., Schmidt, O., et al.: Volume ejected in early systole, a sensitive index of left ventricular performance in coronary artery disease. Circulation 52:378, 1975.

166. Leighton, R.F., Pollack, M.E.M., and Welch, T.G.: Abnormal left ventricular wall motion at mid-ejection in patients with coronary heart disease. Circulation 52:238, 1975.

167. Sniderman, A., Marpole, D., and Fallen, E.: Regional contraction patterns in the normal and ischemic left ventricle in man. Am. J. Cardiol. 31:484, 1973.

168. Slutsky, R., Karliner, J.S., Battler, A., et al.: Comparison of early systolic and holosystolic ejection phase indexes by contrast ventriculography in patients with coronary artery disease. Circulation 61:1083, 1980.

169. Weyman, A.E., Franklin, T.D., Hogan, R.D., et al.: Importance of temporal heterogeneity in assessing the contraction abnormalities associated with acute myocardial ischemia. Circulation 70:102, 1984.

170. Thomas, J.D., Hagege, A.A., Choong, C.Y., et al.: Improved accuracy of echocardiographic endocardial borders by spatiotemporal filtered Fourier reconstruction: Description of the method and optimization of filter cutoffs. Circulation 77:415, 1988.

171. Mancini, G.B.J., DeBoe, S.F., Lefree, M.T., et al.: Quantitative regional curvature: A comparison of shape vs wall motion analysis. (Abstract.) Circulation (Suppl. II):II–498, 1986.

172. Force, T., Kemper, A., Leavitt, M., et al.: Acute reduction in functional infarct expansion with late reperfusion: Assessment with quantitative two-dimensional echocardiography. J. Am. Coll. Cardiol. 11:192, 1988.

173. Heng, M.K., Lang, T.W., Takashi, T., et al.: Quantification of myocardial ischemic damage by two-dimensional echocardiography. (Abstract.) Circulation 56 (Suppl. III):III–125, 1977.

174. Meltzer, R.S., Woythaler, J.N., Buda, A.J., et al.: Non-invasive quantification of experimental canine myocardial infarct size using two-dimensional echocardiography. Eur. J. Cardiol. 11:215, 1980.

175. Weiss, J.L., Bulkley, B.H., Hutchins, G.M., et al.: Two-dimensional echocardiographic recognition of myocardial injury in man: Comparison with postmortem studies. Circulation 63:401, 1981.

176. Weyman, A.E., Franklin, T.D., Egenes, K.M., et al.: Correlation between extent of abnormal regional wall motion and myocardial infarct size in chronically infarcted dogs. Circulation 56 (Suppl. III):III–72, 1977.

177. Lieberman, A.N., Weiss, J.L., Jugdutt, B.J., et al.: Two-dimensional echocardiography and infarct size: Relationship of regional wall motion and thickening to the extent of myocardial infarction in the dog. Circulation 63:739, 1981.

178. Kaul, S., Glasheen, W., Ruddy, T.D., et al.: The importance of defining left ventricular area at risk in vivo during acute myocardial infarction: An experimental evaluation with myocardial contrast two-dimensional echocardiography. Circulation 75:1249, 1987.

179. Guyer, D.E., Foale, R.A., Gillam, L.D., et al.: An echocardiographic technique for quantifying and displaying the extent of regional left ventricular dyssynergy. J. Am. Coll. Cardiol. 8:830, 1986.

180. Guyer, D.E., Gibson, T.C., Gillam, L.D., et al.: A new echocardiographic model for quantifying three-dimensional endocardial surface area. J. Am. Coll. Cardiol. 8:819, 1986.

181. Picard, M.H., Wilkins, G.T., Ray, P.A., et al.: Natural history of left ventricular size and function after acute myocardial infarction: Assessment and prediction by echocardiographic endocardial surface mapping. Circulation 82:484, 1990.

182. Wilkins, G.T., Southern, J.F., Choong, C.Y., et al.: Correlation between echocardiographic endocardial surface mapping of abnormal wall motion and pathologic infarct size in autopsied hearts. Circulation 77:978, 1988.

183. Geiser, E.A., Skorton, D.J., and Conetta, D.A.: Quantification of left ventricular function by two-dimensional echocardiography: Consideration of factors restricting image quality. Am. Heart J. 103:905, 1982.

184. Meister, S.G., Casey, P.R., Jacobs, L., et al.: 2D echo definition of endocardium. Circulation 62 (Suppl. III):III–132, 1980.

185. Fedele, F., Penco, M., and Dagianti, A.: Quantification of left ventricular regional wall thickening in two-dimensional echocardiography: Analysis of a new semiautomated method. J. Cardiovasc. Ultrasonogr. 4:201, 1985.

186. Lima, J.A.C., Becker, L.C., Melin, J.A., et al.: Impaired thickening of nonischemic myocardium during acute regional ischemia in the dog. Circulation 71:1048, 1985.

187. Watanabe, T., Katsume, H., Matsukubo, H., et al.: Estimation of right ventricular volume with two dimensional echocardiography. Am. J. Cardiol. 49:1946, 1982.

188. Sasayama, S., Franklin, D., Ross, J., Jr., et al.: Dynamic changes in left ventricular wall thickness and their use in analyzing cardiac function in the conscious dog. A study based on modified ultrasonic technique. Am. J. Cardiol 38:870, 1976.

189. Heikkila, J., Tabakin, B.S., and Hugenholtz, P.G.: Quantification of function in normal and infarcted regions of the left ventricle. Cardiovasc. Res. 6:516, 1972.

190. Pandian, N.G., and Kerber, R.E.: Two-dimensional echocardiography in experimental coronary stenosis. I. Sensitivity and specificity in detecting transient myocardial dyskinesis: Comparison with sonomicrometers. Circulation 66:597, 1982.

191. Pandian, N.G., Kieso, R.A., and Kerber, R.E.: Two-dimensional echocardiography in experimental coronary stenosis. II. Relationship between systolic wall thinning and regional myocardial perfusion in severe coronary stenosis. Circulation 66:603, 1982.

192. O'Boyle, J.E., Parisi, A.F., Nieminen, M., et al.: Quantitative detection of regional left ventricular contraction abnormalities by two-dimensional echocardiography. Comparison of myocardial thickening and thinning and endocardial motion in a canine model. Am. J. Cardiol. 51:1732, 1983.

193. Pandian, N.G., Koyanagi, S., Skorton, D.J., et al.: Relations between 2-dimensional echocardiographic wall thickening abnormalities, myocardial infarct size and coronary risk area in normal and hypertrophied myocardium in dogs. Am. J. Cardiol. 52:1318, 1983.

194. Ellis, S.G., Henschke, C.I., Sandor, T., et al.: Relation between the transmural extent of acute myocardial contractility and associated myocardial contractility two weeks after infarction. Am. J. Cardiol. 55:1412, 1985.

195. Savage, R.M., Guth, B., White, F.C., et al.: Correlation of regional myocardial blood flow and function with myocardial infarct size during acute myocardial ischemia in the conscious pig. Circulation 64:699, 1981.

196. Garrison, J.B., Weiss, J.L., Maughan, W.L., et al.: Quantitative regional wall motion and thickening in two-dimensional echocardiography with a computer-aided contouring system. In Ostrow, H., and Ripley, K. (eds.): Proceedings of Computers in Cardiology. Long Beach, Calif, IEEE, 1977.

197. Armstrong, W.F., Conley, M.J., Dillon, J.C., et al.: Systolic expansion of infarcted myocardium explains the overestimation of infarct size by wall motion analysis (Abstract.) J. Am. Coll. Cardiol. 3:513, 1984.

198. Bates, J.R., Ryan, T., Rimmerman, C.M., et al.: Color coding of digitized echocardiograms: Description of a new technique and application in detecting and correcting for cardiac transplantation. J. Am. Soc. Echocardiogr. 7:363, 1994.

199. Kagan, A.: Dynamic responses of the right ventricle following extensive damage by cauterization. Circulation 5:816, 1952.

200. Starr, I., Jeffers, W.A., and Meade, R.H., Jr.: The absence of conspicuous increments of venous pressure after severe damage to the right ventricle of the dog, with a discussion of the relationship between clinical congestive heart failure and heart disease. Am. Heart J. 26:291, 1943.

201. Cohn, J.N., Guiha, N.H., Broder, M.I., et al.: Right ventricular infarction. Clinical and hemodynamic features. Am. J. Cardiol. 33:209, 1974.
202. Matsumoto, M., and Matsuo, H.: Echocardiography for the evaluation of the tricuspid valve, right ventricle, and atrium. Prog. Cardiovasc. Dis. 21:1, 1978.
203. Feigenbaum, H.: Echocardiography. Philadelphia, Lea & Febiger, 1986.
204. Popp, R.L., Wolfe, S.B., Hirata, T., et al.: Estimation of right and left ventricular size by ultrasound. A study of the echoes from the interventricular septum. Am. J. Cardiol. 24:523, 1969.
205. Sahn, D.J., DeMaria, A., Kisslo, J., et al.: Recommendations regarding quantitation in M-mode echocardiography: Results of a survey of echocardiographic measurements. Circulation 58:1072, 1978.
206. Bommer, W., Weinert, L., Neumann, A., et al.: Determination of right atrial and right ventricular size by two-dimensional echocardiography. Circulation 60:91, 1979.
207. Aebischer, N.M., and Czegledy, F.: Determination of right ventricular volume by two dimensional echocardiography with a crescentic model. J. Am. Soc. Echocardiogr. 2:110, 1989.
208. Kaul, S., Tei, C., Hopkins, J.M., et al.: Assessment of right ventricular function using two-dimensional echocardiography. Am. Heart J. 107:526, 1984.
209. Levine, R.A., Gibson, T.C., Aretz, T., et al.: Echocardiographic measurement of right ventricular volume. Circulation 69:497, 1983.
210. Ninomiya, K., Duncan, W.J., Cook, D.H., et al.: Right ventricular ejection fraction and volumes after Mustard repair: Correlation of two dimensional echocardiograms and cineangiograms. Am. J. Cardiol. 48:317, 1981.
211. Panidis, I.P., Ren, J.F., Kotler, M.N., et al.: Two-dimensional echocardiographic estimation of right ventricular ejection fraction in patients with coronary artery disease. J. Am. Coll. Cardiol. 2:911, 1983.
212. Saito, A., Ueda, K., and Nakano, H.: Right ventricular volume determination by two-dimensional echocardiography. J. Cardiogr. 11:1159, 1981.
213. Starling, M.R., Crawford, M.H., Sorensen, S.G., et al.: A new two-dimensional echocardiographic technique for evaluating right ventricular size and performance in patients with obstructive lung disease. Circulation 66:612, 1982.
214. Silverman, N.H., and Hudson, S.: Evaluation of right ventricular volume and ejection fraction in children by two-dimensional echocardiography. Pediatr. Cardiol. 4:197, 1983.
215. Trowitzsch, E., Colan, S.D., and Sanders, S.P.: Two-dimensional echocardiographic estimation of right ventricular area change and ejection fraction in infants with systemic right ventricle (transposition of the great arteries or hypoplastic left heart syndrome). Am. J. Cardiol. 55:1153, 1985.
216. Wann, L.S., Stickels, K.R., Bamrah, V.S., et al.: Digital processing of contrast echocardiograms: A new technique for measuring right ventricular ejection fraction. Am. J. Cardiol. 53:1164, 1984.
217. Tomita, M., Masuda, H., Sumi, T., et al.: Estimation of right ventricular volume by modified echocardiographic subtraction method. Am. Heart J. 123:1011, 1992.
218. Force, T.L., Folland, E.D., Aebischer, N., et al.: Echocardiographic assessment of ventricular function. In Marcus, M.L., Schelbert, H.R., Skorton, D.J., et al. (eds.): Cardiac Imaging. Philadelphia, W.B. Saunders, 1991.
219. Jiang, L., Handschumacher, M.D., Hibberd, M.G., et al.: Three-dimensional echocardiographic reconstruction of right ventricular volume: In vitro comparison with two-dimensional methods. J. Am. Soc. Echocardiogr. 7:150, 1994.
220. Jiang, L., Siu, S.C., Handschumacher, M.D., et al.: Three-dimensional echocardiography: In vivo validation of right ventricular volume and function. Circulation 89:2342, 1994.
221. D'Arcy, B., and Nanda, N.C.: Two-dimensional echocardiographic features of right ventricular infarction. Circulation 65:167, 1982.
222. Jugdutt, B.I., Sussex, B.A., Sivaram, C.A., et al.: Right ventricular infarction: Two-dimensional echocardiographic evaluation. Am. Heart J. 107:505, 1984.
223. Panidis, I.P., Kotler, M.N., Mintz, G.S., et al.: Right ventricular function in coronary artery disease as assessed by two-dimensional echocardiography. Am. Heart J. 107:1187, 1984.
224. Sharpe, D.N., Botvinick, E.H., Shamos, D.M., et al.: The noninvasive diagnosis of right ventricular infarction. Circulation 57:483, 1978.
225. Arditti, A., Lewin, R.F., Hellman, C., et al.: Right ventricular dysfunction in acute inferoposterior myocardial infarction. An echocardiographic and isotopic study. Chest 87:307, 1985.
226. Sharkey, S.W., Shelley, W., Carlyle, P.F., et al.: M-mode and two-dimensional echocardiographic analysis of the septum in experimental right ventricular infarction: Correlation with hemodynamic alterations. Am. Heart J. 110:1210, 1985.
227. Bellamy, G.R., Rasmussen, H.H., Nasser, F.N., et al.: Value of two-dimensional echocardiography, electrocardiography, and clinical signs in detecting right ventricular infarction. Am. Heart J. 112:304, 1986.
228. Cecchi, F., Zuppiroli, A., Favilli, S., et al.: Echocardiographic features of right ventricular infarction. Clin. Cardiol. 7:405, 1984.
229. Lopez-Sendon, J., Garcia-Fernandez, M.A., Coma-Canella, I., et al.: Segmental right ventricular function after acute myocardial infarction: Two-dimensional echocardiographic study in 63 patients. Am. J. Cardiol. 51:390, 1983.

CHAPTER

28 Assessment of Systolic Function With Doppler Echocardiography

Alan S. Pearlman, M.D.

RELATIVE ROLE OF ULTRASONIC IMAGING AND DOPPLER TECHNIQUES ___ 325
ASSESSMENT OF LEFT VENTRICULAR SYSTOLIC FUNCTION ___ 325
Measures of Interest ___ 325
Measurement of Ventricular Systolic Function at Rest ___ 327
Measurement of Ventricular Systolic Function After Interventions ___ 329
Doppler Indices of Systolic Performance: Caveats ___ 329
Clinical Role of Doppler Techniques ___ 330
ASSESSMENT OF RIGHT VENTRICULAR SYSTOLIC FUNCTION ___ 331
Measures of Interest ___ 331
Associated Hemodynamics ___ 331
Doppler Hemodynamics: Caveats ___ 331
Clinical Role of Doppler Techniques ___ 333
RELATION BETWEEN SYSTOLIC AND DIASTOLIC VENTRICULAR FUNCTION ___ 333
SUMMARY ___ 333

Among the earliest applications of Doppler echocardiography was its use for the noninvasive evaluation of cardiac function. More than 30 years ago, both Franklin and associates[1] and Yoshida and co-workers[2] independently described how ultrasonic Doppler shifts can be used to study cardiac performance. In the late 1960s and early 1970s, Light and colleagues[3–7] used suprasternal Doppler echocardiography to measure the velocity of blood flow in the ascending aorta to evaluate systolic left ventricular performance quantitatively. In the past 10 to 15 years, many investigators have applied both pulsed-wave and continuous-wave Doppler to assess cardiac performance noninvasively. This chapter reviews the Doppler echocardiographic methods that can be used, the clinical questions that can be studied, and the technical cautions that must be kept in mind by the investigator who uses Doppler echocardiography to evaluate systolic cardiac function.

RELATIVE ROLE OF ULTRASONIC IMAGING AND DOPPLER TECHNIQUES

As described in Chapter 27, echocardiographic imaging is of great value in the assessment of cardiac function. This chapter focuses instead on Doppler echocardiographic techniques for evaluating cardiac function. It seems appropriate to comment on the comparative utility of these related but different ultrasonic techniques. Both imaging and Doppler techniques are important components of "echocardiography." However, these techniques have several fundamental differences between them. In assessing cardiac performance, echocardiographic imaging uses tomographic views of ventricular structure that result from ultrasound *reflected* at myocardial-blood interfaces, whereas Doppler echocardiography uses frequency shifts in ultrasound *backscattered* from moving blood cells to measure blood flow within the cardiac chambers and great vessels. In essence, ultrasonic imaging focuses on the dynamic changes in ventricular chamber size during systole (or diastole) to evaluate the volume and time course of ventricular emptying (or filling), whereas ultrasonic Doppler techniques determine the velocity, timing, and volume of blood flow leaving (or entering) the ventricle directly.

Ultrasonic imaging techniques provide valuable data about both global and regional ventricular performance. However, global measures are somewhat more complicated and generally less accurate when regional abnormalities are present. Although Doppler blood flow measurement techniques cannot quantitate regional ventricular function, they do provide a simple and practical means of measuring global performance that is relatively unaffected by regional nonuniformity. Even though this chapter focuses exclusively on Doppler techniques, it is important to recognize that echocardiographic imaging and Doppler techniques are largely complementary and not competing. These modes are best used together, with the results of one technique interpreted in the context of the findings from the other technique.

Doppler echocardiography can be used to assess both left and right ventricular function. This chapter emphasizes the Doppler techniques and applications used to assess systolic function. Assessment of diastolic function is described in detail in Chapter 29.

ASSESSMENT OF LEFT VENTRICULAR SYSTOLIC FUNCTION

Initially, one of the main uses of Doppler echocardiographic techniques was in evaluating systolic ventricular performance.[3-9] Although important Doppler applications in evaluating valvular disorders and shunt lesions have also evolved,[10-17] assessment of systolic function has remained an area of substantial clinical as well as investigative interest.

Measures of Interest

Various Doppler measures can be used to evaluate ventricular function during the ejection phase (Table 28–1). In general, all these measures are based on determining the velocity of blood flow out of the ventricle during systole, which can be accomplished either with the use of range-gated, pulsed-wave Doppler to examine flow selectively in the left ventricular outflow tract or in the ascending aorta, or with the use of continuous-wave Doppler to examine flow through the aortic valve. The techniques of pulsed-wave and continuous-wave Doppler, and the technical details of

TABLE 28–1. DOPPLER MEASURES OF SYSTOLIC VENTRICULAR FUNCTION

Ejection velocity	Preejection period
Peak	Acceleration time
Mean	Deceleration time
Ejection duration	Systolic velocity-time integral ("stroke distance")
Acceleration	Stroke volume
Maximum	Cardiac output
Average	Ventricular dP/dt

Doppler blood flow velocity measurement, are the subject of Chapter 26.

Representative pulsed-wave and continuous-wave Doppler recordings of systolic left ventricular ejection for a normal subject are illustrated in Figure 28–1. The graphic output shows flow velocity (on the *ordinate*) plotted against time (on the *abscissa*), with signal intensity shown in gray scale. From such tracings, a variety of measurements can be made directly: velocities, time intervals, and velocity-time integrals. When combined with anatomical dimensions, determined by echocardiographic imaging, Doppler measures also can be used to compute flow volumes and flow rates.

Figure 28–2 illustrates systolic left ventricular ejection velocities. The instantaneous velocity can be measured at any desired point during the ejection phase. The duration of ejection, and fractional durations, also can be determined. The area encompassed by the ejection curve, referred to as the systolic velocity-time integral (VTI), can be determined with planimetry, as can fractional integrals. Note that because velocity is a derivative measure, expressing distance per unit time, the integral of velocity (as a function of time) is a measure of distance. Therefore, the systolic velocity-time integral is equivalent to the distance downstream through which a representative blood cell is propelled during systole. The velocity-time integral is often referred to as "stroke distance," which is an intuitively sensible term.

Physiologists have emphasized that volumetric flow rate can be calculated by multiplying the average flow velocity (in centimeters per second) by the area filled by flow (in square centimeters). The product of these two terms is expressed in units of cubic centimeters per second (i.e., milliliters per second). The average flow velocity can be determined by dividing the velocity-time integral by the duration of flow. The stroke volume can be calculated directly as the product of systolic velocity-time integral (in centimeters per beat) and flow cross-sectional area (in square centimeters); this product represents the volume of flow ejected per beat (in milliliters per beat). As illustrated in Figure 28–3, Doppler measures can be combined with anatomical area determinations to calculate volumetric flow.

It is important to recall that area and velocity integral measures must be made at the same anatomical site. Thus, if pulsed-wave Doppler is used to record systolic ejection velocity in the left ventricular outflow tract, then flow area should be measured at that same site.[18-22] When continuous-wave Doppler is used to record ejection velocity, the area should be measured at the narrowest portion of the aorta, since peak instantaneous velocities will be recorded from the narrowest part of the ejection flowstream,[23-26] as long as flow direction and the ultrasound-beam orientation are nearly coaxial. In either case, flow area typically is computed from the measured diameter of the outflow tract or aorta, when one assumes that the area filled by flow is circular in cross section and that the measured anatomical diameter is equivalent to the average diameter of the flow area during systole. The systolic velocity profile is usually recorded from the center of the outflow tract or aorta and is assumed to represent the spatial average velocity of a laminar blunt plug of flow. Experimental observations[22, 27] suggest that these assumptions generally are appropriate.

An additional marker of global systolic left ventricular function is the rate of rise of left ventricular systolic pressure (dP/dt). The

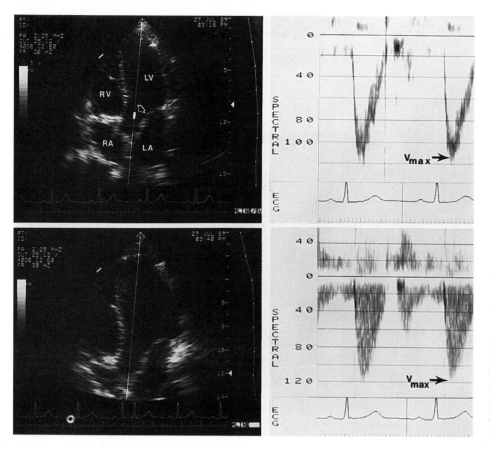

FIGURE 28–1. Left ventricular ejection flow in a normal 30-year-old woman. *Top Panels,* Pulsed-wave Doppler imaging. *Upper Left,* Systolic freeze-frame, apical four-chamber plane. The Doppler sample volume *(open arrow)* is positioned along the Doppler interrogation cursor in the high left ventricular outflow tract, just proximal to the aortic leaflets. Doppler velocities are recorded from blood cells moving through this region. LA = left atrium; LV = left ventricle; RA = right atrium; RV = right ventricle. *Upper Right,* Graphic output of Doppler velocity (*y* axis) as a function of time (*x* axis), with simultaneous electrocardiogram (ECG) recorded for timing. Velocities are calibrated in centimeters per second; small time markers are 0.04 second apart. The narrow band of velocities at each instant in systole denotes organized ejection flow through the region of sampling. Maximum ventricular ejection velocity (Vmax) is indicated. *Bottom Panels,* Continuous-wave Doppler. *Lower Left,* Systolic freeze-frame, apical four-chamber plane. The Doppler cursor is oriented parallel to the direction of ventricular outflow. Doppler velocities are recorded all along this line of interrogation, with the highest instantaneous velocities coming from the region of the aortic valve and proximal ascending aorta. *Lower Right,* Graphic output, same format as above. The broad band of velocities at each instant in systole denotes recording of simultaneous Doppler shifts from blood cells at multiple depths along the cursor line. Maximum ejection velocity (Vmax) is indicated and typically is slightly higher than that measured proximal to the aortic valve.

FIGURE 28–2. Ejection velocities in a normal subject, recorded from the left ventricular outflow tract (apical examining window) with pulsed-wave Doppler. Maximum ejection velocity (Vmax) is 120 cm per second (first complex), and instantaneous velocities also can be determined throughout systole (third complex). The duration of ejection (ET = ejection time) is 0.33 second. The time from onset to peak ejection (at = acceleration time) and from peak to end-ejection (dt = deceleration time) also can be measured. The area enclosed by the velocity curve (VTI = velocity-time integral) can be determined by planimetry and represents the "stroke distance."

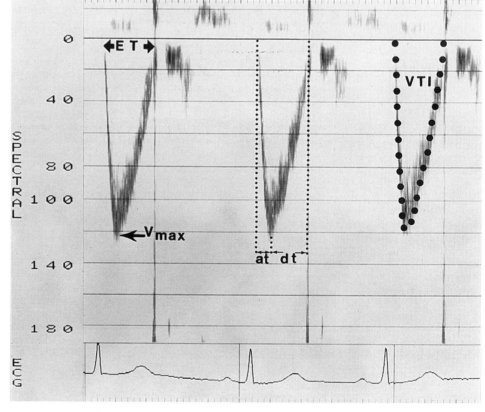

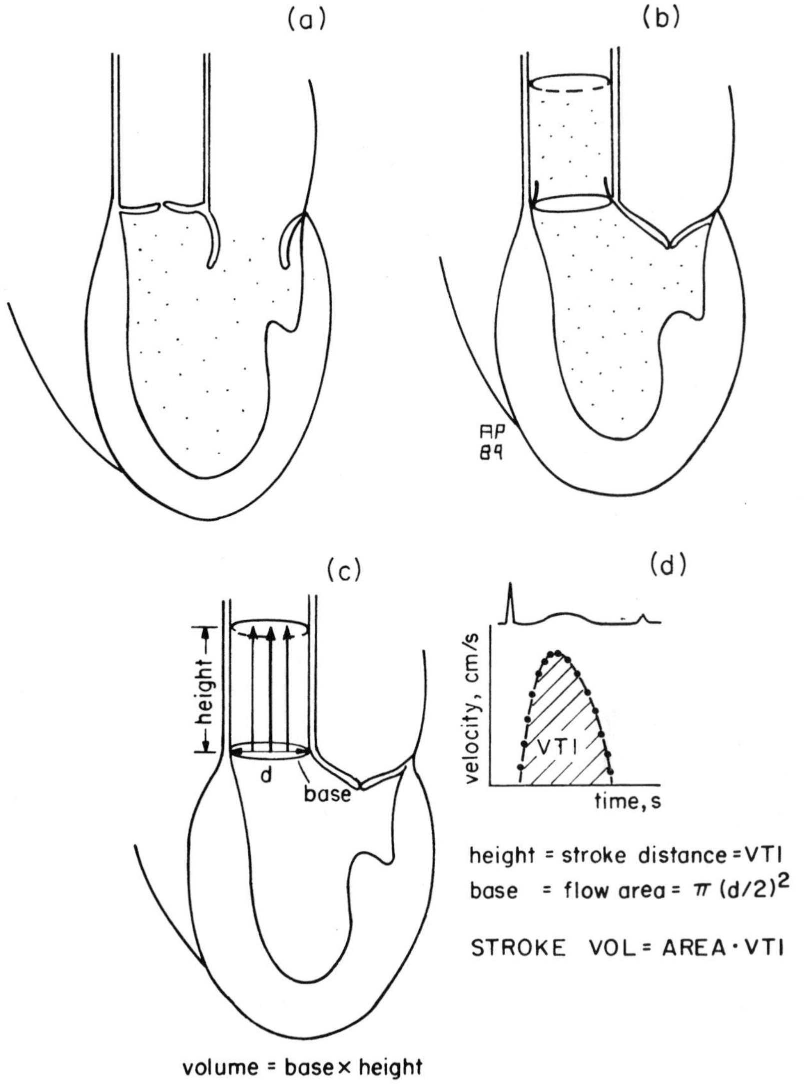

FIGURE 28–3. Diagram illustrating determination of systolic left ventricular stroke volume with Doppler echocardiographic data. *a,* Frontal view showing the left ventricle in diastole; for purposes of illustration, blood in the ventricular cavity is stippled. *b,* In late systole, the ventricle has emptied into the ascending aorta, filling a cylindrical segment of this vessel with stippled blood. *c,* The volume of the cylindrical segment of aorta filled during systole can be measured as the product of its base times height. The area of the base can be calculated from the diameter (*d*) as $\pi(d/2)^2$. *d,* The height of the cylinder is equivalent to the distance downstream through which an average blood cell is propelled during systole (the "stroke distance"). This distance is equivalent to the velocity-time integral (VTI) measured as the area enclosed by the ejection velocity curve. The product of flow area and stoke distance yields stroke volume.

average rate of pressure rise can be estimated noninvasively with the use of Doppler techniques in patients with mitral regurgitation.[28–31] Because left atrial pressure changes relatively little during pre-ejection ventricular systole, the rate of change of mitral regurgitant velocity (which is proportional to the square root of the left ventricular–left atrial pressure difference) is determined primarily by the rate of change of simultaneous left ventricular pressure. Hence, in patients with mitral regurgitation, continuous-wave Doppler recordings of mitral regurgitant velocity can be used to measure the time interval (Δt) in seconds during which mitral regurgitant velocity increases from 1 m per second to 3 m per second (Fig. 28–4). During this interval, the left ventricular–left atrial pressure difference increases from 4 to 36 mm Hg. Accordingly, the average rate of change of pressure is $32/\Delta t$, expressed in millimeters of mercury per second per second. Experimental and clinical hemodynamic studies[29–31] indicate that Doppler measures of dP/dt correspond well to invasive measures using catheter-tip pressure manometry.

Measurement of Ventricular Systolic Function at Rest

Many of the variables just described can be used to assess resting left ventricular systolic function. Stroke volume and cardiac output are perhaps the most popular measures of systolic ventricular function (Fig. 28–5). A number of experimental[9, 13, 32–34] and clinical[12, 18–21, 23–25, 34, 35] studies have demonstrated good agreement between

Doppler and invasive (Fick or indicator dilution) measures of stroke volume and cardiac output.

When Doppler volumetric flow measures are used, several important technical points should be kept in mind. First, Doppler stroke volumes can be determined with the use of either pulsed-wave[13, 19, 21, 32, 35] or continuous-wave[9, 23–25] techniques. A number of measurement sites, including the ascending aorta, left ventricular outflow tract, descending aorta, main pulmonary artery, mitral annulus, and mitral valve leaflet tips, have been described.* Second, although the studies cited have reported high correlations, data points from some individual experimental subjects have demonstrated significant disagreement between the Doppler results and the invasively determined standards of reference. It is important to recognize that stroke volume and cardiac output are dynamic variables that can change from moment to moment; the majority of studies comparing Doppler and invasive measures of volume flow were *not* performed simultaneously. Furthermore, the available standards of reference are not true "gold standards," because cardiac outputs determined by thermodilution, Fick, and angiographic techniques can demonstrate significant disagreement among themselves.[39–42] In fact, duplicate measures show imperfect agreement when a given "reference standard" technique is used to evaluate the same patients. For example, repeat determinations of cardiac output by thermodilution often differ from each other,[39] to the same degree that Doppler and thermodilution methods differ.

---

*See references 3, 12, 13, 18, 19, 21, 23, and 34 to 38.

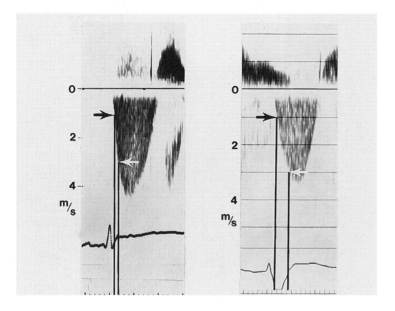

FIGURE 28–4. Mitral regurgitation, continuous-wave Doppler, recorded from the cardiac apex. *Left,* Recording from a 56-year-old man with moderate mitral regurgitation and normal left ventricular systolic function. Regurgitant velocity increases from 1 m per second *(black arrow)* to 3 m per second *(white arrow)* in 0.015 second, corresponding to an average dP/dt of 2133 mm Hg per second. See text for details. *Right,* Recording from a 49-year-old man with an aortic prosthesis, moderate mitral regurgitation, and markedly decreased global left ventricular systolic function (ejection fraction 15 to 20 percent). In this case, regurgitant velocity increases from 1 m per second *(black arrow)* to 3 m per second *(white arrow)* in 0.055 second, corresponding to a depressed average dP/dt of 582 mm Hg per second.

These considerations suggest that whereas Doppler stroke volumes and cardiac outputs do have technical limitations, in practice they may be generally as accurate as other available methods for measuring volumetric flow.

Ejection velocities, systolic time intervals, and velocity-time integrals also provide insight into resting systolic left ventricular function. More than 30 years ago, Rushmer described the ventricles as impulse generators and suggested that "initial ventricular impulse" can be used as an indicator of global systolic ventricular performance.[43] Because ultrasonic Doppler methods were not then available, Rushmer and associates used electromagnetic flowmeters to demonstrate increases in measures of systolic ejection velocity and acceleration induced by treadmill exercise and decreases induced by ischemic systolic dysfunction.[44] The studies of Rushmer and associates also showed that measures of the velocity and timing of blood ejection into the systemic and pulmonary circulations were

indicative of selective experimentally induced changes in left and right ventricular systolic function, respectively.

These observations were extended by Gardin and associates,[45] who used pulsed-wave Doppler echocardiography to study normal subjects and patients with dilated cardiomyopathy, both ischemic and idiopathic in etiology. Measures of peak left ventricular ejection velocity, recorded in the ascending aorta, were found to be significantly lower in patients with cardiomyopathy than in normal subjects. Measures of average flow acceleration and ejection time (Fig. 28–6) were also smaller in cardiomyopathy patients than in normal subjects. Although Gardin and associates reported complete separation in peak velocities between individuals with normal systolic left ventricular function and those with depressed function, the group of cardiomyopathy patients they studied had severely impaired systolic left ventricular function that was obvious clinically, as well as from two-dimensional echocardiographic im-

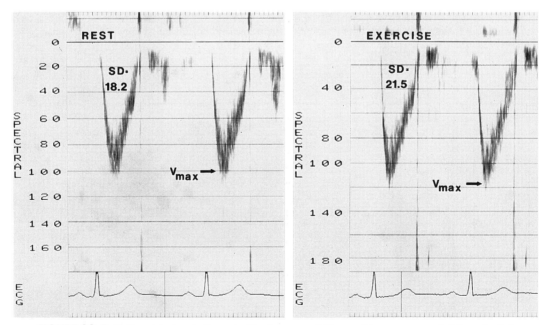

FIGURE 28–5. Left ventricular ejection velocities in a normal 30-year-old woman, recorded from the left ventricular outflow tract (apical examining window) with pulsed-wave Doppler. *Left,* At rest, maximum velocity (Vmax) is 100 cm per second, stroke distance (SD) is 18.2 cm, and calculated stroke volume is 76 mL per beat. Heart rate is 63 beats per minute, and thus cardiac output is 4.8 L per minute. *Right,* After mild exercise, maximum velocity has increased to 120 cm per second, and stroke distance to 21.5 cm. Calculated stroke volume has increased to 89 mL, heart rate to 74 beats per minute, and cardiac output to 6.6 L per minute.

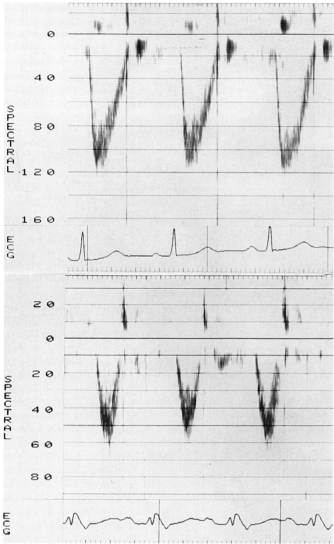

FIGURE 28–6. Left ventricular ejection velocities, recorded from the left ventricular outflow tract (apical examining window) with pulsed-wave Doppler. *Top,* A normal 30-year-old woman with normal ventricular systolic function. Maximum ejection velocity is 115 cm per second, and stroke distance is 18.2 cm. *Bottom,* A 46-year-old man with dilated cardiomyopathy and severe global ventricular systolic dysfunction. Maximum ejection velocity is markedly depressed at 60 cm per second, and stroke distance is 8.0 cm. The ejection duration and acceleration measures also are obviously reduced from normal.

aging (J.M. Gardin, personal communication). Clinical experience has demonstrated that whereas ejection velocities often are depressed in patients with systolic left ventricular dysfunction, there may be overlap between patients with impaired global systolic function and those with normal left ventricular function. Hence, normal systolic left ventricular function at rest does not exclude the possibility of significant heart disease. This caveat has long been recognized as true by advocates of stress testing,[46, 47] and similar cautions pertain to Doppler measures of systolic left ventricular function.

Measures of systolic blood flow acceleration in the ascending aorta have been reported as correlating well with traditional indices of global systolic performance.[48–54] Both experimental[48, 50] and clinical[52] studies have concluded that maximum acceleration may be superior to peak ejection velocity for assessing systolic left ventricular function. Moreover, maximum acceleration is relatively independent of changes in preload but sensitive to altered inotropic state.[48, 50] Hence, this measure may be particularly appealing as a marker of left ventricular contractile performance.

Measurement of Ventricular Systolic Function After Interventions

Because Doppler echocardiographic measures may be normal when made under resting conditions in patients with impaired left ventricular systolic function, the use of Doppler methods to assess ventricular systolic function during, or immediately following, interventions is of great practical interest. A number of investigators have demonstrated exercise-induced increases in left ventricular stroke volume and cardiac output[55–63] that agree well with those measured by means of traditional invasive techniques. These observations suggest that Doppler methods can be used not only to define systolic ventricular function under basal conditions but also to document changes in function resulting from intervention. Significant increases in peak ejection velocity and acceleration have been demonstrated during supine bicycle ergometer exercise[55–57, 59, 61, 63] and during upright bicycle or treadmill exercise[58, 64–67] in patients with normal ventricular systolic function. In contrast, patients with impaired systolic left ventricular function have demonstrated a blunted response or an actual decline in ejection-phase measures. Hence, exercise Doppler measures have been advocated as a means of detecting ischemic heart disease[64–66, 68] and as a useful adjunct to conventional treadmill or bicycle testing.

Doppler methods also can be used to study changes in systolic performance resulting from treatment of depressed ventricular systolic function (Fig. 28–7). Elkayam and associates[69] reported increases in peak ejection velocity and stroke distance (systolic velocity-time integral) in patients with heart failure following treatment with vasodilator agents. These investigators also noted that the magnitude of change in Doppler measures was reasonably predictive of the magnitude of improvement in invasive indicators of systolic ventricular performance. Sabbah and associates[70] also studied patients with congestive heart failure and reported that initially depressed measures of maximum acceleration increased toward normal during treatment of those patients whose heart failure improved but not in the subgroup with failure persisting after drug therapy. Labovitz and associates[71] studied patients undergoing percutaneous transluminal angioplasty and reported evidence of reversible depression of systolic left ventricular function (manifested as a fall in Doppler systolic ejection velocities), resulting from myocardial ischemia caused by angioplasty balloon inflation, which returned toward normal after balloon deflation and coronary reperfusion. Harrison and associates[67] used Doppler techniques to evaluate the hemodynamic effects of cardioactive drugs. These investigators reported increases during exercise in both peak ejection velocity and maximum acceleration, as measured by continuous-wave Doppler. These increases, particularly acceleration, were blunted significantly by propranolol therapy, which was consistent with the negative inotropic effect of this drug. In contrast, acute administration of verapamil did not alter exercise-induced increases in ejection velocity or acceleration. All these studies illustrate how Doppler measures can be used to assess the effect of interventions on global systolic left ventricular performance.

Doppler Indices of Systolic Performance: Caveats

The use of Doppler techniques to assess global left ventricular systolic function is attractive, in part, because the methods are atraumatic, noninvasive, and widely available and, in part, because the measures are physiologically meaningful. Notwithstanding their practical utility, however, Doppler echocardiographic measures of systolic left ventricular function have several notable limitations.

Accurate Doppler measures of flow velocity depend on examining the flowstream of interest with the use of an ultrasound beam that is oriented nearly parallel to the direction of blood flow, but doing so is not always possible. The inability to orient the examining ultrasonic beam coaxial to the direction of blood flow leads to underestimation of velocity, acceleration, and velocity-time integrals. Moreover, Doppler shifts measured from a given area of a

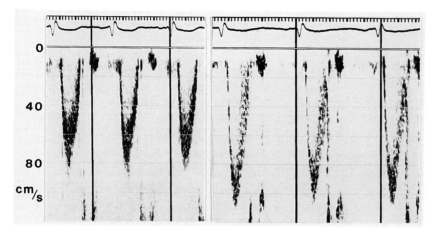

FIGURE 28-7. Left ventricular ejection velocities in a 31-year-old man with an infiltrative cardiomyopathy due to hemochromatosis, recorded from the left ventricular outflow tract (apical examining window) with pulsed-wave Doppler. *Left,* Before treatment, depressed measures of systolic function parallel clinical symptoms and signs of left ventricular failure; maximum ejection velocity is 80 cm per second, stroke distance is 10.9 cm, stroke volume is 54 mL, and cardiac output is 4.3 L per minute. *Right,* After treatment, clinical improvement in ventricular systolic function is accompanied by increases in maximum ejection velocity to 105 cm per second, stroke distance to 15.7 cm, and stroke volume to 77 mL. Although heart rate has slowed, cardiac output has increased to 5.1 L per minute.

cardiac chamber or blood vessel are assumed to be representative of the average behavior of blood flow at that spatial location and at that time during the cardiac cycle. This assumption is legitimate only when the blood flow is laminar and its spatial profile is blunt. Additionally, there are important potential physiologic variations in the actual behavior of blood flow that must be considered. The time course of ventricular ejection, as well as the stroke volume, may vary not only with changes in systolic left ventricular performance but also with changes in heart rate and ventricular loading conditions. Unfortunately, alterations in heart rate or changes in ventricular preload and afterload are not always accompanied by obvious changes in clinical status. Therefore, Doppler echocardiographic measures of flow velocity and stroke distance can change, even though ventricular contractile function does not. Some investigators have suggested that maximum flow acceleration may be a more sensitive indicator of systolic contractile ventricular performance that is less influenced by loading conditions[48, 50]; however, acceleration is not completely afterload-independent.[72] Accordingly, when the physician assesses a patient with suspected impairment of left ventricular systolic function, it is important to consider the hemodynamic milieu as well as the clinical context in which the Doppler measures were obtained.

Because it is possible to use Doppler echocardiography to measure a number of indicators of systolic performance, it is reasonable to ask, "Which measure is best?" To date, this question has not been answered definitively by comparative studies of different diagnostic protocols in the same patients. Accordingly, we cannot assume that what is most appropriate for a given clinical application will necessarily be equally useful for another. Different characteristics may be desirable for particular applications. For example, a measure with high sensitivity would be particularly valuable for detecting systolic dysfunction as an early marker of myocardial ischemia, whereas a measure with narrow confidence limits and excellent reproducibility would be most valuable for demonstrating improvement in function resulting from pharmacologic treatment of impaired ventricular function in heart failure. At present, it is not possible to identify a single Doppler echocardiographic measure that is ideal for particular clinical applications. Further research will be needed to help define the relative clinical utility of different Doppler measures of ventricular systolic function.

Clinical Role of Doppler Techniques

Notwithstanding the preceding cautions, Doppler techniques for assessing left ventricular systolic function have practical value in a number of clinical settings. As noted earlier, Doppler measures of stroke volume and cardiac output provide an accurate assessment of left ventricular pump function. Doppler measures can be made at rest in patients with heart failure to document the degree of functional impairment[23, 45] and can be repeated after the institution of pharmacotherapy to help evaluate the effectiveness of

treatment.[69, 70] In general, Doppler measures would not be used in isolation to evaluate systolic left ventricular function but rather would be employed in combination with qualitative and quantitative two-dimensional echocardiographic imaging (see Chapter 27). For example, in a hypertensive patient presenting with heart failure, two-dimensional echocardiography should be used to evaluate left ventricular chamber size and regional as well as global systolic dynamics. When image quality allows, it is appropriate to measure chamber volume and ventricular mass. Careful regional assessment may help suggest whether the existence of associated coronary artery disease is likely. In this same patient, Doppler techniques should be used to evaluate valvular function and also to assess global systolic (as well as diastolic) ventricular function. Doppler measures might then be used to follow the functional response to medical therapy.

Doppler measures of stroke volume, ejection velocity, and acceleration can be used before, during, or immediately after the induction of stress to detect inducible ischemic systolic left ventricular dysfunction.[64-66, 68] Once again, these Doppler measures would not be used in isolation but rather would be employed in conjunction with the findings on echocardiographic imaging and color flow Doppler studies. For example, consider the patient who complains of exertional breathlessness and in whom a resting comprehensive echo-Doppler study demonstrates normal left ventricular and valvular function, with only mild mitral regurgitation. An exercise echocardiographic study would be useful (1) to document exercise tolerance, (2) to evaluate for inducible segmental, multisegmental, or even global ventricular dysfunction with two-dimensional imaging, (3) to evaluate global function quantitatively by the Doppler measurement of stroke volume, peak ejection velocity and acceleration, and left ventricular positive dP/dt, (4) to examine for worsening of mitral regurgitation induced by exercise, using both color and spectral Doppler modalities, and (5) to assess diastolic function. Many of these issues are also discussed in Chapters 27, 29, 30, and 36.

Doppler assessment of left ventricular systolic performance also can be valuable for guiding clinical management. In patients with symptoms suggesting heart failure, Doppler measures, and concomitant echo imaging results, can help document the presence and define the severity of impaired systolic function,[23, 45] evaluate for disease progression, and assess the response to therapy.[69, 70] In patients with ischemic heart disease or risk factors that suggest its presence, exercise Doppler findings, coupled with echo imaging results, can help document inducible dysfunction and its physiologic extent, especially when the echocardiographic image quality is limited. In patients with valvular disease, Doppler assessment of global systolic left and right ventricular function and of right-sided hemodynamics can provide important clues regarding the etiology of symptoms. Doppler functional assessment also may help one judge the risks and benefits of surgical treatment. In patients with severe mitral regurgitation who underwent surgical valve replacement, Doppler measures of left ventricular dP/dt were found to predict postoperative ejection fraction,[73] thereby helping researchers judge the potential benefit of surgical treatment in patients who had impairment of both ventricular and valvular function. In patients with prosthetic heart valves, Doppler functional assessment may help determine when the signs and symptoms of heart failure are due to ventricular impairment, prosthetic valve dysfunction, or both. Doppler measures of right heart hemodynamics are helpful in a wide range of acquired and congenital cardiac disorders, as well as in patients with pulmonary vascular or parenchymal disease.

The preceding examples illustrate the importance of using Doppler methods for evaluating cardiac performance as part of the integrated, comprehensive echocardiographic assessment of patients with a host of documented or suspected cardiac disorders.

ASSESSMENT OF RIGHT VENTRICULAR SYSTOLIC FUNCTION

Doppler echocardiographic techniques used to evaluate left ventricular systolic function can be adapted to assess global right ventricular systolic performance as well.

Measures of Interest

Systolic ejection velocities can be recorded in both the right ventricular outflow tract and the main pulmonary artery with the use of range-gated pulsed-wave Doppler. Continuous-wave Doppler can also be used to record right ventricular ejection velocities. Measures of systolic flow velocity, acceleration, and deceleration, as well as systolic time intervals and velocity-time integrals, provide insight into global right ventricular function. By combining measures of anatomical diameter, with the use of two-dimensional echocardiographic imaging, and velocity-time integral recorded in the proximal pulmonary artery, right ventricular stroke volume can be calculated noninvasively.[12, 18, 34] A similar approach can be applied to measure the diameter and velocity-time integrals in the right ventricular outflow tract, just proximal to the pulmonic valve.[74] Several groups of investigators have compared echocardiographic measures, with the use of both imaging and Doppler, of right and left ventricular stroke volume in children and adults with intracardiac shunts and have reported pulmonary-to-systemic flow ratios that show good agreement with those determined by conventional invasive techniques.[12, 34, 75–77]

The rate of change of right ventricular pressure (dP/dt) during early systole can be determined in patients with tricuspid regurgitation.[78, 79] By using continuous-wave Doppler to record the velocity of tricuspid regurgitation, it is possible to calculate either the average or the maximum instantaneous positive dP/dt. In general, Doppler measures of right ventricular dP/dt have demonstrated significant agreement with simultaneous determinations made from high-fidelity catheter manometers.[78, 79]

Associated Hemodynamics

Several different Doppler techniques can be used to evaluate pulmonary artery pressure in a wide range of cardiac disorders. Assessment of the time course of flow acceleration by the ejecting right ventricle during early systole provides a simple approach to evaluating pulmonary artery peak systolic pressure. In normal individuals, peak ejection velocity typically occurs in midsystole, and the systolic velocity curve has a relatively parabolic, smoothly "rounded" shape. The time from the onset to the peak of systolic flow velocity, also referred to as "acceleration time," normally is 100 to 120 msec or longer. When pulmonary hypertension is present, right ventricular pressure development occurs more rapidly, so that peak ejection velocity occurs earlier in systole,[80] and

the flow velocity curve often demonstrates an early systolic "spike." When the pulmonary acceleration time is 60 msec or shorter, substantial pulmonary hypertension can be inferred, particularly when the heart rate is less than 100 beats per minute. Several investigators have reported inverse relations between measures of Doppler flow acceleration time and mean pulmonary artery pressure,[80–82] although different investigators do not agree as to which site is ideal for velocity recording, whether it is necessary to normalize for heart rate or pre-ejection period, or whether pressure should be expressed on a logarithmic or linear scale. Many echocardiographers believe that pulmonary acceleration times provide only a semiquantitative assessment of the range of pulmonary artery pressure, rather than a precise numerical measure of peak systolic pressure.

In patients with tricuspid regurgitation, an alternative Doppler approach to calculating pulmonary artery systolic pressure is extremely useful. The peak systolic velocity of tricuspid regurgitation can be used to calculate the maximum systolic pressure difference between the right ventricle and the right atrium, with the use of the simplified Bernoulli equation.[83–85] When the right ventricular–right atrial maximum pressure difference is added to an estimate of mean right atrial pressure, peak right ventricular (and, hence, pulmonary arterial) systolic pressure can be determined.[83, 84] Invasive measures of the maximal right ventricular–right atrial pressure difference with the use of manometer-tipped catheters have demonstrated excellent agreement with simultaneous pressure differences calculated from continuous-wave Doppler peak regurgitant velocity measures.[84] Mean right atrial pressure can be estimated from inspection of the jugular venous-pulse contour, although this approach is not always accurate.[83] An alternative approach entails imaging of the hepatic vein as it empties into the right atrium, with the use of subcostal two-dimensional echocardiographic imaging. When the inferior vena cava is normal in size and shows brisk collapse during rapid inspiration (the "sniff" test), right atrial pressure is relatively low—less than 10 mm Hg. When the inferior vena cava is dilated and its caliber does not change during "sniff," right atrial pressure (which resists inspiratory emptying of the vena cava and hepatic veins) is high—about 20 mm Hg.[86]

Another approach involves measuring the time interval from the cessation of pulmonary artery systolic flow to the onset of diastolic flow through the tricuspid valve. This interval, which can be measured from pulsed-wave or continuous-wave Doppler recordings of flow through the pulmonic and tricuspid valves (with the use of the electrocardiogram as a timing reference), represents the right ventricular isovolumic relaxation time. In the absence of elevated right atrial pressure, the right ventricular isovolumic relaxation time lengthens as pulmonary artery systolic pressure rises. Accordingly, measures of right ventricular isovolumic relaxation time, coupled with heart rate, can be used to determine peak systolic pulmonary artery pressure.[87] A final Doppler approach can be applied to patients with pulmonic regurgitation. In this setting, coaxially oriented recordings of pulmonic regurgitant flow velocity permit computation (with the use of the simplified Bernoulli equation) of the early- and end-diastolic pressure differences between the pulmonary artery and the right ventricle. When these values are coupled with estimates of right atrial pressure, pulmonary artery mean and end-diastolic pressures can be approximated.[88]

Doppler Hemodynamics: Caveats

Most of the Doppler echocardiographic techniques that can be used to evaluate right-sided hemodynamics are influenced by tricuspid regurgitation. Determination of the peak systolic pressure difference between the right ventricle and the right atrium requires that sufficient tricuspid regurgitant volume is present to record its maximal velocity accurately. When minimal tricuspid regurgitation is present (as in most normal subjects and in some patients with pulmonary hypertension), it may be difficult to record peak tricuspid regurgitant velocity accurately. In this setting, it may be useful to enhance Doppler signal strength by using contrast echocardiography.[89, 90] When tricuspid regurgitation is substantial in magnitude, mean right atrial pressure is often elevated. This elevation affects the calculation of right-sided pressures, regardless of whether the tricuspid regurgitant velocity, right ventricular isovolumic relaxation time, or pulmonic regurgitant velocity approaches are used. Hence, the severity of tricuspid regurgitation and the level of right atrial pressure must be considered when one uses any of the preceding Doppler methods—other than the pulmonary acceleration-time approach—to assess right-sided hemodynamics.

The severity of tricuspid regurgitation can be evaluated with the use of either spectral or color flow Doppler techniques, and it is often advantageous to use multiple approaches. The spatial distribution of regurgitant signals within the right atrium[91, 92] can be evaluated with the use of range-gated pulsed-wave Doppler, or color flow imaging techniques. Localized signals imply mild regurgitation, whereas widespread signals indicated severe regurgitation. The systolic flow-velocity pattern recorded from the middle hepatic vein also may be helpful.[93, 94] Normally, the middle hepatic vein empties into the right atrium during ventricular systole, as the ejecting right ventricle "decompresses" the adjacent right atrium. When moderate tricuspid regurgitation is present, the systolic hepatic venous emptying pattern is blunted; when severe tricuspid regurgitation is present, there is usually obvious reversal of systolic

flow in the hepatic veins, implying a large regurgitant volume (Fig. 28–8).

In addition, accurate Doppler velocity recordings (needed to calculate right-sided hemodynamics with the use of the tricuspid-regurgitant or pulmonic-regurgitant velocity curves) also require a coaxial orientation between the examining Doppler ultrasound beam and the regurgitant jet. This orientation may not always be possible, which leads to underestimation of the calculated pressure difference and, hence, underestimation of calculated pulmonary artery pressure. An appropriate intercept angle is less of a problem when time intervals are measured from Doppler velocity curves. However, it should be noted that because the main pulmonary artery is somewhat curved, the profile of flow velocities across this region may not be entirely uniform. Flow acceleration is frequently more rapid along the medial wall of the main pulmonary artery than in the center of the flowstream. When pulmonary artery recordings are made in a medial sampling site, acceleration time may be shorter than normal, even though pulmonary artery pressure is not elevated. This potential problem can often be obviated by recording acceleration time in the right ventricular outflow tract,[81, 82] where flow convergence typically flattens the spatial profile of flow velocities.

All the preceding Doppler approaches for evaluating tricuspid

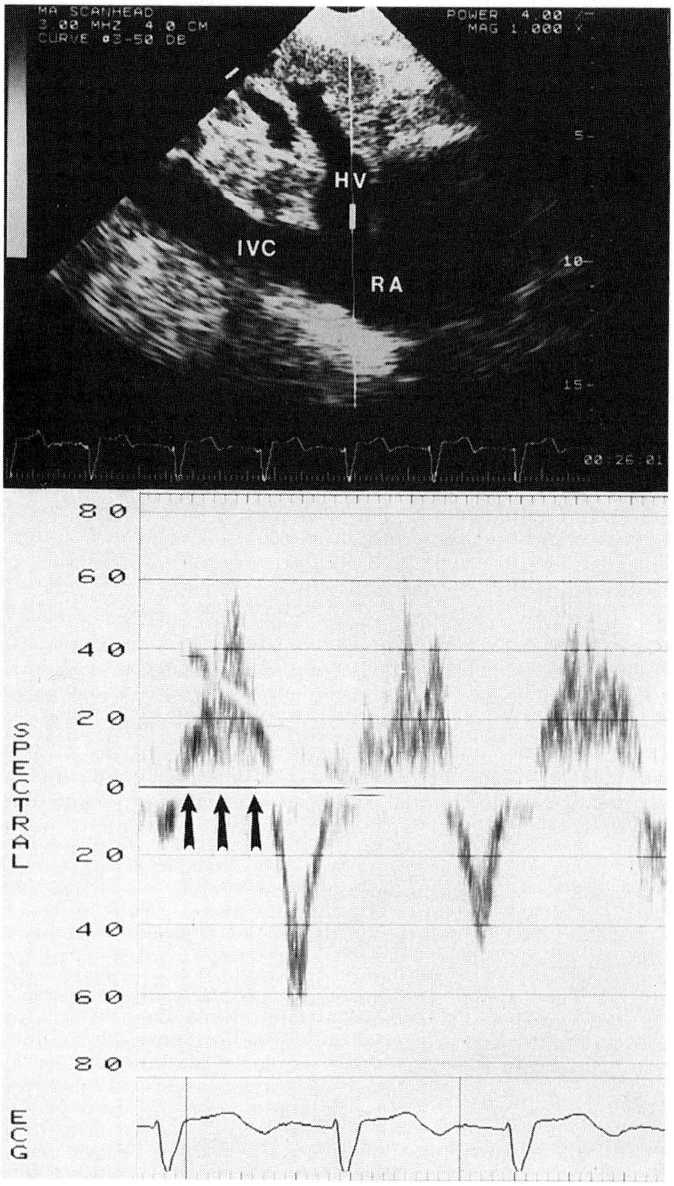

FIGURE 28–8. Right atrial filling velocities in a 71-year-old man with pulmonary hypertension and right ventricular failure. *Top*, Velocity curve recorded (subcostal examining window) from the middle hepatic vein (HV), near its junction with the right atrium (RA), by pulsed-wave Doppler. IVC = inferior vena cava. *Bottom*, Velocity record shows reversed systolic flow (*arrows*) upward into the hepatic vein, followed by diastolic flow out of the hepatic veins and through the right atrium into the right ventricle. Systolic reversal of flow into the systemic veins denotes significant tricuspid regurgitation.

and pulmonary flow do have shortcomings. However, these approaches typically do permit noninvasive assessment of right heart hemodynamics in the large majority of patients[95] and in a wide variety of disorders.

Clinical Role of Doppler Techniques

Doppler measures of global right ventricular systolic function have been reported relatively infrequently. However, it is reasonable to expect that these measures will prove valuable in a number of clinical settings. For example, measurement of right ventricular ejection fraction from two-dimensional echocardiographic images, though feasible,[96] is made difficult because of the complex shape of the right ventricle, which does not lend itself to simple geometric description. Spatial reconstruction of the right ventricle is feasible with the use of three-dimensional echocardiographic methods, and this technique provides accurate volume measurements.[97, 98] However, such sophisticated imaging approaches are not widely available. Instead, it may be possible to use Doppler measures as a more simple means of defining global right ventricular systolic performance. This approach could be used to detect and study the functional consequences of right ventricular infarction,[99] to evaluate right ventricular decompensation in patients with congestive cardiomyopathy[100] or those with cor pulmonale, or to assess right ventricular function in patients with mitral valve disease. Measures of relative right and left ventricular stroke volumes have already proved useful in assessing shunt size in children and adults with atrial septal defect,[12, 34, 76] and similar approaches can be used for other shunt lesions.[37, 76] Doppler measures of pulmonary artery pressure are clearly valuable in helping clinicians evaluate the significance of mitral valve disease, and in assessing the suitability of patients with severe heart failure as potential candidates for cardiac transplantation. Thus, in the assessment of right ventricular systolic performance, Doppler techniques have a number of practical clinical applications.

RELATION BETWEEN SYSTOLIC AND DIASTOLIC VENTRICULAR FUNCTION

This chapter focuses on the evaluation of ventricular systolic function, whereas the next chapter, Chapter 29, focuses specifically on the assessment of diastolic function. It is important to remember that systolic and diastolic function are not "independent" physiologic events. Typically, a ventricle with impaired systolic ejection does not fill normally, and a variety of compensatory mechanisms often are called into play. A normally contracting ventricle that cannot fill properly may not be able to provide sufficient blood flow to meet the needs of vital organs. This situation is quite familiar in patients with tamponade on the basis of metastatic disease or following cardiac surgery. In this setting, patients often present with hypotension and evidence of low output, despite vigorous contraction of the left and right ventricles that eject blood with great efficiency during systole but cannot fill normally and, hence, cannot maintain a normal stroke volume. Accordingly, the comprehensive evaluation of cardiac function requires consideration of *both* systolic and diastolic function in a coordinated fashion, and not as "independent" factors.

SUMMARY

Doppler recordings of flow velocity during ventricular ejection provide an attractive means of quantitating ventricular function during systole. Doppler techniques can be applied to both the left and right ventricles; they are completely noninvasive, atraumatic, and well suited to serial studies. The necessary equipment is widely available, relatively inexpensive compared with other equipment used for cardiac imaging, and fairly robust. Patient acceptance is excellent. Doppler echocardiographic measures of blood-flow velocity provide a direct means of assessing the time course, rate, and volume of ventricular emptying (and filling). Cardiac function can be evaluated with Doppler echocardiography in both inpatient and outpatient settings, under basal conditions, and during interventions. Thus, Doppler echocardiography is well suited for use in studying a wide variety of cardiac disorders in a range of settings.

However, although the concept of "evaluating cardiac function" sounds deceptively simple, ventricular systole is quite complex (and so is diastole). Thus, it probably is naive to expect to use relatively simple Doppler measures to define ventricular function, without considering the hemodynamic context in which the measures are obtained. Systolic ventricular function varies not only with the contractile state of the ventricle but also with ventricular loading conditions, especially afterload, which may change significantly from moment to moment. Other clinical and hemodynamic variables, such as age and heart rate, also influence some indices of systolic ventricular function. The assessment of cardiac function with the use of Doppler techniques requires several assumptions: that blood flow is relatively laminar and blunt in profile, that the cross-sectional area filled by flow is relatively constant, and that the direction of blood flow is stable during the cardiac cycle as well as relatively coaxial with the examining ultrasound beam. Although these assumptions are reasonable in general, they are not always strictly true. Furthermore, Doppler measures cannot demonstrate regional abnormalities; they provide only an assessment of global chamber function. Finally, it may be difficult to judge the "true" accuracy of Doppler measures, since the available standards of reference themselves often are flawed.

While much remains to be learned about the factors that influence cardiac function and how these factors alter ventricular ejection (and filling) velocities, Doppler techniques are of practical utility in evaluating patients with cardiac disease. Functional abnormalities are prevalent and clinically important in a large number of cardiovascular disorders. A practical way of detecting, quantitating, and following these abnormalities during treatment is of considerable clinical interest. Doppler echocardiographic techniques appear to address these needs.

References

1. Franklin, D.L., Schlegel, W., and Rushmer, R.F.: Blood flow measured by Doppler frequency shift of backscattered ultrasound. Science 134:564, 1961.
2. Yoshida, T., Mori, M., Nimura, Y., et al.: Analysis of heart motion with ultrasonic Doppler methods and its clinical application. Am. Heart J. 61:61, 1961.
3. Light, L.H.: Non-injurious ultrasonic technique for observing flow in the human aorta. Nature (London) 224:119, 1969.
4. Light, L.H., and Cross, G.: Cardiovascular data by transcutaneous aortovelography. In Roberts, C. (ed.): Blood Flow Measurement. London, Sector Publishing, 1972, p. 60.
5. Cross, G., and Light, L.H.: Non-invasive intra-thoracic blood velocity measurement in the assessment of cardiovascular function. Biomed. Eng. 9:464, 1974.
6. Light, L.H.: Transcutaneous aortovelography: A new window on the circulation. Br. Heart J. 38:433, 1976.
7. Sequeira, R.F., Light, L.H., Cross, G., et al.: Transcutaneous aortovelography: A quantitative evaluation. Br. Heart J. 38:443, 1976.
8. Huntsman, L.L., Gams, E., Johnson, C.C., et al.: Transcutaneous determination of aortic blood flow velocities in man. Am. Heart J. 89:605, 1975.
9. Colocousis, J.S., Huntsman, L.L., and Curreri, P.W.: Estimation of stroke volume changes by ultrasonic Doppler. Circulation 56:914, 1977.
10. Hatle, L., Angelsen, B., and Tromsdal, A.: Noninvasive assessment of atrioventricular pressure half-time by Doppler ultrasound. Circulation 60:1096, 1979.
11. Hatle, L., Angelsen, B., and Tromsdal, A.: Non-invasive assessment of aortic stenosis by Doppler ultrasound. Br. Heart J. 43:284, 1980.
12. Sanders, S.P., Yeager, S., and Williams, R.G.: Measurement of systemic and pulmonary blood flow and QP/QS ratio using Doppler and two-dimensional echocardiography. Am. J. Cardiol. 51:952, 1983.
13. Valdes-Cruz, L.M., Horowitz, S., Mesel, E., et al.: A pulsed Doppler echocardiographic method for calculation of pulmonary and systemic flow: Accuracy in a canine model with ventricular septal defect. Circulation 68:597, 1983.
14. Callahan, M.J., Tajik, A.J., Su-Fan, Q., et al.: Validation of instantaneous pressure gradient measured by continuous-wave Doppler in experimentally induced aortic stenosis. Am. J. Cardiol. 56:989, 1985.
15. Otto, C.M., Pearlman, A.S., Comess, K.A., et al.: Determination of the stenotic aortic valve area in adults using Doppler echocardiography. J. Am. Coll. Cardiol. 7:509, 1986.
16. Wilkins, G.T., Gillam, L.D., Kritzer, G.L., et al.: Validation of continuous-wave

Doppler echocardiographic measurements of mitral and tricuspid prosthetic valve gradients: A simultaneous Doppler-catheter study. Circulation 74:786, 1986.

17. Pearlman, A.S., and Otto, C.M.: Quantification of valvular regurgitation. Echocardiography 4:271, 1987.

18. Goldberg, S.J., Sahn, D.J., Allen, H.D., et al.: Evaluation of pulmonary and systemic blood flow by 2-dimensional Doppler echocardiography using fast Fourier transform spectral analysis. Am. J. Cardiol. 50:1394, 1982.

19. Lewis, J.D., Kuo, L.C., Nelson, J.G., et al.: Pulsed Doppler echocardiographic determination of stroke volume and cardiac output: Clinical validation of two new methods using the apical window. Circulation 70:425, 1984.

20. Ihlen, H., Amlie, J.P., Dale, J., et al.: Determination of cardiac output by Doppler echocardiography. Br. Heart J. 51:54, 1984.

21. Gardin, J.M., Tobis, J.M., Dabestani, A., et al.: Superiority of two-dimensional measurement of aortic vessel diameter in Doppler echocardiographic estimates of left ventricular stroke volume. J. Am. Coll. Cardiol. 6:66, 1985.

22. Otto, C.M., Pearlman, A.S., Gardner, C.L., et al.: Experimental validation of Doppler echocardiographic measurement of volume flow through the stenotic aortic valve. Circulation 78:435, 1988.

23. Huntsman, L.L., Stewart, D.K., Barnes, S.R., et al.: Noninvasive Doppler determination of cardiac output in man: Clinical validation. Circulation 67:593, 1983.

24. Chandraratna, P.A., Nanna, M., McKay, C., et al.: Determination of cardiac output by transcutaneous continuous-wave ultrasonic Doppler computer. Am. J. Cardiol. 53:234, 1984.

25. Nishimura, R.A., Callahan, M.J., Schaff, H.V., et al.: Noninvasive measurement of cardiac output by continuous-wave Doppler echocardiography: Initial experience and review of the literature. Mayo Clin. Proc. 59:484, 1984.

26. Bouchard, A., Blumlein, S., Schiller, N.B., et al.: Measurement of left ventricular stroke volume using continuous wave Doppler echocardiography of the ascending aorta and M-mode echocardiography of the aortic valve. J. Am. Coll. Cardiol. 9:75, 1987.

27. Burwash, I.G., Forbes, A.D., Sadahiro, M., et al.: Echocardiographic volume flow and stenosis severity measures with changing flow rate in aortic stenosis. Am. J. Physiol. 265:H1734, 1993.

28. Hatle, L., and Angelsen, B.: Doppler Ultrasound in Cardiology: Physical Principles and Clinical Applications. 2nd ed. Philadelphia, Lea & Febiger, 1985, p. 188.

29. Bargiggia, G.S., Bertucci, C., Recusani, F., et al.: A new method for calculation of left ventricular dP/dt by continuous wave Doppler-echocardiography: Validation studies at cardiac catheterization. Circulation 80:1287, 1989.

30. Chen, C., Rodriguez, L., Guerrero, J.L., et al.: Noninvasive estimation of the instantaneous first derivative of left ventricular pressure using continuous-wave Doppler echocardiography. Circulation 83:2101, 1991.

31. Chen, C., Rodriguez, L., Lethor, J.-P., et al.: Continuous wave Doppler echocardiography for noninvasive assessment of left ventricular dP/dt and relaxation time constant from mitral regurgitant spectra in patients. J. Am. Coll. Cardiol. 23:970, 1994.

32. Steingart, R.M., Meller, J., Barovick, J., et al.: Doppler echocardiographic measurement of beat-to-beat changes in stroke volume in dogs. Circulation 62:542, 1980.

33. Magnin, P.A., Stewart, J.A., Myers, S., et al.: Combined Doppler and phased array echocardiographic estimations of cardiac output. Circulation 63:388, 1981.

34. Valdes-Cruz, L.M., Horowitz, S., Mesel, E., et al.: A pulsed Doppler echocardiographic method for calculating pulmonary and systemic blood flow in atrial level shunts: Validation studies in animals and initial human experience. Circulation 69:80, 1984.

35. Labovitz, A.J., Buckingham, T.A., Habermehl, K., et al.: The effect of sampling site on the two-dimensional echo Doppler determination of cardiac output. Am. Heart J. 109:327, 1985.

36. Fisher, D.C., Sahn, D.J., Friedman, M.J., et al.: The mitral valve orifice method for noninvasive two-dimensional echo Doppler determinations of cardiac output. Circulation 67:872, 1983.

37. Sahn, D.J.: Determination of cardiac output by echocardiographic Doppler methods: Relative accuracy of various sites for measurement. J. Am. Coll. Cardiol. 6:663, 1985.

38. Hoit, B.D., Rashwan, M., Watt, C., et al.: Calculating cardiac output from transmitral volume flow using Doppler and M-mode echocardiography. Am. J. Cardiol. 62:131, 1988.

39. Ganz, W., Donoso, R., Marcus, H.S., et al.: A new technique for measurement of cardiac output by thermodilution in man. Am. J. Cardiol. 27:392, 1971.

40. Hodges, M., Downs, J.B., and Mitchell, L.A.: Thermodilution and Fick cardiac index determinations following cardiac surgery. Crit. Care Med. 3:182, 1975.

41. Reddy, P.S., Curtis, E.I., Bell, B., et al.: Determinants of variation between Fick and indicator dilution estimates of cardiac output during diagnostic catheterization. Fick vs. dye cardiac outputs. J. Lab. Clin. Med. 87:568, 1976.

42. Croft, C.H., Lipscomb, K., Mathis, K., et al.: Limitations of qualitative angiographic grading in aortic or mitral regurgitation. Am. J. Cardiol. 53:1593, 1984.

43. Rushmer, R.F.: Initial ventricular impulse: A potential key to cardiac evaluation. Circulation 39:268, 1964.

44. Rushmer, R.F., Watson, N., Harding, D., et al.: Effects of acute coronary occlusion on performance of right and left ventricles in intact unanesthetized dogs. Am. Heart J. 66:522, 1963.

45. Gardin, J.M., Iseri, L.E., Elkayam, U., et al.: Evaluation of dilated cardiomyopathy by pulsed Doppler echocardiography. Am. Heart J. 106:1057, 1983.

46. Bruce, R.A., Blackmon, J.R., Jones, J.W., et al.: Exercise testing in adult normal subjects and cardiac patients. Paediatrics 32:742, 1963.

47. Goldschlager, N., Selzer, A., and Cohn, K.: Treadmill stress tests as indicators of presence and severity of coronary artery disease. Ann. Intern. Med. 85:277, 1976.

48. Noble, M.I.M., Trenchard, D., and Guz, A.: Left ventricular ejection in conscious dogs: Measurement and significance of the maximum acceleration of blood from the left ventricle. Circ. Res. 19:139, 1966.

49. Chandraratna, P.A.N., Silveira, B., and Aronow, W.S.: Assessment of left ventricular function by determination of maximum acceleration of blood flow in the aorta using continuous Doppler ultrasound. Am. J. Cardiol. 45:398, 1980.

50. Bennett, E.D., Barclay, S.A., Davis, A.L., et al.: Ascending aorta blood velocity and acceleration using Doppler ultrasound in the assessment of left ventricular function. Cardiovasc. Res. 18:632, 1984.

51. Wallmeyer, K., Wann, L.S., Sagar, K.B., et al.: The influence of preload and heart rate on Doppler echocardiographic indexes of left ventricular performance: Comparison with invasive indexes in an experimental preparation. Circulation 74:181, 1986.

52. Sabbah, H.N., Khaja, F., Brymer, J.F., et al.: Noninvasive evaluation of left ventricular performance based on peak aortic blood acceleration measured with a continuous-wave Doppler velocity meter. Circulation 74:323, 1986.

53. Sabbah, H.N., Przbylski, J., Albert, D.E., et al.: Peak aortic blood acceleration reflects the extent of left ventricular ischemic mass at risk. Am. Heart J. 113:885, 1987.

54. Stein, P.D., Sabbah, H.N., Albert, D.E., et al.: Continuous wave Doppler for the noninvasive evaluation of aortic blood velocity and rate of change of velocity: Evaluation in dogs. Med. Instrum. 21:177, 1987.

55. Loeppky, J.A., Greene, E.R., Hoekenga, E.D., et al.: Beat-by-beat stroke volume assessment by pulsed Doppler in upright and supine exercise. J. Appl. Physiol. 50:1173, 1981.

56. Rose, J.S., Nanna, M., Rahimtoola, S.H., et al.: Accuracy of determination of changes in cardiac output by transcutaneous continuous-wave Doppler computer. Am. J. Cardiol. 54:1099, 1984.

57. Daley, P.J., Sagar, K.B., and Wann, L.S.: Supine versus upright exercise: Doppler echocardiographic measurement of ascending aortic flow velocity. Br. Heart J. 54:562, 1985.

58. Shaw, J.G., Johnson, E.C., Voyles, W.F., et al.: Noninvasive Doppler determination of cardiac output during submaximal and peak exercise. J. Appl. Physiol. 59:722, 1985.

59. Gardin, J.M., Kozlowski, J., Dabestani, A., et al.: Studies of Doppler aortic flow velocity during supine bicycle exercise. Am. J. Cardiol. 57:327, 1986.

60. Christie, J., Sheldahl, L.M., Tristani, F.E., et al.: Determination of stroke volume and cardiac output during exercise: Comparison of two-dimensional and Doppler echocardiography, Fick oximetry, and thermodilution. Circulation 76:539, 1987.

61. Marx, G.R., Hicks, R.W., Allen, H.D., et al.: Measurement of cardiac output and exercise factor by pulsed Doppler echocardiography during supine bicycle ergometry in normal young adolescent boys. J. Am. Coll. Cardiol. 10:430, 1987.

62. Ihlen, H., Endresen, K., Golf, S., et al.: Cardiac stroke volume during exercise measured by Doppler echocardiography: Comparison with the thermodilution technique and evaluation of reproducibility. Br. Heart J. 58:455, 1987.

63. Maeda, M., Yokota, M., Iwase, M., et al.: Accuracy of cardiac output measured by continuous wave Doppler echocardiography during dynamic exercise testing in the supine position in patients with coronary artery disease. J. Am. Coll. Cardiol. 13:76, 1989.

64. Bryg, R.J., Labovitz, A.J., Mehdirad, A.A., et al.: Effect of coronary artery disease on Doppler-derived parameters of aortic flow during upright exercise. Am. J. Cardiol. 58:14, 1986.

65. Mehta, N., Bennett, D., Mannering, D., et al.: Usefulness of noninvasive Doppler measurement of ascending aortic blood velocity and acceleration in detecting impairment of the left ventricular functional response to exercise three weeks after acute myocardial infarction. Am. J. Cardiol. 58:879, 1986.

66. Mehdirad, A.A., Williams, G.A., Labovitz, A.J., et al.: Evaluation of left ventricular function during upright exercise: Correlation of exercise Doppler with postexercise two-dimensional echocardiographic results. Circulation 75:413, 1987.

67. Harrison, M.R., Smith, M.D., Nissen, S.E., et al.: Use of exercise Doppler echocardiography to evaluate cardiac drugs: Effects of propranolol and verapamil on aortic blood flow velocity and acceleration. J. Am. Coll. Cardiol. 11:1002, 1988.

68. Daley, P.J., Sagar, K.B., Collier, B.D., et al.: Detection of exercise-induced changes in left ventricular performance by Doppler echocardiography. Br. Heart J. 58:447, 1987.

69. Elkayam, U., Gardin, J.M., Berkley, R., et al.: The use of Doppler flow velocity measurement to assess hemodynamic response to vasodilators in patients with heart failure. Circulation 67:377, 1983.

70. Sabbah, H.N., Gheorghiade, M., Smith, S.T., et al.: Serial evaluation of left ventricular function in congestive heart failure by measurement of peak aortic blood acceleration. Am. J. Cardiol. 61:367, 1988.

71. Labovitz, A.J., Lewen, M.K., Kern, M., et al.: Evaluation of left ventricular systolic and diastolic dysfunction during transient myocardial ischemia produced by angioplasty. J. Am. Coll. Cardiol. 10:748, 1987.

72. Berk, M.R., Evans, J., Knapp, C., et al.: Influence of alterations in loading produced by lower body negative pressure on aortic blood flow acceleration. J. Am. Coll. Cardiol. 15:1069, 1990.

73. Pai, R.G., Bansal, R.C., and Shah, P.M.: Doppler-derived rate of left ventricular pressure rise: Its correlation with the postoperative left ventricular function in mitral regurgitation. Circulation 82:514, 1990.

74. Meijboom, E.J., Valdes-Cruz, L.M., Horowitz, S., et al.: A two-dimensional Doppler echocardiographic method for calculation of pulmonary and systemic blood flow in a canine model with a variable-sized left-to-right extracardiac shunt. Circulation 68:437, 1983.

75. Kitabatake, A., Inoue, M., Asao, M., et al.: Noninvasive evaluation of the ratio of

pulmonary to systemic flow in atrial septal defect by duplex Doppler echocardiography. Circulation 69:73, 1984.

76. Barron, J.V., Sahn, D.J., Valdes-Cruz, L.M., et al.: Clinical utility of two-dimensional Doppler echocardiographic techniques for estimating pulmonary to systemic blood flow ratios in children with left to right shunting atrial septal defect, ventricular septal defect or patent ductus arteriosus. J. Am. Coll. Cardiol. 3:169, 1984.

77. Dittmann, H., Jacksch, R., Voelker, W., et al.: Accuracy of Doppler echocardiography in quantification of left-to-right shunts in adult patients with atrial septal defect. J. Am. Coll. Cardiol. 11:338, 1988.

78. Anconina, J., Danchin, N., Selton-Suty, C., et al.: Noninvasive estimation of right ventricular dP/dt in patients with tricuspid valve regurgitation. Am. J. Cardiol. 71:1495, 1993.

79. Imanishi, T., Nakatani, S., Yamada, S., et al.: Validation of continuous wave Doppler-determined right ventricular peak positive and negative dP/dt: Effect of right atrial pressure on measurement. J. Am. Coll. Cardiol. 23:1638, 1994.

80. Dabestani, A., Mahan, G., Gardin, J.M., et al.: Evaluation of pulmonary artery pressure and resistance by pulsed Doppler echocardiography. Am. J. Cardiol. 59:662, 1987.

81. Kitabatake, A., Inoue, M., Asao, M., et al.: Noninvasive evaluation of pulmonary hypertension by a pulsed Doppler technique. Circulation 68:302, 1983.

82. Isobe, M., Yazaki, Y., Takaku, F., et al.: Prediction of pulmonary arterial pressure in adults by pulsed Doppler echocardiography. Am. J. Cardiol. 57:316, 1986.

83. Yock, P.G., and Popp, R.L.: Noninvasive estimation of right ventricular systolic pressure by Doppler ultrasound in patients with tricuspid regurgitation. Circulation 70:657, 1984.

84. Currie, P.J., Seward, J.B., Chan, K.-L., et al.: Continuous wave Doppler determination of right ventricular pressure: A simultaneous Doppler-catheterization study in 127 patients. J. Am. Coll. Cardiol. 5:750, 1985.

85. Berger, M., Haimowitz, A., Van Tosh, A., et al.: Quantitative assessment of pulmonary hypertension in patients with tricuspid regurgitation using continuous wave Doppler ultrasound. J. Am. Coll. Cardiol. 6:359, 1985.

86. Kircher, B.J., Himelman, R.B., and Schiller, N.B.: Noninvasive estimation of right atrial pressure from the inspiratory collapse of the inferior vena cava. Am. J. Cardiol. 66:493, 1990.

87. Hatle, L., Angelsen, B.A., and Tromsdal, A.: Non-invasive estimation of pulmonary artery systolic pressure with Doppler ultrasound. Br. Heart J. 45:157, 1981.

88. Masuyama, T., Kodama, K., Kitabatake, A., et al.: Continuous-wave Doppler echocardiographic detection of pulmonary regurgitation and its application to noninvasive estimation of pulmonary artery pressure. Circulation 74:484, 1986.

89. Beppu, S., Tanabe, K., Shimizu, T., et al.: Contrast enhancement of Doppler signals by sonicated albumin for estimating right ventricular systolic pressure. Am. J. Cardiol. 67:1148, 1991.

90. Himelman, R.B., Stulberg, M., Kircher, B., et al.: Noninvasive evaluation of pulmonary artery pressure during exercise by saline-enhanced Doppler echocardiography in chronic pulmonary disease. Circulation 79:863, 1989.

91. Miyatake, K., Okamoto, M., Kinoshita, N., et al.: Evaluation of tricuspid regurgitation by pulsed Doppler and two-dimensional echocardiography. Circulation 66:777, 1982.

92. Suzuki, Y., Kambara, H., Kadota, K., et al.: Detection and evaluation of tricuspid regurgitation using a real-time, two-dimensional, color-coded, Doppler flow imaging system: Comparison with contrast two-dimensional echocardiography and right ventriculography. Am. J. Cardiol. 57:811, 1986.

93. Pennestri, F., Loperfido, F., Salvatori, M.P., et al.: Assessment of tricuspid regurgitation by pulsed Doppler ultrasonography of the hepatic veins. Am. J. Cardiol. 54:363, 1984.

94. Sakai, K., Nakamura, K., Satomi, G., et al.: Evaluation of tricuspid regurgitation by blood flow pattern in the hepatic vein using pulsed Doppler technique. Am. Heart J. 108:516, 1984.

95. Chan, K.-L., Currie, P.J., Seward, J.B., et al.: Comparison of three Doppler ultrasound methods in the prediction of pulmonary artery pressure. J. Am. Coll. Cardiol. 9:549, 1987.

96. Levine, R.A., Gibson, T.C., Aretz, T., et al.: Echocardiographic measurement of right ventricular volume. Circulation 69:497, 1984.

97. Linker, D.T., Moritz, W.E., and Pearlman, A.S.: A new three-dimensional echocardiographic method of right ventricular volume measurement: In vitro validation. J. Am. Coll. Cardiol. 8:101, 1986.

98. Jiang, L., Handschumacher, M.D., Hibberd, M.G., et al.: Three-dimensional echocardiographic reconstruction of right ventricular volume: In vitro comparison with two-dimensional methods. J. Am. Soc. Echocardiogr. 7:150, 1994.

99. Polack, J.F., Holman, B.L., Wynne, J., et al.: Right ventricular ejection fraction: An indicator of increased mortality in patients with congestive heart failure associated with coronary artery disease. J. Am. Coll. Cardiol. 2:217, 1983.

100. Baker, B.J.: Dilated cardiomyopathy: The role of the right ventricle in determining function capacity. *In* Konstam, M.A., and Isner, J.M. (eds.): The Right Ventricle. Boston, Kluwer, 1988, p. 131.

29 Doppler-Echocardiographic Evaluation of Diastolic Function

James D. Thomas, M.D.
Allan L. Klein, M.D.

**BASIC PHYSIOLOGY OF DIASTOLIC
FUNCTION ____ 336**
**PHYSICS AND PHYSIOLOGY OF DIASTOLIC
FILLING ____ 337**
**DETERMINANTS OF MITRAL
DECELERATION ____ 338**
**OVERALL DETERMINANTS OF THE EARLY FILLING
WAVE ____ 338**
**DETERMINANTS OF THE ATRIAL FILLING
WAVE ____ 342**
**CHARACTERISTIC MITRAL VELOCITY
PATTERNS ____ 342**
**RELATING MITRAL FILLING PATTERNS TO
DIASTOLIC FUNCTION ____ 344**
**PULMONARY VENOUS VELOCITY
PATTERNS ____ 344**
**CLINICAL APPROACH TO DIASTOLIC
FUNCTION ____ 345**
**DOPPLER ECHOCARDIOGRAPHIC
MEASUREMENTS AND SIGNIFICANCE ____ 346**
**CLINICAL FRAMEWORK OF DIASTOLIC FUNCTION
USING COMPREHENSIVE DOPPLER
ASSESSMENT ____ 349**
**PITFALLS OF DIASTOLIC FUNCTION
MEASUREMENTS ____ 349**

SPECIFIC DISEASES ____ 350
Constrictive Pericarditis ____ 350
Cardiac Tamponade ____ 354
**Restrictive Myocardial Disease: Cardiac
Amyloidosis ____ 354**
Hypertrophic Cardiomyopathy ____ 355
Dilated Cardiomyopathy ____ 357
Cardiac Transplantation ____ 357
Hypertensive Heart Disease ____ 357
Coronary Artery Disease ____ 357
**Diastolic Dysfunction in Congenital Heart
Disease ____ 358**
**Estimating Left Ventricular Filling
Pressures ____ 358**
**Prognostic Implications of Doppler
Variables ____ 358**
**OTHER ECHOCARDIOGRAPHIC
MODALITIES ____ 358**
Continuous-Wave Doppler Imaging ____ 358
**Color Doppler M-Mode Recording of Left
Ventricular Inflow ____ 359**
Doppler Tissue Imaging ____ 361
CONCLUSIONS ____ 361

Diastolic dysfunction may be defined as the inability of the ventricle to fill with sufficient blood for normal cardiac output at an acceptably low (<12 mm Hg) mean left atrial pressure. Left ventricular diastolic dysfunction is an important component of cardiac morbidity in a number of disease states and is one of the earliest detectable abnormalities in several pathologic disorders.[1-6]

Doppler echocardiography can be used noninvasively at the bedside to assess left and right ventricular diastolic filling and provide important information about the functional class, management, and prognosis of patients with diastolic dysfunction.[7] In particular, it has been used increasingly to differentiate constrictive pericarditis from restrictive cardiomyopathy[8] and to describe the spectrum of diastolic filling abnormalities in restrictive cardiomyopathy, with cardiac amyloidosis as the prototype.[9] Abnormalities of diastolic function have also been described in hypertrophic cardiomyopathy,[10, 11] dilated cardiomyopathy,[12, 13] hypertensive heart disease,[11, 14] and congenital heart disease.[15, 16] In addition, it has been used to assess the effects of the aging process[17-19] and to assist in the diagnosis of both acute[20] and chronic rejection[21] in cardiac transplantation. Most recently, there has been enthusiasm for using Doppler echocardiography to determine prognosis in dilated[22] and restrictive cardiomyopathies.[23] Finally, Doppler echocardiography can be used to estimate left ventricular filling pressures.[24, 25] From the transthoracic route and increasingly from the transesophageal approach, pulsed Doppler interrogation of the atrioventricular valves and central flow velocities provides a comprehensive approach to diastolic function.[7, 26, 27] Before describing

in detail the clinical Doppler examination for diastolic function, we shall review some basic physiology and fluid dynamics that can be of help in the interpretation of Doppler flow patterns.

BASIC PHYSIOLOGY OF DIASTOLIC FUNCTION

The physiology of ventricular diastolic function is complex, involving interactions at the subcellular, myocyte, myocardial tissue, and whole-chamber levels. Several outstanding reviews of the basic physiology of diastole have recently appeared[28-30] and will be briefly reviewed here. Although an oversimplification, diastole may be thought of as having two distinct features: *relaxation*, the active transition of the myocardium from the end-systolic contraction state, and *compliance*, the pressure-volume relationship of the ventricle in its fully relaxed state.

Relaxation

Myocardial relaxation is an active, energy-requiring process, mediated by intracellular adenosine triphosphate (ATP) and calcium. Released in large quantities from the sarcoplasmic reticulum at the initiation of systole, calcium ion binds to the troponin-tropomyosin complex, removing the inhibitory effect of that complex on the actin myosin myofilaments.[31] Active cross-bridges then form between actin and myosin, with consequent contraction of the myofilaments, continuing until (1) intracellular calcium levels fall enough to reactivate the inhibitory effect of troponin-tropomyosin complex[32] and (2) sufficiently high levels of ATP are present in the cytosol to dissociate the actin and myosin myofibrils.[29] ATP is critical for resequestering calcium from the cytosol and dissociating actin from myosin. Abnormal relaxation and diastolic tone may result from either elevated cytosolic calcium in diastole or inadequate intracellular ATP levels to dissociate actin from myosin, with the two mechanisms often synergistic with each other.[33]

Compliance

The fundamental "springiness" of the myocardium is provided by its stress-strain relationship. *Stress,* given in units of force per unit area (dynes/cm², mm Hg, for example), is a measure of the force pulling on a segment of myocardium. *Strain,* on the other hand, is the proportional stretch in the length of tissue under the influence of a given stress and is, thus, dimensionless. The ratio of stress to strain is *stiffness* (in mechanics, Young's modulus, E), reflecting the residual tone within the myocytes (incomplete relaxation) and the nature and amount of collagen within the myocardium. Collagen transduces myocyte contractile force into intraventricular pressure and helps determine overall ventricular size and shape.[34–36] Collagen has a highly nonlinear stress-strain relationship, coiled around myofibrils so that little force is needed initially to stretch the coil, then revealing its full stiffness above a critical strain so that the overall curve is exponential in shape.[37] When myocardial collagen rises (pressure hypertrophy), overall stiffness increases, whereas a local collagen scar (reparative fibrosis after myocardial infarction) is three-fold stiffer than the surrounding myocardium.[38]

Pressure-Volume Curves in the Intact Ventricle

The pressure-volume curve of the ventricle combines the mechanics of the myocardium with the morphology of the ventricle. A thin-walled sphere with wall thickness h made up of tissue with constant stiffness E has chamber stiffness (dP/dV) of approximately hE. More sophisticated analyses have used nonlinear stress-strain relationships for the myocardium.[39] Below the equilibrium volume of the ventricle (the volume at zero transmural pressure), increasingly negative pressure is required to decrease the volume further, consistent with the storage of energy in parallel elastic elements within the ventricle.[40]

Combined Effect of Relaxation and Compliance

Thus, the instantaneous ventricular stiffness is a complex function of the extent of relaxation and the current chamber volume.

At end-systole, the ventricle has an approximately linear pressure-volume relationship,[41] followed by an approximately exponential pressure drop in isovolumic relaxation.[42, 43] Ventricular stiffness also decreases rapidly as actin myosin cross-bridges are broken, and chamber stiffness is approximately proportional to the instantaneous pressure.[44, 45] Even after ventricular filling begins, continued relaxation makes the ventricle more compliant, which is exemplified by falling of pressure despite rising chamber volume. Once relaxation is complete (generally by mid-diastole), the chamber pressure-volume curve is approximately exponential. Figure 29–1 displays this change schematically from end-systole to end-diastole.

Principal Indices of Diastolic Function

The optimal index to use in characterizing diastolic function is controversial, although mean left atrial pressure appears to correlate best with congestive symptoms. Isovolumic relaxation may be characterized by an exponential curve with either a zero[42] ($P_0 e^{-t/\tau}$) or nonzero[43] ($P_0 e^{-t/\tau} + P_b$) asymptote to measure the time constant of ventricular relaxation, τ. Passive ventricular properties can be characterized by combining intraventricular pressure measurements with volume measurements obtained from radionuclide imaging,[46] contrast angiography,[47] or echocardiography.[48] Fitting an exponential curve to latter diastole can yield the exponential *volume constant* (the volume of blood required to raise ventricular pressure by a factor of e, 2.718) and the end-diastolic stiffness of the ventricle (slope of the pressure-volume curve at this point, dP/dV). None of these indices, however, can account for a parallel shift in the curve as may seen with ischemia[47] or pericardial tamponade. Figure 29–1 shows that chamber stiffness may be increased either by filling at a higher ventricular volume (systolic dysfunction) or by filling along a steeper curve (primary diastolic dysfunction). Even with invasive left ventricular diastolic pressure, characterization of diastolic function is imperfect, a situation compounded in the Doppler echocardiographic assessment of diastolic function, in which direct measurements of intracardiac pressure is not possible.

PHYSICS AND PHYSIOLOGY OF DIASTOLIC FILLING

Before describing the clinical application of Doppler echocardiography in the assessment of diastolic function, it is important to understand the fundamental relationship governing the passage of blood into the ventricle. Armed with this knowledge, one can more easily comprehend interpretation of Doppler filling patterns.

Physical Determinants of Transmitral Flow

All movement of blood within the heart is governed by the Navier-Stokes equations, a coupled set of four partial differential

FIGURE 29–1. A schematic representation of the left ventricular pressure-volume curve from end-systole to end-diastole. At end-systole, the pressure volume relationship is linear, whereas at end-diastole it is sigmoid in shape, with an exponentially rising portion at higher volumes and a concave downward portion below the equilibrium volume of the ventricle. The time is given in milliseconds from end-systole and demonstrates that some relaxation continues well into diastole.

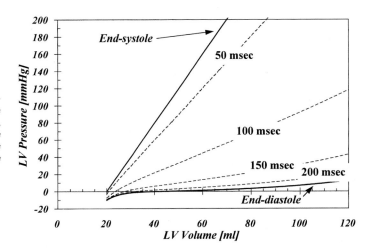

equations relating pressure and the three components of velocity at each point within the heart and each instant in the cardiac cycle. Because these equations are quite complex, consider the simpler schematic anatomy in Figure 29–2, where a column of blood of length L, area A, and density ρ (mass m = ρAL) is accelerated by the transmitral force (pressure gradient ΔP times mitral area A) between the atrium and the ventricle. Newton's second law (force equals mass times acceleration) dictates that the instantaneous acceleration of blood across the mitral valve is as follows:

$$\text{Acceleration} = dV/dt = \frac{F}{m} = \frac{A\Delta p}{\rho AL} = \frac{\Delta p}{\rho L}$$

Here we see that mitral valve area cancels out, leaving inertance (functional mass of blood being accelerated) as the effective length of the blood column within the mitral valve, multiplied by blood density, previously identified by Yellin as a key determinant for transmitral blood acceleration.[49] The impact of inertance was demonstrated in an in vitro model by quantifying the acceleration of blood under conditions of differing pressure gradients and valvular inertance (determined explicitly, in this case, by a physical column within which blood accelerated through an orifice). It was shown that with increasing inertance the peak acceleration slowed for a given pressure gradient.[50] This work suggested that the mitral inertance length is approximately equal to three times the valve diameter, although clinical validation of this measurement is incomplete at present.

Physiologic Determinants of Mitral Acceleration

In the clinical situation, the transmitral pressure gradient ΔP is not established instantaneously but rather rises linearly as left ventricular pressure falls below left atrial pressure with ventricular relaxation, and this rate (dΔP/dt) is thus a principal determinant of E-wave (early diastolic filling wave) acceleration. For exponential isovolumic relaxation (P = $P_0e^{-t/\tau}$), the rate of ventricular pressure decline (-dP_V/dt) at a particular atrial pressure P_a is given by P_a/τ, suggesting that E-wave acceleration should be proportional to left atrial pressure and inversely related to the relaxation time constant. Figure 29–3 shows this interplay between left atrial pressure and τ in determining dΔP/dt, along with animal data by Choong and co-workers, demonstrating in vivo the same interplay between τ and left atrial pressure in determining E-wave acceleration.[51] Their study was particularly elucidating, since left atrial pressure and τ could be manipulated independently of each other by a nonphar-

macologic adjustment of preload and afterload, but numerous other studies have shown concordant results.[52–57]

DETERMINANTS OF MITRAL DECELERATION

Physical Determinants

Even before peak velocity is achieved in the E wave, physical forces begin to decelerate and stop flow into the ventricle because of the reversal of the atrioventricular pressure gradient by blood volume leaving the atrium and entering the ventricle. Because the relationship between chamber volume and pressure is defined by compliance (dV/dP), we anticipate that velocity deceleration will be closely related to chamber stiffness. Two simplified mathematical analyses have been performed to relate deceleration to compliance.

The first[58] analyzed flow through a restrictive orifice, demonstrating that the velocity deceleration rate was inversely proportional to compliance (and directly proportional to mitral valve area): $-dV/dt = A/\rho C_n$. As shown in the in vitro modeling in Figure 29–4, decreasing chamber compliance from 30 to 15 resulted in a doubling of the rate of velocity decline. This relationship is strictly applicable only for restrictive orifices and has proved useful in the analysis of the mitral pressure half-time in mitral stenosis.[59] For normal mitral orifices, it is more appropriate to analyze transmitral flow as an inertial system, similar to a harmonic oscillator. Modeled in this way, the critical mitral parameter to relate to compliance is the deceleration time (DT, the interval from the peak of the E wave until zero velocity), which is predicted to be proportional to the square root of the net compliance of the atrium and ventricle: DT $\propto (C_n)^{1/2}$.[60]

Physiologic Determinants

To apply these analyses to the clinical situation, the meaning of compliance in these equations must be carefully considered. As shown in Figure 29–1, the key parameter is the operating compliance (local slope, dP/dV), which can change either by shifting along a particular pressure volume curve or by changing the curve itself. Compounding the confusion is the fact that the curve itself is not static but rather shifts downward throughout diastole as relaxation proceeds. Atrial compliance adds to this ambiguity but may have relatively little impact because atrial pressure is fairly constant during diastole because of the relative balance between mitral outflow and pulmonary venous inflow. Several studies have demonstrated qualitatively that mitral deceleration time shortens in other situations of reduced ventricular compliance, such as constrictive pericarditis[8, 61] and acute severe aortic insufficiency.[53, 62]

OVERALL DETERMINANTS OF THE EARLY FILLING WAVE (DOPPLER E WAVE)

Figure 29–5 summarizes the interplay between the physical and the physiologic forces that affect mitral acceleration and deceleration. It is also useful for analyzing a more sophisticated mathematical model, where acceleration and deceleration forces can coexist, to assess the impact that diastolic function parameters have on the overall shape of the E wave. This mathematical model (termed a "lumped parameter" model, since distributed quantities, such as atrial and ventricular pressure, are lumped into single numbers) has been described in detail previously,[63, 64] with similar models also reported.[65–71] Additionally, distributed models of two dimensional flow[72–75] and preliminary three dimensional models[76, 77] have also been described, although the computational demands of these latter models have limited their widespread application.

Figure 29–6 shows a series of numerical solutions to this lumped parameter model. In each pair of drawings, the diastolic portion of

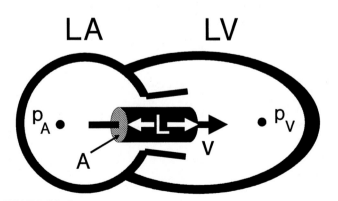

FIGURE 29–2. A schematic diagram that illustrates the physical forces associated with diastolic filling of the ventricle. A mass of blood with area A, length L, and density ρ is accelerated by the transmitral pressure gradient ($P_a - P_v$) to pass at velocity (v) into the ventricle. (From Thomas, J.D., Newell, J.B., Choong, C.Y.P., et al.: Physical and physiologic determinants of transmitral velocity: Numerical analysis. Am. J. Physiol. 260 (5 Pt. 2):H1718, 1991. Reprinted with permission from the American Journal of Physiology.)

FIGURE 29-3. Numerical and animal modeling of the determinants of E-wave acceleration. In the left-hand panel, isovolumic relaxation is modeled as an exponential decay curve for three values of τ (20, 40, and 60 msec) with three levels of left atrial pressure (5, 10, and 20 mm Hg). The middle panels show the growth in the atrioventricular pressure gradient in the first 10 msec after mitral valve opening, as it relates to variations in left atrial pressure (LAP) when τ is constant (*top panel*) and to variations in τ when LAP is constant (*lower panel*). The panels in the right-hand column show corresponding experimental data for mitral filling curves as left atrial pressure (*top*) and τ (*bottom*) are varied while the other is held constant. For exponential decay of isovolumic ventricular pressure, the growth rate of the transmitral pressure gradient (dΔP/dt) is directly proportional to left atrial pressure (the left ventricular pressure at the time of mitral opening) and inversely proportional to τ: dΔP/dt = LAP/τ. Thus, the rise in ΔP is faster when left atrial pressure equals 20 mm Hg than when it equals 5 mm Hg (*middle, top*), reflected in the brisker acceleration and higher peak velocity of the E wave (*right, top*). Conversely, at a given left atrial pressure, ΔP rises faster for τ = 20 msec than for τ = 60 msec (*middle, bottom*), shown also in the experimental data (*right, bottom*). These data predict that mitral acceleration rises with left atrial pressure as τ is held constant and falls with delayed relaxation when left atrial pressure is held constant. (*Left and Middle Panels,* Adapted from Thomas, J.D., and Weyman, A.E.: Echocardiographic Doppler evaluation of left ventricular diastolic function: Physics and physiology. Circulation 84:977, 1991. *Right Panels,* Adapted from Choong, C.Y., et al.: Combined influence of ventricular loading and relaxation in the transmitral flow velocity profile in dogs measured by Doppler echocardiography. Circulation 78:672, 1988. With permission of the American Heart Association.)

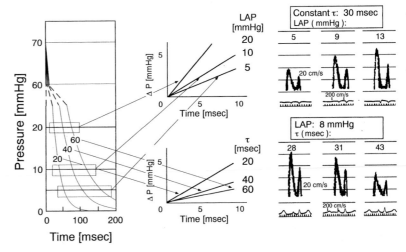

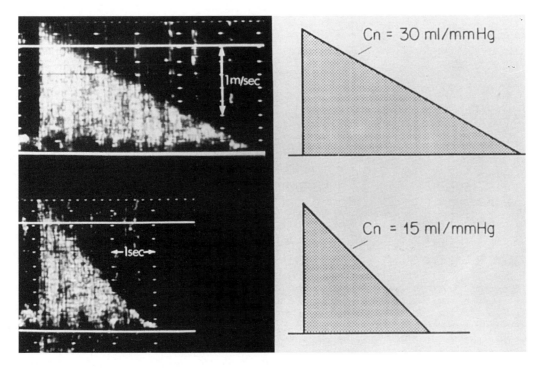

FIGURE 29-4. Continuous-wave Doppler tracings of transmitral flow in an in vitro model. When compliance is reduced from 30 to 15 ml/mm Hg, the slope of the velocity decay is doubled but remains linear. (From Flachskampf, F.A., Weyman, A.E., Guererro, J.L., et al.: Calculation of atrial ventricular compliance from the mitral flow profile: Analytical and in vitro study. J. Am. Coll. Cardiol. 19:998, 1992. Reprinted with permission of the Journal of the American College of Cardiology.)

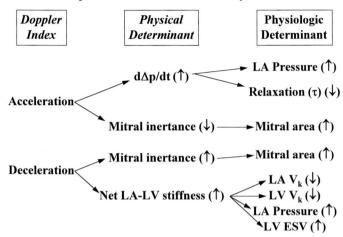

Physical and Physiologic Determinants
of Transmitral Flow Velocity

FIGURE 29–5. Physical parameters that predict acceleration and deceleration of flow across the mitral valve, with the physiologic parameters that determine these physical forces. Up arrows indicate a direct impact on the parameter to the left; down arrows indicate an inverse relationship. (From Thomas, J.D., and Weyman, A.E.: Echocardiographic Doppler evaluation of left ventricular diastolic function: Physics and physiology. Circulation 84:977–990, 1991. Reproduced with permission from the American Heart Association.)

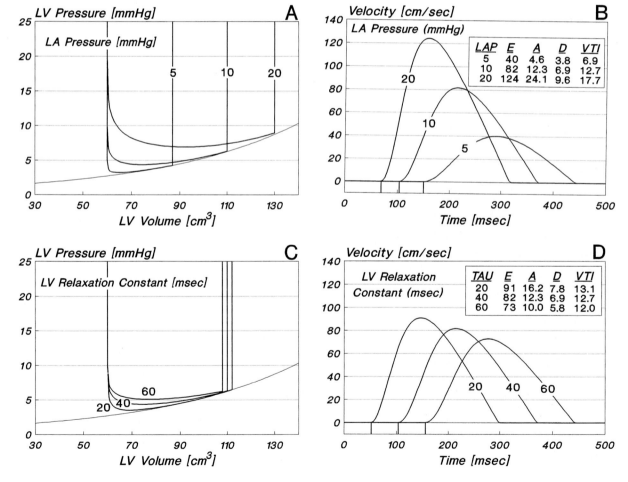

FIGURE 29–6 *See legend on opposite page*

the pressure-volume curve is shown on the left, and the time-velocity curve is shown to the right. In each case, the middle curve represents the same set of parameters in all pairs of figures: left atrial pressure = 10 mm Hg, τ = 40 msec, ventricular volume constant = 60 cm³, and ventricular end-systolic volume = 60 cm³. The other two curves in each pair of figures shows a decrease and an increase in the parameter of interest.

Influence of Atrial Pressure

In Panels A and B of Figure 29–6, increasing atrial pressure has the effect of increasing early acceleration, shortening isovolumic relaxation, and increasing the time-velocity integral of the curve, as more flow is propelled across the mitral valve by the higher left atrial pressure.

Impact of Ventricular Relaxation

Figure 29–6C and D shows that increases in τ cause a delay in filling, as manifested particularly by the prolonged isovolumic

relaxation time (vertical lines in panel D). Peak acceleration rate and maximal velocity are also reduced, consistent with the inverse relationship between dΔP/dt and τ (see Fig. 29–3), but the time velocity integral of the E wave is only slightly reduced, also shown by the minimal change in end-diastolic volume in panel C. Thus, delayed relaxation does not significantly impact total filling, as long as relaxation is ultimately complete before the end of the E wave.

Impact of Intrinsic Chamber Stiffness

Figure 29–6E shows three different ventricular pressure volume curves, reflecting volume constants of 40, 60, and 90 cm³. Reduction in the volume constant leads to a steeper pressure volume curve at all volumes, resulting in more rapid deceleration (compare Fig. 29–4), along with a lower peak velocity and a markedly reduced time-velocity integral and end-diastolic volume.

Impact of End-Systolic Volume

Figure 29–6G and H shows changes similar to those seen in 29–6E and F, but this time the reduction in operating compliance

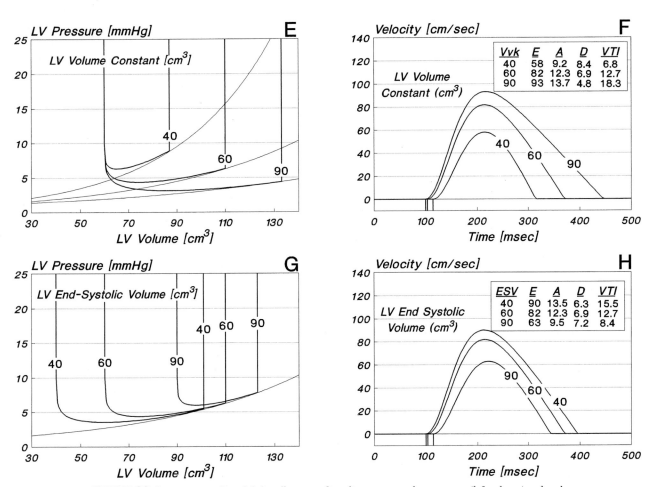

FIGURE 29–6. A numerical model that illustrates diastolic pressure-volume curves (left column) and early transmitral filling wave (right column), depicting the impact of changing atrial pressure (panels A and B), ventricular relaxation time constant (panels C and D), ventricular stiffness (panels E and F), and ventricular end-systolic volume (panels G and H). The middle curve in each pair of graphs represents identical parameter input: left atrial pressure equals 10 mm Hg; relaxation time constant (τ) equals 40 msec; left ventricular volume constant (volume needed to raise left ventricular pressure by a factor of E, 2.718) equals 60 cm³; and left ventricular end-systolic volume equals 60 cm³. Changes above and below these values are indicated in each pair of panels. E = peak velocity of E-wave (cm/sec); A = peak acceleration rate of E wave (m/sec²); D = peak deceleration rate of E wave (m/sec²); VTI = E-wave velocity time integral (cm); LAP = left atrial pressure (mm Hg); V_vk = left ventricular volume constant (cm³); ESV = left ventricular end-systolic volume (cm³). The vertical lines in each right-hand panel represent the isovolumic relaxation time (IVRT). See text for description of results. (From Thomas, J.D., and Weyman, A.E.: Echocardiographic Doppler evaluation of left ventricular diastolic function: Physics and physiology. Circulation 84:977–990, 1991. Reproduced with permission from the American Heart Association.)

is achieved by increasing the end-systolic volume, on which the ventricle must fill. With an elevated end-systolic volume, deceleration is more rapid, and the peak velocity, the time-velocity integral of filling, and the stroke volume (end-diastolic volume minus end-systolic volume) all are reduced.

DETERMINANTS OF THE ATRIAL FILLING WAVE (DOPPLER A WAVE)

The simulations depicted in Figure 29–6 model only the early filling wave, without any provision for atrial contraction. Several other numerical[65, 66, 69, 70] and in vivo[78, 79] studies have investigated the determinants of the atrial filling wave. In essence, the *physical* determinants of the transmitral A wave are identical to those for the E wave: acceleration is produced by an atrioventricular pressure difference (caused by atrial contraction), whereas deceleration results from equilibration of the gradient due to the passive rise in ventricular pressure or the fall in atrial pressure, either because of transfer of blood from the atrium or the end of atrial contraction. The physiology of atrial function has been less studied than early ventricular relaxation but may be broadly divided into preload, afterload, and intrinsic contractility.[26, 80]

Atrial Preload

Prior animal experiments[81, 82] have shown that the strength of atrial contraction is affected by its preload (the volume and pressure at the time of atrial activation), which is analogous to Starling's law, relating myofibril stretch and contractile force in the ventricle, and means that a high left atrial pressure at the time of atrial contraction (because of, for example, delayed ventricular relaxation, elevated heart rate, or first-degree atrioventricular block) leads to a more forceful contraction and a larger A wave.

Atrial Afterload

The second determinant of A-wave magnitude is atrial afterload, in effect, ventricular stiffness shown in advanced cases of restrictive cardiomyopathy, in which even a forceful atrial contraction results in very little transfer to the ventricle because of the extremely steep ventricular pressure-volume curve. The problem is compounded further by volume ejected by the atrium, which may instead go up the pulmonary veins (see below), rather than forward through the mitral valve.

Atrial Systolic Function

Finally, a critical determinant of the forward A wave is atrial contractile performance, which has been shown to vary considerably in health and disease, such as the delayed recovery seen after electrical cardioversion.[83] Decreased atrial systolic function also plays a role in the reduction in forward A wave seen in advanced amyloidosis, in addition to the increased atrial afterload (ventricular stiffness) mentioned earlier.

CHARACTERISTIC MITRAL VELOCITY PATTERNS

Principal Indices of Left Ventricular Filling

A detailed description of mitral filling patterns seen in specific disease states is discussed subsequently, but we shall first present some general observations. The standard Doppler measurements of left- and right-sided filling are shown diagrammatically in Figure

29–7. Left ventricular inflow early filling wave (E) and atrial wave (A) velocities can be measured and the E:A ratio calculated.[9] The darkest portion of the spectral Doppler (modal velocity) can be digitized on-screen or off-line, with the use of a digitizing tablet to obtain time-velocity integrals. The E-wave deceleration time is measured by extrapolating the deceleration slope of the outer edge of the E-wave tracing from peak velocity to the baseline.[61] In addition, the isovolumic relaxation time (IVRT), the time from aortic valve closure to mitral valve opening and an indirect measure of relaxation, may be measured by directing a large pulsed Doppler sample volume to intercept both the mitral and the aortic valves.[26]

"Normal" Filling Pattern

The top panel in Figure 29–8 displays a filling pattern typically observed in young healthy patients, with a briskly accelerating E wave, relatively gradual deceleration, and an A wave smaller in magnitude than the E wave.

"Delayed-Relaxation" Pattern

As a consequence of normal aging and various pathologic states, a pattern like that in Figure 29–8B emerges, the "delayed-relaxation" pattern. One can rationalize its appearance by careful consideration of Figure 29–6. When the relaxation time constant is lengthened, the E wave indeed displays slower acceleration and a lower peak amplitude. To the extent that emptying may not be complete by the end of diastasis, an increased left atrial volume will be present at the time of atrial contraction, leading to a larger A wave, compensating in large part for the smaller E-wave time-velocity integral.

Note, however, that this pattern is not pathognomonic for delayed relaxation. As shown in Figure 29–6B, simple reduction in left atrial pressure produces a reduced E wave, typically out of proportion to any change in the A wave.[56, 84, 85] Nevertheless, this pattern has been reported as a pathologic finding in situations such as hypertrophic cardiomyopathy,[10, 86–88] secondary hypertrophy,[89] morbid obesity,[90] myocardial infarction,[91] acute ischemia due to increased myocardial oxygen demand[92] and transient coronary occlusion,[93–96] and dilated cardiomyopathy,[97] as well as immediately after coronary artery bypass grafting.[98] Reversal of this pattern has even been used to assess the benefit of pharmacologic therapy,[99–101] coronary angioplasty,[102] and septal myomectomy.[103]

Pattern of Restrictive Filling

Figure 29–8C displays a second type of pathologic filling pattern, the "restrictive" filling pattern, which is characterized by a very elevated peak E-wave velocity with extremely rapid deceleration and diminutive (often absent) A wave. Analysis of Figure 29–6 shows that no isolated parameter adjustment will produce a pattern such as that of Figure 29–8C. The key point, of course, is that Figure 29–6 was produced with *isolated* diastolic parameter changes, whereas in the clinical situation, multiple changes often occur simultaneously, either in compensation for a primary change or as part of the disease process. For instance, reduction in filling due to increased ventricular stiffness may be counteracted by increases in heart rate, inotropic state, or, most commonly, left atrial pressure. Figure 29–9 demonstrates the dramatically different effects that a reduction in ventricular compliance has on the shape of the E wave when it is accompanied by a compensatory rise in left atrial pressure, as compared to when one keeps left atrial pressure constant. Preload compensation dramatically changes the morphology of the E wave from a pattern consistent with delayed relaxation (although relaxation was not altered in this model) to one consistent with the restrictive pattern, characterized by a short isovolumic relaxation time, high peak velocity, and very rapid deceleration. In between these two patterns a "pseudonormal" pattern may be seen, with an appearance quite similar to that in Figure

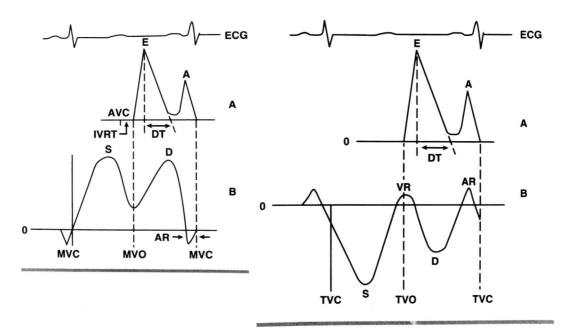

FIGURE 29-7. Standard measurements of left *(left panels)* and right *(right panels)* ventricular filling patterns. *Left panels: A,* Diagram of normal left ventricular inflow velocities, showing biphasic diastolic filling pattern with a greater peak early (E) flow velocity and smaller peak late (A) flow velocity. Deceleration time (DT) is the time required for the E velocity to decline from its peak to the baseline. Isovolumic relaxation time (IVRT) is the time from aortic valve closure (AVC) to mitral valve opening (MVO). *B,* Diagram of normal pulmonary venous flow velocity, showing a biphasic forward filling pattern with slightly greater systolic (S) than diastolic (D) flow velocities and reverse flow with atrial contraction (AR). MVC = mitral valve closure. *Right panels: A,* A diagram of normal right ventricular inflow velocities showing a biphasic diastolic filling pattern with a greater peak early (E) flow velocity and a smaller peak late (A) flow velocity. Deceleration time (DT) is the time interval required for the E velocity to decline from its peak to the baseline. *B,* Diagram of normal superior vena cava or hepatic vein flow velocity showing a biphasic forward filling pattern with greater systolic (S) than diastolic (D) filling and reverse flow during late ventricular systole (VR) and with atrial contraction (AR). Usually, the hepatic vein has more prominent flow reversals than does the superior vena cava. TVC = tricuspid valve closure; TVO = tricuspid valve opening. (From Klein, A.L.: Doppler echocardiographic assessment of constrictive pericarditis, cardiac amyloidosis, and cardiac tamponade. Cleve. Clin. J. Med. 59:279, 280, 1992. Reproduced with permission of the Cleveland Clinic Journal of Medicine.)

FIGURE 29-8. Characteristic transmitral filling patterns. The left panel shows a typical pattern from a healthy young person, with the E wave greater than the A wave, while the center panel (E < A) is termed the delayed relaxation pattern. The right panel, with E >> A is referred to as the restrictive filling pattern.

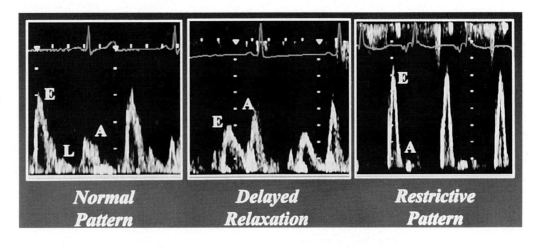

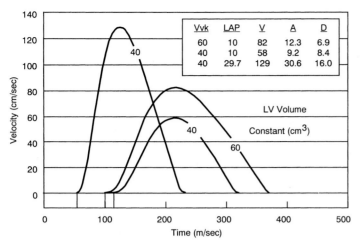

Vvk	LAP	V	A	D
60	10	82	12.3	6.9
40	10	58	9.2	8.4
40	29.7	129	30.6	16.0

FIGURE 29–9. The impact of preload compensation on the E wave. If ventricular stiffness is increased (V_{vk} reduced from 60 to 40 cm³) while atrial pressure is held constant at 10 mm Hg, the E wave is reduced in magnitude in a manner similar to that seen in Figure 29–8, center panel. However, if atrial pressure is allowed to rise close to 30 mm Hg to maintain transmitral filling volume, the resultant E wave has a very high peak velocity with steep deceleration and a short isovolumic relaxation time, similar to the restrictive pattern of Figure 29–8, right panel. (From Thomas, J.D.: Assessment of diastolic heart failure by echocardiography. Heart Failure 7:195, 1991. Reprinted with permission of Le Jacq Communications, Greenwich, CT.)

29–8A. The association between the restrictive filling pattern and the need for elevated filling pressures perhaps explains the poor prognosis connoted by the restrictive pattern.[23]

rect determination of τ) are quite promising and will be discussed at the end of this chapter.

RELATING MITRAL FILLING PATTERNS TO DIASTOLIC FUNCTION

Thus, multiple physiologic parameters may have similar effects on the mitral inflow pattern, making it impossible to relate a given inflow pattern to a specific set of diastolic function parameters. As shown in Figure 29–10, even the simple index of E:A wave ratio demonstrates a characteristic U-shaped curve during the course of normal aging and the development of a restrictive filling pattern, and it is impossible to tell from the E:A ratio, whether one is on the left side or right side of the U-shaped curve, showing the difficulty of solving the "inverse problem" in clinical practice. In the case of mitral filling, it is relatively straightforward to proceed in the "forward" direction (using diastolic function parameters to predict mitral filling patterns, as in Figure 29–6) but generally impossible to use a given mitral filling pattern to predict a unique set of diastolic function parameters. Additional data are needed to determine whether a patient is on the left- or right-hand side of the U-curve in Figure 29–10. The pulmonary venous pattern is an important source of additional information and will be discussed in general terms presently. In addition, several new approaches to the Doppler assessment of diastolic function (e.g., color M-mode, di-

PULMONARY VENOUS VELOCITY PATTERNS

The pulmonary venous velocity pattern provides important adjunctive information to the transmitral pattern, providing important evidence distinguishing the normal transmitral pattern from the "pseudonormal" pattern, while additionally providing important evidence characterizing the severity of mitral regurgitation and left atrial dysfunction. These clinical issues will be discussed subsequently, but first we shall introduce the physical and physiologic determinants of pulmonary venous flow.

Physical Determinants

Like transmitral flow, pulmonary venous flow is dictated physically by Newton's second law, F = ma, where force is the pressure difference between the central pulmonary veins and the left atrium, and the mass relates to the inertance of blood within the distal pulmonary veins. Previous in vitro work suggests that pulmonary venous inertance is approximately equal to the length of the distal pulmonary veins. Alexander and associates investigated the frequency dependence of pulmonary venous impedance, demonstrating in a preliminary study that impedance falls with increasing frequency, reaching a minimum at 6.9 Hz, reflecting the optimal manner for the pulmonary veins to transmit pressure and flow.[104]

Physiologic Determinants

The pulmonary venous velocity pattern typically has three distinct waves associated with particular events in the cardiac cycle (see Fig. 29–7B).[80, 105] The S wave, occurring during ventricular systole, is an antegrade wave (into the left atrium), reflecting the fall in left atrial pressure decreases (x descent) due to atrial relaxation and descent of the mitral annulus during ventricular contraction; these two etiologies for the fall in atrial pressure sometimes lead to a notched S wave. The second major pulmonary venous wave (D wave) occurs during ventricular diastole shortly after the peak of the forward E wave through the mitral valve, reflecting the fall in atrial pressure with atrial emptying into the left ventricle (y descent). During this phase, the left atrium functions largely as a conduit between the pulmonary veins and the left ventricle. The final pulmonary venous wave is the atrial reversal (AR) wave, a retrograde wave (up the pulmonary veins) that occurs with atrial contraction. The clinical interpretation of each of these waves in a variety of disease states will be discussed subsequently. We shall

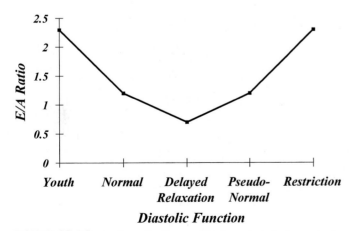

FIGURE 29–10. A schematic diagram showing a typical change in the E:A wave ratio from youth, to healthy old age (middle), to advanced restrictive disease (right side), demonstrating the inability to uniquely determine diastolic function from diastolic flow characteristics.

present here some basic studies that relate the atrial reversal wave to atrial function and left ventricular stiffness.

Physiologic Interpretation of the Transmitral and Pulmonary Venous A Wave

At the time of atrial contraction, blood may exit the atrium either by traveling forward through the mitral valve or retrograde up the pulmonary veins in proportion to the relative impedance to flow presented by the left ventricle versus the pulmonary veins. When we hypothesize pulmonary venous impedance to be relatively constant (an unproven assertion but a reasonable approximation), then the ratio of forward to reversed A wave should relate to the operating compliance of the ventricle at the time of atrial contraction. Furthermore, the sum of the forward and reverse blood velocity should relate to the total stroke volume of atrial contraction and thus reflect, to some degree, atrial systolic function. Figure 29–11 demonstrates the divergent effects that changes in preload and ventricular compliance have on the forward and reversed A waves.[80] When fluid is infused, we see an increase in both the forward A-wave velocity through the mitral valve and the retrograde A-wave velocity of the pulmonary veins, reflecting the increased stroke volume without significant change in ventricular compliance. In contrast, when nitroglycerin is infused, the retrograde A wave falls considerably, in comparison with the forward A wave, reflecting the increased operating compliance of the ventricle at the lower end-diastolic pressure.

Another important index to follow with regard to the A wave is the duration of the pulmonary venous versus mitral A wave. It has been shown previously,[25] in the setting of elevated left ventricular pressure (presumably causing elevated operating stiffness of the left ventricle at end-diastole), the duration of the pulmonary venous reversal wave is prolonged with respect to that of the forward mitral A wave.

We shall now consider the clinical application of transmitral velocity and pulmonary venous flow patterns in the assessment of diastolic function in a variety of clinical settings.

CLINICAL APPROACH TO DIASTOLIC FUNCTION

Doppler-Echocardiographic Examination for Diastolic Function

A comprehensive evaluation of diastolic function includes both structural analysis (by M-mode and two-dimensional echo) and filling analysis of the left and right atria and ventricles by pulsed Doppler.

Two-Dimensional Echocardiography

Two-dimensional echocardiography (transthoracic or transesophageal) can often complement Doppler echocardiography by providing anatomical delineation of the disease type (such as in cardiac amyloidosis) and assessing chamber size and function in diseases with diastolic dysfunction.[7] Key findings are ventricular systolic dysfunction and left atrial enlargement,[106, 107] which may provide a clue as to the chronicity of diastolic dysfunction and provide a simple assessment of the disease progression. In patients with cardiac amyloidosis, abnormal myocardial specular reflections may be seen,[108] while the increased wall thickness of compensatory or cardiomyopathic hypertrophy can be well visualized.[109] In addition, increased pericardial thickness and the abnormal septal bounce characteristic of constrictive pericarditis can be seen,[110] while dilation of the pulmonary and hepatic veins and venae cavae may suggest elevated filling pressures.[111]

Transthoracic Doppler Examination

An integrated approach to diastolic function includes evaluation of filling of both the left[9] and right ventricle.[112] Left ventricular diastolic function can be comprehensively assessed with pulsed Doppler interrogation of the mitral inflow and pulmonary venous flow. Similarly, right ventricular diastolic function can be comprehensively assessed with pulsed Doppler interrogation of tricuspid inflow, hepatic vein, and superior vena cava, as well as inferior vena cava diameter.[27] The phase of respiration is important to

FIGURE 29–11. The impact of fluid infusion (*left panels*) and nitroglycerin infusion (*right panels*) on the transmitral (*top row*) and pulmonary venous (*bottom row*) velocity patterns. With fluid infusion, both forward and reversed A waves increase in amplitude, consistent with an increase in atrial stroke volume, but the ratio of forward to reversed A waves remains similar, consistent with relatively constant ventricular compliance. In contrast, when nitroglycerin is infused, the reversed A wave shrinks, with preservation of the forward A wave, consistent with an increase in the operating compliance of the ventricle in the face of diminished atrial stroke volume. (From Nishimura, R.A., Abel, M.D., Hatle, L.K., et al.: Relation of pulmonary vein to mitral flow velocities by transesophageal Doppler echocardiography: Effect of different loading conditions. Circulation 81:1488, 1990. Reprinted with permission from the American Heart Association.)

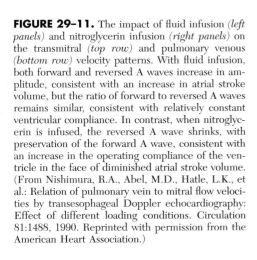
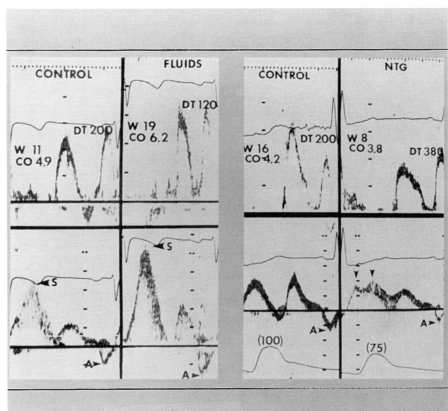

monitor, and it can be assessed simultaneously with Doppler flow velocities with the use of a nasal thermistor to measure the change in temperature between inspiration, expiration, and apnea. These respiratory variations are crucial in differentiating constrictive pericarditis from restrictive cardiomyopathy.[8] The nasal thermistor is connected by a nasal clip to the patient, amplified, and input into the auxiliary port of the Doppler-echocardiography machine. In addition, an accurate electrocardiographic signal is necessary for the proper timing of the Doppler flow events and the cardiac cycle.[7]

Left Heart Filling

With the use of transthoracic imaging from the apical four-chamber view, the pulsed Doppler sample volume is placed at the mitral leaflet tips to measure the maximal flow velocities. Doppler measurements will change as the sample volume is placed at the annulus or left ventricular outflow tract.[113, 114] Initial studies have found that placement of the sample volume at the mitral annulus provides a better volumetric assessment of flow (cardiac output).[7] Often, the sample volume is placed superior to the leaflet tips to detect diastolic mitral regurgitation.[8] Isovolumic relaxation time can be measured by placing a continuous-wave Doppler beam between the left ventricular outflow tract and the left ventricular inflow tract to measure the time from aortic valve closure to mitral valve opening.[9]

Similarly, pulmonary venous flow can be assessed with transthoracic echocardiography by placing the sample volume 1 to 2 cm into the right upper pulmonary vein from the apical four-chamber view.[25] Occasionally, the apical two-chamber view may be necessary to record pulmonary venous flow, or a modified precordial or supraclavicular position.[115] Color flow imaging is often useful in aligning the sample volume parallel to flow to obtain accurate left ventricular inflow and pulmonary venous flow recordings.

Right Heart Filling

Right ventricular inflow can be assessed by placing the sample volume at the leaflet tips of the tricuspid inflow from the apical four-chamber view or the right ventricular inflow view.[112] The inferior vena cava diameter can be measured from the subcostal view and its respiratory variation calculated with M-mode echocardiography.[111] Also from the subcostal position, hepatic venous flow can be recorded by placing the sample volume 1 to 2 cm into the right superior hepatic vein. The patient may have to control the depth of respiration to maintain the sample volume in a stable position. Finally, superior vena cava flow can be measured by placing the sample volume at a depth of 5 to 7 cm into the vein from the supraclavicular position.[112]

Transesophageal Echocardiography

Transesophageal echocardiography can often complement transthoracic echocardiography in the comprehensive assessment of diastolic filling, providing both a physiologic assessment with the use of Doppler echocardiography and excellent anatomical delineation.[116] Increasingly, transesophageal echocardiography has been used when transthoracic imaging is suboptimal because of chronic lung disease, obesity, or poor acoustic windows. With the use of biplane or multiplane imaging of the left and right ventricle from the basal view at 0 or 110 degrees, left ventricular inflow recordings can be obtained with the sample volume at the mitral leaflet tips.[117] In addition, optimal pulmonary venous flow recordings can be obtained with pulsed Doppler in virtually all patients from both the left and the right upper veins from multiple planes.[105] Often, 110 degrees gives the best view of the left upper pulmonary vein, while 70 degrees most optimally images the right upper pulmonary vein. Isovolumic relaxation time measured by continuous-wave Doppler is difficult to record with the transesophageal approach but sometimes can be recorded from the apical five-chamber view from the deep transgastric approach. Similarly, right ventricular inflow measured by pulsed Doppler can be recorded between 70

TABLE 29–1. DIASTOLIC FILLING PARAMETERS

Left Ventricular Filling Dynamics	Right Ventricular Filling Dynamics
Left Ventricular Inflow	*Right Ventricular Inflow*
Peak E (cm/second)	Peak E (cm/second)
Peak A (cm/second)	Peak A (cm/second)
E/A	E/A
DT (milliseconds)	DT (milliseconds)
IVRT (milliseconds)	
Pulmonary Vein	*Superior Vena Cava*
Forward flow	*Hepatic Vein*
Peak S (cm/second)	Forward flow
Peak D (cm/second)	Peak S (cm/second)
Reverse flow	Peak D (cm/second)
Peak AR (cm/second)	Reverse flow
	Peak AR (cm/second)
	Peak VR (cm/second)
	Inferior vena cava size (cm)

DT, deceleration time; IVRT, isovolumic relaxation time; peak A, peak late diastolic flow velocity; peak AR, peak atrial reversal flow velocity; peak D, peak venous diastolic forward flow velocity; peak E, peak early diastolic flow velocity; peak S, peak venous systolic forward flow velocity; peak VR, peak V wave reversal flow velocity.

From Klein, A. L., and Cohen, G. I.: Doppler echocardiographic assessment of constrictive pericarditis, cardiac amyloidosis, and cardiac tamponade. Cleve. Clin. J. Med. 59:279, 1992. Reprinted with permission from Cleveland Clinic Journal of Medicine.

and 90 degrees, and inferior vena cava diameter and hepatic vein flow can be easily assessed from the transverse or longitudinal planes, which can be obtained from views of the coronary sinus and the right atrium and rotating rightward toward the liver. Superior vena cava flow can be well visualized, but the angle of the Doppler sample volume with flow is too large to provide clinically useful information. Similar to transthoracic echocardiography, color flow imaging is necessary to obtain optimal flow recordings.

DOPPLER ECHOCARDIOGRAPHIC MEASUREMENTS AND SIGNIFICANCE

In clinical practice, pulsed Doppler tracings with respiratory monitoring can be recorded on either videotape, a hard copy at either 50 mm per second or 100 mm per second sweep speed, or on an optical disk for digital storage. The important measurements

TABLE 29–2. LEFT VENTRICULAR FILLING DYNAMICS IN NORMAL SUBJECTS

	<50 Years (n = 61)	≥50 Years (n = 56)	P Value
Left Ventricular Inflow			
Peak E (cm/second)	72 ± 14	62 ± 14	<0.01
Peak A (cm/second)	40 ± 10	59 ± 14	<0.01
E/A	1.9 ± 0.6	1.1 ± 0.3	<0.01
DT (milliseconds)	179 ± 20	210 ± 36	<0.01
IVRT (milliseconds)	76 ± 11	90 ± 17	<0.01
Pulmonary Vein	(n = 44)	(n = 41)	
Peak S (cm/second)	48 ± 9	71 ± 9	<0.01
Peak D (cm/second)	50 ± 10	38 ± 9	<0.01
Peak AR (cm/second)	19 ± 4	23 ± 14	<0.01

From Klein, A. L., and Cohen, G. I.: Doppler echocardiographic assessment of constrictive pericarditis, cardiac amyloidosis, and cardiac tamponade. Cleve. Clin. J. Med. 59:281, 1992. Reprinted with permission from Cleveland Clinic Journal of Medicine.

of left and right ventricular diastolic function are shown in Table 29–1. Key indices of mitral inflow have been discussed previously and are shown in Figure 29–7A (see normal values in Table 29–2). Figure 29–12 demonstrates the age-related changes in normal values of left ventricular inflow.

Pulmonary Venous Flow

Peak pulmonary venous flow velocity can be measured in ventricular systole (S wave) and diastole (D wave) and the S:D ratio calculated (see Fig. 29–7B). These are analogous to the x and y descents of the left atrial pressure tracings.[13] Also, the magnitude and duration of the atrial reversal (AR) filling wave, which begins about 60 msec after the P wave on the electrocardiogram, can be measured, providing important insight into ventricular stiffness and atrial contractile function[80] as well as into ventricular filling pressures.[25] There is a strong direct relationship between the timing and the magnitude of the mitral E wave and the pulmonary D wave. Under normal conditions, there is little respiratory variation of pulmonary venous flow (<4 percent).[19] Normal values for pulmonary venous flow with 95 percent confidence intervals are shown in Figure 29–13, while some of the physiologic factors that affect these waves are shown in Table 29–3.

Right Ventricular Inflow

The standard Doppler measurements of right ventricular inflow are shown diagrammatically in Figure 29–7C and are similar to the left ventricular measurements, including the early filling wave (E) and atrial wave (A), E:A ratio, and deceleration time. The right ventricular inflow is more affected by the respiratory cycle and shows increased flow velocities, with inspiration compared to expiration and apnea.[112]

Hepatic Vein and Vena Cava Flow

Normal hepatic vein and superior vena cava velocities are shown in Figure 29–7D. These flow patterns are similar to those of the pulmonary veins, with forward systolic (S) and diastolic (D) waves, analogous to the x and y descents of the right atrial pressure tracings. In addition, small reversals in late ventricular systole (VR) and with atrial contraction (AR) can be seen. Normally, there is greater respiratory variation in hepatic vein and superior vena cava than in the pulmonary vein, with an increase of systolic and diastolic flows in inspiration and more prominent reversals with expiration.[7] Normal values for the right ventricular inflow and vena cava velocities are shown in Table 29–4.

The maximum and minimum diameters of the inferior vena cava can be measured, and normally there is more than a 50 percent collapse of the inferior vena cava from expiration, compared to inspiration. Inferior vena cava plethora is defined as a lack of collapse, which may indicate an elevated right atrial pressure (>15 mm Hg).[111]

Similar to the pulmonary veins, the hepatic vein and superior vena cava flow velocities are closely related to right atrial pressure, and both atrial and ventricular factors can influence the S, D, VR, and AR waves. The S wave (equivalent to the x descent) is related to atrial relaxation and descent of the tricuspid annulus, while the D wave (equivalent to the y descent) is related to the rapid filling of the right ventricle. The late ventricular systolic and atrial reversals are related to right ventricular compliance and right atrial preload, contractility, and afterload.[118]

Effects of Aging

Abnormalities of left ventricular diastolic function have been described as a part of the normal aging process, resulting from intrinsic myocardial changes and hypertrophy of the left ventri-

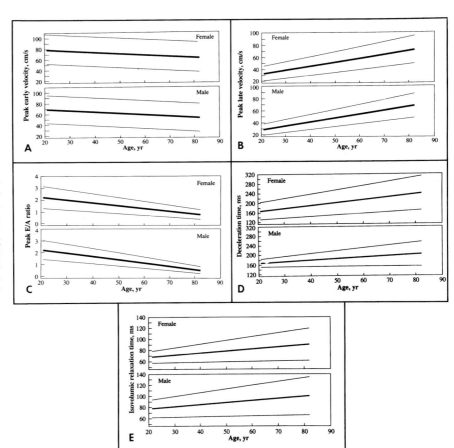

FIGURE 29–12. Peak early velocity (A), peak late velocity (B), peak E:A ratio (early filling velocity to atrial filling velocity) (C), deceleration time (D), and isovolumic relaxation time (E) (*boldface lines* = mean values; *lightface lines* = 95 percent confidence intervals) in female and male subjects, shown by increasing age. (From Klein, A.L., Burstow, D.J., Tajik, A.J., et al.: Effects of age on left ventricular dimensions and filling dynamics in 117 normal persons. Mayo Clin. Proc. 69:219, 1994. Reprinted with permission from the Mayo Clinic Proceedings.)

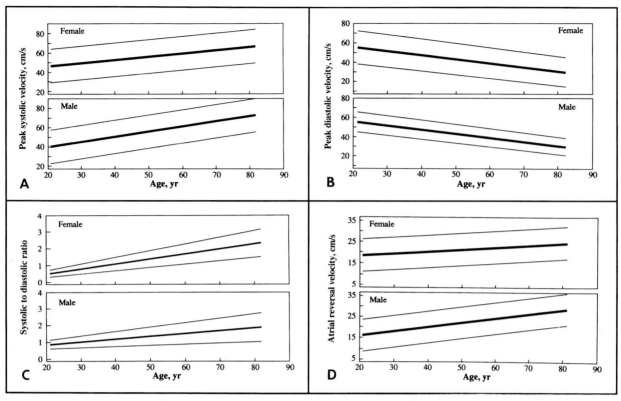

FIGURE 29–13. Pulmonary venous peak systolic velocity (*A*), diastolic velocity (*B*), systolic-to-diastolic ratio (*C*), and atrial reversal velocity (*D*) (*boldface lines* = mean values; *lightface lines* = 95 percent confidence intervals) in female and male subjects, shown by increasing age. (From Klein, A.L., Burstow, D.J., Tajik, A.J., et al.: Effects of age on left ventricular dimensions and filling dynamics in 117 normal persons. Mayo Clin. Proc. 69:217, 1994. Reprinted with permission from the Mayo Clinic Proceedings.)

cle.[119] There have been many studies showing that with the aging process, there is a change in the left ventricular ventricular inflow[17, 18, 120, 121] as well as in pulmonary venous flow. In a recent publication,[19] we showed that young subjects (in the third decade of life) have the highest peak E velocity, the lowest peak A velocity, the highest E:A ratio (2.2), and some of the lowest deceleration times and the shortest isovolumic relaxation times. Middle-aged subjects

(in the fifth decade) have a decreasing E:A ratio (1.6). Thereafter, deceleration time and isovolumic relaxation times are prolonged. Older subjects (in the eighth decade or beyond) have the highest A wave. Thus, with aging there is a spectrum of diastolic filling that is age appropriate and similar to that of the abnormal relaxation pattern seen in younger patients with organic disease. This increased A wave with aging may be adaptive, allowing the heart

TABLE 29–3. FACTORS INFLUENCING PULMONARY VENOUS FLOW

	Atrial Factors	Ventricular Factors
Systolic phase	Left atrial function (contraction)	Ventricular systolic function (mitral annular displacement)
	Left atrial function (relaxation)	Cardiac output
	Left atrial pressure	
	Left atrial compliance	
	Rhythm	
Diastolic phase	Left atrial pressure	Left ventricular compliance
		Left ventricular relaxation
Atrial reversal phase	Left atrial function (contraction)	
	Left atrial function (relaxation)	
	Left atrial compliance	
	Rhythm	

Factors influencing systolic and diastolic and atrial reversal phases of pulmonary venous flow.

From Klein, A. L., and Tajik, A. J.: Doppler assessment of pulmonary venous flow in healthy subjects and in patients with heat disease. J. Am. Soc. Echocardiogr. 4:381, 1991. Reprinted with permission from Mosby–Year Book, Inc., St. Louis, MO.

TABLE 29–4. RIGHT VENTRICULAR FILLING DYNAMICS IN NORMAL SUBJECTS

	<50 Years (n = 61)	≥50 Years (n = 56)	P Value
Right Ventricular Inflow			
Peak E (cm/second)	51±7	41±8	<0.01
Peak A (cm/second)	27±8	33±8	<0.01
E/A	2.0±0.5	1.34±0.4	<0.01
DT (cm/second)	188±22	198±23	<0.01
Superior Vena Cava	(n = 59)	(n = 53)	
Peak S (cm/second)	41±9	42±12	(Not significant)
Peak D (cm/second)	22±5	22±5	(Not significant)
Peak AR (cm/second)	13±3	16±3	<0.01

Peak A, peak late diastolic flow velocity; peak E, peak early diastolic flow velocity; DT, deceleration time; IVRT, isovolumic relaxation times; peak D, peak venous diastolic forward flow; peak S, peak venous systolic forward flow velocity; peak AR, peak atrial reversal flow velocity.

Modified from Klein, A. L., and Cohen, G. I.: Doppler echocardiographic assessment of constrictive pericarditis, cardiac amyloidosis, and cardiac tamponade. Cleve. Clin. J. Med. 59:281–290, 1992. Reprinted with permission from Cleveland Clinic Journal of Medicine.

to maintain a normal left ventricular end-diastolic volume and adequate cardiac output at an acceptably low mean left atrial pressure despite slowed ventricular relaxation.

Similarly, pulmonary venous flow variables are also affected by the aging process with an increased S wave, S:D ratio, and atrial reversal flow velocity. In young subjects (in the third and fourth decades), pulmonary venous S and AR waves are lowest, with the highest D waves noted of any normal subjects. In middle age (fifth decade), the pulmonary venous S wave starts to exceed the D wave. In older subjects (in the seventh decade or beyond), the S and AR waves are the highest, with low D waves, but the peak atrial reversal flow velocity should not exceed 35 cm per second.[107]

The increase in S wave velocity in older subjects may result from marked atrial relaxation after an augmented atrial contraction rather than after apical displacement of the annulus. The relative increase in the D wave in young subjects results from an accentuated mitral E wave because of enhanced ventricular suction and decreased left atrial pressure. The parallel increases in the pulmonary AR and mitral A waves with age suggest that the left atrial and left ventricular compliance are only minimally altered with the normal aging process.

Gender may also have an effect on left ventricular inflow and pulmonary venous flow variables concomitant with the aging process; thus, these variables should be evaluated separately in males and females (see Figs. 29–12 and 29–13). It has also been noted that other variables, such as heart rate, blood pressure, left ventricular cavity size, and left ventricular mass may also have an effect on diastolic function, in addition to age.[19]

CLINICAL FRAMEWORK OF DIASTOLIC FUNCTION USING COMPREHENSIVE DOPPLER ASSESSMENT

The general clinical approach to left and right ventricular diastolic function divides diastolic filling into the three Doppler flow patterns of Figure 29–8, which includes abnormal relaxation, normal or "pseudonormal filling," and restrictive filling. These patterns are not unique to a specific disease but represent a spectrum, which may be influenced by changing hemodynamics.[54] To understand their clinical relevance, these patterns must be compared to age-related normals with 95 percent confidence intervals listed.

Abnormal Relaxation

This pattern (Fig. 29–8B) is characterized by an E:A ratio of less than 1, a prolonged deceleration time (>240 msec), and isovolumic relaxation time of more than 90 msec.[54, 107, 122, 123] Pulmonary and systemic venous flows usually show S > D with prominent atrial reversals.

This pattern is seen in normal aging as well as in patients with early stages of diastolic dysfunction who typically have only mild symptoms or are asymptomatic. Patients usually have only mild enlargement of the left atrium[107] with etiologies such as hypertension, early cardiac amyloidosis, ischemia, and aortic stenosis. Although this pattern may be due to true relaxation abnormalities, such as that due to diastolic calcium overload, it may also be seen in hypovolemia[84, 123] and during the Valsalva maneuver.[124]

Pseudonormalization

The second clinical pattern of diastolic dysfunction can be either truly normal (Fig. 29–8A) or "pseudonormal," a reversal of the delayed relaxation pattern due to elevated left ventricular filling pressures. The key to distinguishing these two possibilities (the left and right sides of the U in Fig. 29–10) is the pulmonary venous AR wave, which in pseudonormal filling displays a prolonged and deep reversal greater than 35 cm per second.[54, 107] Although trans-

thoracic echocardiography can be used to detect this pattern, the AR wave is particularly difficult to quantify from the chest wall, and transesophageal echocardiography may be required. Other findings that suggest "pseudonormalization" include any structural heart disease, moderate left atrial enlargement, a change in the left ventricular inflow from an E:A ratio of 1 to less than 1 with the Valsalva maneuver, and reduced atrial systolic function. Once again, this pseudonormal pattern is not disease specific but has been best characterized in cardiac amyloidosis, in which patients who initially have an abnormal relaxation pattern evolve through this transition, or pseudonormal, stage toward truly restrictive filling.[122]

Restrictive Filling

The last clinical filling pattern (Fig. 29–8C) is termed "restrictive" and is characterized by an increased E:A ratio greater than 2:1, a deceleration time less than 150 msec, and an isovolumic relaxation time of less than 60 msec.[61] In this pattern, there may be an inspiratory decrease in the deceleration times as well as diastolic mitral and tricuspid regurgitation, resulting from ventricular pressure, rising rapidly in a stiff ventricle and exceeding atrial pressure in middle or late diastole. Pulmonary venous flow usually shows markedly blunted systolic flows with large and prolonged atrial reversals[9] unless atrial systolic failure has ensued. Superior vena cava and hepatic venous flow classically show an inspiratory increase in reversals.[112]

The restrictive filling pattern is equivalent to the "square-root sign" or "dip-and-plateau" pattern seen in the ventricular pressure tracing at cardiac catheterization. This pathophysiology is characterized by a rapid increase in ventricular pressure during early diastolic filling, with little additional filling in late diastole, because of chamber stiffness.[61]

This pattern can be seen in patients with advanced stages of diastolic dysfunction due to restrictive, dilated, or ischemic cardiomyopathy, and usually the patients have dyspnea at rest and high New York Heart Association functional class. Severe enlargement and hypocontractility of the left atrium may be seen,[107] and this pattern carries a poor prognosis.[23]

Correlates of Doppler Flow Patterns by Physical Examination

A loud S_4 on physical examination has been shown to indicate abnormal relaxation pattern, while an S_3 has been related to the restrictive filling pattern.[125] In addition, the central venous flows relate directly to the right atrial pressure and jugular venous pulse, as well as the left atrial pressure.

PITFALLS OF DIASTOLIC FUNCTION MEASUREMENTS

There are various technical limitations of Doppler echocardiography that are found in assessing diastolic function, as shown in Table 29–5.[123] In general, attention to detail and sufficient time are required to ensure accurate recordings. The angle (θ) of the ultrasound beam to the blood flow direction must be minimized because Doppler records velocities in proportion to cos θ, leading to underestimation of flow as θ exceeds 30 degrees (cos 30 degrees = 0.866). This phenomenon is especially important during transesophageal recordings of the right ventricular inflow or the right upper pulmonary vein from the transverse imaging plane.[126] Color flow imaging is a useful tool for aligning the sample volume parallel to flow.

Sample Volume Location

The location of the sample volume is also crucial in recording adequate flow velocities, since the left ventricular inflow E:A ratio

TABLE 29–5. TECHNICAL LIMITATIONS OF DOPPLER IN THE ASSESSMENT OF DIASTOLIC FUNCTION

> Angle of the ultrasound beam
> Location of the sample volume
> Filter settings
> Hard copy recording speed
> Normal and abnormal Doppler pattern recognition
> Sufficient time
> Attention to detail
> Standard limitations of cardiac ultrasound

From Grodecki, P. V., and Klein, A. L.: Pitfalls in the echo-Doppler assessment of diastolic dysfunction. Echocardiography 10:216, 1993. Reprinted with permission from Futura Publishing Company, Inc.

is higher and the deceleration time longer at the tips of the mitral valve compared to those of the mitral annulus.[113, 127] The deceleration time also varies across the left ventricular inflow tract and may be shortened when measured medially adjacent to the left ventricular outflow tract.[114, 123]

For time-interval measurements of left ventricular inflow A wave, the sample volume should be on the atrial side of the mitral leaflets to avoid factitious shortening of the A wave as the mitral annulus moves basally during atrial contraction. Similarly, when the sample volume location is too medial, it also results in falsely shortening the A-wave duration.[25] The duration of the atrial reversal of the pulmonary vein can be measured directly, indirectly (the interval between cessation of forward diastolic flow and the start of forward systolic flow), or by referencing the end of the atrial reversal to the R wave of the electrocardiogram. The peak atrial reversal flow velocity may be difficult to measure because of wall motion artifacts during atrial contraction, and optimal tracings may be obtained from a window different from that used to obtain adequate systolic and diastolic flow.[128]

Other Instrument Factors

In general, the lowest filter settings should be used to obtain flow velocities, except for the isovolumic relaxation time in which a higher wall filter may highlight the discrete sounds of aortic valve closure and mitral valve opening. Tracings should be recorded at both 50 and 100 mm per second sweep speed. The 100 mm per second speed may be better for isovolumic relaxation measurements, whereas 50 mm per second may allow more reproducible measurements of deceleration time.

Physiologic Influences

In addition, various physiologic conditions may influence diastolic function, as shown in Table 29–6. The most important of these is preload, which, as was discussed earlier, can have an impact on both mitral inflow and pulmonary venous flow.[80] Heart rate also

TABLE 29–6. PHYSIOLOGICAL INFLUENCES ON DIASTOLIC STUDIES

> Loading conditions
> Baseline filling characteristics
> Heart rate
> Heart rhythm
> Atrioventricular sequence
> Mitral regurgitation
> Normal aging
> Respiratory cycle
> Isovolumic relaxation flow

From Grodecki, P. V., and Klein, A. L.: Pitfalls in the echo-Doppler assessment of diastolic dysfunction. Echocardiography 10:218, 1993. Reprinted with permission from Futura Publishing Company, Inc.

exerts a profound effect on mitral filling patterns. With tachycardia, peak E velocity falls with a reversal of the E:A wave ratio.[129] Again, this change is almost certainly mediated through fundamental changes in diastolic function parameters, such as atrial pressure and τ, and indeed the response of the mitral filling pattern to tachycardia can tell much about changes in diastolic function parameters. For instance, in an animal model that used pacing to produce tachycardia, Appleton and colleagues observed reduction in E wave and fusion between the E and A waves occurring at the relatively low heart rate of 130.[130] However, when tachycardia was induced by isoproterenol infusion, which reduces τ as well as the atrioventricular conduction interval, much less E-wave reduction was noted, and E wave–A wave fusion was not seen until a heart rate of 180 was recorded. It has been suggested that if the E velocity at the time of atrial contraction exceeds 20 cm per second, the E:A ratio should not be used.[107] Carotid sinus massage may be useful to separate these waves.

In atrial fibrillation, with varying cardiac cycles, the mitral deceleration time and isovolumic relaxation time can still be measured, but pulmonary venous systolic flow will be blunted.[123] The atrioventricular sequence will also alter the left ventricular inflow and pulmonary venous flow.[131] A long PR interval results in an increased A wave, since atrial contraction occurs in early diastole, when atrial volume is greater, whereas a short PR results in a decreased A wave because atrial contraction is influenced by ventricular systole. With atrioventricular dissociation (Fig. 29–14), the velocity of the left ventricular inflow and pulmonary venous flow varies depending on the time of atrial contraction.

Mitral regurgitation can also affect pulmonary venous flow and left ventricular inflow.[132] With significant mitral regurgitation, the E wave increases and the A wave decreases, although the deceleration time may still be useful in assessing diastolic filling. The pulmonary venous systolic flow is often blunted or reversed in the presence of severe mitral regurgitation.

SPECIFIC DISEASES

Constrictive Pericarditis

Constrictive pericarditis results from pericardial thickening, with impaired cardiac filling causing severe right heart failure with ascites, peripheral edema, and low cardiac output.[8, 133] The hallmark of the Doppler-echocardiographic diagnosis of constrictive pericarditis is identification of a restrictive filling pattern (due to the steep ventricular pressure-volume relationship) with reciprocal respirophasic changes in atrioventricular and venous velocities between the left and the right sides of the heart, reflecting ventricular interaction due to the fixed intrapericardial volume.[134] It is very important to distinguish between constrictive pericarditis and restrictive cardiomyopathy, since constrictive pericarditis can be cured surgically and has an excellent prognosis, whereas restrictive cardiomyopathy is treated medically and has a poor prognosis.[135, 136] Constrictive pericarditis is characterized hemodynamically by elevated right and left atrial pressures with a preserved x and a prominent y descent and equalization of all chambers with a "dip-and-plateau" pattern.[137, 138]

Two-dimensional echocardiographic criteria for constrictive pericarditis include abnormal septal bounce, a dilated inferior vena cava, and increased pericardial thickness,[110] often with normal systolic function. Transesophageal echocardiography is often useful for assessing the location and magnitude of abnormal pericardial thickness.[116]

Doppler Assessment

Doppler flow velocities in constriction show marked respiratory variation and limitation to filling (Fig. 29–15A to D). The left ventricular inflow shows significant reduction in peak velocity and deceleration time during inspiration and opposite changes in expi-

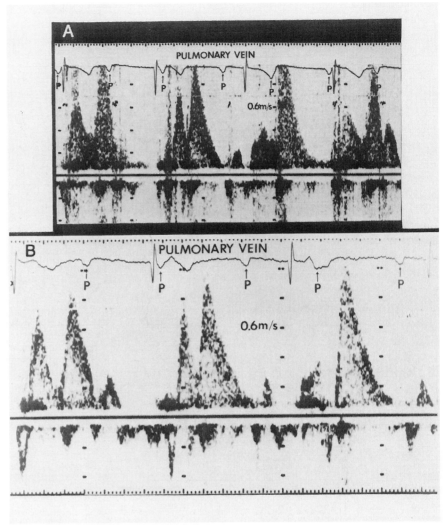

FIGURE 29–14. Pulsed-wave Doppler recordings of pulmonary venous flow in a 10-year-old boy with complete heart block. Note the atrioventricular dissociation, with the P wave marching through the tracing, and the relationship of the P wave to systolic filling of the pulmonary vein. When ventricular systole occurred within 200 msec after the onset of the P wave, systolic filling was accentuated, as shown after the first beat (A). Note also the influence of atrial contraction against a closed valve (during systole) with a prominent atrial reversal in the pulmonary venous tracing (third P wave; B). (From Klein, A.L., and Tajik, A.J.: Doppler assessment of pulmonary venous flow in healthy subjects and in patients with heart disease. J. Am. Soc. Echocardiogr. 4:389, 1991. Reprinted with permission from the Mosby–Year Book, Inc., St. Louis, MO.)

ration. In contrast, the right ventricular inflow shows a marked decrease in the E wave, A wave, and deceleration time in expiration and increases in inspiration. Hatle and co-workers showed that with inspiration, isovolumic relaxation time increased by 50 percent, left ventricular inflow peak E velocity decreased by 33 percent, right ventricular inflow peak E velocity increased by 44 percent, and right ventricular inflow peak A velocity increased by 38 percent. In contrast, patients with restriction and normal volunteers had less than 5 percent variation in the left and right ventricular inflow peak E velocities.[8] The largest change in the left ventricular inflow velocity occurs on the *first* beat after the onset of inspiration, distinguishing these changes from patients with chronic obstructive lung disease, in which there may be a delay in respiratory variation, compared to that of constriction. Also, the depth of respiration may influence the degree of respiratory variation. In a series of seven patients, after pericardiectomy the Doppler respiratory variation disappeared, and the Doppler flow velocity returned to normal.

Complementary data can be obtained from the pulmonary and systemic veins. The systemic venous flow velocities reflect the right atrial pressure tracing, and usually the systolic wave exceeds the diastolic wave.[134, 137] Respiratory variation of the superior vena cava and hepatic vein flow velocities parallel the changes in the right ventricular inflow, increasing with inspiration and decreasing (even reversing) with expiration.[7] Rarely, in severe constriction, there may be increased reversals in inspiration because of the shortened filling, but still there are prominent expiratory reversals. The inspiratory increase in forward flow is more apparent in the hepatic vein than in the superior vena cava, reflecting differences in intra-abdominal pressures on inspiration. Occasionally, the superior vena

cava forward flow actually decreases, with an increase in right atrial pressure during inspiration (Kussmaul's sign), suggesting better filling from the inferior vena cava because of the increase in intra-abdominal pressure.[134]

Respiratory variation in pulmonary venous flow parallels that in left ventricular inflow, decreasing in inspiration, increasing in expiration. Klein and associates showed the usefulness of Doppler transesophageal echocardiography in the measurement of respiratory variation in pulmonary venous flow.[116] In 31 patients with diastolic dysfunction, they demonstrated that a combination of a pulmonary systolic-to-diastolic inspiratory velocity ratio of 0.65 or more and a greater than 40 percent reduction in diastolic flow in inspiration correctly identified 12 of 14 patients with constrictive pericarditis (Fig. 29–16). Another recent study of 28 patients with diastolic dysfunction who underwent exploratory thoracotomy confirmed the usefulness of Doppler echocardiography in diagnosing constrictive pericarditis and predicting the functional response after pericardiectomy.[133]

Physiologic Mechanisms of Doppler Findings

These patterns occur because in constrictive pericarditis, the change in intrathoracic pressure with respiration is not transmitted to the cardiac chambers because of the thickened pericardium. Thus, with inspiration, as intrathoracic pressure falls, there is little effect on left ventricular diastolic pressure, whereas the pulmonary venous pressure decreases significantly, lowering the gradient across the mitral valve. The isovolumic relaxation time is prolonged, since left ventricular isovolumic pressure must fall further before the mitral valve will open.

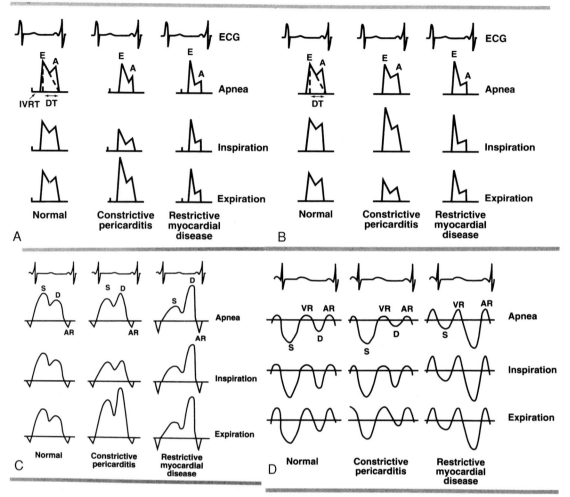

FIGURE 29–15. *A,* Diagram of left ventricular inflow velocities during difference phases in respiration. In normal subjects, there is a little change in E:A ratio, deceleration time (DT), and isovolumic relaxation time (IVRT) during apnea, inspiration, and expiration. In constrictive pericarditis, Doppler flow velocities show marked respiratory variation, with increased peak E and peak A flow velocities and shortened IVRT in expiration versus inspiration, as well as intermediate values for apnea. In restrictive myocardial disease (cardiac amyloidosis), there is an increased E:A ratio, a markedly shortened deceleration time, and a decreased IVRT; however, there is minimal respiratory variation in the Doppler flow velocities. *B,* Diagram of right ventricular inflow velocities during different phases of respiration. In normal subjects there is a mild increase in the peak early (E) and peak late (A) velocities, with inspiration compared with expiration and apnea. In constrictive pericarditis, there is markedly decreased peak E velocity and peak A velocity in expiration, compared with inspiration, with intermediate values for apnea. In restrictive myocardial disease, there is markedly increased E:A ratio, shortened deceleration time (DT) with a further shortening during inspiration. There is no significant change in the E:A ratio with respiration. *C,* Diagram of pulmonary venous flow velocities during different phases of respiration. In normal subjects, there is very little respiratory change in the pulmonary venous flow velocities, with a greater peak systolic (S)-to-diastolic (D) flow velocity ratio and a small reversal flow at atrial contraction (AR). In constrictive pericarditis there is a slight decrease in the peak systolic-to-diastolic flow for all phases of respiration; however, there is a marked increase in the systolic and especially the diastolic flow velocities in expiration, as compared with those of inspiration and apnea. In restrictive myocardial disease, peak diastolic-to-systolic flow ratio is increased, atrial reversal (AR) is markedly increased, and there is only little respiratory change in the flow velocities. *D,* Diagram of hepatic venous flow velocities during different phases of respiration. In normal subjects there is a greater peak systolic-to-diastolic flow velocity ratio, with an increase in forward flow on inspiration, with small reversals of flow associated with a late ventricular systole (VR) AR. The reversals are usually more prominent in expiration compared with inspiration and apnea. In constrictive pericarditis, there is a normal increase in peak systolic-to-diastolic flow velocity ratios in inspiration; however, in expiration, systolic flow velocity decreases and diastolic flow velocities decrease, reflecting decreased flow velocities in the right ventricular inflow. There is also a markedly increased reversal of flow in expiration compared with inspiration and apnea. In restrictive myocardial disease, there is greater peak diastolic-to-systolic flow ratio during all phases of respiration, with increased reversals of flow during inspiration compared with expiration and apnea. (From Klein, A.L., and Cohen, G.I.: Doppler echocardiographic assessment of constrictive pericarditis, cardiac amyloidosis, and cardiac tamponade. Cleve. Clin. J. Med. 59:282–283, 1992. Reprinted with permission from the Cleveland Clinic Journal of Medicine.)

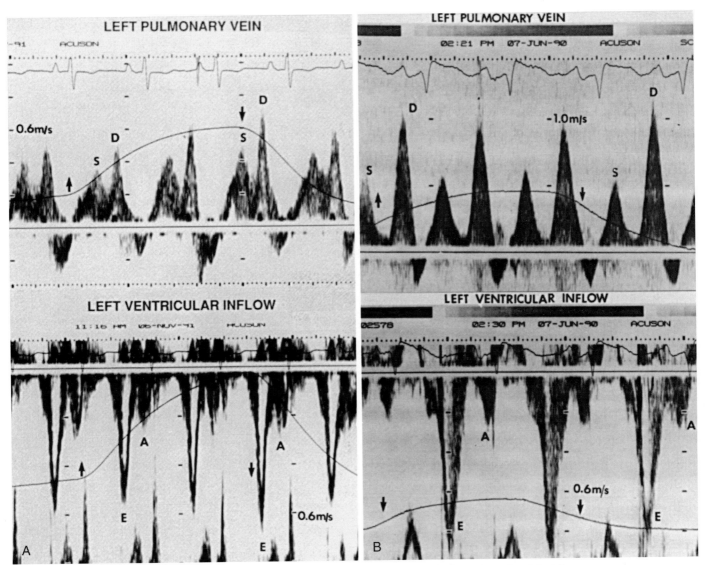

FIGURE 29–16. *A,* Constrictive pericarditis. Doppler transesophageal echocardiography of the left upper pulmonary venous flow *(top)* and left ventricular inflow *(bottom)* in a 30-year-old man with constrictive pericarditis with respiratory monitoring with inspiration *(ascending arrow)* and expiration *(descending arrow).* The systolic-to-diastolic flow ratio is 0.70 for expiration and 0.72 for inspiration. The respiratory variation of pulmonary venous systolic (S) (25 percent) and diastolic (D) (26 percent) flows from expiration to inspiration is marked. The left ventricular inflow peak early (E) filling velocity shows a small respiratory variation (17 percent) from expiration to inspiration. A = late filling velocity. *B,* Restrictive cardiomyopathy. Doppler transesophageal echocardiography of the left upper pulmonary venous flow *(top)* and left ventricular inflow *(bottom)* in a 64-year-old man with restrictive cardiomyopathy secondary to advanced cardiac amyloidosis during inspiration *(ascending arrow)* and expiration *(descending arrow).* Both inspiration and expiration show a markedly decreased systolic-to-diastolic flow ratio of 0.4, and there are no significant respiratory changes in the peak systolic (S) and diastolic (D) flow velocities from expiration to inspiration. Similarly, the left ventricular inflow peak E velocity shows no respiratory variation from expiration to inspiration. (From Klein, A.L., Cohen, G.I., Pietrolungo, J.F., et al.: Differentiation of constrictive pericarditis from restrictive cardiomyopathy by Doppler transesophageal echocardiographic measurements of respiratory variations in pulmonary venous flow. J. Am. Coll. Cardiol. 22:1939, 1993. Reprinted with permission from the American College of Cardiology.)

Reciprocal changes are seen in the right side of the heart, because the pericardial encasement limits the space available for ventricular filling, making total ventricular volume relatively fixed. Thus, during inspiration, when the left ventricular inflow and pulmonary venous flow are decreased, the right ventricular inflow, hepatic vein, and superior vena cava flow are increased. In contrast, during expiration, when the left ventricular inflow and pulmonary venous flows increase, there is a decrease in the right ventricular inflow velocities and a decrease or complete loss of diastolic forward flow in the superior vena cava and hepatic vein.

Pitfalls

There are several pitfalls in the assessment of constrictive pericarditis by Doppler echocardiography. Experience and attention to detail are necessary, and the patient has to be breathing regularly and fairly deeply. When atrial pressures are very high, the respiratory change in intrathoracic pressure may be insufficient to significantly modulate filling velocities; in such a circumstance, reducing preload by examining the patient in the sitting or standing position or with lower body negative pressure may help bring out diagnostic respiratory fluctuations. Conversely, if the filling pressures are very low, constriction may be occult with no respiratory variation detected, requiring volume loading to enhance respiratory changes.[134, 139] Atrial fibrillation introduces its own beat-to-beat velocity fluctuation, and observation of three to six respiratory cycles may be necessary to see the independent changes induced by breathing. Finally, features of mixed constriction and restriction may be detected in some patients, as well as localized constriction, effusive constriction, and restriction with a pericardial effusion. Right ventricular biopsy may be helpful, but there remains a small subset of mixed patients in whom a therapeutic trial of pericardiectomy may be necessary.[7]

Cardiac Tamponade

Cardiac tamponade is characterized by a rising venous pulse, decreasing arterial pressure, a small quiet heart, and evidence of pulsus paradoxus.[137] Hemodynamically, there is equalization of filling pressures, and the right atrial pressure shows a prominent x descent, with an absent or diminished y descent. Diastolic collapse of the right atrium and right ventricle and left atrial collapse have been described as echocardiographic markers of tamponade but are not always reliable.[140–142] Doppler echocardiography with respiratory monitoring may provide a more precise assessment of the hemodynamic changes with pericardial effusion,[7] showing significant respiratory variation in inflow and outflow velocities in cardiac tamponade, which disappear after pericardiocentesis.[143, 144] In a manner similar to that of patients with constrictive pericarditis, patients with tamponade show marked variation in left ventricular inflow velocities from expiration to inspiration: a 34 to 85 percent increase in isovolumic relaxation time, a 34 to 44 percent decrease in peak E velocity, and a 25 percent decrease in peak A velocity. Reciprocal respiratory changes are seen in right ventricular filling because of ventricular interdependence. Superior vena cava and hepatic vein velocities show a predominance of systolic flow (equivalent to the x descent in the right atrial pressure tracing) with the onset of inspiration. On the first beat after the onset of expiration, diastolic flow decreases or disappears, corresponding to the decrease in the right ventricular inflow peak E velocity, and reversed flow increases. In some patients, the respiratory variation does not disappear after pericardiocentesis, which may suggest effusive constriction.[143]

Cardiac tamponade represents a continuum of hemodynamic embarrassment, and respiratory variation is strongly influenced by central venous pressures as well as by the depth of respiration.[144] In one study,[145] there was a close relationship between the degree of respiratory variation (> 22 percent) of left ventricular inflow velocities, collapse of the right atrium and ventricle, and equalization of filling pressures (Fig. 29–17). Therefore, both the two-

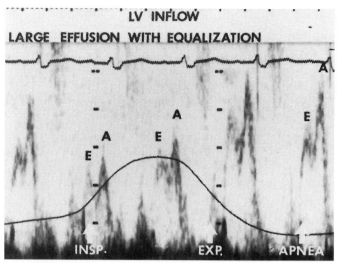

FIGURE 29–17. Pulsed Doppler tracing of left ventricular (LV) inflow of a large pericardial effusion with right-sided equalization, showing a marked decrease in left ventricular inflow early (E) filling velocity from expiration (Exp.) to inspiration (Insp.). (From Schultzman, J.J., Obarski, T.P., Pearce, G.L., et al.: Comparison of Doppler and two-dimensional echocardiography for assessment of pericardial effusion. Am. J. Cardiol. 70:1355, 1992. Reprinted with permission from the American Journal of Cardiology.)

dimensional signs of tamponade and Doppler findings should be used to evaluate patients with pericardial effusion and tamponade, with an appreciation that the etiology (surgical versus medical) and position (loculated versus circumferential) of the effusion may mask some of the usual signs of tamponade.

Restrictive Myocardial Disease: Cardiac Amyloidosis

Restrictive myocardial disease, whether primary (endomyocardial fibrosis, Löffler's endocarditis, and idiopathic) or secondary (amyloidosis and sarcoidosis), is characterized by nondilated but abnormally stiff ventricles, with elevated left and right heart filling pressures, resulting in pulmonary congestion, hepatic congestion, peripheral edema, and ascites.[134, 146] Two-dimensional echocardiography and Doppler interrogation of atrioventricular and central venous flow velocities are important to the diagnosis and characterization of these disorders, with cardiac amyloidosis being the best studied.[9, 23, 112, 147, 148]

The two-dimensional echo appearance in amyloidosis includes small or normal-sized ventricular cavities with diffusely increased wall thickness and biatrial enlargement. The myocardial texture may show a characteristic "speckled" appearance, and a small pericardial effusion and mild thickening of the interatrial septum may also be seen.[108]

While hemodynamic investigations of amyloidosis have traditionally shown a dip-and-plateau pattern similar to constrictive pericarditis,[149, 150] recent Doppler investigations integrating ventricular inflow and venous flow patterns have clarified the diastolic abnormalities in this disease. Klein and co-workers demonstrated a spectrum of filling abnormalities in this disease, related to mean left ventricular wall thickness. The early subgroup (mean wall thickness < 15 mm) usually shows an abnormal relaxation pattern, with a prolonged isovolumic relaxation time, a decreased E:A ratio, and a normal or prolonged deceleration time. The pulmonary venous flow showed an increased systolic-to-diastolic flow ratio (Fig. 29–18).

In contrast, the advanced subgroup (mean wall thickness ≥ 15 mm) showed a restrictive pattern with a markedly shortened deceleration time and increased E:A ratio, whereas the pulmonary venous flow showed a markedly blunted systolic-to-diastolic flow ratio with large atrial reversals (Fig. 29–19). Right ventricular dia-

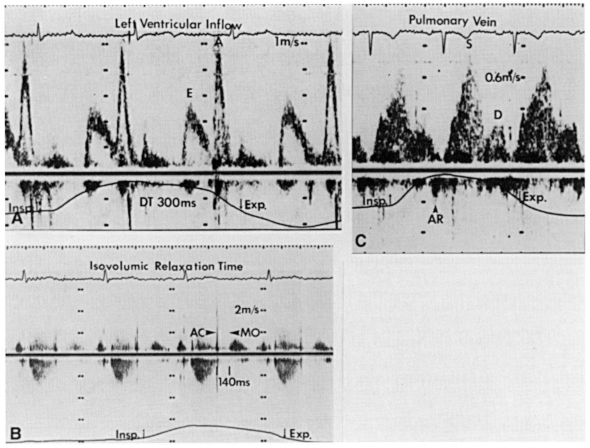

FIGURE 29–18. Abnormal relaxation flow pattern of left ventricular inflow in a subgroup with early cardiac amyloidosis. *A,* Pulsed-wave Doppler recording of a left ventricular inflow profile with decreased peak E velocity and increased peak A velocity. The E:A ratio was decreased (0.5), and deceleration time (DT) was prolonged (300 msec). *B,* Continuous-wave Doppler recording of the aortic valve, with simultaneous mitral valve inflow profile. Note that aortic closure (AC) and mitral opening (MVO) sounds are well defined, and isovolumic relaxation time is markedly prolonged (140 msec). *C,* Pulsed-wave Doppler recording of right lower pulmonary vein flow profile with increased peak forward systolic (S) and decreased diastolic (D) flow velocities and normal reversal of atrial filling (AR). Exp. = expiration; Insp. = inspiration. (From Klein, A.L., Hatle, L.K., Burstow, D.J., et al.: Doppler characterization of left ventricular diastolic function in cardiac amyloidosis. J. Am. Coll. Cardiol. 13:1021, 1989. Reprinted with permission from the American College of Cardiology.)

stolic flow is similarly abnormal in cardiac amyloidosis, with a right ventricular wall thickness of 7 mm dividing patterns of abnormal relaxation from restrictive filling. The superior vena cava and hepatic vein flow velocity showed a decreased systolic-to-diastolic flow ratio (similar to the y descent in the right atrial pressure tracing) and a short deceleration time, across the right ventricular inflow, which decreased with inspiration.[112] In general, progressive amyloidosis leads to predictable change in filling patterns from abnormal relaxation to pseudonormal filling to a restrictive pattern in advanced disease (Fig. 29–20), changes which have important prognostic information.[147] During an 18-month follow-up of patients with cardiac amyloidosis, the risk of cardiac death was five times higher in the restrictive group (deceleration time ≤ 150 msec), compared to a nonrestrictive group (deceleration time > 150 msec). The 1-year survival rate for the restrictive group was 49 percent, compared to 92 percent for the nonrestrictive group. In fact, the best predictors of cardiac death were the E:A ratio and deceleration time, which were more predictive than mean left ventricular wall thickness (Fig. 29–21).[23]

Hypertrophic Cardiomyopathy

This disease is characterized by idiopathic hypertrophy of the myocardium of the left and right ventricles, with evidence of microscopic fiber disarray. Hypertrophy is usually asymmetric and may include septal, midventricular, or apical hypertrophy, which may vary in degree.[151] Diastolic dysfunction may occur secondary to increased chamber stiffness (owing to both increased intrinsic myocardial stiffness and thick walls) as well as abnormal relaxation, which may in part be due to nonuniformity of load and inactivation in time and space, as described by Brutsaert and co-workers[152, 153] and Bonow and colleagues.[154]

Two-dimensional and Doppler echocardiography have been useful in characterizing the outflow tract obstruction, the distribution of the hypertrophy, and the type of diastolic dysfunction in this disease.[155] As with patients having other cardiomyopathies, patients with hypertrophic cardiomyopathy may progress from abnormal relaxation to pseudonormal to restrictive filling patterns. The isovolumic relaxation time often is prolonged but can be shortened with severe obstruction, because of delayed closure of the aortic valve and early opening of the mitral valve because of elevated left atrial pressure. The presence of severe mitral regurgitation may elevate the left ventricular inflow E wave, as may atrial fibrillation, because of the importance of the atrial contribution to filling in hypertrophic cardiomyopathy.[151] Additionally, asymmetric relaxation of the ventricle may lead to abnormal diastolic flow during the isovolumic relaxation phase, with flow from base to apex in cases of midcavity obstruction, and from apex to base with apical hypertrophy.[155]

Several studies have suggested that verapamil is useful for in-

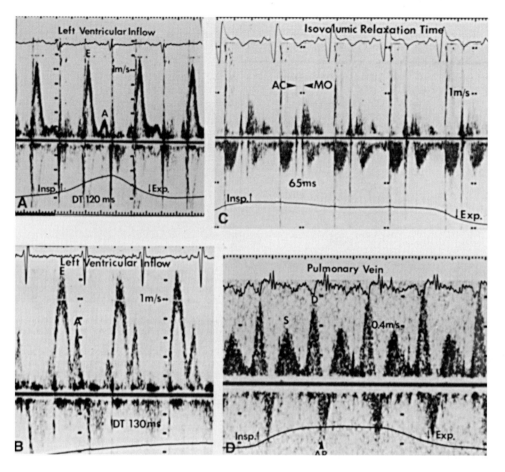

FIGURE 29–19. Restrictive flow patterns of left ventricular inflow in the subgroup with advanced cardiac amyloidosis. *A,* Pulsed-wave Doppler recording of a left ventricular inflow profile with an increased E:A ratio (3.7) and short deceleration time (120 msec). *B,* Pulsed-wave Doppler recording of a left ventricular inflow profile with a normal E:A ratio and short deceleration time (DT) (130 msec). *C,* Continuous-wave Doppler recording of the aortic valve with simultaneous mitral valve flow profile. Note the normal isovolumic relaxation time (65 msec). *D,* Pulsed-wave Doppler recording of a right lower pulmonary vein flow profile with decreased peak forward systolic (S) and increased peak diastolic (D) velocities and reversal of atrial filling (AR). Note that the left-sided flow velocities are influenced minimally by respiration. (From Klein, A.L., Hatle, L.K., Burstow, D.J., et al.: Doppler characterization of left ventricular diastolic function in cardiac amyloidosis. J. Am. Coll. Cardiol. 13:1022, 1989. Reprinted with permission from the American College of Cardiology.)

FIGURE 29–20. Serial left ventricular Doppler inflow recordings 7 months apart in a 55-year-old man with early cardiac amyloidosis. *Left,* Pulsed-wave Doppler recording of left ventricular inflow shows a normal E:A ratio and a normal deceleration time (DT) (190 msec). *Right,* Follow-up recording shows restriction with an increased early (E) to late (A) velocity ratio (2.5) and a shortened deceleration time (140 msec). Calibration marks represent 0.2 m per second. (From Klein, A.L., Hatle, L.K., Taliercio, C.P., et al.: Serial Doppler echocardiographic follow-up of left ventricular diastolic function in cardiac amyloidosis. J. Am. Coll. Cardiol. 16:1139, 1990. Reprinted with permission from the American College of Cardiology.)

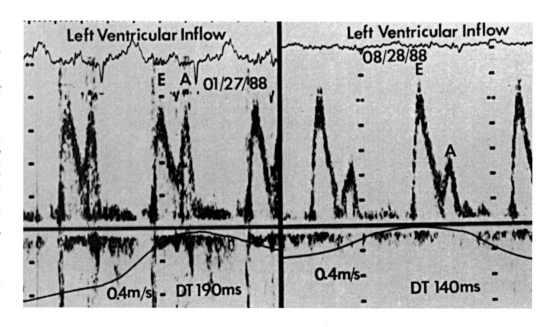

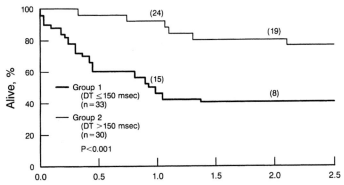

FIGURE 29–21. Survival rate in 63 patients with cardiac amyloidosis, as assessed by the effect of deceleration time (DT) on cardiac death. The 1-year probability of avoiding cardiac death for group 1 patients was significantly less than that for group 2 patients (49 versus 92 percent, $P < .001$). (From Klein, A.L., Hatle, A.L., Taliercio, C.P., et al.: Prognostic significance of Doppler measures of diastolic function in cardiac amyloidosis. Circulation 83:813, 1991. Reprinted with permission from the American Heart Association.)

creasing early ventricular filling in hypertrophic cardiomyopathy.[151, 155, 156] However, in a study of acute treatment with intravenous verapamil, Nishimura and associates[157] have shown that the rise in transmitral E:A ratio actually was associated with a rise in end-diastolic pressure and a prolongation in τ, indicating that the filling pattern was pseudonormal. Dual-chamber pacing has been proposed as decreasing the left ventricular outflow tract gradient in hypertrophic cardiomyopathy by activating the septum asymmetrically,[158] but the ultimate role of this technique and the proper atrioventricular interval to use are still under investigation.

Dilated Cardiomyopathy

Whether idiopathic or secondary to multiple myocardial infarctions, this condition is characterized by dilation of the left and right ventricles with reduced systolic function.[146] It has been noted that patients with idiopathic cardiomyopathy usually have impairment of all four cardiac chambers, in contrast to those with ischemic cardiomyopathy, in whom the right-sided function is often better than that on the left side.[159] Left atrial dilation may indicate chronically elevated filling pressures.[106, 107] Similar to patients having the above conditions, the three filling patterns have been described including (in order of diastolic derangement) abnormal relaxation, pseudonormal filling, or restrictive filling,[61] which has important prognostic information independent of the degree of systolic dysfunction.[160] For example, if a patient has a better diastolic filling (abnormal relaxation) pattern despite a very low ejection fraction, this condition would indicate a relatively high operating compliance of the ventricle, with a better prognosis than that for a patient with a restrictive pattern and a less reduced ejection fraction.

Cardiac Transplantation

Cardiac allograft recipients have had increased survival with the use of cyclosporine therapy, but increased surveillance for acute and chronic rejection with myocardial biopsy is necessary.[20] Recently, two-dimensional and Doppler echocardiography have played an important part in patient management after cardiac transplantation. The two-dimensional echocardiographic signs of acute rejection include an increased left ventricular wall thickness and mass, presence of a pericardial effusion, increased myocardial echogenicity, and a decreased ejection fraction, but these are relatively late findings. Doppler variables of diastolic filling may be more sensitive to early rejection and decrease the need for serial myocardial biopsies, but meticulous measurements are necessary.[161] At Stanford University, the patient has daily serial studies immediately

after transplantation, carefully excluding beats in which the recipient's native atrial contraction interferes with the left ventricular inflow. The Doppler signs for acute rejection include a decrease of 20 percent or more in the deceleration time (restrictive physiology) and isovolumic relaxation time, with a sensitivity of 85 to 90 percent for acute rejection on cardiac biopsy. It is important to note, however, that the restrictive filling pattern may be a normal finding within the first 6 weeks after transplantation,[162] and other groups have reported less success in detecting rejection.[163] In the latter study, there was discordance between restrictive filling and acute rejection, with important correlations to variables such as ischemic time and donor age, suggesting the multitude of factors that influence diastolic filling. Right ventricular inflow and central veins may also show restrictive filling abnormalities during rejection.[61] Doppler echocardiography has also been used to monitor diastolic function in long-term cardiac transplant patients, with restrictive filling noted in as many as 15 percent of long-term cardiac transplant recipients because of either chronic rejection or small vessel coronary artery disease.[21]

Hypertensive Heart Disease

Hypertensive heart disease secondary to systemic arterial hypertension is characterized by left ventricular hypertrophy, which develops as a physiologic adaptation to normalize wall stress.[164, 165] Chamber stiffness may be increased, because of both excessive wall thickness and increased intrinsic myocardial stiffness (due to fibrosis or collagen deposition). Relaxation is typically delayed because of impairment of sarcoplasmic reticulum function and calcium overload, along with nonuniformity of inactivation. With abnormal relaxation, ventricle filling is dependent on atrial contraction to maintain the cardiac output, whereas decreased compliance results in elevated filling pressures and pulmonary congestion.[109] Hypertensive heart disease commonly presents as diastolic dysfunction, accounting for 30 to 40 percent of patients presenting with heart failure, especially among the elderly.[4, 166] Often, exercise testing is needed to elicit abnormalities of diastolic function that are not present at rest.[167]

Like dilated and restrictive cardiomyopathies, progressive diastolic dysfunction in hypertensive heart disease is characterized initially by a delayed relaxation pattern, then, as left atrial pressure rises to compensate for increased ventricular stiffness, pseudonormal and rarely restrictive patterns emerge, with corresponding changes in pulmonary venous patterns.[14, 54, 168, 169] There is an imperfect relationship between absolute blood pressure elevation (increased afterload) and diastolic dysfunction, with important contributions from other variables such as left ventricular hypertrophy, abnormal coronary flow reserve, heart rate, preloading, and aging.[35] Increased mass alone does not cause diastolic dysfunction, as noted in athletes with physiologic hypertrophy.

Treatment of diastolic dysfunction in hypertensive heart disease is directed principally toward the hypertension itself, including β-blockers, calcium-channel blockers, angiotensin-converting enzyme inhibitors, and diuretics with regression of hypertrophy, noted with some of these agents.[35, 170, 171] Unfortunately, simple normalization of inflow filling patterns does not necessarily indicate improved diastolic function, as they may indicate pseudonormalization with elevated left atrial pressure.[157]

Coronary Artery Disease

Coronary artery disease is composed of acute and chronic disease states, which may have abnormal diastolic function—seen in as many as 90 percent of patients—because of the effects of myocardial ischemia or fibrosis. With myocardial ischemia, diastolic dysfunction often precedes systolic dysfunction, because of decreased ATP stores, which influence reuptake of calcium by the sarcoplasmic reticulum, causing impaired and inhomogeneous relaxation. Additionally, the ischemic myocardial region becomes less compliant and pulmonary venous pressure rises; these findings can occur during exercise or pacing-induced angina, during vasospastic angina, and during transient coronary occlusion while the patient is undergoing angioplasty. With acute myocardial infarction, there may be similar mechanical and cellular events described with ischemia, but these progress to irreversible fibrosis and scarring with remodeling of noninfarcted myocardium and chamber dilation, increasing the operating stiffness of the ventricle.[172, 173]

Two-dimensional and Doppler echocardiography can be used to comprehensively evaluate systolic and diastolic dysfunction in patients with coronary artery disease. Like myopathic diseases, the earliest change observed is an age-inappropriate abnormal relaxation filling pattern,[54] with restrictive filling observed with progressive ventricular decompensation. In the acute myocardial infarction setting, the restrictive filling pattern is ominous and is associated with a higher Killip class, increased pulmonary capillary filling pressures, and a poor prognosis.[174] In addition, left atrial size may indicate the chronicity and degree of ventricular diastolic pressure elevation.

Diastolic Dysfunction in Congenital Heart Disease

Diastolic dysfunction has been well described by Doppler echocardiography in children with congenital heart disease.[15, 175–177] In the normal developing fetus, Doppler echocardiography usually shows a greater A-wave velocity in both the left and the right ventricular inflow, shifting in the first 3 weeks of life to the normal elevated E:A ratio of childhood,[178] with this shift occurring in the left ventricle (day 1) earlier than in the right ventricle.[16] Doppler variables in the normal premature infant often resemble those described in full-term infants, not those of the fetal period.[179] In subsequent studies, normal values have been published in children and young adults and are related to age and heart rate and are influenced as well by the respiratory cycle, especially of the right ventricular inflow.[16, 180]

Abnormalities of diastolic function have been described in various congenital heart diseases, including systemic hypertension,[37] hypertrophic cardiomyopathy, and left[15] and right ventricular outflow tract obstruction[176] as well in the postoperative period,[181] with a range of filling patterns noted from abnormal relaxation to restriction, reflecting the severity of the underlying diastolic derangement.[54] Similarly, with left ventricular outflow tract obstruction secondary to aortic stenosis or coarctation, there is a pattern of abnormal relaxation, which persists after relief of the obstruction, suggesting that the filling abnormalities are related to the accompanying hypertrophy and are not simply afterload mismatch. Relief of right ventricular outflow tract obstruction, however, may normalize the previous abnormal relaxation pattern in right ventricular inflow. Also, patients with isolated right ventricular outflow tract obstruction can also have abnormalities of left ventricular filling, which suggests a shift in the ventricular septum and an effect on left ventricular preload.[182] Abnormalities of diastolic function by Doppler echocardiography have also been described after the Fontan procedure[181] and the arterial switch procedure for transposition of the great arteries.[177, 183]

Estimating Left Ventricular Filling Pressures

Doppler echocardiography has been used to estimate left ventricular filling pressures noninvasively.[25, 115] Both mean pulmonary capillary wedge pressure and left atrial pressure, as well as left ventricular end-diastolic pressure, can be estimated. An increased E:A ratio, a shortened isovolumic relaxation and deceleration time, a decreased atrial filling fraction, a decreased pulmonary venous systolic fraction, an elevated and prolonged pulmonary atrial reversal flow velocity, and an increased left atrial volume all are indicative of elevated mean left atrial pressure. Recently, the difference between the duration of the width of the pulmonary venous atrial reversal duration and mitral inflow A-wave duration may indicate

an elevated left ventricular A-wave pressure increase and left ventricular end-diastolic pressures. The difference in duration between pulmonary venous flow atrial reversal and mitral inflow A wave greater than 20 msec suggests an elevated left ventricular end-diastolic pressure greater than 15 mm Hg with a sensitivity of 85 percent and specificity of 79 percent.[25] In addition, this new variable of diastolic function has been shown to be relatively age independent[115] (Fig. 29–22).

Prognostic Implications of Doppler Variables

An increasing number of studies have shown that restrictive filling by Doppler echocardiography is associated with worsening symptoms, New York Heart Association functional class, and higher left ventricular filling pressures and that it is a very important predictor of cardiac death or the need for cardiac transplantation.[22, 23, 184]

OTHER ECHOCARDIOGRAPHIC MODALITIES

Continuous-Wave Doppler Imaging

In patients with mitral regurgitation, it is possible to use continuous-wave Doppler imaging to obtain an approximation of the left ventricular pressure throughout diastole. For example, subtracting the peak left ventricular–left atrial gradient (from the mitral regurgitation jet) from the systolic blood pressure should yield an approximation for left atrial pressure, but although theoretically sound, the inherent errors in measuring the jet velocity and systolic blood pressure tend to overwhelm the accuracy of the left atrial pressure, since it is so much smaller than the other numbers. For this method to yield results more reliable than simple clinical assessment, exquisite care must clearly be taken in acquiring the primary data.

Left Ventricular dP/dt

In contrast to the assessment of absolute left atrial pressure, the measurement of the rate of change of pressure within the left ventricle (dP/dt) is well validated by use of continuous-wave Doppler interrogation of mitral regurgitation. One simple method measures the time interval between a mitral regurgitant velocity of 1 and 3 m per second (corresponding, respectively, to a left ventricular pressure of 4 and 36 mm Hg above left atrial pressure). Because this phenomenon represents a change in pressure of 32 mm Hg, mean dP/dt during this time interval then is given by $32/\Delta t$.[185]

Greater accuracy can be obtained by digitizing the mitral regurgitant spectrum continuously and taking the derivative of the velocity over time, shown in dogs[186] and patients,[187] to avoid the slight but systematic underestimation of left ventricular dP/dt by the 1 to 3 m per second method. Accuracy has also been shown in estimating peak negative dP/dt. Importantly, calculation of left ventricular dP/dt does not require any knowledge of absolute left atrial pressure but requires only an assumption that the rate of change of left atrial pressure is small in comparison to left ventricular dP/dt. This may explain the slight underestimation of the magnitude of negative left ventricular dP/dt, because of the concomitant fall in left atrial pressure during isovolumic relaxation.[186]

Calculation of the Relaxation Time Constant

Figure 29–23 shows how analysis of the mitral regurgitant spectrum during isovolumic relaxation allows calculation of the relaxation time constant, τ.[187–189] The general approach is to translate the ventriculoatrial gradient into left ventricular pressure by adding an assumed or measured left atrial pressure and calculating τ by logarithmic transformation[42] or Marquardt nonlinear parameter estimation. Because these methods assume that left ventricular pressure decays to a zero asymptote, it is critical that a reasonably

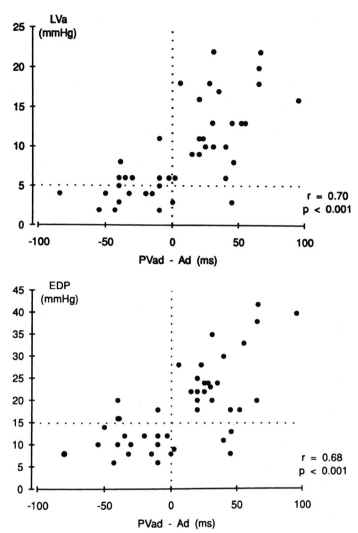

FIGURE 29–22. *Upper Panel,* Peak left ventricular pressure increase at atrial contraction (LVa) versus the difference in duration between reverse pulmonary venous and mitral A waves (PVad − Ad). Horizontal dotted line at 5 mm Hg marks an arbitrary upper normal limit for pressure before atrial contraction. Data points on the right side of the vertical dotted line have a longer duration of pulmonary reverse flow than of mitral forward flow. *Lower Panel,* Left ventricular end-diastolic pressure (EDP) versus the difference in A-wave duration. Horizontal dotted line at 15 mm Hg marks an arbitrary upper normal for end-diastolic pressure. (From Rossvoll, O., and Hatle, L.K.: Pulmonary venous flow velocities recorded by transthoracic Doppler ultrasound: Relation to left ventricular diastolic pressures. J. Am. Coll. Cardiol. 21:1693, 1993. Reprinted with permission from the American College of Cardiology.)

accurate estimate of left atrial pressure be added to the ventriculo-atrial gradient to recover true left ventricular pressure. If left atrial pressure is underestimated (or omitted entirely), then significant underestimation of τ results, by as much as 50 percent. Actual measurement of left atrial pressure (via Swan-Ganz catheter or other measure) provides the estimate for τ, but when true left atrial pressure lies between 5 and 20 mm Hg, an assumed pressure of 10 mm Hg should cause less than a 15 percent error in estimating τ by this method. Nevertheless, the precision with which digitization must be performed and the requirement for some estimation of left atrial pressure have led to relatively limited use of this method for estimating τ. A recent animal experiment suggests that when aortic regurgitation is present, it may be possible to use the upslope of the AR spectrum (during isovolumic relaxation) to estimate τ.[190]

Color Doppler M-Mode Recording of Left Ventricular Inflow

In recent years, a number of investigators have studied the use of the color Doppler M-mode to characterize the spatiotemporal distribution of blood velocity throughout the left ventricular inflow region in diastole. Although this technique is not fully integrated into routine clinical practice, the early results reported are promising enough to suggest that color Doppler M-mode may represent an important new methodology for the noninvasive characterization of diastolic function.

Physics and Instrumentation Issues With Color Doppler M-Mode Echocardiography

Color Doppler echocardiography uses the autocorrelation method to determine blood velocity along the entire extent of a given scanline. By sending out a series of pulses along a single scanline and comparing the phase shifts occurring between pairs of them, it is possible to reconstruct velocity with high spatial, temporal, and velocity resolution. The typical color Doppler M-mode echocardiograph has a temporal resolution of 5 msec and a spatial resolution of 300 μm (although the true effective resolution is likely more on the order of 1 mm), and the velocity output is divided into 32 bins distributed evenly between the forward and the reversed Nyquist limit (typical resolution about 4 cm per second).

Color Doppler M-Mode Filling Patterns

As shown in Figure 29–24, patients in normal sinus rhythm display a characteristic filling pattern consisting of two filling waves, propagating from the left atrium to the left ventricle, corresponding to the E and A waves. Several features are evident. First, it can be seen that the flow stream begins in the atrium and propagates into the ventricle, with the central change in color representing aliasing of the blood velocity during maximal filling. Second, the flow does not propagate instantaneously but rather propagates with a velocity provided by the slope of the leading edge of the blood wave. This parameter, the propagation velocity, has been reported to be altered in conditions of delayed relaxation and ischemia.[191, 192] Third, the

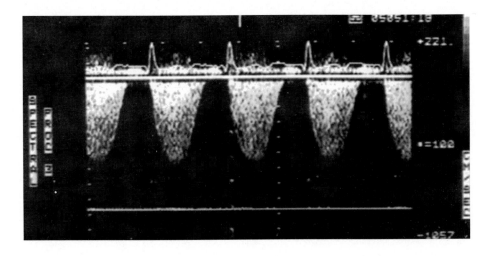

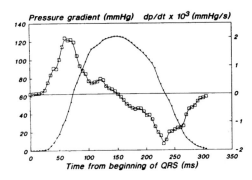

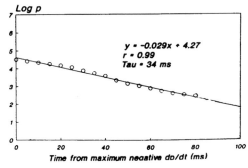

FIGURE 29–23. Calculation of the relaxation time constant τ from a continuous-wave Doppler representation of mitral regurgitation. From the velocity spectrum *(upper panel)*, the ventriculoatrial gradient can be estimated by the simplified Bernoulli equation, $\Delta P = 4v^2$, along with $d\Delta P/dt$ *(lower left panel)*. Adding a measured or estimated left atrial pressure to ΔP allows τ to be calculated with the use of logarithmic transformation with linear regression *(lower right panel)*. (From Chen, C., Rodriguez, L., Levine, R.A., et al.: Noninvasive measurement of the time constant of left ventricular relaxation using the continuous wave Doppler velocity profile of mitral regurgitation. Circulation 86:272–278, 1992. Reproduced with permission from the American Heart Association.)

spatial position of the maximal velocity is closer to the ventricular apex for the E wave than it is for the A wave, perhaps reflecting the fact that the E wave velocity is pulled into the ventricle by the declining left ventricular pressure during the act of relaxation, whereas the A wave is "pushed" into the ventricle against an unfavorable pressure gradient by atrial contraction.[193]

FIGURE 29–24. See Color Plate 3.

Derived Parameters of the Color Doppler M-Mode

Several qualitative and quantitative parameters have been proposed as characterizing transmitral filling by the color Doppler M-mode. Brun and co-workers[191] identified the leading edge of the E wave as representing the propagation velocity. This parameter is measured by identifying the boundary of the leading edge of color as it propagates into the ventricle, drawing a tangent to this line and measuring its slope on the M-mode, which corresponds to the velocity with which this leading edge propagates into the ventricle (Fig. 29–24). Interestingly, there is relatively little correlation between the velocity of propagation of the E wave and the velocities that make up the E wave, with propagation typically occurring with 25 to 50 percent of the speed with which individual blood particles within the E wave are moving. This phenomenon can be explained on the basis of vorticeal formation with higher velocities present within the core of the propagating E wave but vorticeal formation lowering the mean velocity of propagation as the blood rushes into the left ventricle.[194] Brun and co-workers[191] demonstrated a negative correlation between the propagation velocity and the time constant of relaxation, suggesting that more rapid ventricular relaxation promotes propagation of the E wave into the ventricle, per-

haps identifying a noninvasive way of assessing ventricular relaxation.

In another approach to characterizing the color Doppler M-mode, Stuggard and colleagues[192] have identified the propagation of the point of maximal velocity from the mitral valve to the apex over time. They demonstrated that the time for flow to propagate from the mitral annulus to the ventricular apex was delayed significantly during ischemia associated with angioplasty, reverting to normal when the angioplasty balloon was deflated (Fig. 29–25). A recent experimental study[195] has demonstrated a close concordance between the delay in propagation to the apex and reduced ventricular systolic function. Recent preliminary reports have demonstrated that the color M-mode propagation velocity increases during the inotropic stimulation of dobutamine echocardiography, with reduced propagation noted with the onset of ventricular ischemia. Furthermore, it appears that restrictive cardiomyopathy and constrictive pericarditis, which may have quite similar pulsed Doppler mitral profiles, can be well distinguished by analysis of the color M-mode velocity. Constrictive pericarditis is associated with extremely rapid flow propagation, whereas restrictive cardiomyopathy shows distinctly slower propagation velocities than the component E-wave velocities.

FIGURE 29–25. See Color Plate 3.

Quantitative Parameters of the Color Doppler M-Mode

Recent work has been directed at achieving more objective and quantitative characterization of the transmitral color Doppler M-mode. With the use of the digitally output velocity, it is possible to more objectively characterize the propagation velocity by localizing the ventricular centroid (spatial location of the weighted peak velocity point) defined as follows:

$$v_c(t) = \dfrac{\displaystyle\int_{LA}^{LV} s\, v(s,t)\, ds}{\displaystyle\int_{LA}^{LV} v(s,t)\, ds}$$

in which $v(s,t)$ represents the distribution of velocity within the left ventricular inflow track over space (s) and time (t).

To the extent that flow from the left atrium to the left ventricle along the M-mode cursor line may be considered as representing a single streamline, then the spatiotemporal distribution of velocity should obey the Euler equation, a differential form of the Bernoulli equation. The Euler equation relates regional pressure gradients to spatial and temporal velocity gradients throughout the inflow tract:

$$\rho\left[\frac{\partial v}{\partial t} + v\,\frac{\partial v}{\partial s}\right] = -\frac{\partial p}{\partial s}$$

Although only preliminary work has been reported,[196] there is a suggestion that such analysis of the color M-mode data may yield an estimate of actual intraventricular pressure gradients, which occur during active relaxation and ventricular recoil (suction).

Doppler Tissue Imaging

The Doppler techniques described thus far have characterized intracardiac blood velocity, which has been shown to be quite dependent on cardiac loading conditions. Recently, a new imaging modality, Doppler tissue imaging (DTI), has been developed, which instead quantifies the velocities within the ventricular myocardium.[197] Although experience with this new modality is limited, preliminary observations suggest that it may be useful in the assessment of diastolic function.[198–200]

Physics and Instrumentation

Traditional Doppler systems seek to display blood velocity, which is characterized by extremely low amplitude signals but relatively high-velocity motion. In contrast, DTI seeks to display the low-velocity but very high-amplitude Doppler signals that exist in moving muscle. To display these intramyocardial velocities, two alterations in the usual Doppler processing chain are made. First, the high-pass filter (wall filter), which specifically excludes low-velocity wall movement, is eliminated; additionally, much lower gain amplification is used before quadrature demodulation of the Doppler signal, so as to suppress display of the low-amplitude Doppler signals from moving blood within the heart.

Doppler Tissue Imaging Display Modes

The DTI principle can be applied to any of the Doppler display modes, color two-dimensional mapping, color M-mode, and pulsed Doppler. In the two-dimensional color mode, DTI provides a spatial map of velocity within the myocardium throughout the entire sector of interrogation. Figure 29–26 shows a parasternal short-axis view of a patient with amyloidosis with the motion coded in color with a Nyquist velocity of 9 cm per second. During systole the posterior wall moves toward the transducer (red signal), while the septum moves away in a symmetric contraction pattern; the colors reverse themselves in diastole. Although this display mode provides useful qualitative indication of motion, in the absence of parallel processing, the frame rate may be below 10 frames per second, limiting its quantitative use. Better timing and quantification of actual velocities within the myocardium are better achieved by the use of color M-mode and pulsed Doppler echocardiography,

which typically yield temporal resolutions on the order of 5 to 10 msec.

FIGURE 29–26. See Color Plate 3.

Clinical Observations

In a preliminary study of normal myocardial velocity by pulsed DTI, several important observations have emerged.[199] Motion of the posterior wall of the ventricle shows the expected anterior motion during systole with posterior motion during early ventricular filling and again with the filling due to atrial contraction. Also seen are high-velocity, short-duration oscillations, which correspond to isovolumic relaxation and contraction. Indeed, the magnitude of these velocities is similar to that of the major filling and emptying waves of the ventricle. Pulsed DTI is the first methodology available to characterize these extremely high-frequency events. It appears that these signals relate to conformational changes within the ventricle during isovolumic contraction in relaxation and may also relate to the differential timing of emptying of the two ventricles.

Another unique type of data available through use of DTI is quantitation of the motion of the mitral annulus and longitudinal contraction of myocardial fibers (Fig. 29–27), which is performed from the apical window by directing an M-mode cursor through the longitudinal extent of the septum or lateral wall. Color Doppler display here shows the longitudinal motion of these walls throughout the cardiac cycle, whereas placing a pulsed Doppler sample volume at the location of the mitral annulus quantifies movement of this structure throughout the cardiac cycle, with important implications for quantification of systolic and diastolic function. In healthy patients, mitral annular velocity in diastole parallels the transmitral velocity pattern, with a fall in the ratio of the annular E velocity to the annular A velocity with age, as is seen in the left ventricular filling curves.[198] However, this concordance between annular motion and ventricular inflow patterns is disrupted in a number of disease states. For instance, a preliminary study of patients with constriction and restriction demonstrated very similar left ventricular inflow E- and A-wave velocities. However, the patients with constriction had very rapid early diastolic annular velocity, whereas the restriction patients had very slow early diastolic motion of the annulus. Indeed, applying a cutoff velocity of 8 cm per second to the early diastolic annular velocity allowed complete separation between patients with constriction and restriction.[200]

FIGURE 29–27. See Color Plate 4.

While these results are preliminary, they do suggest that important fundamental data is contained in intramyocardial velocity. With further improvements in technology, in particular an increase in the two-dimensional frame rate and the ability to extract actual velocities from the color images, DTI may become an important component in the diagnostic armamentarium for diastolic function.

CONCLUSIONS

In this chapter we have shown how Doppler echocardiography can be used to characterize ventricular diastolic function in health and disease. Through understanding of the physical and physiologic factors that influence ventricular filling, important clinical information can be obtained from analysis of transmitral velocity patterns, although limited in many ways by load dependency and nonuniqueness of the patterns themselves. Fortunately, these limitations can be largely overcome by careful integration of transmitral flow data with the pulmonary venous velocity pattern. Finally, a number of novel echocardiographic methodologies have emerged recently that appear to offer unique insight into important aspects of ventricular mechanical function.

References

1. Hirota, Y.: A clinical study of left ventricular relaxation. Circulation 62:756, 1980.
2. Rousseau, M.F., Pouleur, H., Detry, J.M.R., et al.: Relaxation between changes in left ventricular inotropic state and relaxation in normal subjects and patients with coronary artery disease. Circulation 64:736, 1981.
3. Dougherty, A.H., Naccarelli, G.V., Gray, E.L., et al.: Congestive heart failure with normal systolic function. Am. J. Cardiol. 54:778, 1984.
4. Topol, E.J., Traill, T.A., and Fortuin, N.J.: Hypertensive hypertrophic cardiomyopathy in the elderly. N. Engl. J. Med. 312:277, 1985.
5. Soufer, R., Wohlgelernter, D., Vita, N.A., et al.: Intact systolic left ventricular function in clinical congestive heart failure. Am. J. Cardiol. 53:567, 1984.
6. Aroesty, J.M., McKay, R.G., Heller, G.V., et al.: Simultaneous assessment of the left ventricular systolic and diastolic dysfunction during pacing-induced ischemia. Circulation 71:889, 1985.
7. Klein, A.L., and Cohen, G.I.: Doppler echocardiographic assessment of constrictive pericarditis, cardiac amyloidosis, and cardiac tamponade. (Review.) Cleve. Clin. J. Med. 59:278, 1992.
8. Hatle, L.K., Appleton, C.P., and Popp, R.L.: Differentiation of constructive pericarditis and restrictive cardiomyopathy by Doppler echocardiography. Circulation 79:357, 1989.
9. Klein, A.L., Hatle, L.K., Burstow, D.J., et al.: Doppler characterization of left ventricular diastolic function in cardiac amyloidosis. J. Am. Coll. Cardiol. 13:1017, 1989.
10. Maron, B.J., Spirito, P., Green, K.J., et al.: Noninvasive assessment of left ventricular diastolic function by pulsed Doppler echocardiography in patients with hypertrophic cardiomyopathy. J. Am. Coll. Cardiol. 10:733, 1987.
11. Pearson, A.C., Labovitz, A.J., Mrosek, D., et al.: Assessment of diastolic function in normal and hypertrophied hearts: Comparison of Doppler echocardiography and M-mode echocardiography. Am. Heart J. 113:1417, 1987.
12. St. Gore, F., Masuyama, T., Alderman, E.L., et al.: Left ventricular diastolic dysfunction in end-stage dilated cardiomyopathy: Simultaneous Doppler echocardiography and hemodynamic evaluation. J. Am. Soc. Echocardiogr. 4:349, 1991.
13. Fujita, N., Hartiala, J., O'Sullivan, M., et al.: Assessment of left ventricular diastolic function in dilated cardiomyopathy with cine magnetic resonance imaging: Effect of an angiotensin-converting enzyme inhibitor, benazepril. Am. Heart J. 125:171, 1993.
14. Kitabatake, A., Tanouchi, J., Masuyama, T., et al.: Limited atrial compensation to reduced early diastolic filling in hypertensive patients with advanced left ventricular hypertrophy: A Doppler echocardiographic study. Heart Vessels 5:33, 1989.
15. Meliones, J.N., Snider, A.R., Serwer, G.A., et al.: Pulsed Doppler assessment of left ventricular diastolic filling in children with left ventricular outflow obstruction before and after balloon angioplasty. Am. J. Cardiol. 63:231, 1989.
16. Riggs, T.W., Rodriguez, R., Snider, A.R., et al.: Doppler echocardiographic evaluation of right and left ventricular diastolic function in normal neonates. J. Am. Coll. Cardiol. 13:700, 1989.
17. Van Dam, I., Fast, J., de Boo, T., et al.: Normal diastolic filling patterns of the left ventricle. Eur. Heart J. 9:165, 1988.
18. Spirito, P., and Maron, B.J.: Influence of aging on Doppler echocardiographic indices of left ventricular diastolic function. Br. Heart J. 59:672, 1988.
19. Klein, A.L., Burstow, D.J., Tajik, A.J., et al.: Effects of age on left ventricular dimensions and filling dynamics in 117 normal persons. Mayo Clin. Proc. 69:212, 1994.
20. Valantine, H.A., Fowler, M.B., Hunt, S.A., et al.: Changes in Doppler echocardiographic indexes of left ventricular function as potential markers of acute rejection. Circulation 76(Suppl. V):V86, 1987.
21. Valantine, H.A., Appleton, C.P., Hatle, L.K., et al.: A hemodynamic and Doppler echocardiographic study of ventricular function in long-term cardiac allograft recipients: Etiology and prognosis of restrictive-constrictive physiology. Circulation 79:66, 1989.
22. Pinamonti, B., Di Lenardo, A., Sinagra, G., et al.: Restrictive left ventricular filling pattern in dilated cardiomyopathy assessed by Doppler echocardiography: Clinical, echocardiographic and hemodynamic correlations and prognostic implications. J. Am. Coll. Cardiol. 22:808, 1993.
23. Klein, A.L., Hatle, L.K., Taliercio, C.P., et al.: Prognostic significance of Doppler measures of diastolic function in cardiac amyloidosis: A Doppler echocardiography study. Circulation 83:808, 1991.
24. Mulvagh, S., Quinones, M.A., Kleiman, N.S., et al.: Estimation of left ventricular end-diastolic pressure from Doppler transmitral flow velocity in cardiac patients independent of systolic performance. J. Am. Coll. Cardiol. 20:112, 1992.
25. Rossvoll, O., and Hatle, L.K.: Pulmonary venous flow velocities recorded by transthoracic Doppler ultrasound: Relation to left ventricular diastolic pressures. J. Am. Coll. Cardiol. 21:1687, 1993.
26. Nishimura, R.A., Housmans, P.R., Hatle, L.K., et al.: Assessment of diastolic function of the heart: Background and current applications of Doppler echocardiography. Part I. Physiologic and pathophysiologic features. Mayo Clin. Proc. 64:71, 1989.
27. Nishimura, R.A., Abel, M.D., Hatle, L.K., et al.: Assessment of diastolic function of the heart: Background and current applications of Doppler echocardiography. Part II. Clinical studies. Mayo Clin. Proc. 64:181, 1989.
28. Gaasch, W.H., and LeWinter M.M.: Left ventricular diastolic dysfunction and heart failure. Philadelphia, Lea & Febiger, 1994, pp. 3–140.
29. Katz, A.M.: Physiology of the Heart. New York, Raven Press, 1992, pp. 151–177.
30. Grossman, W. (ed.): Diastolic Relaxation of the Heart. Boston, Martinus-Nijhoff, 1988.
31. Morgan, J.P.: Mechanisms of disease: Abnormal intracellular modulation of calcium as a major cause of cardiac contractile dysfunction. N. Engl. J. Med. 325:625, 1991.
32. Morgan, J.P., Erny, R.E., Allen, P.D., et al.: Abnormal intracellular calcium handling: A major cause of systolic and diastolic dysfunction in ventricular myocardium from patients with heart failure. Circulation 81:21, 1990.
33. Cunningham, M.J., Apstein, C.S., Weinberg, E.O., et al.: Deleterious effect of ouabain on myocardial function during hypoxia. Am. J. Physiol. 256:H681, 1989.
34. Janicki, J.S., and Matsubara, B.B.: Myocardial collagen and left ventricular diastolic function. In Gaasch, W.H., and LeWinter, M.M. (eds.): Left Ventricular Diastolic Dysfunction and Heart Failure. Philadelphia, Lea & Febiger, 1994, pp. 125–140.
35. Robinson, T.F., Factor, S.F., and Sonnenblick, E.H.: The heart as a suction pump. Sci. Am. 254:84, 1986.
36. Matsubara, B.B., Hennigar, J.R., and Janicki, J.S.: Structural and functional role of myocardial collagen. Circulation 84:II-212, 1991.
37. Factor, S.M., Flomenbaum, M., Zhao, M.J., et al.: The effect of acutely increased ventricular cavity pressure on intrinsic myocardial connective tissue. J. Am. Coll. Cardiol. 12:1582, 1988.
38. Lerman, R.H., Apstein, C.S., Kagan, H.M., et al.: Myocardial healing and repair after experimental infarction in the rabbit. Circ. Res. 53:378, 1983.
39. Glantz, S.A., and Kernoff, R.S.: Muscle stiffness determined from canine left ventricular pressure volume curves. Circ. Res. 37:787, 1975.
40. Nikolic, S., Yellin, E.L., Tamura, K., et al.: Passive properties of the canine left ventricle: Diastolic stiffness and restoring forces. Circ. Res. 62:1210, 1988.
41. Suga, H., and Sagawa, K.: Instantaneous pressure-volume relationships and their ratio in the excised, supported canine left ventricle. Circ. Res. 35:117, 1974.
42. Weiss, J.L., Frederikson, J.W., and Weisfeldt, J.L.: Hemodynamic determinants of the time-course of fall in canine left ventricular pressure. J. Clin. Invest. 58:751, 1976.
43. Raaf, G.L., and Glantz, S.A.: Volume loading slows left ventricular relaxation rate. Circ. Res. 48:813, 1981.
44. Templeton, G.H., Donald, I.T.C., Mitchell, J.H., et al.: Dynamic stiffness of papillary muscle during contraction and relaxation. Am. J. Physiol. 224:692, 1973.
45. Templeton, G.H., Ecker, R.R., and Mitchell, J.H.: Left ventricular stiffness during diastole and systole: The influence of changes in volume and inotropic state. Cardiovasc. Res. 6:95, 1972.
46. Udelson, J.E., Bacharach, S.L., Cannon R.O., et al.: Minimum left ventricular pressure during beta adrenergic stimulation in human subjects: Evidence for myocardial recoil and diastolic section in the normal heart. Circulation 82:1174, 1990.
47. Mann, T., Goldberg, S., Mudge, G.H., et al.: Factors contributing to altered left ventricular diastolic properties during angina pectoris. Circulation 59:14, 1979.
48. Gorcsan, J., Ramond, J.A., Mandarino, W.A., et al.: Assessment of left ventricular performance by on-line pressure-area relations using echocardiographic automated border detection. J. Am. Coll. Cardiol. 23:242, 1994.
49. Yellin, E.L.: Mitral valve motion, intracardiac dynamics and flow pattern modelling: Physiology and pathophysiology. In Ghista's Advances in Cardiovascular Physics. Vol. 5. Basel, S. Karger, 1983, pp. 137–161.
50. Flachskampf, F.A., Rodriguez, L.L., Chen, C., et al.: Analysis of mitral inertance: A factor critical for early transmitral filling. J. Am. Soc. Echocardiogr. 6:422, 1993.
51. Choong, C.Y., Abascal, V.A., Thomas, J.D., et al.: The combined effect of ventricular loading and relaxation on the transmitral flow velocity profile in dogs measured by Doppler echocardiography. Circulation 78:672, 1988.
52. Takahashi, T., Iizuka, M., Serizawa, T., et al.: Significance of left atrial pressure and left ventricular relaxation as determinants of left ventricular early diastolic filling in man. Jpn. Heart J. 31:319, 1990.
53. Stoddard, M.F., Pearson, A.C., Kern, M.J., et al.: Influence of alteration in preload on the pattern of left ventricular diastolic filling as assessed by Doppler echocardiography in humans. Circulation 79:1226, 1989.
54. Appleton, C.A., Hatle, L.K., and Popp, R.L.: Relation of transmitral flow velocity patterns to left ventricular diastolic function: New insights from a combined hemodynamic and Doppler echocardiographic study. J. Am. Coll. Cardiol. 12:426, 1988.
55. Davidson, W.R., Pasquale, M.J., and Aronoff, R.D.: Doppler left ventricular filling pattern is closely related to ventricular relaxation abnormalities. (Abstract.) J. Am. Coll. Cardiol. 13:197A, 1989.
56. Burke, M.R., Xie, G.Y., Kwan, O.L., et al.: Reduction of left ventricular preload by lower body negative pressure alters Doppler transmitral filling patterns. J. Am. Coll. Cardiol. 16:1387, 1990.
57. Kyriakides, Z.S., Kremastinos, D.T., Paraskevaides, I.A., et al.: Effect of a preload increase on ventricular filling in coronary artery disease. Cardiology 82:229, 1993.
58. Flachskampf, F.A., Weyman, A.E., Guererro, J.L., et al.: Calculation of atrioven-

tricular compliance from the mitral flow profile: Analytical and in vitro study. J. Am. Coll. Cardiol. 19:998, 1992.

59. Thomas, J.D., Wilkins, G.T., Choong, C.Y., et al.: Inaccuracy of the mitral pressure half-time immediately following percutaneous mitral valvotomy: Dependence on transmitral gradient and left atrial and ventricular compliance. Circulation 78:980, 1988.

60. Ohno, M., Cheng, C.P., and Little, W.C.: Mechanism of altered patterns of left ventricular filling during the development of congestive heart failure. Circulation 89:2241, 1994.

61. Appleton, C., Hatle, L., and Popp, R.: Demonstration of restrictive ventricular physiology by Doppler echocardiography. J. Am. Coll. Cardiol. 11:757, 1988.

62. Oh, J.K., Hatle, L.K., Sinak, L.J., et al.: Characteristic Doppler echocardiographic pattern of mitral inflow velocity in severe aortic regurgitation. J. Am. Coll. Cardiol. 14:1712, 1989.

63. Thomas, J.D., Newell, J.B., Choong, C.Y.P., et al.: Physical and physiological determinants of transmitral velocity: Numerical analysis. Am. J. Physiol. 2605 Pt. 2:H1718, 1991.

64. Thomas, J.D., and Weyman, A.E.: Echocardiographic Doppler evaluation of left ventricular diastolic function: Physics and physiology. Circulation 84:977, 1991.

65. Meissner, J.S., Pajaro, O.E., and Yellin, E.L.: Investigation of left ventricular filling dynamics: Development of a model. Einstein Q. J. Biol. Med. 4:47, 1986.

66. Keren, G., Meisner, J.S., Sherez, J., et al.: Interrelationship of mid-diastolic mitral valve motion, pulmonary venous flow, and transmitral flow. Circulation 74:36, 1986.

67. Kovacs, S.J., Barzilai, B., and Perez, J.E.: Evaluation of diastolic function with Doppler echocardiography: The PDF formalism. Am. J. Physiol. 252(1 Pt. 2):H178, 1987.

68. Bakalyar, D.M., Hauser, A.M., and Timmis, G.C.: Theoretical description of blood flow through the mitral orifice. J. Biomech. Eng. 111:141, 1989.

69. Beyar, R., and Sideman, S.: Atrioventricular interactions: A theoretical simulation study. Am. J. Physiol. 252:H653, 1987.

70. Lau, V.K., and Sagawa, K.: Model analysis of the contribution of atrial contraction to ventricular filling. Ann. Biomed. Eng. 7:167, 1979.

71. Chadwick, R.S., and Brun, P.: A theoretical model of left ventricular filling and interpretation of echographic waveforms. In Cardiovascular Dynamics and Models. Proceedings of the NIH-Inserm Workshops, Colloque Inserm. 183, Inserm, Paris, 1988, pp. 339–348.

72. Peskin, C.S.: Numerical analysis of blood flow in the heart. J. Comput. Phys. 25:220, 1977.

73. McQueen, D.M., Peskin, C.S., and Yellin, E.L.: Fluid dynamics of the mitral valve: Physiologic aspects of a mathematical model. Am. J. Physiol. 242:H1095, 1982.

74. McQueen, D.M., and Peskin, C.S.: Computer-assisted design of pivoting disc prosthetic mitral valves. J. Thorac. Cardiovasc. Surg. 86:126, 1983.

75. Meisner, J.S., McQueen, D.M., Ishida, Y., et al.: Effects of timing of atrial systole on ventricular filling and mitral valve closure: Computer and dog studies. Am. J. Physiol. 249(3 Pt. 2):H604, 1985.

76. Peskin, C.S., and McQueen, D.M.: A three-dimensional computational method for blood flow in the heart. I. Immersed elastic fibers in a viscous incompressible fluid. J. Comput. Phys. 81:372, 1989.

77. McQueen, D.M., and Peskin, C.S.: A three-dimensional computational method for blood flow in the heart. II. Contractile fibers. J. Comput. Phys. 82:289, 1989.

78. Hoit, B.D., Shao, Y., Gabel, M., et al.: In vivo assessment of left atrial contractile performance in normal and pathological conditions using a time varying elastance model. Circulation 89:1829, 1994.

79. Hoit, B.D., Shao, Y., Tsai, L.M., et al.: Altered left atrial compliance after atrial appendectomy: Influence on left atrial and ventricular filling. Circ. Res. 72:167, 1993.

80. Nishimura, R.A., Abel, M.D., Hatle, L.K., et al.: Relation of pulmonary vein to mitral flow velocities by transesophageal Doppler echocardiography: Effect of different loading conditions. Circulation 81:1488, 1990.

81. Alexander, J., Jr., Sunagawa, K., Chang, N., et al.: Instantaneous pressure-volume relation of the ejecting left atrium. Circ. Res. 61:209, 1987.

82. Lau, V.K., Sagawa, K., and Suga, H.: Instantaneous pressure volume relationship of right atrium during isovolumic contraction in the canine heart. Am. J. Physiol. 236:H672, 1979.

83. Manning, W.J., Leeman, D.E., Gotch, P.J., et al.: Pulsed Doppler evaluation of atrial mechanical function after electrical cardioversion of atrial fibrillation. J. Am. Coll. Cardiol. 13:617, 1989.

84. Choong, C.Y.C., Hermann, H.C., Weyman, A.E., et al.: Preload dependence of Doppler-derived indices of left ventricular diastolic function in humans. J. Am. Coll. Cardiol. 10:800, 1987.

85. Ishida, Y., Meisner, J.S., Tsujioka, K., et al.: Left ventricular filling dynamics: Influence of left ventricular relaxation and left atrial pressures. Circulation 74:187, 1986.

86. Takenaka, K., Dabestani, A., Gardin, J.M., et al.: Left ventricular filling in hypertrophic cardiomyopathy: A pulsed Doppler echocardiographic study. J. Am. Coll. Cardiol. 7:1263, 1986.

87. Bryg, R.J., Pearson, A.C., Williams, G.A., et al.: Left ventricular systolic and diastolic flow abnormalities determined by Doppler echocardiography in obstructive hypertrophic cardiomyopathy. Am. J. Cardiol. 59:925, 1987.

88. Pearson, A.C., Gudipati, C.V., and Labovitz, A.J.: Systolic and diastolic flow abnormalities in elderly patients with hypertensive hypertrophic cardiomyopathy. J. Am. Coll. Cardiol. 12:989, 1988.

89. Otto, C.M., Pearlman, A.S., and Amsler, L.C.: Doppler echocardiographic evaluation of left ventricular diastolic filling in isolated valvular aortic stenosis. Am. J. Cardiol. 63:313, 1989.

90. Zarich, S.W., Kowalchuk, G.J., McGuire, M.P., et al.: Left ventricular filling abnormalities in asymptomatic morbid obesity. Am. J. Cardiol. 68:377, 1991.

91. Fujii, J., Yazaki, Y., Sawada, H., et al.: Noninvasive assessment of left and right ventricular filling in myocardial infarction with a two-dimensional Doppler echocardiographic method. J. Am. Coll. Cardiol. 5:1155, 1985.

92. Iliceto, S., Amico, A., Marangelli, V., et al.: Doppler echocardiographic evaluation of the effect of atrial pacing-induced ischemia on left ventricular filling in patients with coronary artery disease. J. Am. Coll. Cardiol. 11:953, 1988.

93. Wind, B.E., Snider, A.R., Buda, A.J., et al.: Pulsed Doppler assessment of left ventricular diastolic filling in coronary artery disease before and immediately after coronary angioplasty. Am. J. Cardiol. 59:1041, 1987.

94. Labovitz, A.J., Lewen, M.K., Kern, M., et al.: Evaluation of left ventricular systolic and diastolic dysfunction during transient myocardial ischaemia produced by angioplasty. J. Am. Coll. Cardiol. 10:748, 1987.

95. de Bruyne, B., Lerch, R., Meier, B., et al.: Doppler assessment of left ventricular diastolic filling during brief coronary occlusion. Am. Heart J. 117:629, 1989.

96. Doria, E., Agostini, P., Loaldi, A., et al.: Doppler assessment of left ventricular filling pattern in silent ischemia in patients with Prinzmetal's angina. Am. J. Cardiol. 66:1055, 1990.

97. Takenaka, K., Dabestani, A., Gardin, J.M., et al.: Pulsed Doppler echocardiographic study of left ventricular filling in dilated cardiomyopathy. Am. J. Cardiol. 58:143, 1986.

98. Wehlage, D.R., Bohrer, H., and Ruffmann, K.: Impairment of left ventricular diastolic function during coronary artery bypass grafting. Anesthesia 45:549, 1990.

99. Iwase, M., Sotobata, I., Takagi, S., et al.: Effects of diltiazem on left ventricular diastolic behavior in patients with hypertrophic cardiomyopathy: Evaluation with exercise pulsed Doppler echocardiography. J. Am. Coll. Cardiol. 9:1099, 1987.

100. Phillips, R.A., Coplan, N.L., Krakoff, L.R., et al.: Doppler echocardiographic analysis of left ventricular filling in treated hypertensive patients. J. Am. Coll. Cardiol. 9:317, 1987.

101. Lee, R.T., Lord, C.P., Plappert, T., et al.: Effects of nifedipine on transmitral Doppler blood flow velocity profile in patients with concentric left ventricular hypertrophy. Am. Heart J. 119:1130, 1990.

102. Snow, F.R., Gorcsan, J., Lewis, S.A., et al.: Doppler echocardiographic evaluation of left ventricular diastolic function after percutaneous transluminal coronary angioplasty for unstable angina pectoris or acute myocardial infarction. Am. J. Cardiol. 65:840, 1990.

103. Masuyama, T., Nellessen, U., Stinson, E.B., et al.: Improvement in left ventricular diastolic filling by septal myectomy in hypertrophic cardiomyopathy. J. Am. Soc. Echocardiogr. 3:196, 1990.

104. Alexander, J., Jr., Nikolic, S., Ghai, P., et al.: Analysis of pulmonary venous admittance: In vivo measurements of pulmonary vein flow. (Abstract.) Circulation 78(Suppl. II):II-248, 1988.

105. Klein, A.L., and Tajik, A.J.: Doppler assessment of pulmonary venous flow in healthy subjects and in patients with heart disease. (Review.) J. Am. Soc. Echocardiogr. 4:379, 1991.

106. Basnight, M.A., Gonzalez, M.S., Kershenovich, S.C., et al.: Pulmonary venous flow velocity: Relation to hemodynamics, mitral flow velocity and left atrial volume, and ejection fraction. J. Am. Soc. Echocardiogr. 4:547, 1991.

107. Appleton, C.P., and Hatle, L.K.: The natural history of left ventricular filling abnormalities: Assessment by two-dimensional and Doppler echocardiography. Echocardiography 9:437, 1992.

108. Cueto, G.L., Reeder, G.S., Kyle, R.A., et al.: Echocardiographic findings in systemic amyloidosis: Spectrum of cardiac involvement and relation to survival. J. Am. Coll. Cardiol. 6:737, 1985.

109. Lorell, B.H., Apstein, C.S., Weinberg, E.O., et al.: Diastolic function in left ventricular hypertrophy: Clinical and experimental relationships. Eur. Heart J. 11(Suppl. G):54, 1990.

110. Himelman, R.B., Lee, E., and Schiller, N.B.: Septal bounce, vena cava plethora, and pericardial adhesion: Informative two-dimensional echocardiographic signs in the diagnosis of pericardial constriction. J. Am. Soc. Echocardiogr. 1:333, 1988.

111. Himelman, R.B., Kircher, B., Rockey, D.C., et al.: Inferior vena cava plethora with blunted respiratory response: A sensitive echocardiographic sign of cardiac tamponade. J. Am. Coll. Cardiol. 12:1470, 1988.

112. Klein, A.L., Hatle, L.K., Burstow, D.J., et al.: Comprehensive Doppler assessment of right ventricular diastolic function in cardiac amyloidosis. J. Am. Coll. Cardiol. 15:99, 1990.

113. Gardin, J.M., Dabestani, A., Takenaka, K., et al.: Effect of imaging view and sample volume location on evaluation of mitral flow velocity by pulsed Doppler echocardiography. Am. J. Cardiol. 57:1335, 1986.

114. Ding, Z.P., Oh, J.K., Klein, A.L., et al.: Effect of sample volume location on Doppler-derived transmitral inflow velocity values. J. Am. Soc. Echocardiogr. 4:451, 1991.

115. Appleton, C.P., Galloway, J.M., Gonzalez, M.S., et al.: Estimation of left ventricular filling pressures using two-dimensional and Doppler echocardiography in adult patients with cardiac disease: Additional value of analyzing left atrial size, left atrial ejection fraction and the difference in duration of pulmonary venous and mitral flow velocity at atrial contraction. J. Am. Coll. Cardiol. 22:1972, 1993.

116. Klein, A.L., Cohen, G.I., Pietrolungo, J.F., et al.: Differentiation of constrictive pericarditis from restrictive cardiomyopathy by Doppler transesophageal echocardiographic measurements of respiratory variations in pulmonary venous flow. J. Am. Coll. Cardiol. 22:1935, 1993.

117. Seward, J.B., Khandheria, B.K., Freeman, W.K., et al.: Multiplane transesophageal echocardiography: Image orientation, examination technique, anatomic correlations, and clinical applications. Mayo Clin. Proc. 68:523, 1993.

118. Zoghbi, W.A., Habib, G.B., and Quinones, M.A.: Doppler assessment of right ventricular filling in a normal population. Circulation 82:1316, 1990.

119. Morley, J.E., and Reese, S.S.: Clinical implications of the aging heart. Am. J. Med. 86:77, 1989.

120. Bryg, R.J., Williams, A., and Labovitz, A.J.: Effect of aging on left ventricular diastolic filling in normal subjects. Am. J. Cardiol. 59:971, 1987.

121. Gardin, J.M., Rohan, M.K., Davidson, D., et al.: Doppler transmitral flow velocity parameters: Relationship between age, body surface area, blood pressure and gender in normal subjects. Am. J. Noninvasive Cardiol. 1:3, 1986.

122. Klein, A.L., and Tajik, A.J.: Doppler assessment of diastolic function in cardiac amyloidosis. Echocardiography 8:233, 1991.

123. Grodecki, P.V., and Klein, A.L.: Pitfalls in the echo-Doppler assessment of diastolic dysfunction. Echocardiography 10:213, 1993.

124. Dumesnil, J.G., Gaudreault, G., Honos, G.N., et al.: Use of Valsalva maneuver to unmask left ventricular diastolic function abnormalities by Doppler echocardiography in patients with coronary artery disease or systemic hypertension. Am. J. Cardiol. 68:515, 1991.

125. Glower, D.D., Murrah, R.L., Olsen, C.O., et al.: Mechanical correlates of the third heart sound. J. Am. Coll. Cardiol. 19:450, 1992.

126. Klein, A.L., Grimm, R.A., Bailey, A.S.: The longitudinal imaging plane by biplane TEE is required for complete assessment of pulmonary venous flow in patients with heart disease. (Abstract.) Circulation 88:I-305, 1994.

127. Delemarre, B.J., Bot, H., Visser, C.A., et al.: Phasic flow in the left ventricular inflow track: The importance of Doppler sample volume position. J. Clin. Ultrasound. 16:227, 1988.

128. Appleton, C.P.: Doppler assessment of left ventricular diastolic function: The refinements continue. (Editorial.) J. Am. Coll. Cardiol. 21:1697, 1993.

129. Airaksinen, K.E.J., Ikaheimo, M.J., Huikuri, H.V., et al.: Effects of isometric exercise and heart rate on left ventricular filling pattern assessed by pulsed Doppler echocardiography. J. Intern. Med. 226:245, 1989.

130. Appleton, C.A., Carucci, M.J., and Henry, C.P.: Influence of incremental changes in heart rate on mitral flow velocity in lightly sedated conscious dogs. J. Am. Coll. Cardiol. 17:227, 1991.

131. Masuyama, T., Kodama, K., Nakatani, S., et al.: Effects of atrial ventricular interval on left ventricular diastolic filling assessed with pulsed Doppler echocardiography. Cardiovasc. Res. 23:1034, 1989.

132. Klein, A.L., Stewart, W.J., Bartlett, J., et al.: Effects of mitral regurgitation on pulmonary venous flow and left atrial pressure: An intraoperative transesophageal echocardiographic study. J. Am. Coll. Cardiol. 20:1345, 1992.

133. Oh, J.K., Hatle, L.K., Seward, J.B., et al.: Diagnostic role of Doppler echocardiography in constrictive pericarditis. J. Am. Coll. Cardiol. 23:154, 1994.

134. Hatle, L.: Diastolic dysfunction in restrictive and constrictive heart disease. In Gaasch, W.H., and LeWinter, M.M. (eds.): Left Ventricular Diastolic Dysfunction and Heart Failure. Philadelphia, Lea & Febiger, 1994, pp. 390–407.

135. Nishimura, R.A., Connolly, D.C., Parkin, T.W., et al.: Constrictive pericarditis: Assessment of current diagnostic procedures. Mayo Clin. Proc. 60:397, 1985.

136. Schiavone, W.A., and Rice, T.W.: Pericardial disease: Current diagnosis and management methods. Clev. Clin. J. Med. 56:639, 1989.

137. Shabetai, R., Fowler, N.O., and Guntheroth, W.G.: The hemodynamics of cardiac tamponade and constrictive pericarditis. Am. J. Cardiol. 26:480, 1970.

138. Benotti, J.R., Grossman, W., and Cohn, P.F.: Clinical profile of restrictive cardiomyopathy. Circulation 61:1206, 1980.

139. Klein, A.L., Al Assaad, A.N., Pietrolungo, J.F., et al.: Does rapid volume loading during transesophageal echocardiography differentiate constrictive pericarditis from restrictive cardiomyopathy. (Abstract.) J. Am. Soc. Echocardiogr. S38:7C, 1994.

140. Gillam, L.D., Guyer, D.E., Gibson, T.C., et al.: Hydrodynamic compression of the right atrium: A new echocardiographic sign of cardiac tamponade. Circulation 68:294, 1983.

141. Schiller, N.B., and Botvinick, E.H.: Right ventricular compression as a sign of cardiac tamponade: An analysis of echocardiographic ventricular dimensions and their clinical implications. Circulation 56:774, 1977.

142. Singh, S., Wann, L.S., Schuchard, G.H., et al.: Right ventricular and right atrial collapse in patients with cardiac tamponade—A combined echocardiographic and hemodynamic study. Circulation 70:966, 1984.

143. Burstow, D.J., Oh, J.K., Bailey, K.R., et al.: Cardiac tamponade: Characteristic Doppler observations. Mayo Clin. Proc. 64:312, 1989.

144. Picard, M.H., Sanfilippo, A.J., Newell, J.B., et al.: Quantitative relation between increased intrapericardial pressure and Doppler flow velocities during experimental cardiac tamponade. J. Am. Coll. Cardiol. 18:234, 1991.

145. Schutzman, J.J., Obarski, T.P., Pearce, G.L., et al.: Comparison of Doppler and two-dimensional echocardiography for assessment of pericardial effusion. Am. J. Cardiol. 70(Nov. 15):1353, 1992.

146. Keren, A., and Popp, R.L.: Assignment of patients into the classification of cardiomyopathies. Circulation 86:1622, 1992.

147. Klein, A.L., Hatle, L.K., Taliercio, C.P., et al.: Serial Doppler echocardiographic follow-up of left ventricular diastolic function in cardiac amyloidosis. J. Am. Coll. Cardiol. 16:1135, 1990.

148. Klein, A.L., Oh, J.K., Miller, F.A., et al.: Two-dimensional and Doppler echocardiographic assessment of infiltrative cardiomyopathy. J. Am. Soc. Echocardiogr. 1:48, 1988.

149. Swanton, R.H., Brooksby, I.A., Davies, M.J., et al.: Systolic and diastolic ventricular function in cardiac amyloidosis. Studies in six cases diagnosed with endomyocardial biopsy. Am. J. Cardiol. 39:658, 1977.

150. Tyberg, T.I., Goodyer, A.V., Hurst, V.W., et al.: Left ventricular filling in differentiating restrictive amyloid cardiomyopathy and constrictive pericarditis. Am. J. Cardiol. 47:791, 1981.

151. Wigle, E.D.: Diastolic dysfunction in hypertropic cardiomyopathy. In Gaasch

152. Brutsaert, D.L., Rademakers, F.E., and Sys, S.U.: Triple control of relaxation: Implications in cardiac disease. Circulation 69:190, 1984.

153. Brutsaert, D.L., Sys, S.U., and Gillebert, T.C.: Diastolic failure: Pathophysiology and therapeutic implications. (Review.) (Published erratum appears in J. Am. Coll. Cardiol. 22(4):1272, 1993.) J. Am. Coll. Cardiol. 22:318, 1993.

154. Bonow, R.O.: Regional left ventricular nonuniformity. Effects on left ventricular diastolic function in ischemic heart disease, hypertrophic cardiomyopathy, and the normal heart. Circulation 81:III54, 1990.

155. Rakowski, H., Sasson, Z., and Wigle, E.D.: Echocardiographic and Doppler assessment of hypertrophic cardiomyopathy. J. Am. Soc. Echocardiogr. 1:31, 1988.

156. Bonow, R.O.: Left ventricular diastolic function in hypertrophic cardiomyopathy. Herz 16:13, 1991.

157. Nishimura, R.A., Schwartz, R.S., Holmes, D.R., Jr., et al.: Failure of calcium channel blockers to improve ventricular relaxation in humans. J. Am. Coll. Cardiol. 21:182, 1993.

158. Fananapazir, L., Cannon, R.O., Tripodi, D., et al.: Impact of dual chamber permanent pacing in patients with obstructive hypertrophic cardiomyopathy with symptoms refractory to verapamil and beta-adrenergic blocker therapy. Circulation 85:2149, 1992.

159. Iskandrian, A.S., Helfield, H., and Lemlek, J.: Differentiation between primary dilated cardiomyopathy based on RV performance. Am. Heart J. 123:768, 1992.

160. Xie, G.Y., Berk, M.R., Smith, M.D., et al.: Prognostic value of Doppler transmitral flow patterns in patients with congestive heart failure. J. Am. Coll. Cardiol. 24:132, 1994.

161. Desruennes, M., Corcos, T., and Cabrol, A.: Doppler echocardiography for the diagnosis of acute cardiac allograft rejection. J. Am. Coll. Cardiol. 12:63, 1988.

162. Valantine, H., Fowler, M., Hatle, L., et al.: Doppler echocardiographic indices of diastolic function as markers of acute cardiac rejection. Transplant. Proc. 19:2556, 1987.

163. Czerska, B., Klein, A.L., Fouad Tarazi, F., et al.: Significance of restrictive cardiac physiology in heart transplant patients. (Abstract.) Eur. J. Cardiac Pacing Electrophysiol. 2:A191, 1992.

164. Lorell, B.H.: Left ventricular hypertrophy and diastolic dysfunction. Hosp. Pract. (Office Ed.), 27:189, 1992.

165. Hoit, B.D., and Walsh, R.A.: Diastolic function in hypertensive heart disease. In Gaasch, W.H., LeWinter, M.M. (eds.): Left Ventricular Diastolic Dysfunction and Heart Failure. Philadelphia, Lea & Febiger, 1994, pp. 354–372.

166. Brogan, W., III, Hillis, L.D., Flores, E.D., et al.: The natural history of isolated left ventricular diastolic dysfunction. Am. J. Med. 92:627, 1992.

167. Kitzman, D.W., Higginbotham, M.B., Cobb, F.R., et al.: Exercise intolerance in patients with heart failure and preserved left ventricular systolic function: Failure of the Frank-Starling mechanism. J. Am. Coll. Cardiol. 17:1065, 1991.

168. Graettinger, W.F., Weber, M.A., Gardin, J.M., et al.: Diastolic blood pressure as a determinant of Doppler left ventricular filling indexes in normotensive adolescents. J. Am. Coll. Cardiol. 10:1280, 1987.

169. Rittoo, D., Monaghan, M., Sadiq, T., et al.: Echocardiographic and Doppler evaluation of left ventricular hypertrophy and diastolic function in black and white hypertensive patients. J. Hum. Hypertens. 4:113, 1990.

170. Lahiri, A., Rodrigues, E.A., Carboni, G.P., et al.: Effects of long-term treatment with calcium antagonists on left ventricular diastolic function in stable angina and heart failure. Circulation 81(Suppl. 2):III 130, 1990.

171. Myreng, Y., and Myhre, E.: Effects of verapamil on left ventricular relaxation and filling dynamics in coronary artery disease: A study by pulsed Doppler echocardiography. Am. Heart J. 117:870, 1989.

172. Gaasch, W.H., Blaustein, A.S., and LeWinter, M.M.: Heart failure and clinical disorders of left ventricular diastolic function. In Gaasch, W.H., and LeWinter, M.M. (eds.): Left Ventricular Diastolic Dysfunction and Heart Failure. Philadelphia, Lea & Febiger, 1994, pp. 245–258.

173. Carroll, J.D., and Carroll, E.P.: Diastolic function in coronary artery disease. Herz 16:1, 1991.

174. Oh, J.K., Ding, Z.P., Gersh, B.J., et al.: Restrictive left ventricular diastolic filling identifies patients with heart failure after acute myocardial infarction. J. Am. Soc. Echocardiogr. 497, 1992.

175. Snider, A.R., Gidding, S.S., Rocchini, A.P., et al.: Doppler evaluation of left ventricular diastolic filling in children with systemic hypertension. Am. J. Cardiol. 56:921, 1985.

176. Vermilion, R.P., Snider, A.R., Meliones, J.N., et al.: Pulsed Doppler evaluation of right ventricular diastolic filling in children with pulmonary valve stenosis before and after balloon valvuloplasty. Am. J. Cardiol. 66:79, 1990.

177. Snider, A.R., Meliones, J.N., and Minich, L.L.: Doppler echocardiographic evaluation of diastolic dysfunction in children. In Gaasch, W.H., and LeWinter, M.M. (eds.): Left Ventricular Diastolic Dysfunction and Heart Failure. Philadelphia, Lea & Febiger, 1994, pp. 408–426.

178. Areias, J.C., Meyer, R., Scott, W.A., et al.: Serial echocardiographic and Doppler evaluation of left ventricular diastolic filling in full-term neonates. Am. J. Cardiol. 66:108, 1990.

179. Johnson, G.L., Moffett, C.B., and Noonan, J.A.: Doppler echocardiographic studies of diastolic ventricular filling patterns in premature infants. Am. Heart J. 116:1568, 1988.

180. Voutilainen, S., Kupari, M., Hippelainen, M., et al.: Factors influencing Doppler indices of left ventricular filling in healthy persons. Am. J. Cardiol. 68:653, 1991.

181. Akagi, T., Benson, L.N., Gilday, D.L., et al.: Influence of ventricular morphology

on diastolic filling performance in double-inlet ventricle after the Fontan procedure. J. Am. Coll. Cardiol. 22:1948, 1993.

182. Sholler, G.F., Colan, S.D., and Sanders, S.P.: Effect of isolated ventricular outflow obstruction on left ventricular function in infants. Am. J. Cardiol. 62:778, 1988.

183. Colan, S.D., Trowitzsch, E., Wernovsky, G., et al.: Myocardial performance after arterial switch operation for transposition of the great arteries with intact ventricular septum. Circulation 78:132, 1988.

184. Vanoverschelde, J.J., Raphael, D.A., Robert, A.R., et al.: Left ventricular filling in dilated cardiomyopathy: Relation to functional class and hemodynamics. J. Am. Coll. Cardiol. 15:1288, 1990.

185. Bargiggia, G.S., Bertucci, C., Recusani, F., et al.: A new method for estimating left ventricular dp/dt by continuous wave Doppler-echocardiography: Validation studies at catheterization. Circulation 80:1287, 1989.

186. Chen, C., Rodriguez, L., Guerrero, J.L., et al.: Noninvasive estimation of instantaneous first derivative of left ventricular pressure using continuous-wave Doppler echocardiography. Circulation 83:2101, 1991.

187. Chen, C., Rodriguez, L., Lethor, J.P., et al.: Continuous wave Doppler echocardiography for noninvasive assessment of left ventricular dP/dt and relaxation time constant from mitral regurgitation spectra in patients. J. Am. Coll. Cardiol. 23:970, 1994.

188. Chen, C., Rodriguez, L., Levine, R.A., et al.: Noninvasive measurement of the time constant of left ventricular relaxation using the continuous wave Doppler velocity profile of mitral regurgitation. Circulation 86:272, 1992.

189. Nishimura, R.A., Schwartz, R.S., Tajik, A.J., et al.: Noninvasive measurement of rate of left ventricular relaxation by Doppler echocardiography. Circulation 88:146, 1993.

190. Yamamoto, K., Masuyama, T., Doi, Y., et al.: Noninvasive assessment of left ventricular relaxation using continuous-wave Doppler aortic regurgitant velocity curve: Its comparative value to the mitral regurgitation method. Circulation 91:192, 1995.

191. Brun, P., Tribouilloy, C., Duval, A.M., et al.: Left ventricular flow propagation during early filling is related to wall relaxation: A color M-mode Doppler analysis. J. Am. Coll. Cardiol. 20:420, 1992.

192. Stuggard, M., Smiseth, O.A., Risoe, C., et al.: Intraventricular early diastolic filling during acute myocardial ischemia: Assessment by multigated color M-mode Doppler echocardiography. Circulation 88:2705, 1993.

193. Thomas, J.D., Aragam, J.R., Rodriguez, L.L., et al.: Spatiotemporal distribution of mitral inflow velocity: Use of the color Doppler M-mode echocardiogram to investigate intracardiac pressure gradients. (Abstract.) Med. Biol. Eng. Comput. 29(Suppl. I):130, 1991.

194. Steen, T., and Steen, S.: Filling of a model left ventricle studied by colour M-mode Doppler. Cardiovasc. Res. 28:1821, 1994.

195. Stugaard, M., Risoe, C., Ihlen, H., et al.: Intracavitary filling pattern in the failing left ventricle assessed by color M-mode echocardiography. J. Am. Coll. Cardiol. 24:663, 1994.

196. Greenberg, N.L., Vandervoort, P.M., and Thomas, J.D.: Estimation of diastolic intraventricular pressure gradients from color Doppler M-mode spatiotemporal velocities: Analytical Euler equation solution. In Proceedings, 1994 Computers in Cardiology, Los Alamitos, CA, IEEE Computer Soc. Press, 1994, p. 465.

197. McDicken, W.N., Sutherland, G.R., Moran, C.M., et al.: Color Doppler velocity imaging of the myocardium. Ultrasound Med. Biol. 18:651, 1992.

198. Rodriguez, L., Garcia, M., Griffin, B.P., et al.: Assessment of mitral annular velocity using Doppler tissue imaging: Comparison with mitral inflow velocity. (Abstract.) J. Am. Soc. Echocardiogr. 7:S41, 1994.

199. Garcia, M., Rodriguez, L., Homa, D., et al.: Intramyocardial motion assessment by Doppler ultrasound: Characteristic findings in normal subjects. (Abstract.) J. Am. Soc. Echocardiogr. 7:S14, 1994.

200. Garcia, M.J., Ares, M.A., Rodriguez, L., et al.: Differentiation of constrictive pericarditis from restrictive cardiomyopathy: Assessment of left ventricular diastolic velocities in the longitudinal axis by Doppler tissue imaging. J. Am. Coll. Cardiol. 1996 (in press).

CHAPTER

30 Valvular Heart Disease

Lyle J. Olson, M.D.
A. Jamil Tajik, M.D.

NATIVE VALVULAR HEART DISEASE ___ 366
Historical Perspective ___ 366
Aortic Stenosis ___ 366
 Doppler Echocardiography in Aortic Stenosis ___ 366
 Role of Echocardiography in Clinical Decision-Making in Aortic Stenosis ___ 369
Aortic Regurgitation ___ 370
 Doppler Echocardiography in Aortic Regurgitation ___ 374
 Role of Echocardiography in Clinical Decision-Making in Aortic Regurgitation ___ 376
Mitral Stenosis ___ 376
 Doppler Echocardiography in Mitral Stenosis ___ 378
 Role of Echocardiography in Clinical Decision-Making in Mitral Stenosis ___ 379
Mitral Regurgitation ___ 380
 Doppler Echocardiography in Mitral Regurgitation ___ 381
 Role of Echocardiography in Clinical Decision-Making in Mitral Regurgitation ___ 383

Tricuspid Stenosis ___ 383
 Doppler Echocardiography in the Evaluation of Tricuspid Stenosis ___ 383
 Role of Echocardiography in Clinical Decision-Making in Tricuspid Stenosis ___ 384
Tricuspid Regurgitation ___ 384
 Doppler Echocardiography in the Evaluation of Tricuspid Regurgitation ___ 385
 Doppler Echocardiographic Estimation of Right Ventricular Systolic Pressure ___ 386
 Role of Echocardiography in the Evaluation of Tricuspid Regurgitation ___ 386
Pulmonary Stenosis and Regurgitation ___ 387
 Doppler Echocardiography in the Evaluation of Pulmonary Valve Disease ___ 387
 Role of Echocardiography in the Evaluation of Pulmonary Valve Disease ___ 387
ASSESSMENT OF VALVE FUNCTION AFTER INTERVENTION ___ 387
Prosthetic Stenosis and Regurgitation ___ 387
Doppler Echocardiography in the Evaluation of Prosthetic Valves ___ 388
Valvuloplasty ___ 389
SUMMARY ___ 389

NATIVE VALVULAR HEART DISEASE

Historical Perspective

The modern era of evaluation and management of valvular heart disease began with the development of cardiac catheterization and surgical intervention more than three decades ago. Cardiac catheterization remains necessary for the detection and assessment of the severity of valvular stenosis and regurgitation in selected cases. However, the development of accurate noninvasive ultrasonic methods for morphologic and hemodynamic assessment and concomitant advances in percutaneous coronary revascularization techniques have directed the primary objectives of the invasive cardiac laboratory to the evaluation and treatment of coronary artery disease. The primary diagnostic role of cardiac catheterization for the evaluation of valvular heart disease has been challenged and in increasingly numerous clinical settings superseded by combined two-dimensional and Doppler echocardiography.

Since the first descriptions of M-mode echocardiography for the evaluation of mitral stenosis more than 40 years ago, echocardiography has evolved from a technique limited to analysis of valve motion to a comprehensive tomographic and hemodynamic method that uses two-dimensional and Doppler echocardiography.[1] The detection and assessment of the cause and hemodynamic severity of stenotic and regurgitant valvular disease now can be reliably performed noninvasively.[2-4] Early diagnosis and accurate characterization of the natural history of valvular heart disease in symptomatic and asymptomatic patients can be accomplished by serial examination without the risk or cost of cardiac catheterization.

This chapter describes the utility and the complementary roles of M-mode, two-dimensional, and spectral and color flow Doppler echocardiography for the evaluation of valvular disease in adult patients, including prosthetic valve dysfunction and valvular disease treated by valvuloplasty. The use of transesophageal echocardiography is also cited in selected clinical settings, and the role of echocardiography in clinical decision-making for patients with valvular heart disease is reviewed.

Aortic Stenosis

The anatomic hallmark of aortic valvular stenosis is reduced orifice dimension, which may be associated with valve calcification and commissural fusion.[5-13] The morphologic appearance of the aortic valve depends on the cause of aortic stenosis. In the past, most cases of fibrocalcific aortic stenosis were considered to be rheumatic in origin,[5-7] but it is now recognized that other causes account for most cases. The three most common causes of aortic stenosis are degenerative (senile) calcification, calcification of a congenital bicuspid aortic valve, and postinflammatory disease.[6, 10, 13, 14] These three causes account for 95 percent of the patients undergoing operation for pure aortic stenosis at the authors' institution.[13, 14] The single most common cause is senile aortic stenosis, which accounts for almost half the cases.[13-15] The increase in relative frequency of senile aortic stenosis has been attributed to the decline in rheumatic fever observed in Western nations.[16, 17]

Senile aortic stenosis is characterized morphologically by a trileaflet aortic valve free of commissural fusion, with calcified nodular excrescences within the valve pockets that restrict motion. The congenitally bicuspid aortic valve is identified by two leaflets of unequal size, the larger of which is conjoined and often contains a fibrous ridge (raphe) at the site of congenital fusion. Calcification of the raphe, annulus, and valve pockets produces a narrowed orifice shaped like an ellipse. Postinflammatory aortic stenosis is characterized by commissural fusion and by cuspid fibrosis and calcification.[13, 14] Stenosis becomes more severe with fusion of more commissures and progressive calcification.

Two-dimensional echocardiography reliably demonstrates valve thickening and calcification and reduced leaflet excursion in systole, thereby qualitatively differentiating valvular stenosis from left ventricular outflow obstruction caused by subvalvular or supravalvular disease.[18-23] This assessment is best performed from the parasternal long-axis view.[24, 25] Typically, severe calcification of the aortic valve leaflets on echocardiographic examination is associated with significant stenosis. However, the severity of calcification is not a reliable predictor of the hemodynamic severity of stenosis, and calcification may be absent, especially in young patients with obstruction caused by congenital or rheumatic disease. Systolic doming of the valve leaflets is frequently observed in association with significant stenosis when calcification is not prominent.[19, 22] Echocardiographic evaluation from the parasternal short-axis view enables characterization of valve leaflet morphology with high sensitivity, including identification of a congenitally bicuspid aortic valve[26, 27] and commissural fusion associated with rheumatic disease (Fig. 30–1). However, dense calcification may make identification of cusp number, and hence morphology, difficult. Assessment of morphology is important for patients considered to be candidates for balloon valvuloplasty, because results of valvuloplasty may be best in elderly patients with senile degenerative disease in which there is no commissural fusion or in patients with rheumatic disease without dense calcification.[28]

Other anatomic abnormalities frequently associated with aortic valvular stenosis demonstrated by two-dimensional echocardiography are left ventricular hypertrophy, poststenotic dilatation of the aorta, other associated valvular heart disease, and subaortic muscular hypertrophy, which may contribute to left ventricular outflow obstruction. Because the risk of aortic dissection is increased in patients with congenitally bicuspid aortic valves, whether or not stenosis is present,[29] patients with a congenitally bicuspid aortic valve should have serial echocardiographic evaluation, including careful evaluation of the aorta.[29a] Echocardiography is used to quantify the dimensions of the aortic root, ventricular wall thickness, and left ventricular cavity dimension in diastole and systole, enabling quantification of left ventricular function (mass and ejection fraction).

The hemodynamic severity of valvular aortic stenosis may be estimated with confidence by two-dimensional echocardiography in some patients.[19-21] In patients with densely calcific aortic stenosis, severely decreased leaflet motion, and left ventricular hypertrophy, two-dimensional echocardiography reliably predicts severe obstruction. Similarly, in patients with minimal aortic valve calcification, normal or nearly normal valve opening, and no left ventricular hypertrophy, two-dimensional echocardiography reliably predicts that aortic stenosis is absent or trivial. However, many patients are not in either of these categories. In these patients, two-dimensional echocardiography is unreliable for prediction of the transvalvular gradient or semiquantitative assessment of the severity of stenosis.[19-21, 30] Definitive assessment of the hemodynamic severity of aortic stenosis requires estimation of the transvalvular pressure gradient and aortic valve area by Doppler echocardiography.

Doppler Echocardiography in Aortic Stenosis

The aim of the Doppler echocardiographic evaluation of the patient with aortic valve stenosis is measurement of both the transvalvular pressure gradient and the aortic valvular orifice area. This may be accomplished in more than 97 percent of patients.[31] Pressure gradient estimation in aortic stenosis by Doppler echocardiography requires measurement of the velocity of blood flow distal to the stenotic valve. This is accomplished by directing the continuous-wave ultrasound beam so that it is within the flow jet and parallel to the velocity vector of transvalvular blood flow. Most often, this is accomplished from an apical transducer position, but occasionally the optimal view is obtained from either the right parasternal or the axillary orientation.[32]

Transvalvular aortic velocity is increased in the presence of aortic stenosis. The measurement of transvalvular aortic velocity by continuous-wave Doppler echocardiography enables estimation of *maximal instantaneous* and mean transvalvular pressure gradients by application of the modified Bernoulli equation.[15, 33-36] The modified Bernoulli equation is expressed as $P = 4V^2$, where P repre-

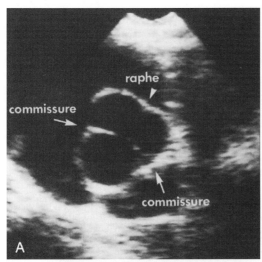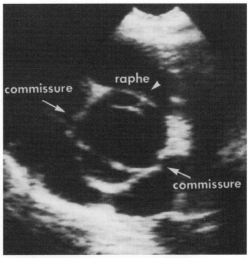

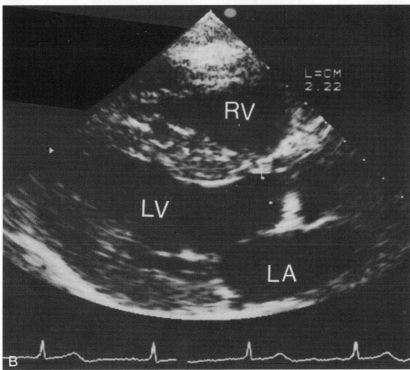

FIGURE 30–1. *A,* Parasternal short-axis view of bicuspid aortic valve in diastole *(left)* and systole *(right).* Commissures are abnormally located at 4 o'clock and nearly 10 o'clock, with a raphe at 1 o'clock *(arrowhead).* Note the oval appearance of the valve during systole. Study of valve opening and closing on real-time two-dimensional echocardiographic examination enables differentiation of the bicuspid from the tricuspid valve. *B,* Parasternal long-axis view in systole from a patient with aortic valvular stenosis. The noncoronary cusp appears thickened and calcified *(arrow).* LA = left atrium; LV = left ventricle; RV = right ventricle. *(A* from Brandenburg, R.O., Jr., Tajik, A.J., Edwards, W.D., et al.: Accuracy of 2-dimensional echocardiographic diagnosis of congenitally bicuspid aortic valve: Echocardiographic-anatomic correlation in 115 patients. Am. J. Cardiol. 51:1469, 1983, with permission of Cahners Publishing Company.)

sents the pressure gradient and V is the velocity of transvalvular blood flow measured by continuous-wave Doppler echocardiography. The pressure gradient is estimated by substituting the measured velocity for V in the modified Bernoulli equation. In addition to providing quantification of the transvalvular gradient, the characteristic Doppler echocardiographic profile aids in the differentiation of valvular or supravalvular stenosis from subvalvular obstruction.[37, 38] The anatomic cause of stenosis is optimally characterized by two-dimensional echocardiography.

Proper interpretation of data obtained by the Doppler echocardiographic method requires appreciation that the maximal instantaneous gradient represents an instantaneous pressure difference between the left ventricle and the aorta, whereas the commonly used peak-to-peak gradient obtained by pull-back of a single catheter at catheterization reflects the difference between peak left ventricular systolic and ascending aortic pressures, which are nonsynchronous[33] (Fig. 30–2). The peak-to-peak gradient is an arbitrary convention; it is not physiologic and therefore is not directly comparable to the Doppler-derived maximal instantaneous gradient. The clinical utility of the catheterization-measured peak-to-peak gradient may be attributed to the fortuitous correlation between peak-to-peak and mean gradients.

The validation of this method for gradient measurement has been proved in simultaneous Doppler echocardiographic and dual

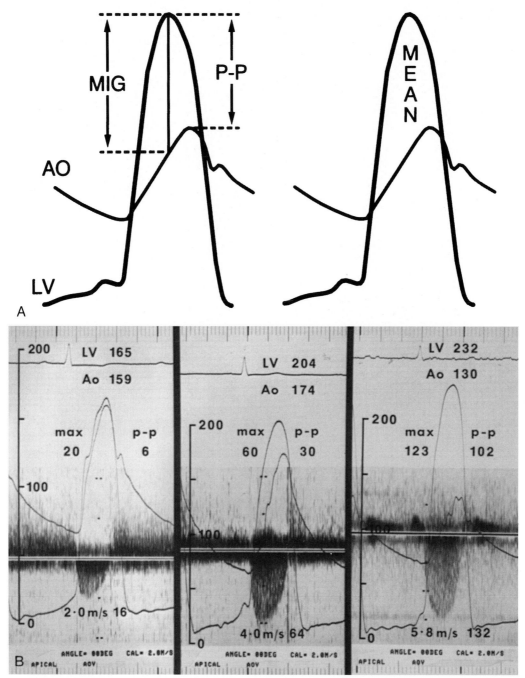

FIGURE 30–2. *A,* Schematic representation of peak-to-peak aortic transvalvular gradients (P-P) and maximal instantaneous gradient (MIG), measured simultaneously, and mean gradient. *Left,* Catheter-determined peak left ventricular systolic pressure and peak aortic systolic pressure are nonsynchronous events; maximal instantaneous pressure gradient determined by continuous-wave Doppler echocardiography reflects simultaneous events. Hence, peak-to-peak and maximal instantaneous pressure measurements do not measure the same gradient, and the maximal instantaneous pressure will always be greater than the peak-to-peak gradient. *Right,* Mean gradient is obtained by planimetry of the area between pressure curves. *B,* Composite of simultaneous Doppler echocardiographic and catheter pressure measurements in three patients with mild, moderate, and severe elevations of transvalvular aortic gradients caused by aortic stenosis. Pressure gradients were measured by dual catheters in the left ventricle and the ascending aorta. The maximal (max) catheter gradient is greater than peak-to-peak (p-p) catheter gradient at each level of stenosis. The maximal Doppler-derived gradients accurately measure the simultaneously recorded maximal catheter gradient but overestimate the peak-to-peak catheter gradient. The Doppler echocardiographic calibrations are in increments of 2 m per second. Ao = ascending aorta; LV = left ventricle. (From Currie, P.J., Seward, J.B., Reeder, G.S., et al.: Continuous-wave Doppler echocardiographic assessment of severity of calcific aortic stenosis: A simultaneous Doppler-catheter study in 100 adult patients. Circulation 71:1162, 1985, with permission of the American Heart Association, Inc.)

cardiac catheterization studies of aortic valve gradients in animals[39, 40] and in humans.[33] They have demonstrated extremely high correlation between maximal instantaneous gradients measured by Doppler echocardiography and those measured by dual catheters in the left ventricle and left aorta. The correlation of mean gradient measurements made by catheterization and by Doppler echocardiography in simultaneous studies has also been extremely high[33] (Fig. 30–3). The hemodynamic severity of aortic valve stenosis as assessed by measurement of catheter pressure gradient is typically expressed as peak-to-peak or mean gradient. The most useful expression for the severity of aortic stenosis by Doppler echocardiography is provided by the mean gradient, because it is directly comparable to the mean gradient estimated by catheterization.

Pressure gradient determination by either Doppler echocardiography or cardiac catheterization provides only partial assessment of the severity of aortic stenosis because of the flow dependence of gradient determinations.[41] Simultaneous Doppler echocardiographic and dual catheter studies have shown that pressure gradient data alone correctly classify the hemodynamic severity of aortic stenosis in fewer than 50 percent of patients, compared with estimates of aortic valve area.[31] It is therefore prudent to determine valve area in all patients with aortic stenosis.

The preferred method for the Doppler echocardiographic determination of aortic valve area is provided by the continuity equation. Although aortic valve area may be determined by the Gorlin formula from data obtained by Doppler echocardiography,[42] the advantages of the continuity equation are that it is completely noninvasive and that it requires only two Doppler echocardiographic velocity measurements. The method is based on the hydraulic principle that laminar flow through a conduit is equal to the mean velocity multiplied by the cross-sectional orifice dimension. At constant flow, the ratio of cross-sectional areas at two different sites is inversely proportional to the ratio of the respective mean velocity at those sites. This relation is expressed by the equation:

$$A_1 \times V_1 = A_2 \times V_2$$

where A_1 is the cross-sectional area of the left ventricular outflow tract, A_2 is the cross-sectional area of the stenotic valve, V_2 is the mean velocity of the obstruction jet, and V_1 is the mean velocity proximal to the obstruction. If the mean velocity at the stenotic valve and the flow are known, the stenotic area can be derived as flow divided by mean velocity of the stenotic jet. Rearrangement of the continuity equation yields the aortic valve area:

$$A_2 = A_1 \times (V_1 \div V_2)$$

In practice, A_1 is determined by two-dimensional echocardiography, and V_1 and V_2 are measured by pulsed and continuous-wave Doppler echocardiography, respectively (Fig. 30–4). If the aortic outflow jet is eccentric, color flow imaging may improve the accuracy of the continuous-wave method for measurement of the aortic velocity by guiding the placement of the continuous-wave ultrasound beam.[43]

Using this method, investigators have consistently demonstrated the accuracy of Doppler echocardiography for the estimation of aortic valve area in adults with aortic stenosis, compared with measurement of aortic valve area by cardiac catheterization using the Gorlin formula[31, 44–47] (Fig. 30–5). For patients in whom it is not possible to reliably measure the left ventricular outflow tract diameter or velocity, the investigator should use, in the absence of mitral regurgitation, the mitral annulus diameter and velocity for calculation of aortic valve area. Another highly sensitive index for the detection of severe aortic stenosis is provided by the ratio of V_1 to V_2. Severe aortic stenosis has been demonstrated to be present in 92 percent of patients in whom V_1/V_2 is less than 0.25.[31] This index is independent of cardiac output and therefore may be used for serial evaluations.

Invasive and Doppler echocardiographic estimates of aortic valve area may yield discordant data.[2, 3] Pitfalls that may contribute to potential discrepancies are associated with either method. Invasive estimates of aortic valve area require precise and accurate measurement of cardiac output by either the Fick or the indicator dilution technique, each of which is subject to considerable error.[48–51] Furthermore, cardiac output may vary substantially during a single invasive procedure, with alterations in sympathetic tone and loading conditions confounding the estimate of valve area because of beat-to-beat variations in cardiac output and gradient, which are not simultaneously measured. In addition, the hydraulic constants of the Gorlin formula[52] are not truly constant, particularly in low-flow states, in which error in estimates of aortic valve area may exceed 50 percent.[53, 54] Finally, the presence of associated more-than-mild aortic regurgitation may cause overestimation of the severity of aortic stenosis.[41]

Advantages of the continuity equation and Doppler echocardiography for estimation of aortic valve area are that the continuity equation does not incorporate any hydraulic constants and that aortic valve area estimates are not affected by aortic regurgitation. However, there are also practical and theoretic limitations to the Doppler echocardiographic method. The measurement of aortic valve gradient depends on the Doppler beam being parallel to blood flow. A small, nonimaging transducer with multiple angulations from various positions is required to obtain peak aortic velocity (Fig. 30–6). Small errors in the measurement of left ventricular outflow tract diameter cause relatively large errors in estimation of aortic valve area, because the diameter is squared in the calculation of area for use in the continuity equation.

Other potential problems are related to assumptions made in the application of the modified Bernoulli equation. Energy loss across the stenosis, pressure recovery distal to the stenosis, acceleration of blood flow, and the velocity of blood flow proximal to the stenosis (V_1) are factors that are neglected when the modified Bernoulli equation is applied. However, neglect of these factors may cause overestimation of the gradient in severe stenosis. In high-output states (e.g., anemia, significant aortic regurgitation), the outflow velocity (V_1) may reach 1.5 to 2.0 m per second, and this should be included in the Bernoulli equation in order to avoid overestimation of gradient.[55] Nevertheless, the performance of the Doppler echocardiographic examination by experienced, well-trained echocardiographers yields reliable hemodynamic data.

Role of Echocardiography in Clinical Decision-Making in Aortic Stenosis

In patients in whom two-dimensional and Doppler echocardiography has established the cause and hemodynamic severity of aortic valvular stenosis, cardiac catheterization for determination of the transvalvular gradient and valve orifice area adds little information to aid clinical decision-making. The authors believe that use of Doppler echocardiography makes cardiac catheterization unnecessary for evaluation of aortic stenosis in those patients. In patients with low cardiac output, it may be difficult to assess the severity of aortic valve stenosis, because both transvalvular gradient and estimated aortic valve area may be low and neither parameter may reflect the intrinsic degree of stenosis. In this setting, dobutamine echocardiography may augment the transvalvular gradient while the aortic valve area remains fixed in patients in whom aortic stenosis is significant.

In the asymptomatic patient with hemodynamically significant aortic stenosis, serial examination is extremely useful for assessment of progression of stenosis.[56] Furthermore, serial assessment by combined two-dimensional and Doppler echocardiography poses no risk to the patient. Echocardiographic evaluation may assist the surgeon by identification of subaortic hypertrophy that requires myectomy and by assessment of aortic root dimension, which may limit the size of the prosthesis used for valve replacement. Preoperative catheterization is indicated only for evaluation of coronary disease or for resolution of discordant clinical and Doppler echocardiographic data. At the authors' institution, the necessity of preoperative invasive hemodynamic investigation (measurement of

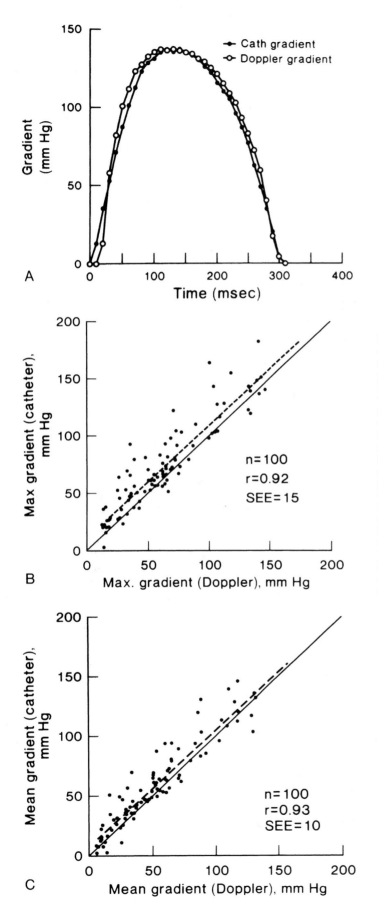

FIGURE 30–3. Validation of maximal instantaneous and mean gradients as estimated by Doppler echocardiography in aortic stenosis with simultaneous catheterization. *A,* Transvalvular instantaneous pressure gradients in experimental aortic stenosis determined at 10-msec intervals throughout systole by simultaneous dual catheters in left ventricle and aorta and by continuous-wave Doppler echocardiography. *B,* Correlation of maximal pressure gradients determined by simultaneous Doppler echocardiographic and catheter measurements in 100 consecutive adult patients. The regression equation is as follows: catheter gradient = 10.3 + 0.97 × Doppler gradient. The dashed line represents the regression line, and the solid line is the line of identity. SEE = standard error of estimation. *C,* Correlation between mean gradients across a stenotic aortic valve derived from Doppler echocardiographic catheter measurements in 100 patients. The mean SEE (estimation of catheter mean gradient from Doppler-derived mean gradient) was 10 mm Hg. (*A* from Callahan, M.J., Tajik, A.J., Su-Fan, Q., et al.: Validation of instantaneous pressure gradients measured by continuous-wave Doppler in experimentally induced aortic stenosis. Am. J. Cardiol. 56:989, 1985. Copyright 1985 by Excerpta Medica Inc. *B and C* from Currie, P.J., Seward, J.B., Reeder, G.S., et al.: Continuous-wave Doppler echocardiographic assessment of severity of calcific aortic stenosis: A simultaneous Doppler-catheter study in 100 adult patients. Circulation 71:1162, 1985, with permission of the American Heart Association, Inc.)

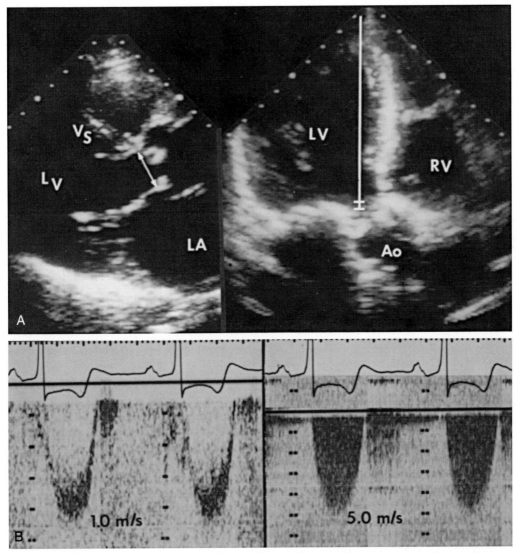

FIGURE 30–4. Determination of aortic valve area by use of the continuity equation. *A, Left,* Parasternal long-axis view of heart in systole. Diameter (d) of the left ventricular outflow tract is measured *(double-headed arrow).* Cross-sectional area of left ventricular outflow tract of the continuity equation is then calculated by the formula, $A = \pi(d/2)^2$. *Right,* Left ventricular outflow velocity (V_1 in the continuity equation) is measured by pulsed-wave Doppler echocardiography with the sample volume in the subvalvular area from an apical position. Ao = aorta; LA = left atrium; LV = left ventricle; RV = right ventricle; VS = ventricular septum. *B,* Velocity profiles of the left ventricular outflow tract *(left)* and aorta *(right)* measured by Doppler echocardiography in a patient with aortic stenosis. (From Olson, L.J., Edwards, W.D., and Tajik, A.J.: Aortic valve stenosis: Etiology, pathophysiology, evaluation, and management. Curr. Probl. Cardiol. 12:455, 1987, with permission of the Mayo Foundation.)

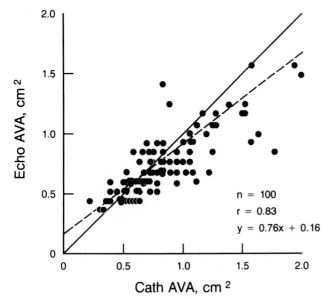

FIGURE 30–5. Correlation between calculations of aortic valve area derived from catheter (Cath AVA) and from Doppler echocardiography (Echo AVA) measurements in 100 patients. Mean standard error of estimation was 0.19 cm². (From Oh, J.K., Taliercio, C.P., Holmes, D.R., Jr., et al.: Prediction of the severity of aortic stenosis by Doppler aortic valve area determination: Prospective Doppler-catheterization correlation in 100 patients. J. Am. Coll. Cardiol. 11:1227, 1988, with permission of the American College of Cardiology.)

gradient and valve area) has been reduced from more than 95 percent of cases in 1984 to 28 percent of cases in 1993.

Aortic Regurgitation

Aortic regurgitation is classified as either acquired or congenital; it is caused by disease of the valve or of the aortic root, or both.[57–59a] Regurgitation is subclassified as acute or chronic, each form with characteristic two-dimensional, M-mode, and Doppler echocardiographic findings. Two-dimensional echocardiography identifies the anatomic abnormality underlying regurgitation and therefore forms the basis of diagnostic classification.

Rheumatic disease of the aortic valve produces leaflet thickening, fibrosis, and retraction and often causes combined regurgitation and stenosis.[59, 60] Leaflet calcification is prominent if stenosis is present.[60] Characteristic echocardiographic features when stenosis is present include leaflet thickening and calcification, reduced leaflet excursion, and leaflet doming, best demonstrated in the parasternal long-axis view. Incomplete diastolic leaflet coaptation may be demonstrated in the parasternal short-axis view, especially with the aid of color flow imaging.

Infectious endocarditis may cause aortic valve regurgitation owing to the presence of vegetations that prevent proper leaflet coaptation or damage to the leaflets that produces perforation or dehiscence. Combined two-dimensional and color flow imaging is used to characterize anatomic abnormalities from the parasternal long-axis and short-axis views. Valvular vegetations less than 3 mm in diameter frequently are not identified by transthoracic two-dimensional echocardiography, especially if there is thickening of the valve leaflets. Transesophageal echocardiography aids in the detection of vegetations because of high image resolution, and, in combination with color flow imaging, it is useful for localization of the regurgitant jet to the valvular orifice or perivalvular region.[61, 62] Transesophageal echocardiography may also demonstrate perivalvular abscess.[63] Less common causes of acquired aortic valvular regurgitation identified by two-dimensional echocardiography are spontaneous dehiscence of an aortic valve leaflet,[64] diastolic leaflet prolapse,[65] and ankylosing spondylitis, which is recognized by aortic root dilatation and characteristic nodules in the vicinity of the aortic-mitral junction with associated leaflet fibrosis and retraction.[66–68]

Enlargement of the aortic root is frequently associated with aortic regurgitation, regardless of cause. Aortic root dilatation may be primary and cause regurgitation, or it may be acquired as a consequence of increased total flow. In chronic aortic regurgitation, idiopathic dilatation of the aortic root is the leading indication for surgical replacement of the aortic valve at the Mayo Clinic.[59] The anatomy of the root and ascending aorta, best evaluated from

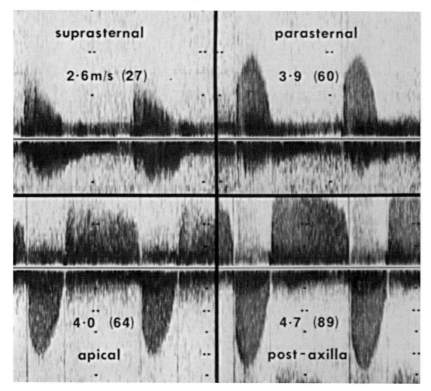

FIGURE 30–6. Underestimation of aortic valve gradient by Doppler echocardiography, illustrated with signals from one patient with aortic stenosis. Maximal velocity varies with position of transducer. The examiner must systematically search for the anatomic window that yields the highest maximal instantaneous velocity. Velocity is given in meters per second (m/sec); instantaneous gradients (mm Hg) determined by Doppler echocardiography are shown in parentheses. (From Olson, L.J., Edwards, W.D., and Tajik, A.J.: Aortic valve stenosis: Etiology, pathophysiology, evaluation, and management. Curr. Probl. Cardiol. 12:455, 1987, with permission of the Mayo Foundation.)

the parasternal long-axis and short-axis views, should be studied systematically in all patients undergoing two-dimensional echocardiography.[69] Careful inspection of the root, ascending aorta, arch, and descending thoracic aorta should be performed in all patients with aortic regurgitation.

Acquired aortic root dilatation causing regurgitation may result from idiopathic dilatation of the annulus and root, with subsequent inadequate aortic valve leaflet coaptation in diastole,[70, 71] disruption of the aortic valve apparatus from aortic dissection,[72] or rupture of a sinus of Valsalva aneurysm.[65] Two-dimensional echocardiography suggests aortic dissection in the presence of aortic dilatation and an associated intraluminal linear echo, which represents the intimal flap separating the true from the false lumen[73] (Fig. 30–7). Typically, the flap moves in unison with the remnant of the aortic wall, and color flow imaging demonstrates flow in the false lumen.[73] Retrograde dissection may disrupt the aortic valve apparatus to produce flail aortic leaflets easily identified by two-dimensional

echocardiography. Dilatation of an aortic sinus associated with a sinus of Valsalva aneurysm may cause prolapse of an aortic leaflet and associated aortic regurgitation, identified echocardiographically by the characteristic appearance of the dilated sinus and diastolic leaflet prolapse.[74]

Congenital disease of the aortic valve or root may produce aortic regurgitation in the young or middle-aged adult. The prevalence of the congenital bicuspid aortic valve is 1 to 2 percent, and it frequently becomes stenotic, regurgitant, or involved by endocarditis.[59, 60, 71, 75] Its characteristic appearance is identified with high sensitivity from the parasternal short-axis view. Similarly, the rare quadricuspid aortic valve may be identified from the parasternal short-axis view and is also frequently associated with aortic regurgitation.[76] Other congenital disorders associated with aneurysms or dilatation of the aortic root and secondary aortic regurgitation are Marfan syndrome,[77] Ehlers-Danlos syndrome,[78] and coarctation of the aorta.[79] In the adult with Marfan syndrome, the aortic root may

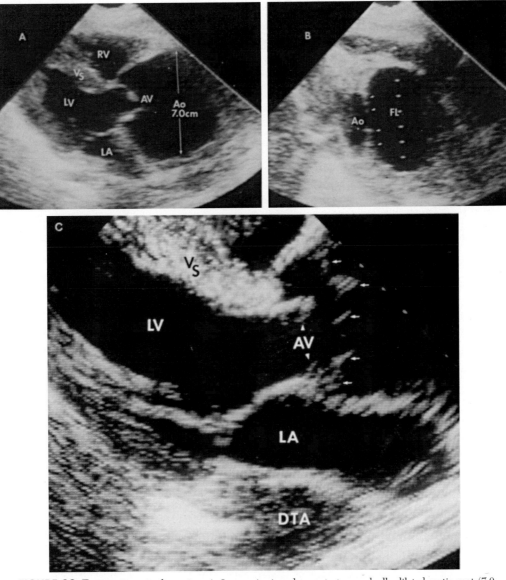

FIGURE 30–7. Type I aortic dissection. *A*, Long-axis view demonstrates markedly dilated aortic root (7.0 cm). *B*, Short-axis view shows intimal flap *(arrowheads)* separating false lumen (FL) from true lumen (Ao). *C*, Systolic frame from another patient. Parasternal long-axis view shows intimal flap *(arrows)* immediately above the aortic valve (AV) in markedly dilated aortic root. DTA = descending thoracic aorta; LA = left atrium; LV = left ventricle; RV = right ventricle; VS = ventricular septum. (From Khandheria, B.K., Tajik, A.J., Taylor, C.L., et al.: Aortic dissection: Review of value and limitations of two-dimensional echocardiography in a six-year experience. J. Am. Soc. Echocardiogr. 2:17, 1989, with permission of the American Society of Echocardiography.)

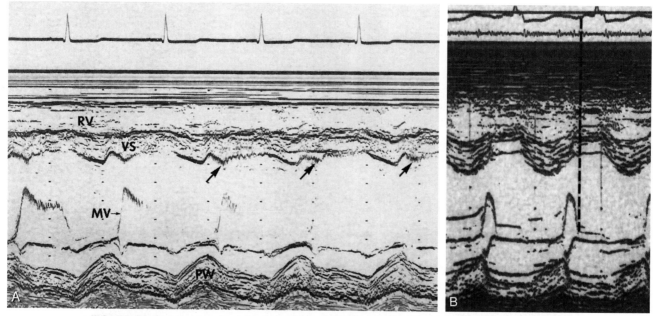

FIGURE 30–8. M-mode echocardiographic features of chronic (*A*) and acute (*B*) aortic regurgitation. *A*, Indirect features of aortic regurgitation include diastolic flutter of mitral valve (MV) and ventricular septum (VS) (*arrows*) and enlarged left ventricle. PW = posterior wall; RV = right ventricle. *B*, Mitral valve closure before onset of QRS complex (*interrupted vertical line*) indicates premature closure of mitral valve, characteristic of acute, severe aortic regurgitation. (*B* from Shub, C.: The role of echocardiography in clinical practice. In Spittell, J.A., Jr. [ed.]: Clinical Medicine. Vol. 6. Philadelphia, Harper & Row, 1982, p. 1, with permission.)

be massively dilated, and the wall appears thin. Dilatation also involves the annulus, sinuses of Valsalva, and aorta. The aortic leaflets are enlarged and yet are often unable to occlude the aortic valve orifice. The dilated root also frequently causes compression of the left atrium, which appears small from the parasternal long-axis view. Mitral valve prolapse is also frequently seen in patients with Marfan syndrome.[80]

In chronic aortic regurgitation, characteristic two-dimensional and M-mode echocardiographic findings are left ventricular volume overload[81, 82] and diastolic fluttering of the anterior leaflet of the mitral valve and interventricular septum.[83–85] In acute severe aortic regurgitation, premature closure of the mitral valve may be observed on M-mode echocardiography; left ventricular cavity size is typically normal or mildly enlarged, and function is normal or hyperdynamic[86] (Fig. 30–8). Echocardiography has proved useful for the serial evaluation of the patient with known aortic regurgitation, for monitoring of left ventricular size and function, and for decision-making about the timing of surgical intervention.[87–96] Although useful for the serial assessment of left ventricular size and systolic function in the patient with known chronic aortic regurgitation, echocardiography has not proved consistently reliable in either the detection or the assessment of the severity of aortic regurgitation, because the findings are nonspecific and are indirectly related to the hemodynamic abnormality. For the direct detection and assessment of severity of aortic regurgitation, Doppler echocardiography is necessary.

Doppler Echocardiography in Aortic Regurgitation

In aortic regurgitation, diastolic reverse flow occurs in the left ventricular outflow tract with a primary velocity vector opposite to normal systolic outflow. Typically, it is holodiastolic and of high velocity, corresponding to the large diastolic pressure gradient between the aorta and the left ventricle. For the detection of aortic regurgitation, pulsed-wave Doppler echocardiography has been shown to be more than 95 percent sensitive and 96 percent specific compared with aortography.[97–99] Continuous-wave and color flow Doppler echocardiography are similarly sensitive.[100, 101] The absence of diastolic regurgitation demonstrated by Doppler echocardiogra-

phy has been reported to be 99 to 100 percent specific for the absence of aortic regurgitation, compared with aortography.[98] Therefore, a discrepancy between Doppler echocardiographic findings and auscultatory evidence of aortic regurgitation by physical diagnosis should be attributed to the limitations of auscultation.

Assessment of the severity of aortic regurgitation may be accomplished by semiquantitative Doppler echocardiographic methods, including demonstration of aortic flow reversal, and by color flow imaging. Determinations of the severity of aortic regurgitation based on pulsed-wave signal depth alone often underestimate the three-dimensional distribution of regurgitant flow and, consequently, the severity of the hemodynamic abnormality.[102, 103]

Detection of thoracic aortic flow reversal by pulsed-wave Doppler echocardiography has been proposed as a semiquantitative method for the assessment of the severity of aortic regurgitation (Fig. 30–9). Quinones and associates showed that if the area of the reverse thoracic aortic flow profile was greater than 30 percent of that of the forward flow profile, pulsed-wave Doppler echocardiography reliably differentiated mild from moderate aortic regurgitation in patients with aortic regurgitation proved by aortography.[104] In a separate study, the detection of reverse flow in the abdominal aorta was observed to correlate well with severe aortic regurgitation demonstrated at aortography, although the number of patients in the study was small.[105] Flow reversal in the descending aorta may also be demonstrated by color flow imaging from the suprasternal notch. The region of brightest color or any region of aliasing may be used to guide the placement of the pulsed-wave Doppler echocardiographic sample volume for recording of flow velocities (Fig. 30–10). The abdominal aorta or iliac and femoral arteries may be examined in similar fashion if the suprasternal window is inadequate. Color M-mode aids in the timing of the regurgitant signal and demonstrates that it is pandiastolic.

FIGURE 30–10. See Color Plate 4.

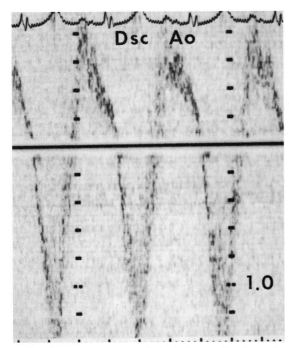

FIGURE 30–9. Velocity profiles of blood flow in the descending aorta (Dsc Ao) in a patient with severe aortic regurgitation. Flow profile above baseline occurs in diastole and represents regurgitant flow, which in this patient is holodiastolic. Flow profile below baseline is systolic and represents forward flow.

Semiquantitative estimation of the severity of aortic regurgitation by color flow imaging is based on the spatial extent of detected regurgitation (Fig. 30–11). Orthogonal imaging planes are used to characterize the severity of regurgitation in both parasternal long- and parasternal short-axis views. Regurgitant flow appears as a jet of mosaic turbulent signals extending from the left ventricular outflow tract into the ventricular cavity during diastole. In clinical practice, measures of the color jet used to estimate severity have included maximal width, area, and length. However, experimental studies comparing known regurgitant volumes with maximal width, area, and length have demonstrated poor correlation. The discrepancies observed in the experimental setting have been attributed to the dependence of the spatial extent of the regurgitant jet on velocity rather than on volume.[103] However, the proximal minimal width of the color jet in the parasternal long-axis view or of the area in the left ventricular outflow tract has been demonstrated to correlate well with quantitative measures of regurgitant volume; this correlation has been attributed to the relation of the proximal width of the color jet to the regurgitant orifice area. Although the minimal proximal width and area of the regurgitant color jet are not direct measures of the volume of regurgitation, correlation with semiquantitative estimates of severity by aortography has also been excellent. Perry and associates, using a ratio of the minimal proximal regurgitant jet width divided by left ventricular outflow width in the parasternal long-axis view, described four grades of aortic regurgitation by color flow imaging. Grade I corresponded to a ratio of less than 0.25; grade II, from 0.25 to 0.46; grade III, from 0.47 to 0.64; and grade IV, 0.65 or greater. By this method, they correctly classified the severity of aortic regurgitation in more than 90 percent of patients, using aortography as the standard.[102]

FIGURE 30–11. See Color Plate 5.

Potential limitations of color flow imaging include variation of the spatial extent of the color jet with transducer frequency, gain

setting, and pulse repetition frequency as well as physiologic factors not directly related to the severity of regurgitation that may affect the dimension of the regurgitant jet, including the driving pressure of the aorta, compliance of the left ventricle, the duration of diastole, and left ventricular end-diastolic pressure.[102] Furthermore, color flow Doppler echocardiography is highly operator-dependent. Small alterations in transducer angulation may substantially influence the dimensions of the regurgitant jet. The dimension of the regurgitant jet must be maximized to avoid underestimation of the severity of the hemodynamic abnormality. Despite these limitations, the semiquantitative estimate of the severity of aortic regurgitation by color flow imaging is widely accepted and used because of its excellent correlation with semiquantitative estimates by aortography. However, it is prudent to use color flow imaging in conjunction with other echocardiographic variables for assessment of the severity of the hemodynamic abnormality.

Continuous-wave Doppler echocardiography is used to measure the velocity of regurgitant blood flow throughout diastole. According to the principles of Bernoulli hydrodynamics, the pressure gradient across a restricting orifice is proportional to the square of the velocity gradient. Therefore, the deceleration slope of the aortic regurgitant signal detected by continuous-wave Doppler echocardiography is a measure of the rate of pressure decay between the aorta and the left ventricle, which reflects the severity of regurgitation in the absence of left ventricular dysfunction or rapid peripheral runoff. In mild aortic regurgitation, aortic diastolic pressure declines slowly, left ventricular pressure rises slowly, and a large pressure gradient persists at end-diastole; accordingly, the Doppler echocardiographic profile of aortic regurgitant velocity also decays slowly. In contrast, in severe aortic regurgitation, there is a rapid decrease in the pressure gradient between the aorta and left ventricle, corresponding to a rapid collapse of aortic diastolic pressure and a simultaneous rapid rise in left ventricular diastolic pressure, manifested by a rapid fall in aortic regurgitant velocity by Doppler echocardiography (Fig. 30–12).

The rate of pressure decline has been demonstrated to be directly related to the severity of regurgitation by measurement of the deceleration slope[106, 107] or derivation of the pressure half-time[108] from the continuous-wave Doppler echocardiographic signal. Generally, a diastolic velocity decay slope of greater than 3 m/sec² is indicative of severe aortic regurgitation. The pressure half-

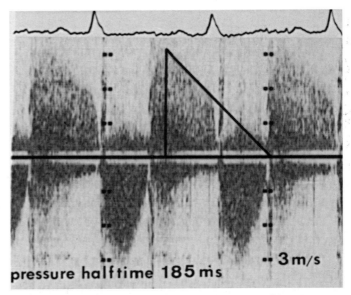

FIGURE 30–12. Severe aortic regurgitation demonstrated by continuous-wave echocardiography. Signals are obtained from the apical window so that regurgitant flow is directed toward the transducer and is displayed above baseline. The slope of deceleration is indicated by solid line. Deceleration rate exceeds 3 m/sec², and pressure half-time is less than 300 msec; each value is consistent with severe aortic regurgitation.

time method was originally described with use of invasive techniques[111]; the use of Doppler echocardiography to derive the pressure half-time has been clinically validated by simultaneous Doppler echocardiography and catheterization studies.[112] Pressure half-time measurements correlate well with the severity of aortic regurgitation as assessed by semiquantitative invasive methods (Fig. 30–13). A pressure half-time of less than 350 msec is usually indicative of severe regurgitation.[110] The method appears to be independent of heart rate, pulse pressure, left ventricular ejection fraction, and the incident angle between the Doppler beam and the regurgitant jet.[110] Potential limitations of the analysis of the continuous-wave profile of regurgitation include acquisition of an analyzable signal, which may not be possible in approximately 10 percent of patients, and increased left ventricular end-diastolic pressure, which may cause overestimation of the severity of aortic regurgitation because of more rapid equalization of aortic and left ventricular diastolic pressures.

Quantitative methods for the assessment of the severity of aortic regurgitation include analysis of the continuous-wave Doppler echocardiographic profile of regurgitation and measurement of regurgitant fraction and regurgitant volume. Doppler echocardiographic methods for the evaluation of regurgitant orifice area have also been described. Quantitative assessment of the severity of aortic regurgitation is possible by the use of combined two-dimensional and Doppler echocardiography for the measurement of either regurgitant fraction, regurgitant volume, or regurgitant orifice dimension.[109, 110]

Calculation of regurgitant fraction or regurgitant volume requires estimation of total stroke volume and forward stroke volume. The difference between the two measurements represents regurgitant stroke volume, and regurgitant fraction is found by dividing the regurgitant stroke volume by the total stroke volume. The total stroke volume is obtained by multiplying the two-dimensional echocardiographic measurement of the left ventricular outflow tract area by the time-velocity integral of left ventricular outflow measured by pulsed-wave Doppler echocardiography; forward stroke volume is similarly measured by evaluation of a second, nondiseased valve. In practice, forward stroke volume is estimated by two-dimensional echocardiographic measurement of the mitral annulus and multiplied by the time-velocity integral of velocity at the annulus measured by pulsed-wave Doppler echocardiography. Limitations of the echocardiographic determination of regurgitant fraction or regurgitant volume include cardiac cycle–dependent variation in annular cross-sectional area, coexistent disease affecting other valves, and intracardiac or extracardiac shunt.[113] Effective regurgitant orifice area may be estimated by dividing regurgitant volume by the regurgitant time-velocity integral. This method is feasible in almost all patients and provides another index of regurgitation severity that correlates well with semiquantitative methods of grading regurgitation, including jet area by color flow imaging, and with invasively determined angiographic grading.[106]

Although echocardiographic methods for the estimation of regurgitant fraction and regurgitant volume have correlated well with invasive techniques, the invasive quantitative methods are not used routinely in clinical practice. This may be attributed to the technical limitations and potential sources of measurement error, including catheter position, volume and rate of injection of contrast medium, left ventricular size, volume of forward flow, ventricular ectopic activity, and the effects of variation in peripheral arterial pressure.[114–117] The chief limitation of the clinical implementation of noninvasive estimates of regurgitant fraction or regurgitant volume has been lack of familiarity with the method in clinical practice, with technical challenges and a definite learning curve for each laboratory. The authors believe that these quantitative measures of the severity of regurgitation will gain acceptance in the routine clinical decision-making process.

Role of Echocardiography in Clinical Decision-Making in Aortic Regurgitation

Doppler echocardiographic information is used in conjunction with M-mode and two-dimensional echocardiographic data for the detection and assessment of the cause and severity of aortic regurgitation. Serial combined M-mode and two-dimensional echocardiography can provide the quantitative assessments of aortic root and left ventricular cavity dimensions and systolic function that are necessary for decisions on the timing of surgery.[84, 88, 89, 91, 93–95]

Doppler echocardiography enables semiquantitative or quantitative assessment of the severity of aortic regurgitation. The availability of several methods makes assessment of the hemodynamic severity of aortic regurgitation possible in virtually all patients. The estimate of the severity of regurgitation may be presumed to be accurate if different methods provide concordant results. As with the evaluation of patients with aortic valvular stenosis, cardiac catheterization for determination of severity of aortic regurgitation adds little to influence clinical decision-making. Transesophageal echocardiography or aortography is indicated for complete preoperative evaluation of patients in whom resection or repair of the aortic root is contemplated. Preoperative coronary angiography is indicated in patients in whom there may be underlying coronary artery disease and aortography in patients in whom echocardiographic data are not optimal.

Mitral Stenosis

Mitral stenosis is characterized by a reduced mitral orifice dimension with associated impairment of left ventricular filling.

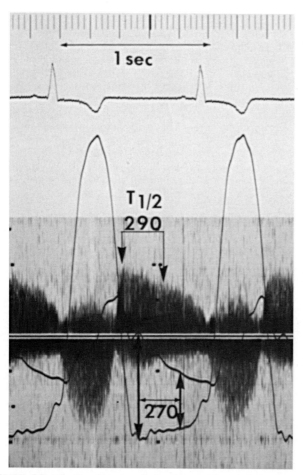

FIGURE 30–13. Simultaneous dual-catheter and Doppler echocardiographic tracings from a patient with aortic regurgitation, illustrating the correlation between diastolic half-times measured by Doppler echocardiography (290 msec) and those measured by catheterization (270 msec). (From Nishimura, R.A., and Tajik, A.J.: Determination of left-sided pressure gradients by utilizing Doppler aortic and mitral regurgitation signals: Validation by simultaneous dual-catheter and Doppler studies. J. Am. Coll. Cardiol. 11:317, 1988, with permission of the American College of Cardiology.)

Rheumatic disease remains the most common cause despite the declining incidence of rheumatic fever in Western nations.[118-120]

Rare causes of valvular obstruction include congenital mitral stenosis and the parachute mitral valve. Other unusual causes of obstruction to left ventricular filling not affecting the mitral valve and easily recognized by two-dimensional echocardiography include tumors, thrombi, dense mitral annulus calcification, cor triatriatum, and supravalvular rings.[121-123]

The echocardiographic features of rheumatic mitral stenosis are best appreciated from the parasternal long-axis and short-axis views and include thickened and deformed leaflets with fusion of the commissures and subvalvular apparatus. Frequently, there is associated calcification of the valvular and subvalvular apparatus.[119, 120, 124, 125] Characteristic motion abnormalities are reduced leaflet excursion in diastole with doming and the so-called hockey-stick deformity of the anterior leaflet, caused by tethering by the subvalvular apparatus (Fig. 30–14). The posterior leaflet is frequently immobile or severely restricted in its motion.

Congenital mitral stenosis is characterized by thickened and fibrotic mitral valve leaflets with fused or absent commissures and fibrotic and shortened chordae and papillary muscles.[126] In contrast to acquired rheumatic mitral stenosis, calcification of the mitral apparatus is not typically seen. Motion abnormalities of the leaflets of the mitral valve are similar to those observed in patients with rheumatic disease. A second form of congenital mitral stenosis is the parachute mitral valve, in which there is a single, large papillary muscle with normal chordae and valve leaflets. The convergence of the chordae to insert on a single papillary muscle may produce obstruction at the subvalvular level.[126-128]

Associated morphologic abnormalities frequently observed by two-dimensional echocardiography in the patient with chronic obstruction to left ventricular filling are left atrial and right heart enlargement. Coexistent left atrial thrombus is not an uncommon finding in the patient with long-standing mitral stenosis, especially in the presence of chronic atrial fibrillation. However, thrombus in the left atrial appendage frequently cannot be demonstrated by transthoracic two-dimensional echocardiography. Transesophageal echocardiography should be performed in patients in whom left atrial thrombus is suspected, especially if transseptal catheterization is anticipated.

Assessment of the hemodynamic severity of mitral valvular stenosis by two-dimensional echocardiography may be performed by direct measurement of the mitral orifice area from the parasternal short-axis view (see Fig. 30–14). The accuracy of the two-dimensional echocardiographic method for the assessment of mitral valve area has been validated by comparison with data obtained at surgery,[129, 130] at pathologic examination,[131] and at cardiac catheterization.[129, 131, 132] The smallest orifice is detected by slow, methodical scanning superiorly to inferiorly, and a reproducible estimate of mitral valve area is possible in 85 to 90 percent of patients. In the remainder of patients, assessment of mitral valve area is either not possible or unreliable because of suboptimal images, dense calcification, prior commissurotomy,[133] or predominant subvalvular obstruction. Whenever possible, estimations of mitral valve area by two-dimensional and Doppler echocardiographic methods should be correlated.

Two-dimensional echocardiography has been used for the identification of patients who may benefit from mitral balloon valvuloplasty. A scoring system based on two-dimensional echocardiographic criteria has been proposed to characterize the suitability of the valve for valvuloplasty.[134] The system assigns a score of grades 1 through 4 to each of four two-dimensional echocardiographic characteristics: valve mobility, valve thickness, valve calcification, and subvalvular thickening. Patients with a total score of 8 or less have a greater than 90 percent chance of a satisfactory result. The most important factors in predicting the initial success and long-term outcome of valvuloplasty are the severity of calcification and subvalvular fibrosis.[134] Evidence of left atrial thrombus is a contrain-

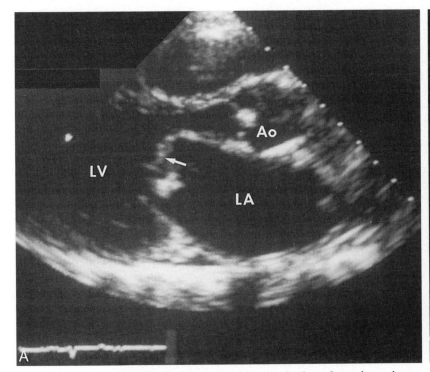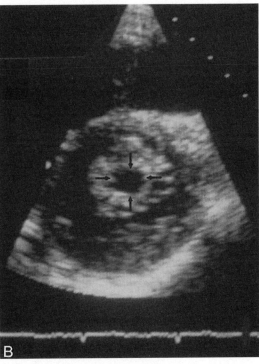

FIGURE 30–14. *A,* Two-dimensional echocardiographic evaluation of rheumatic mitral stenosis. Parasternal long-axis view demonstrates typical appearance of stenotic mitral valve. The anterior leaflet of the mitral valve *(arrow)* has a doming configuration (also referred to as a "hockey-stick" appearance) in diastole. Full excursion of valve leaflet is prevented by tethering effect of subvalvular apparatus. The posterior leaflet is immobile. The left atrium (LA) is enlarged. Ao = aorta; LV = left ventricle. *B,* Parasternal short-axis view of stenotic mitral valve. Restriction of opening of anterior and posterior leaflets causes reduced mitral orifice area *(arrows)*. There is minimal calcification of valve leaflets. The mitral orifice area may be measured directly by planimetry from a freeze-frame image on modern equipment.

dication to the procedure. Because two-dimensional echocardiography usually does not visualize the left atrial appendage, transesophageal echocardiography should be performed to exclude thrombus.

Doppler Echocardiography in Mitral Stenosis

Analysis of the mitral valve inflow velocity profile by Doppler echocardiography provides direct hemodynamic assessment of the severity of obstruction to mitral inflow. The optimal Doppler echocardiographic flow profile is obtained from an apical window and, in the absence of valvular disease, demonstrates low-velocity diastolic flow toward the transducer, with a peak velocity of less than 1.3 m/sec.

Impediment to mitral inflow causes an increase in left atrial pressure, thereby increasing the driving pressure from left atrium to ventricle, and also slows emptying of the left atrium. Continuous-wave Doppler echocardiography is used to assess mitral inflow because velocity aliasing occurs with pulsed-wave Doppler echocardiography in moderate-to-severe stenosis. Continuous-wave Doppler echocardiography demonstrates an increased diastolic flow velocity and a reduced rate of velocity decay corresponding directly to the severity of the pressure gradient throughout diastole.[135–138] Color flow imaging is helpful in optimizing the parallel placement of the continuous-wave cursor by identification of the direction of the jet, which may be eccentric.[139]

The left atrial–left ventricular diastolic pressure gradient is obtained from the mitral inflow velocity profile by application of the modified Bernoulli equation. The instantaneous pressure gradient between the left atrium and the left ventricle can be estimated at any point in diastole. As has been the convention by invasive techniques, hemodynamic severity is assessed by estimation of the transvalvular left atrial–left ventricular peak, mean, and end-diastolic gradients. If the gradient is mild to moderate at rest, the authors' practice is to exercise the patient in the supine position and repeat the Doppler echocardiographic examination immediately after exercise. Because the gradient is flow-dependent, it is also always necessary to estimate mitral valve area.

Mitral valve area may be estimated by three different Doppler echocardiographic methods: estimation of the pressure half-time, measurement of valve area by the continuity equation, or estimation of valve area by the proximal flow convergence method. Estimation of the pressure half-time, originally described by invasive methods,[140] has been adapted for the assessment of mitral valve area by Doppler echocardiography. The rate of decline of the diastolic pressure gradient may be described by the pressure half-time, which is the time required for the initial diastolic gradient to decline by 50 percent. Estimation of mitral valve area is based on the observation that, as the degree of stenosis becomes more severe, the diastolic gradient is maintained for a longer period and the pressure half-time is prolonged. On continuous-wave Doppler echocardiographic examination, this effect is manifested as a reduced rate of decline and prolongation of the diastolic flow-velocity profile.

According to the principles of Bernoulli hydrodynamics, the relation between pressure drop and velocity is quadratic. Accordingly, the pressure half-time is obtained from the Doppler velocity profile by dividing peak velocity by the square root of 2 (to identify the point at which pressure has declined to half its peak value) and then measuring the time from peak velocity to the time of peak velocity divided by the square root of 2. The pressure half-time is directly related to mitral valve area: the more prolonged the half-time, the more severe the reduction in orifice area. Hatle and associates[141] derived an empiric constant that relates pressure half-time to mitral valve area (MVA):

$$MVA = 220 \div \text{pressure half-time}$$

$$MVA \ (cm^2) = \frac{220}{\text{pressure halftime (msec.)}} = \frac{220}{220} = 1.0 \ cm^2$$

FIGURE 30–15. Continuous-wave Doppler echocardiography for the hemodynamic evaluation of mitral stenosis. *A*, Estimation of end-diastolic gradient by continuous-wave Doppler echocardiographic evaluation. End-diastolic velocity measured at peak of electrocardiographic R wave equals 2.3 m per second, yielding an end-diastolic pressure gradient between left atrium and left ventricle of 21 mm Hg. *B*, Initial peak velocity (V_0) is 2.5 m per second. Peak velocity divided by the square root of 2 equals approximately 1.8 m per second. The time elapsed between initial peak velocity of 2.5 m per sec, and half-time velocity of 1.8 m per second equals approximately 220 msec. *C*, Calculation of mitral valve area. Diastolic half-time (220 msec) is divided into the empirically derived constant of 220, yielding an estimated valve area of 1 cm². (From Callahan, M.J., Seward, J.B., Tajik, A.J., et al.: Continuous-wave Doppler echocardiographic assessment of mitral stenosis: Case example and technique. Echocardiography 1:102, 1984, with permission of Futura Publishing Company.)

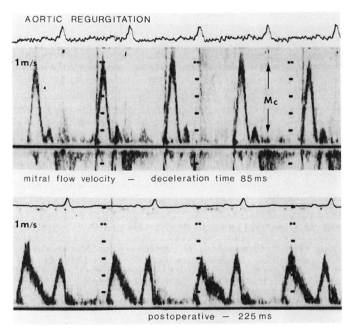

AORTIC REGURGITATION

1m/s

M_c

mitral flow velocity — deceleration time 85 ms

1m/s

postoperative — 225 ms

FIGURE 30–16. Effect of severe aortic regurgitation on the profile of mitral flow velocity obtained by Doppler echocardiography. *Top,* Mitral flow velocity profile in a patient with a normal mitral valve and severe aortic regurgitation. The peak velocity of early mitral inflow is increased, and deceleration time is markedly shortened. Abbreviation of the inflow signal would lead to a shortened half-time estimate and, therefore, overestimate of the mitral valve area. *Bottom,* Same patient after aortic valve replacement. Mitral valve inflow has become normalized.

In normal individuals, pressure half-time is less than 60 msec, whereas it is 100 to 400 msec in patients with mitral stenosis (Fig. 30–15). Mitral valve area determined by the pressure half-time method has been demonstrated to correlate extremely well with mitral valve area determination at cardiac catheterization by the Gorlin formula in patients without other associated valvular disease or coronary artery disease.[141, 142] The pressure half-time method is also independent of heart rate and mitral regurgitation.[143]

Although estimation of mitral valve area by use of the Doppler velocity profile and the pressure half-time method is widely used, it cannot be applied to all patients with mitral stenosis. In patients with a prolonged PR interval, increased velocity from atrial contraction in early diastole makes it impossible to separate the mitral inflow E and A waves, and therefore the pressure half-time cannot be measured. Similar problems are encountered in patients with sinus tachycardia, atrial flutter, and atrial tachycardia.[141] In patients with atrial fibrillation, pressure half-time should be estimated from an average of at least five inflow signals.

Use of the pressure half-time method is also precluded after recent mitral valvuloplasty[144] or if moderate or severe aortic regurgitation is present.[145, 147] In these two situations, estimates of mitral valve area by the half-time method may differ significantly from estimates based on the Gorlin formula. Significant aortic regurgitation is associated with a rapidly rising left ventricular diastolic pressure, which may decrease the transmitral pressure gradient, thereby abbreviating the pressure half-time and causing overestimation of valve area (Fig. 30–16). The discrepancy between valve areas estimated immediately after valvuloplasty by the pressure half-time method and by the Gorlin formula is not entirely explained. Furthermore, it has been demonstrated in experimental models and in patients with mitral stenosis that the pressure half-time depends on chamber stiffness and the peak pressure difference as well as orifice area. Accordingly, in patients with mitral stenosis and coexistent coronary artery disease or aortic valvular stenosis with increased left ventricular stiffness, the pressure half-time method may also overestimate mitral valve area.[148]

The limitations of the pressure half-time method for estimation of mitral valve area may be overcome by use of the continuity equation. The continuity equation may be applied to mitral stenosis to yield valve area estimates that correlate extremely well with Gorlin formula estimates despite coexistent moderate or severe aortic regurgitation.[147] The method assumes that flow volume through the mitral annulus in one cardiac cycle is equal to left ventricular stroke volume. Mitral valve area can be determined as the stroke volume (SV) divided by the time-velocity integral of mitral flow (TVIm):

$$MVA = SV \div TVIm$$

Because stroke volume is the product of the cross-sectional area of the aortic or pulmonary annulus and the time-velocity integral of aortic (TVIa) or pulmonary (TVIp) flow velocity, MVA is equal to the aortic or pulmonary cross-sectional area multiplied by the appropriate time-velocity integral and divided by TVIm. In the presence of significant mitral regurgitation, this method underestimates mitral valve area.

A more recently developed technique for estimation of mitral orifice area, which also relies on the principles of the continuity equation, is the proximal flow convergence method. This method uses color flow imaging to depict a proximal (to the stenotic orifice) isovelocity surface area (PISA) by demonstration of an aliasing interface. Volume flow rate through the orifice is then calculated as the PISA multiplied by the aliasing velocity; for mitral stenosis, an angle correction factor must be applied to account for the restriction imposed by the inlet funnel.[149, 150] This method has been validated clinically by comparison to estimates of mitral valve area by planimetry, by the pressure half-time obtained from the Doppler velocity profile, and by the Gorlin equation.[149, 150] A more complete discussion of the proximal flow convergence method is presented in the section on mitral regurgitation.

In addition to measurement of transvalvular gradients and mitral valve area, complete Doppler echocardiographic evaluation of mitral stenosis requires assessment of pressure in the right side of the heart. Assessment of the pulmonary artery systolic pressure is performed by measurement of the peak tricuspid regurgitant jet velocity by continuous-wave echocardiography and application of the modified Bernoulli equation, which yields the pressure gradient between the right ventricle and the right atrium. The estimated right atrial pressure is added to the measured right ventricular–right atrial gradient to yield right ventricular systolic pressure, which is equivalent to pulmonary artery systolic pressure in the absence of obstruction to right ventricular outflow. Determination of pulmonary artery systolic pressure by this method is possible in approximately 90 percent of patients (see the section on tricuspid regurgitation for details).

Similarly, pulmonary artery end-diastolic pressure may also be estimated by application of the modified Bernoulli equation. Pulmonary regurgitation velocity reflects the diastolic pressure difference between the pulmonary artery and the right ventricle. Pulmonary artery end-diastolic pressure is obtained by adding the right ventricular end-diastolic pressure (which is equal to right atrial pressure) to the gradient between the right ventricle and the pulmonary artery at end-diastole, which is obtained by substituting the measured pulmonary regurgitant end-diastolic velocity into the modified Bernoulli equation. Assessment of right heart pressures should be performed in the resting and postexercise states in patients with mitral stenosis to completely assess the hemodynamic severity of the lesion.[151, 152]

Role of Echocardiography in Clinical Decision-Making in Mitral Stenosis

Combined two-dimensional and Doppler echocardiography is the preferred method for the detection and assessment of severity of mitral stenosis because of proven efficacy and safety. Two-dimensional echocardiography is used for the detection, morphologic characterization, and initial assessment of the hemodynamic severity of obstruction to left ventricular filling. Doppler echocardiography methods are superior to conventional cardiac catheterization in the estimation of the transmitral pressure gradient.[153] Moreover, Doppler echocardiographic methods for estimation of mitral valve area are superior to invasive methods in the presence of mitral or aortic regurgitation. Mitral valve area can be determined by the continuity equation or by the proximal flow convergence method if the pressure half-time method cannot be applied. Serial study enables assessment of the progression of disease. Invasive studies are unnecessary except in the rare patient in whom two-dimensional and Doppler echocardiographic data are unsatisfactory. Cardiac catheterization (coronary angiography) is indicated only in patients who have suspected coronary artery disease.

Mitral Regurgitation

Proper coaptation of the mitral valve leaflets depends on the normal function of the leaflets, chordae tendineae, papillary mus-

cles, and subjacent ventricular myocardium. Dysfunction of any of these components of the mitral valve apparatus may produce mitral regurgitation.[154, 155] Therefore, mitral regurgitation can have many causes.

Structural abnormalities of the valve apparatus are readily identified by two-dimensional echocardiography. The most frequent cause of isolated mitral regurgitation is leaflet prolapse.[118, 146] The prevalence of mitral prolapse, the variability of clinical findings, and the skill required to detect midsystolic clicks or a late systolic murmur have made M-mode and two-dimensional echocardiography extremely important for the detection of mitral prolapse.[146] The two-dimensional echocardiographic diagnosis is based on the demonstration of a systolic arching (billowing) motion of one or both of the valve leaflets above the mitral annulus into the left atrium (Fig. 30–17). However, clinical echocardiographic investigation has demonstrated that M-mode and two-dimensional echocardiography can overdiagnose prolapse. The diagnosis should be limited to patients in whom there is late systolic prolapse by M-mode or two-dimensional echocardiographic evidence of prolapse

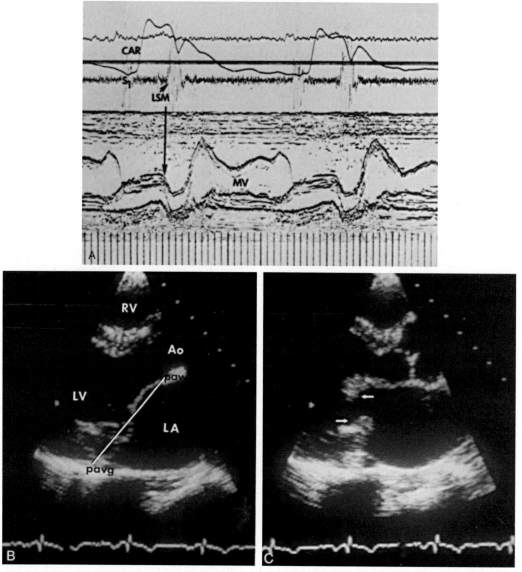

FIGURE 30–17. Mitral valve prolapse. *A*, M-mode echocardiogram demonstrates posterior motion of mitral valve leaflets in late systole. *B*, Two-dimensional echocardiogram from parasternal long-axis view demonstrates prolapse of anterior and posterior mitral valve leaflets into the left atrium (LA) during systole. Prolapse is defined as detection of motion of one or both leaflets superior to an imaginary line drawn between posterior atrioventricular groove (pavg) and posterior aortic wall (paw). Ao = aorta; LV = left ventricle; RV = right ventricle. *C*, Two-dimensional echocardiogram from parasternal long-axis view in diastole demonstrates redundant anterior and posterior leaflets characteristic of mitral valve prolapse *(arrows)*. (*A* from Shub, C.: The role of echocardiography in clinical practice. *In* Spittell, J.A. [ed.]: Clinical Medicine. Vol. 6. Philadelphia, Harper & Row, 1982, p. 18, with permission.)

from the parasternal long-axis view. Two-dimensional echocardiographic evaluation for prolapse from apical views alone is associated with false-positive diagnosis.[156] Prolapse of the valve leaflets is also frequently associated with exaggerated motion of the posterior aspect of the mitral annulus[157, 158] and increased thickness and redundancy of the leaflets.[159, 160]

A great spectrum of anatomic abnormalities is associated with mitral valve prolapse demonstrated by M-mode and two-dimensional echocardiography.[159–162] Routine assessment of severity is based on the magnitude of leaflet prolapse and degree of leaflet thickness.[158, 160] Other patient groups may be identified in whom there is annular and leaflet enlargement.[163] Quantitative assessment of prolapse, leaflet thickness, and leaflet and annular size by combined two-dimensional and M-mode echocardiography has demonstrated that the severity of prolapse is related to subsequent morbid events, including endocarditis, thromboembolism, sudden death, and the need for surgical valve repair or replacement.[159, 160, 163–166] Men and patients older than 45 years appear to be at greatest risk for severe mitral regurgitation.[167]

Chordal rupture is a frequent complication of mitral valve prolapse and may be associated with acute, severe decompensation or chronic progressive regurgitation.[168–173] The most common cause of acute, severe mitral regurgitation is ruptured chordae tendineae; this condition may also be associated with infectious endocarditis, rheumatic disease, myocardial infarction, or trauma, or it may occur in isolation. A ruptured chord is recognized echocardiographically as a highly mobile linear density that may appear to move primarily with the leaflet or subvalvular structures, depending on the site of rupture.[174] It should be sought carefully in all patients with mitral regurgitation associated with exaggerated prolapse or flail segments of the mitral valve. Transesophageal echocardiography establishes the diagnosis when transthoracic echocardiographic findings are indeterminate. Other echocardiographic abnormalities associated with chordal rupture depend on the underlying disease, duration, and hemodynamic severity of mitral regurgitation.

A flail mitral valve leaflet is associated with acute, severe regurgitation caused by disruption of either the chordae tendineae or the papillary muscles. The motion of the flail leaflet is best demonstrated from either the parasternal long-axis or the apical four-chamber view.[175] The motion is exaggerated and not easily missed, because the valve whips between the left ventricular cavity and the left atrium. The portion of the subvalvular apparatus that is affected is usually recognized on transthoracic two-dimensional echocardiographic examination.[175–176] Transesophageal echocardiography is useful in selected cases in which the diagnosis is uncertain.[177]

Papillary muscle dysfunction from any cause may produce mitral regurgitation. Abnormalities of the papillary muscles associated with regurgitation and identified by two-dimensional echocardiography include fibrosis, calcification, dysfunction of the subjacent myocardium, and papillary muscle rupture.[176, 178, 179] Dysfunction of the papillary muscle produces mitral regurgitation because of consequent improper systolic leaflet coaptation.

Infectious endocarditis produces mitral regurgitation by prevention of proper function of the mitral valve apparatus because of damage to the leaflets or subvalvular structures (Fig. 30–18). Complications of infectious endocarditis detected by two-dimensional echocardiography include large vegetations preventing leaflet coaptation, leaflet prolapse, chordal rupture, leaflet perforation, and flail leaflets.[118] The demonstration of vegetations less than 3 mm in diameter is usually not possible.[180] Furthermore, because bacterial endocarditis frequently involves previously diseased valves, it is often impossible to differentiate valvular vegetations from leaflet thickening, calcification, or myxomatous degeneration. Transesophageal echocardiography is useful for identification of small vegetations and characterization of valvular abnormalities, including leaflet perforation, perivalvular abscess, and damage to the subvalvular apparatus.[181]

Mitral annular calcification, a frequent echocardiographic finding in elderly patients, is a degenerative disorder that is often associated with mitral regurgitation. It is recognized echocardiographi-

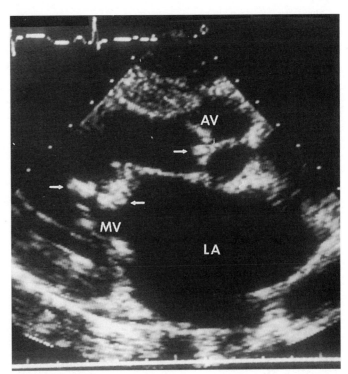

FIGURE 30–18. Parasternal long-axis view in diastole of mitral and aortic valvular vegetations (*arrows*) from a patient with bacterial endocarditis. AV = aortic valve; LA = left atrium; MV = mitral valve.

cally by the presence of dense echoes in the region of the annulus. It may be mild or severe and is typically most severe at the posterior aspect of the annulus.[182] Less commonly, it is associated with obstruction to mitral inflow.[121]

Rheumatic mitral regurgitation is recognized echocardiographically from the parasternal long- and parasternal short-axis views by the presence of thickened, deformed leaflets and subvalvular apparatus with or without associated calcification. Frequently, mitral stenosis and aortic valve disease are associated. In the absence of mitral stenosis, there is little leaflet calcification and no commissural fusion.[183, 184]

A congenital anomaly of the mitral valve that may be responsible for mitral regurgitation in the adult is a cleft of the anterior leaflet, which may be either partial or complete.[185] Accessory chordae from the anterior leaflet attach to the crest of the ventricular septum, effectively preventing coaptation and causing regurgitation. The cleft is best appreciated from the parasternal short-axis view in diastole, is frequently associated with an ostium primum atrial septal defect, and only occasionally occurs as an isolated anomaly.

In the evaluation of the patient with suspected or proved mitral regurgitation, combined two-dimensional and M-mode echocardiography is used to evaluate left atrial and left ventricular size and function and to detect associated valvular heart disease. Serial studies are useful for the longitudinal follow-up of patients with known chronic mitral regurgitation for evaluation of the timing of surgical intervention.[186–188] Two-dimensional echocardiographic assessment of left atrial size and left ventricular size and function are of demonstrated prognostic utility.[189, 190] However, neither M-mode nor two-dimensional echocardiography is useful for the detection or estimation of severity of mitral regurgitation, because the findings are nonspecific and are indirectly related to the severity of the hemodynamic abnormality.

Doppler Echocardiography in Mitral Regurgitation

Mitral regurgitation is detected with very high sensitivity by pulsed-wave[191–193] and color flow Doppler echocardiography.[194, 195] Physiologic mitral regurgitation is detected in more than 40 percent of normal patients by Doppler echocardiography.[196, 197] This does not represent false-positive evidence of mitral regurgitation. Instead, it represents subclinical regurgitation, detected by an extremely sensitive technique. The authors' practice is to describe this as physiologic or trivial regurgitation.

The semiquantitative estimation of significant mitral regurgitation is performed by combined color flow and pulsed-wave Doppler echocardiography. Mitral regurgitant color flow signals characteristically have a mosaic appearance because of turbulence and variance associated with the high-velocity flow that is caused by the large systolic pressure gradient between the left ventricle and atrium (Fig. 30–19A). For regurgitant color flow jets that are not eccentric (centrally directed), more severe grades of regurgitation are associated with larger areas of turbulent systolic flow within the body of the left atrium. Helmcke and colleagues demonstrated high correlation between color flow imaging and semiquantitative grading by angiography, correctly classifying grade I, II, or III mitral regurgitation in 77 of 82 patients.[198] In their study, the spatial extent of the regurgitant jet was analyzed in three different tomographic planes, and severity was expressed as the maximum jet area indexed by left atrial area. A ratio of less than 0.2 corresponded to angiographic grade I (mild), a ratio of between 0.2 and 0.4 represented grade II (moderate), and a ratio greater than 0.4 corresponded to grade III (severe) regurgitation. In the same study, evaluation of the severity of mitral regurgitation by color flow imaging correlated well with invasive estimates of regurgitant fraction. Other investigators have demonstrated acceptable reproducibility and interobserver variability in the quantification of Doppler echocardiographic color flow jet area and correlation with the angiographic grade of mitral regurgitation.[199, 200] However, this method underestimates regurgitant severity if the jets are eccentric and adherent to the walls of the left atrium, directed either toward the atrial septum, posteriorly, or toward the lateral wall because of the Coanda effect.[201]

Color flow imaging of valvular regurgitation is also dependent on gain setting, pulse repetition frequency, field depth, jet direction, and loading conditions. Jet size in color flow imaging must be interpreted in the context of both machine factors and jet geometry related to surrounding solid boundaries.[202] Quantitative methods may also be used to assign a semiquantitative grade of regurgitant severity and are particularly useful for the evaluation of eccentric regurgitant jets.

FIGURE 30–19. See Color Plate 5.

Pulsed-wave mapping of the body of the left atrium is no longer routinely performed in the assessment of mitral regurgitation because it is laborious and time consuming and has been supplanted by color flow imaging. However, pulsed-wave Doppler echocardiographic assessment of pulmonary vein flow is useful for the characterization of hemodynamically severe mitral regurgitation. Detection of systolic flow reversal in the pulmonary veins by pulsed-wave Doppler echocardiography is the hemodynamic equivalent of angiographic reflux into the pulmonary veins on left ventriculography and is characteristic of severe regurgitation. In the assessment of the patient with severe mitral regurgitation, placement of the pulsed-wave Doppler echocardiographic sample volume must be well within the pulmonary vein and not at the orifice of the pulmonary vein, because the latter position may yield systolic flow disturbances as a result of an eccentric mitral regurgitant jet, and not true pulmonary venous systolic flow.

Normal pulmonary venous flow is biphasic, with forward flow in systole and diastole. Alterations of pulmonary venous flow that result from significant mitral regurgitation associated with increased left atrial pressure include diminished systolic flow and reversal of systolic flow. Pulmonary venous systolic flow reversal is consistent with severe regurgitation; diminished antegrade systolic flow is

typical of significant, but less than severe, regurgitation.[203, 204] Discordant flow profiles between right and left upper pulmonary veins may be observed and attributed to various factors, including eccentric mitral regurgitation directed toward either the right or left pulmonary venous orifice, left atrial size, and left lateral decubitus posture during examination.[204]

Continuous-wave Doppler echocardiography enables measurement of the peak mitral regurgitant velocity, which typically is 4 to 5 m/sec. The instantaneous pressure difference between the left ventricle and the left atrium can be measured at any point in systole by application of the modified Bernoulli equation and correlates extremely well with instantaneous pressure gradients measured by simultaneous dual catheterization of the left atrium and left ventricle.[112] However, the maximum instantaneous pressure gradient is not a measure of severity of mitral regurgitation. The gradient is determined chiefly by the left ventricular systolic (driving) pressure and reflects the left ventricular–left atrial gradient in systole, which may have little relation to the severity of regurgitation. Analysis of the time-velocity profile of mitral regurgitation enables estimation of the maximal left ventricular dP/dt, a measure of left ventricular contractile reserve that may be useful in the setting of mitral regurgitation. The time derivative of the left ventricular–left atrial pressure gradient is obtained by differentiating the time course of the ventriculoatrial gradient assessed by continuous-wave Doppler echocardiography. This method has been demonstrated to correlate well with catheter-derived measures and is not substantially affected by orifice size or flow rate;[205] however, dP/dt is load-dependent to a mild degree.[206]

It has been suggested that the severity of mitral regurgitation may be semiquantitatively estimated by analysis of the intensity of the continuous-wave Doppler echocardiographic profile of regurgitation relative to the mitral diastolic inflow signal. By visual inspection, if regurgitation is mild the Doppler echocardiographic signal appears faint, and if regurgitation is severe the signal appears intense. The intensity of the regurgitant signal is proportional to volumetric flow and, after normalization to mitral inflow, enables estimation of regurgitant fraction. The intensity of the mitral regurgitant signal and mitral inflow profile may be measured on-line by computer programs and the regurgitant fraction calculated by the amplitude weighted time-velocity integral method.[207]

Quantitative evaluation of the severity of mitral regurgitation requires estimation of regurgitant volume or regurgitant fraction. Combined pulsed-wave Doppler and two-dimensional echocardiography has been used to calculate regurgitant fraction and volume from the difference between mitral and aortic stroke volume, and the results correlate well with angiographic and scintigraphic estimates.[208] Aortic stroke volume is derived as the product of the aortic time-velocity integral and aortic annular cross-sectional area. Similarly, mitral stroke volume is derived as the product of the mitral time-velocity integral and mitral cross-sectional annulus area. The diameter of the mitral annulus is measured from the apical four-chamber view at maximal diastolic leaflet excursion from the medial inner edge to the lateral inner edge of the annulus just below the insertion of the leaflets. Cross-sectional areas for each valve are calculated as πr^2, assuming circular valve orifices, with r equivalent to one half of the measured diameter. Regurgitant flow is the difference between mitral and aortic flow, and regurgitant fraction is regurgitant flow divided by mitral inflow. This method has been compared with two-dimensional echocardiographic estimation of regurgitant volume using Simpson's biapical method, which demonstrated that quantitative Doppler echocardiographic assessment of mitral regurgitation is feasible in a high proportion of patients and that correlation between the Doppler and two-dimensional echocardiographic methods is excellent.[209]

A Doppler echocardiographic color flow method for the quantitative estimation of regurgitant volume and the severity of valvular regurgitation is based on measurement of volume flow rate proximal to the regurgitant orifice.[210–214] This method differs substantially from previously described Doppler echocardiographic color flow methods in that it does not assess the spatial extent of the jet distal to the regurgitant orifice but instead identifies a proximal (to the regurgitant orifice) isovelocity surface area (PISA) by detection of an aliasing interface (see Fig. 30–19B). Regurgitant volume flow rate in milliliters per second can be calculated as the PISA in square centimeters multiplied by the aliasing velocity in centimeters per second. Assuming that the PISA is a hemispheric shell of accelerating flow proximal to the regurgitant orifice, the mitral regurgitant flow ($Flow_{mr}$) is calculated as

$$Flow_{mr} = 2\pi r^2 \times V_r$$

where $2\pi r^2$ is the area of the PISA having a radius r at the aliasing velocity V_r interface. Because flow is equal to the product of velocity and the area through which it passes,

$$Flow_{mr} = ERO_{mr} \times V_{mr}$$

where ERO_{mr} is the mitral regurgitant effective orifice area (in square centimeters) and V_{mr} is the maximal mitral regurgitant velocity (in centimeters per second) by color flow–directed continuous-wave Doppler echocardiography. By rearranging,

$$ERO_{mr} = Flow_{mr} \div V_{mr}$$

The mitral regurgitant volume (RV_{mr}) in milliliters may then be calculated by

$$RV_{mr} = ERO_{mr} \times TVI_{mr}$$

where TVI_{mr} is the time-velocity integral of the mitral regurgitant signal obtained by continuous-wave Doppler echocardiography. In severe mitral regurgitation, the calculated ERO_{mr} is typically more than 0.4 cm^2 and the RV_{mr} is greater than 50 mL.

In principle, the PISA method may be affected by changes in instrumentation factors and the shape of the regurgitant orifice. However, if a hemispheric model is assumed for the regurgitant orifice, differences in plane or orifice shape do not appear to affect the calculated volume flow rate. Instrumentation factors, including gain, filter settings, frame rate, transmission power, and packet size, do not appear to significantly affect calculations of volume flow rate by this method. In principle, therefore, this method may have advantages over previous Doppler echocardiographic methods in estimation of volume flow rate. However, in contrast to the assessment of orifice dimension for valvular stenosis, there is no reliable reference standard for comparison of regurgitant orifice dimension.

The major limitation of echocardiographic methods for the estimation of regurgitant fraction or volume is the exclusion of patients with other left-sided valvular heart disease. The most important potential sources of error are the measurements of aortic and mitral orifice area, which may lead to estimates of regurgitant fraction as high as 20 percent for normal valves.[215] However, this is similar to the error inherent in measurement of regurgitant fraction by invasive methods.[216] The chief problems or uncertainties with the use of any invasive or noninvasive quantitative method for the assessment of the severity of regurgitation include the learning curve, reproducibility of the techniques in different laboratories, and usefulness of the techniques for decision-making about the timing of valve surgery.

Role of Echocardiography in Clinical Decision-Making in Mitral Regurgitation

Combined two-dimensional and M-mode echocardiography provides anatomic and quantitative information that enables classification of the cause of mitral regurgitation and assessment of cardiac chamber dimension and left ventricular function necessary for longitudinal follow-up in the patient with chronic mitral regurgitation; two-dimensional echocardiographic data is of prognostic utility in selection of patients for mitral valve repair or replacement.[189, 190] Doppler echocardiography enables detection and assessment of the

hemodynamic severity of regurgitation. Complete Doppler echocardiographic assessment should include estimation of pulmonary artery pressure for the assessment of possible pulmonary hypertension (see section on tricuspid regurgitation). Cardiac catheterization is reserved for patients in whom suboptimal data are obtained, clinical and echocardiographic data are discordant, or there is suspected coronary artery disease.

Tricuspid Stenosis

The tricuspid valve is larger and more complex than the mitral valve. It consists of three leaflets, an annular ring, and subvalvular components, including chordae tendineae, papillary muscles, and subjacent right ventricular myocardium. It is differentiated from the mitral valve by its trileaflet structure, multiple separate papillary muscles, and annular insertion inferior to the mitral annulus.[217] Like mitral stenosis, tricuspid stenosis is characterized by reduced orifice dimension, which impairs right ventricular filling. Obstruction to right ventricular inflow may be caused by congenital or acquired disease and may be primarily valvular, subvalvular, or supravalvular in location.[218]

Rheumatic heart disease is the most common cause of tricuspid stenosis.[218, 219] Stenosis is produced by leaflet fibrosis, commissural fusion, and fibrosis and thickening of the chordae; calcification is unusual.[218–220] Tricuspid regurgitation and rheumatic mitral disease are almost always associated. Echocardiographic evaluation of the tricuspid valve is best performed from the right ventricular inflow view, in long- and short-axis orientations. Rheumatic stenosis is recognized by demonstration of thickened and deformed leaflets, abnormal leaflet motion, and reduced orifice dimension. Unlike rheumatic mitral disease, tricuspid stenosis is uncommonly accompanied by calcification. As in other stenotic valvular lesions, abnormal leaflet motion is characterized by doming at maximal excursion.[221]

Less frequent causes of acquired tricuspid valvular stenosis are carcinoid, methysergide toxicity, endomyocardial fibrosis, and endomyocardial fibroelastoma.[218, 222, 223, 228] Each of these disorders is characterized pathologically by deposition of fibrous material on the tricuspid leaflet, producing combined stenosis and regurgitation. Two-dimensional echocardiography demonstrates a thickened valve, shortened supporting structures, and diastolic doming of the leaflets. In severe cases, the tricuspid valve is immobile, fixed in a semiopen position[224] (Fig. 30–20). These disorders are not always easily differentiable from rheumatic disease by echocardiography. However, associated findings suggest specific diagnoses. Mitral valve disease is almost always associated with rheumatic disease, whereas, in carcinoid and methysergide toxicity, combined pulmonary stenosis and regurgitation are frequent and left-sided valvular disease is extremely unusual. Similarly, endomyocardial fibrosis and fibroelastosis are frequently associated with obliteration of the right ventricular apex, easily demonstrated by two-dimensional echocardiography.

The hemodynamic severity of tricuspid stenosis cannot be assessed directly by combined two-dimensional and M-mode echocardiography. Short-axis recording of the tricuspid orifice is seldom possible. For these reasons, estimation of the orifice area cannot be performed routinely, as it is in mitral stenosis. Enlargement of the right atrium, inferior vena cava, and hepatic veins is frequently seen but is an indirect marker of right atrial hypertension. An estimate of the severity of tricuspid stenosis requires Doppler echocardiography.

Doppler Echocardiography in the Evaluation of Tricuspid Stenosis

The tricuspid inflow Doppler echocardiographic signals are best demonstrated in the right ventricular inflow view or the apical four-chamber view. The normal tricuspid valve flow profile is qualitatively similar to that of mitral inflow but of lesser magnitude.

Tricuspid stenosis causes an increased gradient from the right

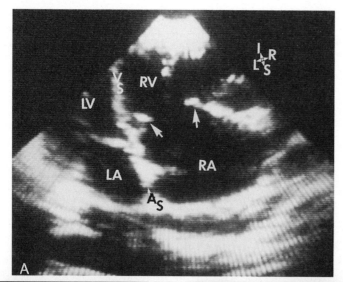

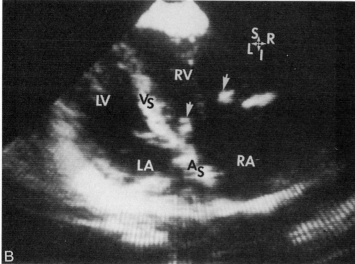

FIGURE 30–20. Carcinoid syndrome. Four-chamber view demonstrates enlarged right ventricle (RV) and right atrium (RA). *A*, Diastolic frame. *B*, Systolic frame. Anterior and septal leaflets of tricuspid valve are thickened, retracted and fixed in a semiopen position. AS = atrial septum; I = inferior; L = left; LA = left atrium; LV = left ventricle; R = right; S = superior; VS = ventricular septum. (From Callahan, J.A., Wroblewski, E.M., Reeder, G.S., et al.: Echocardiographic features of carcinoid heart disease. Am. J. Cardiol. 50:762, 1982, with permission of Cahners Publishing Company.)

atrium to the right ventricle throughout diastole. Pressure gradients by continuous-wave Doppler echocardiography may be reliably estimated. Doppler echocardiography demonstrates increased velocity and slowed decay of the inflow signal, as in mitral stenosis[225, 226] (Fig. 30–21). However, the velocities observed are usually not as high as those in mitral stenosis. The ease of the Doppler echocardiographic method contrasts with the difficulty of verifying the pressure gradient at cardiac catheterization (especially in the presence of atrial fibrillation) because of the effects of respiration, unless right atrial and right ventricular pressures are recorded simultaneously by the dual-catheter technique. The pressure half-time method has been used to estimate tricuspid valve area, as in mitral stenosis, with use of the empiric formula of Hatle and associates[141] described for mitral stenosis. Noninvasive estimates of severity correlate well with invasive methods.[227]

Role of Echocardiography in Clinical Decision-Making in Tricuspid Stenosis

Two-dimensional echocardiography demonstrates the anatomic location and cause of obstruction to right ventricular filling. Evaluation of associated valvular pathologic conditions and of chamber size and function is helpful in determining the cause of disease and provides indirect assessment of hemodynamic severity. Doppler echocardiography confirms the presence and severity of stenosis.

Tricuspid Regurgitation

Tricuspid valve regurgitation may be caused by either intrinsic valvular disease or tricuspid annular dilatation.[228-231] Functional tricuspid regurgitation is caused by right ventricular hypertension of any cause, with associated dilatation of the right ventricle and the tricuspid annulus.

Valvular abnormalities producing tricuspid regurgitation are associated with many diseases, in part because of the anatomic and functional complexity of the valve apparatus. Proper closure of the tricuspid valve requires coordinated function of the leaflets, chordae, papillary muscles, and subjacent ventricular myocardium. Functional or anatomic abnormality of any component of the tricuspid valve apparatus may produce tricuspid regurgitation. Two-dimensional echocardiography identifies the morphologic abnormality causing tricuspid regurgitation and also associated anatomic abnormalities of the right side of the heart.

Valvular disease diagnosed by two-dimensional echocardiography includes leaflet prolapse, endocarditis, carcinoid, and Ebstein anomaly. Prolapse of the tricuspid valve, like mitral prolapse, is recognized by systolic buckling of one or more leaflets beyond the plane of the tricuspid annulus into the right atrium, best appreciated in either the parasternal long-axis view of the right ventricular inflow tract or the apical four-chamber view. Isolated tricuspid valve prolapse is unusual; it occurs most commonly in association with mitral valve prolapse.[232]

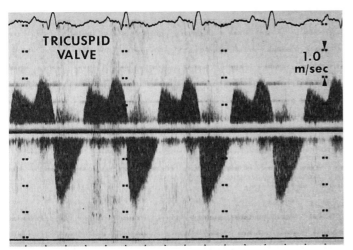

FIGURE 30–21. Combined tricuspid stenosis and regurgitation in a patient with carcinoid evaluated by continuous-wave Doppler echocardiography. Examination was performed from an apical window; signals above the baseline correspond to diastolic antegrade tricuspid flow, and systolic signals below baseline indicate tricuspid regurgitation (2.7 m per second). Peak and mean diastolic gradients measured 16 and 9 mm Hg, respectively. The estimated right ventricular systolic pressure was 42 mm Hg.

Infectious endocarditis of the tricuspid valve is relatively uncommon. As in endocarditis of the left side of the heart, the diagnosis is primarily clinical. Echocardiographic findings characteristic of tricuspid endocarditis include large vegetations with a so-called shaggy appearance. In the presence of severe leaflet and subvalvular damage, there may be flail motion of the valvular apparatus.[233, 234] If chronic disease occurs, there will be associated right atrial and ventricular enlargement.

Echocardiographic characteristics of carcinoid heart disease include thickening and retraction of the leaflets owing to leaflet and subvalvular involvement. The valve leaflets may become fixed in a semiopen position, producing combined tricuspid stenosis and regurgitation.[228, 235, 236] There is frequently associated pulmonary valve involvement. Rarely, an associated myocardial mass caused by carcinoid is observed.[228] Other unusual causes of tricuspid regurgitation are nonpenetrating chest trauma with disruption of the tricuspid chordal apparatus[237–239] and sinus of Valsalva aneurysm.[240]

Ebstein anomaly is a congenital abnormality of the tricuspid valve and right side of the heart characterized by apical displacement of deformed tricuspid leaflets.[241, 242] The characteristic echocardiographic findings have been extensively reviewed[243] and are described here in Chapter 33.

The presence of tricuspid regurgitation is suggested on combined M-mode and two-dimensional echocardiography by valvular anatomic abnormalities and associated dilatation of the right heart chambers and central veins. Volume overload of the right side of the heart also shifts the interventricular septum toward the left side, producing paradoxic systolic septal motion.[244] The severity of tricuspid regurgitation is best evaluated by combined two-dimensional and Doppler echocardiography. In severe tricuspid regurgitation, two-dimensional echocardiography invariably demonstrates right ventricular and right atrial enlargement as well as dilatation of the inferior vena cava and hepatic veins. Doppler echocardiography enables direct detection and assessment of the severity of the flow abnormality.

Doppler Echocardiography in the Evaluation of Tricuspid Regurgitation

Pulsed-wave, continuous-wave, and color flow imaging are all extremely sensitive for the detection of tricuspid regurgitation.[245–248] However, tricuspid regurgitation is detected in at least 60 to 70 percent of normal individuals and is attributed to normal, physiologic but subclinical tricuspid regurgitation.[197] These regurgi-

tant jets are localized and narrow, corresponding to a relatively low volume of regurgitant flow, and are easily differentiated from pathologic regurgitation.

Validation of the accuracy of Doppler echocardiography for the assessment of severity of tricuspid regurgitation has not been possible because there is no reliable reference standard. Ventriculography requires placement of a catheter across the tricuspid orifice, which induces regurgitation. A practical semiquantitative approach uses pulsed-wave Doppler echocardiography and color flow imaging in combination with anatomic assessment by two-dimensional echocardiography for assessment of the severity of regurgitation, whereas continuous-wave Doppler echocardiography is used to estimate right ventricular systolic pressure. If the right heart chambers are of normal dimension, the likelihood of significant tricuspid regurgitation is low. Conversely, patients with moderate-to-severe tricuspid regurgitation typically have enlarged right heart chambers with large-volume tricuspid regurgitation, manifested by color flow imaging as a broad systolic right atrial signal.

Tricuspid regurgitation by color flow imaging has an appearance similar to that of mitral regurgitation (Fig. 30–22). The flow signal originates from the valve annulus and extends into the right atrium. From the apical four-chamber view and the right ventricular inflow view, the regurgitant jet is directed away from the transducer and appears in shades of blue. If tricuspid regurgitation is severe, the right atrium and ventricle essentially function as a single chamber. In this situation, there is a low pressure gradient from the right ventricle to the right atrium, and the color flow image does not demonstrate the aliasing and mosaic colors characteristic of turbulent flow. However, the severity of regurgitation is recognized because the low-velocity regurgitant signals fill most of the right atrium.

FIGURE 30–22. See Color Plate 5.

Assessment of hepatic vein flow by pulsed-wave Doppler echocardiography and color flow imaging is a useful adjunct for the characterization of the severity of regurgitation. Normally, hepatic blood flow is antegrade and toward the right side of the heart, producing a signal below the baseline if examined from the subcostal view[249] (Fig. 30–23). In the presence of severe tricuspid regurgitation, right ventricular systole may produce retrograde flow through the tricuspid orifice into the right atrium, inferior vena cava, and hepatic veins. The detection of systolic flow reversal in the hepatic veins by pulsed-wave Doppler echocardiography or color flow imaging is indicative of severe tricuspid regurgitation.[246, 250] Conversely, the absence of flow reversal in the hepatic

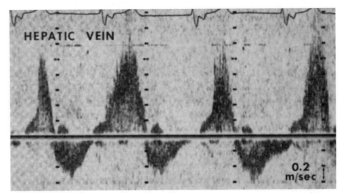

FIGURE 30–23. Pulsed-wave Doppler echocardiographic evaluation of hepatic vein flow in a patient with tricuspid regurgitation. The examination was performed from the subcostal window in short-axis view. Marked systolic flow reversal (flow signals above baseline) is seen, indicative of severe tricuspid regurgitation.

veins does not necessarily imply that tricuspid regurgitation is not severe, especially in the presence of an enlarged and compliant right atrium.

Doppler Echocardiographic Estimation of Right Ventricular Systolic Pressure

Continuous-wave Doppler echocardiographic characterization of tricuspid regurgitation facilitates diagnosis and clinical decision-making in patients with a wide spectrum of cardiac disease by enabling noninvasive quantitative estimation of right ventricular systolic pressure and pulmonary artery pressure.

The velocity of the tricuspid regurgitant jet is related to the systolic right ventricular–right atrial pressure gradient by the principles of Bernoulli hydrodynamics. Estimation of the systolic maximal instantaneous right ventricular–right atrial pressure gradient is performed by application of the modified Bernoulli equation to velocity data obtained by continuous-wave Doppler echocardiography. Currie and colleagues demonstrated high correlation between Doppler echocardiographic estimates and simultaneous dual-catheter measurements of the right ventricular–right atrial pressure gradient in 111 patients with a wide spectrum of cardiac disease, severity of tricuspid regurgitation, and right heart pressures[251] (Fig. 30–24). On the basis of their investigation, simple regression equations were devised that enable accurate assessment of right ventricular systolic pressure. In patients with normal right heart pressures, right ventricular systolic pressure is obtained by the addition of 14 to the right ventricular-right atrial pressure gradient. In patients with moderately or severely elevated right heart pressure, the best

estimate of right ventricular systolic pressure is obtained by the addition of 20 to the right ventricular–right atrial gradient. Other investigators have demonstrated analyzable tricuspid regurgitation signals by continuous-wave Doppler echocardiography in up to 90 percent of patients with congestive heart failure, and in a high proportion of normal patients as well.[252, 253] Therefore, measurement of peak tricuspid regurgitant jet velocity should be attempted routinely in patients undergoing echocardiographic examination.

As in the evaluation of mitral regurgitation by continuous-wave Doppler echocardiography, the magnitude of regurgitant velocity is not a measure of the severity of tricuspid regurgitation. Instead, the velocity is determined primarily by the right ventricular–right atrial pressure gradient.

Role of Echocardiography in the Evaluation of Tricuspid Regurgitation

Combined two-dimensional and color flow imaging provides anatomic and hemodynamic information that enables diagnostic classification and assessment of the severity of tricuspid regurgitation. Echocardiography is the diagnostic method of choice for the evaluation of the patient with tricuspid regurgitation. Invasive methods requiring catheterization induce regurgitation because the catheter must be placed across the tricuspid orifice to perform ventriculography. In the absence of obstruction to right ventricular outflow, estimated peak right ventricular systolic pressure is equivalent to pulmonary artery systolic pressure. Noninvasive assessment of pulmonary artery pressure is useful for the evaluation of patients with a wide spectrum of diseases, including mitral stenosis, mitral

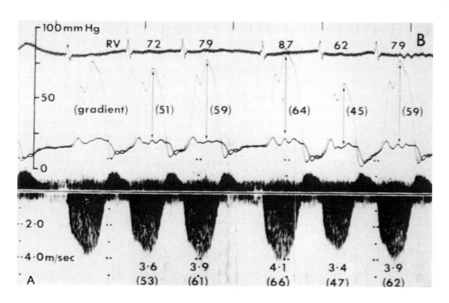

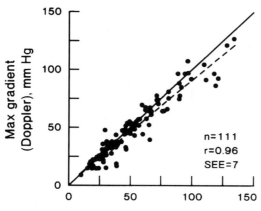

FIGURE 30–24. Assessment of right ventricular–right atrial systolic pressure gradients by continuous-wave Doppler echocardiography. *A,* Simultaneous Doppler echocardiographic and right ventricular and right atrial tracings. The patient was in atrial fibrillation; the fourth beat was chosen for analysis. The right ventricular (RV) systolic pressure was 87 mm Hg, and the maximal catheter right ventricular–right atrial pressure gradient was 64 mm Hg. The maximal Doppler echocardiographic velocity was 4.1 m per second, and maximal Doppler gradient was 66 mm Hg. Note the excellent beat-to-beat correlation between the Doppler echocardiographic and catheter maximal gradients. *B,* Correlation of simultaneous Doppler echocardiographic and right ventricular–right atrial maximal (Max) systolic pressure gradients in 111 patients with tricuspid regurgitation. The dashed line is the regression line, and the solid line is the line of identity. The regression equation is as follows: Doppler gradient = 2.2 + 0.88 × catheter gradient. SEE = standard error of estimation. (From Currie, P.J., et al.: Continuous-wave Doppler determination of right ventricular pressure: A simultaneous Doppler-catheterization study in 127 patients. J. Am. Coll. Cardiol. 6:750, 1985, with permission of the American College of Cardiology.)

regurgitation, and malfunctioning mitral or aortic prostheses. The ability to perform serial noninvasive assessment of right heart pressures at rest and at exercise is extremely useful in these patient groups.

Pulmonary Stenosis and Regurgitation

Acquired pulmonary valve disease is extremely uncommon in adult patients. Most often, pulmonary valve stenosis or significant pulmonary valve regurgitation is associated with congenital heart disease and is recognized in childhood. However, an increasing adult population with treated congenital heart disease may come under the care of the adult cardiologist.

Congenital pulmonary valve stenosis may occur in isolation or in association with other congenital cardiac abnormalities.[254-256] Acquired disease of the pulmonary valve in adult patients is usually associated with combined stenosis and regurgitation caused by rheumatic heart disease or carcinoid.[228, 254-256] Rheumatic disease should be suspected in the patient with typical left-sided valvular abnormalities suggestive of previous rheumatic fever. Carcinoid heart disease is most often isolated to the right side of the heart. Pulmonary valvular regurgitation is most often functional and may be acquired because of underlying pulmonary hypertension of any cause. Endocarditis of the pulmonary valve is relatively rare but may produce isolated regurgitation.[257, 258]

Echocardiographic assessment of the pulmonary valve is performed from the parasternal long-axis, parasternal short-axis, and subcostal long-axis views. Pulmonary valve stenosis is suspected on the basis of two-dimensional echocardiography if systolic doming of the valve leaflets is observed.[259, 260] Doppler echocardiography increases the sensitivity of the detection of pulmonary valve stenosis and provides accurate hemodynamic assessment.[261]

Pulmonary valve regurgitation is suspected on two-dimensional echocardiographic examination if valvular vegetations are demonstrated or if there is rapid oscillatory motion of the free edges of the valve during diastole.[262, 263] In patients with carcinoid heart disease, the pulmonary valve may be relatively fixed in a semiopen position, the leaflets appear retracted, and the pulmonary annulus may be narrowed, producing outflow obstruction. There is usually associated involvement of the tricuspid valve.[224, 228] Another abnormality demonstrated by two-dimensional echocardiography may be right ventricular enlargement, depending on the duration and severity of regurgitation.

Doppler Echocardiography in the Evaluation of Pulmonary Valve Disease

Pulmonary valve stenosis causes alteration in blood flow that is qualitatively similar to that seen in other valvular stenoses. Blood flow accelerates proximal to the valve and flows through the stenotic orifice in a laminar jet. The peak velocity of flow in the jet measured by continuous-wave Doppler echocardiography allows estimation of the transvalvular gradient by application of the modified Bernoulli equation.[264] Gradient estimations of discrete nonvalvular right ventricular outflow obstruction by continuous-wave Doppler echocardiography have been clinically validated by simultaneous invasive examination in several studies.[265, 266] Color flow imaging aids in the assessment of the transvalvular gradient by guiding the placement of the ultrasonic beam to a position parallel to flow. Estimation of pulmonary valve area is possible by the continuity equation, but at present there are no established criteria for estimation of severity of stenosis on the basis of valve area.

Pulmonary valve regurgitation may be detected in most normal patients by Doppler echocardiography, corresponding to the subclinical, physiologic regurgitation that is also seen in normal mitral and tricuspid valves.[267, 268] In the normal population, pulmonary regurgitation is detected by pulsed-wave echocardiography only in the region immediately below the valve, whereas in those with significant pulmonary valve regurgitation, color flow imaging demonstrates a wide regurgitant jet extending deep into the right

ventricle, with associated right ventricular enlargement. The appearance of pulmonary regurgitation by color flow imaging is qualitatively similar to that of aortic regurgitation (Fig. 30–25). It is best demonstrated from the parasternal short-axis view and appears as a pandiastolic jet of red signals extending from the pulmonary valve into the right ventricular outflow tract and cavity. The dimensions of the color jet increase with increasing severity of pulmonary regurgitation.

FIGURE 30–25. See Color Plate 6.

Role of Echocardiography in the Evaluation of Pulmonary Valve Disease

Combined two-dimensional and Doppler echocardiography is reliable for the identification of the cause of pulmonary valve disease and for assessment of hemodynamic severity. Data on abnormalities of valvular structure and cardiac chamber dimensions are helpful in diagnostic classification. Doppler echocardiography provides a definitive assessment of hemodynamic severity.

ASSESSMENT OF VALVE FUNCTION AFTER INTERVENTION

Prosthetic Stenosis and Regurgitation

Prosthetic valves have either bioprosthetic or mechanical components. Bioprosthetic valves are more easily evaluated, because the valve leaflets are composed of tissue and have echocardiographic characteristics somewhat similar to those of native valves. However, the struts and ring to which the leaflets are attached are metallic and therefore cause ultrasonic reverberations and sidelobe artifacts that may obscure anatomic abnormalities. Mechanical valves are composed entirely of inert, highly reflective materials that tend to saturate the recording system and make evaluation more difficult than it is for bioprosthetic valves. Acoustic shadowing from bioprostheses and mechanical valves may limit the usefulness of transthoracic two-dimensional echocardiography for the detection of leaflet vegetations, ring abscess, valve-associated thrombus, and left atrial thrombus.[269]

In the assessment of tissue valves by two-dimensional echocardiography, the bioprosthetic portion of the valve normally moves in concert with the highly echo-reflective struts and sewing ring. Bioprosthetic valves are normally subject to degeneration over a span of 8 to 10 years, and this is clinically manifested as stenosis or regurgitation, or both.[270, 271] Bioprosthetic valve degeneration appears echocardiographically as increased leaflet thickness and calcification.[272] Other abnormalities of the leaflets identified by echocardiography include focal masses, perforations, prolapse, and fluttering caused by endocarditis or thrombosis.[271-275] For mitral prostheses, leaflet motion detected within the body of the left atrium indicates disruption of the leaflet from the valve apparatus, which may result from endocarditis or degeneration.[273] Abnormalities of the sewing ring are also demonstrated by two-dimensional echocardiography, including excessive rocking caused by dehiscence of the sewing ring from the annulus.[273]

Two-dimensional echocardiographic evaluation of mechanical prostheses is more difficult. Although the valves have a characteristic appearance and are easily recognized by two-dimensional echocardiography, the individual components of the valve apparatus are difficult to differentiate because of the highly echo-reflective materials used in their construction. Futhermore, because of acoustic "masking," structures beyond the valve relative to the incident ultrasound beam are poorly visualized, especially in the mitral position.[276, 277] Despite these difficulties, gross evaluation of valve motion, detection of large masses associated with the valve, and detection of perivalvular abnormalities are routinely possible.[271, 273]

Doppler Echocardiography in the Evaluation of Prosthetic Valves

Normal Doppler echocardiographic findings for prosthetic valves have been described and reviewed.[278–280] It has been suggested that the complex and multiple orifices of prosthetic valves may invalidate the assumptions of the modified Bernoulli equation for the evaluation of prosthetic stenosis[281]; in vitro work has indicated that correlation between Doppler-derived and manometric pressure gradients varies with the size and type of prosthesis.[282] Another in vitro investigation has demonstrated the validity of the Doppler echocardiographic method for the evaluation of irregular, tunnel-like obstructions.[283] Furthermore, the use of the modified Bernoulli equation and Doppler echocardiography has been validated by comparison with catheterization for the evaluation of stenosis of a variety of bioprosthetic and mechanical valves.[284, 285]

Close correlation between Doppler-derived and simultaneous catheter-measured gradients in patients with mitral and tricuspid prostheses has been described in small numbers of patients.[284–287]

Nonsimultaneous studies in patients with aortic prostheses have yielded conflicting results.[277, 288, 289] However, simultaneous echocardiographic and dual-catheter study of 42 prosthetic valves, including 20 in the aortic position, has demonstrated extremely high correlation between catheter- and Doppler-derived maximal instantaneous and mean gradients, regardless of prosthetic position or type[284] (Fig. 30–26). Furthermore, in this same study, Doppler echocardiography correlated better with estimation of transmitral prosthetic gradient when direct left atrial measurement was used instead of pulmonary capillary wedge pressure, a result suggesting that overestimation of transmitral gradients may occur if pulmonary capillary wedge pressure is used.[284, 290] As in native valve disease, the transvalvular pressure gradient alone may be insufficient to characterize the severity of prosthetic dysfunction because of the flow dependence of the measured gradients. An estimate of prosthetic valve area is therefore indicated. However, in studies of a limited number of patients with mitral prostheses, correlation between Doppler- and catheter-derived valve areas has been poor.[285] It has been suggested that this may represent a limitation of the Gorlin formula in the assessment of prosthetic valve area.[285]

Aortic prosthetic regurgitation is detected with high sensitivity, and severity is accurately assessed by Doppler echocardiography.[291, 292] In contrast, acoustic "masking" by the inert materials

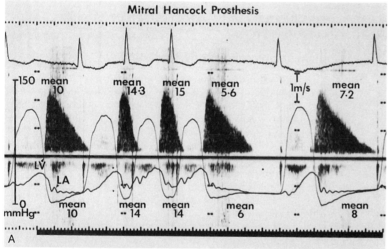

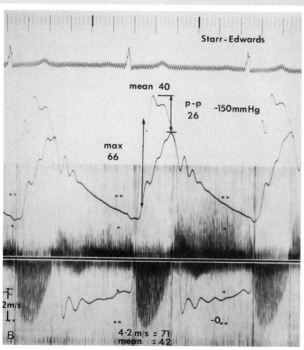

FIGURE 30–26. *A*, Simultaneous Doppler echocardiographic and catheter pressure estimates in a patient with a stenotic mitral Hancock prosthesis. The pressure gradient was measured by the dual-catheter technique, with catheters in the left ventricle (LV) and left atrium (LA). Note the excellent beat-to-beat correlation in estimated mean gradients by Doppler echocardiography and cardiac catheterization. *B*, Simultaneous Doppler and catheter pressure estimates in a patient with a stenotic Starr-Edwards aortic prosthesis. Pressure gradient was measured by the dual-catheter technique, with catheters in the left ventricle and left aorta. Note that the maximal (max) instantaneous and mean gradients exceed the peak-to-peak (p-p) gradient. There is excellent correlation between Doppler echocardiographic and catheter-determined mean gradients.

used in construction of bioprostheses and mechanical valves severely limits the usefulness of transthoracic Doppler echocardiography for the assessment of prosthetic mitral regurgitation.[269, 276, 293] However, transesophageal echocardiography provides an unimpeded ultrasonic window to the left atrium, allowing easy characterization of left atrial anatomy and mitral regurgitation. Furthermore, sensitivity for detection of mitral regurgitation is markedly enhanced compared with conventional transthoracic imaging.[276, 294] In suspected endocarditis, vegetations and perivalvular disease are also identified with much greater sensitivity.[61, 276]

Valvuloplasty

Experience with surgical valvuloplasty preceded the development and use of prosthetic valves.[186] Although surgical valvuloplasty was performed at only a few centers after the development of prosthetic valves, there has been renewed interest in the technique in the past 10 years. Surgical repair, rather than replacement, of the mitral valve is frequently feasible and offers many advantages. Done by experienced surgeons, the procedure is associated with increased survival and improved left ventricular function as well as a lower frequency of valve-related complications.[294a–297] Operative repair of the aortic valve has been performed by mechanical[298] and by ultrasonic[299] decalcification of stenotic valves, with consistent relief of stenosis. Tricuspid annuloplasty is routinely performed at many centers and is generally favored over valve replacement whenever possible. Data obtained by intraoperative transesophageal echocardiographic assessment can guide the surgeon in making the repair; these data are directly comparable with data obtained postoperatively and are useful for follow up.[300] The intraoperative assessment of valvuloplasty by echocardiography is described in Chapter 39.

Combined two-dimensional and Doppler echocardiography has also been used for patient selection and for the assessment of the morphologic and hemodynamic alterations associated with percutaneous aortic, mitral, and pulmonary balloon valvuloplasty.[301–306] Echocardiographic criteria for identification of patients who are optimal candidates for mitral valvuloplasty were described earlier in this chapter. Two-dimensional echocardiography has demonstrated that the mechanism of successful mitral balloon valvuloplasty is the splitting of fusions along one or both leaflets' commissures. This is associated with an increase in the transverse diameter and an increased opening of the angle between the commissures.[144, 307] In patients with calcification of the mitral leaflets or commissures, incomplete splitting of commissures and less increase in the angle of opening are observed, with less associated improvement in mitral valve area.

The pressure half-time method immediately after valvuloplasty has been demonstrated to correlate poorly with Gorlin formula estimates of mitral valve area by invasive techniques.[308] However, the half-time method may be applied with confidence from 24 to 48 hours after valvuloplasty.[308] Doppler echocardiography is also useful for estimation of valve gradient immediately after intervention and for the detection of mitral regurgitation.[309]

Combined two-dimensional and Doppler echocardiography is ideal for long-term follow-up of patients with valvuloplasty, because the techniques are noninvasive and provide accurate morphologic and hemodynamic assessment, including estimates of valve area.[310–313] The discrepancy between estimates of mitral valve area by catheterization and by the Doppler echocardiographic half-time method immediately after valvuloplasty is not observed at 6 months.[314] Restenosis occurs in some patients, and patients at risk are identified by the same two-dimensional echocardiographic scoring system described for the identification of optimal candidates for valvuloplasty.[301, 315]

Echocardiographic evaluation of aortic valvular morphology has not been used for the selection of patents for aortic balloon valvuloplasty. The morphologic abnormalities of the stenotic aortic valve are not as heterogeneous as those in mitral stenosis, so an anatomic scoring system would not be expected to stratify patients. Some experience has suggested that the stenotic valve resulting from degenerative disease may be more successfully dilated than the calcified, congenitally bicuspid or rheumatic aortic valve.[28] However, if calcification is dense, this distinction cannot always be made by two-dimensional echocardiography.

The early postintervention hemodynamic effects of aortic balloon valvuloplasty have been described by Doppler echocardiography. Nishimura and associates reported a significant reduction in the aortic mean gradient and valve area within 24 to 48 hours after the procedure, but restenosis was frequently observed in patients seen at 6-month follow-up.[316] These investigators cautioned against hemodynamic assessment immediately after intervention because of transient left ventricular dysfunction related to the procedure, with associated alterations in cardiac output, gradient, and valve area. However, aortic valve area derived from Doppler echocardiography longer than 24 to 48 hours after balloon valvuloplasty correlates well with valve area determined by invasive methods.[316, 317] Trivial-to-mild aortic regurgitation is frequently observed by Doppler echocardiography after intervention, but significant regurgitation has been described infrequently.[316, 318]

Morphologic alterations of the aortic valve associated with aortic balloon valvuloplasty have been characterized in intraoperative[319, 321] and postmortem[319, 321, 322] studies. The mechanism of successful aortic valvuloplasty has been attributed to fracture of calcific deposits of the aortic valve leaflets, with associated increased leaflet mobility.[28, 319, 321, 322] Small postmortem studies suggest that fracture of fused commissures associated with rheumatic or senile stenosis does not occur.[28] These observations have not been corroborated by two-dimensional echocardiography, probably because most patients who undergo the procedure have senile aortic stenosis and because the detection of fracture of calcium deposits is not possible.

SUMMARY

Echocardiography has become the preferred diagnostic modality for the evaluation of patients with valvular heart disease. Although there are limitations to the techniques, interpretive errors may be avoided by a thorough understanding of the methods. Careful attention to detail on the part of the operator performing the study ensures data of high quality for analysis. Combined two-dimensional and Doppler echocardiography with color flow imaging provides comprehensive, accurate, and noninvasive assessment of the cause and hemodynamic severity of valvular heart disease. Doppler echocardiographic methods have been proved to be extremely accurate for the assessment of valvular stenosis, yielding data that are directly comparable to those obtained by cardiac catheterization. For the evaluation of valvular regurgitation, Doppler echocardiography provides a semiquantitative estimate of hemodynamic severity that compares favorably with semiquantitative invasive estimation by angiography. It is now possible to perform accurate serial quantitative evaluation of the hemodynamic severity of not only stenotic lesions but also regurgitant lesions, allowing greater confidence in determining the progression of valvular heart disease without the cost or risk of cardiac catheterization.

References

1. American College of Cardiology/American Heart Association Task Force on Assessment of Diagnostic and Therapeutic Cardiovascular Procedures: ACC/AHA guidelines for the clinical application of echocardiography. Circulation 82:2323, 1990.
2. Cheitlin, M.D.: Valvular heart disease: Management and intervention: Clinical overview and discussion. Circulation 84:I259, 1991.
3. van den Brink, R.B., Verheul, H.A., Hoedemaker, G., et al.: The value of Doppler echocardiography in the management of patients with valvular heart disease: Analysis of one year of clinical practice. J. Am. Soc. Echocardiogr. 4:109, 1991.
4. Slater, J., Gindea, A.J., Freedberg, R.S., et al.: Comparison of cardiac catheterization and Doppler echocardiography in the decision to operate in aortic and mitral valve disease. J. Am. Coll. Cardiol. 17:1026, 1991.
5. Clawson, B.J.: Rheumatic heart disease: An analysis of 796 cases. Am. Heart J. 20:454, 1940.
6. Davies, M.J.: Pathology of Cardiac Valves. London, Butterworth, 1980, p. 18.

7. Dry, T.J., and Willius, F.A.: Calcareous disease of the aortic valve: A study of two hundred twenty-eight cases. Am. Heart J. 17:138, 1939.

8. Edwards, J.E.: Calcific aortic stenosis: Pathologic features. Mayo Clin. Proc. 36:444, 1961.

9. Edwards, J.E.: Pathology of left ventricular outflow tract obstruction. Circulation 31:586, 1965.

10. Pomerance, A.: Pathogenesis of aortic stenosis and its relation to age. Br. Heart J. 34:569, 1972.

11. Roberts, W.C.: The structure of the aortic valve in clinically isolated aortic stenosis: An autopsy study of 162 patients over 15 years of age. Circulation 42:91, 1970.

12. Roberts, W.C.: The congenitally bicuspid aortic valve: A study of 85 autopsy cases. Am. J. Cardiol. 26:72, 1970.

13. Subramanian, R., Olson, L.J., and Edwards, W.D.: Surgical pathology of pure aortic stenosis: A study of 374 cases. Mayo Clin. Proc. 59:683, 1984.

14. Passik, C.S., Ackermann, D.M., Pluth, J.R., et al.: Temporal changes in the causes of aortic stenosis: A surgical pathologic study of 646 cases. Mayo Clin. Proc. 62:119, 1987.

15. Hegrænæs, L., and Hatle, L.: Aortic stenosis in adults: Non-invasive estimation of pressure differences by continuous wave Doppler echocardiography. Br. Heart J. 54:396, 1985.

16. Annegers, J.F., Pillman, N.L., Weidman, W.H., et al.: Rheumatic fever in Rochester, Minnesota, 1935–1978. Mayo Clin. Proc. 57:753, 1982.

17. DiSciascio, G., and Taranta, A.: Rheumatic fever in children. Am. Heart J. 99:635, 1980.

18. Chang, S., Clements, S., and Chang, J.: Aortic stenosis: Echocardiographic cusp separation and surgical description of aortic valve in 22 patients. Am. J. Cardiol. 39:499, 1977.

19. DeMaria, A.N., Bommer, W., Joye, J., et al.: Value and limitations of cross-sectional echocardiography of the aortic valve in the diagnosis and quantification of valvular aortic stenosis. Circulation 62:304, 1980.

20. Godley, R.W., Green, D., Dillon, J.C., et al.: Reliability of two-dimensional echocardiography in assessing the severity of valvular aortic stenosis. Chest 79:657, 1981.

21. Weyman, A.E., Feigenbaum, H., Dillon, J.C., et al.: Cross-sectional echocardiography in assessing the severity of valvular aortic stenosis. Circulation 52:828, 1975.

22. Weyman, A.E., Feigenbaum, H., Hurwitz, R.A., et al.: Localization of left ventricular outflow obstruction by cross-sectional echocardiography. Am. J. Med. 60:33, 1976.

23. Wong, M., Tei, C., Sadler, N., et al.: Echocardiographic observations of calcium in operatively excised stenotic aortic valves. Am. J. Cardiol. 59:324, 1987.

24. Bansal, R.C., Tajik, A.J., Seward, J.B., et al.: Feasibility of detailed two-dimensional echocardiographic examination in adults: Prospective study of 200 patients. Mayo Clin. Proc. 55:291, 1980.

25. Tajik, A.J., Seward, J.B., Hagler, D.J., et al.: Two-dimensional real-time ultrasonic imaging of the heart and great vessels: Technique, image orientation, structure identification, and validation. Mayo Clin. Proc. 53:271, 1978.

26. Brandenburg, R.O., Jr., Tajik, A.J., Edwards, W.D., et al.: Accuracy of 2-dimensional echocardiographic diagnosis of congenitally bicuspid aortic valve: Echocardiographic-anatomic correlation in 115 patients. Am. J. Cardiol. 51:1469, 1983.

27. Nanda, N.C., and Gramiak, R.: Evaluation of bicuspid valves by two-dimensional echocardiography. (Abstract.) Am. J. Cardiol. 41:372, 1978.

28. Kennedy, K.D., Hauck, A.J., Edwards, W.D., et al.: Mechanism of reduction of aortic valvular stenosis by percutaneous transluminal balloon valvuloplasty: Report of five cases and review of literature. Mayo Clin. Proc. 63:769, 1988.

29. Larson, E.W., and Edwards, W.D.: Risk factors for aortic dissection: A necropsy study of 161 cases. Am. J. Cardiol. 53:849, 1984.

29a. Seward, J.B., and Tajik, A.J.: Noninvasive visualization of the entire thoracic aorta: A new application of wide-angle two-dimensional sector echocardiographic technique. (Abstract.) Am. J. Cardiol. 43:387, 1979.

30. Schwartz, A., Vignola, P.A., Walker, H.J., et al.: Echocardiographic estimation of aortic-valve gradient in aortic stenosis. Ann. Intern. Med. 89:329, 1978.

31. Oh, J.K., Taliercio, C.P., Holmes, D.R., Jr., et al.: Prediction of the severity of aortic stenosis by Doppler aortic valve area determination: Prospective Doppler-catheterization correlation in 100 patients. J. Am. Coll. Cardiol. 11:1227, 1988.

32. Nishimura, R.A., Miller, F.A., Jr., Callahan, M.J., et al.: Doppler echocardiography: Theory, instrumentation, technique, and application. Mayo Clin. Proc. 60:321, 1985.

33. Currie, P.J., Seward, J.B., Reeder, G.S., et al.: Continuous-wave Doppler echocardiographic assessment of severity of calcific aortic stenosis: A simultaneous Doppler-catheter correlative study in 100 adult patients. Circulation 71:1162, 1985.

34. Currie, P.J., Hagler, D.J., Seward, J.B., et al.: Instantaneous pressure gradient: A simultaneous Doppler and dual-catheter correlative study. J. Am. Coll. Cardiol. 7:800, 1986.

35. Hatle, L., Angelsen, B.A., and Tromsdal, A.: Non-invasive assessment of aortic stenosis by Doppler ultrasound. Br. Heart J. 43:284, 1980.

36. Stamm, R.B., and Martin, R.P.: Quantification of pressure gradients across stenotic valves by Doppler ultrasound. J. Am. Coll. Cardiol. 2:707, 1983.

37. Sasson, Z., Yock, P.G., Hatle, L.K., et al.: Doppler echocardiographic determination of the pressure gradient in hypertrophic cardiomyopathy. J. Am. Coll. Cardiol. 11:752, 1988.

38. Yock, P.G., Hatle, L., and Popp, R.L.: Patterns and timing of Doppler-detected intracavitary and aortic flow in hypertrophic cardiomyopathy. J. Am. Coll. Cardiol. 8:1047, 1986.

39. Callahan, M.J., Tajik, A.J., Su-Fan, Q., et al.: Validation of instantaneous pressure gradients measured by continuous-wave Doppler in experimentally induced aortic stenosis. Am. J. Cardiol. 56:989, 1985.

40. Smith, M.D., Dawson, P.L., Elion, J.L., et al.: Correlation of continuous wave Doppler velocities with cardiac catheterization gradients: An experimental model of aortic stenosis. J. Am. Coll. Cardiol. 6:1306, 1985.

41. Carabello, B., and Grossman, W.: Calculation of stenotic valve orifice area. In Grossman, W. (ed.): Cardiac Catheterization and Angiography. Philadelphia, Lea & Febiger, 1986, p. 143.

42. Teirstein, P., Yeager, M., Yock, P.G., et al.: Doppler echocardiographic measurement of aortic valve area in aortic stenosis: A noninvasive application of the Gorlin formula. J. Am. Coll. Cardiol. 8:1059, 1986.

43. Fan, P-H., Kapur, K.K., and Nanda, N.C.: Color-guided Doppler echocardiographic assessment of aortic valve stenosis. J. Am. Coll. Cardiol. 12:441, 1988.

44. Otto, C.M., Pearlman, A.S., Comess, K.A., et al.: Determination of the stenotic aortic valve area in adults using Doppler echocardiography. J. Am. Coll. Cardiol. 7:509, 1986.

45. Otto, C.M., Pearlman, A.S., and Gardner, C.L.: Hemodynamic progression of aortic stenosis in adults assessed by Doppler echocardiography. J. Am. Coll. Cardiol. 13:545, 1989.

46. Skjaerpe, T., Hegrenaes, L., and Hatle, L.: Noninvasive estimation of valve area in patients with aortic stenosis by Doppler ultrasound and two-dimensional echocardiography. Circulation 72:810, 1985.

47. Zoghbi, W.A., Farmer, K.L., Soto, J.G., et al.: Accurate noninvasive quantification of stenotic valve area by Doppler echocardiography. Circulation 73:452, 1986.

48. Selzer, A., and Sudrann, R.B.: Reliability of the determination of cardiac output in man by means of the Fick principle. Circ. Res. 6:485, 1958.

49. Thomasson, B.: Cardiac output in normal subjects under standard conditions: The repeatability of measurements by the Fick method. Scand. J. Clin. Lab. Invest. 9:365, 1957.

50. Visscher, M.B., and Johnson, J.A.: The Fick principle: Analysis of potential errors in its conventional application. J. Appl. Physiol. 5:635, 1953.

51. Van Grondelle, A., Ditchey, R.V., Groves, B.M., et al.: Thermodilution method overestimates low cardiac output in humans. Am. J. Physiol. 245:H690, 1983.

52. Gorlin, R., and Gorlin, S.G.: Hydraulic formula for calculation of the area of the stenotic mitral valve, other cardiac valves, and central circulatory shunts: I. Am. Heart J. 41:1, 1951.

53. Cannon, S.R., Richards, K.L., and Crawford, M.: Hydraulic estimation of stenotic orifice area: A correction of the Gorlin formula. Circulation 71:1170, 1985.

54. Segal, J., Lerner, D.J., Miller, D.C., et al.: When should Doppler-determined valve area be better than the Gorlin formula? Variation in hydraulic constants in low flow states. J. Am. Coll. Cardiol. 9:1294, 1987.

55. Rijsterborgh, H., and Roelandt, J.: Doppler assessment of aortic stenosis: Bernoulli revisited. Ultrasound Med. Biol. 13:241, 1987.

56. Pellikka, P.A., Nishimura, R.A., Bailey, K.R., et al.: The natural history of adults with asymptomatic, hemodynamically significant aortic stenosis. J. Am. Coll. Cardiol. 15:1012, 1990.

57. Edwards, J.E.: Pathologic aspects of cardiac valvular insufficiencies. Arch. Surg. 77:634, 1958.

58. Edwards, J.E.: Pathology of acquired valvular disease of the heart. Semin. Roentgenol. 14:96, 1979.

59. Olson, L.J., Subramanian, R., and Edwards, W.D.: Surgical pathology of pure aortic insufficiency: A study of 225 cases. Mayo Clin. Proc. 59:835, 1984.

59a. Roberts, W.C.: Left ventricular outflow tract obstruction and aortic regurgitation. Monogr. Pathol. 15:110, 1974.

60. Subramanian, R., Olson, L.J., and Edwards, W.D.: Surgical pathology of combined aortic stenosis and insufficiency: A study of 213 cases. Mayo Clin. Proc. 60:247, 1985.

61. Erbel, R., Rohmann, S., Drexler, M., et al.: Improved diagnostic value of echocardiography in patients with infective endocarditis by transoesophageal approach: A prospective study. Eur. Heart J. 9:43, 1988.

62. Stewart, W.J., Agler, D.A., Koch, J.M., et al.: Color flow mapping diagnosis and localization of paravalvular aortic regurgitation. (Abstract.) Circulation 76(Suppl. IV):IV-448, 1987.

63. Daniel, W.G., Mügge, A., Martin, R.D., et al.: Improvement in the diagnoses of abscesses associated with endocarditis by transesophageal echocardiography. N. Engl. J. Med. 324:795, 1991.

64. Silverman, K.J., and Hutchins, G.M.: Spontaneous dehiscence of an aortic commissure complicating idiopathic aortic root dilatation. Am. Heart J. 97:367, 1979.

65. Carter, J.B., Sethi, S., Lee, G.B., et al.: Prolapse of semilunar cusps as causes of aortic insufficiency. Circulation 43:922, 1971.

66. Bulkley, B.H., and Roberts, W.C.: Ankylosing spondylitis and aortic regurgitation: Description of the characteristic cardiovascular lesion from study of eight necropsy patients. Circulation 48:1014, 1973.

67. Stewart, S.R., Robbins, D.L., and Castles, J.J.: Acute fulminant aortic and mitral insufficiency in ankylosing spondylitis. N. Engl. J. Med. 299:1448, 1978.

68. Tucker, C.R., Fowles, R.E., Calin, A., et al.: Aortitis in ankylosing spondylitis: Early detection of aortic root abnormalities with two-dimensional echocardiography. Am. J. Cardiol. 49:680, 1982.

69. DeMaria, A.N., Bommer, W., Neumann, A., et al.: Identification and localization of aneurysms of the ascending aorta by cross-sectional echocardiography. Circulation 59:755, 1979.

70. Davies, M.J.: Pathology of Cardiac Valves. London, Butterworth, 1980, p. 37.

71. Edwards, J.E.: Pathology of aortic incompetence. In Silver, M.D. (ed.): Cardiovascular Pathology. Vol 1. New York, Churchill Livingstone, 1983, p. 619.

72. Roberts, W.C.: Aortic dissection: Anatomy, consequences, and causes. Am. Heart J. 101:195, 1981.

73. Khandheria, B.K., Tajik, A.J., Taylor, C.L., et al.: Aortic dissection: Review of

value and limitations of two-dimensional echocardiography in a six year experience. J. Am. Soc. Echocardiogr. 2:17, 1989.
74. el Haitem, N., Chaara, A., Mesbahi, R., et al.: Rupture traumatique du sinus de Valsalva antéro-droit dans le ventricule droit, associée à une insuffisance aortique. Arch. Mal. Coeur 81:793, 1988.
75. Roberts, W.C., Morrow, A.G., McIntosh, C.L., et al.: Congenitally bicuspid aortic valve causing severe, pure aortic regurgitation without superimposed infective endocarditis: Analysis of 13 patients requiring aortic valve replacement. Am. J. Cardiol. 47:206, 1981.
76. Davia, J.E., Fenoglio, J.J., DeCastro, C.M., et al.: Quadricuspid semilunar valves. Chest 72:186, 1977.
77. Pyeritz, R.E., and McKusick, V.A.: The Marfan syndrome: Diagnosis and management. N. Engl. J. Med. 300:772, 1979.
78. Leier, C.V., Call, T.D., Fulkerson, P.K., et al.: The spectrum of cardiac defects in the Ehlers-Danlos syndrome, types I and III. Ann. Intern. Med. 92:171, 1980.
79. Sahn, D.J., Allen, H.D., McDonald, G., et al.: Real-time cross-sectional echocardiographic diagnosis of coarctation of the aorta: A prospective study of echocardiographic-angiographic correlations. Circulation 56:762, 1977.
80. Pyeritz, R.E., and Wappel, M.A.: Mitral valve dysfunction in the Marfan syndrome: Clinical and echocardiographic study of prevalence and natural history. Am. J. Med. 74:797, 1983.
81. McDonald, I.G.: Echocardiographic assessment of left ventricular function in aortic valve disease. Circulation 53:860, 1976.
82. McDonald, I.G., and Jelinek, V.M.: Serial M-mode echocardiography in severe chronic aortic regurgitation. Circulation 62:1291, 1980.
83. Cope, G.D., Kisslo, J.A., Johnson, M.L., et al.: Diastolic vibration of the interventricular septum in aortic insufficiency. Circulation 51:589, 1975.
84. D'Cruz, I., Cohen, H.C., Prabhu, R., et al.: Flutter of left ventricular structures in patients with aortic regurgitation, with special reference to patients with associated mitral stenosis. Am. Heart J. 92:684, 1976.
85. Johnson, A.D., and Gosink, B.B.: Oscillation of left ventricular structures in aortic regurgitation. J. Clin. Ultrasound 5:21, 1977.
86. Botvinick, E.H., Schiller, N.B., Wickramasekaran, R., et al.: Echocardiographic demonstration of early mitral valve closure in severe aortic insufficiency: Its clinical implications. Circulation 51:836, 1975.
87. Morganroth, J., Perloff, J.K., and Zeldis, S.M.: Acute severe aortic regurgitation: Pathophysiology, clinical recognition, and management. Ann. Intern. Med. 87:223, 1977.
88. Cunha, C.L.P., Guiliani, E.R., Fuster, V., et al.: Preoperative M-mode echocardiography as a predictor of surgical results in chronic aortic insufficiency. J. Thorac. Cardiovasc. Surg. 79:256, 1980.
89. Daniel, W.G., Hood, W.P., Jr., Siart, A., et al.: Chronic aortic regurgitation: Reassessment of the prognostic value of preoperative left ventricular end-systolic dimension and fractional shortening. Circulation 71:669, 1985.
90. Fioretti, P., Roelandt, J., Bos, R.J., et al.: Echocardiography in chronic aortic insufficiency: Is valve replacement too late when left ventricular end-systolic dimension reaches 55 mm? Circulation 67:216, 1983.
91. Gaasch, W.H., Carroll, J.D., Levine, H.J., et al.: Chronic aortic regurgitation: Prognostic value of left ventricular end-systolic dimension and end-diastolic radius/thickness ratio. J. Am. Coll. Cardiol. 1:775, 1983.
92. Henry, W.L., Bonow, R.O., Borer, J.S., et al.: Observations on the optimum time for operative intervention for aortic regurgitation: I. Evaluation of the results of aortic valve replacement in symptomatic patients. Circulation 61:471, 1980.
93. Henry, W.L., Bonow, R.O., Rosing, D.R., et al.: Observations on the optimum time for operative intervention for aortic regurgitation: II. Serial echocardiographic evaluation of asymptomatic patients. Circulation 61:484, 1980.
94. Kumpuris, A.G., Quinones, M.A., Waggoner, A.D., et al.: Importance of preoperative hypertrophy, wall stress and end-systolic dimension as echocardiographic predictors of normalization of left ventricular dilatation after valve replacement in chronic aortic insufficiency. Am. J. Cardiol. 49:1091, 1982.
95. Nishimura, R.A., McGoon, M.D., Schaff, H.V., et al.: Chronic aortic regurgitation: Indications for operation—1988. Mayo Clin. Proc. 63:270, 1988.
96. Bonow, R.O., Lakatos, E., Maron, B.J., et al. Serial long-term assessment of the natural history of asymptomatic patients with chronic aortic regurgitation and normal left ventricular systolic function. Circulation 84:1625, 1991.
97. Ciobanu, M., Abbasi, A.S., Allen, M., et al.: Pulsed Doppler echocardiography in the diagnosis and estimation of severity of aortic insufficiency. Am. J. Cardiol. 49:339, 1982.
98. Grayburn, P.A., Smith, M.D., Handshoe, R., et al.: Detection of aortic insufficiency by standard echocardiography, pulsed Doppler echocardiography, and auscultation: A comparison of accuracies. Ann. Intern. Med. 104:599, 1986.
99. Wautrecht, J.C., Vandenbossche, J.L., and Englert, M.: Sensitivity and specificity of pulsed Doppler echocardiography in detection of aortic and mitral regurgitation. Eur. Heart J. 5:404, 1984.
100. Masuyama, T., Kodama, K., Kitabatake, A., et al.: Noninvasive evaluation of aortic regurgitation by continuous-wave Doppler echocardiography. Circulation 73:460, 1986.
101. Omoto, R., Yokote, Y., Takamoto, S., et al.: The development of real-time two-dimensional Doppler echocardiography and its clinical significance in acquired valvular diseases: With special reference to the evaluation of valvular regurgitation. Jpn. Heart J. 25:325, 1984.
102. Perry, G.J., Helmcke, F., Nanda, N.C., et al.: Evaluation of aortic insufficiency by Doppler color flow mapping. J. Am. Coll. Cardiol. 9:952, 1987.
103. Switzer, D.F., Yoganathan, A.P., Nanda, N.C., et al.: Calibration of color Doppler flow mapping during extreme hemodynamic conditions in vitro: A foundation for a reliable quantitative grading system for aortic incompetence. Circulation 75:837, 1987.
104. Quinones, M.A., Yound, J.B., Waggoner, A.D., et al.: Assessment of pulsed Doppler echocardiography in detection and quantification of aortic and mitral regurgitation. Br. Heart J. 44:612, 1980.
105. Takenaka, K., Dabestani, A., Gardin, J.M., et al.: A simple Doppler echocardiographic method for estimating severity of aortic regurgitation. Am. J. Cardiol. 57:1340, 1986.
106. Grayburn, P.A., Handshoe, R., Smith, M.D., et al.: Quantitative assessment of the hemodynamic consequences of aortic regurgitation by means of continuous wave Doppler recordings. J. Am. Coll. Cardiol. 10:135, 1987.
107. Labovitz, A.J., Ferrara, R.P., Kern, M.J., et al.: Quantitative evaluation of aortic insufficiency by continuous wave Doppler echocardiography. J. Am. Coll. Cardiol. 8:1341, 1986.
108. Teague, S.M., Heinsimer, J.A., Anderson, J.L., et al.: Quantification of aortic regurgitation utilizing continuous wave Doppler ultrasound. J. Am. Coll. Cardiol. 8:592, 1986.
109. Enriquez-Sarano, M., Seward, J.B., Bailey, K.R., et al.: Effective regurgitant orifice area: A noninvasive Doppler development of an old hemodynamic concept. J. Am. Coll. Cardiol. 23:443, 1994.
110. Reimold, S.C., Maier, S.E., Fleischman, K.E., et al.: Dynamic nature of the aortic regurgitant orifice area during diastole in patients with chronic aortic regurgitation. Circulation 89:2085, 1994.
111. Libanoff, A.J.: A hemodynamic measure of aortic regurgitation: Half-time of the rate of fall in aortic pressure during diastole. Cardiology 58:162, 1973.
112. Nishimura, R.A., and Tajik, A.J.: Determination of left-sided pressure gradients by utilizing Doppler aortic and mitral regurgitant signals: Validation by simultaneous dual-catheter and Doppler studies. J. Am. Coll. Cardiol. 11:317, 1988.
113. Rokey, R., Sterling, L.L., Zoghbi, W.A., et al.: Determination of regurgitant fraction in isolated mitral or aortic regurgitation by pulsed Doppler two-dimensional echocardiography. J. Am. Coll. Cardiol. 7:1273, 1986.
114. Arvidsson, H., and Karnell, J.: Quantitative assessment of mitral and aortic insufficiency by angiocardiography. Acta Radiol. 2:105, 1964.
115. Croft, C.H., Lipscomb, K., Mathis, K., et al.: Limitations of qualitative angiographic grading in aortic or mitral regurgitation. Am. J. Cardiol. 53:1593, 1984.
116. Fifer, M.A., and Grossman, W.: Measurement of ventricular volumes, ejection fraction, mass and wall stress. *In* Grossman, W. (ed.): Cardiac Catheterization and Angiography. Philadelphia, Lea & Febiger, 1986, p. 282.
117. Sandler, H., Dodge, H.T., Hay, R.E., et al.: Quantitation of valvular insufficiency in man by angiocardiography. Am. Heart J. 65:501, 1963.
118. Olson, L.J., Subramanian, R., Ackermann, D.M., et al.: Surgical pathology of the mitral valve: A study of 712 cases spanning 21 years. Mayo Clin. Proc. 62:22, 1987.
119. Roberts, W.C.: Morphologic features of the normal and abnormal mitral valve. Am. J. Cardiol. 51:1005, 1983.
120. Rusted, I.E., Scheifley, C.H., and Edwards, J.E.: Studies of the mitral valve: II. Certain anatomic features of the mitral valve and associated structures in mitral stenosis. Circulation 14:398, 1956.
121. Hammer, W.J., Roberts, W.C., and DeLeon, A.C., Jr.: "Mitral stenosis" secondary to combined "massive" mitral anular calcific deposits and small, hypertrophied left ventricles: Hemodynamic documentation in four patients. Am. J. Med. 64:371, 1978.
122. Osterberger, L.E., Goldstein, S., Khaja, F., et al.: Functional mitral stenosis in patients with massive annular calcification. Circulation 64:472, 1981.
123. Weyman, A.E.: Cross-Sectional Echocardiography. Philadelphia, Lea & Febiger, 1982, p. 150.
124. Pomerance, A.: Chronic rheumatic and other inflammatory valve disease. *In* Pomerance, A., Davies, M.J. (eds.): The Pathology of the Heart. London, Blackwell Scientific, 1975, p. 307.
125. Zanolla, L., Marino, P., Nicolosi, G.L., et al.: Two-dimensional echocardiographic evaluation of mitral valve calcification: Sensitivity and specificity. Chest 82:154, 1982.
126. Ruckman, R.N., and Van Praagh, R.: Anatomic types of congenital mitral stenosis: Report of 49 autopsy cases with consideration of diagnosis and surgical implications. Am. J. Cardiol. 42:592, 1978.
127. Snider, A.R., Roge, C.L., Schiller, N.B., et al.: Congenital left ventricular inflow obstruction evaluated by two-dimensional echocardiography. Circulation 61:848, 1980.
128. Shone, J.D., Sellers, R.D., Anderson, R.C., et al.: The developmental complex of "parachute mitral valve," supravalvular ring of left atrium, subaortic stenosis, and coarctation of aorta. Am. J. Cardiol. 11:714, 1963.
129. Glover, M.U., Warren, S.E., Vieweg, W.V.R., et al.: M-mode and two-dimensional echocardiographic correlation with findings at catheterization and surgery in patients with mitral stenosis. Am. Heart J. 105:98, 1983.
130. Henry, W.L., Griffith, J.M., Michaelis, L.L., et al.: Measurement of mitral orifice area in patients with mitral valve disease by real-time, two-dimensional echocardiography. Circulation 51:827, 1975.
131. Wann, L.S., Weyman, A.E., Feigenbaum, H., et al.: Determination of mitral valve area by cross-sectional echocardiography. Ann. Intern. Med. 88:337, 1978.
132. Martin, R.P., Rakowski, H., Kleiman, J.H., et al.: Reliability and reproducibility of two-dimensional echocardiographic measurement of the stenotic mitral valve orifice area. Am. J. Cardiol. 43:560, 1979.
133. Smith, M.D., Handshoe, R., Handshoe, S., et al.: Comparative accuracy of two-dimensional echocardiography and Doppler pressure half-time methods in assessing severity of mitral stenosis in patients with and without prior commissurotomy. Circulation 73:100, 1986.
134. Wilkins, G.T., Weyman, A.E., Abascal, V.M., et al.: Percutaneous balloon dilatation of the mitral valve: An analysis of echocardiographic variables related to outcome and the mechanism of dilatation. Br. Heart J. 60:299, 1988.

135. Holen, J., Aaslid, R., Landmark, K., et al.: Determination of pressure gradient in mitral stenosis with a non-invasive ultrasound Doppler technique. Acta Med. Scand. 199:455, 1976.
136. Hatle, L., Brubakk, A., Tromsdal, A., et al.: Noninvasive assessment of pressure drop in mitral stenosis by Doppler ultrasound. Br. Heart J. 40:131, 1978.
137. Holen, J., and Simonsen, S.: Determination of pressure gradient in mitral stenosis with Doppler echocardiography. Br. Heart J. 41:529, 1979.
138. Knutsen, K.M., Bae, E.A., Sivertssen, E., et al.: Doppler ultrasound in mitral stenosis: Assessment of pressure gradient and atrioventricular pressure half-time. Acta Med. Scand. 211:433, 1982.
139. Khandheria, B.K., Tajik, A.J., Reeder, G.S., et al.: Doppler color flow imaging: A new technique for visualization and characterization of the blood flow jet in mitral stenosis. Mayo Clin. Proc. 61:623, 1986.
140. Libanoff, A.J., and Rodbard, S.: Atrioventricular pressure half-time: Measure of mitral valve orifice area. Circulation 38:144, 1968.
141. Hatle, L., Angelsen, B., and Tromsdal, A.: Noninvasive assessment of atrioventricular pressure half-time by Doppler ultrasound. Circulation 60:1096, 1979.
142. Holen, J., Aaslid, R., Landmark, K., et al.: Determination of effective orifice area in mitral stenosis from non-invasive ultrasound Doppler data and mitral flow rate. Acta Med. Scand. 201:83, 1977.
143. Bryg, R.J., Williams, G.A., Labovitz, A.J., et al.: Effect of atrial fibrillation and mitral regurgitation on calculated mitral valve area in mitral stenosis. Am. J. Cardiol. 57:634, 1986.
144. Reid, C.L., McKay, C.R., Chandraratna, P.A.N., et al.: Mechanisms of increase in mitral valve area and influence of anatomic features in double-balloon, catheter balloon valvuloplasty in adults with rheumatic mitral stenosis: A Doppler and two-dimensional echocardiographic study. Circulation 76:628, 1987.
145. Moro, E., Nicolosi, G.L., Zanuttini, D., et al.: Influence of aortic regurgitation on the assessment of the pressure half-time and derived mitral-valve area in patients with mitral stenosis. Eur. Heart J. 9:1010, 1988.
146. Procacci, P.M., Savran, S.V., Schreiter, S.L., et al.: Prevalence of clinical mitral-valve prolapse in 1169 young women. N. Engl. J. Med. 294:1086, 1976.
147. Nakatani, S., Masuyama, T., Kodama, K., et al.: Value and limitations of Doppler echocardiography in the quantification of stenotic mitral valve area: Comparison of the pressure half-time and the continuity equation methods. Circulation 77:78, 1988.
148. Karp, K., Teien, D., Bjerle, P., et al.: Reassessment of valve area determinations in mitral stenosis by the pressure half-time method: Impact of left ventricular stiffness and peak diastolic pressure difference. J. Am. Coll. Cardiol. 13:594, 1989.
149. Rodriquez, L., Thomas, J.D., Monterosso, V., et al.: Validation of the proximal flow convergence method: Calculation of orifice area in patients with mitral stenosis. Circulation 88:1157, 1993.
150. Deng, Y.B., Matsumoto, M., Wang, X.F., et al.: Estimation of mitral valve area in patients with mitral stenosis by the flow convergence region method: Selection of aliasing velocity. J. Am. Coll. Cardiol. 24:683, 1994.
151. Leavitt, J.I., Coats, M.H., and Falk, R.H.: Effects of exercise on transmitral gradient and pulmonary artery pressure in patients with mitral stenosis or a prosthetic mitral valve: A Doppler echocardiographic study. J. Am. Coll. Cardiol. 17:1520, 1991.
152. Tunick, P.A., Freedberg, R.S., Garginlo, A., et al.: Exercise Doppler echocardiography as an aid to clinical decision making in mitral valve disease. J. Am. Soc. Echocardiogr. 5:225, 1992.
153. Nishimura, R.A., Rihal, C.S., Tajik, A.J., et al.: Accurate measurement of the transmitral gradient in patients with mitral stenosis: A simultaneous catheterization and Doppler echocardiographic study. J. Am. Coll. Cardiol. 24:152, 1994.
154. Perloff, J.K., and Roberts, W.C.: The mitral apparatus: Functional anatomy of mitral regurgitation. Circulation 46:227, 1972.
155. Roberts, W.C., and Perloff, J.K.: Mitral valvular disease: A clinicopathologic survey of the conditions causing the mitral valve to function abnormally. Ann. Intern. Med. 77:939, 1972.
156. Levine, R.A., Stathogiannis, E., Newell, J.B., et al.: Reconsideration of echocardiographic standards for mitral valve prolapse: Lack of association between leaflet displacement isolated to the apical four chamber view and independent echocardiographic evidence of abnormality. J. Am. Coll. Cardiol. 11:1010, 1988.
157. Gilbert, B.W., Schatz, R.A., VonRamm, O.T., et al.: Mitral valve prolapse: Two-dimensional echocardiographic and angiographic correlation. Circulation 54:716, 1976.
158. Mintz, G.S., Kotler, M.N., Segal, B.L., et al.: Two-dimensional echocardiographic evaluation of patients with mitral insufficiency. Am. J. Cardiol. 44:670, 1979.
159. Marks, A.R., Choong, C.Y., Sanfilippo, A.J., et al.: Identification of high-risk and low-risk subgroups of patients with mitral-valve prolapse. N. Engl. J. Med. 320:1031, 1989.
160. Nishimura, R.A., McGoon, M.D., Shub, C., et al.: Echocardiographically documented mitral-valve prolapse: Long-term follow-up of 237 patients. N. Engl. J. Med. 313:1305, 1985.
161. Devereux, R.B., Kramer-Fox, R.B., Shear, M.K., et al.: Diagnosis and classification of severity of mitral valve prolapse: Methodologic, biologic, and prognostic considerations. Am. Heart J. 113:1265, 1987.
162. Pini, R., Greppi, B., Kramer-Fox, R., et al.: Mitral valve dimensions and motion and familial transmission of mitral valve prolapse with and without mitral leaflet billowing. J. Am. Coll. Cardiol. 12:1423, 1988.
163. Pini, R., Devereux, R.B., Greppi, B., et al.: Comparison of mitral valve dimensions and motion in mitral valve prolapse with severe mitral regurgitation to uncomplicated mitral valve prolapse and to mitral regurgitation without mitral valve prolapse. Am. J. Cardiol. 62:257, 1988.
164. Düren, D.R., Becker, A.E., and Dunning, A.J.: Long-term follow-up of idiopathic mitral valve prolapse in 300 patients: A prospective study. J. Am. Coll. Cardiol. 11:42, 1988.
165. MacMahon, S.W., Roberts, J.K., Kramer-Fox, R., et al.: Mitral valve prolapse and infective endocarditis. Am. Heart J. 113:1291, 1987.
166. Wilcken, D.E.L., and Hickey, A.J.: Lifetime risk for patients with mitral valve prolapse of developing severe valve regurgitation requiring surgery. Circulation 78:10, 1988.
167. Devereux, R.B., Hawkins, I., Kramer-Fox, R., et al.: Complications of mitral valve prolapse: Disproportionate occurrence in men and older patients. Am. J. Med. 81:751, 1986.
168. Goodman, D., Kimbiris, D., and Linhart, J.W.: Chordae tendineae rupture complicating the systolic click–late systolic murmur syndrome. Am. J. Cardiol. 33:681, 1974.
169. Grenadier, E., Alpan, G., Keidar, S., et al.: The prevalence of ruptured chordae tendineae in the mitral valve prolapse syndrome. Am. Heart J. 105:603, 1983.
170. Hickey, A.J., Wilcken, D.E.L., Wright, J.S., et al.: Primary (spontaneous) chordal rupture: Relation to myxomatous valve disease and mitral valve prolapse. J. Am. Coll. Cardiol. 5:1341, 1985.
171. Osmundson, P.J., Callahan, J.A., and Edwards, J.E.: Ruptured mitral chordae tendineae. Circulation 23:42, 1961.
172. Oliveira, D.B.G., Dawkins, K.D., Kay, P.H., et al.: Chordal rupture: I. Aetiology and natural history. Br. Heart J. 50:312, 1983.
173. Roberts, W.C., Braunwald, E., and Morrow, A.G.: Acute severe mitral regurgitation secondary to ruptured chordae tendineae: Clinical, hemodynamic, and pathologic considerations. Circulation 33:58, 1966.
174. Mintz, G.S., Kotler, M.N., Segal, B.L., et al.: Two-dimensional echocardiographic recognition of ruptured chordae tendineae. Circulation 57:244, 1978.
175. Erbel, R., Schweizer, P., Bardos, P., et al.: Two-dimensional echocardiographic diagnosis of papillary muscle rupture. Chest 79:595, 1981.
176. Nishimura, R.A., Schaff, H.V., Shub, C., et al.: Papillary muscle rupture complicating acute myocardial infarction: Analysis of 17 patients. Am. J. Cardiol. 51:373, 1983.
177. Himelman, R.B., Kusumoto, F., Oken, K., et al.: The flail mitral valve: Echocardiographic findings by precordial and transesophageal imaging and Doppler color flow mapping. J. Am. Coll. Cardiol. 17:272, 1991.
178. Edwards, J.E.: Pathology of mitral incompetence. *In* Silver, M.D. (ed.): Cardiovascular Pathology. Vol. 1. New York, Churchill Livingstone, 1983, p. 575.
179. Godley, R.W., Wann, L.S., Rogers, E.W., et al.: Incomplete mitral leaflet closure in patients with papillary muscle dysfunction. Circulation 63:565, 1981.
180. Martin, R.P., Meltzer, R.S., Chia, B.L., et al.: Clinical utility of two-dimensional echocardiography in infective endocarditis. Am. J. Cardiol. 46:379, 1980.
181. Daniel, W.G., Schröder, E., Mügge, A., et al.: Transesophageal echocardiography in infective endocarditis. Am. J. Card. Imaging 2:78, 1988.
182. Nestico, P.F., Depace, N.L., Morganroth, J., et al.: Mitral annular calcification: Clinical, pathophysiology, and echocardiographic review. Am. Heart J. 107:989, 1984.
183. Byram, M.T., and Roberts, W.C.: Frequency and extent of calcific deposits in purely regurgitant mitral valves: Analysis of 108 operatively excised valves. Am. J. Cardiol. 52:1059, 1983.
184. Davies, M.J.: Pathology of Cardiac Valves. London, Butterworth, 1980, p. 73.
185. Di Segni, E., and Edwards, J.E.: Cleft anterior leaflet of the mitral valve with intact septa: A study of 20 cases. Am. J. Cardiol. 51:919, 1983.
186. McGoon, D.C.: Repair of mitral insufficiency due to ruptured chordae tendineae. J. Thorac. Cardiovasc. Surg. 39:357, 1960.
187. Zile, M.R., Gaasch, W.H., Carroll, J.D., et al.: Chronic mitral regurgitation: Predictive value of preoperative echocardiographic indexes of left ventricular function and wall stress. J. Am. Coll. Cardiol. 3:235, 1984.
188. Zile, M.R., Gaasch, W.H., and Levine, H.J.: Left ventricular stress-dimension-shortening relations before and after correction of chronic aortic and mitral regurgitation. Am. J. Cardiol. 56:99, 1985.
189. Reed, D., Abbott, R.D., Smucker, M.L., et al.: Prediction of outcome after mitral valve replacment in patients with symptomatic chronic mitral regurgitation: The importance of left atrial size. Circulation 84:23, 1991.
190. Enriquez-Sarano, M., Tajik, A.J., Schaff, H.V., et al.: Echocardiographic prediction of survival after surgical correction of organic mitral regurgitation. Circulation 90:830, 1994.
191. Abbasi, A.S., Allen, M.W., DeCristofaro, D., et al.: Detection and estimation of the degree of mitral regurgitation by range-gated pulsed Doppler echocardiography. Circulation 61:143, 1980.
192. Blanchard, D., Diebold, B., Peronneau, P., et al.: Non-invasive diagnosis of mitral regurgitation by Doppler echocardiography. Br. Heart J. 45:589, 1981.
193. Veyrat, C., Ameur, A., Bas, S., et al.: Pulsed Doppler echocardiographic indices for assessing mitral regurgitation. Br. Heart J. 51:130, 1984.
194. Miyatake, K., Izumi, S., Okamoto, M., et al.: Semiquantitative grading of severity of mitral regurgitation by real-time two-dimensional Doppler flow imaging technique. J. Am. Coll. Cardiol. 7:82, 1986.
195. Miyatake, K., Okamoto, M., Kinoshita, N., et al.: Clinical applications of a new type of real-time two-dimensional Doppler flow imaging system. Am. J. Cardiol. 54:857, 1984.
196. Yoshida, K., Yoshikawa, J., Shakudo, M., et al.: Color Doppler evaluation of valvular regurgitation in normal subjects. Circulation 78:840, 1988.
197. Klein, A.L., Burstow, D.J., Tajik, A.J., et al.: Age-related prevalence of valvular regurgitation in normal subjects: A comprehensive color flow examination of 118 volunteers. J. Am. Soc. Echocardiogr. 3:54, 1990.
198. Helmcke, F., Nanda, N.C., Hsuing, M.C., et al.: Color Doppler assessment of mitral regurgitation with orthogonal planes. Circulation 75:175, 1987.
199. Spain, M.G., Smith, M.D., Grayburn, P.A., et al.: Quantitative assessment of

mitral regurgitation by Doppler color flow imaging: Angiographic and hemodynamic correlations. J. Am. Coll. Cardiol. 13:585, 1989.

200. Smith, M.D., Grayburn, P.A., Spain, M.G., et al.: Observer variability in the quantitation of Doppler color flow jet areas for mitral and aortic regurgitation. J. Am. Coll. Cardiol. 11:579, 1988.

201. Sahn, D.J.: Instrumentation and physical factors related to visualization of stenotic and regurgitant jets by Doppler color flow mapping. J. Am. Coll. Cardiol. 12:1354, 1988.

202. Cape, E.G., Yoganathan, A.P., Weyman, A.E., et al.: Adjacent solid boundaries alter the size of regurgitant jets on Doppler color flow maps. J. Am. Coll. Cardiol. 17:1094, 1991.

203. Castello, R., Pearson, A.C., Lenzen, P., et al.: Effect of mitral regurgitation on pulmonary venous velocities derived from transesophageal echocardiography color-guided pulsed Doppler imaging. J. Am. Coll. Cardiol. 17:1499, 1991.

204. Klein, A.L., Obarski, T.P., Stewart, W.J., et al.: Transesophageal Doppler echocardiography of pulmonary venous flow: A new marker of mitral regurgitation severity. J. Am. Coll. Cardiol. 18:518, 1991.

205. Chung, N., Nishimura, R.A., Holmes, D.R., Jr., et al.: Measurement of left ventricular dP/dt by simultaneous Doppler echocardiography and cardiac catheterization. J. Am. Soc. Echocardiogr. 5:147, 1992.

206. Chen, C., Rodriquez, L., Guerrero, J.L., et al.: Noninvasive estimation of the instantaneous first-derivative of left ventricular pressure using continuous-wave Doppler echocardiography. Circulation 83:2101, 1991.

207. Enriquez-Sarano, M., Kaneshige, A.M., Tajik, A.J., et al.: Amplitude-weighted mean velocity: Clinical utilization for quantitation of mitral regurgitation. J. Am. Coll. Cardiol. 22:1684, 1993.

208. Blumlein, S., Bouchard, A., Schiller, N.B., et al.: Quantitation of mitral regurgitation by Doppler echocardiography. Circulation 74:306, 1986.

209. Enriquez-Sarano, M., Bailey, K.R., Seward, J.B., et al.: Quantitative Doppler assessment of valvular regurgitation. Circulation 87:841, 1993.

210. Chen, C., Wang, Y., Guo, B., et al.: Reliability of the Doppler pressure half-time method for assessing effects of percutaneous mitral balloon valvuloplasty. J. Am. Coll. Cardiol. 13:1309, 1989.

211. Recusani, F., Bargiggia, G.S., Yoganathan, A.P., et al.: A new method for quantification of regurgitant flow rate using color Doppler flow imaging of the flow convergence region proximal to a discrete orifice: An in vitro study. Circulation 83:594, 1991.

212. Bargiggia, G.S., Tronconi, L., Sahn, D.J., et al.: A new method for quantification of mitral regurgitation based on color flow Doppler imaging at flow convergence proximal to regurgitant orifice. Circulation 84:1481, 1991.

212a. Vandervoort, P.M., Rivera, J.M., Mele, D., et al.: Application of color Doppler flow mapping to calculate effective regurgitant orifice area: An in vitro study and initial clinical observations. Circulation 88:1150, 1993.

213. Chen, C., Koschyk, D., Brockhoff, C., et al.: Noninvasive estimation of regurgitant flow rate and volume in patients with mitral regurgitation by Doppler color mapping of accelerating flow field. J. Am. Coll. Cardiol. 21:374, 1993.

214. Vandervoort, P.M., Thoreau, D.H., Rivera, J.M., et al.: Automated flow rate calculations based on digital analysis of flow convergence proximal to regurgitant orifices. J. Am. Coll. Cardiol. 22:535, 1993.

215. Lewis, J.F., Kuo, L.C., Nelson, J.G., et al.: Pulsed Doppler echocardiographic determination of stroke volume and cardiac output: Clinical validation of two new methods using the apical window. Circulation 70:425, 1984.

216. Lopez, J.F., Hanson, S., Orchard, R.C., et al.: Quantification of mitral valvular incompetence. Cathet. Cardiovasc. Diagn. 11:139, 1985.

217. Silver, M.D., Lam, J.H.C., Ranganathan, N., et al.: Morphology of the human tricuspid valve. Circulation 43:333, 1971.

218. Silver, M.D.: Obstruction to blood flow related to tricuspid, pulmonary, and mitral valves. In Silver, M. D. (ed.): Cardiovascular Pathology. Vol. 1. New York, Churchill Livingstone, 1983, p. 551.

219. Hauck, A.J., Freeman, D.P., Ackermann, D.M., et al.: Surgical pathology of the tricuspid valve: A study of 363 cases spanning 25 years. Mayo Clin. Proc. 63:851, 1988.

220. Chopra, P., and Tandon, H.D.: Pathology of chronic rheumatic heart disease with particular reference to tricuspid valve involvement. Acta Cardiol. 32:423, 1977.

221. Daniels, S.J., Mintz, G.S., and Kotler, M.N.: Rheumatic tricuspid valve disease: Two-dimensional echocardiographic, hemodynamic, and angiographic correlations. Am. J. Cardiol. 51:492, 1983.

222. Harley, J.B., McIntosh, C.L., Kirklin, J.J.W., et al.: Atrioventricular valve replacement in the idiopathic hypereosinophilic syndrome. Am. J. Med. 73:77, 1982.

223. Weyman, A.E., Rankin, R., and King, H.: Loeffler's endocarditis presenting as mitral and tricuspid stenosis. Am. J. Cardiol. 40:438, 1977.

224. Callahan, J.A., Wroblewski, E.M., Reeder, G.S., et al.: Echocardiographic features of carcinoid heart disease. Am. J. Cardiol. 50:762, 1982.

225. Hatle, L.K., and Angelsen, B.A.: Doppler Ultrasound in Cardiology: Physical Principles and Clinical Applications. 2nd ed. Philadelphia, Lea & Febiger, 1985, p. 151.

226. Pearlman, A.S.: Role of echocardiography in the diagnosis and evaluation of severity of mitral and tricuspid stenosis. Circulation 84(Suppl. 3):I193, 1991.

227. Denning, K., Henneke, K-H., and Rudolph, W.: Assessment of tricuspid stenosis by Doppler-echocardiography. (Abstract.) J. Am. Coll. Cardiol.(Suppl. A):237A, 1987.

228. Pellikka, P.A., Tajik, A.J., Khandheria, B.K., et al.: Carcinoid heart disease: Clinical and echocardiographic spectrum in 74 patients. Circulation 87:1188, 1993.

229. Edwards, J.E.: The spectrum and clinical significance of tricuspid regurgitation. Pract. Cardiol. 6:86, 1980.

230. Waller, B.F., Moriarty, A.T., Eble, J.N., et al.: Etiology of pure tricuspid regurgitation based on anular circumference and leaflet area: Analysis of 45 necropsy

patients with clinical and morphologic evidence of pure tricuspid regurgitation. J. Am. Coll. Cardiol. 7:1063, 1986.

231. Waller, B.F.: Etiology of pure tricuspid regurgitation. Cardiovasc. Clin. 17:53, 1987.

232. Ogawa, S., Hayashi, J., Sasaki, H., et al.: Evaluation of combined valvular prolapse syndrome by two-dimensional echocardiography. Circulation 65:174, 1982.

233. Banks, T., Fletcher, R., and Ali, N.: Infective endocarditis in drug heroin addicts. Am. J. Med. 55:444, 1973.

234. McKinsey, D.S., Ratts, T.E., and Bisno, A.L.: Underlying cardiac lesions in adults with infective endocarditis: The changing spectrum. Am. J. Med. 82:681, 1987.

235. Okada, R., Ewy, G.A., and Copeland, J.G.: Echocardiography and surgery in tricuspid and pulmonary valve stenosis due to carcinoid syndrome. Cardiovasc. Med. 4:871, 1979.

236. Strickman, N.E., Rossi, P.A., Massumkhani, G.A., et al.: Carcinoid heart disease: A clinical, pathologic, and therapeutic update. Curr. Probl. Cardiol. 6:1, 1982.

237. Berkery, W., Hare, C., Warner, R.A., et al.: Nonpenetrating traumatic rupture of the tricuspid valve: Formation of ventricular septal aneurysm and subsequent septal necrosis. Recognition by two-dimensional Doppler echocardiography. Chest 91:778, 1987.

238. Katz, N.M., and Pallas, R.S.: Traumatic rupture of the tricuspid valve: Repair by chordal replacements and annuloplasty. J. Thorac. Cardiovasc. Surg. 91:P310, 1986.

239. Watanabe, T., Katsume, H., Matsukubo, H., et al.: Ruptured chordae tendineae of the tricuspid valve due to nonpenetrating trauma: Echocardiographic findings. Chest 80:751, 1981.

240. Gibbs, K.L., Reardon, M.J., Strickman, N.E., et al.: Hemodynamic compromise (tricuspid stenosis and insufficiency) caused by an unruptured aneurysm of the sinus of Valsalva. J. Am. Coll. Cardiol. 7:1177, 1986.

241. Lev, M., Liberthson, R.R., Joseph, R.H., et al.: The pathologic anatomy of Ebstein's disease. Arch. Pathol. 90:334, 1970.

242. Zuberbuhler, J.R., Allwork, S.P., and Anderson, R.H.: The spectrum of Ebstein's anomaly of the tricuspid valve. J. Thorac. Cardiovasc. Surg. 77:202, 1979.

243. Shiina, A., Seward, J.B., Tajik, A.J., et al.: Two-dimensional echocardiographic–surgical correlation in Ebstein's anomaly: Preoperative determination of patients requiring tricuspid valve plication vs replacement. Circulation 68:534, 1983.

244. Weyman, A.E., Wann, S., Feigenbaum, H., et al.: Mechanism of abnormal septal motion in patients with right ventricular volume overload: A cross-sectional echocardiographic study. Circulation 54:179, 1976.

245. Miyatake, K., Okamoto, M., Kinoshita, N., et al.: Evaluation of tricuspid regurgitation by pulsed Doppler and two-dimensional echocardiography. Circulation 66:777, 1982.

246. Pennestrí, F., Loperfido, F., Salvatori, M.P., et al.: Assessment of tricuspid regurgitation by pulsed Doppler ultrasonography of the hepatic veins. Am. J. Cardiol. 54:363, 1984.

247. Skjaerpe, T., and Hatle, L.: Diagnosis and assessment of tricuspid regurgitation by Doppler ultrasound. In Rijsterbough, H. (ed.): Echocardiography. The Hague, Martinus-Nijhoff, 1981, p. 299.

248. Waggoner, A.D., Quinones, M.A., Young, J.B., et al.: Pulsed Doppler echocardiographic detection of right-sided valve regurgitation: Experimental results and clinical significance. Am. J. Cardiol. 47:279, 1981.

249. Appleton, C.P., Hatle, L.K., and Popp, R.L.: Superior vena cava and hepatic vein Doppler echocardiography in healthy adults. J. Am. Coll. Cardiol. 10:1032, 1987.

250. Wranne, B., and Marklund, T.: Evaluation of tricuspid regurgitation: A comparison between pulsed Doppler, jugular vein and liver pulse recordings, contrast echocardiography and angiography. In Spencer, M.P. (ed.): Cardiac Doppler Diagnosis. Boston, Martinus-Nijhoff, 1984, p. 255.

251. Currie, P.J., Hagler, D.J., Seward, J.B., et al.: Instantaneous pressure gradient: A simultaneous Doppler and dual-catheter correlative study. J. Am. Coll. Cardiol. 7:800, 1986.

252. Skjærpe, T., and Hatle, L.: Noninvasive estimation of pulmonary artery pressure by Doppler ultrasound in tricuspid regurgitation. In Spencer, M.P. (ed.): Cardiac Doppler Diagnosis. Boston, Martinus-Nijhoff 1984, p. 247.

253. Yock, P.G., and Popp, R.L.: Noninvasive estimation of right ventricular systolic pressure by Doppler ultrasound in patients with tricuspid regurgitation. Circulation 70:657, 1984.

254. Altrichter, P.M., Olson, L.J., Edwards, W.D., et al.: Surgical pathology of the pulmonary valve: A study of 116 cases spanning 15 years. Mayo Clin. Proc. 64:1352, 1989.

255. Davies, M.J.: Pathology of Cardiac Valves. London, Butterworth, 1980, p. 8.

256. Gikonyo, B.M., Lucas, R.V., and Edwards, J.E.: Anatomic features of congenital pulmonary valvular stenosis. Pediatr. Cardiol. 8:109, 1987.

257. Cremieux, A.-C., Witchitz, S., Malergue, M-C., et al.: Clinical and echocardiographic observations in pulmonary valve endocarditis. Am. J. Cardiol. 56:610, 1985.

258. Naidoo, D.P., Seedat, M.A., and Vythilingum, S.: Isolated endocarditis of the pulmonary valve with fragmentation haemolysis. Br. Heart J. 60:527, 1988.

259. Weyman, A.E., Dillon, J.C., Feigenbaum, H., et al.: Echocardiographic differentiation of infundibular from valvular pulmonary stenosis. Am. J. Cardiol. 36:21, 1975.

260. Weyman, A.E., Hurwitz, R.A., Girod, D.A., et al.: Cross-sectional echocardiographic visualization of the stenotic pulmonary valve. Circulation 56:769, 1977.

261. Lima, C.O., Sahn, D.J., Valdes-Cruz, L.M., et al.: Noninvasive prediction of transvalvular pressure gradient in patients with pulmonary stenosis by quantitative two-dimensional echocardiographic Doppler studies. Circulation 67:866, 1983.

262. Berger, M., Delfin, L.A., Jelveh, M., et al.: Two-dimensional echocardiographic findings in right-sided infective endocarditis. Circulation 61:855, 1980.
263. Kramer, N.E., Gill, S.S., Patel, R., et al.: Pulmonary valve vegetations detected with echocardiography. Am. J. Cardiol. 39:1064, 1977.
264. Hatle, L.K., and Angelsen, B.A.: Doppler Ultrasound in Cardiology: Physical Principles and Clinical Applications. 2nd ed. Philadelphia, Lea & Febiger, 1985, p. 109.
265. Fyfe, D.A., Currie, P.J., Seward, J.B., et al.: Continuous-wave Doppler determination of the pressure gradient across pulmonary artery bands: Hemodynamic correlation in 20 patients. Mayo Clin. Proc. 59:744, 1984.
266. Reeder, G.S., Currie, P.J., Fyfe, D.A., et al.: Extracardiac conduit obstruction: Initial experience in the use of Doppler echocardiography for noninvasive estimation of pressure gradient. J. Am. Coll. Cardiol. 4:1006, 1984.
267. Kostucki, W., Vandenbossche, J-L., Friart, A., et al.: Pulsed Doppler regurgitant flow patterns of normal valves. Am. J. Cardiol. 58:309, 1986.
268. Miyatake, K., Okamoto, M., Kinoshita, N., et al.: Pulmonary regurgitation studied with the ultrasonic pulsed Doppler technique. Circulation 65:969, 1982.
269. Sprecher, D.L., Adamick, R., Adams, D., et al.: In vitro color flow, pulsed and continuous wave Doppler ultrasound masking of flow by prosthetic valves. J. Am. Coll. Cardiol. 9:1306, 1987.
270. Cohn, L.H., Mudge, G.H., Pratter, F., et al.: Five to eight-year follow-up of patients undergoing porcine heart-valve replacement. N. Engl. J. Med. 304:258, 1981.
271. Schoen, F.J., Collins, J.J., Jr., and Cohn, L.H.: Long-term failure rate and morphologic correlations in porcine bioprosthetic heart valves. Am. J. Cardiol. 51:957, 1983.
272. Alam, M., Lakier, J.B., Pickard, S.D., et al.: Echocardiographic evaluation of porcine bioprosthetic valves: Experience with 309 normal and 59 dysfunctioning valves. Am. J. Cardiol. 52:309, 1983.
272a. Forman, M.B., Phelan, B.K., Robertson, R.M., et al.: Correlation of two-dimensional echocardiography and pathologic findings in porcine valve dysfunction. J. Am. Coll. Cardiol. 5:224, 1985.
273. Effron, M.K., and Popp, R.L.: Two-dimensional echocardiographic assessment of bioprosthetic valve dysfunction and infective endocarditis. J. Am. Coll. Cardiol. 2:597, 1983.
274. Grenadier, E., Sahn, D.J., Roche, A.H.G., et al.: Detection of deterioration or infection of homograft and porcine xenograft bioprosthetic valves in mitral and aortic positions by two-dimensional echocardiographic examination. J. Am. Coll. Cardiol. 2:452, 1983.
275. Kotler, M.N., Mintz, G.S., Panidis, I., et al.: Noninvasive evaluation of normal and abnormal prosthetic valve function. J. Am. Coll. Cardiol. 2:151, 1983.
276. Nellessen, U., Schnittger, I., Appleton, C.P., et al.: Transesophageal two-dimensional echocardiography and color Doppler flow velocity mapping in the evaluation of cardiac valve prostheses. Circulation 78:848, 1988.
277. Williams, G.A., and Labovitz, A.J.: Doppler hemodynamic evaluation of prosthetic (Starr-Edwards and Björk-Shiley) and bioprosthetic (Hancock and Carpentier-Edwards) cardiac valves. Am. J. Cardiol. 56:325, 1985.
278. Nellessen, U., Masuyama, T., Appleton, C.P., et al.: Mitral prosthesis malfunction: Comparative Doppler echocardiographic studies of mitral prostheses before and after replacement. Circulation 79:330, 1989.
279. Ryan, T., Armstrong, W.F., Dillon, J.C., et al.: Doppler echocardiographic evaluation of patients with porcine mitral valves. Am. Heart J. 111:237, 1987.
280. Reisner, S.A., and Meltzer, R.S.: Normal values of prosthetic valve Doppler echocardiographic parameters: A review. J. Am. Soc. Echocardiogr. 1:203, 1988.
281. Baumgartner, H., Schima, H., and Kuhn, P.: Effect of prosthetic valve malfunction on the Doppler-catheter gradient relation for bileaflet aortic prostheses. Circulation 87:1320, 1993.
282. Yoganathan, A.P., Jones, M., Sahn, D.J., et al.: Bernoulli gradient calculations for mechanical prosthetic aortic valves: In vitro Doppler studies. (Abstract.) Circulation 74(Suppl. II):391, 1986.
283. Teirstein, P.S., Yock, P.G., and Popp, R.L.: The accuracy of Doppler ultrasound measurement of pressure gradients across irregular, dual, and tunnellike obstructions to blood flow. Circulation 72:577, 1985.
284. Burstow, D.J., Nishimura, R.A., Bailey, K.R., et al.: Continuous-wave Doppler echocardiographic measurement of prosthetic valve gradients: A simultaneous Doppler-catheter correlative study. Circulation 80:504, 1989.
285. Wilkins, G.T., Gillam, L.D., Kritzer, G.L., et al.: Validation of continuous-wave Doppler echocardiographic measurements of mitral and tricuspid prosthetic valve gradients: A simultaneous Doppler-catheter study. Circulation 74:786, 1986.
286. Holen, J., Simonsen, S., and Frøysaker, T.: An ultrasound Doppler technique for the noninvasive determination of the pressure gradient in the Björk-Shiley mitral valve. Circulation 59:436, 1979.
287. Holen, J., Simonsen, S., and Fröysaker T.: Determination of pressure gradient in the Hancock mitral valve from noninvasive ultrasound Dopper data. Scand. J. Clin. Lab. Invest. 41:177, 1981.
288. Rothbart, R.M., Smucker, M.L., and Gibson, R.S.: Overestimation by Doppler echocardiography of pressure gradients across Starr-Edwards prosthetic valves in the aortic position. Am. J. Cardiol. 61:475, 1988.
289. Sagar, K.B., Wann, L.S., Paulsen, W.H.J., et al.: Doppler echocardiographic evaluation of Hancock and Björk-Shiley prosthetic valves. J. Am. Coll. Cardiol. 7:681, 1986.
290. Schoenfeld, M.H., Palacios, I.F., Hutter, A.M., Jr., et al.: Underestimation of prosthetic mitral valve areas: Role of transseptal catheterization in avoiding unnecessary repeat mitral valve surgery. J. Am. Coll. Cardiol. 5:1387, 1985.
291. Alam, M., Rosman, H.S., Lakier, J.B., et al.: Doppler and echocardiographic features of normal and dysfunctioning bioprosthetic valves. J. Am. Coll. Cardiol. 10:851, 1987.
292. Panidis, I.P., Ross, J., and Mintz, G.S.: Normal and abnormal prosthetic valve function as assessed by Doppler echocardiography. J. Am. Coll. Cardiol. 8:317, 1986.
293. Come, P.C.: Pitfalls in the diagnosis of periprosthetic valvular regurgitation by pulsed Doppler echocardiography. J. Am. Coll. Cardiol. 9:1176, 1987.
294. Seward, J.B., Khandheria, B.K., Oh, J.K., et al.: Transesophageal echocardiography: Technique, anatomic correlations implementation, and clinical applications. Mayo Clin. Proc. 63:649, 1988.
294a. Bochek, L.I.: Correction of mitral valve disease without mitral valve replacement. Am. Heart J. 104:865, 1982.
295. Carpentier, A.: Cardiac valve surgery: The "French correction." J. Thorac. Cardiovasc. Surg. 86:323, 1983.
296. Galloway, A.C., Colvin, S.B., Baumann, F.G., et al.: Current concepts of mitral valve reconstruction for mitral insufficiency. Circulation 78:1087, 1988.
297. Perier, P., Deloche, A., Chauvaud, S., et al.: Comparative evaluation of mitral valve repair and replacement with Starr, Björk, and porcine valve prostheses. Circulation 70(Suppl. I):187, 1984.
298. King, R.M., Pluth, J.R., Giuliani, E.R., et al.: Mechanical decalcification of the aortic valve. Ann. Thorac. Surg. 42:269, 1986.
299. Freeman, W.K., Schaff, H.V., and Orszulak, T.A.: Ultrasonic aortic valve decalcification: Serial Doppler echocardiographic follow-up. Circulation 78(Suppl. II):379, 1988.
300. Galloway, A.C., Colvin, S.B., Baumann, F.G., et al.: Long-term results of mitral valve reconstruction with Carpentier techniques in 148 patients with mitral insufficiency. Circulation 78(Suppl. I):97, 1988.
301. Block, P.C.: Who is suitable for percutaneous balloon mitral valvotomy? (Editorial.) Int. J. Cardiol. 20:9, 1988.
302. Marantz, P.M., Huhta, J.C., Mullins, C.E., et al.: Results of balloon valvuloplasty in typical and dysplastic pulmonary valve stenosis: Doppler echocardiographic follow-up. J. Am. Coll. Cardiol. 12:476, 1988.
303. Rediker, D.E., Block, P.C., Abascal, V.M., et al.: Mitral balloon valvuloplasty for mitral restenosis after surgical commissurotomy. J. Am. Coll. Cardiol. 11:252, 1988.
304. O'Shea, J.P., Abascal, V.M., Wilkins, G.T., et al.: Unusual sequelae after percutaneous mitral valvuloplasty: A Doppler echocardiographic study. J. Am. Coll. Cardiol. 19:186, 1992.
305. Fatkin, D., Roy, P., Morgan, J.J., et al.: Percutaneous balloon mitral valvotomy with the Inoue single-balloon catheter: Commissural morphology as a determinant of outcome. J. Am. Coll. Cardiol. 21:390, 1993.
306. Reid, C.L., and Rahimtoola, S.H.: The role of echocardiography/Doppler in catheter balloon treatment of adults with aortic and mitral stenosis. Circulation 84(Suppl. 3)I240, 1991.
307. Block, P.C., Palacios, I.F., Jacobs, M.L., et al.: Mechanisms of percutaneous mitral valvotomy. Am. J. Cardiol. 59:178, 1987.
308. Chen, C., Weng, Y., Guo, B., et al.: Reliability of the Doppler pressure half-time method for assessing effects of percutaneous mitral balloon valvuloplasty. J. Am. Coll. Cardiol. 13:1309, 1989.
309. Abascal, V.M., Wilkins, G.T., Choong, C.Y., et al.: Mitral regurgitation after percutaneous balloon mitral valvuloplasty in adults: Evaluation by pulsed Doppler echocardiography. J. Am. Coll. Cardiol. 11:257, 1988.
310. Otto, C.M., Mickel, M.C., Kennedy, J.W., et al.: Three year outcome after balloon aortic valvuloplasty: Insights into prognosis of valvular aortic stenosis. Circulation 89:642, 1994.
311. Anonymous: Multicenter experience with mitral commissurotomy: NHLBI balloon valvuloplasty registry report on immediate and 30-day follow up results. The National Heart, Lung, and Blood Institute balloon valvuloplasty registry participants. Circulation 85:448, 1992.
312. Masura, J., Burch, M., Deanfield, J.E., et al.: Five-year follow-up after balloon valvuloplasty. J. Am. Coll. Cardiol. 21:132, 1993.
313. McCrindle, B.W., and Kan, J.S.: Long-term results after balloon pulmonary valvuloplasty. Circulation 83:1915, 1991.
314. Abascal, V.M., Wilkins, G.T., Choong, C.Y., et al.: Echocardiographic evaluation of mitral valve structure and function in patients followed for at least 6 months after percutaneous balloon mitral valvuloplasty. J. Am. Coll. Cardiol. 12:606, 1988.
315. Palacios, I.F., Block, P.C., Wilkins, G.T., et al.: Follow-up of patients undergoing percutaneous mitral balloon valvotomy: Analysis of factors determining restenosis. Circulation 79:573, 1989.
316. Nishimura, R.A., Holmes, D.R., Jr., Reeder, G.S., et al.: Doppler evaluation of results of percutaneous aortic balloon valvuloplasty in calcific aortic stenosis. Circulation 78:791, 1988.
317. Come, P.C., Riley, M.F., McKay, R.G., et al.: Echocardiographic assessment of aortic valve area in elderly patients with aortic stenosis and of changes in valve area after percutaneous balloon valvuloplasty. J. Am. Coll. Cardiol. 10:115, 1987.
318. Safian, R.D., Warren, S.E., Berman, A.D., et al.: Improvement in symptoms and left ventricular performance after balloon aortic valvuloplasty in patients with aortic stenosis and depressed left ventricular ejection fraction. Circulation 78:1181, 1988.
319. McKay, R.G., Safian, R.D., Lock, J.E., et al.: Balloon dilatation of calcific aortic stenosis in elderly patients: Postmortem, intraoperative, and percutaneous valvuloplasty studies. Circulation 74:119, 1986.
320. Robicsek, F., and Harbold, N.B., Jr.: Limited value of balloon dilatation in calcified aortic stenosis in adults: Direct observations during open heart surgery. Am. J. Cardiol. 60:857, 1987.
321. Safian, R.D., Mandell, V.S., Thurer, R.E., et al.: Postmortem and intraoperative balloon valvuloplasty of calcific aortic stenosis in elderly patients: Mechanisms of successful dilation. J. Am. Coll. Cardiol. 9:655, 1987.
322. Isner, J.M., Samuels, D.A., Slovenkai, G.A., et al.: Mechanism of aortic balloon valvuloplasty: Fracture of valvular calcific deposits. Ann. Intern. Med. 108:377, 1988.

CHAPTER

31 Cardiomyopathies

Arthur J. Labovitz, M.D.

HYPERTROPHIC CARDIOMYOPATHY ____ 395
Echocardiographic Findings ____ 395
   Ventricular Hypertrophy ____ 395
   Left Ventricular Size and Function ____ 396
   Left Ventricular Outflow Obstruction ____ 396
     Systolic Anterior Motion of the Mitral
     Valve ____ 396
Doppler Evaluation ____ 396
   Outflow Obstruction ____ 396
   Diastolic Function ____ 397
     Left Ventricular Relaxation ____ 397
     Compliance ____ 397
   Mitral Regurgitation ____ 398
Hypertensive Hypertrophic Cardiomyopathy of
the Elderly ____ 398

DILATED CARDIOMYOPATHY ____ 399
Echocardiographic Features ____ 400
   Systolic Dysfunction ____ 400
   Left Ventricular Diastolic Function ____ 401
   Mitral Regurgitation ____ 401
   Pulmonary Pressures ____ 401
   Intracavitary Thrombus ____ 402
RESTRICTIVE CARDIOMYOPATHY ____ 402
Infiltrative Cardiomyopathies ____ 402
   Amyloidosis ____ 402
     Echocardiographic Features ____ 402
   Other Infiltrative Cardiomyopathies ____ 402
   Obliterative Cardiomyopathies ____ 402
   Endocardial Fibroelastosis ____ 402
Diastolic Filling ____ 403

The term "cardiomyopathy" was originally proposed to define a group of disorders with a primary abnormality of heart muscle function of unknown cause.[1] Recently, however, the term "cardiomyopathy" has evolved to represent a heterogeneous group of disorders of heart muscle function that are classified on the basis of distinct clinical syndromes, as well as hemodynamic and histopathologic features.[2] The three major categories of cardiomyopathy are hypertrophic cardiomyopathy, dilated cardiomyopathy, and restrictive infiltrative cardiomyopathy. Each of these three categories has distinct structural and functional features that are well described with the use of cardiac ultrasound.

HYPERTROPHIC CARDIOMYOPATHY

Hypertrophic cardiomyopathy is an abnormality characterized by unexplained hypertrophy of the left ventricle. Hypertrophic cardiomyopathy is inherited in its familial form as an autosomal dominant disease in more than 50 percent of the cases.[3, 4] In addition, the relatively high incidence of sporadically occurring cases suggests that spontaneous mutations in the gene for this disease occur commonly. In its classic description, asymmetric and marked hypertrophy occurs in the ventricular septum, which can cause outflow-tract obstruction when associated with systolic anterior motion of the mitral valve. This abnormality has been referred to as "hypertrophic obstructive cardiomyopathy" as well as "idiopathic hypertrophic subaortic stenosis." Histologically, this abnormality is characterized by myocardial fiber disarray.[5] Hypertrophic cardiomyopathy represents one of the most common causes of sudden cardiac death in younger individuals and athletes.[6-8] The symptoms associated with hypertrophic cardiomyopathy include dyspnea on exertion, anginal chest pain, syncope and presyncope, and palpitations. The physical examination is variable, but in those with outflow obstruction a harsh systolic ejection murmur is heard along the left lower sternal border, with radiation to the apex. The murmur characteristically increases in intensity with maneuvers that enhance contractility or reduce preload or afterload.

Echocardiographic Findings

Ventricular Hypertrophy

The most common echocardiographic feature in patients with hypertrophic cardiomyopathy is a marked increase in diastolic wall thickness of the left ventricle. Although this hypertrophy is most commonly confined to the ventricular septum (Fig. 31–1), localized hypertrophy of the cardiac apex and left ventricular free wall occur as well.[7, 9, 10] Concentric hypertrophy may be found in these patients as well, either as a primary cardiomyopathy or, more commonly, as secondary hypertrophy that occurs in response to left ventricular outflow-tract obstruction.

Much of what has been described in the literature concerning hypertrophic cardiomyopathy paralleled the early use of M-mode echocardiography in the evaluation of these patients.[11-15] Accordingly, the criteria established for the presence of hypertrophic cardiomyopathy initially included indices that compared the thickness of intraventricular septum with that of the posterior left ventricular wall.[8] A commonly accepted definition includes an increased interventricular diastolic thickness (>1.3 cm), with a ratio of septal-to-posterior wall thickness of 1.5:1.0. With the widespread application of two-dimensional echocardiography, involvement of regions other than the basal interventricular septum was appreciated.[7-9, 15-17]

Maron reported four types of hypertrophic cardiomyopathy based on the distribution of hypertrophy (Fig. 31–2). In 10 percent of the cases, the anterior ventricular septum alone was involved (type I). The anterior and posterior ventricular septum were thickened in 20 percent of the cases (type II). The majority of patients (52 percent) had septal and anterolateral wall involvement (type III). Type IV (18 percent) consisted of patients with isolated posterior-septal, apical-septal, or anterolateral wall involvement. Patients classified as Maron's type IV would not have been detected by M-mode echocardiography.

Concentric hypertrophy was found to be relatively rare in Maron's population. Similarly, Wigle and co-workers found concentric hypertrophy in only a minority (5 percent) of the patients studied.[10] However, in their series, 90 percent of the patients had asymmetric septal hypertrophy. That patients with hypertrophic cardiomyopathy constitute a heterogeneous group is highlighted by the incidence of asymmetric septal hypertrophy and concentric hypertrophy reported by different investigators. Shapiro and McKenna reported on a group of 89 patients with hypertrophic cardiomyopathy, in which 31 percent had concentric left ventricular hypertrophy and 14 percent had apical hypertrophy.[18] Despite these differences, two-dimensional echocardiography provides an ideal

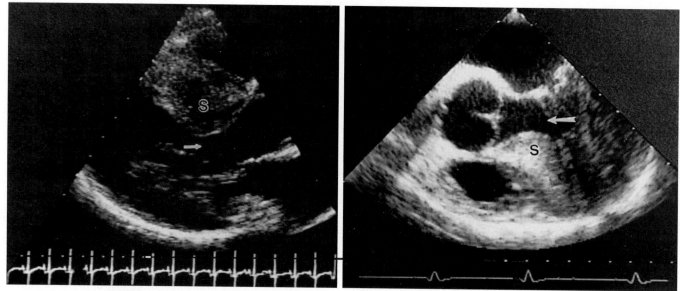

FIGURE 31-1. Two-dimensional echocardiographic image obtained by transthoracic (*left*) and transesophageal (*right*) echocardiography in a patient with hypertrophic cardiomyopathy. Note the asymmetric septal hypertrophy (S), causing narrowing of the left ventricular outflow tract (*arrow*).

method by which the extent of left ventricular hypertrophy can be determined in patients with hypertrophic cardiomyopathy. There is ample evidence that the extent of hypertrophy correlates with patients' symptomatology as well as prognosis.

Several authors have noted a distinct pattern of hypertrophy in elderly patients, with hemodynamic abnormalities virtually identical to those of younger patients with hypertrophic cardiomyopathy.[19-22] These patients are found much more commonly to have the concentric variety of hypertrophy and much more frequently to have a history of systemic hypertension. The degree of hypertrophy, however, appears markedly out of proportion to that typically associated with systemic hypertension. This group of patients has been referred to as having "hypertrophic hypertensive cardiomyopathy of the elderly," as well as "hypertrophic cardiomyopathy with hypertension." Although a similar prevalence of left ventricular outflow obstruction and diastolic filling abnormalities are seen in this more elderly group of patients, it has been suggested that preservation of the normal septal curvature, which is often reversed in younger patients with hypertrophic cardiomyopathy, might be one distinguishing characteristic.

A somewhat unique pattern of acoustic reflectance has been described in the ventricular septum of patients with hypertrophic cardiomyopathy.[16] This so-called "ground-glass" appearance, found most commonly in parasternal views, has been noted to support the diagnosis of hypertrophic cardiomyopathy. Similar findings, however, have been reported in patients with infiltrative diseases such as amyloidosis.

Left Ventricular Size and Function

Patients with hypertrophic cardiomyopathy will often have supernormal indices of left ventricular systolic function. Elevated left ventricular ejection fraction and increased contractility, as evidenced by increased shortening fraction and velocity of circumferential shortening, are common findings in this group of patients. Although it has been suggested that systolic thickening of the interventricular septum might be decreased in this group of patients, overall contractility appears to be increased. Smaller cavity size with increased wall thickness to left ventricular cavity ratio is also commonly observed.

Left Ventricular Outflow Obstruction

The vast majority of patients with hypertrophic cardiomyopathy have either resting or provokable gradients across the left ventricu-

lar outflow tract (Fig. 31-3). In general, maneuvers that increase contractility as well as those that decrease preload or afterload result in increases in the subaortic gradients. Early studies of patients with hypertrophic cardiomyopathy focused on this gradient as a factor primarily responsible for morbidity and mortality in these patients. It is now clear, however, that abnormalities of diastolic function, as well as life-threatening arrhythmias, are of at least equal clinical importance and may occur in the absence of significant outflow-tract obstruction. Nevertheless, studies investigating the mechanism of left ventricular outflow-tract obstruction have enhanced our understanding of hypertrophic cardiomyopathy and remain as useful diagnostic markers in this group of patients.

Systolic Anterior Motion of the Mitral Valve

Early studies using M-mode echocardiography demonstrated a characteristic finding of systolic anterior motion of the mitral valve, with or without septal contact, in patients with obstructive hypertrophic cardiomyopathy (Fig. 31-4). Various theories, including altered geometry and Venturi effect, as well as pressure differences between the left atrium and the left ventricle, have been proposed as a mechanism by which systolic anterior motion of the mitral valve occurs.

In normal individuals, blood is ejected from the ventricular apex through the aortic valve across a wide-open left ventricular outflow tract, in which the distance between the mitral valve and the interventricular septum offers no obstruction to flow. In patients with hypertrophic cardiomyopathy, on the other hand, the increased septal thickness narrows the distance between the mitral valve and the interventricular septum, thus creating a dynamic systolic gradient. The mitral valve is then drawn further in proximity to the septum by the Venturi effect, further increasing left ventricular outflow-tract obstruction. Accordingly, patients with more marked upper septal thickness or states of increased contractility and/or decreased ventricular filling will exhibit a larger pressure gradient.

Several studies that used simultaneous pressure measurements and M-mode echocardiography have demonstrated that the more prolonged the mitral valve-septal contact, the more significant the left ventricular outflow-tract gradient.[23, 24]

Doppler Evaluation

Outflow Obstruction

Continuous-wave Doppler from the cardiac apex currently represents the technique of choice for evaluating left ventricular outflow-

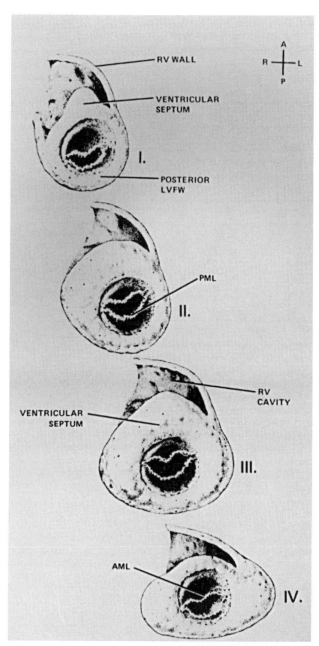

FIGURE 31–2. Schematic representation of the four patterns of hypertrophy identified with two-dimensional echocardiography in 125 patients with hypertrophic cardiomyopathy. Only cross-sectional planes are shown at the level of the mitral valve. AML = anterior mitral leaflet; LVFW = left ventricular free wall; PML = posterior mitral leaflet; RV = right ventricular. (From Maron, B.J., Gottdiener, J.S., and Epstein, S.E.: Patterns and significance of distribution of left ventricular hypertrophy in hypertrophic cardiomyopathy. Am. J. Cardiol. 48:418–428, 1981, with permission.)

tract gradient associated with hypertrophic cardiomyopathy. Pulsed and, more recently, color flow Doppler techniques allow localization of acceleration of flow just proximal to the point of maximal obstruction.[25–27] This situation typically occurs at the point of mitral leaflet and septal contact; however, it may occur at the midventricular or even apical regions of the left ventricle, depending on the location of hypertrophied muscle (Fig. 31–5). Color flow Doppler can be extremely helpful in directing the continuous-wave beam through the outflow jet, as mitral regurgitation commonly occurs in these patients. Continuous-wave Doppler can accurately measure left ventricular outflow tract gradient when the continuous-wave beam is aligned parallel to flow. The continuous-wave spectral recording will usually be displayed as a characteristic late-peaking

pattern, although occasionally the contour may be similar to that seen in valvular aortic stenosis (Fig. 31–6). Obviously, in patients with calcified aortic valves, the outflow-tract and subvalvular regions must be carefully examined to determine whether the resultant gradient is secondary to valvular aortic stenosis or dynamic left ventricular outflow-tract obstruction. One can apply the simplified Bernoulli equation to the peak velocity obtained with continuous-wave Doppler to estimate the left ventricular outflow-tract gradient. It is important to keep in mind that this method measures the peak instantaneous pressure gradient (i.e., the largest pressure difference across the obstruction at any instant in time). This value would typically be somewhat higher than the peak-to-peak gradient traditionally measured with simultaneous fluid-filled catheters. Likewise, the phenomenon of pressure recovery will often elevate Doppler estimated pressure gradients beyond those typically measured in the catheter laboratory.

FIGURE 31–5. See Color Plate 6.

Several conditions associated with hypercontractile states have been reported to be associated with a late-peaking contour, with or without an associated gradient. These conditions might include hypovolemia-dehydration and catecholamine excess with or without concentric hypertrophy, often in conjunction with tachycardia.[28]

Transesophageal echocardiography has been shown to be helpful in localizing the site of obstruction, as well as enabling measurement of left ventricular outflow-tract gradient in a parallel fashion in patients with hypertrophic cardiomyopathy.[29] Transesophageal echocardiography is also useful in the intraoperative assessment of these patients.

Diastolic Function

Abnormalities of left ventricular diastolic function have been well described in patients with hypertrophic cardiomyopathy.[30] These abnormalities are apparent in two distinct components of diastolic function: relaxation and compliance.

Left Ventricular Relaxation

Diastolic left ventricular relaxation is a complex, energy-dependent process that is reflected by changes early in diastole. Several studies have shown the rate of relaxation in patients with hypertrophic cardiomyopathy to be prolonged,[25, 31] as evidenced by a prolonged isovolumic relaxation time and a reduced rate of decrease of left ventricular diastolic pressure, or tau. Relaxation is a complex process that is dependent on many factors, including loading conditions, wall stress, systolic function, and coronary blood flow, many of which may be abnormal in patients with hypertrophic cardiomyopathy. Accordingly, evaluation of left ventricular relaxation by means of Doppler interrogation of transmitral flow frequently demonstrates findings consistent with abnormal relaxation, including prolonged isovolumic relaxation time, reduced early diastolic filling, and increased dependence of filling on atrial systole, which results in a reversed E:A ratio with a prolonged deceleration time (Fig. 31–7).

Compliance

Patients with hypertrophic cardiomyopathy frequently also demonstrate abnormal compliance, particularly in the later stages of the disease. This abnormal increase in wall stiffness reflects an abnormality of the elastic properties of myocardium secondary to hypertrophy or fibrosis, or both. In patients with abnormal left ventricular compliance, measurement of the pressure-volume relationship shows abnormally steep slopes, in which small increases in ventricular volume result in abnormally marked increases in left ventricular diastolic pressure. Examination of transmitral flow reflects the findings common to patients with abnormal left ventric-

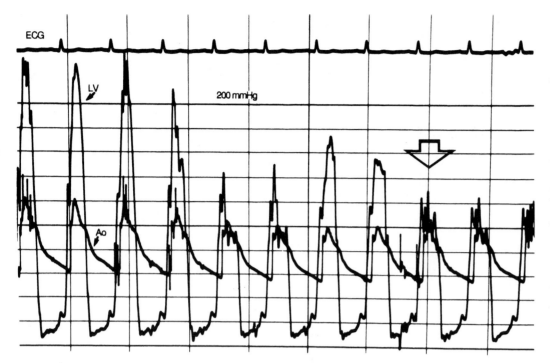

FIGURE 31–3. Simultaneous left ventricular (LV) and aortic (Ao) pressures in a patient with obstructive hypertrophic cardiomyopathy during pullback of the catheter from the distal portion of the left ventricle. LV systolic pressure matches aortic pressure during catheter pullback before the catheter is pulled out of the left ventricle. There is no true aortic valve gradient. The left ventricular–aortic gradient is located in the middle left ventricular wall beneath the aortic valve. The arrow indicates the matching of aortic and left ventricular systolic pressures in the proximal chamber. (From Kern, M.J. [ed.]: The Cardiac Catheterization Handbook. St. Louis, Mosby–Year Book, 1995, with permission.)

ular compliance, which include augmented early diastolic flow (increased E wave) and a diminution of atrial contractile function (reduced A wave). This pattern of increased E:A ratio is exaggerated in the presence of elevated left atrial and left ventricular filling pressures, and significant mitral regurgitation, which also leads to increased early diastolic flow in many of these patients.

The relative impact of abnormalities in relaxation and compliance on transmitral diastolic velocity recordings may well have contrasting effects and, therefore, mask the actual degree of diastolic dysfunction. Evaluation of pulmonary venous flow may be helpful in such instances.

Mitral Regurgitation

Mitral regurgitation is present in the majority of patients with hypertrophic cardiomyopathy. Both the abnormal geometry and

intraventricular pressure gradient appear to contribute to the development of mitral regurgitation, particularly in the presence of systolic anterior motion of the mitral valve. Treatment aimed at decreasing left ventricular outflow-tract obstruction frequently results in a decrease in the degree of mitral regurgitation.

Hypertensive Hypertrophic Cardiomyopathy of the Elderly

As mentioned earlier, a group of elderly individuals with long-standing hypertension and marked concentric hypertrophy has been described in which many of the abnormal hemodynamics of hypertrophic cardiomyopathy are present.[19–22, 32, 33] These individuals frequently have demonstrable outflow-tract gradients as well as

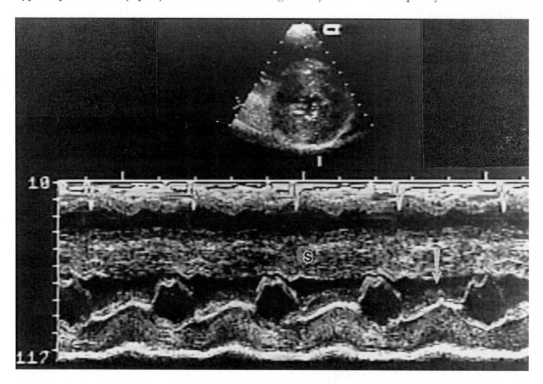

FIGURE 31–4. M-mode echocardiogram, demonstrating asymmetric septal hypertrophy (S) and systolic anterior motion of the mitral valve (*arrow*).

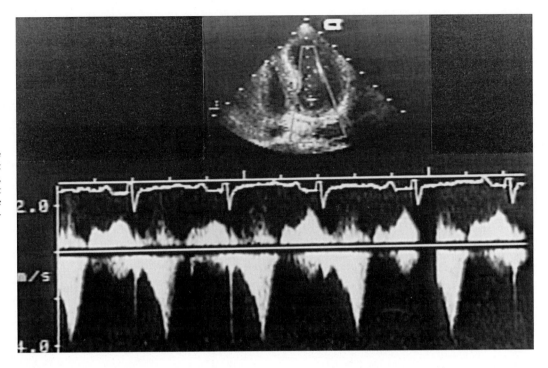

FIGURE 31–6. Characteristic late peaking systolic flow in a patient with hypertrophic cardiomyopathy, with a peak velocity across the left ventricular outflow tract of 4 msec and a resting intraventricular gradient of 64 mm Hg.

abnormalities in diastolic function very similar to those of younger individuals with primary hypertrophic cardiomyopathy. It is likely that in these elderly patients, hypertrophy has developed secondary to long-standing hypertension and perhaps later in the course of their disease, because of the development of left ventricular outflow-tract obstruction secondary to hypertrophy. Although these individuals do not have the classic myocardial fiber disarray found in the younger cohort with classic hypertrophic cardiomyopathy, medical therapy in the two groups may well be similar (i.e., β- or calcium blockers).

DILATED CARDIOMYOPATHY

The term "dilated" or "congestive cardiomyopathy" refers to the clinical syndrome characterized by primary impairment of left ventricular systolic function. Typically, categorization of patients with the diagnosis of dilated cardiomyopathy excludes those with significant coronary artery disease. Patients with ischemic heart disease and diffuse or extensive left ventricular dysfunction are sometimes referred to as having "ischemic dilated cardiomyopathy." The nonischemic causes of dilated cardiomyopathy are multiple,

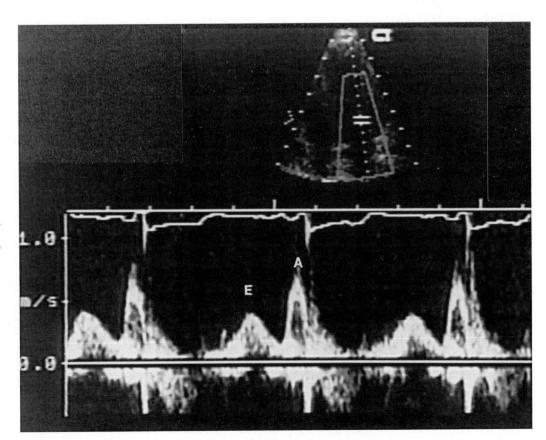

FIGURE 31–7. Pulsed Doppler recording of transmitral flow in a patient with hypertrophic cardiomyopathy, with abnormal relaxation and "reversed" E:A ratio.

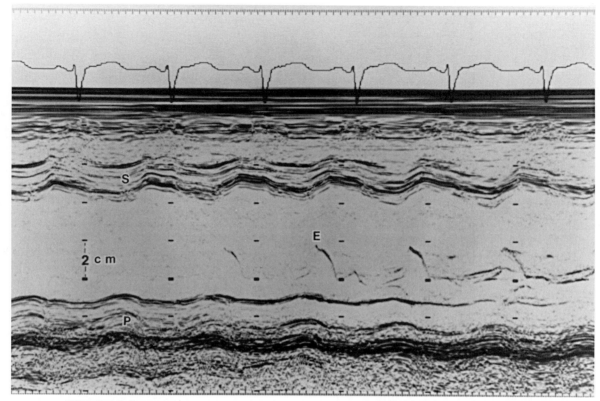

FIGURE 31–8. M-mode echocardiographic recording of a patient with a dilated left ventricular cavity, as well as an increased distance from the mitral early diastolic opening (E) to the intraventricular septum (S). P = left ventricular posterior wall.

although an underlying etiology is frequently not determined, and the diagnosis of dilated cardiomyopathy refers to the group of patients with end-stage left ventricular dysfunction and extensive fibrosis. Documented etiologies of dilated cardiomyopathy include a variety of underlying causes, including an inherited variety, nutritional deficiencies, toxic agents such as alcohol and anthracycline, and chemotherapeutic agents, as well as viral, inflammatory, and degenerative causes. The clinical syndrome of patients with dilated cardiomyopathy most often manifests with signs and symptoms of congestive heart failure, including pulmonary edema and peripheral interstitial edema. These patients may also present with symptoms of decreased forward cardiac output, including fatigue and decreased exercise tolerance.

Echocardiographic Features

The echocardiographic features of patients with dilated cardiomyopathy are those common to most patients with end-stage cardiac disease.

Systolic Dysfunction

The patient with dilated cardiomyopathy most commonly presents with an enlarged and globally hypokinetic left ventricle.[34, 35] Frequently, the right ventricle is involved as well. Left ventricular wall thickness is typically normal or decreased; however, left ventricular diastolic size is increased significantly, leading to an increase in left ventricular mass (left ventricular hypertrophy) in most patients.

The M-mode echocardiogram shows characteristic changes, including increased left ventricular diastolic and systolic diameters (Fig. 31–8), a decreased left ventricular shortening fraction (<25 percent), and increases in the E-point septal separation.[36]

The two-dimensional echocardiogram shows a dilated left ventricular chamber and, frequently, increased right ventricular, left atrial, and right atrial chamber size as well (Fig. 31–9). A global or

diffuse involvement of the left ventricle, rather than segmental left ventricular dysfunction, is typically present in patients with dilated cardiomyopathy and may be helpful in differentiating patients with coronary artery disease from those with dilated cardiomyopathy as an etiology of the left ventricular dysfunction. This is not always the case, however, and patients with dilated cardiomyopathy in the absence of significant epicardial coronary artery disease may present with isolated segmental wall motion abnormalities.[37, 38] Papillary muscle dysfunction may also be present and recognized on the

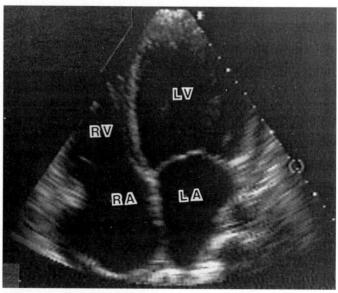

FIGURE 31–9. Two-dimensional echocardiographic image in a patient with dilated cardiomyopathy. There is enlargement of all four chambers.

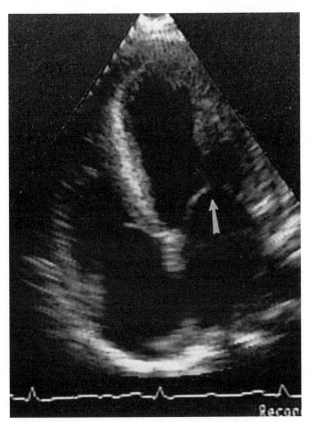

FIGURE 31-10. End-systolic frame in a patient with dilated cardiomyopathy and severe mitral insufficiency secondary to papillary muscle dysfunction. Note ventricular displacement of the mitral valve leaflet coaptation point, suggestive of papillary muscle dysfunction *(arrow).*

two-dimensional echocardiogram as incomplete closure of the mitral valve leaflets (Fig. 31–10).[39]

Doppler characteristics of impaired systolic function include decreased left ventricular outflow-tract and aortic velocities, secondary to decreased cardiac output.[40] When mitral regurgitation is present, the time to peak regurgitant velocity, or acceleration slope, is prolonged, reflecting impaired left ventricular systolic function,[41] which correlates well with abnormally depressed dP/dt.

Several studies have demonstrated that echocardiographic indices of left ventricular systolic function provide important prognostic information in patients with dilated cardiomyopathy.[34, 41–43] These include the M-mode measurements of left ventricular chamber size, wall thickness–to–cavity ratio, and E-point septal separation, as well as the left ventricular ejection fraction measured from the two-dimensional echocardiogram.

Left Ventricular Diastolic Function

As previously described, left ventricular diastolic function represents a complex series of events. Diastolic function has traditionally been characterized by assessing the components of relaxation, an early diastolic event that is an active energy-dependent process, and compliance, which reflects to a larger extent, the passive elastic characteristics of the receiving chamber. Evaluation of transmitral diastolic flow with Doppler echocardiography may provide some information concerning the diastolic function of patients with dilated cardiomyopathy.[44, 45] Abnormalities of diastolic relaxation, characterized by diminished early filling and prolonged isovolumic relaxation time, have been well described in patients with relatively mild abnormalities of systolic function early in the course of their disease. More commonly, patients with chronic or long-standing dilated cardiomyopathy develop pseudonormalization of transmitral flow patterns and increased early filling velocities with a decreased deceleration slope and decreased volume of flow during atrial

systole (Fig. 31–11). This so-called restrictive transmitral flow pattern also reflects, to some extent, abnormally elevated left ventricular diastolic pressure as well as less compliant walls secondary to fibrosis. This abnormal pattern of increased early diastolic filling velocities has also been shown to be associated with a poor prognosis and a decreased rate of survival.[46, 47]

Mitral Regurgitation

Mitral regurgitation is a common finding in patients with dilated cardiomyopathy. Ventricular dilatation, papillary muscle dysfunction, and incomplete leaflet coaptation all contribute to the development of mitral insufficiency in patients with dilated cardiomyopathy. Mitral regurgitation can be readily assessed with Doppler echocardiography. Pulsed, continuous-wave and color flow Doppler techniques all can be used to quantitate the degree of mitral regurgitation (for a detailed discussion see Chapter 30). The slope of the mitral regurgitant velocity in continuous-wave Doppler imaging during the preejection period is directly related to the left ventricular contractile reserve.[41]

Pulmonary Pressures

Assessment of pulmonary vascular pressures and left ventricular diastolic pressure is an important factor in the evaluation of patients with dilated cardiomyopathy. Most patients with some degree of pulmonary hypertension have Doppler-detectable tricuspid insufficiency.[48] One can then apply the Bernoulli equation to this velocity to derive an estimate of right ventricular–to–right atrial gradient, and then add the estimated right atrial pressure to determine right ventricular pressure and pulmonary artery systolic pressure.[49, 50] Likewise, measurement of the acceleration time (time from onset to peak systolic flow) in the right ventricular outflow tract can be used to assess pulmonary artery mean pressure.[51] Several reports have indicated that application of the Bernoulli equation to the end-diastolic velocity in patients with pulmonic insufficiency provides an estimate of the pulmonary artery diastolic pressure.[52]

Several methods have been described in which both mitral and pulmonary venous flow velocities have been used to determine left ventricular end-diastolic pressure.[53]

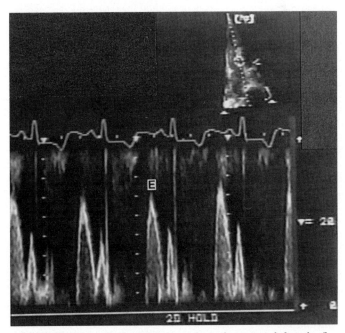

FIGURE 31-11. Pulsed Doppler recording of transmitral diastolic flow pattern in 60-year-old with idiopathic dilated cardiomyopathy. Note the "pseudonormalized" restrictive pattern of increased early (E) diastolic flow velocities, with a rapid deceleration slope. This finding suggests elevated left ventricular filling pressures and a poor prognosis.

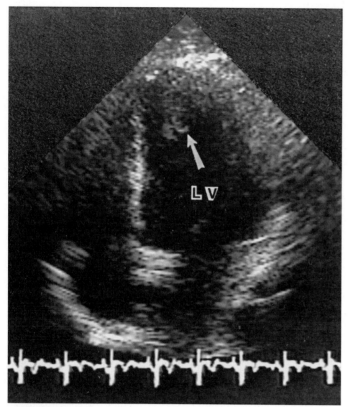

FIGURE 31–12. Apical four-chamber view in a patient with severe left ventricular (LV) dysfunction and a pedunculated apical mural thrombus (*arrow*).

Intracavitary Thrombus

Patients with dilated cardiomyopathy have an annual incidence of embolic complications of between 3 and 5 percent per year,[54] which is secondary to the formation of thrombus in the heart that is favored by the low-flow conditions present. Two-dimensional echocardiography is an excellent method for diagnosing left ventricular thrombus (sensitivity >90 percent),[55] the vast majority of which are located in the left ventricular apex (Fig. 31–12). Recent studies that used transesophageal echocardiography have demonstrated that patients with dilated cardiomyopathy also have a high incidence of left atrial thrombus as well as of left atrial spontaneous echo contrast, both of which have been associated with increased embolic phenomena.

RESTRICTIVE CARDIOMYOPATHY

The term "restrictive cardiomyopathy" refers to a heterogeneous group of disorders that share the common features of abnormally restricted ventricular diastolic filling and normal or only mildly reduced systolic ventricular function. Pathologically, the restrictive cardiomyopathies can be classified into two groups: the infiltrative cardiomyopathies, such as amyloidosis and hemochromatosis, and the obliterative cardiomyopathies, which involve the endomyocardium, of which endomyocardial fibrosis is the most common.[1, 2]

Infiltrative Cardiomyopathies

Amyloidosis

Amyloidosis is the most common of the restrictive cardiomyopathies in the United States and is characterized by the deposition of an abnormal protein (amyloid) in various tissues throughout the body. In the heart, this abnormal deposition occurs between myo-

cardial fibers, initially causing functional abnormalities, the most prominent of which is restriction to filling. As the disease progresses, left ventricular systolic dysfunction becomes increasingly more prominent.

Echocardiographic Features

The characteristic echocardiographic findings in patients with advanced amyloidosis include symmetric left ventricular hypertrophy, frequently associated with increases in the right ventricular wall thickness, and atrial enlargement.[56, 57] A characteristic speckled appearance of the myocardium is frequently seen (Fig. 31–13). It has been postulated that this characteristic results from the acoustic interface between myocardial fibers and amyloid material. Left ventricular systolic function as well as left ventricular size is typically normal early in the course of the disease, despite signs and symptoms consistent with congestive heart failure. In patients with advanced amyloidosis, left ventricular dilation as well as impaired left ventricular systolic function more is commonly found.

Other Infiltrative Cardiomyopathies

A variety of infiltrative cardiomyopathies share many features of amyloid heart disease. Both hemochromatosis and sarcoidosis result in cardiac infiltration, and although restrictive hemodynamics can be observed, left ventricular dilation and systolic dysfunction are often prominent in advanced disease. Many of the inherited cardiomyopathies occur in the presence of metabolic storage diseases, with resultant accumulation of glycogen, lipids, and mucopolysaccharides. This may result in asymmetric or symmetric ventricular hypertrophy and a clinical picture of restrictive cardiomyopathy.

Obliterative Cardiomyopathies

Endocardial Fibroelastosis

Although rare in the United States, endomyocardial fibroelastosis is commonly seen in certain endemic regions.[1, 2] This abnormality is characterized by progressive thickening or fibrosis of the endo-

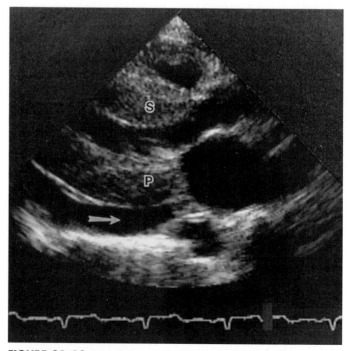

FIGURE 31–13. Two-dimensional echocardiographic image in a patient with biopsy-proven amyloid heart disease. Note the hypertrophy of both the septum (S) and the posterior wall (P), along with the highly echogenic appearance of the myocardium. This patient also has a moderate-sized pericardial effusion (*arrow*).

cardium in both the left and the right ventricles. Superimposed thrombus formation is a common finding. Both the mitral and the tricuspid valves may be thickened and insufficient.

Diastolic Filling

By definition, patients with restrictive cardiomyopathy exhibit abnormalities of ventricular diastolic filling. In general, patients with these abnormalities exhibit abnormally rapid increases in diastolic pressure during the early rapid-filling phase of diastole, which results in the dip and plateau, or "square-root sign," frequently seen in these patients with catheter measurement of ventricular pressure.[58] Characterizing a specific filling pattern by means of Doppler evaluation of transmitral flow, however, is a bit more difficult, as both abnormalities of relaxation and compliance predominate at various phases of the disease process. In general, early in the course of the disease, patients with restrictive cardiomyopathy display patterns consistent with abnormal relaxation.[59, 60] In general, these patients have preserved left ventricular systolic function. Doppler evaluation of transmitral flow shows prolonged isovolumic relaxation time, decreased early filling velocities, decreased deceleration time, and a relatively low E:A ratio. These patients also have a decreased peak filling rate and increased time to peak filling rate.

As the disease progresses, increased chamber stiffness and abnormal compliance become more prominent features, resulting in a more classic restrictive pattern of transmitral diastolic flow. Isovolumic relaxation time shortens, and with increased diastolic pressures the early diastolic velocities (E-wave) increase relative to the A-wave velocities. This restrictive pattern in patients with cardiac amyloidosis has been shown to be a strong predictor of cardiac death in such patients and an accurate marker of advanced disease.[61]

References

1. WHO/ISFC Task Force: Report of the WHO/ISFC Task Force on the definition and classification of cardiomyopathies. Br. Heart J. 44:672, 1980.
2. Abelmann, W.H., and Lorell, B.H.: The challenge of cardiomyopathy. J. Am. Coll. Cardiol. 13:1219, 1989.
3. Maron, B.J.: The genetics of hypertrophic cardiomyopathy. Ann. Intern. Med. 105:610, 1986.
4. Greaves, S.C., Roche, A.H.G., Neutze, J.M., et al.: Inheritance of hypertrophic cardiomyopathy: A cross-sectional and M-mode echocardiographic study of 50 families. Br. Heart J. 58:259, 1987.
5. Maron, B.J., and Roberts, W.C.: Hypertrophic cardiomyopathy and cardiac muscle cell disorganization revisited: Relation between the two and significance. Am. Heart J. 102:95, 1981.
6. McKenna, W., Deanfield, J., Farugui, A., et al.: Prognosis in hypertrophic cardiomyopathy: Role of age and clinical, electrocardiographic and hemodynamic features. Am. J. Cardiol. 47:532, 1981.
7. Maron, B.J., Bonow, R.O., Cannon, R.O., et al.: Hypertrophic cardiomyopathy: Interrelations of clinical manifestations, pathophysiology and therapy (first of two parts). N. Engl. J. Med. 316:780, 1987.
8. Maron, B.J., Bonow, R.O., Cannon, R.O., et al.: Hypertrophic cardiomyopathy: Interrelations of clinical manifestations, pathophysiology and therapy (second of two parts). N. Engl. J. Med. 316:844, 1987.
9. Maron, B.J., Gottdiener, J.S., and Epstein, S.E.: Patterns and significance of distribution of left ventricular hypertrophy in hypertrophic cardiomyopathy: A wide angle, two dimensional echocardiographic study of 125 patients. Am. J. Cardiol. 48:418, 1981.
10. Wigle, E.D., Sasson, Z., Henderson, M.A., et al.: Hypertrophic cardiomyopathy. The importance of the site and the extent of hypertrophy. A review. Prog. Cardiovasc. Dis. 28:1, 1985.
11. Rodger, J.C.: Motion of mitral apparatus in hypertrophic cardiomyopathy with obstruction. Br. Heart J. 38:732, 1976.
12. Popp, R.L., and Harrison, D.C.: Ultrasound in the diagnosis and evaluation of therapy of idiopathic hypertrophic subaortic stenosis. Circulation 40:905, 1969.
13. Shah, P.M., Gramiak, R., and Kramer, D.H.: Ultrasound localization of left ventricular outflow obstruction in hypertrophic obstructive cardiomyopathy. Circulation 40:3, 1969.
14. Henry, W.L., Clark, C.E., and Epstein, S.E.: Asymmetric septal hypertrophy: Echocardiographic identification of the pathognomonic anatomic abnormality of IHSS. Circulation 47:225, 1973.
15. Gilbert, B.W., Pollick, C., Adelman, A.G., et al.: Hypertrophic cardiomyopathy: Subclassification by M mode echocardiography. Am. J. Cardiol. 45:861, 1980.
16. Martin, R.P., Rakowski, H., French, J., et al.: Idiopathic hypertrophic subaortic stenosis viewed by wide-angle, phased-array echocardiography. Circulation 59:1206, 1979.
17. Keren, G., Belhassen, B., Sherez, J., et al.: Apical hypertrophic cardiomyopathy: Evaluation by non-invasive and invasive techniques in 23 patients. Circulation 71:45, 1985.
18. Shapiro, L.M., and McKenna, W.J.: Distribution of left ventricular hypertrophy in hypertrophic cardiomyopathy: A two-dimensional echocardiographic study. J. Am. Coll. Cardiol. 2:437, 1983.
19. Pearson, A.C., Gudipati, C.V., and Labovitz, A.J.: Systolic and diastolic flow abnormalities in elderly patients with hypertensive hypertrophic cardiomyopathy. J. Am. Coll. Cardiol. 12:989, 1988.
20. Lever, H.M., Karam, R.F., Currie, P.J., et al.: Hypertrophic cardiomyopathy in the elderly: Distinctions from the young based on cardiac shape. Circulation 79:580, 1989.
21. Karam, R., Lever, H.M., and Healy, B.P.: Hypertensive hypertrophic cardiomyopathy or hypertrophic cardiomyopathy with hypertension?: A study of 78 patients. J. Am. Coll. Cardiol. 13:580, 1989.
22. Lewis, J.F., and Maron, B.J.: Elderly patients with hypertrophic cardiomyopathy: A subset with distinctive left ventricular morphology and progressive clinical course late in life. J. Am. Coll. Cardiol. 13:36, 1989.
23. Pollick, C., Morgan, C.D., Gilbert, B.W., et al.: Muscular subaortic stenosis: The temporal relationship between systolic anterior motion of the anterior mitral leaflet and the pressure gradient. Circulation 66:1087, 1982.
24. Pollick, C., Rakowski, H., and Wigle, E.D.: Muscular subaortic stenosis: The quantitative relationship between systolic anterior motion and the pressure gradient. Circulation 69:43, 1984.
25. Bryg, R.J., Pearson, A.C., Williams, G.A., et al.: Left ventricular systolic and diastolic flow abnormalities determined by Doppler echocardiography in obstructive hypertrophic cardiomyopathy. Am. J. Cardiol. 59:925, 1987.
26. Pearson, A.C., and Labovitz, A.J.: Color flow imaging in hypertrophic obstructive cardiomyopathy. Dynamic CV Imaging 1:187, 1987.
27. Sasson, Z., Yock, P.G., Hatle, L.K., et al.: Doppler echocardiographic determination of the pressure gradient in hypertrophic cardiomyopathy. J. Am. Coll. Cardiol. 11:752, 1988.
28. Sakurai, S., Tanaka, H., Yoshimura, H., et al.: Production of systolic anterior motion of the mitral valve in dogs. Circulation 71:805, 1985.
29. Grigg, L.E., Wigle, E.D., Williams, W.G., et al.: Transesophageal Doppler echocardiography in obstructive hypertrophic cardiomyopathy: Clarification of pathophysiology and importance in intraoperative decision making. J. Am. Coll. Cardiol. 20:42, 1992.
30. Spirito, P., Maron, B.J., Chiarella, F., et al.: Diastolic abnormalities in patients with hypertrophic cardiomyopathy: Relation to magnitude of left ventricular hypertrophy. Circulation 72:310, 1985.
31. Takenaka, K., Dabestani, A., Gardin, J.M., et al.: Left ventricular filling in hypertrophic cardiomyopathy: A pulsed Doppler echocardiographic study. J. Am. Coll. Cardiol. 7:1263, 1986.
32. Topol, E.J., Traill, T.A., and Fortuin, N.J.: Hypertensive hypertrophic cardiomyopathy of the elderly. N. Engl. J. Med. 312:277, 1985.
33. Agatston, A.S., Polakoff, R., Hippogoankar, R., et al.: The significance of increased left ventricular outflow tract velocities in the elderly measured by continuous wave Doppler. Am. Heart J. 117:1320, 1989.
34. Shah, P.M.: Echocardiography in congestive or dilated cardiomyopathy. J. Am. Soc. Echocardiogr. 1:20, 1988.
35. Louie, E.K.: Congestive cardiomyopathy: Doppler echocardiographic assessment of structure and function. Echocardiography 4:119, 1987.
36. Massie, B.M., Schiller, N.B., Ratshin, R.A., et al.: Mitral-septal separation: New echocardiographic index of left ventricular function. Am. J. Cardiol. 39:1008, 1977.
37. Wallis, D.E., O'Connell, J.B., Henkin, R.E., et al.: Segmental wall motion abnormalities in dilated cardiomyopathies: A common finding and good prognostic sign. J. Am. Coll. Cardiol. 4:674, 1984.
38. Medina, R., Panidis, I.P., Morganroth, J., et al.: The value of echocardiographic regional wall motion abnormalities in detecting coronary artery disease in patients with or without a dilated left ventricle. Am. Heart J. 109:799, 1985.
39. Godley, R.W., Wann, L.S., Rogers, E.W., et al.: Incomplete mitral leaflet closure in patients with papillary muscle dysfunction. Circulation 63:565, 1981.
40. Gardin, J.M., Iseri, L.T., Elkayam, U., et al.: Evaluation of dilated cardiomyopathy by pulsed Doppler echocardiography. Am. Heart J. 106:1057, 1983.
41. Chen, C., Rodriguez, L., Guerrero, J.L., et al.: Noninvasive estimation of the instantaneous first derivative of left ventricular pressure using continuous-wave Doppler echocardiography. Circulation 83:2101, 1991.
42. Rihal, C.S., Nishimura, R.A., Hatle, L.K., et al.: Systolic and diastolic dysfunction in patients with clinical diagnosis of dilated cardiomyopathy: Relation to symptoms and prognosis. Circulation 90:2772, 1994.
43. Galderisi, M., Lauer, M.S., and Levy, D.: Echocardiographic determinants of clinical outcome in subjects with coronary artery disease (the Framingham Heart Study). Am. J. Cardiol. 70:971, 1992.
44. Stoddard, M.F., Pearson, A.C., Kern, M.J., et al.: Left ventricular diastolic function: Comparison of pulsed Doppler echocardiographic and hemodynamic indexes in subjects with and without coronary artery disease. J. Am. Coll. Cardiol. 13:327, 1989.
45. Stoddard, M.F., Pearson, A.C., Kern, M.J., et al.: Influence of alteration in preload on the pattern of left ventricular diastolic filling as assessed by Doppler echocardiography in humans. Circulation 79:1226, 1989.
46. Xie, G.Y., Berk, M.R., Smith, M.D., et al.: Prognostic value of Doppler transmitral flow patterns in patients with congestive heart failure. J. Am. Coll. Cardiol. 24:132, 1994.

47. Werner, G.S., Schaefer, C., Dirks, R., et al.: Doppler echocardiographic assessment of left ventricular filling in idiopathic dilated cardiomyopathy during a one-year follow-up: Relation to the clinical course of disease. Am. Heart J. 126:1408, 1993.
48. Berger, M., Haimowitz, A., Van Tosh, A., et al.: Quantitative assessment of pulmonary hypertension in patients with tricuspid regurgitation using continuous-wave Doppler ultrasound. J. Am. Coll. Cardiol. 6:359, 1985.
49. Currie, P.J., Seward, J.B., Chan, K.L., et al.: Continuous wave Doppler determination of right ventricular pressure: A simultaneous Doppler-catheterization study in 127 patients. J. Am. Coll. Cardiol. 6:75, 1985.
50. Yock, P., and Popp, R.: Non-invasive measurement of right ventricular systolic pressure by Doppler ultrasound in patients with tricuspid regurgitation. Circulation 70:657, 1984.
51. Isobe, M., Yazaki, Y., Takaku, F., et al.: Prediction of pulmonary arterial pressure in adults by pulsed Doppler echocardiography. Am. J. Cardiol. 57:316, 1986.
52. Masuyama, T., Kodama, K., Kitabatake, A., et al.: Continuous-wave Doppler echocardiographic detection of pulmonary regurgitation and its application to noninvasive estimation of pulmonary artery pressure. Circulation 74:484, 1986.
53. Brunazzi, M.C., Chirillo, F., Pasqualini, M., et al.: Estimation of left ventricular diastolic pressures from precordial pulsed-Doppler analysis of pulmonary venous and mitral flow. Am. Heart J. 128:293, 1994.
54. Resnikov, L., Chediak, J., Hirsh, J., et al.: Antithrombotic agents in coronary artery disease. Chest 95 (Suppl.): 52, 1989.
55. Stratton, J.R., Lighty, G.W., Pearlman, A.S., et al.: Detection of left ventricular thrombus by two-dimensional echocardiography: Sensitivity, specificity, and causes of uncertainty. Circulation 66:156, 1982.
56. Hongo, M., and Ikeda, S.I.: Echocardiographic assessment of the evolution of amyloid heart disease: A study with familial amyloid polyneuropathy. Circulation 73:249, 1986.
57. Cueto-Garcia, L., Reeder, G.S., Kyle, R.A., et al.: Echocardiographic findings in systemic amyloidosis: Spectrum of cardiac involvement and relation to survival. J. Am. Coll. Cardiol. 6:737, 1985.
58. Benotti, J.R., Grossman, W., and Cohn, P.F.: Clinical profile of restrictive cardiomyopathy. Circulation 61:1206, 1980.
59. Klein, A.L., Hatle, L.K., Burstow, D.J., et al.: Doppler characterization of left ventricular diastolic function in cardiac amyloidosis. J. Am. Coll. Cardiol. 13:1017, 1989.
60. Spirito, P., Lupi, G., Melevendi, C., et al.: Restrictive diastolic abnormalities identified by Doppler echocardiography in patients with thalassemia major. Circulation 82:88, 1990.
61. Klein, A.L., Hatle, L.K., Taliercio, C.P., et al.: Prognostic significance of Doppler measures of diastolic function in cardiac amyloidosis: A Doppler echocardiography study. Circulation 83:808, 1991.

CHAPTER

32 Echocardiography in Pericardial Diseases

Bibiana Cujec, M.D.

Gary M. Brockington, M.D.

Steven L. Schwartz, M.D.

Natesa G. Pandian, M.D.

ECHOCARDIOGRAPHIC APPEARANCE AND ANATOMY OF THE NORMAL PERICARDIUM _____ 404
PERICARDIAL EFFUSION _____ 405
Detection of Pericardial Effusion _____ 405
Localization of Pericardial Fluid _____ 405
Quantitation of the Amount of Pericardial Fluid _____ 408
Assessment of the Contents of Pericardial Effusion _____ 408
Conditions That May Mimic Pericardial Effusion _____ 408
CARDIAC TAMPONADE _____ 409
Pathophysiology _____ 409

Echocardiographic Signs of Tamponade _____ 409
Echocardiography During Pericardiocentesis _____ 412
CONSTRICTIVE PERICARDITIS _____ 413
ECHOCARDIOGRAPHIC FINDINGS IN CERTAIN SPECIFIC DISORDERS _____ 416
Acute and Chronic Pericarditis _____ 416
Neoplastic Pericardial Disease _____ 416
Traumatic Pericardial Disease _____ 416
Pericardial Hematoma Following Cardiac Surgery _____ 417
Pericardial Cysts _____ 417
Absence of Pericardium _____ 417
CONCLUSION _____ 418

Pericardial involvement in disease processes is manifested in a multitude of ways, ranging from innocuous, trivial pericardial effusion to life-threatening cardiac tamponade. Echocardiography has proved highly valuable in evaluating pericardial disorders. This technique aids in the detection, localization, and quantitation of pericardial effusion as well as in the diagnosis of cardiac tamponade and constrictive pericarditis, in the evaluation of pericardial neoplasms, and in the detection of congenital abnormalities of the pericardium, such as absence of the pericardium and pericardial cysts. All the different modalities of cardiac ultrasound, including two-dimensional echocardiography, M-mode echocardiography, pulsed-wave and continuous-wave Doppler, color flow imaging, and transesophageal echocardiography are used in the comprehensive evaluation of patients with pericardial disease. In this chapter, we review the utility and limitations of echocardiography in the evaluation of pericardial disease.

ECHOCARDIOGRAPHIC APPEARANCE AND ANATOMY OF THE NORMAL PERICARDIUM

The appearance of the pericardium in M-mode and two-dimensional echocardiography is that of a bright, dense layer of echoes inseparable from the epicardial echo. This echo layer covers the entire surface of the heart, except for the posterior aspect of the left atrium, and is composed of signals from the epicardium, or visceral pericardium, and the parietal pericardium. Signals generated by this layer are generally the brightest signals originating from the heart. Figure 32–1 illustrates that even when the ultrasound gain is low and the signals from other cardiac structures are not apparent, the pericardial echo is often persistent. Although the morphologic thickness of the normal pericardium is 1 mm or less, the pericardial echo on transthoracic echocardiography usually appears thicker because of ultrasound reverberation and image "blooming" related to the strong pericardial reflection. The motion of the pericardial echo is congruent with that of the posterior left ventricular wall throughout the cardiac cycle. In the presence of a pericardial effusion, there is decreased pericardial motion relative to the epicardium.

The pericardial sinuses are blind outpouchings of the parietal pericardium.[1] Pericardial fluid may accumulate in these potential spaces. The superior pericardial sinus extends in a semicircular fashion around the anterior wall of the ascending aorta from the aortic root to the origin of the right innominate artery. It connects with the transverse pericardial sinus, which is situated between the posterior wall of the ascending aorta and the anterior walls of the right pulmonary artery and the left atrium. The postcaval pericardial sinus surrounds the anterolateral circumference of the superior vena cava and is an extension of the superior sinus. The oblique pericardial sinus, situated behind the left atrium, is formed by the parietal pericardial reflections over the pulmonary veins and the inferior vena cava.

PERICARDIAL EFFUSION

Detection of Pericardial Effusion

Echocardiography is the most sensitive technique for the detection of fluid in the pericardial space.[2] Pericardial fluid is seen on two-dimensional echocardiographic images and M-mode recordings as a relatively echo-free space between the epicardium and the pericardium (Figs. 32–2 to 32–4).[2-4] If the fluid contains clots or fibrinous material, granular, strand-like, or masses of echo signals can be visualized on the two-dimensional echocardiogram (Fig. 32–5).[5] Although M-mode echocardiography is useful in the detection of an effusion, two-dimensional echocardiography is the method of choice for assessing a pericardial effusion, since it presents a two-dimensional spatial display of the pericardial fluid. If the effusion is trivial, the echo-free space between the epicardial and the pericardial echoes is apparent only during systole. In the presence of a small effusion, a small echo-free space is seen during both diastole and systole. The size of the echo-free space varies with the amount of fluid present, as demonstrated in Figure 32–4, which shows images recorded from patients with small, moderate-sized, and large pericardial effusions. It is essential to use varying ultrasound gain and gray-scale (compression) settings to accurately detect pericardial effusions and any masses within the effusion.

Localization of Pericardial Fluid

Most pericardial effusions are circumferential, as seen in Figure 32–4. The majority of small effusions are only seen posteriorly because this region is most dependent during the routine echocardiographic study performed with the patient in the supine position. Moderate-sized and large effusions result in echo-free spaces both anteriorly and posteriorly in the parasternal long-axis view and circumferentially in the parasternal short-axis and apical views (see Fig. 32–4). Small pericardial effusions generally are not seen behind the left atrium unless there is preferential accumulation of fluid in the oblique pericardial sinus. Fluid confined to the anterior region is uncommon; posteriorly loculated effusions are more frequently encountered. Posterior loculation is particularly common in patients after cardiac surgery.[6] In these patients, the right ventricular epicardium and pericardium are often adherent to the inner surface of the chest wall, and thus pericardial fluid collection

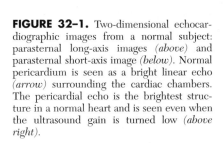

FIGURE 32–1. Two-dimensional echocardiographic images from a normal subject: parasternal long-axis images *(above)* and parasternal short-axis image *(below)*. Normal pericardium is seen as a bright linear echo *(arrow)* surrounding the cardiac chambers. The pericardial echo is the brightest structure in a normal heart and is seen even when the ultrasound gain is turned low *(above right)*.

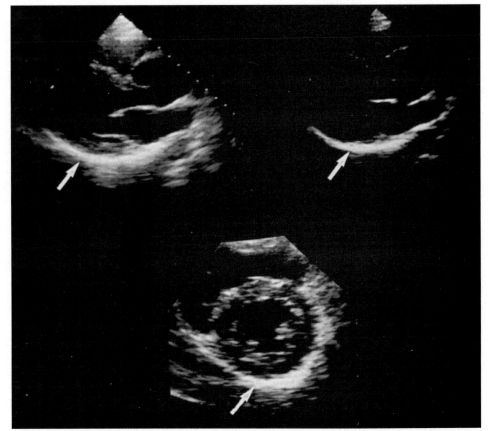

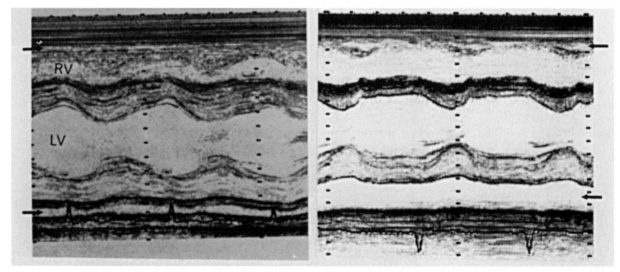

FIGURE 32–2. An M-mode echocardiographic tracing from two patients with pericardial effusion. In the recording at the left, a small echo-free space is seen between the epicardium and the pericardium both anteriorly and posteriorly *(arrows)*. In the recording on the right, from a patient with a moderate-sized effusion, a larger anterior and posterior space is noted *(arrows)*. LV = left ventricle; RV = right ventricle.

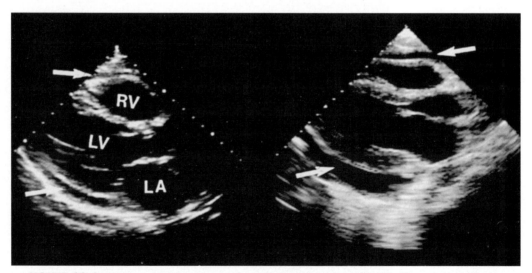

FIGURE 32–3. Parasternal long-axis images from two patients with pericardial effusions. A small echo-free space surrounding both the right and the left ventricles is seen *(arrows)*, indicating the presence of a pericardial effusion. A larger effusion is noted in the image on the right. RV = right ventricle; LV = left ventricle; LA = left atrium.

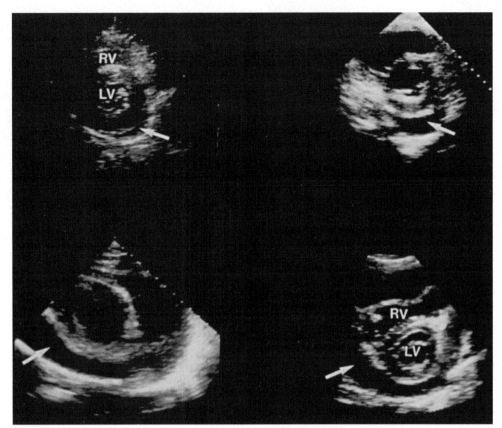

FIGURE 32–4. Short-axis images from four patients with pericardial effusions display different amounts and distributions of pericardial fluid. *Top Left,* A very small echo-free space is seen in the posterior region without any fluid anteriorly. *Top Right,* A relatively larger space is seen posteriorly, and there is no anterior pericardial effusion. *Bottom Left,* A large pericardial effusion surrounds the heart, with the exception of the anterior region. *Bottom Right,* A very large pericardial effusion surrounds the entire heart. RV = right ventricle; LV = left ventricle; arrows = pericardial effusion.

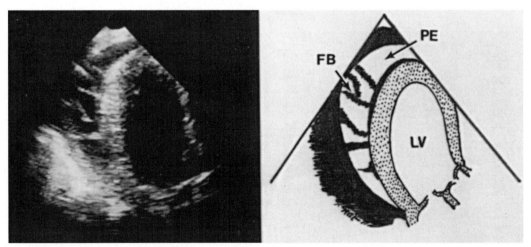

FIGURE 32–5. An apical long-axis image from a patient with an organized pericardial effusion. A moderate-sized pericardial effusion is seen posteriorly and around the cardiac apex. Within the effusion, multiple linear band-like echoes indicate the presence of fibrinous bands within the pericardial cavity. PE = pericardial effusion; FB = fibrinous band; LV = left ventricle.

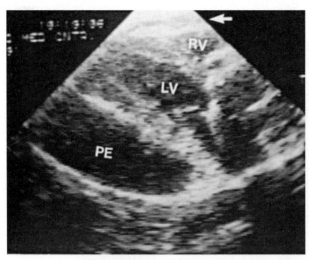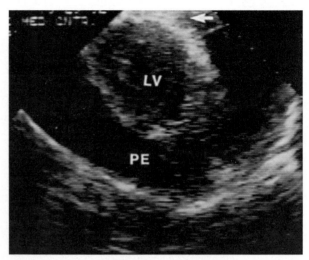

FIGURE 32–6. Parasternal long-axis *(left)* and parasternal short-axis *(right)* images from a patient with a postoperative pericardial effusion. A large echo-free space is seen posteriorly and laterally in this patient, but no fluid is seen anteriorly. The anterior right ventricular wall *(arrow)* adheres to the chest wall, which is usually the case in postoperative pericardial effusions. RV = right ventricle; LV = left ventricle; PE = pericardial effusion.

does not accumulate in this region. Figure 32–6 illustrates these findings in a patient who had recently undergone bypass surgery.

Quantitation of the Amount of Pericardial Fluid

The sensitivity of echocardiography is such that as little as 20 mL of pericardial fluid can be detected if proper ultrasound techniques are used. Since even healthy individuals occasionally may have as much as 50 mL of pericardial fluid, echocardiographic visualization of a small amount of pericardial fluid in an otherwise healthy individual should not be cause for concern.[7, 8] Accurate quantitation of pericardial fluid is not possible with echocardiography or any noninvasive technique, but echocardiography allows discrimination among small, moderate-sized, and large quantities of fluid.[8, 9] The images seen in Figure 32–4 are examples of how two-dimensional echocardiography can be used to semiquantify the

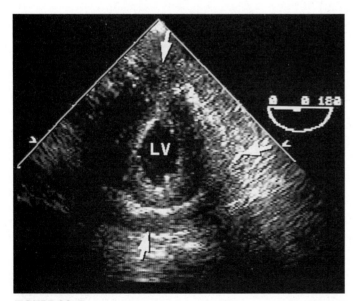

FIGURE 32–7. A transesophageal transgastric short-axis image of the left ventricle *(LV)* in a patient who became hypotensive after removal of epicardial pacing wires following coronary artery bypass surgery. The arrows point to the hemopericardium. Note that the echogenicity of the clotted blood within the pericardial cavity is similar to that of the myocardium.

volume of an effusion. In general, if a circumferential effusion is seen clearly, it indicates the presence of an effusion usually exceeding 300 mL. If the average width of the space circumferentially exceeds 1 cm, the effusion is likely to be larger than 500 mL; if the average width is close to 2 cm, the fluid collection is likely to be more than 700 mL.[8]

Assessment of the Contents of Pericardial Effusion

It is not possible to assess the character of pericardial fluid accurately with echocardiography. Serous effusions, purulent effusions, unclotted blood in the pericardial space, and chylopericardium all may appear as similar clear spaces. Clotted blood in the pericardium produces granular echoes that are of similar or even greater acoustic density than the myocardium.[10] This ambiguity may lead to misinterpretation of clotted hemopericardium as an absence of pericardial effusion.[11] Figure 32–7 illustrates the increased echogenicity of clotted hemopericardium in a patient following coronary artery bypass surgery. Fibrous strands may be observed in both purulent and nonpurulent pericardial effusions.[5] Figure 32–5 illustrates these strands, which appear as small linear bands that in real time may exhibit mobility. In neoplastic disease, solid masses of echoes caused by metastatic deposits may occasionally be visualized within the pericardial cavity.[12] Frequently, the masses are seen to be adherent to the epicardial surface, as shown in Figure 32–8.

Conditions That May Mimic Pericardial Effusion

Certain conditions and pitfalls in echocardiographic examination techniques may result in apparently echo-free spaces that may mimic the presence of a pericardial effusion.[11, 13–17] A prominent epicardial fat pad may sometimes be mistaken for pericardial fluid. Layers of fat, although more common on the anterior surface of the heart, can surround both ventricles. Space caused by a fat pad may be devoid of echo signals but often contains granular echoes, whereas a pericardial effusion causes a clear echo-free space.[17] An organized effusion, however, can exhibit echo signals within the pericardial space and may appear similar to an epicardial fat pad. Close observation of the motion of the pericardial echo layer, appropriate adjustment of the gain, and examination from various views are often helpful in differentiating a pericardial effusion from an epicardial fat pad. Similar maneuvers would help in the

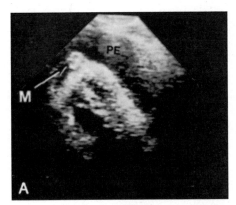
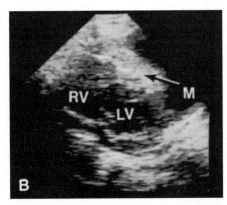
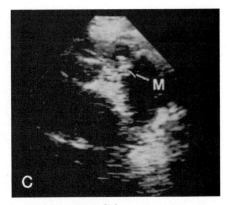

FIGURE 32–8. Two-dimensional echocardiographic images from a patient with neoplastic pericardial disease, showing a pericardial effusion and tumor deposits at the left ventricular apex (A), along the anterior left ventricle (B), and near the right ventricular outflow tract area (C). RV = right ventricle; LV = left ventricle; PE = pericardial effusion; M = mass.

discrimination of an effusion from certain tumors that may encircle the heart.[18]

Left pleural effusions may occasionally be difficult to distinguish from pericardial fluid collections. In the parasternal long-axis view, a pericardial effusion results in an echo-free space that separates the posterior left atrial wall from the anterior wall of the descending aorta (Fig. 32–9).[14] In contrast, a left pleural effusion extends posteriorly to the descending thoracic aorta. Other conditions that may be confused with pericardial effusions include pericardial cysts, mediastinal tumors, pericardial masses, pneumopericardium, and diaphragmatic hernias.[13, 18, 19] Most of the difficulties in differentiating these entities can be eliminated by optimizing the technical and practical aspects of ultrasound imaging. Transesophageal echocardiography allows improved resolution and spatial reconstruction of pericardial and mediastinal abnormalities and may be a useful supplement to transthoracic echocardiography in select patients. Care must also be taken with transesophageal echocardiography to avoid misinterpretation of the transverse pericardial sinus as the left main coronary artery[20] or pericardial masses in the transverse sinus as left atrial appendage thrombi.

CARDIAC TAMPONADE

Pathophysiology

The output of both ventricles depends on adequate diastolic filling. Normally, intrapericardial pressure is zero or slightly negative, and there is a positive transmural pressure gradient across the myocardium during diastole that aids ventricular filling. With increasing pericardial pressure, the transmural pressure gradient decreases, and ventricular filling and therefore stroke volume and cardiac output fall, resulting in cardiac tamponade.[21–27] Pulsus paradoxus, an important clinical sign of tamponade, is observed because inspiration increases the filling gradient across the right side of the heart but does not increase it across the left side of the heart. The augmented right ventricular filling occurs at the expense of reduced filling and stroke output of the left ventricle. These pathophysiologic alterations in tamponade are also responsible for the many echocardiographic findings.[6, 25–33]

Echocardiographic Signs of Tamponade

Two-dimensional echocardiography is useful in assessing cardiac tamponade. Besides demonstrating the presence and distribution of pericardial fluid, two-dimensional echocardiography provides two useful signs in tamponade: right ventricular diastolic collapse and right atrial collapse, which are illustrated in Figures 32–10 and 32–11.[22, 27, 32, 34, 35] In normal individuals and in patients with pericardial effusion without tamponade, the free walls of the cardiac chambers maintain a rounded contour. During tamponade, a transient invagination (or collapse) of the right ventricular and right atrial free wall occurs when intracavitary pressures are lowest: early diastole for the right ventricle and late diastole or early systole for the right atrium (see Fig. 32–11)[22, 32, 34, 36] In the presence of right atrial and right ventricular collapse, the cardiac walls are acting as visual transducers of the transmural pressure gradient. Since this gradient is the basis of cardiac tamponade, it is not surprising that collapse of the right atrium or right ventricle is more reliable in the diagnosis of tamponade than are clinical signs. In general, right

FIGURE 32–9. Parasternal long-axis images from two patients demonstrating the presence of both pericardial and pleural effusions. The pericardial effusion is seen posterior to the left ventricle aligned with the anterior aspect of the descending thoracic aorta (arrows); the pleural effusion extends beyond the posterior aspect of the left ventricle and is aligned with the posterior aspect of the descending thoracic aorta. LV = left ventricle; LA = left atrium; PE = pericardial effusion; PLE = pleural effusion.

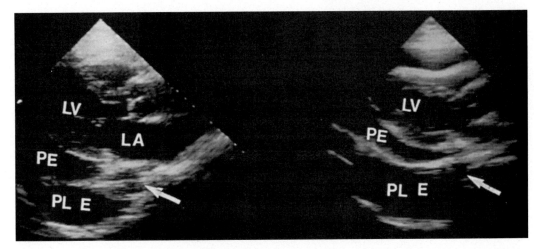

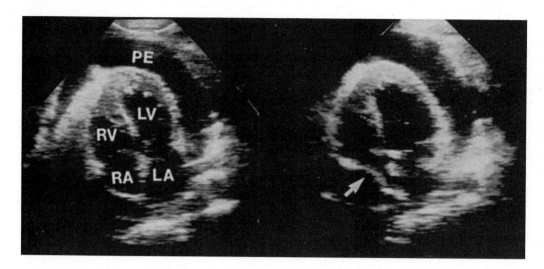

FIGURE 32–10. Apical four-chamber images from a patient with cardiac tamponade. A large pericardial effusion is noted surrounding almost the entire heart. The right atrial wall has a rounded contour during mid-diastole *(left)* but exhibits indentation during late diastole. The arrow points to right atrial collapse. RV = right ventricle; LV = left ventricle; RA = right atrium; LA = left atrium; PE = pericardial effusion.

atrial collapse is highly sensitive (100 percent) but relatively less specific for the diagnosis of tamponade.[32] The specificity is improved when the duration of right atrial collapse occupies a longer portion of the cardiac cycle. Right ventricular diastolic collapse is a more specific sign of tamponade than is right atrial collapse and is also highly sensitive.[22, 27, 32] Diastolic collapse of the right ventricle has been found to develop when tamponade causes a decline of 20 percent in cardiac output. Right atrial and right ventricular collapse may precede the development of pulsus paradoxus; both occur prior to the reduction of mean arterial pressure.[32] The presence of both these signs almost always indicates that the effusion is hemodynamically significant. These signs are present even in the setting of low-pressure tamponade, since the transient relative changes in the pressure gradients between the pericardial cavity

and the chambers persist despite low absolute pressures.[37] If tamponade is caused by a large or posteriorly localized effusion, the left atrial free wall also may manifest an inward motion, which is referred to as left atrial collapse (see Fig. 32–11).[35]

In patients who have had cardiac surgery, the right ventricular and right atrial walls are often adherent to the inner chest wall, in which case collapse of these chambers may not be evident despite tamponade. In these patients, pericardial fluid is often in a posterior location. If such an effusion causes regional tamponade, even the thick-walled left ventricle can be deformed and can collapse during diastole.[6] This sign, left ventricular diastolic collapse, is useful in the diagnosis of postoperative tamponade caused by a loculated pericardial effusion (Fig. 32–12). Localized compression of a single cardiac chamber (most commonly the anterior or lateral

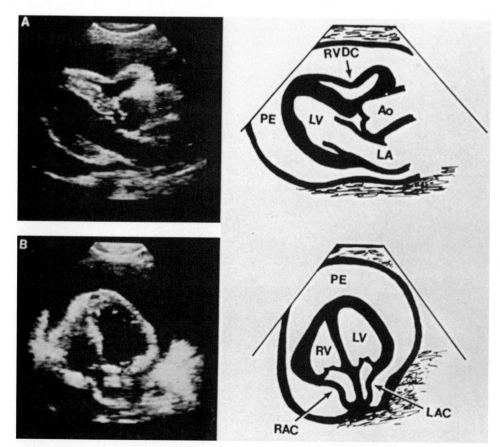

FIGURE 32–11. Parasternal long-axis *(A)* and apical four-chamber *(B)* images from a patient with cardiac tamponade, demonstrating the presence of right ventricular diastolic collapse and right atrial collapse. In this patient, even the left atrium is seen to collapse because of tamponade. LV = left ventricle; LA = left atrium; Ao = aorta; PE = pericardial effusion; RVDC = right ventricular diastolic collapse; RAC = right atrial collapse; LAC = left atrial collapse.

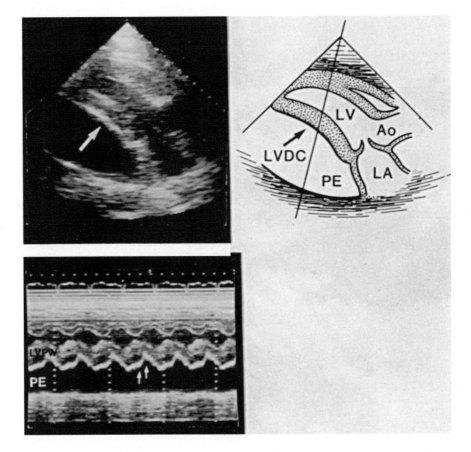

FIGURE 32–12. A low parasternal long-axis image from a patient with postoperative pericardial effusion and cardiac tamponade demonstrates a large posterior effusion and the presence of left ventricular diastolic collapse. Anteriorly, the right ventricular wall is adherent to the chest wall. The left ventricular posterior wall exhibits an invagination during early ventricular diastole (*large arrow*). Left ventricular diastolic collapse is seen in the M-mode echocardiographic recording as well (*second small arrow*). The first arrow points to the end of ventricular systole. LV = left ventricle; LA = left atrium; Ao = aorta; LVPW = left ventricular posterior wall; LVDC = left ventricular diastolic collapse; PE = pericardial effusion.

right atrium) by pericardial hematoma may also produce a syndrome similar to tamponade without the presence of right ventricular diastolic collapse, as demonstrated in Figure 32–13. This can readily be identified with transesophageal echocardiography.[38, 39] Right ventricular diastolic collapse may also be absent despite tamponade when the right ventricular wall is thickened and stiff or when pulmonary hypertension is present. Elevation of right atrial pressure in patients with cardiac tamponade results in an ancillary echocardiographic sign. Inferior vena cava plethora, defined as dilation or engorgement of the inferior vena cava associated with an inspiratory reduction in diameter of less than 50 percent, is a sensitive sign for the presence of cardiac tamponade, although it is nonspecific.[40]

Respiration profoundly influences cardiac hemodynamics and intracardiac flow dynamics. Normally, inspiration causes less than a 20 percent increase in systemic venous, tricuspid valvular, and pulmonary valvular blood flow velocities and a corresponding decrease in pulmonary venous, mitral valvular, and aortic blood flow velocities.[41–43] A minimal inspiratory change in blood flow velocities is noted in patients with hemodynamically insignificant pericardial effusions as well.[44] In the setting of cardiac tamponade, however, there is a pronounced increase in the magnitude of inspiratory change in blood flow velocity. With inspiration, right-sided flow velocities are increased by more than 40 percent, whereas left-sided flow velocities are decreased by more than 40 percent. Figures 32–14 and 32–15 demonstrate this finding, which is known as flow velocity paradoxus.[29, 43, 44] Another measurement that can be derived from spectral Doppler tracings is the isovolumic relaxation time, which is prolonged during inspiration in patients with tamponade. This feature is a result primarily of an inspiratory decrease in the pressure gradient between pulmonary capillary wedge pressure and left ventricular diastolic pressure.[44] Color flow Doppler mapping can also demonstrate the changes in blood flow velocity caused by cardiac tamponade. Right-sided filling is greatest during inspiration. The tricuspid flow jet as seen by color Doppler imaging appears correspondingly larger during inspiration than during expiration. Conversely, the mitral flow jet is smaller during inspiration.[31] Thus, the various Doppler modalities are useful in instantly showing the flow variations associated with respiration during tamponade. However, an exaggerated inspiratory change in blood flow velocities may be noted in patients with obstructive pulmonary disease or even in normal individuals if respiration is highly labored.

FIGURE 32–13. A transesophageal echocardiogram, transverse plane. A large echodense pericardial hematoma (*arrows*) selectively compresses the right atrium (*RA*) in this patient with cardiac tamponade following mitral repair. RV = right ventricle; PE = pericardial effusion.

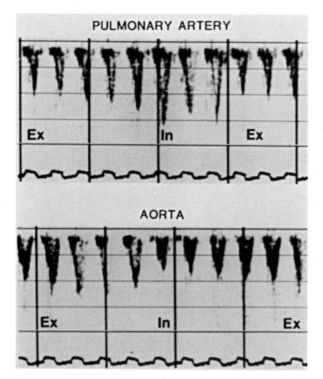

FIGURE 32–14. Pulmonary artery and aortic blood flow velocity recordings in cardiac tamponade. There is a marked increase in the pulmonary flow velocity during inspiration. Simultaneously, there is a marked decrease in aortic flow velocity. In = inspiration, Ex = expiration.

A comprehensive cardiac ultrasound examination involving all modalities is necessary to make the diagnosis of tamponade with maximal confidence. By its ability to detect early tamponade, echocardiography is an extremely valuable tool in assessing the hemodynamic significance of a pericardial effusion.

Echocardiography During Pericardiocentesis

Once the diagnosis of tamponade has been made, echocardiography may be instrumental in aiding with therapeutic modalities to relieve hemodynamic compromise.[6, 45, 46] Pericardiocentesis is the preferred procedure for relieving hemodynamic compromise, since previous studies have indicated that temporizing measures (i.e., fluid loading) may not be effective.[47]

When pericardiocentesis is contemplated, it is important to obtain a two-dimensional echocardiographic image of the planned path of the aspiration needle to confirm the presence of fluid in that orientation. Two-dimensional echocardiography is also frequently used to guide pericardiocentesis. Proper needle and catheter position in the pericardial cavity can be confirmed with confi-

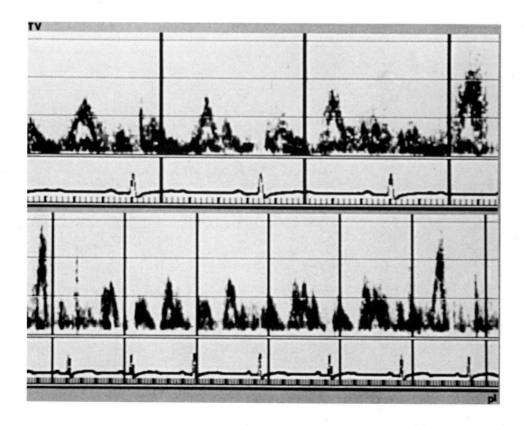

FIGURE 32–15. Tricuspid flow velocity recordings from a patient with cardiac tamponade, recorded at a fast paper speed on top and at a slower paper speed on the bottom. Both tracings exhibit a marked variation in tricuspid flow velocity during expiration but an increase in flow velocity during inspiration. TV = tricuspid valve.

dence, as shown in Figure 32–16.[48–50] It is particularly useful during drainage of loculated effusions.[46] Figure 32–17 shows images before and after pericardiocentesis and illustrates how echocardiography can confirm resolution of chamber compression, indicate the efficacy of drainage, and delineate residual fluid.

CONSTRICTIVE PERICARDITIS

Constrictive pericarditis is associated with two fundamental abnormalities, one anatomical and the other physiologic. The fundamental anatomical feature is a thickened pericardium; the physiologic abnormality is filling dysfunction.[24, 25, 51–54] Several M-mode echocardiographic patterns can be consistent with pericardial thickening. They include a single, thick, echo-dense line, a double line of echoes moving synchronously, multiple parallel moving lines, and multiple parallel nonmoving lines (Fig. 32–18).[55–57] None of these, however, has proved reliably diagnostic of thickened pericar-

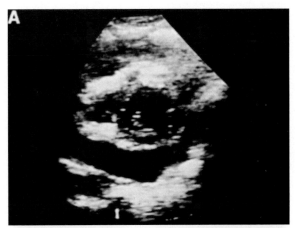

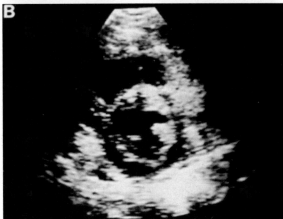

FIGURE 32–17. Parasternal short-axis images from a patient with cardiac tamponade before *(A)* and after *(B)* pericardiocentesis. A large pericardial effusion is seen prior to pericardiocentesis. The image obtained following the procedure demonstrates absence of fluid in the pericardial cavity.

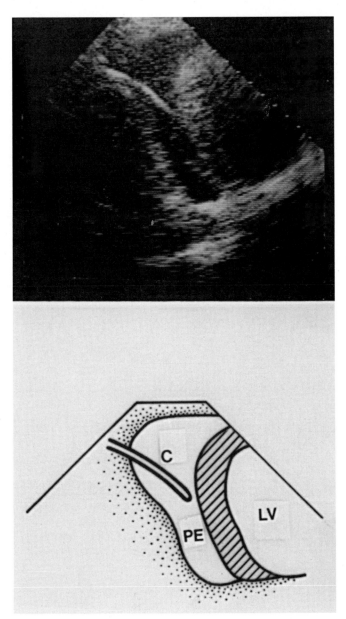

FIGURE 32–16. A two-dimensional echocardiographic image obtained during pericardiocentesis. A large effusion is seen surrounding the left ventricle. A catheter that has been introduced into the pericardial cavity is seen as a bright linear echo. LV = left ventricle; PE = pericardial effusion; C = catheter.

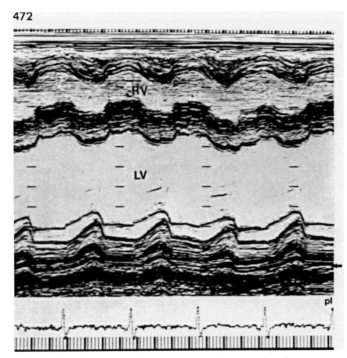

FIGURE 32–18. An M-mode echocardiographic recording from a patient with constrictive pericarditis. The pericardial echo *(arrow)* is seen as multiple dense layers moving in concert. The left ventricular posterior wall demonstrates a rapid relaxation at early diastole but appears flattened during the rest of diastole. RV = right ventricle; LV = left ventricle.

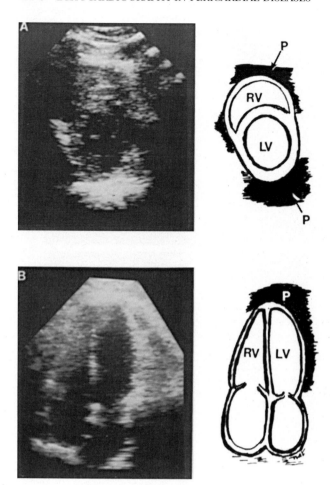

FIGURE 32–19. Parasternal short-axis (A) and apical four-chamber (B) two-dimensional echocardiographic images from a patient with constrictive pericarditis. In both images, the pericardium appears bright and thickened. Computed tomography in this patient demonstrated a markedly thickened pericardium. RV = right ventricle; LV = left ventricle; P = pericardium.

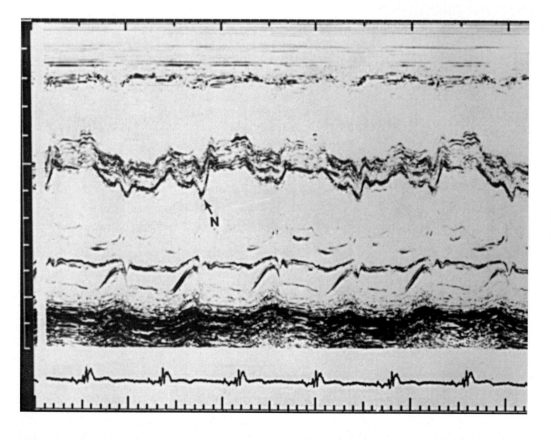

FIGURE 32–20. An M-mode echocardiographic tracing in a patient with constrictive pericarditis. An early diastolic notch (N) is evident on the interventricular septum.

dium or constrictive pericarditis. Two-dimensional echocardiography may show a bright, thick pericardial echo in patients with thickened pericardium (Fig. 32–19).[58] In patients with advanced calcific constrictive pericarditis, the pericardium may appear like a shell encompassing the heart. Accurate assessment of pericardial thickness, however, is not possible with M-mode or two-dimensional transthoracic echocardiographic techniques.[59] Instrument settings such as gain and gray scale profoundly influence the echocardiographic appearance of this structure and make it difficult to assess the presence of a thickened pericardium. In general, transthoracic two-dimensional echocardiography tends to overestimate the thickness of the pericardial layer. Transesophageal echocardiography may allow more accurate measurement of pericardial thickness.[60] Computed tomography is an alternative approach to quantifying pericardial thickness.[53]

Echocardiographic techniques are more useful in defining the filling impairment associated with constrictive pericarditis. The physiologic abnormality in constriction is an impediment to filling during the middle and late periods of diastole, when ventricular diastolic expansion is suddenly restricted by the thick, noncompliant pericardium. Consequently, most of the filling occurs early in diastole.[53, 61, 62] Various qualitative M-mode echocardiographic findings have been reported to be consistent with constrictive physiology. Figure 32–18 shows an example of one of these signs. After normal rapid early diastolic outward motion, the left ventricular posterior wall demonstrates flattening during the rest of diastole.[53, 55, 59] Other M-mode echocardiographic findings reported in constrictive pericarditis include a rapid E-F slope in the mitral valve echogram, paradoxical septal motion, diastolic notching of the interventricular septum (Fig. 32–20), and premature opening of the pulmonic valve (Fig. 32–21).[52, 53, 63–65] These signs are, in general, nonspecific and insensitive for constrictive pericarditis.[53, 63–65]

Two-dimensional echocardiography in patients with constriction usually demonstrates a normal-sized heart with preserved left and right ventricular systolic function. A repeated finding in patients with constriction is a brisk, early diastolic bouncing motion of the interventricular septum, evident particularly during inspiration.[40, 58] This finding has been reported to have 93 percent specificity and 62 percent sensitivity. Plethora of the inferior vena cava with decreased inspiratory collapse is another two-dimensional echocardiographic sign noted in constrictive pericarditis.

Both the filling dysfunction of constrictive pericarditis and the abnormal respiratory influence on filling are reflected in the pattern of intracardiac and venous flows. Doppler echocardiography allows evaluation of such abnormalities, as illustrated in Figure 32–22. Examination of the mitral flow velocity in constrictive pericarditis shows a markedly increased early diastolic filling velocity (E velocity) with a rapid deceleration and a decreased late diastolic filling velocity following atrial contraction (A velocity), resulting in an increased E:A ratio.[42, 51, 61, 62] This finding, however, is not specific for constriction and may be noted with restrictive cardiomyopathy or with severe mitral regurgitation. Such analysis of mitral flow may be difficult in patients who are tachycardic, and it is not possible in the presence of atrial fibrillation. Nevertheless, in a patient known to have a thickened pericardium who has sinus rhythm and does not have severe mitral regurgitation, the observation of an increased E:A ratio and a rapid deceleration slope of the early filling wave strongly suggests constrictive physiology.

The filling dysfunction in constrictive pericarditis results in elevated ventricular diastolic pressures. If right ventricular diastolic pressure exceeds right atrial pressure, diastolic tricuspid regurgitation can occur. Right ventricular diastolic pressure may also transiently exceed pulmonary artery pressure. This reversal of the usual pressure gradient leads to premature opening of the pulmonary valve, with resulting diastolic antegrade flow into the pulmonary artery (see Fig. 32–21).[42] Diastolic mitral regurgitation may also be

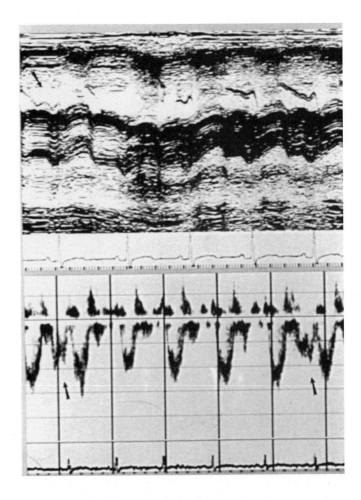

FIGURE 32–21. An M-mode recording of the pulmonary valve and pulsed Doppler recording of pulmonary artery blood flow velocity. The pulmonary valve shows premature opening, and the pulmonary blood flow velocity recording shows intermittent diastolic antegrade flow into the pulmonary artery *(arrows)*. This diastolic flow pattern occurred during inspiration.

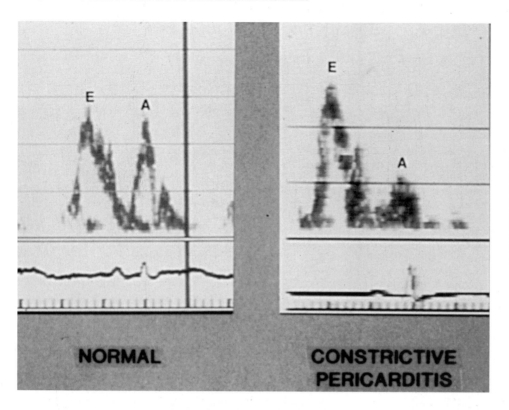

FIGURE 32–22. Pulsed Doppler recording of mitral flow velocity from a normal subject and from a patient with constrictive pericarditis. Compared to the normal pattern, the pattern of the patient with constrictive pericarditis exhibits a markedly increased early diastolic velocity (E), a rapid deceleration of the early diastolic velocity, and a markedly reduced late diastolic flow velocity (A).

found in some patients. These findings, however, are encountered in patients with restrictive cardiomyopathy as well.[66]

Another feature noted in patients with constrictive pericarditis is an exaggerated respiratory variation in the velocity of right-sided and left-sided flows, with a more than 25 percent difference between inspiratory and expiratory values.[61, 62] During inspiration, there is an increase in right-sided flow velocities and a corresponding decrease in left-sided flow velocities. The mitral flow velocity tracings shown in Figure 32–23 demonstrate these changes. Respiratory variation is seen in the left ventricular isovolumic relaxation time as well; this parameter decreases during expiration and increases during inspiration in patients with constrictive pericarditis. Patients with restrictive cardiomyopathy do not exhibit these exaggerated respiratory changes in flow velocities and isovolumic relaxation time.[61] Sampling of the pulmonary vein flow with transesophageal echocardiography reveals more respiratory variation in systolic and diastolic velocities and a higher systolic-to-diastolic pulmonary venous flow ratio in patients with constrictive pericarditis when compared with those with restrictive cardiomyopathy.[33, 67] Analysis of superior vena cava and hepatic vein flow velocity recordings is also useful in differentiating constriction from restriction. In patients with constriction, the systolic component of the systemic venous flow velocity is increased, corresponding to the deep x descent on pressure tracings. Alternatively, the diastolic antegrade component, which corresponds to the y descent, is prominent in restrictive cardiomyopathy.[68]

In effusive-constrictive pericarditis, echocardiography demonstrates the presence of a clear or organized pericardial effusion. There are usually echocardiographic features consistent with cardiac tamponade or constriction. In contrast to tamponade, in which the flow abnormalities registered by Doppler imaging typically resolve after pericardiocentesis, there is persistent evidence of elevated diastolic pressures in patients with effusive-constrictive pericarditis.

ECHOCARDIOGRAPHIC FINDINGS IN CERTAIN SPECIFIC DISORDERS

Acute and Chronic Pericarditis

The causes of acute pericarditis are legion, including viral, bacterial, and mycobacterial infections; myocardial infarction; connective tissue diseases; and drugs. Acute pericarditis also occurs following cardiotomy and radiation.[69–78] Pericardial effusion may be noted in patients with acute pericarditis, but its absence does not exclude the diagnosis. When present, the effusion is usually small, but occasionally a large amount of fluid accumulates, and cardiac tamponade may result. The size of the effusion and the presence of tamponade can be evaluated with echocardiography, based on the features previously described. However, the cause of the effusion cannot be determined echocardiographically. The inflammatory process may progress and lead to constrictive pericarditis.[79–80]

Neoplastic Pericardial Disease

Pericardial involvement in malignant disease can occur via contiguous spread or metastatic implants. Carcinoma of the breast and lung, leukemia, lymphoma, and melanoma have the highest incidence of cardiac involvement. Primary malignant tumors of the heart, including angiosarcoma, mesothelioma, fibrosarcoma, and rhabdomyoma, may involve the pericardium. This structure is the predominant site of neoplasm in 85 percent of patients with cardiac malignancies.[81] Pericardial effusion with or without tamponade is the major manifestation of neoplastic pericardial disease. In addition, solid tumor masses occupying the pericardial cavity have been visualized with two-dimensional echocardiography, as shown in Figure 32–8.[12] Besides revealing the presence of pericardial effusion and offering guidance during pericardiocentesis, repeat studies following pericardiocentesis are useful because the fluid frequently reaccumulates. Cardiac constriction secondary to encasement of the heart by a tumor may occur, and this can also be identified.[18] Thus, echocardiography provides diagnostic information regarding pericardial neoplasms and can be instrumental in facilitating their treatment.

Traumatic Pericardial Disease

Cardiac tamponade and constrictive pericarditis may result from chest trauma.[82] Since the echocardiographic findings in these disorders were mentioned earlier, attention here is only given to traumatic entities that were not previously discussed. Penetrating wounds of the chest or inadvertent surgical disruption of the thoracic duct can result in a chylous effusion that is echocardiographically indistinct from other effusions.[81] As always, analysis of the fluid is necessary to confirm the diagnosis. Pneumopericardium can be seen secondary to penetrating wounds of the chest, esophageal rupture, gastric rupture, or infections involving gas-producing organisms and may result in cardiac tamponade.[83] Echocardiography may demonstrate an "air gap" in the pericardium, although on a plain chest film air can usually be seen between the heart and the pericardium.[84]

Pericardial Hematoma Following Cardiac Surgery

Loculated blood in the pericardium following cardiac surgery is of variable acoustic impedance and may be echo-free, simulating blood in a cardiac chamber, or as echo-reflective as the myocardium (see Fig. 32–13). Hematomas may selectively compress a cardiac chamber, most commonly the right atrium[38, 39] and less frequently the right ventricle or the left atrium. Loculated pericardial hematomas may not be visualized with transthoracic echocardiography, which is frequently of suboptimal quality because of surgical dressings and drainage tubes, mechanical ventilation, and immobilization of the patient in the immediate postoperative period. Transesophageal echocardiography allows rapid and accurate diagnosis of pericardial hematomas, which can cause significant hemodynamic compromise and require prompt surgical evacuation.[38, 39]

Pericardial Cysts

Pericardial cysts are round, smooth-walled outpouchings of the parietal pericardium with loss of visible communication with the pericardial cavity. They contain varying amounts of pericardial fluid. The congenital type is most often located at the right cardiophrenic angle but can be seen in almost any position.[85] Acquired cysts can be caused by neoplastic infiltration of the pericardium, trauma, or infection. The pericardial cyst may resemble a ventricular aneurysm, cardiac mass, mediastinal tumor, or hiatal hernia on a plain chest film. Confirmation of a fluid-filled pericardial mass seen echocardiographically allows a cyst to be diagnosed (Fig. 32–24).[19, 86] Calcium deposits in the cyst wall may also be noted.[87] Occasionally, such cysts rupture and therefore are not present on follow-up studies.[88]

Absence of Pericardium

Complete absence of pericardium is a rare congenital anomaly. Most of these patients are asymptomatic despite the loss of the stabilizing effect of the pericardium.[89] In individuals with complete absence of the pericardium, echocardiographic imaging reveals apparent enlargement of the right ventricle and paradoxical septal motion, mimicking right ventricular volume overload.[90] These signs are due to the marked leftward displacement and lateral rotation of the heart and may also be present in patients who have undergone surgical removal of the pericardium. Congenital absence of the left pericardium, although rare, does occur more frequently than absence of the entire pericardium. Pericardial dropout associated with localized bulging of the inferior left ventricular wall through the pericardial defect has been reported on two-dimensional echocardiography in patients with absence of the left pericardium.[91, 92] Protrusion of the left atrial appendage through the left-sided pericardial defect may lead to expansion or aneurysm formation of the left atrium, which can also be visualized on the two-dimensional echocardiogram.[93] Rare cases of strangulation or herniation of portions of the heart, or both, have been reported in patients with partial absence of the pericardium.[94, 95]

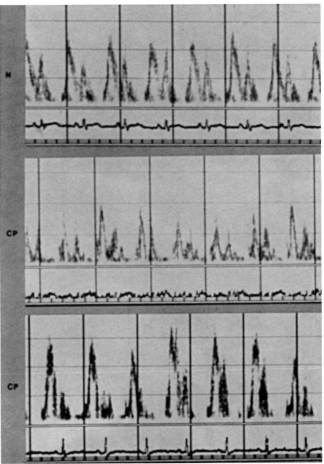

FIGURE 32–23. Mitral flow velocity recordings from a normal subject *(N)* and from two patients with constrictive pericarditis *(CP)*. In contrast with the minimal respiratory variation in mitral flow velocity seen in the normal patient, a markedly exaggerated variation in the mitral flow velocity is noted in the patients with constrictive pericarditis.

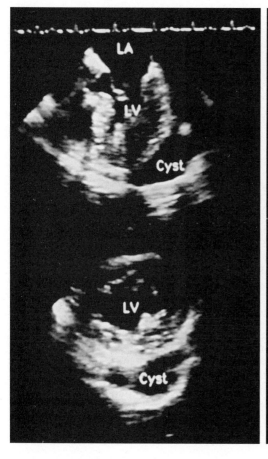
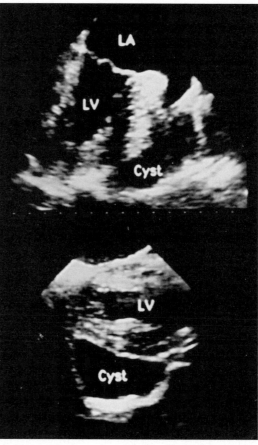

FIGURE 32–24. A biplane transesophageal echocardiogram. The left panels are transverse imaging planes, and the right panels are longitudinal imaging planes. The lower panels are transgastric views. A large pericardial cyst is seen as an echo-free loculated mass adjacent to the anterolateral wall of the left ventricle (LV) that does not communicate with the cardiac chambers. LA = left atrium.

CONCLUSION

Echocardiography has become the technique of choice for the assessment of most disorders involving the pericardium. A comprehensive examination with multiple echocardiographic modalities is necessary for proper delineation of the morphologic and physiologic abnormalities associated with pericardial disease. In addition to its diagnostic capability, echocardiography contributes by guiding and monitoring therapeutic interventions.

References

1. Choe, Y.H., Im, J.-G., Han, M.C., et al.: The anatomy of the pericardial space: A study in cadavers and patients. AJR 149:693, 1987.
2. Feigenbaum, H. (ed.): Echocardiography. 5th ed. Philadelphia, Lea & Febiger, 1993, p. 556.
3. Feigenbaum, H., Waldhauser, J.A., and Hyde, L.P.: Ultrasonic diagnosis of pericardial effusion. J.A.M.A. 191:107, 1965.
4. Matuso, H., Matsumoto, M., Hamarrha, Y., et al.: Rotational excursion of the heart in massive pericardial effusion studied by phased-array echocardiography. Br. Heart J. 41:513, 1979.
5. Martin, R.P., Bowden, R., Filly, K., et al.: Intrapericardial abnormalities in patients with pericardial effusion: Findings by two-dimensional echocardiography. Circulation 61:568, 1980.
6. Chuttani, K., Pandian, N.G., Mohanty, P.K., et al.: Left ventricular diastolic collapse: An echocardiographic sign of regional cardiac tamponade. Circulation 83:1999, 1991.
7. Braunwald, E. (ed.): Heart Disease: A Textbook of Cardiovascular Medicine. 4th ed. Philadelphia, W.B. Saunders, 1992, p. 102.
8. Horowitz, M.S., Schully, C.S., Stinson, E.B., et al.: Sensitivity and specificity of echocardiographic diagnosis of pericardial effusion. Circulation 50:239, 1974.
9. D'Cruz, I.A., Cohen, H.C., Prabbu, R., et al.: Potential pitfalls in quantification of pericardial effusion by echocardiography. Br. Heart J. 39:529, 1977.
10. Lopez-Sendon, J., Garcia-Fernandez, M.A., Coma-Canella, I., et al.: Identification of blood in the pericardial cavity in dogs by two-dimensional echocardiography. Am. J. Cardiol. 53:1194, 1984.
11. Yousem, D., Traill, T.T., Wheeler, P.S., et al.: Illustrative cases in pericardial effusion misdetection: Correlation of echocardiography and CT. Cardiovasc. Intervent. Radiol. 10:162, 1987.
12. Chandraratna, P.A., and Aronow, W.S.: Detection of pericardial metastasis by cross-sectional echocardiography. Circulation 63:54, 1981.
13. Cummings, R.G., Wesley, R.L.R., Adams, D.H., et al.: Pneumopericardium resulting in cardiac tamponade. Ann. Thorac. Surg. 37:511, 1984.
14. Lewandowski, B.J., Jaffer, N.M., and Winsberg, F.: Relationship between the pericardial and pleural spaces in cross sectional imaging. J. Clin. Ultrasound 9:272, 1981.
15. Millman, A., Meller, J., Motro, M., et al.: Pericardial tumor or fibrosis mimicking pericardial effusion by echocardiography. Ann. Intern. Med. 86:434, 1977.
16. Ratshin, R.A., Smith, M.K., and Hood, W.P., Jr.: Possible false-positive diagnosis of pericardial effusion by echocardiography in the presence of large left atrium. Chest 65:112, 1974.
17. Rifkin, R.D., Isner, J.M., Carter, B.L., et al.: Combined posteroanterior subepicardial fat simulating the echocardiographic diagnosis of pericardial effusion. J. Am. Coll. Cardiol. 3:1333, 1984.
18. Lin, T.K., Stech, J.M., Echert, W.G., et al.: Pericardial angiosarcoma simulating pericardial effusion by echocardiography. Chest 73:881, 1978.
19. Nasser, W.K.: Congenital disease of the pericardium. Cardiovasc. Clin. 7:271, 1976.
20. Stoddard, M.F., Liddell, N.E., Longaker, R.A., et al.: Transesophageal echocardiography: Normal variants and mimickers. Am. Heart J. 124:1587, 1992.
21. Gaffney, F.A., Keller, A.M., Perchock, R.M., et al.: Pathophysiologic mechanisms of cardiac tamponade and pulsus alternans shown by echocardiography. Am. J. Cardiol. 53:1662, 1984.
22. Schiller, N.B., and Botvinich, E.H.: Right ventricular compression as a sign of cardiac tamponade: An analysis of echocardiographic ventricular dimensions and their clinical implications. Circulation 56:774, 1977.
23. Settle, H.P., Adolph, R.J., Fowler, N.O., et al.: Echocardiographic study of cardiac tamponade. Circulation 56:951, 1977.
24. Shabetai, R.: The pathophysiology of cardiac tamponade and constriction. Cardiovasc. Clin. 7:67, 1976.
25. Shabetai, R., Fowler, N.O., and Guntheroth, W.G.: The hemodynamics of cardiac tamponade and constrictive pericarditis. Am. J. Cardiol. 26:480, 1970.
26. Shiina, S., Yagirymat, T., Kondo, K., et al.: Echocardiographic evaluation of inpending cardiac tamponade. J. Cardiogr. 9:555, 1979.
27. Singh, S., Wann, S., Schuchard, G.H., et al.: Right ventricular and right atrial collapse in patients with cardiac tamponade: A combined echocardiographic and hemodynamic study. Circulation 68:294, 1983.
28. Leimbruger, P.P., Klopfenstein, S., Wann, L.S., et al.: The hemodynamic derangement associated with right ventricular collapse in cardiac tamponade: An experimental echocardiographic study. Circulation 689:612, 1983.
29. Pandian, N.G., Rifkin, R.D., and Wang, S.S.: Flow velocity paradoxus: A Doppler echocardiographic sign of cardiac tamponade. Exaggerated respiratory variation in pulmonary and aortic blood flow velocities. (Abstract.) Circulation 70(Suppl. II):II-381, 1984.

30. Pandian, N.G., Wang, S.S., McInerney, K., et al.: Doppler echocardiography in cardiac tamponade abnormalities in tricuspid and mitral flow response to respiration in experimental and clinical tamponade. (Abstract.) J. Am. Coll. Cardiol. 5:485, 1985.

31. Pandian, N.G., Wang, S.S., Moten, M., et al.: Color Doppler study of tricuspid and mitral flow changes in cardiac tamponade. (Abstract.) Circulation 76(Suppl. IV):IV-525, 1987.

32. Rifkin, R.D., Pandian, N.G., Funai, J.T., et al.: Sensitivity of right atrial collapse and right ventricular diastolic collapse in the diagnosis of graded cardiac tamponade. Am. J. Noninvas. Cardiol. 1:73, 1987.

33. Schiavone, W.A., Calafiore, P.A., and Salcedo, E.E.: Transesophageal Doppler echocardiographic demonstration of pulmonary venous flow velocity in restrictive cardiomyopathy and constrictive pericarditis. Am. J. Cardiol. 63:1286, 1989.

34. Gillam, L.D., Guyer, D.E., Gibson, T.E., et al.: Hydrodynamic compression of the right atrium: A new echocardiographic sign of cardiac tamponade. Circulation 68:294, 1983.

35. Kronzon, I., Cohen, M.L., and Winer, H.E.: Diastolic atrial compression: A sensitive echocardiographic sign of cardiac tamponade. J. Am. Coll. Cardiol. 2:770, 1983.

36. Martins, J.B., and Kerber, R.E.: Can cardiac tamponade be diagnosed by echocardiography? Experimental studies. Circulation 60:733, 1979.

37. Labib, S., Udelson, J., and Pandian, N.G.: Echocardiography in low-pressure cardiac tamponade. Am J. Cardiol. 63:1156, 1989.

38. Beppu, S., Tanaka, N., Nakatani, S., et al.: Pericardial clot after open heart surgery: Its specific localization and haemodynamics. Eur. Heart J. 14:230, 1993.

39. Kochar, G.S., Jacobs, L.E., and Kotler, M.N.: Right atrial compression in postoperative cardiac patients: Detection by transesophageal echocardiography. J Am. Coll. Cardiol. 16:511,1990.

40. Himelman, R.B., Lee, E., and Schiller, N.B.: Septal bounce, vena cava plethora and pericardial adhesion: Informative two-dimensional echocardiographic signs in the diagnosis of pericardial constriction. J. Am. Soc. Echocardiogr. 1:333, 1988.

41. Dabestani, A., Takenak, K., Allen, B., et al.: Effects of spontaneous respiration on diastolic left ventricular filling assessed by pulsed Doppler echocardiography. Am. J. Cardiol. 61:1356, 1988.

42. King, W.S., Pandian, N.G., and Gardin, J.M.: Doppler echocardiographic findings in pericardial tamponade and constriction. Echocardiography 5:361, 1988.

43. Leeman, D.E., Levine, M.J., and Come, P.C.: Doppler echocardiography in cardiac tamponade: Exaggerated respiratory variation in transvalvular flow velocity integrals. J. Am. Coll. Cardiol. 11:572, 1988.

44. Appleton, C.P., Hatle, L.K., and Popp, R.L.: Cardiac tamponade and pericardial effusion: Respiratory variation in transvalvular flow velocities studied by Doppler echocardiography. J. Am. Coll. Cardiol. 11:1020, 1988.

45. Kopecky, S.L., Callahan, J.A., Tajik, A.J., et al.: Percutaneous pericardial catheter drainage: Report of 42 consecutive cases. Am. J. Cardiol. 50:633, 1986.

46. Pandian, N.G., Brockway, B., Simonetti, J., et al.: Pericardiocentesis under two-dimensional echocardiographic guidance in loculated pericardial effusion. Ann. Thorac. Surg. 45:99, 1988.

47. Kerber, R.E., Gascho, J.A., Litchfield, R., et al.: Hemodynamic effects of volume expansion and nitroprusside compared with pericardiocentesis in patients with acute cardiac tamponade. N. Engl. J. Med. 307:929, 1982.

48. Callahan, J.A., Seward, J.B., and Tajik, A.J.: Pericardiocentesis assisted by two-dimensional echocardiography. J. Thorac. Cardiovasc. Surg. 85:877, 1983.

49. Callahan, J.A., Seward, J.B., and Tajik, A.J.: Cardiac tamponade pericardiocentesis directed by two-dimensional echocardiography. Mayo Clin. Proc. 60:344, 1985.

50. Santos, G.H., and Rrater, R.W.M.: The subxyphoid approach in the treatment of pericardial effusion. Ann. Thorac. Surg. 23:467, 1977.

51. Agatson, A.S., Rao, A., Price, R.J., et al.: Diagnosis of constrictive pericarditis by pulsed Doppler echocardiography. Am. J. Cardiol. 54:929, 1984.

52. Hancock, W.E.: On the elastic and rigid forms of constrictive pericarditis. Am. Heart J. 100:917, 1980.

53. Isner, J.M., Pandian, N.G., McInerney, K.P., et al.: The pericardial tourniquet: Evaluation of the anatomic and physiologic features of constrictive pericarditis by combined use of computed tomography and cardiac ultrasound. Echocardiography 2:197,1985.

54. Marsa, R., Mehta, S., Willis, W., et al.: Constrictive pericarditis after myocardial revascularization: Report of 3 cases. Am. J. Cardiol. 44:177, 1979.

55. Engel, P.J., Fowler, N.O., Tei, C., et al.: M-mode echocardiography in constrictive pericarditis. J. Am. Coll. Cardiol. 6:471, 1985.

56. Horowitz, M.S., Rossen, R., and Harrison, D.C.: Echocardiographic diagnosis of pericardial disease. Am. Heart J. 97:420, 1979.

57. Schnittger, I., Bowden, R.E., Abrams, J., et al.: Echocardiography: Pericardial thickening and constrictive pericarditis. Am. J. Cardiol. 42:388, 1978.

58. Pandian, N.G., Skorton, D.J., Kiesco, R.A., et al.: Diagnosis of constrictive pericarditis by two-dimensional echocardiography: Studies in a new experimental model and in patients. J. Am. Coll. Cardiol. 4:1164, 1984.

59. Hinds, S.W., Reisner, S.A., Amico, A.F., et al.: Diagnosis of pericardial abnormalities by 2D-echo: A pathology-echocardiography correlation in 85 patients. Am. Heart J. 123:143, 1992.

60. Hsu, T.-L., Chen, C.-H., Weintraub, A., et al.: Utility of transesophageal echocardiography in the detailed depiction of simple and complex pericardial disorders: Comparison with transthoracic imaging. (Abstract.) J. Am. Soc. Echocardiogr. 4:290, 1991.

61. Hatle, L.K., Appleton, C.P., and Popp, R.L.: Differentiation of constrictive pericarditis and restrictive cardiomyopathy, by Doppler echocardiography. Circulation 79:357, 1989.

62. Oh, J.K., Hatle, L.K., Seward, J.B., et al.: Diagnostic role of Doppler echocardiography in constrictive pericarditis. J. Am. Coll. Cardiol. 23:154, 1994.

63. Candell-Riera, J., DelCastillo, A.G., Dermanger-Miralda, G., et al.: Echocardiographic features of the interventricular septum in chronic constrictive pericarditis. Circulation 57:1154, 1978.

64. Elkayam, U., Kotler, M.N., Segal, B., et al.: Echocardiographic findings in constrictive pericarditis: A case report. J. Med. Sci. 12:1308, 1976.

65. Tanaka, C., Nishimoto, M., Takeudi, K., et al.: Presystolic pulmonary valve opening in constrictive pericarditis. Jpn. Heart J. 20:419, 1979.

66. Klein, A.L., Hatle, L.K., Burstow, D.J., et al.: Doppler characterization of left ventricular function in cardiac amyloidosis. J. Am. Coll. Cardiol. 13:1017, 1989.

67. Klein, A.L., Cohen, G.I., Pietrolungo, J.F., et al.: Differentiation of constrictive pericarditis from restrictive cardiomyopathy by Doppler transesophageal echocardiographic measurements of respiratory variations in pulmonary venous flow. J. Am. Coll. Cardiol. 22:1935, 1993.

68. Appleton, C.P., Hatle, L.K., and Popp, R.L.: Central venous flow velocity patterns can differentiate constrictive pericarditis from restrictive cardiomyopathy. (Abstract.) J. Am. Coll. Cardiol. 9(Suppl. A):119A, 1987.

69. Applefield, M.M., Cole, J.F., Pollack, S.H., et al.: The late appearance of chronic pericardial disease in patients treated by radiotherapy for Hodgkin's disease. Ann. Intern. Med. 94:338, 1981.

70. Baldwin, J.J., and Edwards, J.E.: Uremic pericarditis as a cause of cardiac tamponade. Circulation 53:896, 1976.

71. Berger, H.W., and Seckler, S.G.: Pleural and pericardial effusions in rheumatoid disease. Ann. Intern. Med. 64:1291, 1966.

72. Botti, R.E., Driscol, T.E., Pearson, O.H., et al.: Radiation myocardial fibrosis simulating constrictive pericarditis. Cancer 22:1254, 1968.

73. Corey, G.R., Campbell, P.T., Van Trigt, P., et al.: Etiology of large pericardial effusions. Am. J. Med. 95:209, 1993.

74. Hochberg, M.S., Merrill, W.H., Bruber, M., et al.: Delayed cardiac tamponade associated with prophylactic anticoagulation in patients undergoing coronary bypass grafting: Early diagnosis with two-dimensional echocardiography. J. Thorac. Cardiovasc. Surg. 75:777, 1978.

75. John, T.J., Hough, A., and Sergent, J.S.: Pericardial disease in rheumatoid arthritis. Am. J. Med. 66:383, 1979.

76. Rooney, J.J., Crocco, J.A., and Lynon, H.A.: Tuberculous pericarditis. Ann. Intern. Med. 64:1291, 1966.

77. Thadani, U., Ivenson, J.M.I., and Wright, V.: Cardiac tamponade, constrictive pericarditis and pericardial resection in rheumatoid arthritis. Medicine 54:261, 1975.

78. Yurchak, P.M., Levine, S.A., and Gorlin, R.: Constrictive pericarditis complicating disseminated lupus erythematosus. Circulation 31:113, 1965.

79. Cameron, J., Osterle, S.N., Baldwon, J.C., et al.: The etiologic spectrum of constrictive pericarditis. Am. Heart J. 113:354, 1987.

80. Cohen, M.V., and Greenberg, M.A.: Constrictive pericarditis: Early and late complication of cardiac surgery. Am. J. Cardiol. 43:657, 1979.

81. Eagle, K.A., Haber, E., DeSanctis, R.W., et al. (eds.): The Practice of Cardiology. 2nd ed. Boston, Little, Brown, 1989, p. 977.

82. Pandian, N.G., Weintraub, A., Kusay, B.S., et al.: Emergency echocardiography. Echocardiography 6:1, 1989.

83. Bedotto, J.B., McBride, W., Abraham, M., et al.: Echocardiographic diagnosis of pneumopericardium and hydropneumopericardium. J. Am. Soc. Echocardiogr. 1:359, 1988.

84. Reid, C.L., Chandraratna, A.W., Kawanishi, D., et al.: Echocardiographic detection of pneumomediastinum and pneumopericardium: The air gap sign. J. Am. Coll. Cardiol. 1:916, 1983.

85. Feigin, D.S., Fenoglio, J.J., McAllister, H.A., et al.: Pericardial cysts: A radiologic pathologic correlation and review. Radiology 15:125, 1977.

86. Hynes, J.K., Tajik, A.J., Osborn, M.J., et al.: Two-dimensional echocardigraphic diagnosis of pericardial cyst. Mayo Clin. Proc. 58:60, 1983.

87. Pugatch, R.D., Braner, J.H., Robbins, A.H., et al.: CT diagnosis of pericardial cysts. AJR 131:515, 1978.

88. King, J.F., Corby, I., Pugh, D., et al.: Rupture of pericardial cyst. Chest 60:611, 1971.

89. Southworth, H., and Stevenson, C.S.: Congenital defects of the pericardium. Arch. Intern. Med. 61:223, 1938.

90. Payvandi, N.M., and Kerber, R.E.: Echocardiography in congenital and acquired absence of the pericardium. Circulation 53:86, 1976.

91. Candan, I., Erol, C., and Sonel, A.: Cross sectional echocardiographic appearance in presumed congenital absence of the left pericardium. Br. Heart J. 55:405, 1986.

92. Kansal, S., Roitman, D., and Sheffield, L.T.: Two-dimensional echocardiography of congenital absence of the pericardium. Am. Heart J. 109:912,1985.

93. Altman, C.A., Ettedgui, J.A., Wozney, P., et al.: Noninvasive diagnostic features of partial absence of the pericardium. Am. J. Cardiol. 16:1536, 1989.

94. Cassosla, L., and Katz, J.A.: Management of cardiac herniation after intrapericardial pneumonectomy. Anesthesiology 60:362, 1984.

95. Minocha, G.K., Falicon, R.E., and Nyensohn, E.: Partial right-sided congenital pericardial defect with herniation of the right atrium and right ventricle. Chest 76:484, 1979.

33 Two-Dimensional and Doppler Echocardiography in the Evaluation of Congenital Heart Disease

A. Rebecca Snider, M.D.

ACYANOTIC CONGENITAL HEART DISEASE WITH INCREASED PULMONARY BLOOD FLOW ____ 420
Ventricular Septal Defects ____ 420
Atrial Septal Defects ____ 423
Patent Ductus Arteriosus ____ 424
Atrioventricular Septal Defects ____ 427
Doppler Quantitation of Left-to-Right Shunts ____ 430
CONGENITAL HEART DISEASE WITH VENTRICULAR OUTFLOW OBSTRUCTION ____ 431
Left Ventricular Outflow Obstruction ____ 431
Right Ventricular Outflow Obstruction ____ 435
CONGENITAL HEART DISEASE WITH CYANOSIS AND DECREASED PULMONARY VASCULARITY ____ 436
Defects With a Right-to-Left Shunt at Ventricular Level ____ 436
Defects With a Right-to-Left Shunt at Atrial Level ____ 437

CONGENITAL HEART DISEASE WITH CYANOSIS AND INCREASED PULMONARY VASCULARITY ____ 438
Increased Pulmonary Arterial Markings ____ 438
Increased Pulmonary Venous Markings ____ 440
ECHOCARDIOGRAPHIC APPROACH TO COMPLEX CONGENITAL HEART DISEASE ____ 441
Echocardiographic Approach to the Segmental Analysis of the Heart ____ 441
Echocardiographic Features of Frequently Encountered Complex Congenital Heart Defects ____ 445
l-Transposition of the Great Arteries ____ 445
Univentricular Heart ____ 448
Dextrocardias ____ 449
TRANSESOPHAGEAL ECHOCARDIOGRAPHY IN CONGENITAL HEART DISEASE ____ 449
SUMMARY ____ 450

In recent years, the noninvasive technique of echocardiography has had a major influence on the diagnostic and therapeutic management of children with congenital heart disease. M-mode echocardiography provided a method for the assessment of wall thickness, chamber size, and valve motion. The development of two-dimensional echocardiography provided a technique for spatial anatomical display of cardiac structures and, thus, led to more exact definition of cardiac anatomy, even in the more complex congenital cardiac defects. Recent advances in equipment and image processing have allowed improved visualization of cardiac structures—even in small preterm infants. The addition of Doppler ultrasonography to the two-dimensional echocardiographic examination has provided a technique for the quantitative assessment of valve gradients, cardiac output, and shunt size. Because of these rapid advances in technology, two-dimensional and Doppler echocardiography have allowed cardiac catheterization for diagnostic purposes to be eliminated in many instances and, in other cases, to be postponed until the infant or child is better able to withstand this invasive procedure.

In this chapter, we shall review the echocardiographic findings in the more common congenital cardiac defects and discuss briefly the echocardiographic approach to the segmental diagnosis of complex congenital cardiac abnormalities.

ACYANOTIC CONGENITAL HEART DISEASE WITH INCREASED PULMONARY BLOOD FLOW

Ventricular Septal Defects

Children with a large ventricular septal defect and normal pulmonary vascular resistance show evidence of left ventricular volume overload (enlarged left atrium and left ventricle) on the two-dimensional echocardiogram. Because of the increase in left ventricular diastolic filling, left ventricular stroke volume is increased, and septal and posterior wall motion is exaggerated. On the two-dimensional echocardiogram, ventricular septal defects can be imaged directly as areas of echocardiographic dropout in the ventricular septum.[1] These defects can occur in any of the four portions of the ventricular septum that have different embryologic derivations but usually are found along the fusion lines between the different portions of the septum.[2] The different portions of the ventricular septum are (1) the membranous septum, which is subaortic and beneath the septal leaflet of the tricuspid valve; (2) the muscular or trabeculated septum, which includes the inferior two thirds of the septum; (3) the outlet or infundibular septum, which is subaortic and subpulmonic; and (4) the inlet or sinus septum, which is the superior and posterior one third of the septum between the atrioventricular valves (Figs. 33–1 and 33–2). With two-dimensional

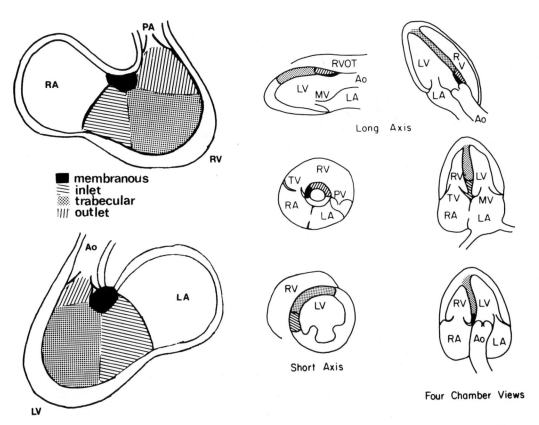

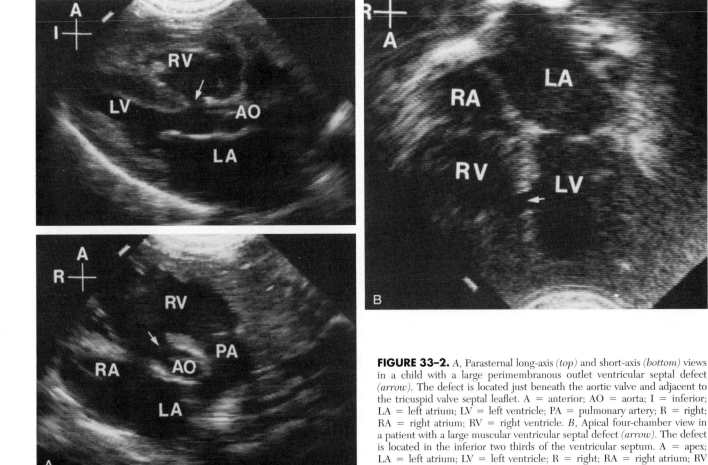

FIGURE 33–1. *Left*, Diagrammatic representation of the parts of the ventricular septum, as viewed from the right ventricle *(above)* and left ventricle *(below)*. *Right*, Diagrammatic representation of the parts of the ventricular septum, as viewed in the long-axis, short-axis, and four-chamber views. Ao = aorta; LA = left atrium; LV = left ventricle; MV = mitral valve; PA = pulmonary artery; PV = pulmonary valve; RA = right atrium; RV = right ventricle; RVOT = right ventricular outflow tract; TV = tricuspid valve. (From Silvermann, N.H., and Snider, A.R.: Two-Dimensional Echocardiography in Congenital Heart Disease. Norwalk, CT, Appleton-Century-Crofts, 1982, pp. 71–72, with permission.)

FIGURE 33–2. A, Parasternal long-axis *(top)* and short-axis *(bottom)* views in a child with a large perimembranous outlet ventricular septal defect *(arrow)*. The defect is located just beneath the aortic valve and adjacent to the tricuspid valve septal leaflet. A = anterior; AO = aorta; I = inferior; LA = left atrium; LV = left ventricle; PA = pulmonary artery; R = right; RA = right atrium; RV = right ventricle. B, Apical four-chamber view in a patient with a large muscular ventricular septal defect *(arrow)*. The defect is located in the inferior two thirds of the ventricular septum. A = apex; LA = left atrium; LV = left ventricle; R = right; RA = right atrium; RV = right ventricle.

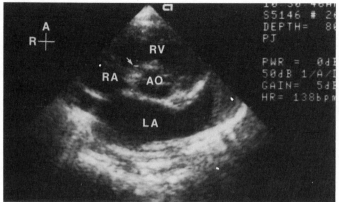

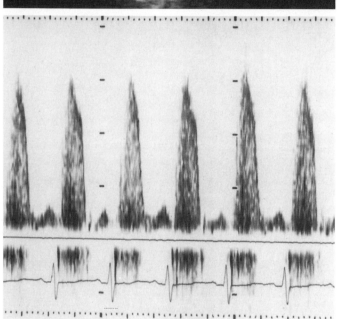

FIGURE 33–3. Simultaneous two-dimensional image and continuous-wave Doppler recording from a child with a membranous ventricular septal defect. The parasternal short-axis view *(top)* shows the position of the continuous-wave beam *(arrow)* at the time of the Doppler recording. The Doppler tracing *(bottom)* shows a high-velocity jet in systole, directed toward the transducer and above the baseline. The peak velocity of the jet is 3.2 m per second, which predicts a pressure gradient of 40 mm Hg across the septal defect. A = anterior; AO = aorta; LA = left atrium; R = right; RA = right atrium; RV = right ventricle.

echocardiography, defects are classified as entirely within a portion of the ventricular septum (i.e., muscular defects) or as on a fusion line between two or more portions of the ventricular septum (i.e., perimembranous outlet defects, perimembranous inlet defects).

Two-dimensional echocardiography has been reported to be 100 percent sensitive in the detection of outlet and inlet ventricular septal defects. In infants younger than 1 year of age, the sensitivity for detecting membranous ventricular septal defects has ranged from 74 to 87 percent.[1, 3, 4] Muscular ventricular septal defects are the most difficult to detect with two-dimensional echocardiography, and sensitivity has been reported to be as low as 30 percent in some prospective studies. Several factors make direct visualization of muscular ventricular septal defects very difficult. First, these defects can occur anywhere in the wide area of the septum that is the muscular septum. Second, these defects are often serpiginous, so the right septal surface of the defect may not be visualized simultaneously with the left septal surface of the defect. Third, these defects may change size and virtually be obliterated in systole. Finally, these defects may be hidden on the right septal surface by septoparietal muscle bundles within the right ventricle.

With the introduction of pulsed, continuous-wave, and color flow

Doppler techniques, the sensitivity for detection of ventricular septal defects has improved considerably. In children with a ventricular septal defect and left ventricular pressure higher than right ventricular pressure, a systolic jet can be recorded in the right ventricle on the Doppler examination (Fig. 33–3).[5–8] Usually, the jet extends throughout systole and has a very high peak velocity, because left ventricular systolic pressure is much higher than right ventricular systolic pressure; however, with very large defects and systemic right ventricular pressure, systolic velocities may be low (less than 2.5 m per second) or may not be recorded at all.[9] In patients with a very large left-to-right ventricular shunt, Doppler examination of the main pulmonary artery shows an increased velocity (because of increased flow) and spectral broadening (owing to the persistence of disturbed flow downstream from the defect).

Color flow Doppler mapping has had a major application in the rapid detection of septal defects (Fig. 33–4). With this technique, blood flow can be seen crossing defects that are too small to be visualized directly on the two-dimensional echocardiogram. In a recent study, the abilities of color Doppler imaging and angiography to detect multiple muscular ventricular septal defects were compared. The color Doppler technique correctly identified 72 percent of all patients proven by angiography to have multiple muscular defects. No false-positive diagnoses were made with the color Doppler technique.[10]

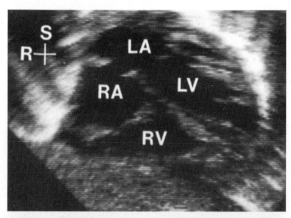

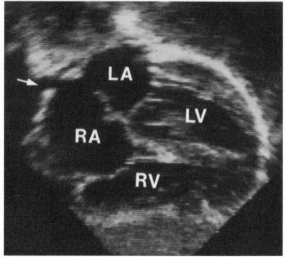

FIGURE 33–5. *Top,* Subcostal four-chamber view in a patient with a secundum atrial septal defect. The secundum atrial septal defect appears as an area of echocardiographic dropout in the midportion of the atrial septum. *Bottom,* Subcostal four-chamber view in a child with a sinus venosus atrial septal defect and anomalous drainage of the right upper pulmonary vein *(arrow).* The sinus venosus atrial septal defect is seen as an area of echocardiographic dropout in the superior portion of the atrial septum. The right upper pulmonary vein drains just to the right of the atrial septal defect. LA = left atrium; LV = left ventricle; R = right; RA = right atrium; RV = right ventricle; S = superior.

FIGURE 33–4. See Color Plate 6.

In patients with a ventricular septal defect and no right or left ventricular outflow obstruction, the pressure difference between the left and the right ventricles can be calculated from the peak velocity of the systolic jet.[5] For this calculation, a simplified Bernoulli equation is used:

$$\text{Pressure gradient} = 4 \times (\text{peak velocity})^2$$

If the arm blood pressure is obtained at the time of the Doppler examination, the right ventricular (RV) systolic pressure can be calculated as follows:

$$\text{RV systolic pressure} = \\ \text{systolic arm blood pressure} - 4 \times (\text{peak velocity})^2$$

With the use of this equation, good correlations have been found between Doppler and cardiac catheterization measurements of right ventricular systolic pressure.[9, 11] If an adequate recording of the peak velocity of the jet through the ventricular septal defect cannot be obtained, the right ventricular systolic pressure can be estimated from the peak velocity of the tricuspid insufficiency jet with the use of the following equation:

$$\text{RV systolic pressure} = \\ 4 \times (\text{peak velocity})^2 + \text{right atrial pressure}$$

Most children, and especially those with right ventricular hypertension, have at least a small tricuspid insufficiency jet that can be used to estimate right ventricular systolic pressure. Right atrial pressure can be estimated from the amount of jugular venous distention, can be assumed to be normal (8 to 10 mm Hg), or can be measured when a central venous line is in place.

Atrial Septal Defects

Children with a large atrial septal defect show evidence of right ventricular volume overload (right atrial and right ventricular dilation, paradoxical septal motion) on the two-dimensional echocardiogram. Atrial septal defects can be visualized directly as an area of echocardiographic dropout in the atrial septum (Fig. 33–5). These defects can occur in the midportion of the atrial septum (ostium secundum defect), in the lower third of the atrial septum adjacent to the atrioventricular valves (ostium primum defect), or in the posterior portion of the atrial septum near the superior or inferior venae cavae (sinus venosus defect). The low parasternal and subcostal four-chamber views are the best views for direct visualization of septal defects because the atrial septum is perpendicular to the plane of sound in these views.[12]

On Doppler examination of the right atrium (from either a subcostal or a right parasternal position), the left-to-right shunt across an atrial septal defect causes disturbed flow above the baseline (toward the transducer) in midsystole, extending into early diastole (Fig. 33–6). Maximal velocity generally occurs in late systole. A second short period of left-to-right shunt appears as disturbed flow above the baseline during atrial contraction. In addition, all simple atrial septal defects have a short period of right-to-left shunting, which produces disturbed flow signals directed away from the transducer (below the baseline) in early systole. Variations in the pressure differences between the left and right atria throughout the cardiac cycle account for these variations in the direction of shunt flow.[5, 13–17]

Usually, the peak velocity of the left-to-right shunt in late systole is between 1 and 1.5 m per second, indicating a peak pressure gradient between the atria of about 5 mm Hg. With a restrictive atrial communication and a large pressure difference between the

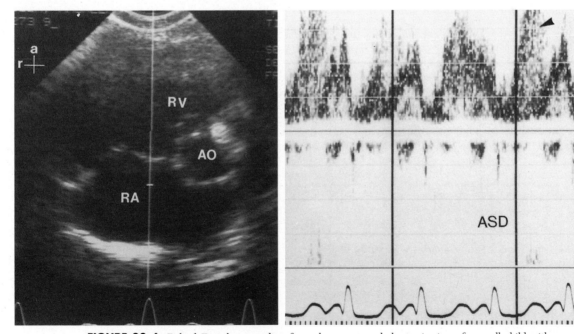

FIGURE 33–6. Pulsed Doppler recording from the parasternal short-axis view of a small child with an atrial septal defect. The freeze-frame image (*left*) shows the position of the sample volume in the right atrium (RA) at the time of the Doppler recording. The Doppler tracing (*right*) shows disturbed flow above the baseline (toward the transducer), beginning in midsystole and extending into early diastole. This flow reaches its peak velocity in late systole (*arrowhead*). A second short period of left-to-right shunting appears as disturbed flow above the baseline at the time of atrial contraction. a = anterior; AO = aorta; r = right; RV = right ventricle. (From Snider, A.R.: Doppler echocardiography in congenital heart disease. *In* Berger, M. [ed.]: Doppler Echocardiography in Heart Disease. New York, Marcel Dekker, 1987, p. 271, with permission.)

atria (i.e., stretched-open patent foramen ovale), a high-velocity jet can be recorded across the atrial septum.

In patients with an atrial septal defect, the increased volume of flow through the right heart chambers causes an increase in flow velocity across the tricuspid and pulmonary valves.[5, 17] Often, flow velocities across the mitral and aortic valves are decreased. Close correlations have been found between the ratios of right-and-left-sided flow velocities (i.e., pulmonary artery-aorta and tricuspid-mitral) and the pulmonary-to-systemic flow ratio measured at cardiac catheterization.[5]

Color flow Doppler mapping techniques can be used to detect shunting across an atrial septal defect (Fig. 33–7). This technique is particularly useful for confirming the presence of an atrial septal defect in patients in whom direct imaging of the atrial septum is technically inadequate and in distinguishing a true atrial septal defect from artifactual echocardiographic dropout in the thin region of the fossa ovalis.

FIGURE 33–7. See Color Plate 7.

Patent Ductus Arteriosus

Patent ductus arteriosus, a communication between the main pulmonary artery and descending aorta, is a common cardiac abnormality that can occur as an isolated defect or in association with various congenital cardiac defects. The medical and surgical management of infants with a patent ductus arteriosus requires knowledge of the direction and magnitude of the ductal shunts.[18, 19] In most instances, two-dimensional echocardiography can accurately define the presence and morphologic characteristics of the patent ductus arteriosus; however, the hemodynamic characteristics of the patent ductus arteriosus cannot usually be defined with two-dimensional echocardiography alone. Doppler echocardiography provides a method for diagnosing the direction and magnitude of ductal shunts, for assessing the relative pulmonary and systemic vascular resistances, and for estimating pulmonary artery systolic, mean, and diastolic pressures.

As pulmonary vascular resistance decreases after birth, the left-to-right shunt through the patent ductus arteriosus increases, leading to increased pulmonary blood flow, increased pulmonary venous return, and, consequently, left atrial and left ventricular volume overload. On the two-dimensional echocardiogram of children with a large patent ductus arteriosus, the left atrium is considerably larger than the right atrium or the aortic root, and the atrial septum bulges toward the right because of left atrial dilation. The left ventricle is dilated and hypercontractile, and the descending aorta pulsations are increased.[18, 20]

The patent ductus arteriosus can be imaged directly from left parasternal, high left parasternal, and suprasternal locations.[19] In the parasternal short-axis view, the patent ductus arteriosus is seen connecting the main pulmonary artery and the descending aorta (Fig. 33–8). In this view, visualization of the patent ductus arteriosus can often be optimized by rotating the transducer slightly clockwise toward a long-axis plane. This maneuver allows one to visualize more of the descending aorta and, usually, the entire length of the patent ductus arteriosus. The patent ductus arteriosus is imaged in the direction of the lateral resolution of the equipment in this view; thus, even with the use of a high-frequency transducer, such as a 7.5-MHz probe, a ductus lumen of 1 mm or less will not be visualized directly by two-dimensional echocardiography.

In most cases of isolated patent ductus arteriosus, the ductus cannot be imaged in the suprasternal long-axis view without tilting the plane of sound toward the left pulmonary artery. In this projection, the patent ductus arteriosus is seen between the origin of the left pulmonary artery and descending aorta (see Fig. 33–8). In patients without a patent ductus arteriosus, one must be careful not to mistakenly diagnose the area where the left pulmonary artery crosses over the descending aorta as a patent ductus arteriosus.

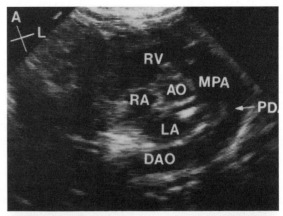

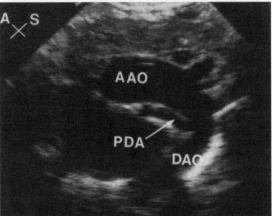

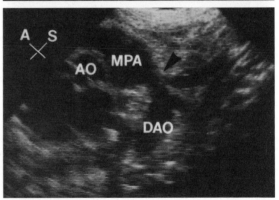

FIGURE 33–8. *Top,* Parasternal short-axis view in an infant with a large patent ductus arteriosus (PDA). In this view, the PDA is seen connecting the main pulmonary artery (MPA) and the descending aorta (DAO). The bright echos in the left atrium (LA) arise from an umbilical venous catheter, which was inadvertently placed across the foramen ovale into the LA. *Middle,* Suprasternal long-axis view in a child with pulmonary atresia and a PDA. Note the long tortuous appearance of the PDA and the lack of aortic isthmus narrowing that is commonly seen in children with severe right ventricular outflow tract obstruction. *Bottom,* High left parasternal view (also known as the ductus view) in a child with a large PDA *(arrow).* The PDA is seen communicating between the MPA and the DAO. This view is obtained by placing the transducer in a parasternal short-axis position and sliding the transducer up toward the suprasternal notch. A = anterior; AAO = ascending aorta; AO = aorta; L = left; LA = left atrium; RA = right atrium; RV = right ventricle; S = superior.

Figure 33–8 contains a high left parasternal view of a patent ductus arteriosus. This view is obtained by sliding the transducer down from the suprasternal notch toward the left parasternal position. The plane of sound is oriented in the same direction as a suprasternal long-axis view.

Doppler interrogation of the main pulmonary artery was the first technique used to confirm the presence of a left-to-right shunt through the patent ductus arteriosus. Several different flow patterns can be seen on the Doppler examination of the main pulmonary artery. If the Doppler sample volume is positioned distally in the main pulmonary artery near the origin of the left pulmonary artery, one can see continuous disturbed flow directed toward the transducer, above the baseline.[21, 22] These signals represent the shunt flow throughout systole and diastole. When the sample volume is placed in the main pulmonary artery adjacent to the pulmonary valve, the systolic portion of the left-to-right shunt may be directed away from the sample volume. Instead, signals arising from the forward flow through the pulmonary valve are seen below the baseline. Signals from the diastolic portion of the left-to-right shunt are seen above the baseline when the pulmonary valve closes. With the sample volume positioned in the midportion of the main pulmonary artery, it is even possible to record diastolic flow signals below the baseline. Presumably, these signals arise as the jet flow from the patent ductus arteriosus strikes the closed pulmonary valve in diastole and swirls back on itself, giving rise to Doppler signals directed away from the transducer.[23]

Following the initial descriptions of the main pulmonary artery Doppler findings in patients with a patent ductus arteriosus, several investigators reported the results of direct interrogation of the ductus arteriosus with pulsed and continuous-wave Doppler.[24, 25]

Direct Doppler interrogation of the ductus arteriosus has many advantages over pulmonary artery Doppler interrogation. First, a small patent ductus arteriosus shunt can be missed by sampling only in the pulmonary artery. Second, direct ductus examination has the advantage of being able to differentiate a patent ductus arteriosus from other defects that cause disturbed diastolic flow in the pulmonary artery (e.g., aortopulmonary window, anomalous origin of a coronary artery from the pulmonary artery, bronchial collateral vessels). Third, Doppler sampling in the main pulmonary artery does not permit detection of a right-to-left ductus shunt.

Several different flow patterns can be observed when the patent ductus arteriosus is sampled directly with the use of pulsed or continuous-wave Doppler.[26] Patients with an isolated left-to-right patent ductus arteriosus shunt and no other cardiac abnormalities have a continuous positive flow with a peak velocity in late systole (Fig. 33–9). Peak systolic pressure gradients across the patent ductus arteriosus can be calculated by substituting the peak velocity in late systole in the simplified Bernoulli equation. If one measures the blood pressure at the time of the Doppler examination, the pulmonary artery systolic pressure can be calculated as the systolic blood pressure minus the Doppler peak gradient.

Patients with an isolated right-to-left patent ductus arteriosus shunt (such as may occur in infants with aortic arch interruption and severe pulmonary hypertension) have a continuous negative flow away from the transducer with a peak velocity in early systole.

Bidirectional ductal shunting is detectable in infants with patent ductus arteriosus and very severe pulmonary artery hypertension (Fig. 33–10). In these cases, the right-to-left shunt occurs as a negative deflection in systole, and the left-to-right shunt occurs as a positive deflection, beginning in late systole and extending into late diastole.[27] Patients with no oxygen-saturation differences above and below the patent ductus arteriosus have a right-to-left shunt that peaks in early systole, whereas those patients with a difference in oxygen saturation of 5 to 30 percent above and below the patent ductus arteriosus have a right-to-left shunt that peaks in middle to late systole. When diagnosing a right-to-left ductal shunt (especially when using continuous-wave Doppler), one must take care not to confuse normal systolic flow in the adjacent left pulmonary artery with a right-to-left patent ductus arteriosus shunt.

In patients with bidirectional patent ductus arteriosus shunt and high pulmonary vascular resistance (Fig. 33–11), the right-to-left shunt begins in diastole, abbreviates the left-to-right diastolic shunt, and extends into early systole as a high-velocity reverse flow. The left-to-right shunt (if present) is present in late systole to early diastole.

Pulsed and continuous-wave Doppler interrogation of the descending aorta is also useful for assessing the magnitude of the left-to-right patent ductus arteriosus shunt. With a large patent ductus arteriosus and low pulmonary artery diastolic pressures, blood flows from the aorta into the pulmonary artery in diastole. Evidence of a diastolic runoff, or "steal," of blood from the aorta can be seen on the Doppler examination of the aorta.[28–32] When

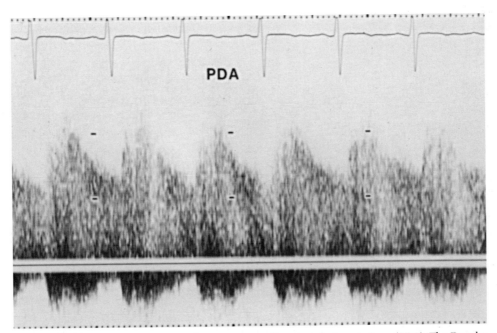

FIGURE 33–9. Continuous-wave Doppler examination of a patent ductus arteriosus (PDA). The Doppler transducer is placed in the second left intercostal space and is aimed toward the pulmonary artery. High-velocity, continuous disturbed flow is seen above the baseline, indicating flow through a restricted PDA toward the transducer. The peak velocity of the flow in early systole is greater than 4 m per second indicating a pressure difference of more than 64 mm Hg between the aorta and the pulmonary artery in systole. This pattern of continuous disturbed flow directed toward the transducer is typical of a PDA with a pure left-to-right shunt.

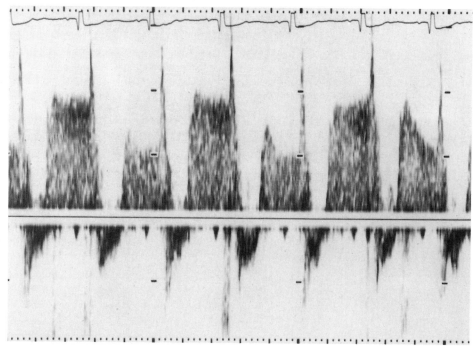

FIGURE 33–10. Continuous-wave Doppler examination of an infant with a patent ductus arteriosus, severe pulmonary artery hypertension, and bidirectional ductal shunting. The left-to-right shunt occurs as a positive deflection (above the baseline), beginning in late systole and extending into late diastole. Note that the peak velocity of the left-to-right shunt is approximately 1 m per second, indicating no pressure difference between the aorta and the pulmonary artery at this time in the cardiac cycle. The right-to-left shunt is seen as a negative deflection below the baseline in systole.

the Doppler sample volume is positioned in the descending aorta below the ductus arteriosus, forward flow signals are seen in systole below the baseline. In diastole, flow signals are seen above the baseline, indicating flow up the descending aorta toward the ductus

arteriosus and main pulmonary artery (Fig. 33–12). Good correlation has been found between clinical estimates of the shunt size and the ratio of the retrograde flow area to the forward flow area.[32]

Color flow Doppler imaging has improved the ease and

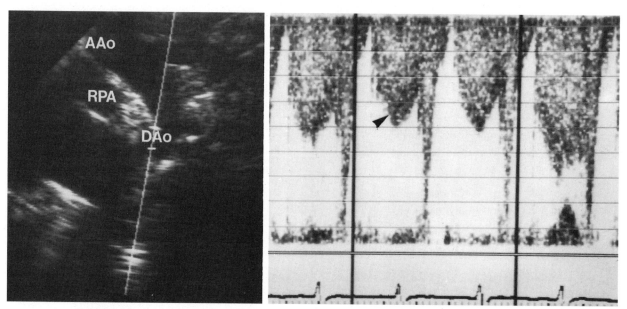

FIGURE 33–11. Doppler spectral recording from the suprasternal notch view of an infant with a patent ductus arteriosus, markedly elevated pulmonary vascular resistance, and a pure right-to-left ductal shunt. The freeze-frame image on the left shows the position of the sample volume at the descending aorta (DAo) end of the patent ductus arteriosus at the time of the Doppler recording. The Doppler spectral tracing on the right shows evidence of forward flow in systole down the descending aorta. In diastole, there are Doppler flow signals below the baseline (*arrowhead*), indicating a right-to-left shunt from the ductus arteriosus to the DAo. AAo = ascending aorta; RPA = right pulmonary artery. (From Snider, A.R.: Doppler echocardiography in congenital heart disease. *In* Berger, M. [ed.]: Doppler Echocardiography in Heart Disease. New York, Marcel Dekker, 1987, p. 294, with permission.)

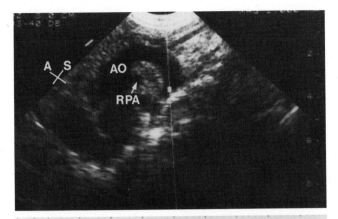

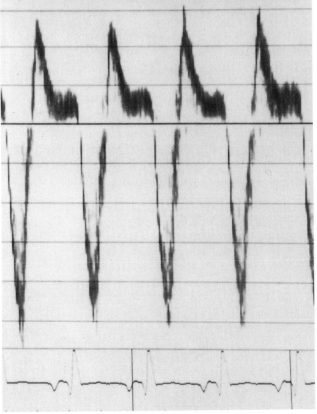

FIGURE 33–12. Pulsed Doppler recording from the suprasternal long-axis view from an infant with a large patent ductus arteriosus. The freeze-frame image at the top shows the position of the sample volume in the descending aorta (AO) at the time of the Doppler recording. The Doppler spectral tracing (*bottom*) shows normal forward flow down the aorta (away from the transducer and below the baseline) in systole. In diastole, there are flow signals above the baseline, indicating retrograde flow up the descending AO toward the transducer. These retrograde diastolic flow signals are caused by a steal of blood in diastole from the AO to the pulmonary artery. A = anterior; RPA = right pulmonary artery; S = superior.

quickness with which one can visualize the patent ductus arteriosus. With color flow Doppler imaging, flow can be detected in a patent ductus arteriosus that is too small to be imaged clearly on the two-dimensional echocardiogram (Fig. 33–13). With the color Doppler display of the patent ductus arteriosus jet, one can obtain better alignment of the pulsed or continuous-wave Doppler beam with the jet flow and, thus, can improve the estimation of pulmonary artery pressures. One limitation of two-dimensional color flow mapping is that it lacks the temporal resolution to identify clearly the exact timing of bidirectional patent ductus arteriosus shunts.

FIGURE 33–13. See Color Plate 7.

Atrioventricular Septal Defects

Atrioventricular septal defects occur because of failure of partitioning of the embryonic atrioventricular canal. This phenomenon results in a confluent defect that involves the ostium primum, atrioventricular canal, and interventricular foramen. Atrioventricular septal defects have a common atrioventricular valve that contains superior (anterior) and inferior (posterior) bridging leaflets as well as left lateral, right lateral, and right accessory leaflets.[33] The common atrioventricular valve can have an undivided common orifice or can be divided into right- and left-sided orifices by a tongue of tissue connecting the superior and inferior bridging leaflets. The common atrioventricular valve can be displaced downward into the ventricle and anchored to the crest of the muscular septum, thus allowing left-to-right shunting to occur only above the valve at atrial level (so-called partial form) or can float freely in the septal defect, allowing shunting to occur above and below the valve at atrial and ventricular levels (the so-called complete form). In addition, intermediate forms of atrioventricular septal defects (incomplete forms) can occur, depending on the position and attachments of the valve leaflets.[34]

Two-dimensional echocardiography has been particularly useful for definition of the morphology and attachments of the atrioventricular valve leaflets, determination of the anatomical level of the left-to-right shunt, and estimation of the sizes of the right and left ventricles (Figs. 33–14 to 33–16).[35] Some two-dimensional echocardiographic findings common to all variants of atrioventricular septal defect include (1) deficiency of the inlet portion of the ventricular septum, (2) displacement of the atrioventricular valve inferiorly, (3) lack of two separate fibrous valve rings at different distances from the cardiac apex, and (4) attachment of the left half of the common atrioventricular valve to the ventricular septum, with resulting orientation of the valve into the left ventricular outflow tract.

From a surgical viewpoint, one of the most important anatomical questions about an atrioventricular septal defect is whether the common atrioventricular valve has a common orifice or is divided by a connecting tongue of tissue into two separate orifices.[36] This determination can be made with the use of a subcostal view of the atrioventricular valve en face.[37] From the standard subcostal four-chamber view, the plane of sound is rotated 30 to 45 degrees clockwise until the atrioventricular valve is seen en face (Fig. 33–16). The plane of sound is then tilted from a superior to an inferior direction to examine cross-sectional views of the atrioventricular valve from the inferior margin of the atrial septum to the superior margin of the ventricular septum. These imaging planes allow direct visualization of all five atrioventricular valve leaflets, as well as the attachments of the anterior bridging leaflet to the anterosuperior muscular (infundibular) septum and the attachments of the posterior bridging leaflet to the posterosuperior muscular (inlet) septum. In real time, the atrioventricular valve is seen opening, either with a common orifice and no bridging tongue connecting the anterior and posterior leaflets or with two separate orifices created by the presence of a bridging tongue of tissue connecting the anterior and posterior leaflets. Determination of the number of atrioventricular valve orifices is made simpler with the use of the slow-motion review mode of the videotape player or the on-line memory loop function of the ultrasound system.

The common atrioventricular valve with a single orifice can be further classified as described by Rastelli and colleagues,[38] based on the amount of bridging and the chordal attachments of the anterior bridging leaflet. In the Rastelli type A valve, the anterior bridging leaflet is nearly completely committed to the left ventricle, and there is minimal bridging of the leaflet into the right ventricle. As a result, the commissure between this leaflet and the right anterosuperior leaflet is lined up with the ventricular septum and

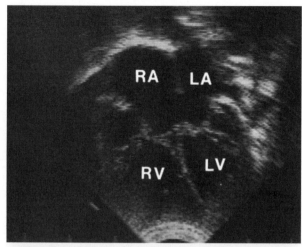

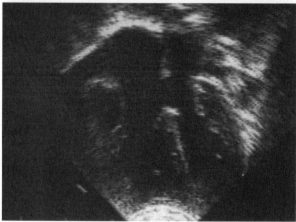

FIGURE 33–14. Apical four-chamber views during systole *(above)* and diastole *(below)* in a patient with a primum atrial septal defect. The primum atrial septal defect is seen as an area of echocardiographic dropout in the lower portion of the atrial septum adjacent to the atrioventricular valve. In this case, the common atrioventricular valve is tethered to the crest of the ventricular septum, so no shunting can occur at ventricular level. Note that there are not separate atrioventricular valve fibrous rings at separate levels, but, rather, there is a single atrioventricular valve ring with the leaflets positioned lower in the heart than usual. LA = left atrium; LV = left ventricle; RA = right atrium; RV = right ventricle.

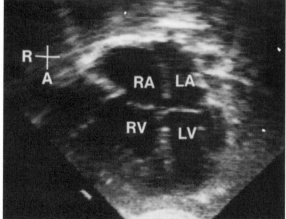

FIGURE 33–15. Apical four-chamber views during systole *(above)* and diastole *(below)* in a child with the so-called complete form of an atrioventricular septal defect. When the common atrioventricular valve is closed in systole, shunting can occur at atrial and ventricular levels. When the atrioventricular valve is open in diastole, a large central confluent defect is seen in the atrioventricular septum. Note the deficiency of the ventricular septum in this view. A = apex; LA = left atrium; LV = left ventricle; R = right; RA = right atrium; RV = right ventricle.

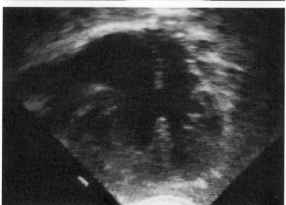

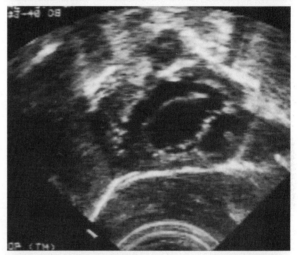

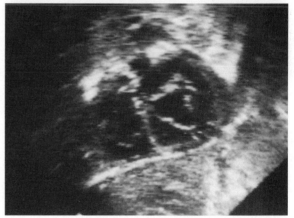

FIGURE 33–16. Subcostal views at the level of the common atrioventricular valve in two patients with atrioventricular septal defect. The top frame shows the atrioventricular valve *(arrowheads)* of one patient in the closed position in systole. The middle frame shows the atrioventricular valve of the same patient in the open position in diastole. Note that the common atrioventricular valve bridges from the right ventricle (RV) to the left ventricle (LV). In this patient, the common atrioventricular valve has a common orifice. The bottom frame is a subcostal view from a different patient with an atrioventricular septal defect. In this patient, the common atrioventricular valve is divided by a bridging tongue of tissue into two separate valve orifices. These frames show how the two-dimensional echocardiogram can be used to determine the morphology of the common atrioventricular valve in patients with atrioventricular septal defect. AO = aorta; R = right; S = superior. (From Snider, A.R.: Two-dimensional and Doppler echocardiographic evaluation of heart disease in the neonate and fetus. Clin. Perinatol. 15:534, 1988, with permission.)

chordae of the anterior bridging leaflet insert into the crest of the septum. In the Rastelli type B valve, there is more bridging of the anterior bridging leaflet into the right ventricle. The commissure moves rightward over the anterior wall of the right ventricle, and chordal attachments of the leaflet insert into papillary muscles in the right ventricle. In the Rastelli type C valve, there is maximum bridging of the anterior bridging leaflet, so the commissure is situated along the right ventricular lateral wall, and chordal attachments of the leaflet insert into the right ventricular lateral wall, rather than into the crest of the ventricular septum (so-called "free-floater").

Another important anatomical variation that occurs in hearts with atrioventricular septal defect is the relationship between the bridging leaflets, the connecting tongue of tissue, and the atrial and ventricular septa. When the leaflets and the bridging tongue of tissue are firmly attached to the crest of the ventricular septum,

shunting through the atrioventricular septal defect is possible only at the atrial level (see Fig. 33–14). In contrast, if the leaflets are firmly attached to the undersurface of the atrial septum, shunting is possible only at the ventricular level. Finally, varying degrees of tethering of the bridging leaflets to the ventricular septum can occur. For example, the leaflets can float freely above the septum, allowing a large nonrestrictive ventricular communication. Although most of these hearts have a common-orifice atrioventricular valve, a large ventricular septal defect can also rarely occur with a two-orifice atrioventricular valve. Alternatively, the leaflets can be closely adherent to the ventricular septum, allowing only a small restrictive ventricular shunt through the interchordal spaces. This type of relationship is usually associated with a two-orifice common atrioventricular valve. Frequently, the systolic pressure gradient between the two ventricles causes the bridging tongue of tissue to protrude into the right ventricle in systole, producing the so-called "tricuspid-pouch" lesion. Thus, by definition, visualization of a tricuspid pouch establishes the diagnosis of a two-orifice common atrioventricular valve.

Another important aspect of the relationship between the leaflets and the septa is how the atrioventricular junction is shared between the two ventricles. If the junction is shared equally, there is a "balanced" situation, and the ventricles are nearly equal in size. Occasionally, the left side of the heart is reduced in size compared with the right side of the heart (Fig. 33–17). Hypoplasia of the left-sided chambers, or right ventricular dominance, is usually associated with either severe aortic coarctation or interruption of the aortic arch. Its counterpart is left ventricular dominance, in which the right-sided chambers are hypoplastic, usually in association with pulmonary stenosis or atresia. Chamber dominance can occur with either a two-orifice or a common-orifice atrioventricular valve. In the latter case, malalignment of the atrial and the ventricular septa is often present.

Pulsed and color flow Doppler techniques have been especially useful for defining the complex patterns of intracardiac shunting and valve regurgitation that occur in patients with atrioventricular septal defects (Figs. 33–18 and 33–19). Deformities of the common atrioventricular valve are such that insufficiency jets can be directed anywhere in the left or right atria. Color flow mapping has provided a technique for the rapid visualization of these eccentric jets.

FIGURES 33–18 and 33–19. See Color Plate 7.

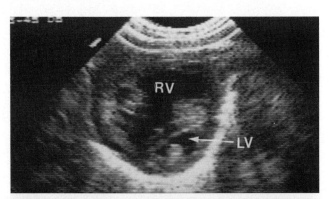

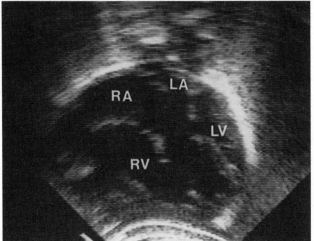

FIGURE 33–17. Parasternal short-axis *(top)* and apical four-chamber *(bottom)* views in a patient with an atrioventricular septal defect and a small left ventricle (LV). This patient had a single papillary muscle in the LV. In addition, only a small portion of the common atrioventricular valve orifice was committed to the LV. LA = left atrium; RA = right atrium; RV = right ventricle. (From Snider, A.R., and Serwer, G.A.: Echocardiography in Pediatric Heart Disease. Chicago, Mosby–Year Book, 1990, p. 155, with permission.)

Doppler Quantitation of Left-to-Right Shunts

Both systemic and pulmonary blood flows can be calculated from the two-dimensional and Doppler echocardiograms in patients with a left-to-right shunt, using these equations for volumetric flow.[39-42]

$$SV = \frac{V \times CSA \times RR}{1000 \text{ mL/L}}$$

where SV = stroke volume (mL/beat), V = mean velocity (cm/s), CSA = vessel cross-sectional area (cm²), and RR = R-to-R interval (s/beat).

Since the cardiac output equals the stroke volume times the heart rate, and heart rate equals 60/RR interval, the following is true:

$$\text{Volumetric Flow (L/min)} = \frac{V \times CSA \times 60 \text{ s/min}}{1000 \text{ mL/L}}$$

Commonly, the pulmonary artery mean velocity and diameter are used to calculate pulmonary blood flow, and the ascending aorta mean velocity and diameter are used to calculate systemic blood flow; however, other sites can be used, depending on the location of the left-to-right shunt. The magnitude of the left-to-right shunt can be calculated directly as pulmonary blood flow minus systemic blood flow, or it can be assessed indirectly by calculating the ratio of the pulmonary and systemic blood flows, or the Qp:Qs.

The calculation of volumetric flow requires measurement of the mean velocity and the vessel cross-sectional area. In measuring the mean velocity, one fundamental assumption made is that flow is laminar and organized and that the velocity profile is uniform across the vessel or valve inlet. Under these circumstances, a single sampling of the flow velocity in the center of the vessel is recorded. Care is taken to align the Doppler beam parallel with flow in the vessel so that the maximal velocities are recorded and no correction for intercept angle need be made. The mean velocity is then calculated as the integrated area under the Doppler curve, or the velocity time integral, divided by the flow period of the traced beats. With the use of a computer program, the Doppler velocity curve is integrated by tracing the densest area of the Doppler curve or the modal velocity over several consecutive cardiac cycles.

For systemic blood flow, aortic velocity can be recorded from many windows, including suprasternal, apical, and subcostal approaches. In most cases, the apical view is preferable because it is easily obtainable in most patients and because one can position the sample volume parallel with flow across the aortic annulus and close to the valve leaflets. In the suprasternal view, it is often not possible to sample aortic flow just at the valve leaflets at an acceptable angle, and often flow has to be sampled in the ascending aorta several centimeters above the valve. If aortic mean velocity is measured in the ascending aorta, the vessel cross-sectional area should be measured at the same location. It is not easy to measure the aortic diameter accurately at this location because of difficulties in imaging the anterior aortic wall from the suprasternal notch and because the aortic diameter is measured in the direction of the lateral resolution of the equipment. The pulmonary blood flow is calculated in a manner similar to the systemic blood flow but using the pulmonary artery Doppler tracing and cross-sectional area. Usually, acceptable pulmonary artery Doppler tracings can be obtained from the parasternal short-axis view or the subcostal view of the right ventricular outflow tract. Frequently, with a large shunt or a shunt whose location is close to the pulmonary artery (i.e., ventricular septal defect), the Doppler tracing shows spectral broadening or signs of disturbed flow. In these instances, one cannot assume a uniform velocity profile in the main pulmonary artery, and another site should be chosen to calculate pulmonary blood flow (i.e., mitral valve for ventricular septal defect). Also, the main pulmonary artery Doppler tracing cannot be used to calculate pulmonary blood flow when there is any pulmonary stenosis accompanying the shunt because, in this instance as well, the velocity profile is not uniform across the vessel lumen.

The vessel cross-sectional area is usually calculated by measuring the vessel diameter from the two-dimensional echocardiogram and assuming that the vessel is circular, so vessel cross-sectional area equals $\pi(d^2)/4$. There are many different techniques for measuring vessel diameters. It is recommended that the aorta and pulmonary artery be measured from inner edge to inner edge in early systole at the level of the valve annulus. The inner edge measurements should be used because they provide the closest approximation of the actual flow diameter. It is known that systolic expansion accounts for a 5 to 10 percent change in aortic cross-sectional area and a 2 to 18 percent change in pulmonary artery cross-sectional area throughout systole. The increase in cross-sectional area occurs early in systole, simultaneously with the upstroke of the pressure curve, so the majority of the flow in the aorta or pulmonary artery occurs when the vessel is at or near its peak systolic dimension. The vessel diameter is measured at the valve annulus because the annulus is the smallest area, or the flow-limiting point in the vessel, where maximal flow velocity should theoretically occur.[40]

For the aorta, the parasternal long-axis view provides a diameter that is measured in the direction of the axial resolution of the equipment. For the pulmonary artery flow diameter, the parasternal long-axis view of the right ventricle can be used. In this view, it is easier to visualize the origin of the pulmonary valve leaflets and the left lateral wall of the main pulmonary artery away from the lung. Accurate measurement of the pulmonary artery diameter is much more difficult than that of the aortic diameter. First, it is usually not possible to image the pulmonary artery in a view that allows one to measure the diameter in the direction of the axial resolution. Second, it may be difficult to visualize the left lateral border of the main pulmonary artery because of the adjacent lung tissue. Placing the patient in a steep left lateral decubitus position optimizes visualization of the left border of the pulmonary artery. Third, Stewart and colleagues have shown that with increasing volumetric flow, pulmonary artery diameter increases to a far greater extent than does aortic diameter.[40] With increasing volume flow from 0.5 to 1 L per minute, aortic mean velocity increased linearly and aortic diameter increased very slightly. No further changes were observed with increasing flow rates from 2 to 5 L per minute. With increasing pulmonary blood flow, there was a consistent increase in pulmonary artery diameter throughout the entire range of flows. Pulmonary artery mean velocity increased as well, but the percent increase in pulmonary artery mean velocity was less than the percent increase in aortic mean velocity for the same change in volumetric flow. Thus, there is far greater variability in pulmonary artery diameter at different volume flows than there is in aortic diameter. Pulmonary artery diameter, then, can never be assumed to be constant in a given patient when one assesses serial changes in pulmonary blood flow.

In patients with a ventricular septal defect, systemic blood flow can be calculated at the aortic and tricuspid valve sites, and pulmonary blood flow can be calculated at the pulmonary and mitral valve sites. With an atrial septal defect, mitral and aortic valve flow reflects systemic output, and tricuspid and pulmonary valve flow reflects pulmonary blood flow. In the case of a patent ductus arteriosus, the left-to-right shunt is downstream from the pulmonary valve; therefore, the pulmonary and tricuspid valve sites reflect systemic blood flow, and the mitral and aortic valve sites reflect pulmonary blood flow.

In general, in patients with left-to-right shunts, Doppler-derived values for pulmonary and systemic blood flows and Qp/Qs have correlated well with the same values determined at cardiac catheterization with the use of the Fick technique.[43, 44] For systemic blood flow, correlation coefficients in several clinical studies have ranged from 0.78 to 0.91, and standard errors of the estimate have ranged from 0.60 to 0.81 L per minute. For pulmonary blood flow, correlation coefficients have ranged from 0.72 to 0.88, and standard

errors from 1.11 to 2.4 L per minute. For Qp/Qs, correlation coefficients have been 0.85, with standard errors of around 0.48. There are several possible explanations for the errors or discrepancies noted between Doppler calculations of shunt magnitude and those measured at cardiac catheterization. Errors can occur in the measurement of the mean velocity from the Doppler spectral tracing. Gardin and colleagues have shown that, in general, there is good reproducibility in measurement of the aortic mean velocity.[45] For the aortic mean velocity, intraobserver variability in their study was 3.2 ± 2.9 percent, interobserver variability was 5.4 ± 3.4 percent, and day-to-day variability was 3.8 ± 3.1 percent. Potential sources of error in measuring the Doppler mean velocity include errors in determining the intercept angle and the lack of a uniform velocity profile across the vessel lumen. Determination of vessel cross-sectional area is the largest source of error in the Doppler technique. Errors can occur in determination of vessel cross-sectional area because the instrument's gain settings may be too high or too low to optimize visualization of the vessel walls; the vessel cross-sectional area changes throughout the cardiac cycle (especially the main pulmonary artery), and these changes depend on factors such as pressure, flow, and elasticity in the vessel; and finally, it may be necessary to measure the vessel in the direction of the lateral resolution of the equipment.

Errors in the calculation of flow also can occur because of the presence of additional defects. For example, an additional undetected shunt, such as a patent ductus arteriosus located downstream from the pulmonary artery sampling site, will lead to an underestimation of the total pulmonary flow and Qp:Qs ratio. Semilunar valve regurgitation results in an overestimation of flow because of failure to measure the regurgitant volume. Finally, discrepancies can occur between the Doppler and the catheterization measurements of flow because of errors in the use of the Fick technique as the "gold standard." Variability in the measurement of blood flow by the Fick technique occurs because this technique requires the patient to be in a steady state for several minutes, which does not often occur, and because the Fick technique is influenced by the patient's ventilatory rate, the room temperature, the barometric pressure, and the patient's respiratory exchange ratio.

CONGENITAL HEART DISEASE WITH VENTRICULAR OUTFLOW OBSTRUCTION

Ventricular outflow obstruction that causes signs and symptoms in childhood is usually hemodynamically severe, and children with these defects are often critically ill. Two-dimensional and Doppler echocardiography provide a noninvasive technique for the rapid diagnosis of the anatomical type of obstruction and its degree of severity. In many cases, the noninvasive techniques have eliminated the need for diagnostic cardiac catheterization prior to surgical therapy. This approach has been especially useful in the care of sick infants with severe left ventricular obstruction in whom dye injections at the time of cardiac catheterization may be poorly tolerated because of low systemic output and poor renal perfusion.[46, 47]

Left Ventricular Outflow Obstruction

Left ventricular outflow obstruction can occur beneath the aortic valve (subvalvular), at the level of the aortic valve (valvular), or above the aortic valve (supravalvular aortic stenosis, coarctation, and interruption of the aorta). In its most severe form, the entire left side of the heart can be underdeveloped, a condition known as hypoplastic left heart syndrome. On the two-dimensional echocardiogram, all these defects can cause left ventricular hypertrophy and decreased left ventricular shortening fraction (caused by increased afterload). Often, left atrial and pulmonary venous distention develops as left ventricular compliance decreases.

Aortic valve stenosis can occur with a normal valve annulus size and fused commissures or with a small valve annulus and dysplastic leaflets (Figs. 33–20 to 33–22).[48] The aortic valve can be tricuspid, bicuspid, or unicuspid, and the left ventricle can be dilated and poorly contractile, small and somewhat underdeveloped, or concentrically hypertrophic. Often, bright echoes arising from areas of endocardial fibroelastosis can be seen in the bases of the papillary muscles or throughout the endocardium. Doppler echocardiography is especially useful for estimating the peak systolic pressure gradient across the aortic valve (Fig. 33–23). For this calculation,

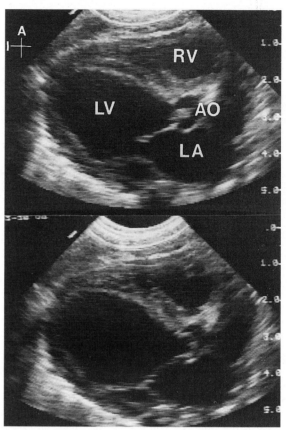

FIGURE 33–21. Parasternal long-axis views during diastole *(top)* and systole *(bottom)* in a newborn with critical aortic valvular stenosis. In this patient, the aortic valve leaflets are thickened and domed, and a clear systolic opening cannot be seen. The left ventricle (LV) is markedly dilated and has a diminished shortening fraction. A = anterior; I = inferior; LA = left atrium; RV = right ventricle. (From Snider, A.R., and Serwer, G.A.: Echocardiography in Pediatric Heart Disease. Chicago, Mosby–Year Book, 1990, p. 247, with permission.)

Doppler recordings of the systolic jet through the aortic valve are obtained from apical, right parasternal, and suprasternal notch transducer positions. The highest value of the peak velocity is used in the simplified Bernoulli equation ($4V^2$) to predict the peak instantaneous pressure gradient across the aortic valve. The Doppler peak gradient is larger than the catheterization-measured peak-to-peak pressure gradient. The difference between the two is greatest in mild aortic stenosis and is less marked in severe aortic stenosis. Nevertheless, excellent correlations have been found between Doppler peak gradients and peak-to-peak pressure gradients measured at cardiac catheterization.[49–53] One should keep in mind that in the presence of myocardial dysfunction and low cardiac output, the peak gradient may not reflect the severity of the aortic stenosis.

The Doppler mean gradient is another useful noninvasive estimate of the severity of aortic stenosis. The Doppler mean pressure gradient is directly comparable to the mean pressure gradient measured at cardiac catheterization. The mean pressure gradient is calculated by tracing the Doppler spectral recording of the aortic stenosis jet along its outermost border, using commercially available computer software. The computer then calculates the instantaneous pressure gradient every few milliseconds. The mean gradient is the average of all the instantaneous gradients throughout systole.

In a group of children with aortic valve stenosis, Bengur and colleagues found that all children with a Doppler mean gradient higher than 27 mm Hg had a catheterization peak-to-peak pressure gradient of 75 mm Hg or more and required intervention.[54] All children with a Doppler mean gradient lower than 17 mm Hg had a catheterization peak-to-peak pressure gradient lower than 50 mm

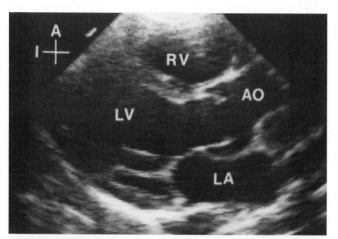

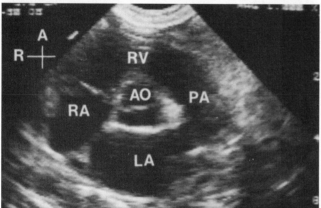

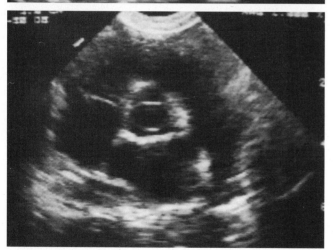

FIGURE 33–20. *Top,* Parasternal long-axis view in a child with aortic valve stenosis. In this view, the aortic valve is thickened and domed in systole. *Middle and Bottom,* Parasternal short-axis views in the same patient. In this view, the aortic valve is bicuspid, forms a single closure line in the closed position, and is "fish-mouthed" in shape in the open position. A = anterior; AO = aorta; I = inferior; LA = left atrium; LV = left ventricle; PA = pulmonary artery; R = right; RA = right atrium; RV = right ventri-

Hg and did not require intervention. Children with Doppler mean gradients between 17 and 27 mm Hg constituted an intermediate group, with peak-to-peak pressure gradients of 50 mm Hg or more and of less than 75 mm Hg. In this group, Doppler mean gradient alone was not sufficient information to predict which child would need intervention; however, the presence of signs or symptoms or an abnormal exercise test provided the additional information necessary for an accurate noninvasive assessment of the severity of the aortic stenosis.

The Doppler mean pressure gradient has several advantages over the Doppler peak instantaneous pressure gradient as a noninvasive indicator of the hemodynamic severity of the obstruction. First, the Doppler mean gradient is directly comparable to the catheterization mean pressure gradient. No such catheterization reference standard exists for the Doppler peak instantaneous pressure gradient. Second, the Doppler mean gradient is the average of all the instantaneous gradients throughout systole and is, therefore, not so dependent on a clear recording of the peak velocity. Doppler peak instantaneous pressure gradient is solely dependent on an accurate recording of the peak systolic velocity and is more sensitive to small measurement errors. Last, the mean transvalvular pressure gradient is the basis for calculation of valve area with the use of the Gorlin equation. Thus, for a normal stroke volume and heart rate, the Doppler mean pressure gradient has a more direct relationship to aortic valve area than the Doppler peak instantaneous pressure gradient.

Both the Doppler mean and peak pressure gradients are dependent on transvalvular flow and are not as reliable as the aortic valve area in indicating the severity of the aortic stenosis. Aortic valve area can be calculated from the Doppler examination with the use of the continuity equation. In a study of children with aortic valve stenosis, Doppler valve areas correlated well with valve areas measured at cardiac catheterization with the use of the Gorlin equation ($r = 0.73$).[55] In this study, predictions of the severity of aortic stenosis from Doppler aortic valve area and Doppler mean gradient were in agreement in most patients. For example, when a Doppler valve area of less than 0.7 cm²/m² and a Doppler mean gradient of more than 27 mm Hg were used to indicate severe

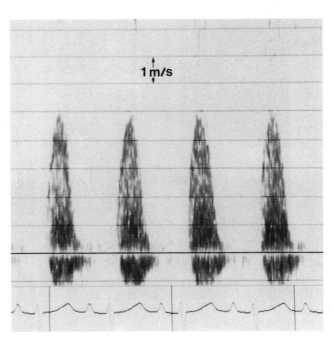

FIGURE 33–23. Continuous-wave Doppler examination from the suprasternal notch of a newborn infant with severe aortic valve stenosis. A high-velocity jet that peaks in late systole is present. The peak velocity of the jet is 5 m per second, which indicates a pressure gradient of 100 mm Hg across the valve.

aortic stenosis requiring intervention, agreement in assessment of the severity of stenosis between these two measurements occurred in 74 percent of the patients. Among the patients in whom the two indicators were not in agreement, the disparity could be explained on the basis of altered transvalvular flow in most patients. Thus, when the Doppler mean gradient is a borderline value or is affected by altered transvalvular flow, calculation of the Doppler aortic valve area is an essential part of the comprehensive noninvasive estimate of the severity of the aortic stenosis.

Aortic valve stenosis that causes symptoms in the neonatal period is usually hemodynamically severe, and infants with this defect are critically ill. Two-dimensional and Doppler echocardiography provide a technique for the rapid, noninvasive diagnosis of the anatomical type of obstruction and its severity. In infants with valvular aortic stenosis and a dilated, poorly contractile left ventricle (see Fig. 33–21), the distinction between aortic stenosis and cardiomyopathy may not be readily apparent. Usually, infants with cardiomyopathy have a normal aortic valve, no poststenotic dilation, and no systolic flow disturbance in the ascending aorta.

In infants with severe aortic stenosis, dilation of the right ventricle may give the hypertrophic left ventricle the appearance of being small or even hypoplastic (see Fig. 33–22). Difficulty may then arise in distinguishing aortic stenosis from a hypoplastic left ventricle. Usually, infants with critical aortic stenosis have a left ventricular cross-sectional area of 1.7 cm² or more in the parasternal long-axis view and an aortic annulus of 5 mm or more.[56] In the presence of severe right ventricular dilation, the shape of the left ventricle may be useful. In critical aortic stenosis, the left ventricle is ellipsoid and extends to the cardiac apex in the four-chamber views. The hypoplastic ventricle is a muscle-bound, globular chamber that usually does not extend to the cardiac apex.[57]

Subvalvular aortic stenosis can occur as a discrete membrane (Fig. 33–24) or as a long area of muscular thickening (tunnel type). Subaortic stenosis can be an isolated defect but most often occurs in association with other cardiac defects (i.e., along with multiple left heart obstructive lesions or along with ventricular septal defect and double-chambered right ventricle). As with valvular aortic stenosis, the severity of discrete membranous subaortic stenosis can be estimated from the simplified Bernoulli equation. The

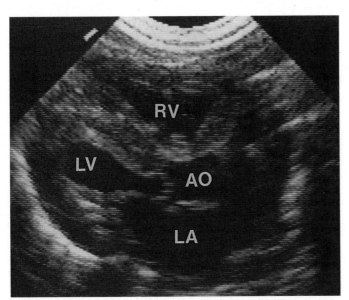

FIGURE 33–22. Parasternal long-axis view from an infant with critical aortic valvular stenosis. The aortic valve annulus is small, and the valve leaflets are thickened and domed. A clear systolic opening cannot be visualized. The left ventricular (LV) cavity is small and smooth walled. The LV is markedly hypertrophied; the echo-bright areas throughout the endocardium represent endocardial fibroelastosis. AO = aorta; LA = left atrium; RV = right ventricle. (From Snider, A.R., and Serwer, G.A.: Echocardiography in Pediatric Heart Disease. Chicago, Mosby–Year Book, 1990, p. 246, with permission.)

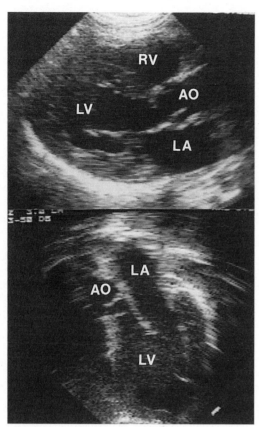

FIGURE 33–24. Parasternal *(top)* and apical *(bottom)* long-axis views in a patient with subvalvular aortic stenosis caused by a discrete fibrous membrane in the left ventricular (LV) outflow tract just beneath the aortic (AO) valve. LA = left atrium; RV = right ventricle. (From Snider, A.R., and Serwer, G.A.: Echocardiography in Pediatric Heart Disease. Chicago, Mosby–Year Book, 1990, p. 252, with permission.)

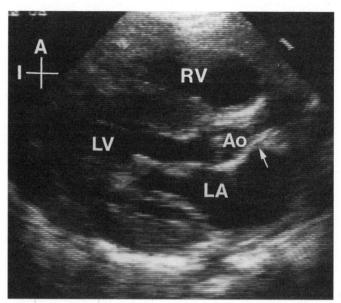

FIGURE 33–25. Parasternal long-axis view in a child with severe supravalvular aortic stenosis. In this view, an area of severe narrowing can be seen above the aortic valve *(arrow)*. Note the marked concentric hypertrophy of the left ventricle (LV). A = anterior; Ao = aorta; I = inferior; LA = left atrium; RV = right ventricle.

highest value for the peak velocity of the subaortic stenosis jet is usually recorded from an apical transducer position. An accurate estimate of the pressure drop across a long tunnel-type subaortic stenosis cannot be obtained with the use of the simplified Bernoulli equation because this equation neglects the pressure drop caused by viscous friction along the flow path.

Supravalvular aortic stenosis occurs in three anatomical forms: (1) a discrete membrane above the aortic sinuses of Valsalva, (2) an hourglass constriction in the ascending aorta, and (3) a long tubular hypoplasia of the ascending aorta.[33] Usually, the exact location and extent of the obstruction can be visualized on the two-dimensional echocardiogram from parasternal and suprasternal views (Fig. 33–25). Because the simplified Bernoulli equation does not apply to a pressure drop across a long tubular narrowing, it can be successfully used only to predict the pressure gradient when the supravalvular obstruction is a discrete membrane.

Supravalvular aortic stenosis is often associated with bilateral, severe peripheral pulmonary artery stenosis. Thus, when one uses a continuous-wave Doppler transducer without image orientation to estimate the severity of supravalvular aortic stenosis, care must be taken not to mistake a high-velocity jet from a peripheral pulmonary artery for the jet flow in the ascending aorta.

The suprasternal notch views have been especially useful for the diagnosis of coarctation and interruption of the aorta.[58–63] In the suprasternal long-axis view, coarctation of the aorta can be visualized as a narrowing in the descending aorta just beyond the left subclavian artery, caused by a prominent posterior endothelial shelf (Fig. 33–26). Poststenotic dilation of the descending aorta is seen just distal to the narrowed area. Unless there is a large right-to-left shunt through a patent ductus arteriosus, descending aorta pulsations are decreased. Interruption of the aorta is seen as an area of

discontinuity between the ascending and the descending aorta in the suprasternal long-axis view. If the plane of sound is tilted slightly leftward of the standard suprasternal long-axis view, then the main pulmonary artery can be seen connecting to the descending aorta via the patent ductus arteriosus. In the newborn infant, the suprasternal views can be obtained by placing the transducer directly over the manubrium sternum, which is not heavily ossified at this age. With this transducer position, there is no need to hyperextend the neck—a maneuver that can be risky in an intubated infant.

In coarctation of the aorta, a high-velocity jet usually can be recorded in the descending aorta when the transducer is positioned

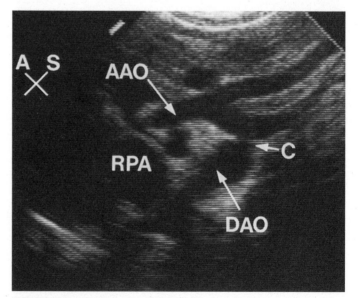

FIGURE 33–26. Suprasternal long-axis view in an infant with a severe coarctation of the aorta. The coarctation (C) is seen as a discrete narrowing just beyond the takeoff of the left subclavian artery. Distal to the coarctation, there is poststenotic dilation of the descending aorta (DAO). A = anterior; AAO = ascending aorta; RPA = right pulmonary artery; S = superior.

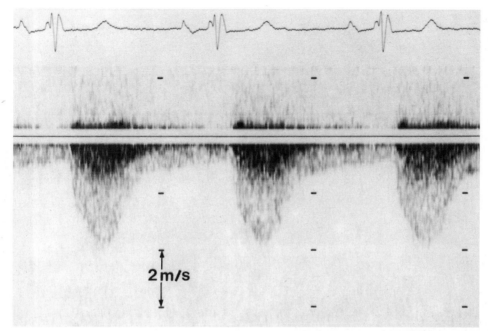

FIGURE 33–27. Continuous-wave Doppler examination from the suprasternal notch of an adolescent female with a severe coarctation of the aorta. There is a high-velocity jet in systole with a peak velocity of nearly 4 m per second. This predicts a pressure gradient of 64 mm Hg down the descending aorta. Forward flow continues throughout diastole in this patient, indicating a very severe coarctation of the aorta with a pressure gradient across the coarctation that persists throughout diastole. Note the darker, low-velocity signals in systole superimposed on the signals from the jet flow. These low-velocity signals indicate normal flow in the descending aorta proximal to the coarctation.

in the suprasternal notch. Figure 33–27 is a continuous-wave Doppler tracing from the suprasternal notch of a patient with severe coarctation. The lower velocity signals from the descending aorta proximal to the obstruction are seen superimposed on the higher velocity signals from the jet flow distal to the obstruction. In this patient, the peak velocity of 4 m per second predicts a 64 mm Hg gradient across the coarctation. If the peak velocity proximal to the coarctation is greater than 1 m per second, the expanded Bernoulli equation (pressure gradient = $4V_2^2 - 4V_1^2$) should be used to obtain an accurate estimate of the pressure gradient across the coarctation. Because a high percentage of patients with aortic coarctation have a bicuspid aortic valve and aortic valve stenosis, the peak velocity proximal to the coarctation is likely to be increased and should be measured (with pulsed Doppler).

With a mild coarctation, the high-velocity jet extends throughout systole only. With increasing severity of the obstruction, the jet extends throughout diastole as well. This finding occurs because, with severe obstruction, the pressure above the coarctation remains elevated throughout diastole.[5]

The most severe form of left ventricular outflow obstruction is hypoplastic left heart syndrome. This defect has many anatomic variations but, in the most common form, both the aortic and the mitral valves are atretic, and the left ventricle is a small, slit-like cavity with no obvious contractions in real-time (Fig. 33–28). The ascending aorta is extremely small, and a coarctation is usually present.[64, 65]

Right Ventricular Outflow Obstruction

Right ventricular outflow obstruction can occur beneath the pulmonary valve (subvalvular), at the level of the pulmonary valve (valvular), or above the pulmonary valve (supravalvular pulmonary stenosis and peripheral or branch pulmonary stenosis). On the two-dimensional echocardiogram, severe right ventricular outflow obstruction results in right ventricular hypertrophy, right atrial dilation (because of decreased right ventricular compliance), and

decreased right ventricular fractional shortening (from increased afterload).

In children with valvular pulmonary stenosis, the two-dimensional echocardiogram shows thickened valve leaflets with restricted lateral mobility (doming). The pulmonary valve annulus varies in size from small to normal (Fig. 33–29), and there is poststenotic dilation of the main pulmonary artery. Doppler echocardiography can be used to record the peak velocity of the pulmonary stenosis jet and, thus, estimate the peak instantaneous pressure gradient across the pulmonary valve. The parasternal and subcostal views provide the best positions for recording the peak velocity of the jet.[51, 66, 67]

Subvalvular pulmonary stenosis is most commonly found in association with a ventricular septal defect in the setting of tetralogy of Fallot, which will be discussed in a later section of this chapter. The most common form of isolated subvalvular pulmonary stenosis is double-chambered right ventricle, a defect in which an anomalous muscle bundle traverses the right ventricular cavity and causes obstruction to forward flow out the right ventricle. The anomalous muscle bundle can be located high in the infundibulum of the right ventricle (so-called napkin-ring type) or low in the body of the right ventricle (Fig. 33–30). Double-chambered right ventricle is often associated with ventricular septal defect and discrete membranous subaortic stenosis.

Because of the fetal circulatory patterns, the pulmonary artery branches are considerably smaller in diameter than the main pulmonary artery at birth.[68] This normal discrepancy in size between the main and the branch pulmonary arteries should not be mistaken for pathologic peripheral pulmonary stenosis. When there is uniform hypoplasia of both pulmonary artery branches, the diagnosis depends on an accurate measurement of the branch pulmonary artery diameter from the two-dimensional echocardiogram and a comparison of this measurement to normal values for the branch pulmonary artery diameter at various body-surface areas. Localized areas of branch stenosis are more easily diagnosed with two-dimensional echocardiography, because they appear as a discrete area of

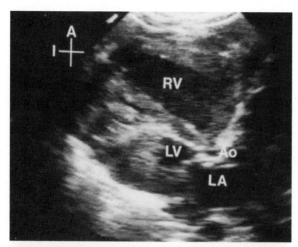

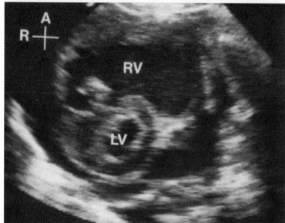

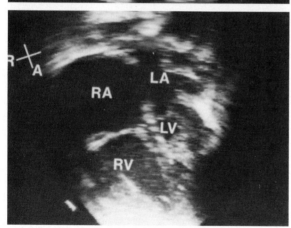

FIGURE 33–28. Parasternal long-axis *(top)*, short-axis *(middle)*, and four-chamber *(bottom)* views in a newborn infant with hypoplastic left heart syndrome. The ascending aorta (Ao) is diminutive, and the left ventricle (LV) is a small muscle-bound chamber. A = anterior; I = inferior; LA = left atrium; R = right; RA = right atrium; RV = right ventricle.

CONGENITAL HEART DISEASE WITH CYANOSIS AND DECREASED PULMONARY VASCULARITY

Infants who present with cyanosis and decreased pulmonary vascularity on chest radiograph have some form of right ventricular

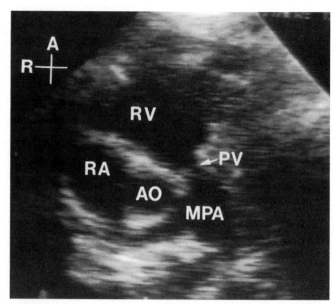

FIGURE 33–29. Parasternal short-axis view in a child with stenosis of the pulmonary valve (PV). There is narrowing of the PV annulus and poststenotic dilation of the main pulmonary artery (MPA). A = anterior; AO = aorta; R = right; RA = right atrium; RV = right ventricle.

outflow obstruction associated with a right-to-left shunt at the atrial or ventricular level. Two-dimensional echocardiography is especially useful for defining the anatomical type of outflow obstruction and the level of intracardiac shunt.

Defects With a Right-to-Left Shunt at Ventricular Level

Decreased pulmonary blood flow and a right-to-left ventricular shunt are characteristic features of several different anatomical types of cyanotic congenital heart disease. One group of defects is characterized by the following anatomical features: (1) anterior discontinuity between the septum and the anterior aortic root, (2) an outlet ventricular septal defect, (3) underdevelopment of the entire right ventricular outflow tract (subvalvular, valvular, and

narrowing in the pulmonary artery branch, followed distally by poststenotic dilation.

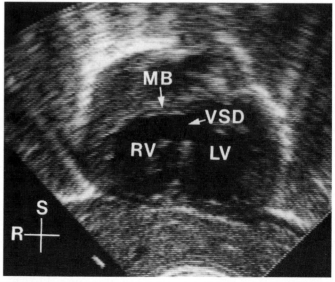

FIGURE 33–30. Subcostal sagittal view of a child with a large ventricular septal defect (VSD) and an anomalous muscle bundle (MB), obstructing the right ventricle (RV). LV = left ventricle; R = right; S = superior.

branch pulmonary stenosis), and (4) severe right ventricular hypertrophy. Defects that belong to this category include tetralogy of Fallot, pulmonary atresia with a ventricular septal defect, and double-outlet right ventricle with normally related great arteries and severe pulmonary stenosis. These defects have in common several two-dimensional echocardiographic features, including (1) a dilated dextraposed aorta that overrides the ventricular septum (Fig. 33–31); (2) a large-outlet ventricular septal defect; (3) a narrowed infundibulum, pulmonary valve annulus, main pulmonary artery, and branches; and (4) severe hypertrophy of the right ventricular anterior wall and septum.[69] These defects each have several distinguishing echocardiographic features. In tetralogy of Fallot and pulmonary atresia with a ventricular septal defect, the posterior aortic root and anterior mitral valve leaflet are in fibrous continuity, and the aorta is committed primarily to the left ventricle. In the parasternal short-axis view in tetralogy of Fallot, the pulmonary valve is small but patent (see Fig. 33–31), and there is antegrade flow, as shown on Doppler examination of the main pulmonary artery. In the parasternal short-axis view in pulmonary atresia–ventricular septal defect, no pulmonary valve leaflet motion can be detected, and Doppler examination of the main pulmonary artery shows no evidence of antegrade blood flow. Usually, an imperforate membrane occupies the position where the pulmonary valve would normally be found; however, occasionally, the right ventricular

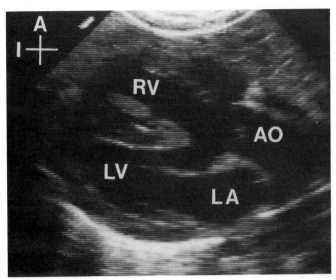

FIGURE 33–32. Parasternal long-axis view from an infant with double-outlet right ventricle. There is anterior discontinuity between the septum and the anterior aortic (AO) root. In addition, there is posterior discontinuity between the anterior leaflet of the mitral valve and the aortic valve. The fibrous area between these two structures represents persistent subaortic conus. A = anterior; I = inferior; LA = left atrium; LV = left ventricle; RV = right ventricle.

outflow tract ends blindly, and there is no evidence of a main pulmonary artery segment. Pulmonary blood flow is supplied by way of a patent ductus arteriosus or bronchial collateral vessels. In both these defects, the two-dimensional echocardiogram is particularly useful for assessing the exact anatomy and measurements of the pulmonary artery branches and for determining whether the branches are confluent. In addition, in tetralogy of Fallot, the two-dimensional echocardiogram is useful for detecting associated lesions (i.e., additional muscular ventricular septal defects or anomalous origin of the left anterior descending coronary artery from the right coronary artery) prior to complete repair. In double-outlet right ventricle and normally related great arteries, the aorta arises predominantly from the right ventricle, and there is, in addition, lack of continuity between the aortic valve and the anterior mitral valve leaflet because of persistent conus tissue beneath the aortic valve (Fig. 33–32). In the parasternal short-axis view, the great arteries are seen in cross-section as double circles side by side. Both semilunar valves are anterior to the level of the ventricular septum and are at the same heights above the ventricles (Fig. 33–33).

Tricuspid atresia with normally related great arteries, small ventricular septal defect, and pulmonary stenosis is another example of a cyanotic defect with a right-to-left ventricular shunt. In the apical and subcostal four-chamber views, the atretic tricuspid valve, small right ventricular chamber, ventricular septal defect, and large right atrium can be visualized (Fig. 33–34). The two-dimensional echocardiogram is useful for assessment of the adequacy of the atrial septal defect and for detection of commonly associated abnormalities (i.e., left juxtaposition of the right atrial appendage, right aortic arch, persistent left superior vena cava to the coronary sinus).

Defects With a Right-to-Left Shunt at Atrial Level

Several cyanotic congenital heart defects are characterized by having severe right ventricular outflow obstruction, an intact ventricular septum, and a right-to-left atrial shunt. Included in this category of defects are Ebstein malformation of the tricuspid valve, critical pulmonary stenosis, and pulmonary atresia with an intact ventricular septum.

In Ebstein malformation, the tricuspid valve apparatus is dis-

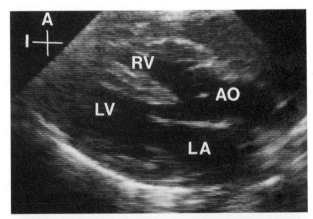

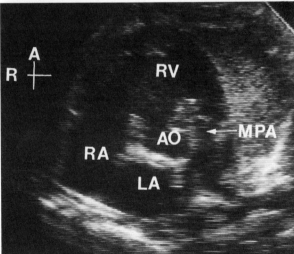

FIGURE 33–31. Parasternal long-axis (*top*) and short-axis (*bottom*) views in an infant with tetralogy of Fallot. Note the lack of anterior continuity between the septum and the anterior aortic (AO) root. This represents aortic override. In the short-axis view, a large ventricular septal defect is seen, extending from the membranous to the outlet septum. The right ventricular outflow tract, main pulmonary artery (MPA), and pulmonary artery branches are small. The pulmonary valve is clearly seen. A = anterior; I = inferior; LA = left atrium; LV = left ventricle; R = right; RA = right atrium; RV = right ventricle.

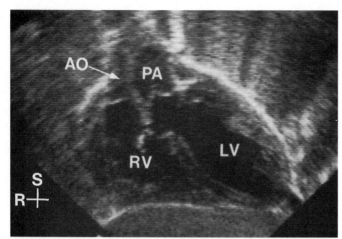

FIGURE 33–33. Subcostal view in a coronal body plane from a child with double-outlet right ventricle and d-transposition of the great arteries. The aorta (Ao) is entirely committed to the right ventricle (RV). The pulmonary artery (PA) overrides the ventricular septum, and there is a large subpulmonary ventricular septal defect. Note that the aortic and pulmonic valves are at the same heights above the ventricles because of the persistence of bilateral conus beneath the semilunar valves. LV = left ventricle; R = right; S = superior.

placed downward, away from the annulus fibrosis. The tricuspid valve septal leaflet can be seen in the apical four-chamber view, arising from the ventricular septum near the cardiac apex and away from the annulus (Fig. 33–35).[70] The anterior leaflet of the tricuspid valve, which usually arises normally from the fibrous annulus, is large and sail-like and spirals downward and outward toward the right ventricular outflow tract. The large redundant anterior leaflet can obstruct forward flow out the right ventricle and, thus, cause pulmonary stenosis. In the most severe cases, there may be true anatomical pulmonary atresia. In infants with a widely patent ductus arteriosus and severe tricuspid insufficiency, the main pulmonary artery systolic pressure can exceed right ventricular systolic pressure, causing a functional pulmonary atresia. In these patients,

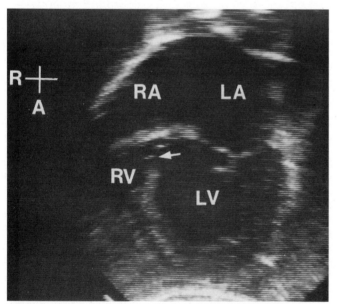

FIGURE 33–34. Apical four-chamber view in a child with tricuspid atresia, normally related great vessels, and severe pulmonary stenosis. An imperforate thick membrane is seen in the area which would normally be occupied by a tricuspid valve. The right ventricle (RV) is extremely small, and there is a moderate-sized inlet ventricular septal defect (arrow). A = apex; LA = left atrium; LV = left ventricle; R = right; RA = right atrium.

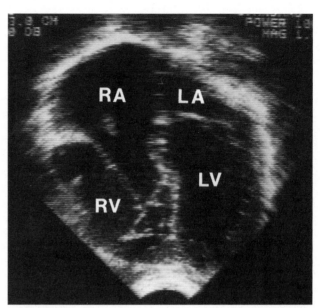

FIGURE 33–35. Apical four-chamber view in a child with Ebstein deformity of the tricuspid valve. The anterior leaflet of the tricuspid valve arises normally from the fibrous annulus; however, the septal leaflet of the tricuspid valve is displaced inferiorly in the right ventricle (RV) and arises from the lower portion of the ventricular septum. This displacement results in atrialization of a large portion of the RV and loss of total functioning RV mass. LA = left atrium; LV = left ventricle; RA = right atrium.

no pulmonary valve leaflet motion can be detected on the two-dimensional echocardiogram, and no antegrade flow across the pulmonary valve can be detected on the Doppler examination. Under these circumstances, it can be very difficult to distinguish true anatomical pulmonary atresia from functional pulmonary atresia by echocardiographic examination.

Additional valuable information that can be obtained from the two-dimensional and Doppler echocardiographic examination in patients with Ebstein malformation includes (1) the size of the atrialized portion of the right ventricle, (2) the size of the functioning portion of the right ventricle, (3) the size of the atrial septal defect, (4) the presence and severity of tricuspid insufficiency, and (5) the presence of a patent ductus arteriosus.

Pulmonary atresia and an intact ventricular septum (hypoplastic right heart syndrome) is another defect with right ventricular obstruction and right-to-left atrial shunting. On the two-dimensional echocardiogram in these infants (Fig. 33–36), the right ventricle is severely hypertrophic and has bright endocardial echoes (fibroelastosis). The right ventricular cavity varies in size from diminutive to nearly normal, and large sinusoids are frequently seen connecting the cavity of the right ventricle to the coronary arteries. Usually, the tricuspid valve is thickened and immobile, and its annulus size is smaller than normal. The right atrium is enlarged and the amount of tricuspid insufficiency, when present, varies considerably. There is also a great deal of variability in the size of the right ventricular infundibulum, main pulmonary artery, and pulmonary artery branches.

CONGENITAL HEART DISEASE WITH CYANOSIS AND INCREASED PULMONARY VASCULARITY

Increased Pulmonary Arterial Markings

Children with cyanosis and increased pulmonary arterial markings on chest radiograph have mixing of venous and arterial blood, increased pulmonary blood flow, and no significant pulmonary ste-

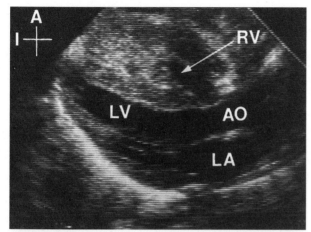

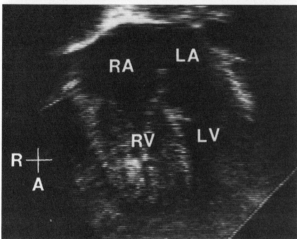

FIGURE 33–36. Parasternal long-axis *(top)* and apical four-chamber *(bottom)* views in an infant with pulmonary atresia and an intact ventricular septum. Note that the right ventricle (RV) is very hypertrophic and has a diminutive cavity. A = anterior; AO = aorta; I = inferior; LA = left atrium; LV = left ventricle; R = right; RA = right atrium. (From Snider AR: Two-dimensional and Doppler echocardiographic evaluation of heart disease in the neonate and fetus. Clin. Perinatol. 15:547, 1988, with permission.)

nosis. Some of the more common congenital heart defects that fall into this category are d-transposition of the great arteries, truncus arteriosus, single ventricle, and single atrium.

In simple or d-transposition of the great arteries, there are concordant atrioventricular connections (right atrium connected to the morphologic right ventricle) and discordant ventriculoarterial connections (aorta arising from the morphologic right ventricle). The morphology of the cardiac chambers is readily determined on the two-dimensional echocardiogram. The techniques for determining cardiac chamber morphology are discussed in detail in a later section. Multiple echocardiographic views are necessary for a complete diagnosis of d-transposition; however, the subcostal views are especially useful for demonstrating the abnormal ventriculoarterial connections. In these views, the aorta is identified as the vessel that arches, and the pulmonary artery is identified as the vessel that bifurcates (Fig. 33–37).[71] d-Transposition of the great arteries is caused by lack of rotation of the embryonic conotruncus; therefore, the great arteries exit the heart in a parallel fashion, rather than being coiled around one another. This abnormal parallel arrangement of the great arteries can be seen in the parasternal long- and short-axis views. In the short-axis view, the great vessels are seen as double circles in cross section with the aorta anterior and rightward of the pulmonary artery.[72]

In severely cyanotic and acidotic newborn infants, the diagnosis of d-transposition can be made rapidly and safely with the use

of two-dimensional echocardiography. To improve mixing of the systemic and pulmonary venous returns, balloon atrial septostomy can be performed at the bedside or in the catheterization laboratory with the use of echocardiographic visualization for guidance (Fig. 33–38). The arterial switch procedure has gained widespread

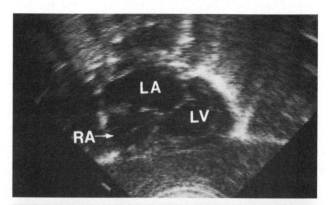

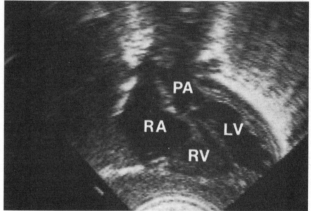

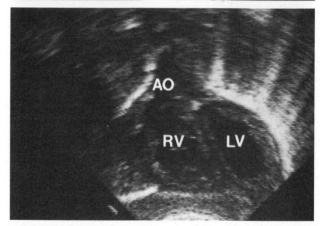

FIGURE 33–37. Subcostal views in coronal body planes from a newborn infant with d-transposition of the great arteries. From top to bottom, these frames represent a progressive tilt of the plane of sound from a posterior to a very anterior position. The top frame is a coronal view taken with the plane of sound oriented posteriorly through the inlet of the heart. The eustachian valve can be imaged in the morphologic right atrium (RA), and the pulmonary veins can be seen draining to the morphologic left atrium (LA). The echocardiographic dropout in the atrial septum represents a secundum atrial septal defect. The middle frame represents a slight anterior tilt of the plane of sound so that the entire left ventricular (LV) outflow tract can be imaged. The pulmonary artery (PA) and its bifurcation into two pulmonary artery branches can be seen arising from the LV. Imaging of a vessel that bifurcates arising from the LV is echocardiographic proof of discordant ventriculoarterial connection or transposition of the great arteries. The bottom frame represents the most anterior coronal plane. In this plane, a vessel that does not bifurcate and is, therefore, the aorta (AO) is seen arising from the right ventricle (RV).

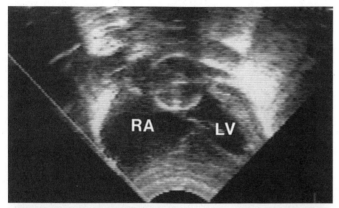

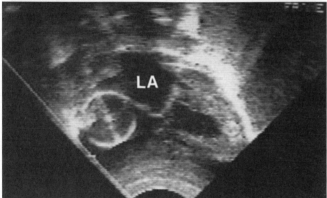

FIGURE 33–38. Subcostal four-chamber views obtained from an infant with d-transposition of the great arteries at the time of atrial septostomy. *Top,* The catheter has been positioned in the left atrium (LA), and the balloon has been inflated. *Bottom,* The balloon has been pulled back across the atrial septum into the right atrium (RA). LV = left ventricle. (From Snider, A.R., and Serwer, G.A.: Echocardiography in Pediatric Heart Disease. Chicago, Mosby–Year Book, 1990, p. 173, with permission.)

acceptance as the preferred surgical repair of transposition in the first month of life. Part of the success of this operation is based on a clear identification of coronary artery anatomy. Coronary artery anatomy can be correctly diagnosed by two-dimensional echocardiography in most infants with simple transposition of the great arteries.[73]

In persistent truncus arteriosus, a large artery exits the heart from both ventricles and gives rise to the aortic arch, coronary arteries, and pulmonary arteries. On the two-dimensional echocardiogram, the truncus arteriosus overrides the ventricular septum, and there is discontinuity between the anterior truncal wall and the ventricular septum (Fig. 33–39).[69] Usually, the truncal valve is in fibrous continuity with the anterior mitral valve leaflet. A large-outlet ventricular septal defect is usually present. The right ventricle is hypertrophic, and the pulmonary valve is absent. The parasternal short-axis views and the suprasternal views are useful for identifying the connections of the pulmonary arteries to the truncus arteriosus. In truncus arteriosus type I, the pulmonary artery branches arise via a short main pulmonary segment from the left lateral aspect of the ascending aorta (Fig. 33–40). In truncus arteriosus type II, the two pulmonary artery branches arise from the posterior wall of the ascending aorta via separate (but side-by-side) orifices. In truncus arteriosus type III, the pulmonary artery branches arise from the truncal vessel via two widely separated orifices.

In children with truncus arteriosus, the two-dimensional echocardiogram is especially useful for detecting associated abnormalities, including (1) the presence of a right aortic arch, present in about one third of patients with truncus arteriosus; (2) the number of truncal valve cusps (quadricuspid truncal valves are common); (3) the presence of a patent ductus arteriosus; and (4) the presence

of additional muscular ventricular septal defects. The Doppler examination is particularly helpful for determining (1) whether the truncal valve is stenotic and, if so, the degree of stenosis; (2) whether the truncal valve is insufficient and, if so, the severity of the insufficiency; and (3) whether the pulmonary artery branches are stenotic at their origins.

Increased Pulmonary Venous Markings

Cyanotic infants with increased pulmonary venous markings on chest radiograph have intracardiac right-to-left shunting and obstruction to pulmonary venous return. The most common defect in this category is total anomalous pulmonary venous return, a condition in which the pulmonary veins join to form a confluence that drains back to the right atrium, rather than to the left atrium. Clinically, this defect can be difficult to differentiate from persistent pulmonary artery hypertension or pulmonary disease of the newborn; prior to the use of echocardiography, cardiac catheterization was often required for a definitive diagnosis. With two-dimensional and Doppler echocardiography, total anomalous pulmonary venous return usually can be diagnosed rapidly and with certainty. Thus, potentially risky cardiac catheterizations can be avoided in unstable newborn infants with lung disease or primary pulmonary hypertension.

Total anomalous pulmonary venous return can be diagnosed on the two-dimensional echocardiogram by identifying the pulmonary venous confluence that is situated posterior to and separated from the left atrium (Fig. 33–41).[2] Usually, the final site of drainage of the pulmonary venous confluence into the right atrium can be visualized.[74] In total anomalous pulmonary venous return to the coronary sinus (intracardiac type), the pulmonary venous confluence can be seen connecting to a very dilated coronary sinus in the parasternal long- and short-axis views.[75] In total anomalous pulmonary venous return to the superior vena cava by way of a left vertical vein and innominate vein (supracardiac type), the entire anomalous connection can be seen in the suprasternal short-axis view (Fig. 33–42).[61]

In infradiaphragmatic total anomalous pulmonary venous return (infracardiac type), the common pulmonary vein can be visualized in the subcostal views as it leaves the pulmonary venous confluence,

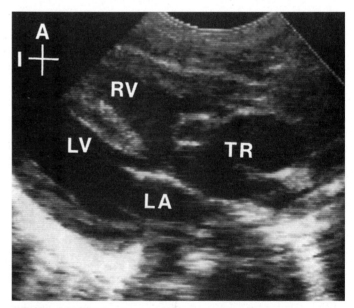

FIGURE 33–39. Parasternal long-axis view in an infant with truncus arteriosus. The discontinuity between the septum and the anterior wall of the truncus arteriosus (TR) represents a large outlet ventricular septal defect. The truncal vessel overrides the ventricular septum so that both the right ventricle (RV) and the left ventricle (LV) eject into the truncus arteriosus. A = anterior; I = inferior; LA = left atrium.

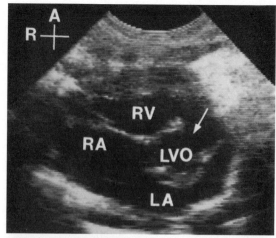

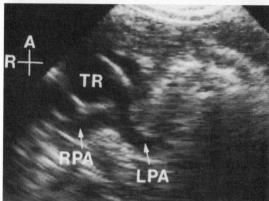

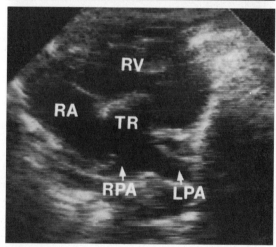

FIGURE 33–40. Parasternal short-axis views in several infants with truncus arteriosus. *Top,* The short-axis view at the base of the heart shows a large ventricular septal defect *(arrow)* in the outlet portion of the ventricular septum. The position of the defect in this patient is very typical of that found in truncus arteriosus. *Middle,* A cross section through the truncal vessel (TR) of an infant with truncus arteriosus type I. In this form of truncus arteriosus, there is a short main pulmonary artery segment that arises from the left lateral aspect of the TR and gives rise to both right and left pulmonary artery branches (RPA and LPA). *Bottom,* A short-axis view through the truncal vessel of an infant with type II truncus arteriosus. In type II truncus arteriosus, both great arteries arise from the posterior aspect of the truncal vessel by way of side-by-side but separate orifices. A = anterior; LA = left atrium; LVO = left ventricular outflow tract; R = right; RA = right atrium; RV = right ventricle.

passes anterior to the aorta through the diaphragm, and drains into a systemic vein in the abdomen—usually the hepatic portal venous system (see Fig. 33–42).[76] In children with total anomalous pulmonary venous return, pulsed and color flow Doppler interrogation of

the left vertical vein or common pulmonary vein show venous flow directed away from the heart (Fig. 33–43). Thus, the Doppler examination is useful for confirming that the unusual venous structure seen on the two-dimensional echocardiogram is the common pulmonary vein and not some other anomalous systemic vein (in which flow would be directed toward the heart).[77]

FIGURE 33–43. See Color Plate 7.

ECHOCARDIOGRAPHIC APPROACH TO COMPLEX CONGENITAL HEART DISEASE

Two-dimensional echocardiography has had a major impact on our ability to diagnose complex congenital heart defects. With this technique, one can image detailed structural anatomy even more precisely than with cardiac catheterization in the majority of patients. The echocardiographic approach to the diagnosis of complex congenital heart disease is a very logical and systematic approach that requires a basic knowledge of how cardiac chambers are identified on the two-dimensional echocardiogram.

Echocardiographic Approach to the Segmental Analysis of the Heart

The echocardiographic approach to the diagnosis of complex congenital heart disease involves a segmental analysis of the heart. In this type of analysis, one can think of the heart as being much like a house. To describe a house completely, one must describe where the rooms or chambers are on each floor. For the cardiac house, then, one must describe where each atrium is located on the ground floor, where the ventricles are located on the second story, and where each great artery is positioned at the top of the house. In addition, one must describe where the staircases are that connect the floors. In other words, one must describe the atrioventricular connections and the ventriculoarterial connections. If ones does not describe the atria correctly, then the entire house comes tumbling down.

Thus, the approach to the echocardiographic diagnosis of the patient with complex congenital heart disease begins with a deter-

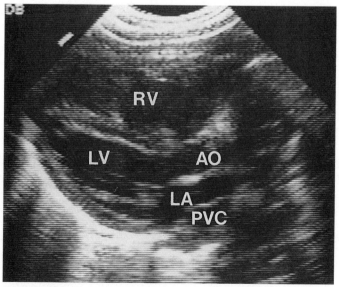

FIGURE 33–41. Parasternal long-axis view in an infant with total anomalous pulmonary venous connection. The pulmonary veins come together to form a confluence (PVC) that is located behind and separate from the left atrium (LA). AO = aorta; LV = left ventricle; RV = right ventricle.

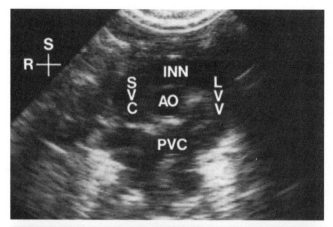

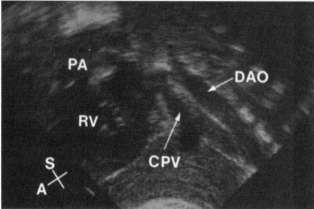

FIGURE 33–42. *Top,* Suprasternal short-axis view in an infant with total anomalous pulmonary venous return to the right superior vena cava (SVC) by way of a left vertical vein (LVV) and innominate vein (INN). In this view, the pulmonary venous confluence (PVC) can be seen draining to the LVV and eventually to the SVC. This anomalous pulmonary venous connection surrounding the aorta (AO) creates the appearance of a snowman-shaped heart on the chest radiograph. *Bottom,* Subcostal sagittal view in an infant with infradiaphragmatic total anomalous pulmonary venous connection. In this view, the pulmonary veins drain together to form a common pulmonary vein (CPV) that then drains anterior to the descending aorta (DAO), through the diaphragm, and into the abdomen. Once in the abdomen, the CPV immediately turned anteriorly and drained into the left hepatic vein. A = anterior; PA = pulmonary artery; R = right; RV = right ventricle; S = superior.

mination of atrial situs. In atrial situs solitus, the morphologic right atrium is on the right, and the morphologic left atrium is on the left. In situs inversus, the morphologic left atrium is on the right, and the morphologic right atrium is on the left. In situs ambiguus, the atria do not differentiate into right and left atria. Instead, both atria can have features of a morphologic right atrium, a condition called asplenia, or both atria can have features of a morphologic left atrium, a condition called polysplenia. The echocardiographic findings used to identify the morphology of the atria will be reviewed later in this section.

The next step in diagnosing complex congenital heart disease is determination of the bulboventricular loop. The bulboventricular loop describes the locations of the ventricles. In a d-loop (dextroloop), the morphologic right ventricle is on the right, and the morphologic left ventricle is on the left. In an l-loop (levo-loop), the morphologic right ventricle is on the left, and the morphologic left ventricle is on the right. These definitions of d- and l-loop apply, regardless of what the atrial situs is.

The final step in the diagnosis of complex congenital heart disease is a description of the great artery connections. In normal or concordant connections, the pulmonary artery arises from the right ventricle, and the aorta arises from the left ventricle. Transpo-

sition is the situation in which the aorta arises from the morphologic right ventricle, and the pulmonary artery arises from the morphologic left ventricle. Transposition is a discordant ventriculoarterial connection. Other types of great artery connections include double-outlet right ventricle, double-outlet left ventricle, and single outlet from the heart. Three common forms of single outlet from the heart include truncus arteriosus, aortic atresia, and pulmonary atresia.

Concordant or normal connections between the atria and ventricles (right atrium to right ventricle, left atrium to left ventricle) occur when there is situs solitus with a d-loop or situs inversus with an l-loop. Discordant or abnormal connections between the atria and ventricles (right atrium to left ventricle, left atrium to right ventricle) occur when there is situs solitus with an l-loop or situs inversus with a d-loop. Before reviewing how cardiac chambers are identified on the two-dimensional echocardiogram, we should review the "rule of 50 percent." The rule of 50 percent states that a chamber is a ventricle when it receives 50 percent or more of an inlet. A chamber need not have an outlet to be a ventricle. For example, the left ventricle in double-outlet right ventricle is a ventricle because it receives the mitral valve, even though it does not have an outlet. Second, if 50 percent or more of a great artery arises above a chamber, it is defined as being connected to that chamber. Rudimentary chambers are chambers that receive less than 50 percent of an inlet and, therefore, do not qualify to be ventricles. There are two types of rudimentary chambers. An outlet chamber is a chamber that has less than 50 percent of an inlet but has 50 percent or more of an outlet or great artery. A trabeculated pouch is a chamber that has less than 50 percent of an inlet and less than 50 percent of an outlet.[78]

To diagnose complex congenital heart disease, one must know how cardiac chambers are identified on the two-dimensional echocardiogram. The cardiac chambers are defined largely by the anatomical landmarks on their septal surfaces. The right atrium has a septal surface that receives the tendinous insertion of the eustachian valve and has the limbus of the fossa ovalis. The eustachian valve crosses the floor of the right atrium from the orifice of the inferior vena cava and inserts into the septum primum (the lower portion of the atrial septum adjacent to the atrioventricular valves). This tendinous insertion is along the lower border of the fossa

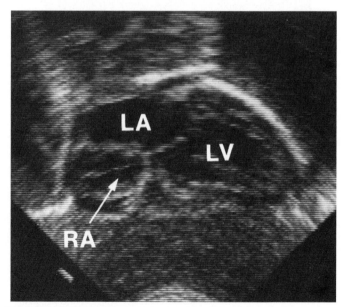

FIGURE 33–44. Subcostal four-chamber view through the inlet of the heart in a normal patient. The eustachian valve can be seen crossing the floor of the right atrium (RA) from its origin at the orifice of the inferior vena cava to its insertion in the lowermost portion of the atrial septum. The eustachian valve is an anatomical marker of a morphologic right atrium. LA = left atrium; LV = left ventricle.

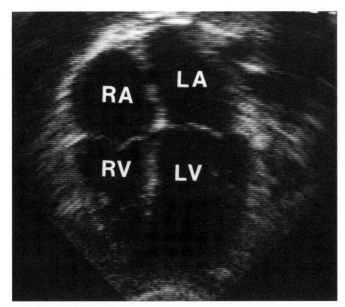

FIGURE 33–45. Apical four-chamber view in a normal patient. The ventricle on the patient's right has an atrioventricular valve that is closer to the cardiac apex and has heavy trabeculations crossing from the septum to the parietal free wall. These anatomical features indicate that the right-sided ventricle is a morphologic right ventricle (RV). The ventricle on the patient's left has a smooth septal surface and no muscle bundles coursing from the septum to the parietal free wall. In addition, its atrioventricular valve is farther from the cardiac apex. These features are landmarks of a morphologic left ventricle (LV). LA = left atrium; RA = right atrium.

ovalis and is called the inferior limbic band (Fig. 33–44). In real time, the eustachian valve moves rapidly back and forth in the right atrium and can be visualized in virtually all infants and in many older children and adults.

The left atrial septal surface has the flap valve of the fossa ovalis. This is the septum primum tissue that covers the foramen ovale and seals it closed after birth. The flap valve can be seen on the two-dimensional echocardiogram protruding into the left atrium in the fetus when the foramen ovale is open; and, often, the flap valve can be seen after infancy lying against the septum secundum.

The right ventricle is the chamber whose septal surface has prominent muscle bundles crossing from the septum to the parietal free wall (Fig. 33–45). The largest of these septoparietal muscle bundles is the moderator band. In addition, the septal surface of the right ventricle receives chordal insertions from the tricuspid valve septal leaflet (Fig. 33–46).

The left ventricle is the chamber whose septal surface is smooth. There are no septoparietal free-wall muscle bundles, and the mitral valve normally has no chordal insertions into the septum.

Another anatomical feature that is useful in identifying the cardiac chambers is that the atrioventricular valve always belongs to the appropriate ventricle. Thus, the tricuspid valve is always found in the morphologic right ventricle, and the mitral valve is always found in the morphologic left ventricle. The tricuspid valve is closer to the cardiac apex (see Fig. 33–45), has three leaflets, and has chordal insertions into the ventricular septum (see Fig. 33–46). The mitral valve is farther from the cardiac apex, is a fish-mouthed bicuspid valve, and has chordal insertions only into two papillary muscles in the left ventricle.

Systemic and pulmonary venous return can be helpful in identifying the atria. The pulmonary veins usually drain to the left atrium; however, this is not a constant feature of the left atrium, as the pulmonary veins can drain anomalously. If three or more pulmonary veins are visualized draining by separate orifices to a chamber and there is no evidence of a pulmonary venous confluence, that chamber is most likely a morphologic left atrium. The inferior vena cava usually drains to the morphologic right atrium. This

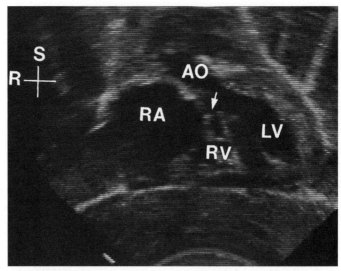

FIGURE 33–46. Subcostal coronal view through the left ventricular (LV) outflow tract of a child with a large membranous ventricular septal defect (*arrow*). Note that the tricuspid valve has chordal insertions into the right ventricular side of the ventricular septum at the lower border of the ventricular septal defect. This anatomical feature identifies the morphologic right ventricle (RV). AO = aorta; R = right; RA = right atrium; S = superior.

relationship is constant in the majority of cases, except in patients with situs ambiguus. The superior vena cava usually drains to the right atrium; however, this relationship is not constant, as the superior vena cava can drain to either or both atria (Figs. 33–47 to 33–49).

The morphology of the atrial appendages can be helpful in identifying the atria. The right atrial appendage is short and stout (resembling "Snoopy's" nose) and the left atrial appendage is long and finger-like (resembling "Snoopy's" ear) (Fig. 33–50).

In addition, the situs of the abdomen may be helpful in de-

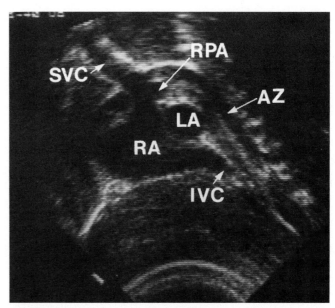

FIGURE 33–47. Subcostal sagittal view in a normal patient, showing the normal pattern of systemic venous return. This view was obtained by positioning the plane of sound in a sagittal body plane and orienting the transducer toward the patient's right atrium (RA). The superior vena cava (SVC) and inferior vena cava (IVC) can be seen draining to the RA. Posteriorly, the azygous vein (AZ) can be seen entering the SVC posterior and superior to the right pulmonary artery (RPA). LA = left atrium.

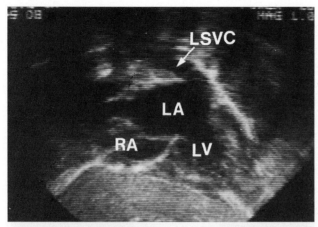

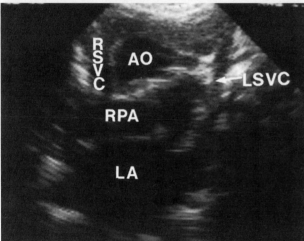

FIGURE 33–48. Subcostal four-chamber *(top)* and suprasternal short-axis *(bottom)* views in a patient with a persistent left superior vena cava (LSVC) draining directly to the left atrium (LA). In these views, the persistent LSVC-to-LA communication can be seen. In addition, this patient also had a right superior vena cava (RSVC). AO = aorta; LV = left ventricle; RA = right atrium; RPA = right pulmonary artery.

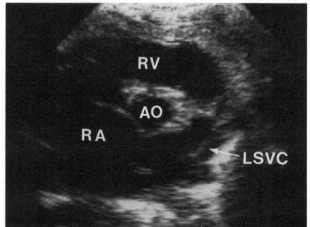

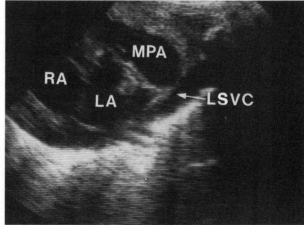

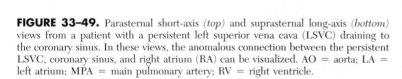

FIGURE 33–49. Parasternal short-axis *(top)* and suprasternal long-axis *(bottom)* views from a patient with a persistent left superior vena cava (LSVC) draining to the coronary sinus. In these views, the anomalous connection between the persistent LSVC, coronary sinus, and right atrium (RA) can be visualized. AO = aorta; LA = left atrium; MPA = main pulmonary artery; RV = right ventricle.

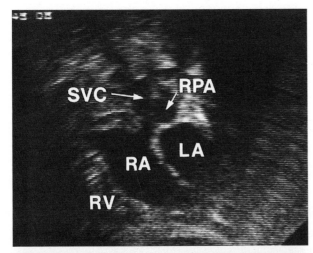

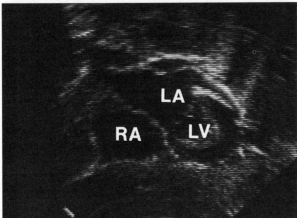

FIGURE 33–50. Subcostal sagittal (*top*) and four-chamber (*bottom*) views in a normal patient, demonstrating the morphology of the atrial appendages. *Top,* The right atrial (RA) appendage can be seen anteriorly as a broad, blunt-shaped structure, resembling "Snoopy's" nose. *Bottom,* The left atrial (LA) appendage can be seen as a long finger-like structure, resembling "Snoopy's" ear. The left atrial appendage can be distinguished from the left lower pulmonary vein by the fact that it is imaged in the plane of the mitral valve and left ventricular (LV) cavity. RPA = right pulmonary artery; RV = right ventricle; SVC = superior vena cava.

termining the atrial situs. In atrial situs solitus, the inferior vena cava is to the right of the spine, the descending aorta is to the left of the spine, the stomach bubble is on the left, and the liver is on the right. In atrial situs inversus, the inferior vena cava is usually to the left of the spine, and the descending aorta is usually to the right of the spine. The stomach bubble is on the right, and the liver is on the left (Fig. 33–51). In situs ambiguus, there are several types of anomalies of systemic venous drainage that are often present.[79, 80] For example, in asplenia, the inferior vena cava and aorta may be on the same side of the spine (Fig. 33–52). Also, in situs ambiguus (especially polysplenia), it is common to find an interrupted inferior vena cava. In this case, the hepatic veins usually drain to the right side of the common atrium, and inferior vena cava drainage is usually by way of an azygous or a hemiazygous vein (Fig. 33–53).

Echocardiographic Features of Frequently Encountered Complex Congenital Heart Defects

l-Transposition of the Great Arteries

l-Transposition of the great arteries is a condition in which there is atrioventricular discordance as well as ventriculoarterial discordance. In situs solitus, the morphologic right atrium on the

patient's right is connected to the morphologic left ventricle on the patient's right which, in turn, is connected to the pulmonary artery. On the left, the morphologic left atrium is connected to the morphologic right ventricle, which is connected to the aorta.[81, 82] This defect is called situs solitus, l-loop, l-transposition, or, simply, l-transposition. The "l" in the third term describes the spatial relations of the aortic and pulmonic valves. In the majority of cases, the aortic valve is to the left, hence the use of the "l." Because discordant connections are present at two levels, the circulation is hemodynamically correct (systemic venous blood flows to the pulmonary artery and pulmonary venous blood flows to the aorta); some investigators have called this defect corrected transposition of the great arteries. Because of the confusion in distinguishing this defect from surgically corrected d-transposition, we prefer not to use this terminology.

As with d-transposition, the echocardiographic diagnosis of l-transposition is based on demonstrating abnormal connections between the right ventricle and aorta and also between the atria and the ventricles. The spatial relationships of the great arteries may provide supportive evidence of the diagnosis; however, spatial relationship is never used as the sole diagnostic criterion.

The morphology of the atria, ventricles, and great arteries is determined on the echocardiogram with the use of the criteria outlined in this chapter. As with d-transposition, the connections of the chambers and great vessels can be seen in multiple echocardiographic views; the subcostal views, however, are particularly useful because, by simply tilting the transducer in one view, one can obtain images of all cardiac chambers, great vessels, and connections. In the subcostal four-chamber view shown in Figure 33–54, the atrium on the patient's left receives the four pulmonary veins and is the morphologic left atrium. The ventricle on the patient's left has characteristic features of a morphologic right ventricle (tricuspid valve, prominent septoparietal muscle bundles) and gives rise to a vessel that arches and is, therefore, the aorta. On the right, the morphologic right atrium is connected to a ventricle that has the anatomical features of a left ventricle (a smooth septal surface, a mitral valve, and two papillary muscles). The morphologic left ventricle on the patient's right is connected to a vessel that bifurcates into two branches and is, therefore, the pulmonary artery. These anatomical features are diagnostic of l-transposition of the great arteries.

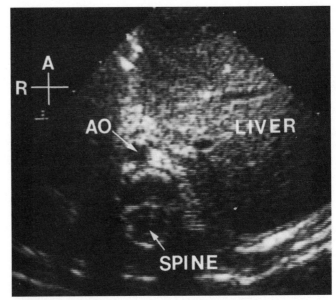

FIGURE 33–51. Subcostal short-axis view of the abdomen of a patient with situs inversus of the atria. In this patient, findings of situs inversus of the abdomen are a clue that there is probably situs inversus of the atria. Note that the liver is on the patient's left, as is the inferior vena cava. The aorta (AO) is to the right of the spine. A = anterior; R = right.

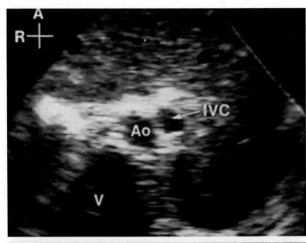

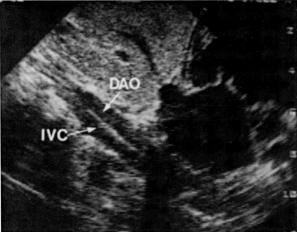

FIGURE 33–52. Subcostal short-axis *(top)* and long-axis *(bottom)* views of two patients with situs ambiguus (asplenia). In these two patients, the inferior vena cava (IVC) was on the same side of the vertebral body (V) as the descending aorta (DAO). The IVC is anterior and to the left of the DAO. This arrangement of the vessels in the abdomen is frequently seen in patients with situs ambiguus. A = anterior; R = right.

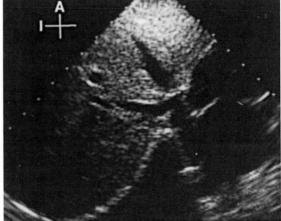

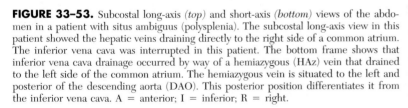

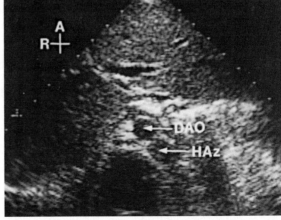

FIGURE 33–53. Subcostal long-axis *(top)* and short-axis *(bottom)* views of the abdomen in a patient with situs ambiguus (polysplenia). The subcostal long-axis view in this patient showed the hepatic veins draining directly to the right side of a common atrium. The inferior vena cava was interrupted in this patient. The bottom frame shows that inferior vena cava drainage occurred by way of a hemiazygous (HAz) vein that drained to the left side of the common atrium. The hemiazygous vein is situated to the left and posterior of the descending aorta (DAO). This posterior position differentiates it from the inferior vena cava. A = anterior; I = inferior; R = right.

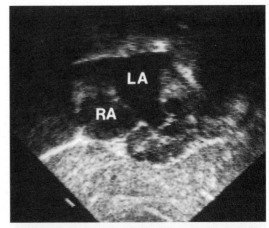

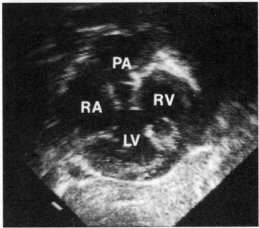

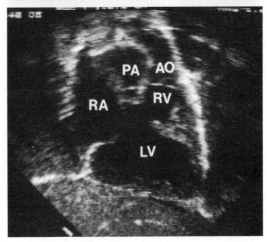

FIGURE 33–54. Subcostal coronal views in a child with situs solitus, l-loop, l-transposition of the great arteries, a large ventricular septal defect, and severe subvalvular and valvular pulmonary stenosis. From top to bottom, these frames represent a progressive tilt of the plane of sound from a posterior to an anterior position. The top frame was obtained with the transducer tilted posteriorly toward the inlet of the heart. In this view, the pulmonary veins can be seen draining to the left-sided atrium, indicating that it is a morphologic left atrium (LA). This finding suggests atrial situs solitus. In the middle frame, the plane of sound has been tilted somewhat more anteriorly. Now, a vessel that bifurcates into two branches, and is therefore a pulmonary artery (PA), is seen arising from the right-sided ventricle. The ventricle on the patient's right side has a smooth septal surface and a shape that suggests that it is a morphologic left ventricle (LV). Note the severe subvalvular and valvular pulmonary stenosis and poststenotic dilation of the PA. Also present is a large ventricular septal defect. In the bottom frame, the plane of sound has been tilted far anteriorly. Now, one can see that the ventricle on the patient's left side has prominent septal-parietal free wall muscle bundles and is triangular. These findings suggest that the left-sided ventricle is a morphologic right ventricle (RV) and that there is therefore an l-loop. A vessel that arches, and is thus an aorta (AO), is seen arising from the morphologic RV. This finding indicates transposition of the great arteries. In summary, this patient has atrial situs solitus, l-loop (discordant atrioventricular connections), and l-transposition of the great arteries (discordant ventriculoarterial connections). RA = right atrium.

As in d-transposition, the ventricular outflow tracts and great arteries in l-transposition exit the heart in a parallel fashion, instead of wrapping around one another. Unlike the normal heart or the heart with d-transposition, however, the right ventricle is usually not anterior to the left ventricle in l-transposition. Typically, the ventricles are positioned side by side, and the ventricular septum is oriented in a straight line perpendicular to the frontal plane through the thorax. In some cases, the ventricles are arranged in a superoinferior manner, with the morphologic right ventricle superior.[83]

Abnormalities of the left-sided tricuspid valve occur in about 90 percent of children with l-transposition of the great arteries.[81] The common malformation is an Ebstein-type deformity, in which the origin of the valve leaflet is displaced downward so that the basal attachment of the leaflets are from the systemic ventricular wall below the annulus fibrosus. Typically, the anterior leaflet is the least malformed, and the septal and posterior leaflets are the most malformed.

Ventricular septal defect occurs in about 70 percent of patients with l-transposition[81] and is usually perimembranous in location. However, ventricular septal defects can occur in any portion of the septum. In l-transposition, ventricular septal defects are frequently accompanied by other malformations. For example, perimembranous inlet defects may be associated with tricuspid valve straddle, whereas anterior outlet defects may be associated with mitral valve straddle.

Left ventricular outflow tract obstruction occurs in approximately 40 percent of patients with l-transposition. Usually, the stenosis is subvalvular—either a subvalvular diaphragmatic ring or an aneurysm of fibrous tissue that protrudes into the left ventricular outflow tract. This fibrous tissue can originate from the membranous septum, the mitral valve, the tricuspid valve, or the pulmonary valve.

Univentricular Heart

The ventricles of the normal heart possess an inlet component, a trabecular component, and an outlet or infundibular component.[84] The inlet component extends from the atrioventricular annulus to the insertions of the papillary muscles and need not contain a perforate atrioventricular valve. The trabecular component comprises the body of the ventricle distal to the insertion of the papillary muscles and extends to the cardiac apex. The outlet component supports a semilunar valve. In the normal heart, each trabecular zone receives its own inlet; however, both atrioventricular inlets can be committed to one trabecular portion, which is the generally accepted definition of a single ventricle.[85] According to common usage, to be classified as a ventricle, a chamber must have 50 percent or more of an inlet portion. As stated previously, chambers receiving less than 50 percent of an inlet are termed rudimentary chambers.

Another important point in the morphology and echocardiographic diagnosis is the nature of the septum that separates the ventricles and rudimentary chambers. Because the ventricles are considered as possessing inlet, trabecular, and outlet portions, the

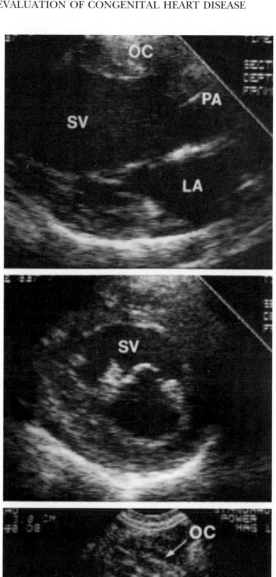

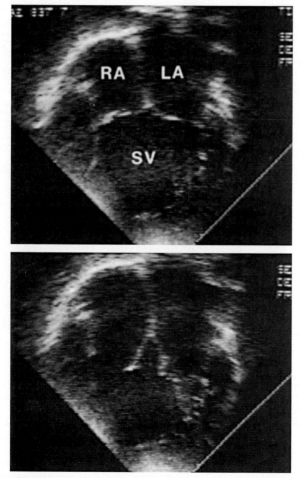

FIGURE 33–55. Apical four-chamber views during systole *(above)* and diastole *(below)* in a child with a single ventricle (SV) of the left ventricular type, l-transposition of the great arteries, and an outlet chamber situated at the left basal aspect of the heart, giving rise to the aorta. In the apical four-chamber views, both atrioventricular valves can be seen emptying into a large posterior single ventricle with no septum oriented toward the crux of heart between the atrioventricular valves. LA = left atrium; RA = right atrium.

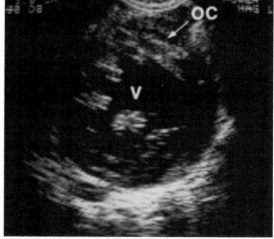

FIGURE 33–56. Parasternal long-axis *(top)* and short-axis *(middle and bottom)* views from the same patient as in Figure 33–55. In the parasternal long-axis view, the single ventricle (SV) can be seen communicating with the outlet chamber (OC) by way of the bulboventricular foramen. The pulmonary artery (PA) is seen arising from the posterior single ventricle. Other views showed the aorta arising from the OC. The middle frame shows that both atrioventricular valves empty into the SV. The bottom frame shows that the OC is located at the left basal aspect of the heart. With these views, it is obvious that the OC does not receive any portion of an inlet and therefore does not qualify to be a ventricle. LA = left atrium.

septum separating them can be considered as possessing inlet, trabecular, and outlet portions. In the univentricular heart, both inlets are committed to only one chamber; hence, by definition, the inlet septum is absent, which means that the septum separating the ventricle from the rudimentary chamber must be the trabecular septum. The position and orientation of the trabecular septum in the ventricular mass is a key feature in the echocardiographic differentiation of rudimentary chambers from hypoplastic ventricles.[84]

For example, in univentricular heart of the left ventricular type, both inlets are committed to a chamber with a left ventricular trabecular zone (Figs. 33–55 and 33–56). The rudimentary chamber has a right ventricular trabecular pattern and is located anterosuperiorly in the ventricular mass. The rudimentary chamber is separated from the main ventricle by an anterior trabecular septum, which courses to the acute or obtuse margin of the heart, rather than to the crux of the heart. Both atrioventricular valves lie posterior to the trabecular septum and have no intervening inlet septum.[78, 86, 87]

From the parasternal short-axis view, one can determine whether the rudimentary chamber lies to the right or left basal aspect of the heart. Most commonly, the rudimentary chamber lies to the left (l-loop), and the trabecular septum courses obliquely and somewhat posteriorly toward the acute margin of the heart. When the rudimentary chamber lies to the right (d-loop), the trabecular septum courses obliquely and somewhat posteriorly toward the obtuse margin of the heart.

In univentricular heart of the right ventricular type, the rudimentary chamber possesses the left ventricular trabecular portion and is, thus, located posteriorly. Likewise, the trabecular septum runs posteriorly to the crux of the heart. Visualization of the atrioventricular connections anterior to the trabecular septum is diagnostic of univentricular heart of the right ventricular type.

With the univentricular heart, any ventriculoarterial connection can occur, including concordant connections, discordant connections, double-outlet from the main or outlet chambers, and single-outlet from the heart. However, certain combinations of univentricular heart and ventriculoarterial connections are commonly associated with one another and, therefore, should be mentioned. A high percentage of patients with univentricular heart of the left ventricular type have discordant ventriculoarterial connections, that is, the aorta arises from the outlet chamber and the pulmonary artery arises from the main ventricle. In univentricular heart of the right ventricular type, the ventriculoarterial connections are usually double outlet from the main chamber or single outlet from the heart with pulmonary atresia.

Dextrocardias

The term dextrocardia indicates that the heart is located primarily in the right chest and implies that one of three conditions is present.[83, 88] First, dextrocardia can occur because the heart is displaced into the right chest, either because of a space-occupying mass in the left chest or the absence of normal lung volume filling the right chest. This form of dextrocardia is commonly called dextroposition. Second, dextrocardia can occur because the cardiac apex fails to pivot to the left (Fig. 33–57). This condition, known as dextroversion, is frequently associated with atrioventricular discordance.[89] Third, dextrocardia can occur in association with abnormal atrial situs (i.e., situs inversus or situs ambiguus). The most common condition in this category is situs inversus totalis, in which the heart is located in the mirror image position of normal. A variety of cardiac abnormalities can occur in the context of atrial situs inversus. Figure 33–58 illustrates how the two-dimensional echocardiogram can be used to diagnose cardiac defects associated with situs inversus.

TRANSESOPHAGEAL ECHOCARDIOGRAPHY IN CONGENITAL HEART DISEASE

Over the past decade, transesophageal echocardiography has rapidly gained acceptance as a diagnostic approach in adults in whom an adequate precordial ultrasound examination is impossible

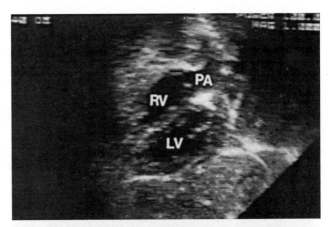
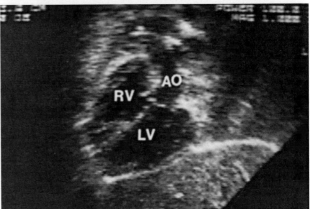

FIGURE 33–57. Subcostal coronal views in a patient with dextrocardia. In these views, the cardiac apex is seen pointing toward the patient's right. The top frame shows that the right-sided ventricle has a prominent moderator band and is therefore a morphologic right ventricle (RV). It gives rise to a vessel that bifurcates and is therefore a pulmonary artery (PA). The bottom frame shows that the left-sided ventricle has a smooth septal surface and is a morphologic left ventricle (LV). This ventricle gives rise to a vessel that arches and is therefore the aorta (AO). Other echocardiographic views in this patient demonstrated atrial situs solitus. In summary, the patient has atrial situs solitus, d-loop, and normally related great vessels. This patient had normal atrioventricular connections and normal ventriculoarterial connections with isolated dextroversion of the cardiac apex.

because of lung disease, chest deformity, or mechanical ventilation. The "explosion" in the use of transesophageal echocardiography in adults has been slow to affect pediatric cardiology for several reasons. First, the examination cannot be performed without general anesthesia in most children younger than 10 years of age, and for children and adolescents older than 10 years of age, general anesthesia or heavy sedation is usually required.[90] Second, with the use of high-frequency transducers and the availability of multiple imaging windows, complete diagnostic information can be obtained in virtually all infants and young children, and recourse to a transesophageal approach is rarely required in this age group.

The use of transesophageal echocardiography in pediatric patients has been spurred on by specific imaging needs in specific situations. For example, in the operating room, a noninvasive technique is required for immediate evaluation of the results of some cardiac surgeries.[91-93] Immediately after cardiac surgery, transesophageal echocardiography performed in the intensive care unit provides an imaging approach unaffected by bandages and chest tubes.[92] Another application for transesophageal imaging in pediatric cardiology is in the catheterization laboratory to monitor and assist in the performance of interventional catheterization procedures (Figs. 33–59 and 33–60).[94, 95] In the late postoperative period, identification of residual cardiac defects may be impaired by chest

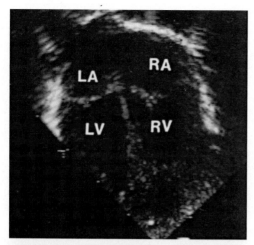

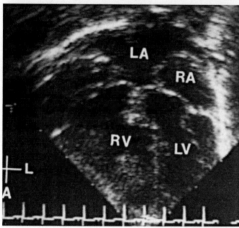

FIGURE 33–58. *Top,* Apical four-chamber view in a patient with situs inversus of the atria, l-loop, and normally connected great arteries. In this patient, the pulmonary veins are seen draining to the right-sided atrium, suggesting that this atrium is a morphologic left atrium (LA). The ventricle on the patient's left has an atrioventricular valve closer to the cardiac apex and has a prominent moderator band. These findings suggest that the left-sided ventricle is a morphologic right ventricle (RV). Thus, the patient has atrial situs inversus with an l-loop. *Bottom,* Apical four-chamber view in a patient with atrial situs inversus, d-loop, and d-transposition of the great arteries. In this patient, the pulmonary veins are seen draining to the right-sided atrium, indicating that it is a morphologic LA. The ventricle on the patient's right side has prominent muscle bundles coursing from the septum to the parietal free wall and has an atrioventricular valve with chordal insertions into the ventricular septum. These findings suggest that the ventricle on the patient's right side is a morphologic RV and that there is a d-bulboventricular loop. Thus, the patient has atrial situs inversus with a d-loop (discordant atrioventricular connections). Note the large inlet ventricular septal defect in this patient. A = apex; L = left; RA = right atrium; LV = left ventricle.

FIGURES 33–59 and 33–60. See Color Plate 8.

There are some aspects of performing the transesophageal echocardiographic examination that are unique to pediatric patients. First, the approach to sedation for the examination in children is different from that in adults. Because endoscopy is poorly tolerated by children, even when they are sedated, most centers recommend performing the transesophageal examination with the patient under general anesthesia with endotracheal intubation in all children younger than 10 years of age. Some investigators have extended this approach to include anyone younger than 15 years of age. If general anesthesia is not used, it is recommended that heavy sedation with an amnestic agent, such as a benzodiazepine, plus a narcotic medication, such as meperidine, be used. Benzodiazepines are short-acting, and the effects of the narcotic drug can be quickly reversed with naloxone.[90]

Probe insertion and manipulation in pediatric patients is often different from that in adult patients. Because most pediatric patients are intubated, probe insertion is best accomplished with direct laryngoscopic visualization of the esophagus. Nasogastric tubes, esophageal stethoscopes, and the like should be removed, or their placement delayed, until the transesophageal probe is in place. In addition, it is often necessary to deflate the cuff of the endotracheal tube during probe insertion. In very small children, the inferosuperior movement of the transesophageal probe should be limited to minimize hypopharyngeal irritation. During the pediatric transesophageal examination, it is recommended that heart rate, blood pressure, and oxygen saturation, especially in cyanotic children, be continuously monitored.[90]

In conflicting reports, the incidence of bacteremia with endoscopy has ranged from 4 to 8 percent. Two recent reports place the incidence of bacteremia in blood cultures obtained within 10 minutes of completing the transesophageal echocardiographic examination at 7 to 17 percent.[96, 97] Because the incidence of penicillin anaphylaxis is 0.015 to 0.04 percent, it seems prudent to use endocarditis prophylaxis in all but the lowest risk patients. This is especially true in pediatric patients, in whom the probe fits tightly against the mucosal surfaces of the esophagus, thus leading to an increased risk of microscopic tears and, theoretically, an increased risk of endocarditis. The Society of Pediatric Echocardiography has recommended that antibiotic prophylaxis in children should follow the American Heart Association guidelines for endoscopy.[90, 98]

Several indications and limitations of transesophageal echocardiography have become apparent from experiences with pediatric patients.[92, 99, 100] In patients with congenital heart disease, transesophageal echocardiography has been particularly useful for delineating (1) abnormalities of systemic and pulmonary venous return; (2) atrial lesions such as septal defects and cor triatriatum; (3) atrial baffle function; (4) the Fontan connection; (5) atrioventricular valve morphology and function; (6) crisscross hearts; (7) chordal straddle; (8) left ventricular outflow tract obstruction; (9) ascending aorta pathology, such as supravalvular aortic stenosis and aortic root dilation in Marfan syndrome; and (10) descending aorta pathology.

Transesophageal echocardiography has several limitations in pediatric patients. Because of large distances between the esophagus and the apical or anterior structures, the right ventricular outflow tract and apical muscular septum are often poorly visualized. On the transesophageal echocardiographic examination, structures can be masked by interposition of the bronchial tree or prosthetic material, such as patches. Finally, without continuous-wave Doppler capabilities, limited hemodynamic information is available.

deformities, fibrous adhesions, prosthetic material, or thoracotomy scars. In addition, ultrasound imaging of complex congenital heart disease becomes more difficult with advancing age because of increased chest and cardiac size and a natural reduction in the available ultrasound windows. Thus, the adolescent or young adult with congenital heart disease can present many imaging difficulties.

SUMMARY

Two-dimensional and Doppler echocardiography provide important noninvasive techniques for the diagnosis and subsequent management of children with congenital heart disease. The spatial anatomical display of cardiac structures provided by two-dimensional echocardiography has led to a more exact definition of cardiac anatomy, even in the most complex congenital cardiac defects. The addition of Doppler echocardiography has provided a noninvasive method for quantitation of the size of intracardiac shunts and the severity of ventricular outflow obstructions. These rapid developments in ultrasound technology have allowed cardiac catheterization for diagnostic purposes to be eliminated in most instances and, in other cases, to be postponed until the infant or child is better able to tolerate this invasive procedure.

References

1. Canale, J.M., Sahn, D.J., Allen, H.D., et al.: Factors affecting real-time cross-sectional echocardiographic imaging of perimembranous ventricular septal defects. Circulation 63:689, 1981.
2. Silverman, N.H., and Snider, A.R.: Two-Dimensional Echocardiography in Congenital Heart Disease. Norwalk, Conn., Appleton-Century-Crofts, 1982, p. 142.
3. Bierman, F.Z., Fellows, K., and Williams, R.G.: Prospective identification of ventricular septal defects in infancy using subxiphoid two-dimensional echocardiography. Circulation 62:807, 1980.
4. Cheatham, J.P., Latson, L.A., and Gutgesell, H.P.: Ventricular septal defect in infancy: Detection with two-dimensional echocardiography. Am. J. Cardiol. 47:85, 1981.
5. Hatle, L., and Angelsen, B.: Doppler Ultrasound in Cardiology. Philadelphia, Lea & Febiger, 1985.
6. Hatle, L., and Rokseth, R.: Noninvasive diagnosis and assessment of ventricular septal defect by Doppler ultrasound. Acta Med Scand 645(Suppl.):47, 1981.
7. Magherini, A., Azzolina, G., Wiechmann, V., et al.: Pulsed Doppler echocardiography for diagnosis of ventricular septal defects. Br Heart J 43:143, 1980.
8. Stevenson, J.G., Kawabori, I., Dooley, T., et al.: Diagnosis of ventricular septal defect by pulsed Doppler echocardiography: Sensitivity, specificity, and limitations. Circulation 58:322, 1978.
9. Murphy, D.J., Jr, Ludomirsky, A., and Huhta, J.C.: Continuous-wave Doppler in children with ventricular septal defect: Noninvasive estimation of inter-ventricular pressure gradient. Am. J. Cardiol. 57:428, 1986.
10. Ludomirsky, A., Huhta, J.C., Vick, G.W., III, et al.: Color Doppler detection of multiple ventricular septal defects. Circulation 74:1317, 1986.
11. Skjaerpe, T., Hegrenaes, L., and Hatle, L.: Noninvasive estimation of right ventricular pressure by Doppler ultrasound in VSD. (Abstract.) Fifth Symposium on Echocardiology, Rotterdam, 1983. Ultrasonar. Bull. 92, 1983.
12. Bierman, F.Z., and Williams, R.G.: Subxiphoid two-dimensional imaging of the interatrial septum in infants and neonates with congenital heart disease. Circulation 60:80, 1979.
13. Alexander, J.A., Reinbert, J.C., Sealy, W.C., et al.: Shunt dynamics in experimental atrial septal defects. J. Appl. Physiol. 39:281, 1975.
14. Goldberg, S.J., Areias, J.C., Spitaels, S.E.C., et al.: Use of time interval histographic output from echo-Doppler to detect left-to-right atrial shunts. Circulation 58:147, 1978.
15. Kalmanson, D., Veyrat, C., Derai, C., et al.: Non-invasive technique for diagnosing atrial septal defect and assessing shunt volume using directional Doppler ultrasound. Br. Heart J. 34:981, 1972.
16. Levin, A.R., Spach, M.S., Boineau, J.P., et al.: Atrial pressure-flow dynamics in atrial septal defects (secundum type). Circulation 37:476, 1968.
17. Minagoe, S., Tei, C., Kisanuki, A., et al.: Noninvasive pulsed Doppler echocardiographic detection of the direction of shunt flow in patients with atrial septal defect: Usefulness of the right parasternal approach. Circulation 71:745, 1985.
18. Goldberg, S.J., Allen, H.D., and Sahn, D.J.: Echocardiographic detection and management of patent ductus arteriosus in neonates with respiratory distress syndrome: A two- and one-half year prospective study. J. Clin. Ultrasound. 5:161, 1977.
19. Sahn, D.J., and Allen, H.D.: Real-time cross-sectional echocardiographic imaging and measurement of the patent ductus arteriosus in infants and children. Circulation 58:343, 1978.
20. Silverman, N.H., Lewis, A.B., Heymann, M.A., et al.: Echocardiographic assessment of ductus arteriosus shunt in premature infants. Circulation 50:821, 1974.
21. Gentile, R., Stevenson, G., Dooley, T., et al.: Pulsed Doppler echocardiographic determination of time of ductal closure in normal newborn infants. J. Pediatr. 98:443, 1981.
22. Stevenson, J.G., Kawabori, I., and Guntheroth, W.G.: Pulsed Doppler echocardiographic diagnosis of patent ductus arteriosus: Sensitivity, specificity, limitations, and technical features. Cathet. Cardiovasc. Diagn. 6:255, 1980.
23. Daniels, O., Hopman, J.C.W., Stelinga, G.B.A., et al.: Doppler flow characteristics in the main pulmonary artery and LA/Ao ratio before and after ductal closure in healthy newborns. Pediatr. Cardiol. 3:99, 1982.
24. Hiraishi, S., Horiguchi, Y., Misawa, H., et al.: Noninvasive Doppler echocardiographic evaluation of shunt flow dynamics of the ductus arteriosus. Circulation 75:1146, 1987.
25. Musewe, N.N., Smallhorn, J.F., Benson, L.N., et al.: Validation of Doppler-derived pulmonary arterial pressure in patients with ductus arteriosus under different hemodynamic states. Circulation 76:1081, 1987.
26. Cloez, J.L., Isaaz, K., and Pernot, C.: Pulsed Doppler flow characteristics of ductus arteriosus in infants with associated congenital anomalies of the heart or great arteries. Am. J. Cardiol. 57:845, 1986.
27. Stevenson, J.G., Kawabori, I., and Guntheroth, W.G.: Noninvasive detection of pulmonary hypertension in patent ductus arteriosus by pulsed Doppler echocardiography. Circulation 60:355, 1979.
28. Alverson, D.C., Eldridge, M., Aldrich, M., et al.: Effect of patent ductus arteriosus on lower extremity blood flow velocity patterns in preterm infants. Am. J. Perinatol. 1:216, 1984.
29. Feldman, R.W., Andrassy, R.J., Alexander, J.A., et al.: Doppler ultrasonic flow detection as an adjunct in the diagnosis of patent ductus arteriosus in premature infants. J. Thorac. Cardiovasc. Surg. 72:288, 1976.
30. Martin, C.G., Snider, A.R., Katz, S.M., et al.: Abnormal cerebral blood flow patterns in preterm infants with a large patent ductus arteriosus. J. Pediatr. 101:587, 1982.
31. Perlman, J., Hill, A., and Volpe, J.: The effect of patent ductus arteriosus on flow velocity in the anterior cerebral arteries: Ductal steal in the premature newborn infant. J. Pediatr. 99:767, 1981.
32. Serwer, G.A., Armstrong, B.E., and Anderson, P.A.W.: Noninvasive detection of retrograde descending aortic flow in infants using continuous wave Doppler ultrasonography. J. Pediatr. 97:394, 1980.
33. Goor, D.A., and Lillihei, C.W.: Congenital Malformations of the Heart. New York, Grune & Stratton, 1975.
34. Becker, A.E., and Anderson, R.H.: Atrioventricular septal defects: What's in a name? J. Thorac. Cardiovasc. Surg. 83:461, 1982.
35. Hagler, D.J., Tajik, A.J., Seward, J.B., et al.: Real-time wide-angle sector echocardiography: Atrioventricular canal defects. Circulation 59:140, 1979.
36. Ebels, T.: Echocardiography and surgery for atrioventricular septal defect. Int. J. Cardiol. 13:353, 1986.
37. Minich, L.A., Snider, A.R., Bove, E.L., et al.: Echocardiographic evaluation of atrioventricular orifice anatomy in children with atrioventricular septal defect. J. Am. Coll. Cardiol. 19:149, 1992.
38. Rastelli, G.C., Kirklin, J.W., and Titus, J.L.: Anatomic observations on complete form of persistent common atrioventricular canal with special reference to atrioventricular valves. Mayo Clin. Proc. 41:296, 1966.
39. Goldberg, S.J., Sahn, D.J., Allen, H.D., et al.: Evaluation of pulmonary and systemic blood flow by 2-dimensional Doppler echocardiography using fast Fourier transform spectral analysis. Am. J. Cardiol. 50:1394, 1982.
40. Stewart, W.I., Jiang, L., Mich, R., et al.: Variable effects of changes in flow rate through the aortic, pulmonary, and mitral valves on valve area and flow velocity: Impact on quantitative Doppler flow calculations. J. Am. Coll. Cardiol. 6:653, 1985.
41. Valdes-Cruz, L.M., Horowitz, S., Mesel, E., et al.: A pulsed Doppler echocardiographic method for calculating pulmonary and systemic blood flow in atrial level shunt: Validation studies in animals and initial human experience. Circulation 69:80, 1984.
42. Valdes-Cruz, L.M., Horowitz, S., Mesel, E., et al.: A pulsed Doppler echocardiographic method for calculation of pulmonary and systemic flow accuracy in a canine model with ventricular septal defect. Circulation 68:597, 1983.
43. Barron, J.V., Sahn, D.J., Valdes-Cruz, L.M., et al.: Clinical utility of two-dimensional Doppler echocardiographic techniques for estimating pulmonary to systemic blood flow ratios in children with left to right shunting atrial septal defect, ventricular septal defect, or patent ductus arteriosus. J. Am. Coll. Cardiol. 3:169, 1984.
44. Sanders, S.P., Yeager, S., and Williams, R.G.: Measurement of systemic and pulmonary blood flow and Qp/Qs ratio using Doppler and two-dimensional echocardiography. Am. J. Cardiol. 51:952, 1983.
45. Gardin, J.M., Tobis, J.M., Dabestani, A., et al.: Superiority of two-dimensional measurement of aortic vessel diameter in Doppler echocardiographic estimates of left ventricular stroke volume. J. Am. Coll. Cardiol. 6:66, 1985.
46. Huhta, J.C., Glasow, P., Murphy, D.J., et al.: Surgery without catheterization for congenital heart defects: Management of 100 patients. J. Am. Coll. Cardiol. 9:823, 1987.
47. Krabill, K.A., Ring, S., Foker, J.E., et al.: Echocardiographic versus cardiac catheterization diagnosis of infants with congenital heart disease requiring cardiac surgery. Am. J. Cardiol. 60:351, 1987.
48. Weyman, A.E., Feigenbaum, H., Hurwitz, R.A., et al.: Cross-sectional echocardiographic assessment of the severity of aortic stenosis in children. Circulation 55:773, 1977.
49. Berger, M., Berdoff, R.L., Gallerstein, P.E., et al.: Evaluation of aortic stenosis by continuous wave Doppler ultrasound. J. Am. Coll. Cardiol. 3:150, 1984.
50. Hatle, L., Angelsen, B.A., Tromsdal, A.: Non-invasive assessment of aortic stenosis by Doppler ultrasound. Br. Heart J. 43:284, 1980.
51. Snider, A.R., Stevenson, J.G., French, G.W., et al.: Comparison of high pulse repetition frequency and continuous-wave Doppler for velocity measurement and gradient prediction in children with valvular and congenital heart disease. J. Am. Coll. Cardiol. 7:873, 1986.
52. Stamm, R.B., and Martin, R.P.: Quantification of pressure gradients across stenotic valves by Doppler ultrasound. J. Am. Coll. Cardiol. 2:707, 1983.
53. Young, D.B., Quinones, M.A., Waggoner, A.D., et al.: Diagnosis and quantification of aortic stenosis with pulsed Doppler echocardiography. Am. J. Cardiol. 45:987, 1980.
54. Bengur, A.R., Snider, A.R., Serwer, G.A., et al.: Usefulness of Doppler mean gradient in evaluation of children with aortic valve stenosis and comparison to gradient at catheterization. Am. J. Cardiol. 64:756, 1989.
55. Bengur, A.R., Snider, A.R., Meliones, J.N., et al.: Doppler evaluation of aortic valve area in children with aortic stenosis. J. Am. Coll. Cardiol. 18:1499, 1991.
56. Latson, L.A., Cheatham, J.P., and Gutgesell, H.P.: Relation of the echocardiographic estimate of left ventricular size to mortality in infants with severe left ventricular outflow obstruction. Am. J. Cardiol. 48:887, 1981.
57. Huhta, J.C., Carpenter, R.J., Jr., Moise, K.J., Jr., et al.: Prenatal diagnosis and postnatal management of critical aortic stenosis. Circulation 75:573, 1987.
58. Morrow, W.R., Huhta, J.C., Murphy, D.J., et al.: Quantitative morphology of the aortic arch in neonatal coarctation. J. Am. Coll. Cardiol. 8:616, 1986.
59. Nihoyannopoulos, P., Karas, S., Sapsford, R.N., et al.: Accuracy of two-dimensional echocardiography in the diagnosis of aortic arch obstruction. J. Am. Coll. Cardiol. 10:1072, 1987.
60. Sahn, D.J., Allen, H.D., McDonald, G., et al.: Real-time cross-sectional echocar-

diographic diagnosis of coarctation of the aorta. A prospective study of echocardiographic-angiographic correlations. Circulation 56:762, 1977.

61. Snider, A.R., and Silverman, N.H.: Suprasternal notch echocardiography: A two-dimensional technique for evaluating congenital heart disease. Circulation 63:165, 1981.

62. Weyman, A.E., Caldwell, R.L., Hurwitz, R.A., et al.: Cross-sectional echocardiographic characterization of aortic obstruction. 1. Supravalvar aortic stenosis and aortic hypoplasia. Circulation 57:491, 1978.

63. Weyman, A.E., Caldwell, R.L., Hurwitz, R.A., et al.: Cross-sectional echocardiographic detection of aortic obstruction. 2. Coarctation of the aorta. Circulation 57:498, 1978.

64. Bash, S.E., Huhta, J.C., Vick, G.S., III, et al.: Hypoplastic left heart syndrome: Is echocardiography accurate enough to guide surgical palliation? J. Am. Coll. Cardiol. 7:610, 1986.

65. Lange, L.W., Sahn, D.J., Allen, H.D., et al.: The utility of cross-sectional echocardiography in the evaluation of hypoplastic left ventricle syndrome—Echocardiographic/angiographic/anatomic correlations. Pediatr. Cardiol. 1:287, 1980.

66. Johnson, G.L., Kwan, O.L., Handshoe, S., et al.: Accuracy of combined two-dimensional echocardiography and continuous wave Doppler recordings in the estimation of pressure gradient in right ventricular outlet obstruction. J. Am. Coll. Cardiol. 3:1013, 1984.

67. Lima, C.O., Sahn, D.J., Valdes-Cruz, L.M., et al.: Noninvasive prediction of transvalvular pressure gradients in patients with pulmonary stenosis by quantitative two-dimensional echocardiographic Doppler studies. Circulation 67:866, 1983.

68. Snider, A.R., Enderlein, M.E., Teitel, D.F., et al.: Two-dimensional echocardiographic determination of aortic and pulmonary artery sizes from infancy to adulthood in normal subjects. Am. J. Cardiol. 53:218, 1984.

69. Hagler, D.J., Tajik, A.J., Seward, J.B., et al.: Wide-angle two-dimensional echocardiographic profiles of conotruncal abnormalities. Mayo Clin. Proc. 55:73, 1980.

70. Ports, T.A., Silverman, N.H., and Schiller, N.B.: Two-dimensional echocardiographic assessment of Ebstein's anomaly. Circulation 58:336, 1978.

71. Bierman, F.Z., and Williams, R.G.: Prospective diagnosis of d-transposition of the great arteries in neonates by subxiphoid two-dimensional echocardiography. Circulation 60:1496, 1979.

72. Henry, W.L., Maron, B.J., Griffith, J.M., et al.: Differential diagnosis of anomalies of the great arteries by real-time two-dimensional echocardiography. Circulation 51:283, 1975.

73. Pasquini, L., Sanders, S.P., Parness, I.A., et al.: Diagnosis of coronary artery anatomy by two-dimensional echocardiography in patients with transposition of the great arteries. Circulation 75:557, 1987.

74. Sahn, D.J., Allen, H.D., Lange, L.W., et al.: Cross-sectional echocardiographic diagnosis of the sites of total anomalous pulmonary venous drainage. Circulation 60:1317, 1979.

75. Snider, A.R., Ports, T.A., and Silverman, N.H.: Venous anomalies of the coronary sinus: Detection by M-mode, two-dimensional and contrast echocardiography. Circulation 60:721, 1980.

76. Snider, A.R., Silverman, N.H., Turley, K., et al.: Evaluation of infradiaphragmatic total anomalous pulmonary venous connection with two-dimensional echocardiography. Circulation 66:1129, 1982.

77. Smallhorn, J.F., and Freedom, R.M.: Pulsed Doppler echocardiography in the pre-operative evaluation of total anomalous pulmonary venous connection. J. Am. Coll. Cardiol. 8:1413, 1986.

78. Huhta, J.C., Seward, J.B., Tajik, A.J., et al.: Two-dimensional echocardiographic

79. Sapire, D.W., Ho, S.Y., Anderson, R.H., et al.: Diagnosis and significance of atrial isomerism. Am. J. Cardiol. 58:342, 1986.

80. Sharma, S., Devine, W., Anderson, R.H., et al.: Identification and analysis of left atrial isomerism. Am. J. Cardiol. 60:1157, 1987.

81. Allwork, S.P., Bentall, H.H., Becker, A.E., et al.: Congenitally corrected transposition: A morphologic study of 32 cases. Am. J. Cardiol. 38:910, 1976.

82. Ellis, K., Morgan, B.C., Blumenthal, S., et al.: Congenitally corrected transposition of the great vessels. Radiology 79:35, 1962.

83. Calcaterra, G., Anderson, R.H., Lau, K.C., et al.: Dextrocardia: Value of segmental analysis in its categorization. Br. Heart J. 42:497, 1979.

84. Anderson, R.H., Tynan, M., and Becker, A.E.: Echocardiography of the univentricular heart. In Lundstrom, N-R. (ed.): Pediatric Echocardiography—Cross Sectional, M-mode, and Doppler. Amsterdam, Elsevier/North Holland Biomedical Press, 1980, pp. 129–146.

85. Anderson, R.H., Tynan, M., Freedom, R.M., et al.: Ventricular morphology in univentricular heart. Herz 4:184, 1979.

86. Freedom, R.M., Picchio, F., Duncan, W.J., et al.: The atrioventricular junction in the univentricular heart: A two-dimensional echocardiographic analysis. Pediatr. Cardiol. 3:105, 1982.

87. Rigby, M.L., Anderson, R.H., Gibson, D., et al.: Two-dimensional echocardiographic categorization of the univentricular heart. Ventricular morphology, type and mode of atrioventricular connection. Br. Heart J. 46:603, 1981.

88. Van Praagh, R., Van Praagh, S., Vlad, P., et al.: Anatomic types of congenital dextrocardia: Diagnostic and embryologic implications. Am. J. Cardiol. 13:510, 1964.

89. Stanger, P., Rudolph, A.M., and Edwards, J.E.: Cardiac malpositions: An overview based on study of sixty-five necropsy specimens. Circulation 56:159, 1977.

90. Fyfe, D.A., Ritter, S.B., Snider, A.R., et al.: Guidelines for transesophageal echocardiography in children. J. Am. Soc. Echocardiogr. 5:640, 1992.

91. Abel, M.D., Nishimura, R.A., Callahan, N.J., et al.: Evaluation of intraoperative transesophageal two-dimensional echocardiography. Anesthesiology 66:64, 1987.

92. Ritter, S.B.: Transesophageal real-time echocardiography in infants and children with congenital heart disease. J. Am. Coll. Cardiol. 18:569, 1991.

93. Roberson, D., Muhuideen, I., Silverman, N., et al.: Intraoperative transesophageal echocardiography in infants and children with congenital cardiac shunt lesions. J. Am. Soc. Echocardiogr. 3:213, 1990.

94. Minich, L.L., and Snider, A.R.: Echocardiographic guidance during placement of the buttoned double-disk device for atrial septal defect closure. Echocardiography 10:567, 1993.

95. van der Velde, M.E., Perry, S.B., and Sanders, S.P.: Transesophageal echocardiography with color Doppler during interventional catheterization. Echocardiography 8:721, 1991.

96. Denning, K., Seldmayer, V., Selig, B., et al.: Bacteremia with transesophageal echocardiography. (Abstract.) Circulation 80:II-473, 1989.

97. Gorge, G., Erbel, R., Henrichs, J., et al.: Positive blood cultures during transesophageal echocardiography. Am. J. Cardiol. 65:1404, 1990.

98. Dajani, A., Bisno, A., and Chung, K.: Prevention of bacterial endocarditis—recommendations by the American Heart Association. J.A.M.A. 264:2919, 1990.

99. Stumper, O.F.W., Elzenga, N.J., Hess, J., et al.: Transesophageal echocardiography in children with congenital heart disease: An initial experience. J. Am. Coll. Cardiol. 16:433, 1990.

100. Weintraub, R., Shiota, T., Elkadi, T., et al.: Transesophageal echocardiography in infants and children with congenital heart disease. Circulation 86:711, 1992.

CHAPTER

34 Cardiac and Extracardiac Masses: Echocardiographic Evaluation

Daniel G. Blanchard, M.D.

Anthony N. DeMaria, M.D.

NORMAL VARIANTS ____ 453
MASSES OF UNCERTAIN SIGNIFICANCE ____ 457
INTRACARDIAC DEVICES, PROSTHETIC MATERIALS, AND FOREIGN BODIES ____ 459
INTRACARDIAC THROMBI ____ 463
Right Atrium ____ 463
Right Ventricle ____ 465

Left Atrium ____ 465
Left Ventricle ____ 466
METASTATIC (SECONDARY) TUMORS OF THE HEART AND PERICARDIUM ____ 468
EXTRACARDIAC MASSES ____ 468
PRIMARY CARDIAC TUMORS ____ 468
PRIMARY BENIGN TUMORS ____ 469

Myxomas _____ 469
Other Primary Tumors _____ 471
    Rhabdomyomas _____ 471
    Fibromas _____ 471
    Papillary Fibroelastomas _____ 473
    Cardiac Lipomas _____ 473

Other Benign Tumors and Masses _____ 474
PRIMARY MALIGNANT TUMORS _____ 475
    Angiosarcoma _____ 475
    Rhabdomyosarcomas _____ 476
    Extraskeletal Cardiac Osteosarcomas _____ 476
    Primary Cardiac Lymphosarcoma _____ 476

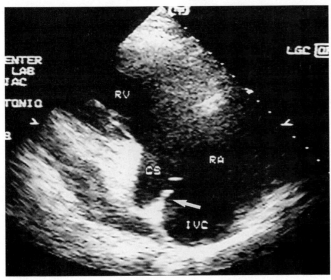

FIGURE 34–1. A modified parasternal right atrial–right ventricular image of a prominent eustachian valve *(arrow)*. RV = right ventricle; RA = right atrium; CS = coronary sinus; IVC = inferior vena cava.

Echocardiography has become the procedure of choice for the detection and evaluation of cardiac masses.[1–8] Transthoracic and transesophageal ultrasonic imaging studies are accurate, widely available, portable, and relatively inexpensive. Transthoracic echocardiography is totally noninvasive and often sufficient for complete evaluation. Transesophageal echocardiography (TEE) provides superior diagnostic imaging of cardiac masses[4] and can often aid in management as well.[9] Pericardial and extracardiac masses also can be visualized with echocardiography, but additional diagnostic modalities, such as computed tomography and magnetic resonance imaging, may be required to define thoracic and abdominal extension of disease processes.[10]

Echocardiography is an invaluable tool for defining size, mobility, shape, and location of cardiac masses, but it cannot describe tissue histologic features. Therefore, the clinician must make inferences using echocardiographic information to arrive at the most likely diagnosis. This chapter discusses the spectrum of echocardiographic mass lesions: normal variants and masses of uncertain significance; artifacts that may be misinterpreted as abnormalities; intracardiac devices, prosthetic materials, and foreign bodies; primary cardiac tumors (benign and malignant); metastatic cardiac and pericardial tumors; paracardiac masses; intracardiac thrombi; and miscellaneous masses. Infective endocarditis and vegetations are discussed in Chapter 30.

NORMAL VARIANTS

Several normal intracardiac structures can mimic pathologic mass lesions. For example, most young children and many adults have persistence of the eustachian valve, a thin structure at the junction of the inferior vena cava and the right atrium.[11–14] This remnant of the embryonic right sinus venosus valve is a thin ridge of tissue that directs inferior vena cava blood flow through the fossa ovalis in the fetal circulation.[15] The eustachian valve is often somewhat mobile and is best visualized in a parasternal right ventricular long-axis view (Fig. 34–1) or in the apical four-chamber view. Rarely, a large eustachian valve may partially obstruct caval flow into the right atrium, simulate a tumor, or trap embolic material.[12, 13] The appearance in multiple imaging planes and TEE, when necessary, may be helpful in distinguishing a eustachian valve from a pathologic right atrial mass.

The Chiari network is another right atrial embryonic remnant seen in 2 to 3 percent of normal hearts (Fig. 34–2).[16–19] A highly mobile, filamentous membrane that extends from the area of the inferior vena cava and coronary sinus to the interatrial septum and tricuspid annulus, the Chiari network is usually best visualized in the parasternal right ventricular long-axis, apical four-chamber, and subcostal long-axis views. Because of its dense reflectances and

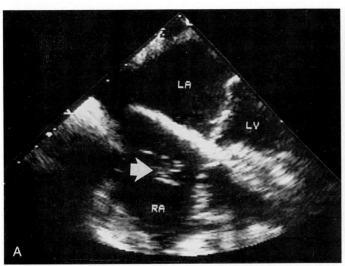
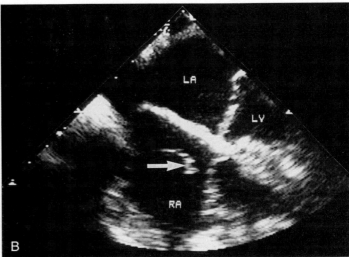

FIGURE 34–2. *A* and *B,* Transesophageal images of a Chiari network *(arrows)* taken several seconds apart, demonstrating the structure's mobility. RA = right atrium; LA = left atrium; LV = left ventricle.

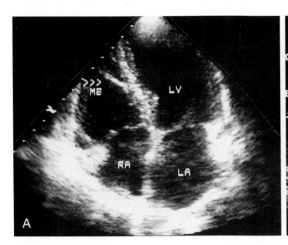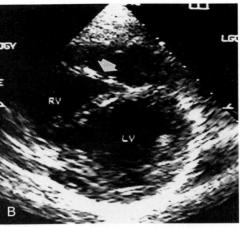

FIGURE 34–3. Apical four-chamber (A) and parasternal short-axis (B) views of moderator bands (MB, arrows). RA = right atrium; LA = left atrium; LV = left ventricle.

mobility, a Chiari network is often striking in appearance. Despite this, the structure is basically unimportant, although rare cases of thrombus formation within a network have been reported.[20] It is essential that a Chiari network be recognized as a benign variant and not misinterpreted as a right atrial thrombus or tumor, tricuspid valve vegetation, or flail tricuspid valve chordae tendineae.[18, 19] Chiari networks occur in the posterior right atrium, are not attached to the tricuspid valve or chordae, and are thin and non-nondular. TEE is useful when the diagnosis is uncertain.[21, 22]

The moderator band of the right ventricle is a muscular structure through which the fibers of the right bundle branch run. It extends from the midinterventricular septum through the cavity of the right ventricle and attaches near the base of the anterior tricuspid papillary muscle (Fig. 34–3). The moderator band is best visualized in the apical four-chamber view, although it may be readily apparent in parasternal views when hypertrophied. It is especially prominent in patients with right ventricular enlargement or hypertrophy, or both (additional muscular trabeculations in the distal right ventricle are also seen in these cases). Although the moderator band is present in most normal individuals,[23] it may be mistaken for a right ventricular tumor or thrombus.

Left ventricular false tendons, or "false chordae," occur as normal variants in a minority of the population.[24–27] As opposed to true chordae tendineae, which extend from papillary muscles to valve leaflets, false tendons originate from and insert into the left ventricular endomyocardium. False tendons cause no symptoms and are not associated with embolic events, but they have been

alleged to cause innocent murmurs occasionally.[24–30] On echocardiography, the tendons are linear, often highly reflective, and sometimes multiple (Fig. 34–4). Although false tendons may be mobile, they are attached to endomyocardium at both ends. They must be distinguished from flail chordae tendineae, subaortic membranes, and other lesions.

Another anomaly found occasionally is a dilated coronary sinus. It may occur with right atrial hypertension, total anomalous pulmonary venous return with coronary sinus drainage, anomalous hepatic venous drainage into the coronary sinus, and coronary arteriovenous fistula. The most common congenital cause, however, is persistent left superior vena cava with drainage into the coronary sinus. This anomaly is seen in approximately 0.5 percent of normal individuals (3 to 10 percent of patients with congenital heart disease)[31–33] and has no clinical significance as an isolated lesion (Fig. 34–5A and B). The diagnosis, which should be suspected whenever the coronary sinus is dilated, can be confirmed by injection of sonicated saline into a left arm vein (see Fig. 34–5C).[34]

TEE has advanced our ability to detect and characterize cardiac abnormalities, but the enhanced echocardiographic sensitivity may sometimes cause misinterpretation of normal cardiac structures as cardiac mass lesions.[35–37] For example, transverse images through the base of the heart can result in the appearance of a "pseudomass" on the aortic valve (Fig. 34–6). This image is caused by oblique imaging of the left coronary cusp. Careful back-and-forth movement of the probe (or multiplane imaging) reveals continuity of the pseudomass with the left coronary cusp. On magnified views

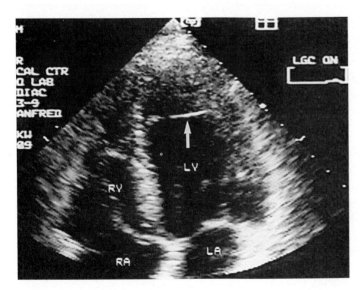

FIGURE 34–4. An apical four-chamber view of a left ventricular false tendon (arrow). RA = right atrium; LA = left atrium; LV = left ventricle; RV = right ventricle.

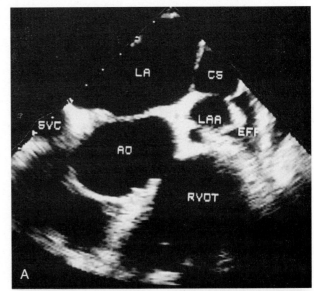

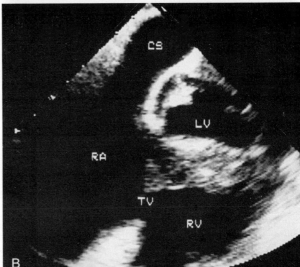

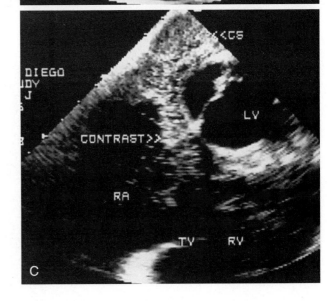

FIGURE 34–5. *A*, A transesophageal image at the level of the aortic root (transverse plane), demonstrating a dilated coronary sinus (*CS*) in a patient with a persistent left superior vena cava. *B*, A transesophageal image (transverse plane) at the level of the gastroesophageal junction in the same patient. *C*, An image at the same plane as that in *B* showing agitated saline entering the right atrium through the coronary sinus after injection into the left antecubital vein. RVOT = right ventricular outflow tract; SVC = superior vena cava; AO = aorta; LA = left atrium; EFF = small pericardial effusion; LAA = left atrial appendage; TV = tricuspid valve; LV = left ventricle; RV = right ventricle.

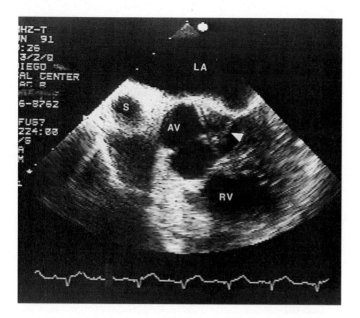

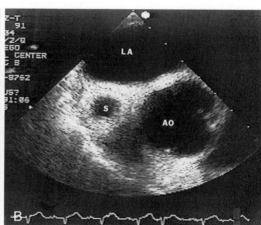

FIGURE 34–6. A transesophageal view (transverse plane) at the level of the aortic valve (AV) showing a "pseudomass" (arrowhead), actually the left coronary cusp. LA = left atrium; S = superior vena cava; RV = right ventricle. (From Blanchard, D.G., and Dittrich, H.C.: Problems and pitfalls. In Dittrich, H.C. [ed.]: Clinical Transesophageal Echocardiography. St. Louis, Mosby–Year Book, 1992, with permission.)

FIGURE 34–7. Transverse transesophageal images at the level of the aortic valve (AV) (A) showing a "mass" (arrowhead) at the lateral border of the right atrium. Withdrawal of the probe (B) demonstrates continuity of this density with the superior vena cava (S). LA = left atrium; AO = aorta. (From Blanchard, D.G., and Dittrich, H.C.: Problems and pitfalls. In Dittrich, H.C. [ed.]: Clinical Transesophageal Echocardiography. St. Louis, Mosby–Year Book, 1992, with permission.)

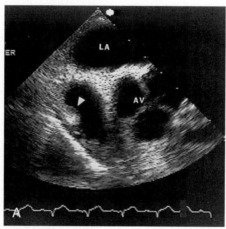

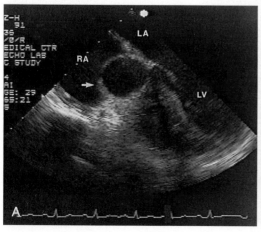

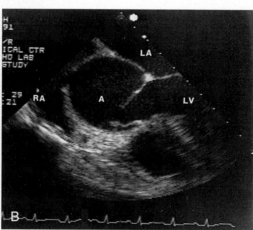

FIGURE 34–8. A, A transverse transesophageal image (four-chamber view) of an apparent cyst (arrow) in the right atrium (RA). B, Withdrawal of the probe demonstrates continuity of the "cyst" with a dilated aortic root (A). LA = left atrium; LV = left ventricle. (From Blanchard, D.G., Dittrich, H.C., Mitchell, M., and McCann, H.A.: Diagnostic pitfalls in transesophageal echocardiography. J. Am. Soc. Echocardiogr. 5:525, 1992, with permission.)

of the aortic valve, small echodensities are sometimes seen on the leaflet tips. In the absence of other findings, these densities probably represent Lambl's excrescences. These normal variants, common in the elderly, are rarely seen on transthoracic echocardiography.

A bright, rounded echodensity is often seen by TEE in the superior portion of the right atrium. This "mass" is the tissue reflection at the junction of the superior vena cava and the right atrium and should not be misinterpreted as a thrombus or tumor (Fig. 34–7). In the presence of a dilated aortic root, the base of the aorta can invaginate the right atrial septal wall, simulating a cystic mass (Fig. 34–8). Another common finding is fat in the atrioventricular groove. This normal variant may appear as a mass or tumor near the tricuspid valve.

TEE is often used to examine the left atrial appendage, a structure that is not well seen from transthoracic windows. The left atrial appendage is lined with small, fairly equally spaced muscular pectinate ridges (Fig. 34–9). These ridges have a homogeneous, medium echodensity, are noncalcified, and do not span the lumen of the appendage at its maximal diameter. These ridges must be distinguished from thrombi. The junction of the left upper pulmonary vein and the left atrium can also appear abnormal and mimic a thrombus, especially when viewed in an oblique plane (Fig. 34–10). With single-plane (transverse) imaging, the left atrial appendage is best visualized at the level of the left coronary artery. If the probe is withdrawn too far and fluid is present in the transverse sinus, the superior wall, or "roof," of the true appendage may be mistaken for a left atrial mass or thrombus (Fig. 34–11).

Other findings that may simulate an abnormal cardiac mass on transthoracic or transesophageal imaging include hiatal hernia, pectus excavatum, esophageal carcinoma, hypertrophied papillary muscles, asymmetric left ventricular apical hypertrophy, and atrial suture lines after cardiac transplantation (Figs. 34–12 to 34–14).[38, 39]

MASSES OF UNCERTAIN SIGNIFICANCE

Aneurysms of the interatrial septum are reasonably common, affecting about 1 percent of adults at autopsy (Fig. 34–15A).[40, 41] It is unclear whether these aneurysms are acquired or congenital, but the cause is thought to be bulging of the septum primum through the foramen ovale. The coexistence of a probe-patent foramen ovale is substantial in affected patients.[40] Atrial septal aneurysm

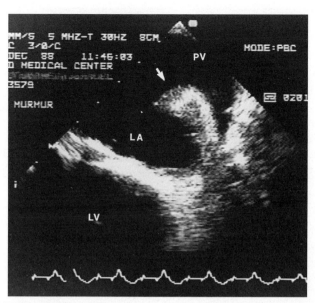

FIGURE 34–10. A transesophageal image (oblique view) of the normal tissue reflection *(arrow)* at the junction of the left upper pulmonary vein *(PV)* and the left atrium *(LA)*. LV = left ventricle. (From Blanchard, D.G., and Dittrich, H.C.: Problems and pitfalls. *In* Dittrich, H.C. [ed.]: Clinical Transesophageal Echocardiography. St. Louis, Mosby–Year Book, 1992, with permission.)

has been associated with atrial arrhythmias, systolic clicks, mitral valve prolapse, and, most important, embolic events.[42] A number of studies have demonstrated an increased incidence of atrial septal aneurysm in patients with unexplained stroke.[43–45] The mechanism of embolization may be in situ thrombus formation with subsequent embolism or paradoxical embolization, as many affected patients have interatrial shunting through the patent foramen ovale detected with intravenous sonicated contrast injection.[43, 46]

Two-dimensional echocardiography is well suited for character-

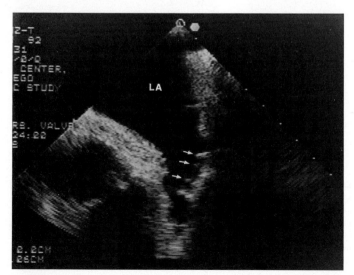

FIGURE 34–9. A transesophageal image of a normal left atrium *(LA)* and appendage. Note the small pectinate ridges *(arrows)* in the appendage. (From Blanchard, D.G., Dittrich, H.C., Mitchell, M., and McCann, H.A.: Diagnostic pitfalls in transesophageal echocardiography. J. Am. Soc. Echocardiogr. 5:525, 1992, with permission.)

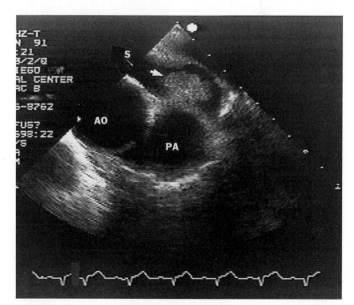

FIGURE 34–11. A transesophageal view of a "pseudomass" *(arrow)* in a patient with a small pericardial effusion. The probe has been withdrawn to the level of the pulmonary artery, and the "roof" of the normal left atrium *(arrow)* may be confused with an appendage clot. S = transverse sinus; AO = aorta; PA = pulmonary artery. (From Blanchard, D.G., and Dittrich, H.C.: Problems and pitfalls. *In* Dittrich, H.C. [ed.]: Clinical Transesophageal Echocardiography. St. Louis, Mosby–Year Book, 1992, with permission.)

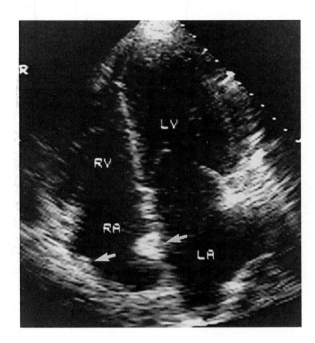

FIGURE 34–12. An apical four-chamber view after heart transplantation. Arrows mark suture line echodensities. RA = right atrium; RV = right ventricle; LA = left atrium; LV = left ventricle.

FIGURE 34–13. Apical three-chamber *(left)* and four-chamber *(right)* views in a patient with a large hiatal hernia that simulated a left atrial mass *(M)*. LV = left ventricle; LA = left atrium. (From D'Cruz, I.A., Feghali, N., and Gross, C.M.: Echocardiographic manifestations of mediastinal masses compressing or encroaching on the heart. Echocardiography 11:523, 1994, with permission.)

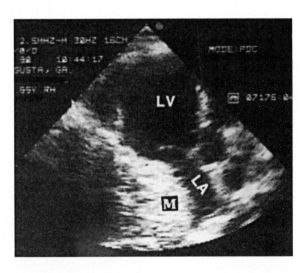 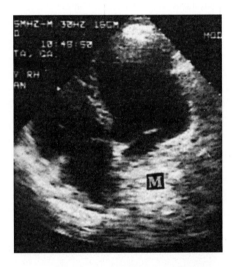

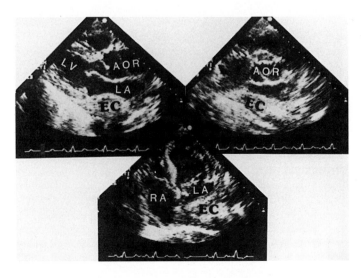

FIGURE 34–14. Transthoracic echocardiographic views taken from a patient with esophageal carcinoma *(EC)*. This mass is seen compressing the left atrium *(LA)*. AOR = aorta; LV = left ventricle; RA = right atrium. (From D'Cruz, I.A., Feghali, N., and Gross, C.M.: Echocardiographic manifestations of mediastinal masses compressing or encroaching on the heart. Echocardiography 11:523, 1994, with permission.)

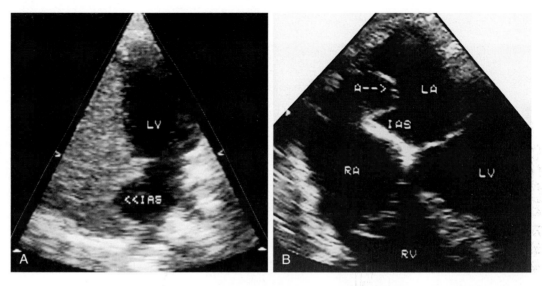

FIGURE 34–15. *A,* An apical four-chamber view (during intravenous injection of sonicated saline to opacify the right side of the heart) of a prominent interatrial septal aneurysm *(arrowheads, IAS). B,* A transesophageal four-chamber view of an interatrial septal aneurysm *(A).* LV = left ventricle; RA = right atrium; RV = right ventricle; LA = left atrium; LV = left ventricle; IAS = interatrial septum.

ization of atrial septal aneurysms, and transesophageal imaging has been reported to be more sensitive than transthoracic techniques (see Fig. 34–15B).[43, 47–50] One large study observed a prevalence of approximately 0.2 percent in a group of patients undergoing transthoracic echocardiography.[42] In a more recent study using TEE, the incidence of atrial septal aneurysm was 4 percent in adults without evidence of embolism compared with 15 percent in patients referred because of unexplained stroke.[43] Echocardiographically, atrial septal aneurysm has been defined as a protrusion of the interatrial membrane at least 1.5 cm from the plane of the atrial septum into the right or left atrium.[42, 51] Although atrial septal aneurysm was initially described in autopsy series, most recent clinical studies rely on echocardiographic criteria for its diagnosis and classification.[42] The aneurysmal membrane is usually freely mobile and sometimes may involve the entire atrial septum rather then the fossa ovalis alone. Its position usually varies with respiration. It is typically thin and sometimes fenestrated, and adherent thrombi within the aneurysm have been observed by echocardiography.[46]

Calcification of the mitral annulus is fairly common in elderly patients; tricuspid annular and papillary muscle calcification are more rare. Mitral annular calcification (MAC) often begins in the posterior aspect of the annulus and extends to involve the posterior mitral valve leaflet as well. On echocardiography, there is characteristic high-intensity thickening of the mitral annulus and the proximal insertion of the posterior mitral valve leaflet (Fig. 34–16).[52, 53] By definition, MAC is fixed and immobile, and this helps differentiate the entity from calcified mitral vegetations and echodense tumors. Although MAC is usually an incidental finding, cases of associated calcific debris embolization have been reported, and MAC is therefore probably not a true "normal variant." Focal calcification of papillary muscles is also fairly common, especially in the elderly, and is in general a benign variant (Fig. 34–17).

As mentioned previously, adipose tissue can accumulate within and around the heart. Epicardial fat may infiltrate the interatrial septum, causing thickening and echodensity of this structure. Lipomatous hypertrophy of the interatrial septum is generally benign, although it has been associated with atrial arrhythmias.[54] It routinely spares the fossa ovalis, creating a distinctive "dumb-bell" echocardiographic appearance (Fig. 34–18A).[55–60] The thickened interatrial septum and thin fossa ovalis are best visualized in the subcostal four-chamber view, but they can also be seen in apical and parasternal imaging planes. When transthoracic images are suboptimal, TEE usually is diagnostic (see Fig. 34–18B).[60]

A more rare "mass" of variable clinical significance is a congenital left atrial membrane (cor triatriatum sinister) (Fig. 34–19). If the membrane obstructs the free flow of blood from the pulmonary veins into the left atrium, symptoms similar to those of mitral stenosis will result.[61–63] Occasionally, nonobstructive or fenestrated membranes may be detected fortuitously in asymptomatic patients who undergo echocardiography for an unrelated indication.

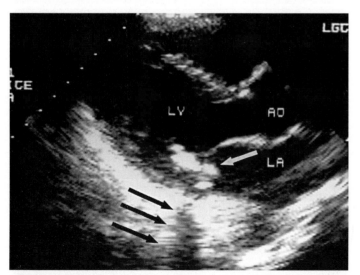

FIGURE 34–16. A parasternal long-axis view of mitral annular calcification *(white arrow)* affecting primarily the posterior aspect of the mitral annulus and the posterior mitral valve leaflet. Ultrasonic shadowing from the calcification is present *(black arrows).* LA = left atrium; LV = left ventricle; AO = aorta.

INTRACARDIAC DEVICES, PROSTHETIC MATERIALS, AND FOREIGN BODIES

Ultrasonic "mass lesions" related to devices, prosthetic materials, or foreign bodies are common and must not be misinterpreted as pathologic cardiac masses. Transvenous right heart catheters and pacemaker wires, the most common examples, are easily visualized with echocardiography (Fig. 34–20).[64–71] They appear as curvilinear, bright echodensities in the right atrium and right ventricle and typically cast both reverberations and an ultrasonic shadow (Fig. 34–21). They may also have thrombi, masses, or vegetations attached (Fig. 34–22).[72–75]

Echocardiography can sometimes detect perforation of a pace-

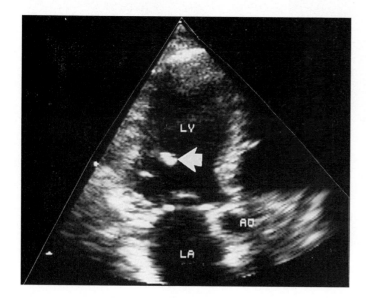

FIGURE 34–17. An apical three-chamber view of a calcified left ventricular (*LV*) papillary muscle (*arrow*). LA = left atrium; AO = aorta.

FIGURE 34–18. *A,* A modified subcostal view from a patient with lipomatous hypertrophy of the interatrial septum (*arrows*). *B,* A transesophageal four-chamber view (transverse plane) of lipomatous hypertrophy of the interatrial septum (*AS, large arrowheads*), with sparing of the fossa ovalis (*small arrows*). RA = right atrium; RV = right ventricle; LA = left atrium; LV = left ventricle; MV = mitral valve; VS = interventricular septum. (From Seward, J.B., Khanderia, B.K., Oh, J.K., et al.: Critical appraisal of transesophageal echocardiography: Limitations, pitfalls, and complications. J. Am. Soc. Echocardiogr. 5:288, 1992, with permission.)

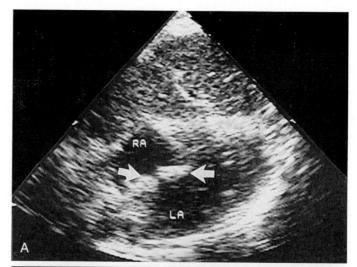

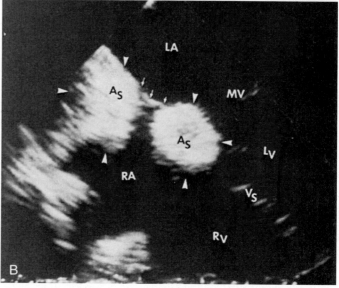

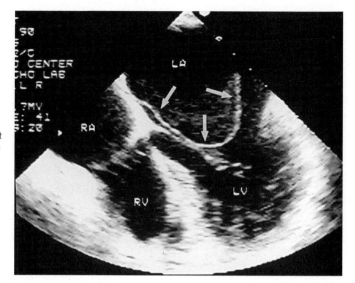

FIGURE 34–19. A transesophageal transverse four-chamber view of a left atrial membrane (cor triatriatum sinister) *(arrows)*. RA = right atrium; RV = right ventricle; LA = left atrium; LV = left ventricle.

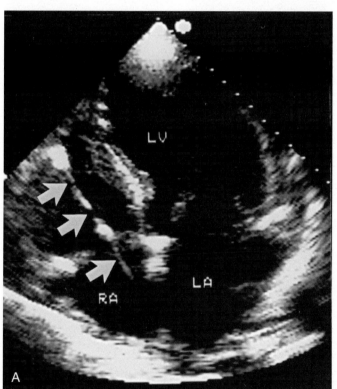

FIGURE 34–20. *A*, An apical four-chamber view of a right ventricular permanent pacemaker lead *(arrows)*. *B*, A transesophageal image of a Swan-Ganz catheter *(arrows)* in the right ventricle *(R)*. RA = right atrium; LA = left atrium; LV = left ventricle; LA = left atrium; A = aorta; P = pulmonary artery.

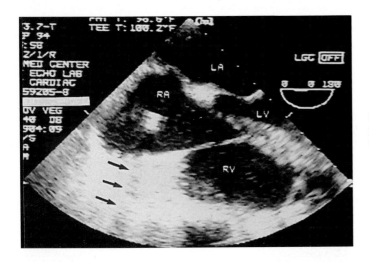

FIGURE 34–21. A transesophageal transverse four-chamber view in a patient with a right atrial pacing lead (echodensity in right atrium). Echo shadowing is present *(arrows)*. RA = right atrium; RV = right ventricle; LA = left atrium; LV = left ventricle.

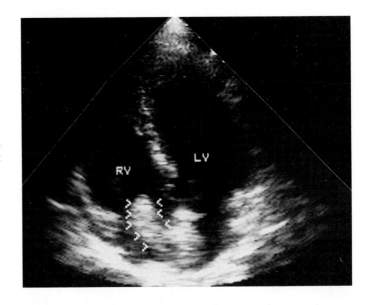

FIGURE 34–22. An apical four-chamber view of a large, infected right atrial mass *(arrowheads)* attached to an indwelling Hickman catheter (not seen). RV = right ventricle; LV = left ventricle.

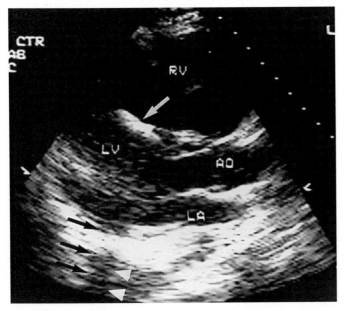

FIGURE 34–23. A parasternal long-axis view of an echo-dense ventricular septal defect patch *(white arrow)* in a patient with Ebstein anomaly and an enlarged right ventricle *(RV)*. The patch casts an echo shadow *(black arrows and white arrowheads)*. AO = aorta; LA = left atrium; LV = left ventricle.

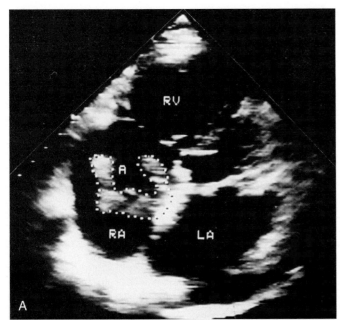

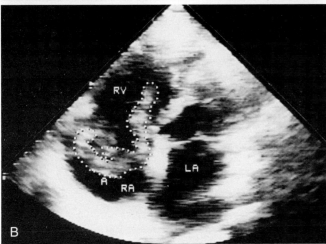

FIGURE 34–24. *A* and *B*, A modified apical four-chamber view of two images taken within several seconds in a patient with a large, mobile, serpentine right atrial thrombus (*A*). RA = right atrium; RV = right ventricle; LA = left atrium; LV = left ventricle.

maker catheter through the interventricular septum or right ventricular free wall by demonstrating extension of the wire into the left ventricle or pericardial space.[76, 77] It can be used to guide bioptome positioning during endomyocardial biopsy and also to delineate size, anatomical location, and possible loculation of pericardial effusions prior to pericardiocentesis.[78–80] In this way, echocardiography can help guide pericardiocentesis, especially when effusions vary with positioning or are not concentric.[78] Evidence of previous cardiac surgery can sometimes be detected: Figure 34–23 shows the heart of a patient with Ebstein anomaly and a repaired ventricular septal defect. The ventricular septal repair is seen as an echodense patch in the ventricular septum. Finally, the imaging of bullets, pellets, nails, and other foreign bodies lodged in the heart has been described with echocardiography.[81–86]

INTRACARDIAC THROMBI

Right Atrium

Low cardiac output states, cardiac injury, and blood stasis predispose to in situ right atrial thrombi.[87, 88] Rheumatic tricuspid steno-

sis, tricuspid valve replacement, atrial fibrillation, transvenous catheter ablation procedures, cardiac surgery, and cardiomyopathy are all associated with right atrial thrombi.[89–91] In situ right atrial clots tend to adhere to the atrial wall and are relatively immobile (although frond-like excrescences can occur). Right atrial thrombi also can form on indwelling cardiac catheters, such as pacemaker leads, Swan-Ganz catheters, ventriculoatrial shunts (for hydrocephalus), and Hickman catheters (see Fig. 34–22).[73, 92] These thrombi are a nidus for infection and may become large.

The most frequent sources of right atrial thrombi are venous thromboemboli that lodge, sometimes transiently, in the right atrium.[93–100] Echocardiographically, these thrombi are mobile and serpentine and often are not attached to the atrial wall. They may prolapse or span across the tricuspid valve into the right ventricle (Fig. 34–24).[94, 96] These mobile thrombi can lead to pulmonary embolism and right-sided heart failure and should be treated aggressively.[101] Right atrial thrombi can be mistaken for vegetations, tumors, and Chiari networks; accurate distinction among these entities is usually possible with TEE (Fig. 34–25).[93, 102, 103]

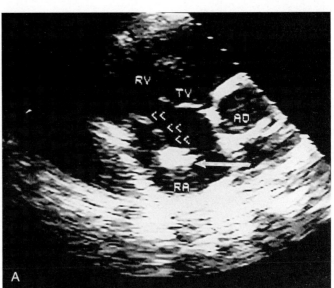

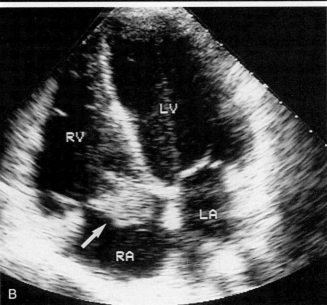

FIGURE 34–25. *A*, A modified parasternal view of a prolapsing tricuspid vegetation (*large arrow*). The affected tricuspid leaflet (*arrowheads*) is flail. *B*, An apical four-chamber view of a large vegetation adherent to the tricuspid valve. RA = right atrium; RV = right ventricle; TV = tricuspid valve; AO = aorta; LA = left atrium; LV = left ventricle.

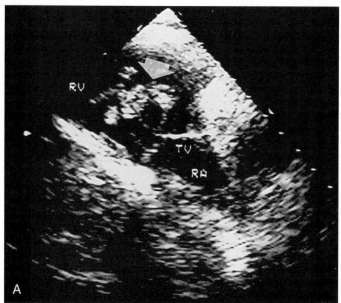

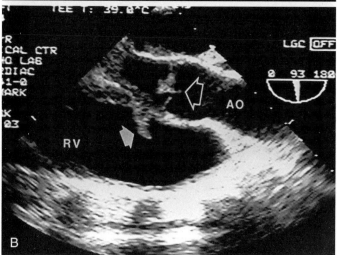

FIGURE 34–26. *A*, A parasternal right atrial–right ventricular view of a cluster of right ventricular thrombi *(arrow)* entrapped in the tricuspid chordal apparatus. *B*, A transesophageal view of a small mass *(solid arrow)* adherent to the right ventricular aspect of the interventricular septum (outflow portion). This mass was not a thrombus but an extension of staphylococcal endocarditis affecting the aortic valve *(open arrow)*, aortic root, and high interventricular septum. RA = right atrium; RV = right ventricle; TV = tricuspid valve; AO = aorta.

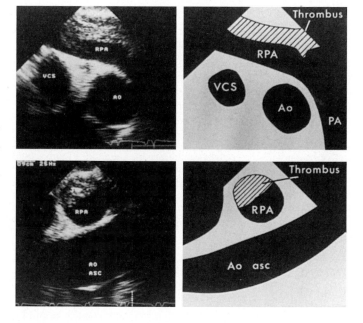

FIGURE 34–27. Transverse *(above)* and longitudinal *(below)* transesophageal views of a right pulmonary artery thromboembolus. Ao = ascending aorta; VCS = superior vena cava; PA = pulmonary artery; RPA = right pulmonary artery; asc = ascending. (From Wittlich, N., Erbel, R., Eichler, A., et al.: Detection of central pulmonary artery thromboemboli by transesophageal echocardiography in patients with severe pulmonary embolism. J. Am Soc. Echocardiogr. 5:515, 1992, with permission.)

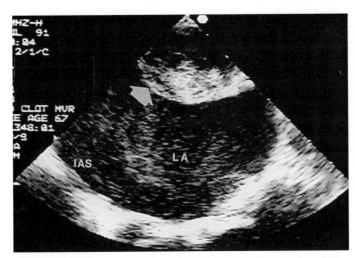

FIGURE 34–28. A transesophageal view of a smooth, protruding thrombus (*arrow*) attached to the posterior wall of the left atrium (*LA*). IAS = interatrial septum.

Right Ventricle

Right ventricular thrombi are rare. They are seen in the same clinical settings as are right atrial thrombi (low cardiac output states, right-sided heart failure, venous thromboembolism, cardiomyopathy), but they also occur with right ventricular infarction, endomyocardial fibrosis, Loeffler's endocarditis, and cardiac trauma.[104–106] Thrombi generated in situ are usually adherent to the ventricular wall and are immobile, whereas embolic thrombi are typically mobile and are sometimes trapped within the tricuspid chordae (Fig. 34–26A). These thrombi can embolize into the pulmonary circulation and may cause right ventricular outflow obstruction;[107] therefore, it is prudent to rule out right ventricular thrombi with echocardiography in cases of pulmonary embolus. Right ventricular thrombi may mimic vegetations (see Fig. 34–26B) and tumors, both of which are much more common.

Pulmonary arterial thrombus is a life-threatening condition that, unfortunately, is not often visualized by transthoracic echocardiography.[108–111] Because of the proximity of the esophagus to the main pulmonary arteries, TEE is a more sensitive technique for recognizing pulmonary clots (Fig. 34–27).[100, 112–114] Both chronic and acute pulmonary emboli may be imaged by TEE if located proximally, although they may simulate the appearance of a tumor.

Exploratory surgery is occasionally required to differentiate the two.

Left Atrium

Left atrial thrombi usually occur in the setting of stagnant blood flow and/or left atrial enlargement. Specific predisposing conditions include atrial fibrillation (both chronic and intermittent), mitral valvular disease (usually mitral stenosis rather than regurgitation), mitral valve prostheses, and cardiomyopathy.[115, 116] Left atrial clots often adhere to the atrial wall (frequently the posterior wall or left atrial appendage) and can be laminar or protruding (Fig. 34–28).[117–119] Less commonly, they are unattached and freely mobile, presumably having detached from the atrial wall. An unattached left atrial thrombus is seen primarily in rheumatic mitral stenosis; the thrombus may act as a ball valve, causing flow obstruction and, rarely, sudden death.[120, 121] Figure 34–29 demonstrates a left atrial ball thrombus that transiently obstructs left ventricular inflow (see Fig. 34–29C). Note the area of echolucency in the thrombus, suggesting central liquefaction (see Fig. 34–29B). Left atrial thrombi may embolize, with disastrous results; therefore, their detection can greatly influence clinical decisions regarding anticoagulation, cardioversion for atrial fibrillation, cardiac surgery, and percutaneous mitral balloon valvuloplasty.[122–127]

Transthoracic echocardiography can detect left atrial thrombi,[116, 117] but because of the distance between the probe and the left atrium (and the difficulty in visualizing the left atrial appendage), it is not a particularly sensitive technique (diagnostic sensitivity of 30 to 50 percent).[116, 128, 129] Large, mobile clots are generally easy to visualize, but laminar thrombi in the posterior left atrium (see Fig. 34–28) or atrial appendage (where up to 50 percent of left atrial clots occur)[116] may go undetected by transthoracic echocardiography.[117] The appendage is usually best visualized in a parasternal short-axis view with angulation toward the base, but it is not well defined in most patients. Thrombi should be suspected when the posterior wall of the left atrium is thickened, especially if the echodensity of the thickened area appears heterogeneous or distinct from surrounding portions of the left atrial wall.

TEE has enhanced our ability to examine the left atrium and atrial appendage[122, 130, 131] and is the procedure of choice to rule out masses in this area (Fig. 34–30). TEE is recommended for patients with suspected left atrial thrombi if transthoracic echocardiography is nondiagnostic. The possibility of a left atrial clot should not be excluded based on transthoracic echocardiography alone, especially when factors that increase the risk of left atrial thrombi (mitral stenosis, left atrial enlargement, severe cardiomyopathy, atrial fi-

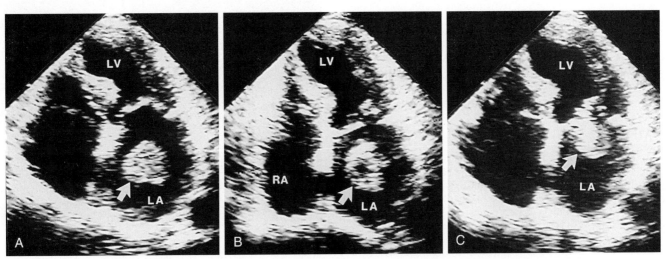

FIGURE 34–29. *A* to *C*, Three images in succession (apical four-chamber view) of a left atrial ball thrombus (*arrow*, *A*) in a patient with rheumatic mitral stenosis. Central liquefaction is seen in *B*, transient left ventricular inflow obstruction is seen in *C*. RA = right atrium; LA = left atrium; LV = left ventricle.

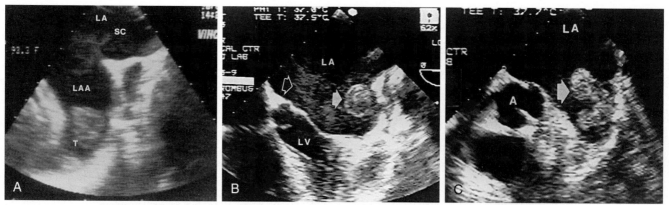

FIGURE 34–30. *A*, A transesophageal image of a thrombus (T) in the left atrial appendage (LAA). Note the spontaneous contrast (SC), which swirls in motion on real-time imaging. *B*, A free-floating left atrial thrombus *(solid arrow)* with spontaneous contrast in the left atrium *(open arrow)*. *C*, A transesophageal image of a large, irregular thrombus *(arrow)* in the left atrial appendage of a patient with severe mitral stenosis. LA = left atrium; LV = left ventricle; A = aorta. (*A* from Camp, A., and Labovitz A.J.: Evaluation of cardiac sources of emboli. *In* Dittrich, H.C. [ed.]: Clinical Transesophageal Echocardiography. St. Louis, Mosby-Year Book, 1992, with permission.)

brillation, prosthetic mitral valve) are present.[132] Left atrial thrombi may be mistaken for myxomas or other tumors. The underlying clinical scenario (and presence of risk factors for thrombus) can aid in the diagnosis. In some cases, magnetic resonance imaging and ultrasonic tissue characterization may help distinguish clot from tumor.[133–135]

Left atrial thrombi appear as discrete masses that are fairly homogeneous in echodensity. Clots in the left atrial appendage may be difficult to distinguish from small muscle bundles (pectinate muscles), which often appear as discrete protuberances on the wall of the appendage. Occasionally, the appendage may be multilobed, and the tissue separating these lobes must be distinguished from thrombi.

Left atrial thrombi are often accompanied by spontaneous echocardiographic contrast (see Fig. 34–30). Spontaneous contrast, or "smoke," is seen when blood flow stagnates; it probably is caused by interaction and transient aggregation of red blood cells and plasma proteins in low-flow states.[136] Spontaneous contrast can appear as discrete echo signals or as wavy, mobile, jelly-like images. It can be seen in any or all cardiac chambers as well as in the aorta (Fig. 34–31). Smoke in the left atrium may predispose patients to thromboembolic events, especially with atrial fibrillation and in cases of mitral stenosis or mitral valve replacement.[137–140] Although TEE is superior to transthoracic echocardiography for detection of left atrial spontaneous contrast,[141] visualization is somewhat operator-dependent, as improper gain settings can lead to both false-negative and false-positive results. Typically, spontaneous contrast is in constant motion, "swirling" in the left atrium and appendage. Suspected contrast that does not move is probably artifactual.[142] Anticoagulation alone usually does not lessen or resolve spontaneous contrast, but platelet disaggregatory agents may decrease the effect in some cases.[143, 144]

Left Ventricle

As in other cardiac chambers, left ventricular thrombi form when regional stasis of blood flow is present. Mural thrombi nearly never occur in a normally functioning ventricle.[145] The most common settings in which left ventricular thrombi occur include acute myocardial infarction, chronic left ventricular aneurysm, and dilated cardiomyopathy.[146–149] Accurate detection of these thrombi is clinically important because of the risk of subsequent peripheral embolization. Autopsy-confirmed left ventricular thrombi are present in up to one half of patients with myocardial infarction and are more common in larger infarctions with regional dyskinesis.[150–152] They form early in the course of myocardial necrosis (usually within the

first 10 days), occur more frequently in anterior infarctions (30 to 40 percent of affected patients), and are seen most often in or near the left ventricular apex. Mural thrombi are relatively uncommon in inferior and posterior infarctions (less than 5 percent of cases).[147, 148]

Echocardiography is the procedure of choice for detecting left ventricular clots[153–155] and is superior to both contrast ventriculography and radionuclide angiography.[149, 156, 157] Although early, smaller echocardiographic trials reported high sensitivity and specificity for detection of ventricular thrombi, the true levels are somewhat less clear, as most large studies do not have pathologic correlation (and ventriculographic comparison cannot be considered a "gold standard").[149, 156] Left ventricular thrombi have various appearances—sometimes echodense and laminar, sometimes speckled and protruding, sometimes filamentous and mobile. On occasion, thrombi undergo central liquefaction and may demonstrate considerable inhomogeneity or even a cystic appearance. Studies suggest that "immature" thrombi are often filamentous with irregular borders, whereas older thrombi tend to be more echodense and fixed.[154] When the echodensity of the thrombus is different from that of the underlying myocardium, detection is fairly simple. Un-

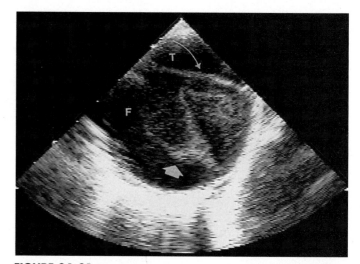

FIGURE 34–31. A transverse transesophageal image of an aortic dissection with spontaneous contrast *(large arrow)* in the false lumen (F). The intimal flap *(small arrow)* is visible as well. T = true lumen. (From Blanchard, D.G., Kimura, B.J., Dittrich, H.C., and DeMaria, A.N.: Transesophageal echocardiography of the aorta. J.A.M.A. 272:546, 1994. Copyright 1994, American Medical Association.)

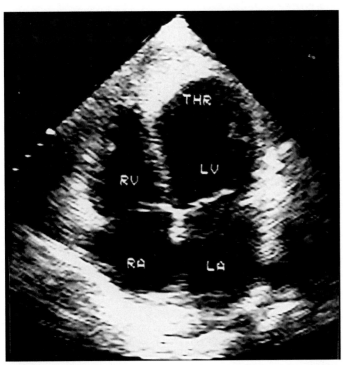

FIGURE 34–32. An apical four-chamber view of an echodense, laminar, apical thrombus (THR). RA = right atrium; RV = right ventricle; LA = left atrium; LV = left ventricle.

fortunately, many clots—particularly laminar, mural thrombi—tend to have a density similar to that of the myocardium and therefore are difficult to visualize. Apical mural thrombi are especially problematic, as near-field artifacts may limit satisfactory imaging in this area and simulate thrombi. When compared with artifacts, however, thrombi have a discrete shape and a definite border. Prominent apical muscular trabeculations, papillary muscles, false tendons, and tumors can also mimic thrombi.[158] True left ventricular clots are attached to, but are discrete from, the underlying myocardium, are visible in multiple imaging planes, and move concordantly with the ventricular wall.[159] As mentioned previously, suspected masses

in areas of normally functioning myocardium are rarely thrombi. Modified imaging planes are helpful in equivocal cases. Figures 34–32 and 34–33 demonstrate laminar, nonmobile apical thrombi in patients who have had recent myocardial infarctions. Figure 34–34 shows a protruding left ventricular thrombus that was quite mobile on real-time imaging. In Figure 34–35, the same patient was imaged serially after myocardial infarction. One week after the event, a laminar apical thrombus was noted (top of figure). Despite

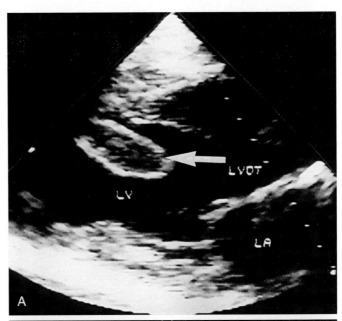

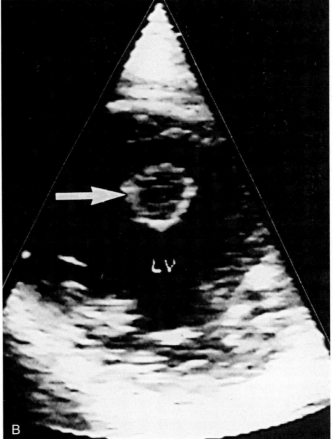

FIGURE 34–34. Parasternal long-axis (A) and short-axis views (B) of a protruding, mobile left ventricular thrombus (arrows). LVOT = left ventricular outflow tract; LA = left atrium; LV = left ventricle.

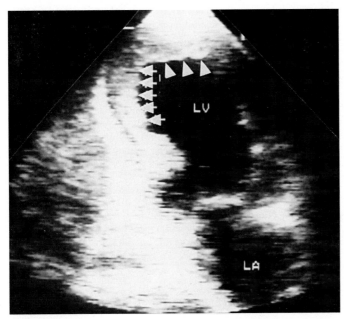

FIGURE 34–33. An apical two-chamber view of an apical laminar thrombus (arrowheads). LA = left atrium; LV = left ventricle.

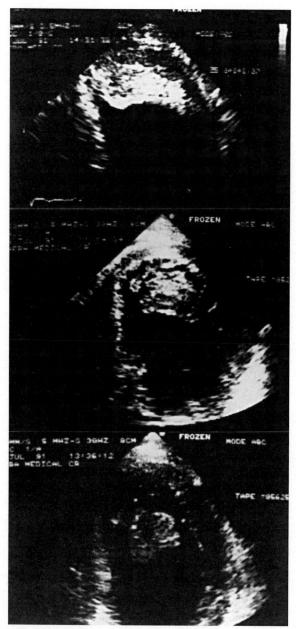

FIGURE 34–35. Evolution of an apical thrombus following myocardial infarction (see text for description). (From Glikson, M., Agranat, O., Ziskind, Z., et al.: From swirling to a mobile, pedunculated mass: The evolution of left ventricular thrombus despite full anticoagulation: Echocardiographic demonstration. Chest 103:281, 1993, with permission.)

heparin therapy, the thrombus began to protrude into the left ventricle by the following day (middle of figure). Several days later, the thrombus had evolved into a pedunculated globular mass (bottom of figure).

Peripheral embolization occurs in up to 10 percent of acute myocardial infarctions, mainly in patients with anterior wall infarction. For this reason, anticoagulation is recommended for 3 to 6 months following large, transmural anterior wall myocardial infarction.[160] The echocardiographic characteristics of thrombi appear to influence the risk of cardiogenic emboli.[161, 162] Irregularly shaped, protruding, and mobile thrombi are more likely to embolize than are laminar, immobile clots.[155, 157, 159, 162] Left ventricular thrombi in chronic aneurysms may also cause embolization, but the risk is lower than in acute myocardial infarction.[149] A mural, laminated thrombus noted in an apical aneurysm is not an absolute indication for anticoagulation per se, but most authorities would recommend it for a mobile, protruding clot.[163, 164]

METASTATIC (SECONDARY) TUMORS OF THE HEART AND PERICARDIUM

Metastatic tumors to the heart and pericardium occur 20 to 40 times more frequently than do primary cardiac tumors.[165] Nearly all types of malignancies (except primary central nervous system tumors) have been reported to metastasize to the heart, and autopsy series of patients with malignancies report cardiac involvement in approximately 5 percent of cases.[165, 166] Malignancies with the highest rates of cardiac and pericardial involvement include melanoma, leukemia and lymphoma, lung carcinoma, breast carcinoma, and renal cell carcinoma. Because of their high prevalence, lung and breast cancers constitute the largest number of cases, but melanoma and lymphoma both have higher rates of cardiac metastasis.[167–169] In general, cardiac metastases indicate wide spread of the primary malignancy, as isolated cardiac or pericardial involvement is uncommon.[170, 171] Tumors can reach the heart via the bloodstream or lymphatics;[165, 167, 168] less commonly, there can be extension of tumor through the vena cavae (with renal cell carcinoma, hepatoma, Wilms tumor, and uterine leiomyoma) or the pulmonary veins.[165, 172] Direct invasion of the heart by mediastinal, pulmonary, or subdiaphragmatic tumors is more rare. Metastatic disease affects the pericardium much more frequently than the heart, occurring in 5 to 15 percent of patients with malignancies at autopsy.[165, 166, 173] Not surprisingly, pericardial effusion is the most common echocardiographic finding in patients with metastatic cardiac disease. Tumors involving the heart itself most often occur in the myocardium and are seen less frequently in the endocardium or valves.[165, 166] Clinical signs and symptoms of cardiac metastases include pericarditis and pericardial effusion, cardiac tamponade, arrhythmias, heart failure, and nonspecific electrocardiographic changes.

Echocardiography is well suited for detecting and characterizing cardiac metastatic disease (Figs. 34–36 and 34–37). Intracavitary and pericardial tumors are usually well visualized as echodense protrusions in the cardiac chambers or pericardial space. Intramural metastases are sometimes more difficult to image, especially if their echodensity is similar to that of the surrounding myocardium. Intracardiac tumors may cause emboli, heart failure and, occasionally, outflow tract obstruction.[165, 174] Pericardial tumors can adhere to the visceral or parietal pericardium (see Fig. 34–36A) but may also involve the pericardium diffusely and cause symptoms of constriction.[175] Metastatic cardiac tumors may be misinterpreted as primary cardiac tumors, vegetations, thrombi, and prominent muscular trabeculations. The distinction among these entities is sometimes difficult, and associated symptoms and echocardiographic findings may be helpful.

EXTRACARDIAC MASSES

A variety of extracardiac masses has been described by echocardiography, including lymphoma, lung carcinoma, esophageal carcinoma, sarcoma, teratoma, thymoma, hematoma, hiatal hernia, pancreatic pseudocyst, pleural tumors, and pericardial cyst.[176–180] These masses range in severity from incidental findings to life-threatening causes of cardiac compression (Figs. 34–38 to 34–40).[181] Superior mediastinal masses may lead to a superior vena cava syndrome, and compressive tumors may mimic cardiac tamponade or constriction.[178, 182, 183] Echocardiography (including TEE)[184, 185] may help define these masses, but computed tomography and magnetic resonance imaging are often required for complete characterization.

PRIMARY CARDIAC TUMORS

Although cardiac tumors are uncommon in general, primary cardiac tumors are even more rare, accounting for less than 0.1

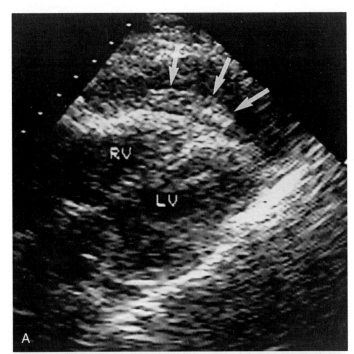

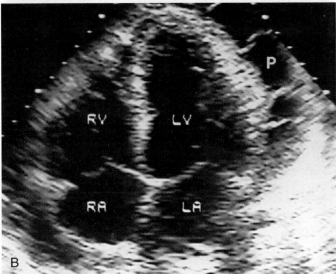

FIGURE 34–36. *A,* A modified subcostal view of a laminar metastasis adherent to the epicardium in a patient with widespread breast carcinoma. *B,* An apical four-chamber view from a patient with diffuse epicardial and pericardial involvement from metastatic lung cancer. Fibrinous strands are apparent in the pericardial space (P). RA = right atrium; RV = right ventricle; LA = left atrium; LV = left ventricle.

when the echodensity of the suspected tumor differs from that of the surrounding tissues.

PRIMARY BENIGN TUMORS

Myxomas

Myxomas are the most common primary cardiac tumors, accounting for about 25 percent of all cardiac tumors and 30 to 50 percent of the histologically benign subgroup.[165, 166, 189–192] Myxomas occur most frequently in patients aged 30 to 60 years and may be more common in women.[193, 194] These tumors are usually isolated findings, but associated skin and endocrine abnormalities ("NAME" syndrome) and familial occurrence have been reported.[195–198] Myxomas can occur in any cardiac chamber or valve, but three quarters

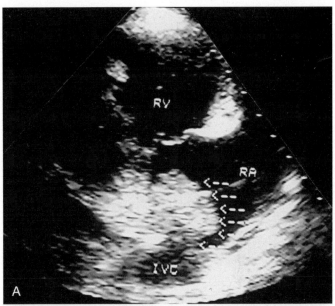

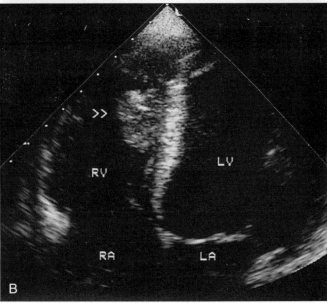

FIGURE 34–37. *A,* A modified parasternal view of a metastatic renal cell carcinoma *(arrows)* that had spread to the heart via the inferior vena cava *(IVC)*. *B,* An apical four-chamber view of a lymphoma *(arrowheads)* that had metastasized to the right ventricle *(RV)*. RA = right atrium; LA = left atrium; LV = left ventricle.

percent of all tumors at autopsy.[186] Three quarters of primary cardiac tumors are benign pathologically (Tables 34–1 and 34–2),[187] but this does not always imply a benign clinical course.[188] The clinical importance of a cardiac tumor varies with its histologic characteristics, rate of growth, propensity toward embolization, and anatomical location. A histologically nonmalignant tumor that embolizes or obstructs ventricular inflow or outflow can cause disastrous complications and even sudden death. Because this is anything but benign, accurate detection of cardiac tumors and masses is extremely desirable.

Cardiac neoplasms involving the ventricles are usually intramural, but atrial tumors are typically intracavitary.[165, 174] In general, extracardiac and intracavitary tumors and cysts are simpler to detect echocardiographically. Intramural tumors should be suspected when there is localized thickening of the myocardium, especially

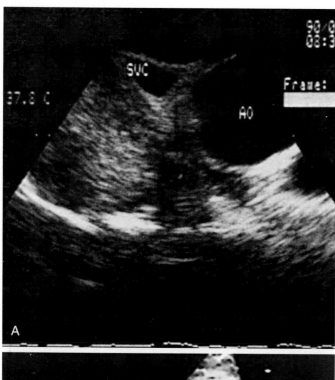

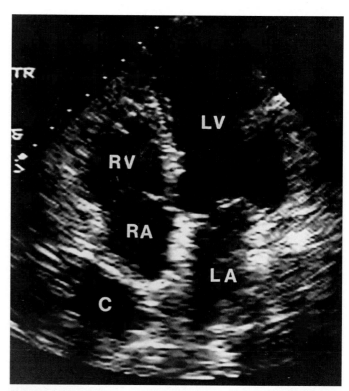

FIGURE 34–39. An apical four-chamber view taken from a patient with a pericardial cyst (C). LA = left atrium; LV = left ventricle; RA = right atrium; RV = right ventricle.

percent of patients have multiple myxomas at diagnosis.[165, 166, 202] Although smaller tumors are fixed to the septum and are immobile, larger myxomas become pedunculated, remaining attached to the septum by a stalk of variable length. Longer stalks may permit the mass to prolapse through the mitral annulus into the left ventricle during diastole, with subsequent movement back into the atrium during systole. Myxomas may be spherical and smooth, or they may develop villous projections. Intramural hemorrhage and necrosis are fairly common (causing the appearance of tissue heterogene-

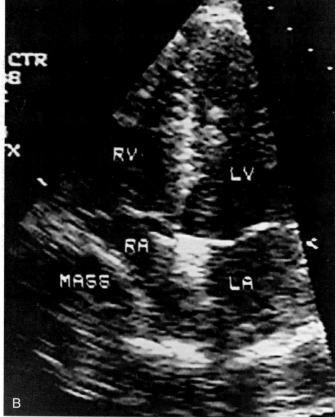

FIGURE 34–38. *A*, A transesophageal view of a non-Hodgkin lymphoma infiltrating the aortic wall and superior vena cava. *B*, An apical four-chamber view of a mediastinal malignant melanoma (MASS) compressing the right atrium (RA). SVC = superior vena cava; AO = aorta; RV = right ventricle; LA = left atrium; LV = left ventricle. (*A* from Faletra, F., Ravini, M., Moreo, A., et al.: Transesophageal echocardiography in the evaluation of mediastinal masses. J. Am. Soc. Echocardiogr. 5:178–186, 1992, with permission.)

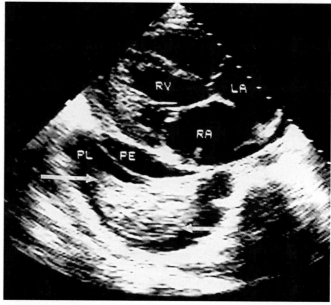

FIGURE 34–40. A modified four-chamber view of atelectatic lung (*arrows*) simulating an extracardiac mass. PL = pleural effusion; PE = pericardial effusion; RA = right atrium; RV = right ventricle; LA = left atrium.

are found in the left atrium. Most of the rest occur in the right atrium.[165, 199–201]

Approximately 90 percent of atrial myxomas grow from the interatrial septum, usually on or near the fossa ovalis, and about 5

TABLE 34–1. CLASSIFICATION OF PRIMARY AND SECONDARY CARDIAC TUMORS

Primary		Secondary		
Benign	*Malignant*	*Direct Extension*	*Venous Extension*	*Metastatic Spread*
Myxoma	Sarcoma	Lung carcinoma	Renal cell carcinoma	Melanoma
Pericardial cyst	Mesothelioma	Breast carcinoma	Adrenal carcinoma	Leukemia
Fibroelastoma	Lymphoma	Esophageal carcinoma	Liver carcinoma	Lymphoma
Rhabdomyoma	Other	Mediastinal tumors	Thyroid carcinoma	Genitourinary tumors
Fibroma			Lung carcinoma	Gastrointestinal tumors
Other			Uterine sarcoma	

Modified from Salcedo, E.E., Cohen, G.I., White, R.D., and Davison, M.B.: Cardiac tumors: Diagnosis and management. Curr. Probl. Cardiol. 17:79, 1992, with permission.

ity), but significant calcification is rare.[199, 203] Only 10 percent of myxomas are sessile and nonpedunculated.[202]

The clinical manifestations of a myxoma depend on its size, mobility, location, and friability. The classic triad of symptoms includes intermittent obstruction of blood flow, peripheral embolization, and constitutional signs and symptoms (e.g., fever, weight loss, malaise, anemia, elevated erythrocyte sedimentation rate, and leukocytosis).[205] Patients are sometimes misdiagnosed with mitral stenosis, as the myxoma may cause both a diastolic rumble at the apex and an early diastolic sound ("tumor plop") which is similar to an opening snap. Cardiac myxomas tend to grow rapidly, and prompt surgical removal is indicated after diagnosis.[206, 207] The tumor, its stalk, and the site of attachment (with wide margins) should be excised to prevent recurrence.[208, 209]

Echocardiographically, myxomas appear as gelatinous, roughly spherical masses attached to the endocardial surface by a pedicle (Figs. 34–41 to 34–44). Although most myxomas attach to the interatrial septum, they may originate from the posterior atrial wall, anterior atrial wall, atrial appendage, or even cardiac valves. Myxomas in these unusual locations may be mistaken for other tumors or thrombi.[204] Myxomas often appear speckled, and frond-like projections and internal echolucent areas (representing hemorrhage) are sometimes seen. Larger tumors are almost always mobile to some degree, and therefore a sizable left atrial mass that appears fixed to the endocardial surface is probably not a myxoma.

Myxomas were originally imaged with M-mode echocardiography, but two-dimensional imaging clearly is superior. Large tumors are usually visible in all transthoracic viewing planes, but detection of smaller myxomas may be more difficult and limited to the apical and subcostal planes. TEE provides clear, detailed visualization of myxomas, especially those in the atria, and usually identifies the site of origin.[210, 211] Doppler echocardiography is useful for evaluating valvular stenosis and regurgitation due to atrial myxomas that prolapse through the mitral (or tricuspid) annulus.[212, 213]

Several other masses may mimic the echocardiographic appearance of myxomas, including thrombi, vegetations, other benign tumors, and malignant tumors. The presence of characteristic echocardiographic features are often diagnostic for myxomas, and the clinical setting also may be helpful. In some cases, however, surgery is required for a definitive diagnosis.

TABLE 34–2. PROPORTIONS OF BENIGN AND MALIGNANT PRIMARY CARDIAC TUMORS

Benign	Malignant
Myxoma 32%	Sarcoma 73%
Pericardial cyst 20%	Mesothelioma 15%
Lipoma 11%	Lymphoma 6%
Fibroelastoma 10%	Other 6%
Rhabdomyoma 9%	

Modified from Salcedo, E.E., Cohen, G.I., White, R.D., and Davison, M.B.: Cardiac tumors: Diagnosis and management. Curr. Probl. Cardiol. 17:79, 1992, with permission.

Other Primary Tumors

The remaining primary cardiac tumors are rare.

RHABDOMYOMAS. These lesions are the most common benign cardiac tumors in children, accounting for 60 percent of all pediatric cardiac tumors.[214] In approximately 90 percent of affected patients, multiple rhabdomyomas are present, occurring in the right and left ventricles with equal frequency. Rhabdomyomas vary greatly in size and can occasionally grow large enough to cause inflow or outflow obstruction as well as conduction abnormalities and ventricular arrhythmias.[215, 216] Rhabdomyomas are strongly associated with tuberous sclerosis, occurring in 30 to 50 percent of affected patients. Because of this, screening echocardiography is recommended for these individuals. Interestingly, the tumors may regress, and surgical excision is not always required.[217]

On two-dimensional echocardiography (Fig. 34–45), rhabdomyomas characteristically appear as multiple intracavitary and intramural masses with a greater echodensity than the surrounding myocardium. When only one mass is present, the diagnosis is more difficult and biopsy may be necessary. Echocardiography may help guide surgical therapy[11] and is also well suited for serial examinations.[218] Doppler interrogation can assess outflow gradients in patients with obstructing tumors.

FIBROMAS. These are the second most frequent benign pediatric cardiac neoplasms and are three times more common in children than in adults.[165, 219] These firm, nonencapsulated tumors range in diameter from several millimeters to 10 cm, but most are 4 to 7 cm. They occur most frequently in the left ventricle and less

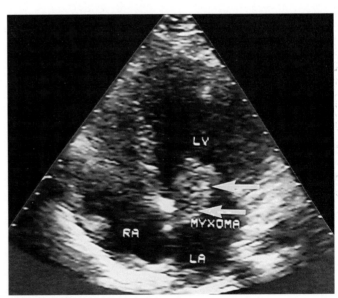

FIGURE 34–41. An apical four-chamber view of a moderate-sized left atrial myxoma (*arrows*), seen prolapsing into the left ventricle during diastole. LA = left atrium; LV = left ventricle; RA = right atrium.

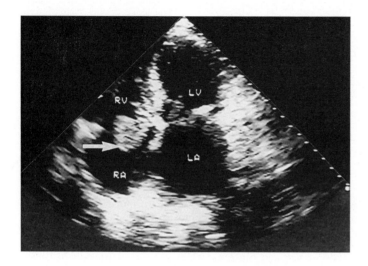

FIGURE 34–42. An apical four-chamber view of a right atrial myxoma (*arrow*) attached near the tricuspid annulus. LA = left atrium; LV = left ventricle; RA = right atrium; RV = right ventricle.

FIGURE 34–43. A parasternal long-axis view of an aortic valvular myxoma (*arrows*). AO = aorta; LA = left atrium; LV = left ventricle.

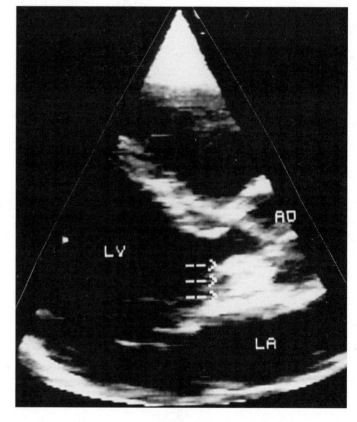

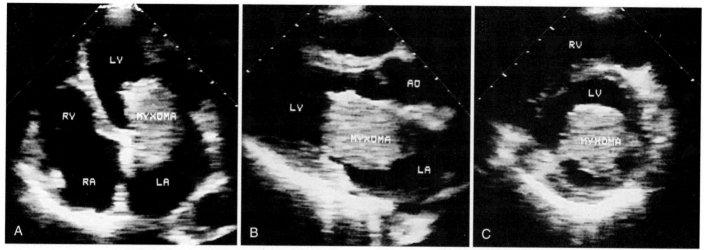

FIGURE 34-44. Apical four-chamber (A), parasternal long-axis (B), and parasternal short-axis (C) views of a large left atrial myxoma that partially obstructs left ventricular inflow. LV = left ventricle; RV = right ventricle; RA = right atrium; LA = left atrium; Ao = aorta.

often in the interventricular septum, right ventricle, and atrioventricular ring. Fibromas are rarely found in the right or left atrium.[220, 221] They may cause outflow or inflow obstruction, arrhythmias, and sudden death.[222-224] On echocardiography, the tumors are echodense with occasional central calcification. They may be homogeneous but can also appear as areas of localized hypertrophy within the ventricular wall. The affected wall segment is usually hypokinetic and heterogeneous in ultrasonic texture.[225] Fibromas are usually single, distinguishing them from most cases of rhabdomyoma (Fig. 34-46). An apical fibroma may mimic apical thrombus or hypertrophy: Differentiation is sometimes difficult, as both apical thrombi and fibroma are associated with abnormal wall motion and heterogeneous echodensity.[226] Echocardiography can aid in tumor localization prior to surgery and in postoperative follow-up as well.[227]

PAPILLARY FIBROELASTOMAS. These lesions can arise from any part of the heart but are most often attached to cardiac valves.[228-230] These pedunculated tumors are usually less than 1 cm in diameter and consist of a central core with multiple small fronds.

Before the advent of two-dimensional echocardiography, these tumors were diagnosed most often at autopsy, as they rarely cause cardiac dysfunction or murmurs. However, this type of tumor seems prone to embolization, leading to stroke, myocardial infarction, and sudden death.[231, 232] Surgical removal is recommended for symptomatic patients to prevent recurrent embolization.[188] Echocardiographically, these tumors are small, mobile, homogeneous masses that are usually attached to cardiac valves or chordae (Fig. 34-47). This attachment distinguishes them from most myxomas, but differentiation from vegetations is problematic.

CARDIAC LIPOMAS. These tumors can occur anywhere in the heart and pericardium but are statistically more prevalent in the right atrium and left ventricle.[165, 166] These benign polypoid tumors vary in size (from small to massive) and may be pedunculated or sessile (Fig. 34-48). Valvular lipomas are distinctly rare.[233] Lipomas usually cause no symptoms but occasionally cause flow obstruction, murmurs, pericardial effusion, and arrhythmias.[234] Diagnosis by echocardiography alone is unlikely, as lipomas may mimic myxomas, fibromas, thrombi, and papillary fibroelastomas.

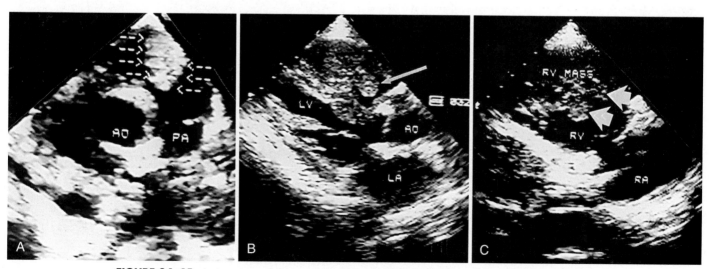

FIGURE 34-45. A, A parasternal short-axis view through the base of the heart in a patient with tuberous sclerosis and a large rhabdomyoma in the right ventricular outflow tract (arrows). Parasternal long-axis (B) and right atrial–right ventricular (C) views of a large right ventricular rhabdomyoma (arrows). AO = aorta; PA = pulmonary artery; LA = left atrium; LV = left ventricle; RA = right atrium; RV = right ventricle.

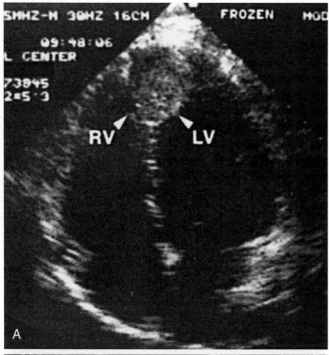

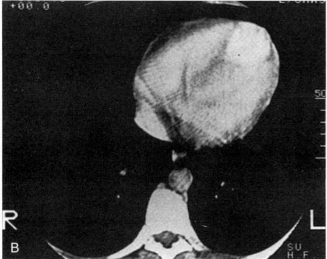

FIGURE 34–46. *A,* An apical four-chamber view of a fibroma in the distal interventricular septum *(arrowheads). B,* An axial computed tomogram of the chest from the same patient following contrast injection, demonstrating the fibroma near the apex. RV = right ventricle; LV = left ventricle. (From Parmley, L.F., Salley, R.K., Williams, J.P., et al.: The clinical spectrum of cardiac fibroma with diagnostic and surgical considerations: Noninvasive imaging enhances management. Ann. Thorac. Surg. 45:455, 1988. Reprinted with permission from the Society of Thoracic Surgeons.)

Because magnetic resonance imaging can distinguish fatty tissue, it can suggest the diagnosis, but biopsy may be necessary.

OTHER BENIGN TUMORS AND MASSES. Teratoma (which occurs mostly in infants), hemangioma, benign mesothelioma of the atrioventricular node (which may cause heart block),[235] lymphangioma, neurofibroma, Purkinje cell tumor,[216] granular cell tumor,[236] pericardial cyst (see Fig. 34–39), blood cysts, and echinococcal cysts are other benign tumors and masses. The heart is rarely involved in echinococcosis (<2 percent of cases), but intracardiac or intrapericardial rupture of a cyst may be disastrous, causing anaphylaxis and cardiac tamponade, respectively.[237–239] Most echinococcal cysts occur in the left ventricular free wall and interventricular septum; few occur in the right side of the heart and the left atrium. Echocardiography is useful for diagnosing

cardiac echinococcal disease (Figs. 34–49 and 34–50), and detection of multiseptated cysts in the left ventricle or interventricular septum is pathognomonic.[240, 241]

Pericardial cysts generally are asymptomatic and are discovered on routine chest radiography. They usually occur in the right costophrenic angle, less often in the left angle, and rarely in the posterior or anterior mediastinum.[242] These cysts are important mainly because they may be mistaken for primary or metastatic malignant tumors. As the cysts rarely cause symptoms and have a benign prognosis,[243, 244] accurate differentiation is essential. Typically, these structures are completely fluid-filled, and do not have internal masses or complex loculations. As opposed to pericardial and paracardiac tumors, pericardial cysts usually do not compress the heart to any significant degree, and they never invade the myocardial wall. Echocardiography, computed tomography, and magnetic resonance imaging are all helpful for visualizing pericar-

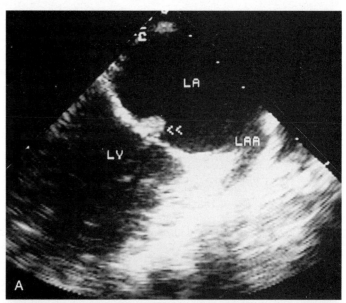

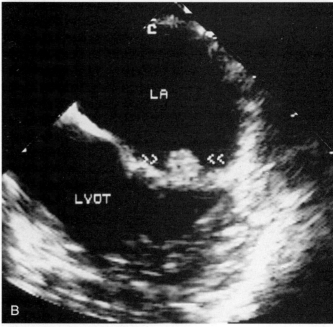

FIGURE 34–47. *A* and *B,* Transesophageal views taken from a patient with peripheral emboli. Images of the mass *(arrowheads)* are characteristic of a small papillary fibroelastoma attached to the mitral valve. LA = left atrium; LV = left ventricle; LAA = left atrial appendage; LVOT = left ventricular outflow tract; RV = right ventricle. (Courtesy of William D. Keen, Jr., M.D.)

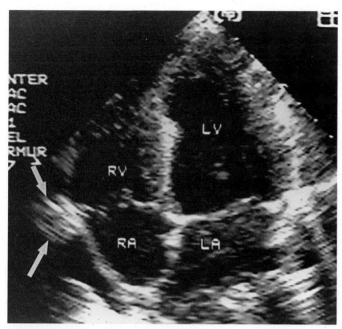

FIGURE 34–48. An apical four-chamber view of a small lipoma in the right atrioventricular groove (arrows). LA = left atrium; LV = left ventricle; RA = right atrium; RV = right ventricle.

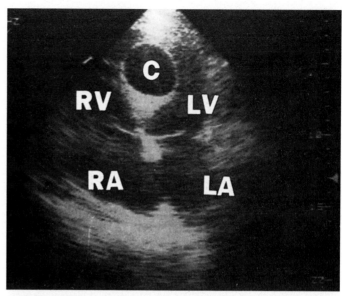

FIGURE 34–50. An apical four-chamber view of a large echinococcal cyst (C) in the interventricular septum. LA = left atrium; LV = left ventricle; RA = right atrium; RV = right ventricle. (From Lanzoni, A.M., Barrios, V., Moya, J.L., et al.: Dynamic left ventricular outflow obstruction caused by cardiac echinococcosis. Am. Heart J. 124:1083, 1992, with permission.)

dial cysts (see Fig. 34–39), and once diagnosed, patients can be assured of a benign outcome.

PRIMARY MALIGNANT TUMORS

Primary malignant tumors of the heart are rare, accounting for about 25 percent of all primary cardiac tumors. They involve the right side of the heart more often than the left side and occur more frequently in adults than in children.[165] The majority of primary cardiac malignancies are sarcomas, and of these, angiosarcomas and rhabdomyosarcomas are the most common. Extraskeletal osteosarcomas, lymphosarcomas, fibrosarcomas, liposarcomas, and leiomyosarcomas are more rare. Most primary cardiac malignancies are intramural and tend to grow rapidly, invading the pericardium and surrounding structures. They metastasize often and are almost always lethal.

ANGIOSARCOMA. This tumor is the most common primary cardiac sarcoma and occurs more often in men than in women.[245] The right atrium is involved most often (Fig. 34–51). Symptoms of

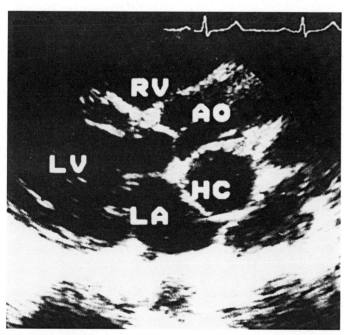

FIGURE 34–49. A parasternal long-axis view of an intrapericardial echinococcal cyst (HC) on the superior wall of the left atrium. RV = right ventricle; LV = left ventricle; AO = aorta; LA = left atrium. (From Rey, M., Alfonso, F.L., Torricella, E.G., et al.: Diagnostic value of two-dimensional echocardiography in cardiac hydatid disease. Eur. Heart J. 12:1300, 1991, with permission.)

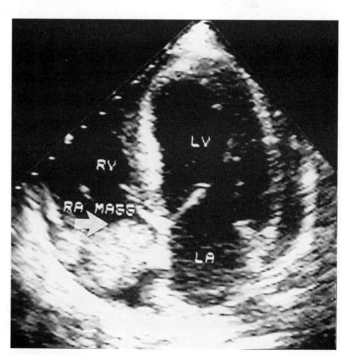

FIGURE 34–51. An apical four-chamber view of a large sarcomatous mass in the right atrium (arrow). LA = left atrium; LV = left ventricle; RA = right atrium; RV = right ventricle.

right-sided heart failure or pericardial disease predominate, although a few patients present with constitutional symptoms. Metastases are common, and the median survival after diagnosis is only 3 months.[246]

RHABDOMYOSARCOMAS. These lesions involve the left and right side of the heart with equal frequency, and multiple intracardiac tumors are common at diagnosis (Figs. 34–52 and 34–53). Most often, patients present with chest pain (of a pleuritic or pericarditic nature), peripheral embolization, and dyspnea.[247] Valvular obstruction and stenosis have been reported as has hypertrophic osteoarthropathy, eosinophilia, and polyarthritis.[247]

EXTRASKELETAL CARDIAC OSTEOSARCOMAS. These tumors often occur in the posterior portion of the left atrium near the junctions of the pulmonary veins.[165] The tumor mass can extend from the left atrium into the pulmonary veins, and this finding is useful in distinguishing osteosarcoma from left atrial myxoma.

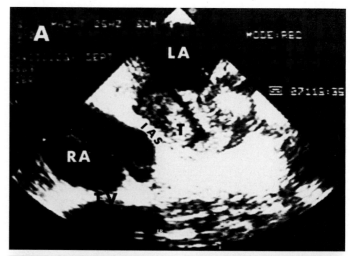

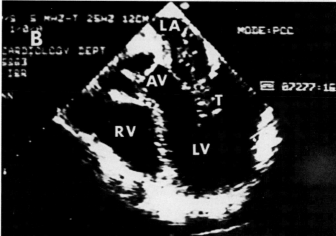

FIGURE 34–53. *A*, A transesophageal echocardiographic view of an intracardiac rhabdomyosarcoma involving the left atrium. *B*, A less magnified view showing prolapse of the tumor through the mitral valve. LA = left atrium; T = tumor; LV = left ventricle; RA = right atrium; TV = tricuspid valve; RV = right ventricle; IAS = interatrial septum; AV = aortic valve. (From Awad, M., Dunn, B., Al Halees, Z., et al.: Intracardiac rhabdomyosarcoma: Transesophageal echocardiographic findings and diagnosis. J. Am. Soc. Echocardiogr. 5:199, 1992, with permission.)

PRIMARY CARDIAC LYMPHOSARCOMA. These lesions may cause heart failure, outflow or inflow obstruction, conduction abnormalities, and pericardial effusion.[248, 249] Both sides of the heart are affected equally, and the tumors may be nodular and multiple or single and large. Nonsarcomatous primary cardiac neoplasms include malignant mesothelioma (the most common primary pericardial malignancy), malignant teratoma, and malignant fibrous histiocytoma.

Echocardiography may help diagnose primary cardiac tumors[11, 250] and evaluate their response to therapy.[251] Although pulmonary venous involvement suggests primary extraskeletal osteosarcoma, most echocardiographic findings are nonspecific, and biopsy is usually required for accurate diagnosis.[252] Intramyocardial infiltration by tumor may cause focal wall thickening, hypokinesis, and heterogeneous echo reflectivity. Because of their invasive nature, these tumors can extend directly into cardiac valves, pericardium, and adjacent structures.[253–255]

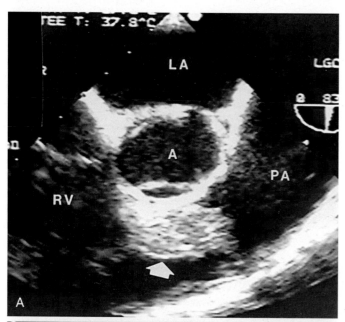

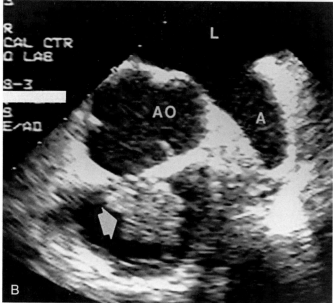

FIGURE 34–52. *A*, A longitudinal transesophageal view of a rhabdomyosarcoma in the right ventricular outflow tract *(arrow)*. *B*, A transverse view in the same patient. LA = left atrium; A = aorta; PA = pulmonary artery; RV = right ventricle; AO = aorta; L = left atrium; A = left atrial appendage.

References

1. Mügge, A., Daniel, W.G., Haverlich, A., et al.: Diagnosis of noninfective cardiac mass lesions by two-dimensional echocardiography. Circulation 83:70, 1991.
2. Herrera, C.J., Mehlman, D.J., Hartz, R.S., et al.: Comparison of transesophageal and transthoracic echocardiography for diagnosis of right sided cardiac lesions. Am. J. Cardiol. 70:964, 1992.

3. Alam, M., Sun, I., and Smith, S.: Transesophageal echocardiographic evaluation of right atrial mass lesions. J. Am. Soc. Echocardiogr. 4:331, 1991.
4. Reeder, G.S., Khandheria, B.K., Seward, J.B., et al.: Transesophageal echocardiography and cardiac masses. Mayo Clin. Proc. 66:1101, 1991.
5. Black, J.W., Hopkins, A.P., Lee, L.C.L., et al.: Role of transesophageal echocardiography in evaluation of cardiogenic embolism. Br. Heart J. 66:302, 1991.
6. Alam, M., and Sun, I.: Transesophageal echocardiographic evaluation of left atrial mass lesions. J. Am. Soc. Echocardiogr. 4:323, 1991.
7. Edwards, L.C., III, and Louie, E.K.: Transthoracic and transesophageal echocardiography for the evaluation of cardiac tumors, thrombi, and valvular vegetations. Am. J. Cardiac Imaging 8:63, 1994.
8. Dressler, F.A., and Labovitz, A.J.: Systemic arterial emboli and cardiac masses: Assessment with transesophageal echocardiography. Cardiol. Clin. 11:447, 1993.
9. Aru, G.M., Falchi, S., Cardu, G., et al.: The role of transesophageal echocardiography in the monitoring of cardiac mass removal: A review of 17 cases. J. Cardiovasc. Surg. (Torino) 8:554, 1993.
10. Kupferwasser, I., Mohr-Kahaly, S., Erbel, R., et al.: Three-dimensional imaging of cardiac mass lesions by transesophageal echocardiographic computed tomography. J. Am. Soc. Echocardiogr. 7:561, 1994.
11. Marx, G.R., Bierman, F.Z., Mathews, E., et al.: Two-dimensional echocardiographic diagnosis of intracardiac masses in infancy. J. Am. Coll. Cardiol. 3:827, 1984.
12. Limacher, M.C., Gutgesell, H.P., Vick, G.W., et al.: Echocardiographic anatomy of the eustachian valve. Am. J. Cardiol. 57:363, 1986.
13. Orita, Y., Meno, H., Kanaide, H., et al.: Echocardiographic features of persistent right sinus venosus valve in adults. J. Clin. Ultrasound 10:461, 1982.
14. Battle-Diaz, J., Stanley, P., Kratz, C., et al.: Manifestations of persistence of right sinus venosus valve. Am. J. Cardiol. 43:850, 1979.
15. Reller, M.D., McDonald, R.W., Gerlis, L.M., et al.: Cardiac embryology: Basic review and clinical correlations. J. Am. Soc. Echocardiogr. 4:519, 1991.
16. Cloez, J.L., Neimann, J.L., Chivoret, G., et al.: Echocardiographic rediscovery of an anatomical structure: The Chiari network: A propos of 16 cases. Arch. Mal. Coeur. 76:1284, 1983.
17. Chiari, H.: Ueber Netzbildungen im rechten vorhofe des herzens. Beitr. Pathol. Anat. 22:1, 1897.
18. Panidis, I.P., Kotler, M.N., Mintz, G.S., et al.: Clinical and echocardiographic features of right atrial masses. Am. Heart J. 107:745, 1984.
19. Werner, J.A., Cheitlin, M.D., Gross, B.W., et al.: Echocardiographic appearance of the Chiari network: Differentiation from right-heart pathology. Circulation 63:1104, 1981.
20. Goldschlager, A., Goldschlager, N., Brewster, H., et al.: Catheter entrapment in a Chiari network involving an atrial septal defect. Chest 62:345, 1972.
21. Katz, E.S., Fredberg, R.S., Rutkovsky, L., et al.: Identification of an unusual right atrial mass as a Chiari network by biplane transesophageal echocardiography. Echocardiography 9:273, 1992.
22. Cujec, B., Mycyk, T., and Khouri, M.: Identification of Chiari's network with transesophageal echocardiography. J. Am. Soc. Echocardiogr. 5:96, 1992.
23. Keren, A., Billingham, M.E., and Popp, R.L.: Echocardiographic recognition and implications of ventricular hypertrophic trabeculations and aberrant bands. Circulation 70:836, 1984.
24. Perry, L.W., Ruckman, R.N., Shapiro, S.R., et al.: Left ventricular false tendons in children: Prevalence as detected by two dimensional echocardiography and clinical significance. Am. J. Cardiol. 52:1264, 1983.
25. Vered, Z., Melzer, R.S., Benjamin, P., et al.: Prevalence and significance of false tendons in the left ventricle as determined by echocardiography. Am. J. Cardiol. 53:330, 1984.
26. Malouf, J., Gharzuddine, W., and Kutayli, F.: A reappraisal of the prevalence and clinical importance of left ventricular false tendons in children and adults. Br. Heart J. 55:587, 1986.
27. Suwa, M., Hirota, Y., Kaku, K., et al.: Prevalence of the coexistence of left ventricular false tendons and premature ventricular complexes in apparently healthy subjects: A prospective study in the general population. J. Am. Coll. Cardiol. 12:910, 1988.
28. Nishimura, T., Kondo, M., Umadome, H., et al.: Echocardiographic features of false tendons in the left ventricle. Am. J. Cardiol. 48:177, 1981.
29. Luetmer, P.H., Edwards, W.D., Seward, J.B., et al.: Incidence and distribution of left ventricular false tendons: An autopsy study of 483 normal human hearts. J. Am. Coll. Cardiol. 8:179, 1986.
30. Brenner, J.I., Baker, K., Ringel, R.E., et al.: Echocardiographic evidence of left ventricular bands in infants and children. J. Am. Coll. Cardiol. 3:1515, 1984.
31. Fraser, R.S., Dvorkin, J., Rossal, R.E., et al.: Left superior vena cava: A review of associated congenital heart lesions. Catheterization data and roentgenologic findings. Am. J. Med. 31:711, 1961.
32. Mantini, E., Grondin, C.M., Lillehei, C.W., et al.: Congenital anomalies involving the coronary sinus. Circulation 33:317, 1966.
33. Cha, E.M., and Khoury, G.H.: Persistent left superior vena cava. Radiology 103:375, 1972.
34. Chaudry, F., and Zabalgoita, M.: Persistent left superior vena cava diagnosed by contrast transesophageal echocardiography. Am. Heart J. 122:1175, 1991.
35. Blanchard, D.G., Dittrich, H.C., Mitchell, M., and McCann, H.A.: Diagnostic pitfalls in transesophageal echocardiography. J. Am. Soc. Echocardiogr. 5:525, 1992.
36. Stoddard, M.F., Liddell, N.E., Longaker, R.A., et al.: Transesophageal echocardiography: Normal variants and mimickers. Am. Heart J. 124:1587, 1992.
37. Seward, J.B., Khanderia, B.K., Oh, J.K., et al.: Critical appraisal of transesophageal echocardiography: Limitations, pitfalls, and complications. J. Am. Soc. Echocardiogr. 5:288, 1992.
38. Starling, R.C., Baker, P.B., Hirsch, S.C., et al.: An echocardiographic and anatomic description of the donor-recipient atrial anastomosis after orthotopic cardiac transplantation. Am. J. Cardiol. 64:109, 1989.
39. Movsowitz, H.D., Jacobs, L.E., Movsowitz, C., et al.: Transesophageal echocardiographic evaluation of a transthoracic echocardiographic pitfall: A diaphragmatic hernia mimicking a left atrial mass. J. Am. Soc. Echocardiogr. 6:104, 1993.
40. Silver, M.D., and Dorsey, J.S.: Aneurysms of the septum primum in adults. Arch. Pathol. Lab. Med. 102:62, 1978.
41. Wysham, D.G., McPherson, D.D., and Kerber, R.E.: Asymptomatic aneurysm of the interatrial septum. J. Am. Coll. Cardiol. 4:1311, 1984.
42. Hanley, P.C., Tajik, A.J., Hynes J.K., et al.: Diagnosis and classification of atrial septal aneurysm by two-dimensional echocardiography: Report of 80 consecutive cases. J. Am. Coll. Cardiol. 6:1370, 1985.
43. Pearson, A.C., Nagelhout, D., Castello, R., et al.: Atrial septal aneurysm and stroke: A transesophageal echocardiographic study. J. Am. Coll. Cardiol. 18:1223, 1991.
44. Comess, K.A., DeRook, F.A., Deach, K.W., et al.: Transesophageal echocardiography and carotid ultrasound in patients with cerebral ischemia: Prevalence of findings and recurrent stroke risk. J. Am. Coll. Cardiol. 23:1598, 1994.
45. Belkin, R.N., Hurwitz, B.J., and Kisslo, J.: Atrial septal aneurysm: Association with cerebrovascular and peripheral embolic events. Stroke 18:856, 1987.
46. Zabalgoitia-Reyes, M., Herrera, C., Gandhi, D.K., et al.: A possible mechanism for neurologic ischemic events in patients with atrial septal aneurysm. Am. J. Cardiol. 66:761, 1990.
47. Pearson, A.C., Labovitz, A.J., Tatineni, S., et al.: Superiority of transesophageal echocardiography in detecting cardiac sources of embolism in patients with cerebral ischemia of uncertain etiology. J. Am. Coll. Cardiol. 17:66, 1991.
48. Kong, C.W., and Chan, W.: The echocardiographic features of an aneurysm of the inter-atrial septum. Angiology 35:188, 1984.
49. Canny, M., Drobinski, G., Thomas, D., et al.: Interatrial septal aneurysm. Echocardiographic diagnosis. Arch. Mal. Coeur. 77:337, 1984.
50. Schneider, B., Hanrath, P., Vogel, P., et al.: Improved morphologic characterization of atrial septal aneurysm by transesophageal echocardiography: Relation to cerebrovascular events. J. Am. Coll. Cardiol. 16:1000, 1990.
51. Vanderbossche, J.L., and Englert, M.: Effects of respiration on atrial septal aneurysm of the fossa ovale shown by echocardiography study. Am. Heart J. 103:922, 1982.
52. Dashkoff, N., Karacuschansky, M., Come, P.C., et al.: Echocardiographic appearance of mitral annular calcification. Am. Heart J. 94:585, 1977.
53. D'Cruz, I.A., Devaraj, N., Hirsch, L.J., et al.: Unusual echocardiographic appearance attributable to submitral calcification simulating left ventricular "masses." Clin. Cardiol. 3:260, 1980.
54. Hutter, A.M., and Page, D.L.: Atrial arrhythmias and lipomatous hypertrophy of the cardiac interatrial septum. Am. Heart J. 82:16, 1971.
55. Simons, M., Cabin, H.S., and Jaffe, C.C.: Lipomatous hypertrophy of the atrial septum: Diagnosis by combined echocardiography and computerized tomography. Am. J. Cardiol. 54:465, 1984.
56. Fyke, F.E., III, Tajik, A.J., Edwards, W.D., et al.: Diagnosis of lipomatous hypertrophy of the interatrial septum by two-dimensional echocardiography. J. Am. Coll. Cardiol. 1:1352, 1983.
57. Jornet, A., Batalla, J., Ulson, M., et al.: Lipomatous hypertrophy of the interatrial septum. Echocardiography 9:501, 1992.
58. Kindman, L.A., Wright, A., Tye, T., et al.: Lipomatous hypertrophy of the interatrial septum: Characterization by transesophageal and transthoracic echocardiography, magnetic resonance imaging, and computed tomography. J. Am. Soc. Echocardiogr. 1:450, 1988.
59. Applegate, P.M., Tajik, A.J., Ehman, R.L., et al.: Two-dimensional echocardiographic and magnetic resonance imaging observations in massive lipomatous hypertrophy of the atrial septum. Am. J. Cardiol. 59:489, 1987.
60. Pochis, W.T., Saeian, K., and Sager, K.B.: Usefulness of transesophageal echocardiography in diagnosing lipomatous hypertrophy of the atrial septum with comparison to transthoracic echocardiography. Am. J. Cardiol. 70:396, 1992.
61. Schülter, M., Langenstein, B.A., Their, W., et al: Transesophageal two-dimensional echocardiography in the diagnosis of cor triatriatum in the adult. J. Am. Coll. Cardiol. 2:1011, 1983.
62. Ludomirsky, A., Erickson, C., Vick, G.W., et al.: Transesophageal color flow Doppler evaluation of cor triatriatum in an adult. Am. Heart J. 120:451, 1990.
63. van Son, J.A.M., Danielson, G.K., Schaff, H.V., et al.: Cor triatriatum: Diagnosis, operative approach, and late results. Mayo Clin. Proc. 68:854, 1993.
64. Kendrick, M.H., Harrington, J.J., Sharma, G.V., et al.: Ventricular pacemaker wire simulating a right atrial mass. Chest 72:649, 1977.
65. Charuzi, Y., Kraus, R., and Swan, H.J.C.: Echocardiographic interpretation in the presence of Swan-Ganz intracardiac catheters. Am. J. Cardiol. 40:989, 1977.
66. Drinkovic, N.: Subcostal echocardiography to determine right ventricular pacing catheter position and control advancement of electrode catheters in intracardiac electrophysiologic studies: M-mode and two-dimensional studies. Am. J. Cardiol. 47:1260, 1981.
67. Meier, B., and Felner, J.M.: Two-dimensional echocardiographic evaluation of intracardiac transvenous pacemaker leads. J. Clin. Ultrasound 10:421, 1982.
68. Chazal, R.A., and Feigenbaum, H.: Two-dimensional echocardiographic identification of epicardial pacemaker wire perforation. Am. Heart J. 107:165, 1984.
69. Iliceto, S., DiBiase, M., Antonelli, G., et al.: Two-dimensional echocardiographic recognition of a pacing catheter perforation of the interventricular septum. PACE 5:934, 1982.
70. Tobin, A.M., Grodman, R.S., Fisherkeller, M., et al.: Two-dimensional echocardiographic localization of a malpositioned pacing catheter. PACE 6:291, 1983.
71. Zehender, M., Buchner, C., Geibel, A., et al.: Diagnosis of hidden pacemaker

lead sepsis by transesophageal echocardiography and a new technique for lead extraction. Am. Heart J. 118:1050, 1989.

72. VanCamp, G., and Vandenbossche, J.L.: Recognition of pacemaker lead infection by transesophageal echocardiography. Br. Heart J. 65:229, 1991.

73. Cohen, G.I., Klein, A.L., Chan, K.-L., et al.: Transesophageal echocardiographic diagnosis of right-sided cardiac masses in patients with central lines. Am. J. Cardiol. 70:925, 1992.

74. Mügge, A., Gulba, D.C., Jost, S., et al.: Dissolution of a right atrial thrombus attached to pacemaker electrodes: Usefulness of recombinant tissue-type plasminogen activator. Am. Heart J. 119:1437, 1990.

75. Vilacosta, I., Zamorano, J., Camino, A., et al.: Infected transvenous permanent pacemakers: Role of transesophageal echocardiography. Am. Heart J. 125:904, 1993.

76. Gondi, B., and Nanda, N.C.: Real-time two dimensional echocardiographic features of pacemaker perforation. Circulation 64:97, 1981.

77. Iliceto, S., Antonelli, G., Sorino, M., et al.: Two-dimensional echocardiographic recognition of complications of cardiac invasive procedures. Am. J. Cardiol. 53:846, 1984.

78. Chandraratna, P.A.N., Reid, C.L., Nimalasuriya, A., et al.: Application of two-dimensional contrast studies during pericardiocentesis. Am. J. Cardiol. 52:1120, 1983.

79. Bierard, L., El Allaf, D., D'Orio, V., et al.: Two-dimensional echocardiographic guiding of endomyocardial biopsy. Chest 85:759, 1984.

80. French, J.W., Popp, R.L., and Pitlick, P.T.: Cardiac localization of transvascular biotome using two-dimensional echocardiography. Am. J. Cardiol. 52:219, 1983.

81. Fyfe, D.A., Edgerton, J.R., Chaikhouni, A., et al.: Preoperative localization of an intracardiac foreign body by two-dimensional echocardiography. Am. Heart J. 113:210, 1987.

82. Reeves, W.C., Movahed, A., Chitwood, R., et al.: Utility of precordial, epicardial and transesophageal two-dimensional echocardiography in the detection of intracardiac foreign bodies. Am. J. Cardiol. 64:406, 1989.

83. Giyanani, V.L., Fertel, D., and Eggerstedt, J.: Use of ultrasound for localization of a foreign object in the heart. J. Clin. Ultrasound 17:379, 1989.

84. Brathwaite, C.E., Weiss, R.L., Baldino, W.A., et al.: Multichamber gunshot wounds of the heart. The utility of transesophageal echocardiography. Chest 101:187, 1992.

85. Potek, I.J., and Wright, J.S.: Needle in the heart. Br. Heart J. 45:325, 1981.

86. Sakai, K., Hoshimo, S., and Osawa, M.: Needle in the heart: Two-dimensional echocardiographic findings. Am. J. Cardiol. 53:1482, 1984.

87. Lim, S.P., Hakim, S.Z., and Van der Bel-Kahn, J.M.: Two-dimensional echocardiography for detection of primary right atrial thrombus in pulmonary embolism. Am. Heart J. 108:1546, 1984.

88. Redish GA, and Anderson A.L.: Echocardiographic diagnosis of right atrial thromboembolism. J. Am. Coll. Cardiol. 1:1167, 1983.

89. Amsel, B.J., Dion, R., and Gillebert, T.C.: Right heart thromboembolism after cardiac surgery. Eur. Heart J. 7:86, 1986.

90. Boulay F., Danchin N., Neimann J.L., et al.: Echocardiographic features of right atrial thrombi. J. Clin. Ultrasound 14:601, 1986.

91. Kunze, K.P., Schluter, M., Costard, A., et al.: Right atrial thrombus formation after transvenous catheter ablation of the atrioventricular node. J. Am. Coll. Cardiol. 6:1428, 1985.

92. Schmaltz, A.A., Huenges, R., and Heil, R.P.: Thrombosis and embolism complicating ventriculo-atrial shunt for hydrocephalus: Echocardiographic findings. Br. Heart J. 43:241, 1980.

93. Felner, J.M., Churchwell, A.L., and Murphy, D.A.: Right atrial thromboemboli: Clinical, echocardiographic, and pathophysiologic manifestations. J. Am. Coll. Cardiol. 4:1041, 1984.

94. Cameron, J., Pohlner, P.G., Stafford, E.G., et al.: Right heart thrombus: Recognition, diagnosis and management. J. Am. Coll. Cardiol. 5:1239, 1985.

95. Rosenzweig, M.D., and Nanda, N.C: Two-dimensional echocardiographic detection of circulating right atrial thrombi. Am. Heart J. 103:435, 1982.

96. Starkey, I.R., and DeBano, D.P.: Echocardiographic identification of right-sided intracavitary thromboembolus in massive pulmonary thromboembolism. Circulation 66:1322, 1982.

97. Ouyang, P., Camara, E.J., Jain, A., et al.: Intracavitary thrombus in the right heart associated with multiple pulmonary emboli. Chest 84:296, 1983.

98. Spirito, P., Bellotti, P., Chiarella, F., et al.: Right atrial thrombus detected by two-dimensional echocardiography after acute pulmonary embolism. Am. J. Cardiol. 54:467, 1984.

99. Goldberg, S.M., Pizzarello, R.A., Goldman, M.A., et al.: Echocardiographic diagnosis of right atrial thromboembolism resulting in massive pulmonary embolization. Am. Heart J. 108:1371, 1984.

100. Hunter, J.J., Johnson, K.R., Karagianes, T.G., et al.: Detection of massive pulmonary embolus-in-transit by transesophageal echocardiography. Chest 100:1210, 1991.

101. Torbicki, A., Pasierski, T., Uchman, B., and Miskiewicz, Z.: Right atrial mobile thrombi: Two-dimensional echocardiographic diagnosis and clinical outcome. Cor Vasa 29:293, 1987.

102. Pasierski, T.J., Alton, M.E., Van Fossen, D.B., et al.: Right atrial mobile thrombus: Improved visualization by transesophageal echocardiography. Am. Heart J. 123:802, 1992.

103. Obeid, A.I., Mudamgha, A.A., and Smulyan, H.: Diagnosis of right atrial mass lesions by transesophageal and transthoracic echocardiography. Chest 103:1447, 1993.

104. Stowers, S.A., Leiboff, R.H., Wasserman, A.G., et al.: Right ventricular thrombus formation in association with acute myocardial infarction: Diagnosis by 2-dimensional echocardiography. Am. J. Cardiol. 52:912, 1983.

105. Wiseman, M.N., Giles, M.S., and Camm, A.J.: Unusual echocardiographic appearance of intracardiac thrombi in a patient with endomyocardial fibrosis. Br. Heart J. 56:179, 1986.

106. Kessler, K.M., Mallon, S.M., Bolooki, H., et al.: Pedunculated right ventricular thrombus due to repeated blunt chest trauma. Am. Heart. J. 102:1064, 1981.

107. Woolridge, J.D., and Healey, J.: Echocardiographic diagnosis of right ventricular thromboembolism. Am. Heart J. 106:590, 1983.

108. Evans, B.H., and Maurer, G.: Echocardiographic diagnosis of pulmonary embolus. Am. Heart J. 120:1236, 1990.

109. Gabrielsen, F., Schmidt, A., Eggeling, T., et al.: Massive main pulmonary artery embolism diagnosed with two-dimensional echocardiography. Clin. Cardiol. 15:545, 1992.

110. Johnson, M.E., Furlong, R., and Schrank, K.: Diagnostic use of emergency department echocardiogram in massive pulmonary emboli. Ann. Emerg. Med. 21:760, 1992.

111. Zaidi, S.J.: Two-dimensional echocardiographic detection of asymptomatic pulmonary thromboembolism. Echocardiography 9:17, 1992.

112. Klein, A.L., Stewart, W.C., Cosgrove, D.M., III, et al.: Visualization of acute pulmonary emboli by transesophageal echocardiography. J. Am. Soc. Echocardiogr. 3:412, 1990.

113. Guindo, J., Montagud, M., Carreras, F., et al.: Fibrinolytic therapy for superior vena cava and right atrial thrombosis: Diagnosis and follow-up with biplane transesophageal echocardiography. Am. Heart J. 124:510, 1992.

114. Popovic, A.D., Milovanovic, B., Neskovic, A.N., et al.: Detection of massive pulmonary embolism by transesophageal echocardiography. Cardiology 80:94, 1992.

115. Jordan, N.A., Scheifly, C.H., and Edwards, J.E.: Mural thrombus and arterial embolism in mitral stenosis. Circulation 3:363, 1951.

116. Schweizer, P., Bardos, P., Erbel, R., et al.: Detection of left atrial thrombi by echocardiography. Br. Heart J. 45:148, 1981.

117. Herzog, C.A., Bass, K., Kane, M., et al.: Two-dimensional echocardiographic imaging of left atrial appendage thrombi. J. Am. Coll. Cardiol. 3:1340, 1984.

118. Hsu, T.L., Chen, C.C., Chen, C.Y., et al.: Two-dimensional echocardiographic features of floating left atrial thrombus. Am. J. Cardiol. 57:701, 1986.

119. Tabak, S.W., and Maurer, G.: Echocardiographic detection of free-floating left atrial thrombus. Am. J. Cardiol. 53:374, 1984.

120. Gottdiener, J.S., Temeck, B.K., Patterson, R.H., et al.: Transient ("hole-in-one") occlusion of the mitral valve orifice by a free-floating left atrial ball thrombus: Identification by two-dimensional echocardiography. Am. J. Cardiol. 53:1730, 1984.

121. Wrisley, D., Giambartolomei, A., Lee, T., et al.: Left atrial ball thrombus: Review of clinical and echocardiographic manifestations with suggestions for management. Am. Heart J. 121:1784, 1991.

122. Hwang J.-J., Kuan, P., Lin S.-C., et al.: Reappraisal by transesophageal echocardiography of the significance of left atrial thrombi in the prediction of systemic arterial embolization in rheumatic mitral valve disease. Am. J. Cardiol. 70:769, 1992.

123. Manning, W.J., Reis, G.J., and Douglas, P.S.: Use of transesophageal echocardiography to detect left atrial thrombi before percutaneous balloon dilation of the mitral valve: A prospective study. Br. Heart J. 67:170, 1992.

124. Olson, J.D., Goldenberg, I.F., Pedersen, W., et al.: Exclusion of atrial thrombus by transesophageal echocardiography. J. Am. Soc. Echocardiogr. 5:52, 1992.

125. Grimm, R.A., Stewart, W.J., Black, I.W., et al.: Should all patients undergo transesophageal echocardiography before electrical cardioversion of atrial fibrillation? J. Am. Coll. Cardiol. 23:533, 1994.

126. Kronzon, I., Tunick, P.A., Glassman, E., et al.: Transesophageal echocardiography to detect atrial clots in candidates for percutaneous transseptal mitral balloon valvuloplasty. J. Am. Coll. Cardiol. 16:1320, 1990.

127. Feltes, T.F., and Friedman, R.A.: Transesophageal echocardiographic detection of atrial thrombi in patients with nonfibrillation atrial tachyarrhythmias and congenital heart disease. J. Am. Coll. Cardiol. 24:1365, 1994.

128. Bansal, R.C., Heywood, J.T., Applegate, P.M., et al.: Detection of left atrial thrombi by two-dimensional echocardiography and surgical correlation in 148 patients with mitral valve disease. Am. J. Cardiol. 64:243, 1989.

129. Herzog, C.A., Bass, D., Kane, M., et al.: Two-dimensional echocardiographic imaging of left atrial appendage thrombi. J. Am. Coll. Cardiol. 3:1340, 1984.

130. Aschenberg, W., Schluter, M., Kremer, P., et al.: Transesophageal two-dimensional echocardiography for the detection of left atrial appendage thrombus. J. Am. Coll. Cardiol. 7:163, 1986.

131. Taams, M.A., Gussenhoven, E.J., and Lancee, C.T.: Left atrial vascularised thrombus diagnosed by transesophageal cross-sectional echocardiography. Br. Heart J. 58:669, 1987.

132. Brickner, M.E., Friedman, D.B., Cigarroa, C.G., et al.: Relation of thrombus in the left atrial appendage by transesophageal echocardiography to clinical risk factors for thrombus formation. Am. J. Cardiol. 74:39, 1994.

133. Green, S.E., Joynt, L.F., Fitzgerald, P.J., et al.: In vivo ultrasonic tissue characterization of human intracardiac masses. Am. J. Cardiol. 51:231, 1983.

134. McPherson, D.D., Knosp, B.M., Kieso, R.A., et al.: Ultrasound characterization of acoustic properties of acute intracardiac thrombi: Studies in a new experimental model. J. Am. Soc. Echocardiogr. 1:254, 1988.

135. Mikell, F.L., Asinger, R.W., Elsperger, K.J., et al.: Tissue acoustic properties of fresh left ventricular thrombi and visualization by two dimensional echocardiography: Experimental observations. Am. J. Cardiol. 49:1157, 1982.

136. Merino, A., Hauptman, P., Badimon, L., et al.: Echocardiographic "smoke" is produced by an interaction of erythrocytes and plasma proteins modulated by shear forces. J. Am. Coll. Cardiol. 20:1661, 1992.

137. Leung, D.Y.C., Black, I.W., Cranney, G.B., et al.: Prognostic implications of left

atrial spontaneous echo contrast in nonvalvular atrial fibrillation. J. Am. Coll. Cardiol. 24:755, 1994.

138. Castello, R., Pearson, A.C., and Labovitz, A.J.: Prevalence and clinical implications of atrial spontaneous contrast in patients undergoing transesophageal echocardiography. Am. J. Cardiol. 65:1149, 1990.

139. Black, I.W., Hopkins, A.P., Lee, L.C.L., et al.: Left atrial spontaneous echo contrast: A clinical and echocardiographic analysis. J. Am. Coll. Cardiol. 18:398, 1991.

140. Daniel, W.G., Nellessen, U., Schröder, E., et al.: Left atrial spontaneous echo contrast in mitral valve disease: An indicator for an increased thromboembolic risk. J. Am. Coll. Cardiol. 11:1204, 1988.

141. Erbel, R., Stern, H., Ehrenthal, W., et al.: Detection of spontaneous echocardiographic contrast within the left atrium by transesophageal echocardiography. Clin. Cardiol. 9:245, 1986.

142. Blanchard, D.G., and Dittrich, H.C.: Problems and pitfalls. In Dittrich, H.C. (ed.): Clinical Transesophageal Echocardiography. St. Louis, Mosby–Year Book, 1992.

143. Mahony, C., Sublett, K.L., and Harrison, M.R.: Resolution of spontaneous contrast with platelet disaggregatory therapy (trifluoperizine). Am. J. Cardiol. 63:1009, 1989.

144. Hoffman, R., Lambertz, H., Kreis, A., et al.: Failure of trifluoperizine to resolve spontaneous echo contrast evaluated by transesophageal echocardiography. Am. J. Cardiol. 66:648, 1990.

145. Chin, W.W., VanTosh, A., Hecht, S.R., et al.: Left ventricular thrombus with normal left ventricular function in ulcerative colitis. Am. Heart J. 116:562, 1988.

146. Keating, E.C., Gross S.A., Schlamowitz, R.A., et al.: Mural thrombi in myocardial infarctions: Prospective evaluations by two-dimensional echocardiography. Am. J. Med. 74:989, 1983.

147. Asinger, R.W., Mikell, F.L., Elsperger, J., et al.: Incidence of left ventricular thrombosis after acute transmural myocardial infarction: Serial evaluation by two-dimensional echocardiography. N. Engl. J. Med. 305:297, 1981.

148. Visser, C.A., Kan, G., David, G.K., et al.: Two-dimensional echocardiography in the diagnosis of left ventricular thrombus: A prospective study of 67 patients with anatomic validation. Chest 83:228, 1983.

149. Reeder, G.S., Lengyel, M., Tajik, A.J., et al.: Mural thrombus in left ventricular aneurysm: Incidence, role of angiography, and relation between anticoagulation and embolization. Mayo Clin. Proc. 56:77, 1981.

150. Dubnow, M.H., Burchell, H.B., and Titus, J.L.: Post-infarction ventricular aneurysm: A clinicopathologic and electrocardiographic study of 80 cases. Am. Heart J. 70:753, 1965.

151. Abrams, D.L., Edelist, A., Luria, M.H., et al.: Ventricular aneurysm: A reappraisal based on a study of sixty-five consecutive autopsied cases. Circulation 27:164, 1965.

152. Weinreich, D.J., Burke, J.F., and Pauletto, F.J.: Left ventricular mural thrombi complicating acute myocardial infarction: Long-term follow-up serial echocardiographically. Ann. Intern. Med. 100:789, 1984.

153. Arvan, S.: Mural thrombi in coronary artery disease. Recent advances in pathogenesis, diagnosis and approaches to treatment. Arch. Intern. Med. 144:13, 1984.

154. DeMaria, A.N., Bommer, W., Neumann. A., et al.: Left ventricular thrombi identified by cross-sectional echocardiography. Ann. Intern. Med. 90:14, 1979.

155. Meltzer, R.S., Visser, C.A., Kan, G., et al.: Two-dimensional echocardiographic appearance of left ventricular thrombi with systemic emboli after myocardial infarction. Am. J. Cardiol. 53:1511, 1984.

156. Takamoto, T., Kim, D., Murie, P., et al.: Comparative recognition of left ventricular thrombi by echocardiography and cineangiography. Br. Heart J. 53:36, 1985.

157. Stratton, J.R., Lighty, G.W., Pearlman, A.S., et al.: Detection of left ventricular thrombi by two-dimensional echocardiography: Sensitivity specificity, and causes of uncertainty. Circulation 66:156, 1982.

158. Visser, C.A., Kan, G., Meltzer, R.S., et al.: Embolic potential of left ventricular thrombus after myocardial infarction: A two-dimensional echocardiographic study of 199 patients. J. Am. Coll. Cardiol. 5:1276, 1985.

159. Asinger, R.W., Midell, F.L., Sharma, B., et al.: Observations on detecting left ventricular thrombus with two-dimensional echocardiography: Emphasis on avoidance of false-positive diagnosis. Am. J. Cardiol. 47:145, 1981.

160. Veterans Administration Cooperative Study Group: Anticoagulants in acute myocardial infarction: Results of a cooperative clinical trial. J.A.M.A. 225:724, 1973.

161. DeGroat, T.S., Parameswaran, R., Popper, R.M., et al.: Left ventricular thrombi in association with normal left ventricular wall motion in patients with malignancy. Am. J. Cardiol. 56:827, 1985.

162. Haugland, J.M., Asinger, R.W., Mikell, F.L., et al.: Embolic potential of left ventricular thrombi detected by two-dimensional echocardiography. Circulation 70:588, 1984.

163. Meltzer, R.S., Visser, C.A., and Fuster, V.: Intracardiac thrombi and systemic embolization. Ann. Intern. Med. 104:689, 1986.

164. Stratton, J.R., Nemanich, J.W., Johannessen, K.A., et al.: Fate of left ventricular thrombi in patients with remote myocardial infarction or idiopathic cardiomyopathy. Circulation 78:1388, 1988.

165. McAllister, H.A., and Fenoglio, J.J.: Tumors of the cardiovascular system. In Atlas of Tumor Pathology. Washington, D.C., Armed Forces Institute of Pathology, Fascicle 15, Series 2, 1978, p.1.

166. Heath, D.: Pathology of cardiac tumors. Am. J. Cardiol. 21:315, 1968.

167. Roberts, W.C., Glancy, D.L., and DeVita, V.T.: Heart in malignant lymphoma (Hodgkin's disease, lymphosarcoma, reticulum cell sarcoma and mycosis fungoides): A study of 196 autopsy cases. Am. J. Cardiol. 22:85, 1968.

168. Glancy, D.L., and Roberts, W.C.: The heart in malignant melanoma: A study of 70 autopsy cases. Am. J. Cardiol. 21:555, 1968.

169. Roberts, W.C., Bouley, C.P., and Wertlake, P.T.: The heart in acute leukemia: A study of 420 autopsy cases. Am. J. Cardiol. 21:388, 1968.

170. Lagrange, J.-L., Despins, P., Spielman, M., et al.: Cardiac metastasis: Case report on an isolated cardiac metastasis of a myxoid liposarcoma. Cancer 58:2333, 1986.

171. Itoh, K., Matsubara, T., Yanagisawa, K., et al.: Right ventricular metastasis of cervical squamous cell carcinoma. Am. Heart J. 108:1369, 1984.

172. Riggs, T., Paul, M.H., DeLeon, S., and Ilbawi, M.: Two-dimensional echocardiography in evaluation of right atrial masses: Five cases in pediatric patients. Am. J. Cardiol. 48:961, 1981.

173. Hanfling, S.M.: Metastatic cancer to the heart. Circulation 22:474, 1960.

174. Goodwin, J.F.: The spectrum of cardiac tumors. Am. J. Cardiol. 21:307, 1968.

175. Kralstein, J., and Frishman, W.: Malignant pericardial diseases: Diagnosis and treatment. Am. Heart J. 113:785, 1987.

176. Canedo, M.I., Otken, L., and Stefadouros, M.A.: Echocardiographic features of cardiac compression by a thymoma simulating cardiac tamponade and obstruction of the superior vena cava. Br. Heart J. 39:1038, 1977.

177. Yoshikawa, J., Sabah, I., and Yanagihara, K.: Cross-sectional echocardiographic diagnosis of a large left atrial tumor and extracardiac tumor compressing the left atrium. Am. J. Cardiol 42:853, 1978.

178. Shah, A., and Schwartz, H.: Echocardiographic features of cardiac compression by mediastinal pancreatic pseudocyst. Chest 77:440, 1980.

179. Chandraratna, P.A.N., Littman, B.B., Serafini, A., et al.: Echocardiographic evaluation of extracardiac masses. Br. Heart J. 40:741, 1978.

180. Faletra, F., Ravini, M., Moreo, A., et al.: Transesophageal echocardiography in the evaluation of cardiac masses. J. Am. Soc. Echocardiogr. 5:178, 1992.

181. Breall, J.A., Goldberger, A.L., Warren, S.E., et al.: Posterior mediastinal masses: Rare causes of cardiac compression. Am. Heart J. 124:523, 1992.

182. Gottdiener, J.S., and Maron, B.J.: Posterior cardiac displacement by anterior mediastinal tumor. Chest 77:784, 1980.

183. Percy, R.F., Conetta, D.A., and Miller, A.B.: Esophageal compression of the heart presenting as an extracardiac mass on echocardiography. Chest 85:826, 1984.

184. Lestuzzi, C., Nicolosi, G.L., Mirno, R., et al.: Usefulness of transesophageal echocardiography in evaluation of paracardiac neoplastic masses. Am. J. Cardiol. 70:247, 1992.

185. D'Cruz, I.A., Feghali, N., and Gross, C.M.: Echocardiographic manifestations of mediastinal masses compressing or encroaching on the heart. Echocardiography 11:523, 1994.

186. Borgren, H.C., DeMaria, A.N., and Mason, D.T.: Imaging procedures in the detection of cardiac tumors with emphasis on echocardiography: A review. Cardiovasc. Intervent. Radiol. 3:107, 1980.

187. Errichetti, A., and Weyman, A.E.: Cardiac tumors and masses. In Weyman, A.E. (ed.): Principles and Practice of Echocardiography. 2nd ed. Philadelphia, Lea & Febiger, 1994.

188. Salcedo, E.E., Cohen, G.I., White, R.D., et al.: Cardiac tumors: Diagnosis and management. Curr. Probl. Cardiol. 17:79, 1992.

189. Griffiths, G.D.: A review of primary tumors of the heart. Prog. Cardiovasc. Dis. 7:465, 1965.

190. Meller, J., Teichholz, L.E., Pichard, A.D., et al.: Left ventricular myxoma: Echocardiographic diagnosis and review of the literature. Am. J. Med. 63:816, 1977.

191. Peters, M.N., Hall, R.J., Cooley, D.A., et al.: The clinical syndrome of atrial myxomas. JAMA 230:695, 1974.

192. Synder, S.N., Smith, D.C., Lau, F.Y., et al.: Diagnostic feature of right ventricular myxoma. Am. Heart J. 91:240, 1976.

193. Hudson, R.E.B.: Cardiovascular Pathology. London, Edward Arnold, 1965.

194. Aldridge, H.E., and Greenwood, W.F.: Myxoma of the left atrium. Br. Heart J. 22:189, 1960.

195. Rees, J.R., Ross, F.G.M., and Keen, G.: Lentiginosis and left atrial myxoma. Br. Heart J. 35:874, 1973.

196. Carney, J.A., Gordon, H., Carpenter, P.C., et al.: The complex of myxomas, spotty pigmentation and endocrine overactivity. Medicine (Baltimore) 64:270, 1985.

197. McCarthy, P.M., Piehler, J.M., Schaff, H.V., et al.: The significance of multiple, recurrent, and "complex" cardiac myxomas. J. Thorac. Cardiovasc. Surg. 91:389, 1986.

198. Farah, M.G.: Familial atrial myxoma. Ann. Intern. Med. 83:358, 1975.

199. Gosse, P., Herpin, D., Roudault, R., et al.: Myxoma of the mitral valve diagnosed by echocardiography. Am. Heart J. 111:803, 1986.

200. Suri, R.K., Pattnkar, V.L., Singh, H., et al.: Myxoma of the tricuspid valve. Aust. N.Z. J. Surg. 48:429, 1978.

201. Devig, P.M., Clark, T.A., and Aron, B.L.: Cardiac myxoma arising from the inferior vena cava. Chest 78:784, 1980.

202. St. John Sutton, M.G., Mercier, L.A., Giuliani, E.R., et al.: Atrial myxomas: A review of clinical experience in 40 patients. Mayo Clin. Proc. 55:371, 1980.

203. Smellie, H.: Myxoma of the left atrium. Proc. R. Soc. Med. 55:226, 1962.

204. Lee, Y.C., and Magran, M.Y.: Nonprolapsing left atrial tumor: The M-mode echocardiographic diagnosis. Chest 78:332, 1980.

205. Goodwin, J.F.: Diagnosis of left atrial myxoma. Lancet 1:464, 1963.

206. Malekzadeh, S., and Roberts, W.C.: Growth rate of left atrial myxoma. Am. J. Cardiol. 64:1075, 1989.

207. Hake, U., Iversen, S., Schmidt, F., et al.: Urgent indications for surgery in primary or secondary cardiac neoplasm. Scand. J. Thorac. Cardiovasc. Surg. 23:111, 1989.

208. Bortolotti, U., Maraglino, G., Rubino, M., et al.: Surgical excision of intracardiac myxomas: A 20-year follow-up. Ann. Thorac. Surg. 49:449, 1990.

209. Nazer, Y.A., Iyer, K.S., Kaul, U., et al.: Surgical experience with intracardiac myxomas. Int. J. Cardiol. 18:371, 1988.

210. Obeid, A.I., Marvasti, M., Parker, F., et al.: Comparison of transthoracic and

transesophageal echocardiography in diagnosis of left atrial myxoma. Am. J. Cardiol. 63:1006, 1989.

211. Reeves, W.C., and Chitwood, W.R., Jr.: Assessment of left atrial myxoma using transesophageal two-dimensional echocardiography and color flow Doppler. Echocardiography 6:547, 1989.

212. Goli, V.D., Thadani, U., Thomas, S.R., et al.: Doppler echocardiographic profiles in obstructive right and left atrial myxomas. J. Am. Coll. Cardiol. 9:701, 1987.

213. Gorcsan, J., III, Blanc, M.S., Reddy, P.S., et al.: Hemodynamic diagnosis of mitral valve obstruction by left atrial myxoma with transesophageal continuous wave Doppler. Am. Heart J. 124:1109, 1992.

214. Fenoglio, J.J., McAllister, H.A., and Fernas, V.J.: Cardiac rhabdomyoma: A clinicopathologic and electron microscopic study. Am. J. Cardiol. 38:241, 1976.

215. Corno, A., deSimone, G., Catena, G., et al.: Cardiac rhabdomyoma: Surgical treatment in the neonate. J. Thorac. Cardiovasc. Surg. 87:725, 1984.

216. Murphy, M.C., Sweeney, M.S., Putnam, J.B., et al.: Surgical treatment of cardiac tumors: A 25-year experience: Discussion. Ann. Thorac. Surg. 49:612, 1990.

217. Smythe, J.F., Dick, J.D., Smallhorn, J.F., et al.: Natural history of cardiac rhabdomyoma in infancy and childhood. Am. J. Cardiol. 66:1247, 1990.

218. Biancaniello, T.M., Meyer, R.A., Gaum, W.E., et al.: Primary benign intramural ventricular tumors in children: Pre- and postoperative electrocardiographic, echocardiographic, and angiocardiographic evaluation. Am. Heart J. 103:852, 1982.

219. Burke, A.P., Rosado-de-Christenson, M., Templeton, P.A., et al.: Cardiac fibroma: Clinicopathologic correlates and surgical treatment. J. Thorac. Cardiovasc. Surg. 108:862, 1994.

220. deRuiz, M., Potter, J.L., and Stavinoha, J.: Real-time ultrasound diagnosis of cardiac fibroma in a neonate. J. Ultrasound Med. 4:367, 1985.

221. Parmley, L.F., Salley, R.K., Williams, J.P., et al.: The clinical spectrum of cardiac fibroma with diagnostic and surgical considerations: Noninvasive imaging enhances management. Ann. Thorac. Surg. 45:455, 1988.

222. Reul, G.J., Howell, J.F., Rubio, P.A., et al.: Successful partial excision of an intramural fibroma of the left ventricle. Am. J. Cardiol. 36:262, 1975.

223. Oliva, P.B., Breckinridge, J.C., Johnson, M.L., et al.: Left ventricular outflow obstruction produced by a pedunculated fibroma in a newborn: Clinical, angiographic, echocardiographic, and surgical observations. Chest 74:590, 1978.

224. Geha, A.S., Weidman, W.H., Soule, E.H., et al.: Intramural ventricular cardiac fibroma: Successful removal in two cases and review of the literature. Circulation 36:420, 1967.

225. Takahashi, K., Imamura, Y., Ochi, T., et al.: Echocardiographic demonstration of an asymptomatic patient with left ventricular fibroma. Am. J. Cardiol. 53:981, 1984.

226. Keren, A., Takamoto, T., Harrison, D.C., et al.: Left ventricular apical masses: Noninvasive differentiation of rare from common ones. Am. J. Cardiol. 56:697, 1985.

227. Brown, I.W., McGoldrick, J.P., Robles, A., et al.: Left ventricular fibroma: Echocardiographic diagnosis and successful surgical excision in three cases. J. Cardiovasc. Surg. 31:536, 1990.

228. Shub, C., Tajik, A.J., Seward, J.B., et al.: Cardiac papillary fibroelastomas. Two-dimensional echocardiographic recognition. Mayo Clin. Proc. 56:629, 1981.

229. Ong, L.S., Nanda, N.C., and Barold, S.S.: Two dimensional echocardiographic detection and diagnostic features of left ventricular papillary fibroelastoma. Am. Heart J. 103:917, 1982.

230. Almagro, U.A., Perry, L.S., Choi, H., et al.: Papillary fibroelastoma of the heart. Report of six cases. Arch. Pathol. Lab. Med. 106:318, 1982.

231. Topol, E.J., Biern, R.O., and Reitz, B.A.: Cardiac papillary fibroelastoma and stroke. Am. J. Med. 80:129, 1986.

232. Fowles, R.E., Miller, D.C., Fitzgerald, J.W., et al.: Systemic embolization from a mitral valve papillary endocardial fibroma detected by two-dimensional echocardiography. Am. Heart J. 102:128, 1981.

233. Esteves, J.M., Thompson, D.S., and Levinson, J.P.: Lipoma of the heart: A review of the literature and report of two autopsied cases. Arch. Pathol. 77:638, 1964.

234. Olsen, R.E., and Tangchai, P.: Large lipoma of the left ventricle. Arch. Pathol. 72:58, 1961.

235. James, T.N.: Fatal electrical instability of the heart associated with benign congenital polycystic tumour of the atrioventricular node. Circulation 58:667, 1977.

236. Schnittger, I.: Cardiac and Extracardiac Masses: Echocardiographic Evaluation. In Marcus, M.L., Schelbert, H.R., Skorton, D.J., and Wolf, G.L. (eds.): Cardiac Imaging. Philadelphia, W.B. Saunders, 1991.

237. Denos, M., Brochet, E., Cristofini, P., et al.: Polyvisceral echinococcosis with cardiac involvement imaged by two-dimensional echocardiography, computed tomography and nuclear magnetic resonance imaging. Am. J. Cardiol. 59:383, 1987.

238. Picchio, E., Giovannini, E., Siolari, F., et al.: Cardiac echinococcosis. Two dimensional echocardiographic diagnosis. G. Ital. Cardiol. 11:1327, 1981.

239. Limacher, M.C., McEntee, C.W., Attar, M., et al.: Cardiac echinococcal cyst: Diagnosis by two dimensional echocardiography. J. Am. Coll. Cardiol. 3:574, 1983.

240. Oliver, J.M., Benito, L.P., Ferrufino, O., et al.: Cardiac hydatid cyst diagnosed by two-dimensional echocardiography. Am. Heart J. 104:164, 1982.

241. Rey, M., Alfonso, F., Torricella, E.G., et al.: Diagnostic value of two-dimensional echocardiography in cardiac hydatid disease. Eur. Heart J. 12:1300, 1991.

242. McAllister, H.A., Jr.: Primary tumors and cysts of the heart and pericardium. Curr. Probl. Cardiol. 4:1, 1979.

243. Feigin, D.S., Fenoglio, J.J., McAllister, H.A., et al.: Pericardial cysts: A radiologic-pathologic correlation and review. Radiology 125:15, 1977.

244. Wychulis, A.R., Connolly, D.C., and McGoon, D.C.: Pericardial cysts, tumors, and fat necrosis. J. Thorac. Cardiovasc. Surg. 62:294, 1971.

245. Janigan, D.T., Husain, A., and Robinson, N.A.: Cardiac angiosarcomas: A review and a case report. Cancer 57:852, 1986.

246. Strobl, K.P.: Angiosarcoma of the heart. Arch. Intern. Med. 136:928, 1976.

247. Hui, K.S., Green, L.K., and Schmidt, W.A.: Primary cardiac rhabdomyosarcoma: Definition of a rare entity. Am. J. Cardiovasc. Pathol. 2:19, 1988.

248. Chou, S.T., Arkles, L.B., Gill, G.D., et al.: Primary lymphoma of the heart: A case report. Cancer 52:744, 1983.

249. Gelman, K.M., Ben-Ezra, J.M., Steinschneider, M., et al.: Lymphoma with primary cardiac manifestations. Am. Heart J. 111:808, 1986.

250. Duncan, W.J., Rowe, R.D., and Freedom, R.M.: Space-occupying lesions of the myocardium: Role of two-dimensional echocardiography in detection of cardiac tumors in children. Am. Heart J. 104:780, 1982.

251. Ludomirsky, A., Vargo, T.A., Murphy, D.J., et al.: Intracardiac undifferentiated sarcoma in infancy. J. Am. Coll. Cardiol. 6:1362, 1985.

252. Mich, R.J., Gillam, L.D., and Weyman, A.E.: Osteogenic sarcomas mimicking left atrial myxomas: Clinical and two-dimensional echocardiographic features. J. Am. Coll. Cardiol. 6:1422, 1985.

253. Caralis, D.G., Kennedy, H.L., Bailey, I., et al.: Primary right cardiac tumor. Detection by echocardiographic and radiotopic studies. Chest 77:100, 1980.

254. Lin, T.U., Stech, J.M., Ecbert, W.G., et al.: Pericardial angiosarcoma simulating pericardial effusion by echocardiography. Chest 73:881, 1978.

255. Shih, W.-J., McCullough, S., and Smith, M.: Diagnostic imagings for primary cardiac fibrosarcoma. Int. J. Cardiol. 39:157, 1993.

CHAPTER

35 Myocardial Perfusion and Other Applications of Contrast Echocardiography

Sanjiv Kaul, M.D.

CONTRAST AGENTS AND ECHOCARDIOGRAPHIC
    SYSTEMS ___ 481
ASSESSMENT OF MYOCARDIAL
    PERFUSION ___ 485
Detection of Acute Myocardial Infarction and
    Estimation of Risk Area and Success of
    Reperfusion ___ 485

Determination of Myocardial
    Viability After Acute Myocardial
    Infarction ___ 486
Quantification of Myocardial
    Perfusion ___ 489
Assessment of Flow Reserve and Detection of
    Coronary Artery Stenosis ___ 494

Intraoperative Assessment of the Myocardial Distribution of Cardioplegia and Success of Bypass Graft Placement ____ 495
Assessment of Microvascular Function ____ 498
NONMYOCARDIAL APPLICATIONS ____ 499
Intracardiac and Extracardiac Shunts ____ 499

Doppler Signal Enhancement ____ 499
Regional and Global Left Ventricular Function ____ 501
Miscellaneous Uses ____ 501
SUMMARY ____ 501

This flow of creation, from where did it arise
Whether it was ordered or was not,
He, the Observer, in the highest heaven,
He alone knows, unless . . . He knows it not.

From the Rig-Veda, 3000 BC

Used as a diagnostic technique since it was first described in 1968,[1] contrast echocardiography is based on the principle that gas-containing microbubbles introduced into the cardiac chambers, great vessels, or coronary circulation will result in contrast enhancement of these regions during simultaneously performed ultrasound examination. This chapter discusses contrast echocardiography under three major categories: (1) contrast agents and echocardiographic equipment, (2) assessment of myocardial perfusion, and (3) nonmyocardial applications.

CONTRAST AGENTS AND ECHOCARDIOGRAPHIC SYSTEMS

The contrast effect seen on echocardiography is based on the liquid-gas interface provided by bubbles that act as scatterers of ultrasound, causing opacification when they enter cardiac chambers or the coronary microcirculation. Microbubbles produced in almost any innocuous and biologically inert liquid medium can be used as a contrast agent. The differences among contrast agents are related to the size, stability, and concentration of the bubbles.

For the initial animal studies aimed at defining myocardial perfusion, the bubbles used were relatively large and were made with nonstandardized procedures such as hand agitation[2] and chemical reactions with blood.[3] Although these bubbles produced excellent opacification, their size and toxicity precluded their use in humans. One of the early attempts at standardizing microbubble size and concentration was the technique of sonication, in which high-energy sound transforms the air within liquid media into microbubbles.[4] Although bubbles were produced in different media with the use of this technique,[4] two important limitations remained: longevity of the bubbles and the toxicity of the liquids in which they were produced. The life of the microbubbles was too short (seconds to minutes) for them to be of major use in the clinical setting,[4] and the liquids in which they were prepared, such as dextrose solutions or iodinated radiopaque contrast agents, were relatively toxic. Thus, the intracoronary injection of microbubbles produced in these media caused significant, albeit transient, changes in coronary and systemic hemodynamics as well as in coronary blood flow.[5, 6] Importantly, however, it was demonstrated that the hemodynamic effects noted were due to the toxic effects of the liquids themselves and were not related to the introduction of microbubbles of air.[6, 7]

These limitations were overcome with the sonication of 5 percent human albumin solutions, which produce no changes in coronary or systemic hemodynamics when injected directly as a small bolus into the coronary arteries.[8, 9] The production of heat during sonication also denatures proteins that form a shell around the bubbles,[10] thus prolonging their shelf life for up to 2 years if they are refrigerated.[10] This shell is 15 nm thick and is composed of insoluble denatured human albumin with intermolecular disulfide bonds.[11]

When injected intravenously, these microbubbles are entrapped mostly within the reticuloendothelial system of the liver (Kupffer cells) after their first pass, and 80 percent are cleared from the blood within 2 minutes.[12] In comparison, when injected into pigs, 90 percent of the microbubbles are engulfed by the pulmonary macrophages.[13] Release of histamine by these macrophages may explain the pulmonary hypertension noted when these microbubbles are injected into pigs.[13] Humans and rats do not possess pulmonary macrophages in such numbers.

These sonicated albumin microbubbles are the first commercial product available for contrast echocardiography (Albunex, Molecular Biosystems, Inc., San Diego, CA), although the indication for their clinical use approved by the United States Food and Drug Administration is for left ventricular cavity opacification from a venous injection.[14] When injected directly into the coronary arteries, these microbubbles produce no or minimal coronary and systemic hemodynamic effects in both dogs[15] and humans.[16] In studies that used high-powered microscopic examination of the hamster cheek pouch, the intravascular rheologic characteristics have been demonstrated as similar to those of red blood cells.[17] More recently, the myocardial transit of these microbubbles has also been shown to be similar to that of red blood cells in both the beating canine[18] and human hearts.[19]

Although it is possible to produce myocardial opacification from direct injection of Albunex into the coronary circulation or the aorta,[20] myocardial opacification is not seen consistently when it is injected intravenously, which is related to three main factors affecting the microbubbles: transpulmonary passage, systemic pressures, and concentration in the myocardium.

The effect of transpulmonary passage on the bubbles mainly pertains to two bubble variables: size and gas content. If the bubbles are too large (>10 μm), they get entrapped within the pulmonary circulation, with the pulmonary capillaries acting as a filter. In the case of Albunex, although less than 5 percent of the microbubbles are greater than 10 μm in size, since the reflectance of a bubble is related to the sixth power of the radius,[21] filtering of these bubbles by the lungs causes a greater than twofold decrease in the video intensity of this agent.[22] Similar principles apply to other intravenous contrast agents such as SHU-508A (Levovist, Schering AG Berlin).[23]

The diffusiveness of the gas in the microbubbles also determines their in vivo survival. Since their exposure to blood is prolonged during transpulmonary passage, microbubbles tend to become smaller as these gases escape from the bubbles into the blood, which contains a lower concentration of the same gases. In this regard, air is highly diffusible, and microbubbles containing air are likely to lose part of their reflectance simply because of a decrease in size due to loss of air as they pass through the lungs. Since the reflectance of a bubble is exponentially related to its size,[21] even a small decrease in size can result in a significant decrease in reflectance. Figure 35–1 illustrates the relationship between microbubble size and echocardiographic reflectance. Bubbles containing high molecular weight gases, such as H_2S_6[24] and perfluorocarbons,[25] which are less diffusible, are less likely to undergo significant changes in size during transpulmonary passage and thus retain their original reflectance. The ambient pressure also affects bubbles with diffusible gases, such as Albunex. A decrease in contrast effect is noted within the left ventricular cavity during systole.[26, 27] This effect has not been seen with the newer contrast agents containing high molecular weight gases.

The concentration of microbubbles entering the coronary circulation also determines the degree of myocardial opacification, and

Supported in part by grants from the National Institutes of Health, Bethesda, Maryland (R01-HL48890), and from the American Heart Association, Dallas, Texas, and its Virginia affiliate, Glen Allen. Dr. Kaul is an Established Investigator of the American Heart Association, Dallas, Texas.

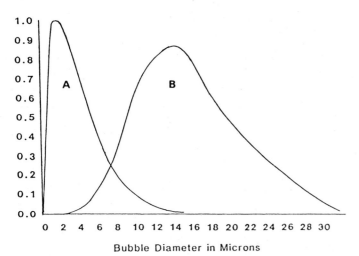

FIGURE 35–1. The relationship between microbubble size (*A*) and reflected power (*B*). Note that the majority of reflected power occurs from the minority of the larger microbubbles. Calculations are based on data from Albers.[21] A = microbubble size distribution αde^{-dk}, where k = 0.5 and average d = 4 µm; B = reflected power $\alpha(de^{-dk})d^6$. (From Kaul, S.: Quantitation of regional myocardial perfusion using myocardial contrast two-dimensional echocardiography. *In* Meerbaum, S., and Meltzer, R. [eds.]: Myocardial Contrast Two-Dimensional Echocardiography. Dordrecht, The Netherlands, Kluwer Academic Publishers, 1989, p. 117, with permission.)

this property is particularly important for venous injections, since at rest only 4 percent of the left ventricular stroke volume enters the coronary circulation. Therefore, the higher the concentration of microbubbles entering the coronary microcirculation, the more likely that myocardial opacification is noted. This principle was proved by demonstrating successful myocardial opacification from venous injections of highly concentrated air-filled albumin microbubbles.[28] When these highly concentrated bubbles were injected during dipyridamole-induced coronary hyperemia, the success rate of myocardial opacification from a venous injection was even higher. Since the percentage of left ventricular stroke volume that enters the coronary circulation during coronary hyperemia is significantly greater than 4 percent (as high as 15 to 20 percent), more microbubbles enter the myocardium and are, therefore, more easily detected on echocardiography.

There are several new agents being developed and tested that are capable of myocardial opacification from a venous injection. These agents are engineered based on some of the principles enumerated earlier. Although none of them are currently approved for human use as a myocardial perfusion agent, their properties will be briefly discussed because they hold promise in this regard.

A second-generation contrast agent (FS-069) manufactured by Molecular Biosystems Inc. consists of albumin microspheres containing perfluoropropane.[29] In closed-chest dogs, 1 to 2 mL of this agent injected intravenously results in consistent myocardial opacification without changing systemic, left-sided heart, or pulmonary hemodynamics. There are no changes noted in pulmonary oxygen exchange, regional myocardial blood flow, or regional wall thickening.[29] This agent is capable of defining the presence of occluded or stenotic coronary arteries when injected intravenously.[30, 31]

A similar agent (Aerosomes, MRX-115) manufactured by ImaRx Pharmaceuticals (Tucson, AZ) also contains perfluoropropane, and the shell of the bubble is a phospholipid with a thickness of 8 nm.[32] The mean microbubble size is 2.5 µm, and it can produce myocardial opacification from a venous injection without any appreciable hemodynamic effects.[32] Another similar agent, Imagent-US, manufactured by Alliance Pharmaceutical Corp. (Costa Mesa, CA), has also been shown to produce myocardial opacification when injected intravenously in dogs.[33]

Another agent (EchoGen) manufactured by Sonus Pharmaceuticals (Bothell, WA) uses phase-shift technology for microbubble formation.[34, 35] When a liquid emulsion of dodecafluoropentane is injected into the body, the liquid is converted into microbubbles of gas at a boiling point of 28.5° C. The persistence of these microbubbles is several thousand–fold greater than that of air-filled bubbles so that myocardial opacification lasts for several minutes to about half an hour after at least 0.6 mL/kg of this agent is injected intravenously.[34, 35] Because it persists in the myocardium after it has disappeared from the left ventricular cavity, this agent overcomes the problem of posterior wall attenuation caused by the presence of contrast material within the left ventricular cavity. Also, because of the same reason, multiple views can be obtained from the same injection. The same property of persistence is also a potential disadvantage and results in significant hemodynamic disturbances at the doses required for myocardial opacification.[34, 35] Both the persistence and hemodynamic disturbances are probably related to the slow transit of these bubbles as they pass through

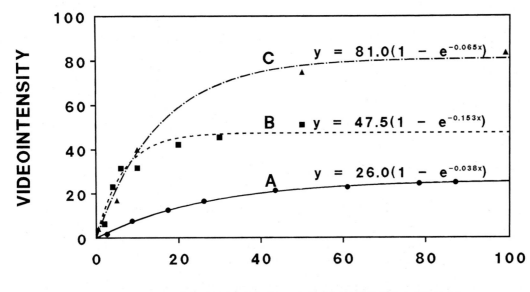

FIGURE 35–2. Relationships between microbubble concentration (*x*-axis) and video intensity (*y*-axis) for three commercially available ultrasound systems (*A* to *C*). The relationships are exponential. (See text for details.) (From Jayaweera, A.R., Skyba, D.M., and Kaul, S.: Technical factors that influence the determination of microbubble transit rate during contrast echocardiography. J. Am. Soc. Echocardiogr. 8:198, 1995, with permission.)

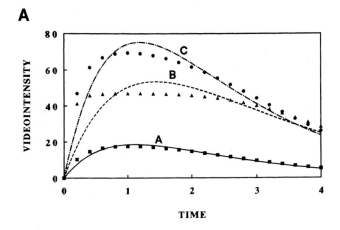

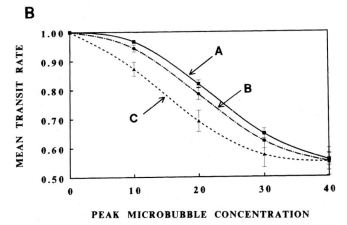

FIGURE 35–3. *A,* Computer-simulated time-intensity plots obtained with the use of the microbubble concentration versus video-intensity relationships shown in Figure 35–2 with a peak microbubble concentration of 30 x 10³/mL. Time to peak was set at 1 second. (See text for details.) *B,* Values for mean microbubble transit rate (with corresponding standard errors) obtained by fitting a γ-variate function to computer-simulated time-intensity data, such as depicted in *A*. The values are obtained at different microbubble concentrations. At higher concentrations, the transit rates deviate from the true value of 1 per second (*A* to *C*). (From Jayaweera, A.R., Skyba, D.M., Kaul, S.: Technical factors that influence the determination of microbubble transit rate during contrast echocardiography. J. Am. Soc. Echocardiogr. 8:198, 1995, with permission.)

the coronary microcirculation.[36] An intravenous injection of the agent can define the risk area during coronary occlusion and infarct size during reperfusion.[37]

In addition to newer contrast agents, engineering modifications of echocardiographic systems are also required to maximize the potential of contrast echocardiography. The two most important modifications pertain to the development of systems with a linear relationship between microbubble concentration and video intensity and systems that can detect microbubbles within the myocardium at concentrations that are generally not detectable with the use of current systems.

Figure 35–2 illustrates the relationship between microbubble concentration and video intensity for three commonly used echocardiographic systems.[38] The saturation level and the rate at which the intensity approaches the saturation level (the exponential factor b) are different for each system. Figure 35–3*A* depicts computer-simulated time-intensity curves from the three echocardiographic systems at a peak microbubble concentration of 30 x 10³/mL with the use of data from Figure 35–2. The plot derived with the use of the microbubble concentration versus video-intensity relationship from system A on the figure provides a reasonably good fit to

a γ-variate function, the plot derived with the use of system B does not provide a good fit to this function, whereas the plot from system C provides an intermediate fit.[38]

Thus, for echocardiographic systems, the concentration of microbubbles in tissue or blood affects their measured mean transit rate (see Fig. 35–3*B*). As can be expected from Figure 35–2, the higher the microbubble concentration, the greater the error in the mean microbubble transit rate. At any given peak concentration, the mean microbubble transit rate derived using system A is the closest to the true mean transit rate (1 per second), that derived from system B is the farthest, and the one using system C is in between.[38]

These findings underscore the importance of a linear relationship between tissue or blood concentration of microbubbles and video intensity. Without such a relationship, mean microbubble transit rate cannot be used to reflect the rheologic character of microbubbles consistently. Although all systems saturate at greater than a certain microbubble concentration (see Fig. 35–2), the longer the relationship between microbubble concentration and video intensity remains linear prior to system saturation, the more likely the time-intensity curve will reflect the true mean microbubble transit rate.

Among the factors that also affect the range over which the relationship between microbubble concentration and video intensity remains linear is the sensitivity of the echocardiographic system. When contrast material is injected into the left atrium to produce myocardial opacification, the transit rate decreases as the dose increases and reaches a plateau at 2 mL of Albunex (Fig. 35–4).[39] The transit rate of a tracer should be independent of the dose injected, and the data in Figure 35–4 indicate that because of low system sensitivity, the time-intensity plots are truncated at lower doses, making the curves narrower and, hence, resulting in an artificial increase in mean transit rates (Fig. 35–5).[39]

Since the sensitivity of the current echocardiographic systems is relatively low, small amounts of microbubbles within the myocardium cannot be visually detected with these systems. Image processing techniques have therefore been used to better demonstrate

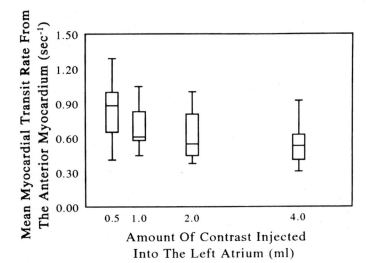

FIGURE 35–4. The relationship between the amount of sonicated albumin microbubbles (Albunex) injected (in milliliters) into the left atrium and the microbubble transit rate obtained from the anterior myocardium. The data are depicted as box plots in which the horizontal line in each box plot denotes the median; the upper and lower margins of the box denote the upper and lower quartiles (levels containing 25 percent of the data above and below the median), whereas the tails depict the upper and lower ranges of the data, respectively. The transit rate decreases exponentially, with "flattening" occurring when the 2-mL dose is exceeded. (From Skyba, D.M., Jayaweera, A.R., Goodman, N.C., et al.: Quantification of myocardial perfusion with myocardial contrast echocardiography during left atrial injection of contrast: Implication for venous injection. Circulation 90:1513, 1994, with permission.)

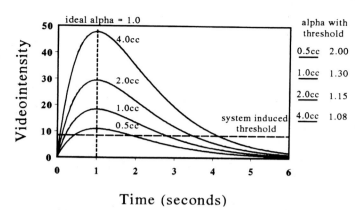

FIGURE 35–5. A diagram depicting the influence of "thresholding" of the echocardiographic system on estimation of mean microbubble transit rate. The ideal alpha is 1 and changes with the dose of contrast material used. With low doses of contrast material and when peak intensity is low, thresholding causes a major overestimation of transit rate, since it makes the curve look narrower. This effect is minimized at higher doses of contrast medium, producing myocardial opacification within the linear range of the system. (From Skyba, D.M., Jayaweera, A.R., Goodman, N.C., et al.: Quantification of myocardial perfusion with myocardial contrast echocardiography during left atrial injection of contrast: Implication for venous injection. Circulation 90:1513, 1994, with permission.)

the presence of microbubbles within the myocardium.[28, 40] Averaging of postcontrast frames and similar precontrast frames has been employed, followed by digital subtraction of the precontrast from the postcontrast averaged image (Fig. 35–6).[28] In Figure 35–6A, contrast medium is seen in the right ventricle and has not yet appeared in the left ventricle. In Figure 35–6B, contrast material is seen in the left ventricular cavity and has resulted in posterior wall attenuation. Subtle opacification is noted in the anterior, medial, and lateral walls. When digital subtraction is performed, the opacification is much more apparent (see Fig. 35–6C). When frames later in the injection sequence are digitally subtracted, the initially attenuated posterior region also demonstrates contrast enhancement (see Fig. 35–6D).[28]

Since the eye can perceive only a limited number of shades of gray but many more hues of color, color coding has also been used

as a means of displaying different levels of contrast within the myocardium.[28, 40] One such approach uses a heated object algorithm whereby a piece of iron placed over a flame successively turns red, orange, yellow, and then white, with these successive colors indicating increasing levels of contrast. Figure 35–7 illustrates the same images as in Figure 35–6 after color coding in which the contrast effect becomes even more visually apparent and is exemplified by the appearance of yellow in the anterior, medial, and lateral walls early after injection (see Fig. 35–7B, which corresponds to Fig. 35–6C). This effect is also noted in the posterior wall after resolution of posterior wall attenuation (see Fig. 35–7C, which corresponds to Figure 35–6D).

FIGURE 35–7. See Color Plate 8.

Although these computer manipulations of images are helpful in displaying video-intensity data that may not be readily apparent visually, more fundamental modifications of the echocardiographic system are required for the detection of small amounts of contrast material within the myocardium, especially after venous injection. Two approaches that are currently being investigated for this purpose seem promising. The first exploits the ability of bubbles to resonate when exposed to ultrasound of a unique frequency, termed the "resonating frequency," which is characteristic of each class of microbubble depending, among other factors, on their size distribution and shell thickness. When these bubbles resonate, in addition to the usual backscatter resulting from the gas-liquid interface (the "first harmonic"), they also generate a frequency of their own at twice the imaging frequency applied.[41] This frequency is unique only to the bubbles and is termed the "second harmonic" frequency. Images obtained with the use of this approach, therefore, utilize signals that emanate only from the microbubbles and can be used to detect very small amounts of microbubbles within tissue that is not affected by noise from the tissue itself.[33]

A second approach uses the ability of the microbubbles to cause a phase shift in the mean imaging frequency, which presumably occurs because of absorption of some of the energy as the sound waves impinge on the bubbles.[42] The mean frequency of the backscatter signal is, therefore, not the same as the imaging frequency.

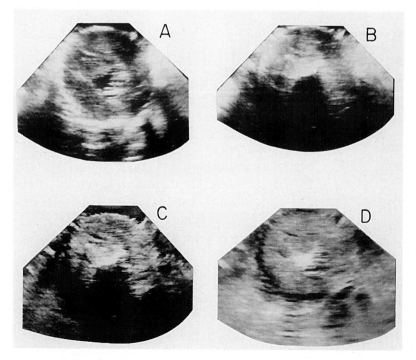

FIGURE 35–6. Echocardiograms after right atrial injection of contrast material in a dog. *A,* Contrast is seen in the right ventricle. *B,* Contrast is seen in the left ventricular cavity, which attenuates the posterior myocardium. The myocardium also shows contrast enhancement. *C,* The image obtained after subtracting *A* from *B.* This subtraction image shows clear myocardial opacification that was not as readily noted in the unsubtracted image (*B*). After a few cycles, when contrast in the left ventricular cavity is not enough to attenuate the posterior wall, a subtraction image still shows homogeneous myocardial opacification. (From Villanueva, F.S., Glasheen, W.P., Sklenar, J., et al.: Successful and reproducible myocardial opacification during two-dimensional echocardiography from right heart injection of contrast. Circulation 85:1557, 1992, with permission.)

Since the phase shift is small, the method of detection has to be sensitive, and thus radiofrequency rather than video-intensity data are used. A fast-Fourier transform is performed in the frequency domain for both the imaging and backscatter ultrasound waves, and these transforms are compared to detect the phase shift.[42]

ASSESSMENT OF MYOCARDIAL PERFUSION

Assessment of myocardial perfusion with contrast echocardiography has gained wider application over the past decade. The initial purpose of these studies was to yield mechanistic information regarding coronary pathophysiology. Given the complexity of coronary pathophysiology, the use of myocardial contrast echocardiography in the clinical setting has heretofore been somewhat slow but has recently increased at a more rapid pace. The advent of venous contrast agents capable of myocardial opacification and the development of new echocardiographic systems will make the use of this technique more common for the assessment of myocardial perfusion. This section discusses the use of contrast echocardiography in the context of coronary artery disease.

Detection of Acute Myocardial Infarction and Estimation of Risk Area and Success of Reperfusion

When a coronary artery is suddenly occluded, such as during acute myocardial infarction, there is an instantaneous decrease of flow through it. The risk area is the zone of the myocardium supplied by the occluded artery, which is likely to undergo necrosis if the occlusion is maintained indefinitely.[43, 44] It is important not to use the terms "perfusion territory of a coronary artery" and "risk area" interchangeably. The former is defined in anatomical terms and is constant in a fully developed heart. It can be defined by contrast echocardiography during injection of contrast material subselectively into the coronary artery at pressures that do not change the hemodynamics within that vessel. Risk area, however, is dynamic and is influenced by the collateral driving pressure.[45, 46] In some instances of chronic coronary artery disease, for example, a large coronary artery may become occluded without any myocardial necrosis or wall motion abnormality. In such cases, the risk area is negligible because of the development of abundant collateral vessels within the myocardium. Thus, the risk area at the time of coronary occlusion can be defined as the zone of the myocardium that is likely to undergo necrosis provided that the hemodynamics in the occluded and remote vessels remain more or less constant during the period of occlusion. In such a case, the risk area can be defined in functional terms as the perfusion territory of the occluded coronary artery minus the region receiving adequate collateral perfusion. The term "adequate" is important, since during coronary occlusion there is seldom zero flow to any region of the myocardium; rather, some level of flow is noted in every segment of the occluded region, with higher flows present in the epicardial and lateral zones. Since necrosis occurs at flows less than or equal to 0.2 to 0.3 mL/g/min,[43, 44] and since at this level of flow microbubbles are generally not detected in the myocardium when injected proximal to the site of occlusion,[47] the functional risk area by contrast echocardiography is usually well defined in the canine model as the region not showing any opacification (Fig. 35–8).[48–51]

When extensive collateral flow is present, such as in patients with chronic coronary artery disease, a pattern of contrast enhancement different from that noted in dogs is seen.[52–54] Figure 35–9 illustrates images from a patient with a recent inferior myocardial infarction and an occluded right coronary artery.[52] Immediately after injection of contrast material into the left main artery, a hypoperfused zone with clearly defined borders (see Fig. 35–8A) is noted. After a few beats, however, contrast material begins to appear within this hypoperfused zone, which slowly fills almost completely and denotes collateral perfusion. Because this patient had a myocardial infarction, the level of collateral flow obviously was not adequate to prevent necrosis. Furthermore, since it took longer for the contrast material to appear in the occluded bed when compared with the normal bed, the collateral flow to the occluded bed was significantly lower than that to the normal bed (see the discussion of the relationship between myocardial microbubble transit rate and blood flow further on). Thus, it is probably prudent to define the risk area in this patient as the region with hypoperfusion in the first frame with contrast enhancement (see Fig. 35–8A) rather than a later frame (see Fig. 35–8B). This area includes the perfusion bed of the occluded vessel minus the most developed collaterals that are present in the lateral borders.

There has been both controversy and confusion regarding the lateral borders of risk areas. Since myocardial capillaries are end

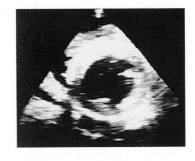
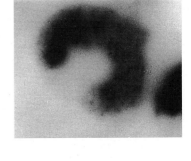
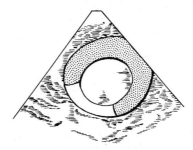
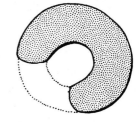

A Contrast Echocardiography   **B** Technetium Autoradiography

FIGURE 35–8. The demonstration of risk area by myocardial contrast echocardiography (A), which corresponds to that measured by technetium autoradiography (B). (From Kaul, S., Pandian, N.G., Okada, R.D., et al.: Contrast echocardiography in acute myocardial ischemia. I. In vivo determination of total left ventricular "area at risk." J. Am. Coll. Cardiol. 4:1272, 1984. Reprinted with permission from the American College of Cardiology.)

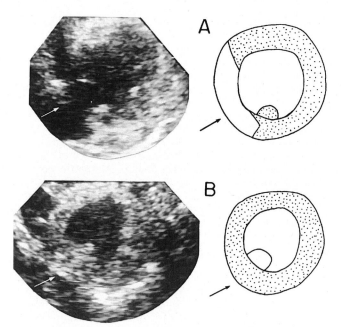

FIGURE 35–9. End-diastolic frames after left main arterial injection of contrast material in a patient with an occluded right coronary artery. Although the first frame (*A*) does not show any contrast effect within the occluded bed, the seventh frame (*B*) does, suggesting moderate collateral flow to the occluded bed. (See text for details.) (From Sabia, P.J., Powers, E.R., Jayaweera, A.R., et al.: Functional significance of collateral blood flow in patients with recent acute myocardial infarction: A study using myocardial contrast echocardiography. Circulation 85:2080, 1992, with permission.)

vessels and those arising from one arteriole do not connect with those arising from another (Fig. 35–10), it has been argued that lateral borders cannot exist.[55] This argument has been further supported by the finding that when necrosis occurs, there is a negligible area of ischemic tissue between the necrotic and normal myocardium.[56] Although end-arterioles do not connect with each other within the myocardium, the vessels they arise from connect with each other on the epicardial surface of the heart (see Fig. 35–10), with the result that an arteriolar unit does not exist in isolation from its surrounding neighbors. Thus, any change in pressure or flow in one unit can affect the direction and degree of flow in the neighboring unit despite no direct connections between them within the myocardium.[45, 46]

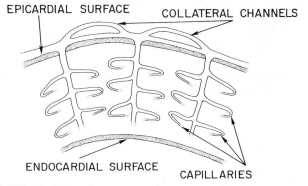

FIGURE 35–10. A diagrammatic representation of end-capillary loops from different arterioles. Although the capillaries arising from different arterioles are not directly interconnected, they are connected to each other via epicardial and endocardial (not shown here) collateral channels. (From Kaul, S., Glasheen, W.P., Oliner, J.D., et al.: Relation between anterograde blood flow through a coronary artery and the size of the perfusion bed it supplies: Experimental and clinical implications. J. Am. Coll. Cardiol. 17:1403, 1991. Reprinted with permission from the American College of Cardiology.)

Because of this anatomical configuration, in the event of coronary occlusion the final boundaries of the risk area are determined by the hemodynamics of not only the occluded artery but also the other nonoccluded arteries.[45, 46] The boundaries may approximate each other and result in a smaller risk area when pressure within the neighboring arteries is significantly higher than that in the occluded artery.[45, 46] In comparison, if the other vessels also have stenoses resulting in lower distal coronary pressures or the systemic pressure is low, the boundaries of the risk area are likely to be farther apart, resulting in larger risk areas.[52, 53] Based on the relative hemodynamics of the occluded and nonoccluded arteries, the risk area can change acutely by approximately 20 percent in either direction[45, 46] in the acute canine model of coronary occlusion. When the collateral vessels are highly developed, such as in patients with chronic coronary artery disease, the risk area could change by even a larger magnitude depending on the relative hemodynamics of the coronary arteries.

When coronary blood flow is re-established, perfusion is noted in regions that did not demonstrate it during coronary occlusion (unless there is necrosis and microvascular damage within the entire risk area [see further on]).[57–61] If necrosis and microvascular damage are extensive, as discussed further on, perfusion will not be seen in the entire revascularized bed. The presence of any perfusion in the heretofore occluded bed, however, indicates that at least some degree of reperfusion has been achieved.[61] Figure 35–11 illustrates an example of reperfusion in a dog who underwent transient occlusion of the left anterior descending coronary artery. Contrast echocardiography, which uses left atrial injection of contrast medium during occlusion, shows a risk area indicated by an anterior transmural relative color defect (see Fig. 35–11*A*), which parallels the risk area on technetium autoradiography (see Fig. 35–11*B*). During reflow, contrast enhancement now occurs in this previously hypoperfused area (see Fig. 35–11*C*), indicated by oranges and yellows. Tissue staining indicates no evidence of infarction (see Fig. 35–11*D*).[61] In comparison, an example of nontransmural infarction is depicted in Figure 35–12. Contrast echocardiography and autoradiography concordantly show a transmural anterior defect (risk area) during left anterior descending artery occlusion (see Fig. 35–12*A* and *B*, respectively). During reperfusion (see Fig. 35–12*C*), the contrast defect persists, but it is no longer transmural (see further on). The subendocardial contrast defect corresponds to a nontransmural infarction indicated in Figure 35–12*D*.[61]

FIGURES 35–11 and 35–12. See Color Plate 9.

Determination of Myocardial Viability After Acute Myocardial Infarction

During coronary occlusion, there are regions with different levels of blood flow within the occluded bed. Regions with severe reduction in flow (<0.2 to 0.3 mL/min/g) will rapidly undergo necrosis (within 45 minutes to 1 hour) if adequate perfusion is not re-established.[43, 44] When systemic hemodynamics are normal, such regions usually lie within the center of the risk area and mainly involve the endocardium. Areas surrounding this severely ischemic region usually have intermediate levels of flow, which prevents necrosis from occurring. In the instance of reduced coronary driving pressure resulting from a decrease in the systemic blood pressure or an increase in right atrial pressure, or in the event of increased myocardial oxygen demand, these zones with intermediate flows are also likely to undergo necrosis. Finally, if there is little residual blood flow within the risk area because of poor collateral channels, virtually the entire risk area is subject to necrosis unless reperfusion is rapidly established.[43, 44]

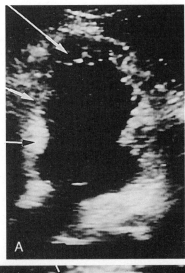

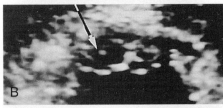

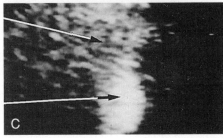

FIGURE 35–13. *A* to *C,* Three different perfusion patterns in the same bed in a patient with a recent anteroseptal infarction and an open left anterior descending artery. The upper septum shows normal homogeneous perfusion, the middle to lower septum depicts patchy perfusion, whereas no perfusion is noted in the apex. (From Ragosta, M., Camarano, G.P., Kaul, S., et al.: Microvascular integrity indicates myocellular viability in patients with recent myocardial infarction: New insights using myocardial contrast echocardiography. Circulation 89:2562, 1994, with permission.)

In addition to cellular necrosis after reperfusion, there is microvascular damage in regions with myocardial infarction. The microvascular damage can take the form of capillary disruption, vascular plugging with white cells and other debris, or vascular obliteration resulting from interstitial edema.[62–64] The areas of vascular damage are located within the borders of the infarct and approximate the size of the infarct.[62–64] Regions within the risk area that do not undergo necrosis during coronary occlusion because they have at least an intermediate level of flow (>0.3 mL/min/g) also do not have microvascular damage.[62–64] Thus, the spatial extent of microvascular damage reflects the extent of cellular damage, and regions without microvascular damage indicate the presence of viable myocardium.

This principle has been employed to define infarct size and the extent of myocardial viability after reperfusion with contrast echocardiography.[57–61] It has been demonstrated that regions showing "low reflow" or "no reflow" with this technique do not improve their thickening despite an open infarct-related artery.[57–61] In comparison, regions showing adequate flow after reperfusion have been demonstrated to improve their thickening if the infarct-related artery remains patent.[57–61] Figure 35–13 depicts a patient with an anteroapical infarction who received thrombolytic therapy.[58] Six

days later, angiography revealed good flow in the left anterior descending artery. Injection of microbubbles into the left main artery, however, showed lack of tissue perfusion in the apex and low tissue perfusion in the middle and lower interventricular septum, whereas the upper interventricular septum demonstrated adequate perfusion. One month later, the upper interventricular septum showed marked improvement in function and the middle and lower interventricular septum demonstrated some improvement, whereas the apex did not depict any improvement.[58] Figure 35–14 illustrates baseline and 1-month wall motion scores in 90 patients who had adequate flow established to the infarct-related artery. The *x*-axis in this figure denotes the perfusion score within the infarct zone (1 = entire infarct zone shows perfusion, 0 = no area of the infarct shows perfusion), whereas the *y*-axis denotes the wall motion score (1 = normal wall motion, 5 = dyskinesia). Although the baseline wall motion score is similar for all degrees of microvascular perfusion within the infarct, the 1-month wall motion score is inversely related to the perfusion score.[58] The results of these studies indicate that the spatial extent of microvascular perfusion as assessed with contrast echocardiography reflects the extent of myocellular viability after reperfusion in patients with acute myocardial infarction.

The data just discussed[58–61] are from patients studied 1 day to 4 weeks after myocardial infarction, when hyperemia in those with reflow had abated. The information obtained from contrast echocardiography immediately after reflow is established is more complex because of reactive hyperemia. It takes several hours or even a day after reflow has been established for reactive hyperemia to abate. The degree of hyperemia is inversely related to the amount of microvascular damage. Thus, if there is severe necrosis and microvascular damage, the ability to mount a hyperemic response (which is modulated by the intact microvasculature) is greatly diminished, and contrast echocardiography may more closely reflect the degree of myocardial damage. Conversely, if microvascular damage is only moderate, significant reactive hyperemia may occur and contrast echocardiography may underestimate the degree of myocardial necrosis. The issue is further complicated by the degree of residual stenosis present in the infarct-related artery. If the stenosis is critical and completely attenuates the hyperemic re-

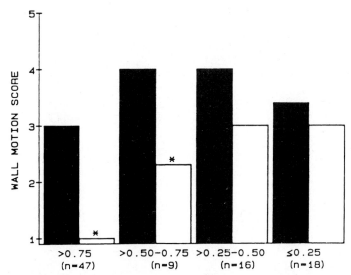

FIGURE 35–14. Bar graphs demonstrating relationships between the contrast score index on the *x*-axis and median baseline and 1-month wall motion scores on the *y*-axis, where *1* = normal, *2* = mild hypokinesia, *3* = severe hypokinesia, *4* = akinesia, and *5* = dyskinesia. Function at 1 month was significantly better (*P* < .01 indicated by asterisks in the figure) in groups with a higher contrast score index. Note that lower scores indicate better regional function. (From Ragosta, M., Camarano, G.P., Kaul, S., et al.: Microvascular integrity indicates myocellular viability in patients with recent myocardial infarction: New insights using myocardial contrast echocardiography. Circulation 89:2562, 1994, with permission.)

sponse, contrast echocardiography will accurately define the region of necrosis. Conversely, if the stenosis is not critical, the degree of hyperemic attenuation may be variable and may underestimate tissue necrosis by a variable amount.

This principle is clearly demonstrated in Figure 35–15 in which myocardial blood flow was measured with radiolabeled microspheres in dogs undergoing left anterior descending artery occlusion anywhere from 2 to 6 hours followed by reperfusion.[65] It can be noted that blood flow within the infarct zone (normalized to the left circumflex bed) can vary over a wide range 15 minutes after reflow. This variability is due to different degrees of microvascular damage in different dogs. Additionally, flow to the infarct region fluctuates randomly over the next few hours. When microbubbles are injected into the left main artery, the perfusion bed size at 45 minutes and 3 hours after reperfusion appears significantly smaller than the actual infarct (see Fig. 35–15A and B).[65] Thus, in the absence of a flow-limiting lesion, contrast echocardiography under-estimates infarct size for several hours after reflow because of reactive hyperemia.

Despite relative hyperemia within the infarct zone after reflow, since microvascular damage has occurred, the hyperemia noted is less than could be mounted within the normal myocardium.[66, 67] This principle can be exploited to define infarct size accurately in the few hours after reflow despite the presence of hyperemia within the infarct zone.[65] When a coronary vasodilator, such as dipyridamole, is infused intravenously, flow in the normal bed (posterior myocardium in Fig. 35–16) increases maximally (approximately four to fivefold), whereas the flow within the infarct bed cannot increase any further.[65] Thus, relative to the normal bed, the infarct bed is now seen to have reduced flow (see Fig. 35–16C). This region of reduced relative flow is almost identical to the region of infarction as determined by triphenyltetrazolium chloride staining of the myocardium (see Fig. 35–16D).[65] As previously described, the color-coding algorithm used ascribes white to the pixel with maximal intensity, and all other pixels are assigned colors that indicate lower intensities.[40] In this manner, all intensities are relative to the brightest pixel within the myocardium. It is for this reason that the infarct zone is seen as an area with relatively low flow. The same maneuver was used to define infarct size immediately after reperfusion in the presence of dipyridamole with the use of left atrial injection of contrast material (see Figs. 35–11C and 35–12C).

FIGURE 35–16. See Color Plate 9.

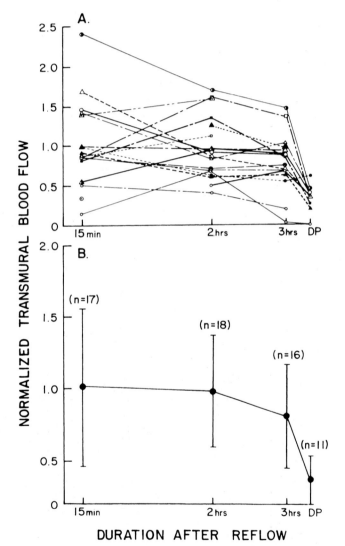

FIGURE 35–15. The temporal sequence of radiolabeled microsphere-derived transmural blood flow within the risk area expressed as a percentage of transmural blood flow in the normal posterior wall on the y-axis and the interval after reperfusion depicted on the x-axis. DP represents measurements made during the infusion of dipyridamole after 3 hours of reflow. (See text for details.) Panel A depicts data in individual dogs, and panel B depicts mean ± 1 SD data. (From Villanueva, F.S., Glasheen, W.D., Sklenar, J., et al.: Assessment of risk area during coronary occlusion and infarct size after reperfusion with myocardial contrast echocardiography using left and right atrial injections of contrast. Circulation 88:2596, 1993, with permission.)

In patients who have not received thrombolytic therapy or who do not have an open infarct-related artery despite thrombolytic therapy, contrast echocardiography can still be used to define myocardial viability following acute myocardial infarction.[68] Since viability can be present only in tissue with some residual flow (>0.3 mL/g/min),[43, 44] it follows that detection of residual flow to the infarct zone via collaterals can indicate regions that are likely to be viable. Conversely, regions not receiving adequate tissue perfusion via collaterals are not likely to survive prolonged periods of coronary occlusion. Because of the low number of bubbles entering the microvasculature, no contrast effect is seen at flows less than 0.15 mL/g/min.[47] Thus the presence of contrast material within the infarct zone usually defines regions with residual blood flow at levels capable of maintaining myocellular viability.[68] The regions within an infarct zone that opacify during coronary occlusion are the same regions that opacify after reflow, which implies that myocardium that receives adequate collateral flow during occlusion tends to have preserved microvasculature and thus intact myocellular viability after reperfusion.[58]

Figure 35–17 illustrates right (see Fig. 35–17A) and left (see Fig. 35–17B) main coronary injections of contrast medium in a patient with a recent anterior infarction and akinesia within the infarct zone.[52] Right coronary artery injection of contrast material demonstrates opacification not only in the bed supplied by that artery but also in the medial half of the occluded left anterior descending arterial bed (see Fig. 35–7A). Similarly, injection of contrast material into the left main artery demonstrates opacification not only of the left circumflex artery, which is patent, but also of the lateral half of the occluded left anterior descending arterial bed (see Fig. 35–17B). In this patient, therefore, contrast echocardiography demonstrates the presence of both right-to-left (see Fig. 35–17A) and left-to-left (see Fig. 35–17B) collaterals.[68] The demonstration of collateral perfusion is more accurate with contrast echocardiography than with coronary angiography,[68] since the latter can only define vessels greater than 100 μm,[69] whereas most collateral channels are much smaller.[70] The correlation between the spatial extent of collateral perfusion within an infarct zone by contrast echocardiography and angiographic collaterals is therefore poor.[68]

A. PRE-PTCA (RCA INJECTION)

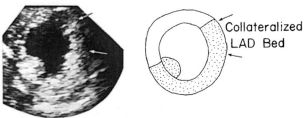

Collateralized
LAD Bed

B. PRE-PTCA (L. MAIN INJECTION)

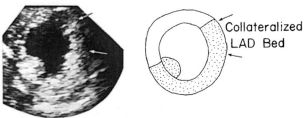

Collateralized
LAD Bed

FIGURE 35–17. Right-to-left collaterals *(arrows)* noted when microbubbles are injected into the right coronary artery *(A)*, and left-to-left collaterals *(arrows)* noted when microbubbles are injected into the left main artery *(B)* in a patient with a recent anteroseptal infarction and an occluded left anterior descending artery. (See text for details.) PTCA = percutaneous transluminal coronary angioplasty; RCA = right coronary artery; LAD = left anterior descending artery. (From Sabia, P.J., Powers, E.R., Ragosta, M., et al.: Functional significance of collateral blood flow in patients with recent acute myocardial infarction. Circulation 85:2080, 1992, with permission.)

Regions that demonstrate adequate collateral perfusion during coronary occlusion by contrast echocardiography improve their function after anterograde flow is restored.[68] Figure 35–18 illustrates the correlation between the 1-month postreperfusion wall motion score and the spatial extent of collateral perfusion during coronary occlusion in patients with recent myocardial infarction.[68]

Interestingly, as long as there is adequate residual collateral perfusion within the infarct zone, function improves even when anterograde flow is established days to weeks after acute myocardial infarction. These data indicate that in addition to the duration of coronary occlusion, the extent of residual collateral perfusion as assessed by contrast echocardiography is a major determinant of infarct size. Thus, myocardial regions that suffer an infarction and do not undergo immediate reperfusion are still likely to be viable if they have adequate residual collateral perfusion. These segments are also likely to show improvement in function even when anterograde flow is re-established days to weeks after the index event.[68]

Quantification of Myocardial Perfusion

Unlike other techniques used for myocardial perfusion imaging, in which the tracer is either extracted by myocytes (e.g., thallium-201 or technetium-99 sestamibi used for nuclear myocardial imaging) or enters the extravascular space (radiopaque dyes used for radiologic imaging), microbubbles of air act as true intravascular tracers that remain within the intravascular space during their transit through the myocardium.[17] The transit rate of these microbubbles through tissue is, therefore, proportional to the flow-to-volume ratio of the tissue.[71] When either flow or volume is constant, the transit rate directly reflects the change in the other.[71]

In an experimental study, the left anterior descending coronary artery in dogs was ligated and cannulated to perfuse it with blood from the carotid artery.[18] Flow was altered to the coronary artery with a roller pump and was measured with a calibrated extracorporeal flow meter. In this model, autoregulation was largely abolished because of the arterial ligation, as evidenced by no change in coronary vascular resistance after direct intracoronary infusion of adenosine. Thus the myocardial blood volume of the left anterior descending arterial bed was unaltered despite changes in flow. When radiolabeled red blood cells were injected as a discrete bolus directly into the left anterior descending artery in this situation, the transit rate was linearly related to the flow to the myocardial bed supplied by that vessel. The myocardial transit of Albunex microbubbles injected at the same flow rate was similar to that of radiolabeled red blood cells (Fig. 35–19).[18]

Likewise, when flow is held constant and myocardial blood volume changes, these changes are reflected as changes in microbub-

FIGURE 35–18. Correlation between wall motion score 1 month after successful angioplasty (where *1* = normal, *2* = mild hypokinesia, and *3* and *4* are severe hypokinesia and akinesia, respectively) and percentage of the infarct bed supplied by collateral blood flow as defined by myocardial contrast echocardiography before angioplasty. (See text for details.) (From Sabia, P.J., Powers, E.R., Ragosta, M., et al.: An association between collateral blood flow and myocardial viability in patients with recent myocardial infarction. N. Engl. J. Med. 327:1825, 1992, with permission. Copyright 1992, Massachusetts Medical Society.)

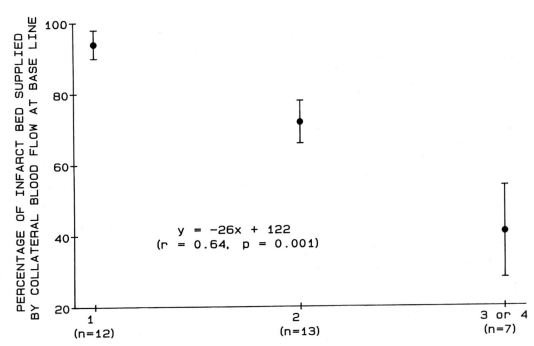

$$y = -26x + 122$$
$$(r = 0.64, \; p = 0.001)$$

PERCENTAGE OF INFARCT BED SUPPLIED BY COLLATERAL BLOOD FLOW AT BASE LINE

WALL MOTION SCORE ONE MONTH AFTER SUCCESSFUL ANGIOPLASTY

1 (n=12) 2 (n=13) 3 or 4 (n=7)

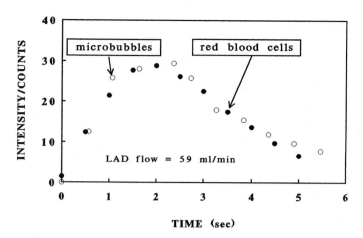

FIGURE 35–19. Microbubble time-intensity and red blood cell time-activity plots obtained from the anterior myocardium in an in vivo beating dog heart at the same left anterior descending arterial (LAD) flow rate. (From Jayaweera, A.R., Edwards, N., Glasheen, W.P., et al.: In vivo myocardial kinetics of air-filled albumin microbubbles during myocardial contrast echocardiography: Comparisons with radiolabeled red blood cells. Circ. Res. 74:1157, 1994, with permission.)

ble transit rate. An experimental model of increasing myocardial blood volume in the presence of constant blood flow is the creation of varying degrees of subcritical coronary stenoses. With each increase in the severity of stenosis, more of the microvascular reserve is exhausted to maintain constant flow until the stenosis is so severe as to completely exhaust flow reserve, at which time the flow within the vessel starts decreasing with increasing degrees of stenosis.[72] When contrast medium is injected as a bolus directly into the artery with a stenosis using such a model, the transit rate of microbubbles correlates with the pressure gradient across the stenosis as long as flow in the artery remains constant.

There are several technical issues that relate to the measurement of mean microbubble transit rate through tissue, which will be discussed briefly in this section. In addition to flow through tissue, the input function (duration of injection) will also influence the output function (width of the time-intensity plot obtained from the myocardium).[71] For example, if the injection is made over a longer period, thus spreading out the input function, the output function will also become more spread out despite the flow rate remaining constant. The manner in which the input function can affect the output function is depicted in Figure 35–20. Figure 35–20A illustrates several reservoirs of the same volume connected in series. Water is flowing through them at the same flow rate. If dye is injected as an instantaneous bolus in the first reservoir (reservoir a on figure), it will demonstrate a logarithmic decay as depicted in Figure 35–20B. By the time the dye appears in reservoir b, it will assume a γ-variate form as illustrated in Figure 35–20B. When the

dye enters the third reservoir (reservoir c), the form of the curve will be unchanged, but it will be more spread out as shown in Figure 35–20B. If the input function for each reservoir (which is the output function of the preceding reservoir) were not known, the different shapes of the curves from the different reservoirs could easily be mistaken for different flow rates or volumes of those reservoirs when, in fact, the different shapes are due to different input functions.[71]

If the input function is known, it can be deconvolved from the output function, thus providing an accurate estimation of the transfer function, which denotes the mean myocardial transit rate or the spread of the bolus within the myocardium itself.[18] In this context, it is important to note that the spread in the myocardium should be greater than the width of the input function, or the calculation of the transfer function is meaningless. Similarly, if the site and duration of injection are always the same, the input function is always the same and the output function will correlate linearly with the flow-to-volume ratio. Consequently, in such a situation, it is not necessary to deconvolve the input from the output functions.[18] This principle has special bearing for assessment of microbubble transit rate during myocardial contrast echocardiography in which the bolus of contrast material injected into a coronary artery cannot itself be imaged. Thus, it becomes imperative to have a constant method of injection to obtain meaningful microbubble transit rates through the myocardium.

There is a great degree of spatial heterogeneity in the video intensity within cardiac images. Thus, larger regions-of-interest

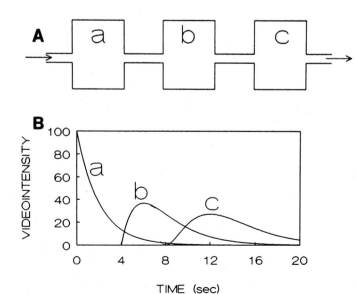

FIGURE 35–20. A model that describes the effect of the input function on the output function. The letters a, b, and c denote compartments of equal volume connected in series. (See text for details.) (From Jayaweera, A.R., Sklenar, J., and Kaul S.: Quantification of images obtained during myocardial contrast echocardiography. Echocardiography 11:385, 1994, with permission.)

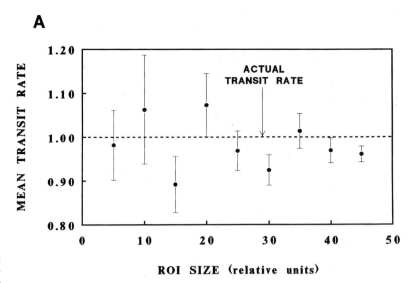

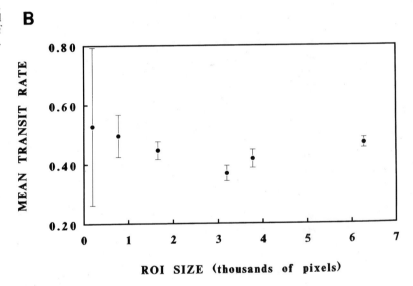

FIGURE 35–21. The impact of the size of the region-of-interest *(ROI)* on the calculation of mean microbubble transit rate for *(A)* computer-simulated data and *(B)* in vivo experimental data. The dashed line represents the true mean transit rate in the computer-simulated data. As the size of the region of interest increases, the estimated transit rate better approximates the true value. Furthermore, the error in the estimation of transit rate also decreases as the size of the region of interest increases. (See text for details.) (From Jayaweera, A.R., Skyba, D.M., and Kaul, S.: Technical factors that influence the determination of microbubble transit rate during contrast echocardiography. J. Am. Soc. Echocardiogr. 8:198, 1995, with permission.)

placed over the myocardium to obtain time-intensity plots should generate less noisy data, resulting in a more accurate estimate of mean transit rates.[38] Figure 35–21 illustrates the influence of the size of the region-of-interest on the estimation of the mean microbubble transit rate. In the simulated data (see Fig. 35–21A), the estimated transit rate approaches the true value (dashed line on figure) as the size of the region-of-interest increases and the error in the estimation of the transit rate, depicted as standard errors, also decreases with an increase in the size of the region-of-interest. Similarly, the errors in the experimental in vivo data (see Fig. 35–21B) rapidly diminish to a fairly constant value when the size of the region-of-interest is greater than approximately 1600 pixels.[38]

Similar to the sample size in the spatial domain (size of region-of-interest), the sample size in the temporal domain (number of data points in the time-intensity plot) will also determine the accuracy of the estimation of transit rate.[38] Figure 35–22 shows the effect of sampling rate (temporal resolution of the data) on the estimation of mean microbubble transit rates. The estimated transit rate in the simulated data (see Fig. 35–22A) approaches the true value (dashed line on figure) as the sampling rate increases and the error in the estimation of transit rates, depicted as error bars, also decreases with an increase in the sampling rate. The results from the in vivo experimental data (see Fig. 35-22B) also show the same phenomenon.[38]

The mean transit rate can be derived with the use of a direct numerical calculation or by fitting the data to a mathematical model.[38] Since it is dependent on integrating finite areas between the baseline and the points within the time-intensity plots, the former method can produce errors when there are a limited number of data points.[38] Figure 35–23A depicts the dependence of a numerically calculated mean transit rate on the sampling rates that were obtained by sequentially deleting alternate points from the computer-simulated time-intensity plots. The dashed line in Figure 35–23A depicts the true transit rate, which is approximated only when the sampling rate is high. Figure 35–23B depicts better approximation of the curve with rectangles when the sampling rate is high, whereas Figure 35–23C illustrates a suboptimal approximation of the curve with the use of rectangles when the sampling rate is low. In comparison, the use of a mathematical model proscribes the shape of the curve, which can be approximated even if all data points are not present. In addition, because of the stochastic nature of ultrasound, smoothing of data, which fitting a mathematical model can provide, can be quite useful. Furthermore, although they are approximations, mathematical models provide a framework for the understanding of the rheologic characterstics of bubbles. Finally, as stated earlier, the echocardiographic equipment used also affects the measurement of the transit rate, the principal system-related factor being the relationship between microbubble

A

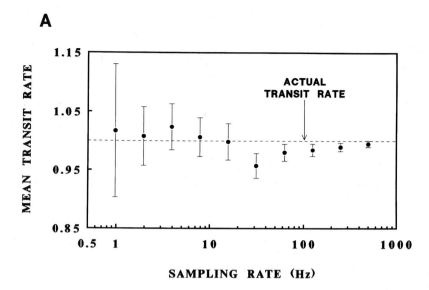

B

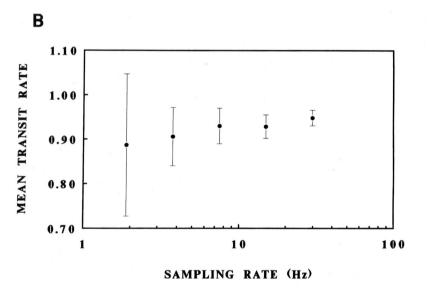

FIGURE 35–22. The impact of sampling rate on estimation of mean microbubble transit rate using (*A*) computer-simulated and (*B*) in vivo experimental data. The dashed line in *A* represents the true transit rate during computer simulation. As the sampling rate increases, the error in the estimation of transit rate decreases. (See text for details.) (From Jayaweera, A.R., Skyba, D.M., and Kaul, S.: Technical factors that influence the determination of microbubble transit rate during contrast echocardiography. J. Am. Soc. Echocardiogr. 8:198, 1995, with permission.)

concentration and video intensity specific for a given echocardiographic system (see Figs. 35–2 and 35–3).[38] Furthermore, both the level of system saturation and system sensitivity affect the measurement of the transit rate (see Figs. 35–4 and 35–5).[38] These issues have been discussed in greater detail elsewhere.[38, 73]

At this point, it may be useful to provide a brief description of the steps involved in derivation of time-intensity plots during myocardial contrast echocardiography. A detailed description is provided elsewhere.[71, 74] Once the data are acquired, end-diastolic frames are selected (either manually or by means of an electrocardiogram-triggered gating algorithm) and aligned with the use of computer cross-correlation. Regions-of-interest are then placed over the myocardium from which serial changes in intensity produced by contrast injection are measured to obtain time-intensity plots. Any of the registered images can be used for the placement of the regions-of-interest. The average video intensity within each of these regions is then calculated automatically for every frame beginning five to six frames prior to the appearance of contrast material and continuing until its disappearance from the myocardium.

The next step after the generation of the time-intensity plots is background subtraction, which is achieved by calculating the average video intensity for each region-of-interest from the five to six frames prior to contrast appearance and subtracting this value from all subsequent frames. A least-squares curve (usually γ-variate,[75] except in the operating room, as described later) is then fit to the time-intensity data, and the parameters of the curve, such as width (or transit rate), amplitude, and area under the curve, are derived.[71, 74]

As described earlier, when microbubbles are injected as a bolus directly into a coronary artery and either myocardial blood flow or volume is selectively altered (without an alteration in both), changes in the mean transit rate of microbubbles reflect changes in either flow or volume, respectively.[71] When contrast medium is injected into a peripheral vein, however, the bolus spreads as it passes through the right side of the heart, the lungs, and the left side of the heart. The input function, therefore, is longer in duration than the mean myocardial transit time of the microbubbles, which means that even if the input function is known, it cannot be deconvolved from the output function to derive the mean myocardial transit rate. Further, after a venous injection, the microbubbles are detected in the myocardium during only a small portion of the time they are in the left ventricular cavity because although the number of bubbles within the left ventricular cavity is high enough to be detected (and even cause attenuation), the number in the myocardium is low, since only a small fraction of stroke volume

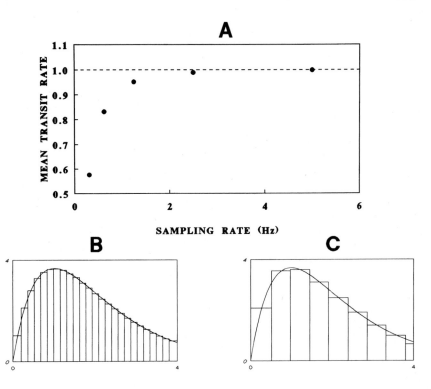

FIGURE 35–23. The effect of sampling rate on direct numerical calculation of mean microbubble transit rate. The dashed line in *A* depicts the true transit rate, which is approximated only when the sampling rate is high. *B* depicts better approximation of the curve using rectangles when the sampling rate is high (more rectangles with more samples), whereas *C* illustrates a suboptimal approximation of the curve using rectangles when the sampling rate is low (less rectangles with less samples). (See text for details.) (From Jayaweera, A.R., Skyba, D.M., and Kaul, S.: Technical factors that influence the determination of microbubble transit rate during contrast echocardiography. J. Am. Soc. Echocardiogr. 8:198, 1995, with permission.)

constitutes myocardial blood flow.[39] This thresholding effect is, therefore, principally related to the paucity of bubbles per unit volume of myocardial tissue compared with unit volume of blood in the left ventricular cavity, and the microbubbles are detected within the myocardium only when their concentration in the left ventricular cavity exceeds a certain value (Fig. 35–24).[39]

A different approach for the quantification of myocardial perfusion involves the assessment of myocardial blood volume rather than blood flow. Myocardial blood volume denotes the volume of blood within the myocardial microvasculature (arterioles, capillaries, and venules) and under resting conditions constitutes approximately 6 to 15 mL/100 g of the left ventricular myocardium.[76] Since, as previously stated, microbubbles remain exclusively within the intravascular space,[17] their concentration per unit of tissue can be used to assess myocardial blood volume.[39] Most imaging techniques used for the detection of coronary artery disease also adopt some form of cardiac stress to increase myocardial blood flow, which can take the form of inotropic stimulation of the heart (such as exercise or dobutamine infusion) or the use of coronary vasodilators. In both instances, myocardial blood flow increases

consequent to an increase in myocardial blood volume.[76] During the infusion of catecholamines, an increase in myocardial blood flow is closely associated with an increase in myocardial blood volume.[39] Consequently, a linear relationship is also found between peak video intensity and myocardial blood flow as long as the linear portion of the relationship between microbubble concentration and video intensity (see Fig. 35–2) is used.[39]

Attempts have been made to measure the endocardial-to-epicardial blood flow ratio with myocardial contrast echocardiography.[61, 65, 77–79] When the endocardial microvasculature is damaged, such as after myocardial infarction, an endocardial-to-epicardial flow ratio can be calculated by measuring the video intensities within these zones. As stated earlier, these video intensities reflect blood volumes within these zones which, in turn, reflect the microvascular densities in these regions. The endocardial-to-epicardial ratio is best reflected during pharmacologically induced hyperemia when the disparity in blood volumes in the two zones is maximized.[61, 65]

It is another thing to measure the endocardial-to-epicardial flow ratio during ischemia induced by coronary stenosis. In the initial stages of stenosis, autoregulation is invoked with resulting dilatation

FIGURE 35–24. A diagram depicting left ventricular and myocardial time-intensity plots after a venous injection of contrast material. The *y*-axis on the left indicates left ventricular cavity video intensity, whereas the *y*-axis on the right denotes myocardial video intensity. Myocardial opacification is detected only during a small portion of the time when contrast material is present in the left ventricular cavity. (See text for details.) (From Skyba, D.M., Jayaweera, A.R., Goodman, N.C., et al.: Quantification of myocardial perfusion with myocardial contrast echocardiography during left atrial injection of contrast: Implication for venous injection. Circulation 90:1513, 1994, with permission.)

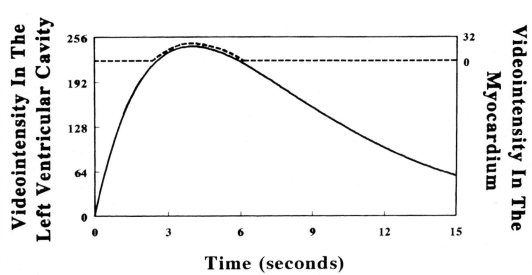

of the microvessels distal to the stenosis. Because of increased severity of ischemia in the endocardium, vasodilatation is more marked in that region. Thus, if anything, video intensity within the ndocardium should be higher than that in the epicardium. The measurement of endocardial-to-epicardial video-intensity ratios can be further complicated by attenuation of the endocardium from microbubbles present within the epicardium, resulting in an apparent decrease in endocardial video intensities.[79]

Taken together, these results indicate that the endocardial-to-epicardial blood flow ratio can be assessed when microvascular damage is present in the endocardium. In the absence of such damage, this ratio cannot be measured because of directionally opposite changes in myocardial blood flow and blood volume within this region during coronary ischemia.

Assessment of Coronary Flow Reserve and Detection of Coronary Artery Stenosis

Coronary flow reserve has historically been used to provide an assessment of the physiologic significance of coronary artery stenosis.[80–82] Either flow or velocity of blood is measured in an artery prior to and following an infusion of a coronary vasodilator in high enough doses to cause maximal hyperemia. Flow reserve is then expressed as hyperemic flow divided by normal flow. In normal individuals, flow through a vessel can increase fourfold to fivefold after infusion of a coronary vasodilator.[72] The degree of attenuation in flow reserve is said to reflect the degree of coronary stenosis.[72]

As discussed previously, attenuation in the measured flow reserve in the presence of coronary artery disease is due to changes induced in the coronary microvasculature by virtue of the presence of a stenosis.[72] Thus, regions of the myocardium subserved by more stenotic vessels have less microvascular reserve than those supplied by less stenotic or normal vessels.[72] Consequently, when a coronary vasodilator is given, the regions with less reserve show a smaller increase in flow than do regions with more reserve.[72] The changes in flow occur, however, from changes in the microvasculature (either dilation or recruitment[83–85]), which are reflected as changes in myocardial blood volume. A measurement of peak video intensity within the myocardium before and after administration of a coronary vasodilator will, therefore, provide an assessment of the changes induced in myocardial blood flow. Since flow and volume are quadratically related, however, the changes in volume and, hence, video intensity will be less than changes in flow.[39]

The other advantage of measuring myocardial blood volume rather than flow or velocity within a vessel is that when autoregulation is abolished during coronary vasodilation, myocardial blood flow becomes dependent on the coronary driving pressure.[86] Changes in coronary flow may, therefore, reflect changes in the coronary driving pressure rather than microvascular responsiveness, which is the subject of interest when flow reserve is assessed. A minor increase or decrease in aortic pressure, for instance, will provide very different values for coronary flows or velocities in the presence of a coronary vasodilator.[87] In contradistinction, since peak video intensity reflects microbubble concentration in tissue, it will always reflect changes induced in myocardial blood volume through microvascular responsiveness and may, therefore, more accurately reflect flow reserve.[87]

The same principles applied to the estimation of myocardial blood volume can be used to detect the presence of coronary stenoses. Most stenoses that cause ischemia in patients are not flow-limiting at rest but become flow-limiting when the myocardial blood flow increases during exercise and other forms of stress.[72] This principle forms the basis of stress testing, be it with exercise or pharmacologic agents, which results in flow mismatch between regions supplied by vessels that limit the increase in coronary blood flow by different degrees. As stated earlier, increases in coronary blood flow normally result from changes that occur in the coronary microvasculature.

If microbubbles are mixed adequately with blood, their relative concentrations within different regions of the myocardium reflect the relative blood volumes within these regions. When a coronary stenosis limits an increase in blood volume and flow within a specific myocardial region in the presence of a pharmacologic vasodilator, the concentration of bubbles in that region will be lower than in another region in which flow and volume have increased. Myocardial contrast echocardiography can be used for detecting this mismatch and determining the presence of flow-limiting lesions during pharmacologic stress.

This principle was first elucidated during intracoronary injections of sonicated diatrizoate (Renografin-76).[88] When a stenosis, which did not limit resting flow, was placed on either a left anterior descending or a left circumflex artery in a dog and contrast material was injected into the left main artery, no difference in the myocardial opacification was noted in the two beds (Fig. 35–25B). In the presence of dipyridamole, however, the opacification was significantly greater in the bed supplied by the normal vessel and less in that supplied by the stenotic vessel (see Fig. 35–25C). Similar results were noted in patients.[88–91]

Obviously, these findings have even greater application when contrast material is injected into a mixing chamber proximal to the aorta to mimic the setting in which an intravenous injection of contrast medium can be administered.[92] Figure 35–26 illustrates digitally subtracted color-coded images from four stages in a dog after left atrial injection of contrast material in which the microbubbles were thoroughly mixed with blood prior to their entry into the coronary circulation. Figure 35–26A and B shows images at baseline and during hyperemia; an increased preponderance of whites and oranges in Figure 35–26B suggest more microbubbles in the myocardium during hyperemia. In the presence of pharmacologic stress, a stenosis was positioned on the left anterior descending artery, which limited hyperemic flow but did not reduce flow below the baseline level in that artery. A lack of oranges and whites is noted in that bed (arrow on figure) when compared with the left circumflex bed (see Fig. 35–26C). Also in the presence of pharmacologic stress, a stenosis was positioned on the left circumflex artery. This stenosis limited hyperemic flow in that vessel but did not reduce flow below baseline level. This time, a lack of oranges, yellows, and whites (arrow on figure) is noted in the left circumflex bed (see Fig. 35–26D) when compared with the left anterior descending arterial bed. The spatial extent of perfusion defects on contrast echocardiography noted in Figure 35–26 also correlates with the spatial extent of relative hypoperfusion measured with radiolabeled microspheres; hence, not only the magnitude but also the spatial extent of pharmacologically induced flow mismatch can be measured by means of contrast echocardiography.[92]

FIGURE 35–26. See Color Plate 10.

The changes in video intensity noted in Figures 35–25 and 35–26 are due to different myocardial blood volumes in the different vascular beds during pharmacologic stress.[92] The video-intensity values in these frames are adjusted in relation to the brightest pixel in each frame and thus represent relative blood volumes.[39, 40] It is also important to note that since the relationship between video intensity and microbubble concentration is different for different commercially available echocardiographic systems, the slope of the relationship between video-intensity and myocardial blood volume ratios may also be different for different systems. Furthermore, since only the initial portion of the relationship between video intensity and microbubble concentration is linear for most systems (see Fig. 35–2), relative myocardial blood volumes can be accurately defined only at low microbubble concentrations, which are just high enough to be barely detectable on echocardiography in its current form. Similar results have also been obtained from the

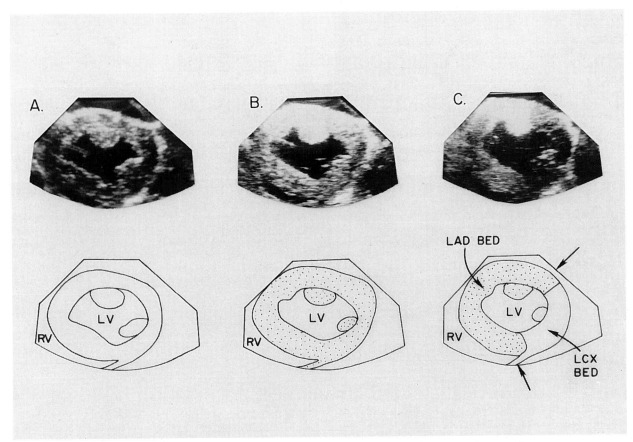

FIGURE 35–25. Two-dimensional echocardiograms *(A)* following placement of critical stenosis but prior to injection of contrast material, *(B)* after injection of contrast medium alone showing homogeneous opacification of the entire left ventricular myocardium, and *(C)* after injection of both papaverine and contrast material, showing significantly greater opacification in the left anterior descending *(LAD)* arterial bed. The size of the less opacified left circumflex *(LCX)* bed *(arrows)* can be easily measured. (See text for details.) RV = right ventricle; LV = right ventricle. (From Keller, M.W., Smucker, M.L., Burwell, L., et al.: Myocardial contrast echocardiography in humans. II. Assessment of coronary blood flow reserve. J. Am. Coll. Cardiol. 12:925, 1988. With permission from the American College of Cardiology.)

new contrast agents that are capable of opacifying the myocardium following venous administration.[30]

Intraoperative Assessment of the Myocardial Distribution of Cardioplegia and Success of Bypass Graft Placement

When coronary artery bypass surgery is performed, two main routes of cardioplegia delivery are used: anterograde and retrograde. Anterograde cardioplegia delivery is achieved by cross-clamping the aortic root and administering cardioplegia into the root, from which point it travels via the coronary arteries to the myocardial tissue. In comparison, retrograde cardioplegia delivery is achieved by placing an occlusive balloon catheter in the coronary sinus and administering cardioplegia through it, from which point it travels to myocardial tissue via venules. In either instance, the goal is to achieve cardiac arrest and cessation of myocellular function by use of a hyperkalemic perfusate during the operative procedure. Failure to achieve cessation of myocellular function can lead to perioperative infarction, since no blood reaches the myocardial tissue during the period of operation. During anterograde delivery, coronary stenoses may severely limit perfusion of tissue by the cardioplegic solution, whereas during retrograde delivery, occlusion of one or more venous draining sites by the balloon placed in the coronary sinus may do the same. To obtain optimal surgical results, it would therefore be useful to know intraoperatively whether cardioplegia is being delivered to different myocardial regions adequately.

Myocardial contrast echocardiography has been demonstrated to be a reliable intraoperative method of on-line monitoring of tissue delivery of cardioplegia during bypass surgery.[93–97] In a canine model of variable left anterior descending artery stenosis, Albunex was introduced into the cardioplegia line during simultaneously performed echocardiography.[95] The input function was unchanged for each dog, since the location of the aortic cross-clamp, cardioplegia flow rate, and duration of injection were held constant during the experiment. Although the rate of appearance of microbubbles within the myocardium distal to the left anterior descending artery stenosis in this model correlated with actual tissue flow as determined by radiolabeled microspheres (Fig. 35–27), the rate of microbubble washout did not correlate with tissue flow.[95] The time-intensity plots obtained from the myocardium depicted in Figure 35–27 do not resemble the ones obtained from the blood-perfused beating heart.[95] For the same tissue flow rate, the washout of the bubbles is markedly prolonged during crystalloid cardioplegia compared with blood perfusion (Fig. 35–28), which cannot be explained on the basis of a difference in input function alone (coronary artery versus aortic root injection).[95] In a separate study that used high-powered microscopy of the hamster cremaster muscle, it was found that in the presence of cardioplegia, the washout of the Albunex bubbles is delayed because of their adherence to the venules.[98] The time to appearance of contrast material can, however, still be used during cardioplegia to quantitatively assess tissue perfusion.[95] Since the shape of the time-intensity plots do not resemble a γ-variate form, a general exponential function is better suited to describe the plots and derive parameters from them.

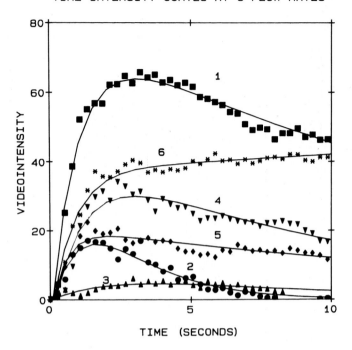

FIGURE 35–27. Time-intensity curves generated from the left anterior descending arterial bed at six different crystalloid cardioplegia flow rates through the left anterior descending coronary artery. Contrast material was injected at each stage into the cross-clamped aortic root during the time of cardioplegia delivery. The time-to-peak effect correlated with radiolabeled microsphere-derived tissue flows. The radiolabeled microsphere-derived flows (in milliliters per minute per gram) corresponding to each of the curves are as follows: curve *1* = 1.7, curve *2* = 0.5, curve *3* = 0.2, curve *4* = 0.8, curve *5* = 1.1, and curve *6* = 1.3. (From Keller, M.W., Spotnitz, W.D., Matthew, T.L., et al.: Intraoperative assessment of regional myocardial perfusion using quantitative myocardial contrast echocardiography: An experimental evaluation. J. Am. Coll. Cardiol. 16:1267, 1990. Reprinted with permission from the American College of Cardiology.)

In the case of retrograde perfusion, contrast echocardiography can demonstrate the spatial distribution of cardioplegia within the myocardium.[99] Figure 35–29*B* illustrates a short-axis view in which contrast material is not present in the interventricular septum (indicated by arrows on the figure) after it was introduced with cardioplegia through a coronary sinus balloon in a dog. Radiolabeled microspheres confirm relative hypoperfusion of this region by cardioplegic solution (also indicated by arrows in Fig. 35–29*A*). Figure 35–29*B* also illustrates the intramyocardial distribution of cardioplegic solution, which appears as spokes of a wheel, consistent with the intramyocardial distribution of veins. Unlike the situation in which it is injected into the aortic root, contrast material is readily noted in the myocardium during retrograde cardioplegia, even when the epicardial coronary arteries are severely stenotic or occluded.[99]

Myocardial contrast echocardiography has also provided unique insights into the "physiology" of retrograde cardioplegia delivery and demonstrates how it is different from that of anterograde cardioplegia delivery.[100] Radiolabeled microspheres (11 μm) under-

estimate the actual flow delivered into the coronary sinus but accurately predict the flow delivered into the cross-clamped aorta. Furthermore, isotopes that are extracted by myocytes, such as technetium-99m and thallium-201, which also provide an accurate estimation of anterograde cardioplegia flow, underestimate retrograde cardioplegia flow even more than do microspheres. In comparison, the rate of contrast appearance in the myocardium provides an accurate estimation of organ flow during both anterograde and retrograde cardioplegia delivery.

The fact that the "physiology" of retrograde cardioplegia delivery is different from that of anterograde cardioplegia delivery can be explained on the basis of differences in the arteriolar and venular level microvascular architecture (Fig. 35–30).[100] During anterograde cardioplegia delivery, essentially all microspheres are entrapped in precapillary arterioles (see Fig. 35–30*A*). Consequent to this anatomical arrangement, whatever transits the epicardial vessels reaches the arterioles and capillaries as well and therefore microspheres are necessarily accurate markers of all three levels of anterograde cardioplegia flow: total, arteriolar, and capillary.[100]

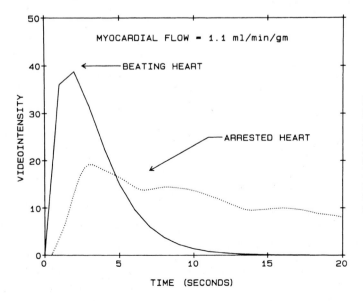

FIGURE 35–28. Time-intensity curves from the blood-perfused beating heart and from a cardioplegia-arrested heart at the same flow rate (1.1 mL/g/min). Note the delayed washout of contrast material from the cardioplegia-arrested heart compared with the blood-perfused beating heart, which cannot be explained on the basis of the differences in the input function alone. (See text for details.) (From Keller, M.W., Spotnitz, W.D., Matthew, T.L., et al.: Intraoperative assessment of regional myocardial perfusion using quantitative myocardial contrast echocardiography: An experimental evaluation. J. Am. Coll. Cardiol. 16:1267, 1990. Reprinted with permission from the American College of Cardiology.)

A

MICROSPHERE FLOW

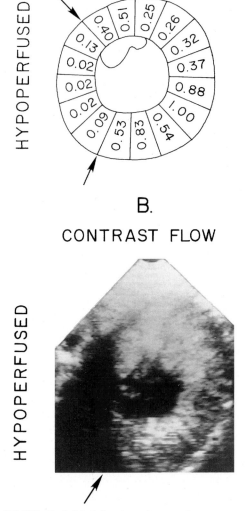

B.

CONTRAST FLOW

Intraoperative contrast echocardiography has been found to be successful for the comparison of myocardial perfusion prior to and after bypass graft placement in humans.[94-97] Quantification of myocardial perfusion can be performed on-line in the operating room with the use of microcomputers.[95] Multiple regions of interest can be placed over the myocardium prior to injection of contrast medium with the transducer held in the same position until contrast material disappears. Because the heart is arrested during cardioplegia delivery, there is no need for image alignment. A frame grabber is used to capture images from which average video intensities within myocardial regions of interest are calculated. Background is subtracted from each video-intensity value, and time-intensity plots are generated. A general exponential function is applied to the plots, and parameters of the curves are automatically calculated. Prebypass and postbypass curves, along with the derived parameters, are simultaneously displayed and compared.[95]

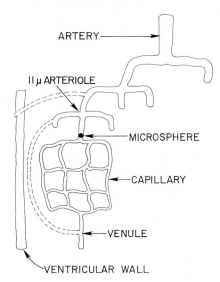

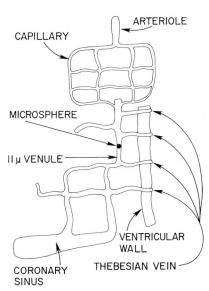

FIGURE 35–29. Radiolabeled microsphere and contrast echocardiographic data from a dog in which microspheres and contrast medium were introduced through the coronary sinus. *A* depicts normalized blood flow data, in which the arrows indicate the regions receiving less than 15 percent of maximal flow. *B* depicts echocardiographic data, showing that the absence of contrast material is noted in exactly the same regions showing less than 15 percent of flow. (From Villanueva, F.S., Kaul, S., Glasheen, W.P., et al.: Intraoperative assessment of the distribution of retrograde cardioplegia using myocardial contrast echocardiography. Surg. Forum 41:252, 1990, with permission.)

In the case of retrograde perfusion, however, thebesian veins interpose between veins and capillaries (see Fig. 35–30*B*), and as the cardioplegia traverses the venous system, a significant portion drains via these channels into the cardiac chambers prior to microsphere entrapment. Furthermore, thebesian veins or other venovenular channels may exist even beyond sites of microsphere entrapment in venules less than 11 μm. Microsphere-derived flow in this situation, therefore, actually overestimates the extent of retrograde capillary permeation. In comparison, flow measured on contrast echocardiography provides an accurate estimation of total cardiac retrograde cardioplegia flow, since the myocardial transit of all the microbubbles (even those ultimately lost from the myocardium) is detected with this technique.[100]

FIGURE 35–30. A diagram that explains differences in the physiology of anterograde *(A)* and retrograde *(B)* cardioplegia delivery based on the microvascular differences between coronary arterial and venous architectures. (See text for details.) (From Villanueva, F.S., Spotnitz, W.D., Glasheen, W.P., et al.: Physiology of retrograde cardioplegia delivery: Comparison with anterograde delivery with respect to myocardial cooling and nutrient blood flow. Am. J. Physiol. 268:H1555, 1995.)

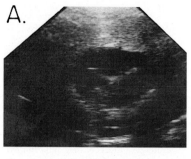

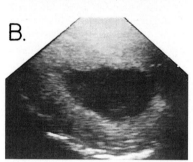

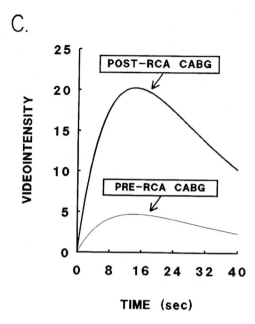

FIGURE 35–31. *A* depicts lack of myocardial perfusion in the posterior wall in a patient with a severely stenotic right coronary artery (RCA) during cardioplegia delivery, which improves dramatically after bypass to the right coronary artery (*B*). *C* shows better perfusion after bypass based on time-intensity curves obtained from the myocardium. (From Villanueva, F.S., Spotnitz, W.D., Jayaweera, A.R., et al.: Myocardial contrast echocardiography in humans: On-line intraoperative quantitation of regional myocardial perfusion during coronary artery bypass graft operations. J. Thorac. Cardiovasc. Surg. 104:1524, 1992, with permission.)

Figure 35–31 is an example of contrast echocardiographic images obtained during cardioplegia delivery into the aortic root prior to and after bypass graft placement distal to a severely stenosed right coronary artery in a patient without a previous myocardial infarction.[97] At baseline, contrast material is noted only in the anterior myocardium, indicating poor cardioplegia delivery to the posterior myocardium (see Fig. 35–31A). After a graft is placed beyond the stenosis and a proximal aortic anastomosis is performed, contrast echocardiography repeated during aortic root cardioplegia delivery shows excellent opacification of the posterior myocardium as well (see Fig. 35–31B). Time-intensity curves (see Fig. 35–31C) show the better time-to-peak contrast effect after bypass surgery. This example shows how contrast echocardiography can demonstrate both adequacy of cardioplegia delivery and graft patency on-line.[97]

Assessment of Microvascular Function

The prolonged washout of microbubbles in the cardioplegia-arrested heart discussed previously first indicated that contrast echocardiography could be used as a tool to assess microvascular function, particularly that relating to the endothelium.[96] Since then it has been determined that microbubble transit through the myocardium during anterograde cardioplegia delivery can be altered if blood is mixed with it.[101] The greater the amount of blood within the cardioplegic solutions, the faster the microbubble transit rate at the same cardioplegia flow rate.[101] This effect is independent of the temperature, osmolality, protein, and potassium concentrations and the oxygen tension of the perfusate.[101] The exact mechanism of this phenomenon is unclear at present but could be related to some aspect of endothelial function modulated by one or more components of blood.

Another piece of evidence linking microbubble washout rates to endothelial function was derived from experiments conducted to determine the mechanism of the changes in conducting properties of tissue after radiofrequency catheter ablation. It is well known that an arrhythmia may not be abolished immediately after attempted radiofrequency catheter ablation but may abate a few hours later, which implies that the injury inflicted at the time of

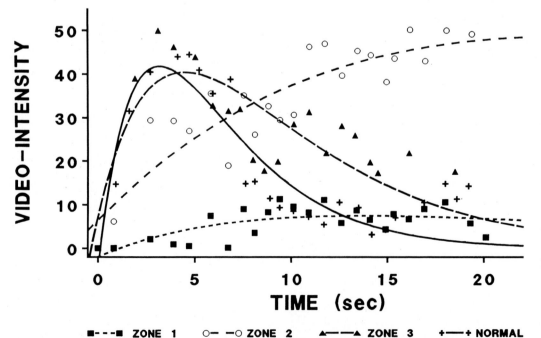

FIGURE 35–32. Time-intensity plots from different myocardial zones after myocardial injury inflicted during radiofrequency catheter ablation. The zones are depicted in Figure 35–33. The zones closer to the necrotic myocardium depict slower microbubble washout, which on electron microscopy was associated with greater endothelial damage. (From Nath, S., Whayne, J.G., Kaul, S., et al.: Effects of radio-frequency catheter ablation on regional myocardial blood flow: Possible mechanism for late electrophysiologic outcome. Circulation 89:2667, 1994, with permission.)

■ – – ■ ZONE 1   ○ – – ○ ZONE 2   ▲ –– ▲ ZONE 3   + —— + NORMAL

ablation may become progressively irreversible. To test this hypothesis, contrast echocardiography was performed before and after catheter ablation of the anterior myocardium, which received constant blood flow through a roller pump.[102] In the central zone of necrosis, no opacification was noted, but opacification was seen in the tissue surrounding the area of necrosis. The rate of microbubble washout, however, was slower closer to the region of necrosis, which on electron microscopy showed evidence of endothelial injury. Figure 35–32 shows time-intensity curves from various zones around a lesion in one dog that correspond to those on the scaled postmortem tissue shown in Figure 35–33. It is evident that the contrast washout is slowest in the area immediately adjacent to the necrotic zone.

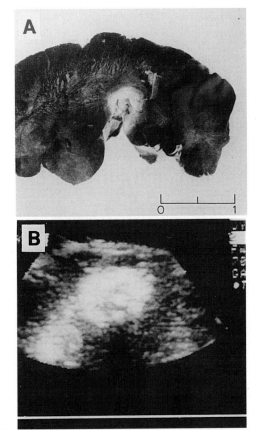

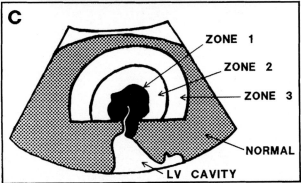

FIGURE 35–33. *A,* A postmortem slice of radiofrequency lesion from the anterior myocardium stained with nitroblue tetrazolium. *B,* An echocardiographic image of the lesion displayed at the same scale as the postmortem slice after injection of contrast material, showing persistence of contrast around the lesion. *C,* A diagrammatic representation of the zones around the lesion from which the time-intensity plots in Figure 35–32 are generated. LV = left ventricular. (From Nath, S., Whayne, J.G., Kaul, S., et al.: Effects of radiofrequency catheter ablation on regional myocardial blood flow: Possible mechanism for late electrophysiologic outcome. Circulation 89:2667, 1994, with permission.)

The current approach for assessing endothelial function in humans is measuring the changes in flow and dimension mediated via smooth muscle relaxation in large vessels. There is no method of directly measuring microvascular endothelial function. The data discussed earlier indicate that contrast echocardiography could offer unique insights into microvascular endothelial function in vivo. This could have even greater implications if, as suggested by preliminary findings, contrast echocardiography offers insights into endothelial function that is not influenced by the effect of the endothelium on large vessel blood flow and dimension.

NONMYOCARDIAL APPLICATIONS

The nonmyocardial applications of contrast echocardiography preceded the myocardial applications by more than a decade. The advent of intravenous contrast agents capable of transpulmonary passage has broadened the scope of these applications.

Intracardiac and Extracardiac Shunts

Although Doppler velocity (color, pulsed, and continuous-wave) mapping has replaced much of the earlier applications of contrast echocardiography in the assessment of cardiac shunts, contrast echocardiography is still useful in demonstrating atrial and ventricular septal defects when Doppler either is not available or the signals are of poor quality.[103–105] Right-to-left shunts show contrast medium in the left-sided chambers from a venous injection,[104] whereas left-to-right shunts show a "negative" contrast effect in the right-sided chambers.[105] Figure 35–34 illustrates an apical four-chamber view before and after an intravenous injection of Albunex in a patient with Eisenmenger syndrome in whom an atrial septal defect was not visualized either on two-dimensional or color Doppler imaging. The simultaneous appearance of contrast material in the chambers of both the right and left sides of the heart (latter indicated by arrow on figure) indicates a right-to-left shunt at the atrial level.

Patent foramen ovale is being increasingly implicated as a cause of paradoxical embolism in younger patients presenting with stroke. Contrast echocardiography prior to and during a Valsalva procedure can document the presence or absence of a patent foramen ovale during transesophageal echocardiography. Similarly, small atrial septal defects not readily apparent during color Doppler imaging can be detected with contrast echocardiography.

An application of contrast echocardiography that is gaining wider recognition is the detection of pulmonary arteriovenous connections.[106] When hand-agitated saline is injected into a peripheral vein and appears in the right ventricle, it is usually not seen in the left ventricle unless there is a right-to-left intracardiac shunt (see Fig. 35–34). In the case of pulmonary arteriovenous connections, the bubbles go out into the pulmonary artery and return to the left-sided heart chambers where they are seen five to six beats after their appearance in the right ventricle. Liver transplant patients can demonstrate these connections as part of their hepatopulmonary syndrome.[106, 107] Because of oxygen desaturation that results from these abnormalities, patients may be mistakenly diagnosed with significant pulmonary disease, which may preclude their being offered liver transplantation. Documentation of these connections by contrast echocardiography can rule out significant lung disease and make the patient a more likely candidate for transplantation.[107]

Doppler Signal Enhancement

Prior to the advent of Doppler techniques, contrast echocardiography was used for the detection and quantification of tricuspid regurgitation.[108–110] The tricuspid regurgitant jet peak velocity on continuous wave Doppler is now routinely used to estimate pulmonary artery pressure.[111] In patients with insignificant jets or poor

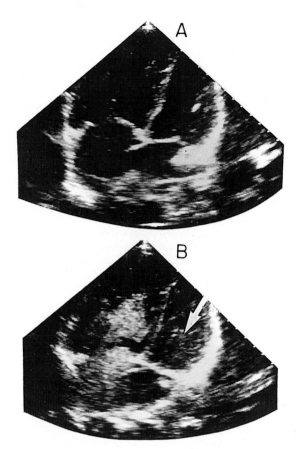

FIGURE 35–34. *A,* An apical four-chamber view of a patient with Eisenmenger syndrome in whom an intracardiac shunt was not demonstrated on two-dimensional and color Doppler imaging. *B,* The simultaneous appearance of microbubbles in the cavities of the right and left sides of the heart *(arrow)* after a peripheral venous injection of contrast material indicates the presence of a right-to-left shunt at the atrial level.

signals, assessment of pulmonary artery pressure may be difficult with the use of this technique. In such patients, contrast echocardiography can be used to enhance the tricuspid regurgitation signal and assess pulmonary artery pressure noninvasively.[112] Figure 35–35 is an example of a poorly defined tricuspid jet (see Fig. 35–35*A*), which is defined much better after peripheral venous injection of 0.2 mL of Albunex diluted with 0.8 mL of saline (see Fig. 35–35*B*).

This ability to enhance the spectral Doppler signal has been found useful in situations involving the left side of the heart, such as aortic stenosis, in which contrast echocardiography has been shown to produce a clearer and more reliable signal that correlates better with hemodynamic data obtained during cardiac catheterization than does the signal without contrast.[113] Similarly, the jet of mitral regurgitation can be better defined to measure hemodynamic variables such as dP/dt. An instance in which the enhancement of the spectral Doppler signal has been useful is in the case of pulmonary venous flow velocities. Obtaining these velocities from the apical four-chamber view during transthoracic echocardiography can be particularly difficult because of a poor signal-to-noise ratio at a greater image depth. Use of venous contrast agents that can enhance these signals after their transpulmonary passage can be a useful adjunct to Doppler echocardiography.

The enhancement of color Doppler signals has also been demonstrated with contrast echocardiography. Since the signal-to-noise ratio is markedly improved with contrast agents, jets that are not well seen or are barely detectable can be more clearly defined, and a sample volume can be placed more precisely within the jet to obtain a pulsed Doppler signal. This is true for any valve and any lesion (stenosis or regurgitation), but it is most useful in the case of tricuspid and mitral regurgitation, particularly when the jets are

not clearly seen or are eccentric. As already stated, this approach is particularly useful for defining the spatial distribution of flow velocities within the pulmonary veins during transthoracic echocardiography.

Unlike the spectral Doppler signals in which the introduction of contrast agents does not change the mean or peak Doppler gradient but only enhances the signal, in the case of color Doppler, the jet areas become larger with the use of these agents.[114] There is, therefore, a tendency to assess the severity of regurgitation as greater after introduction of contrast material. It must be remembered, however, that the reason that the jets appear larger is because of enhancement of the low-velocity signals within the jet by the microbubbles; this underscores the fact that the signal-to-noise ratio is just another of many variables that can influence jet area size. The potentially more useful application of contrast enhancement in the case of color Doppler is better definition of the proximal isovelocity surface area; however, this phenomenon needs to be demonstrated.

Another area in which enhancement of the color Doppler signal can be useful is when coronary flow velocity is being measured, especially during transesophageal echocardiography.[23] Similarly, the differentiation of false from true lumen during aortic dissection could also be performed with contrast enhancement of the color Doppler signal. Abnormalities in flow within surgically created

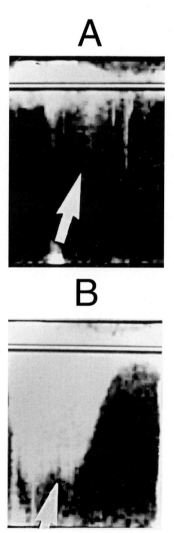

FIGURE 35–35. Spectral Doppler tracings of a tricuspid regurgitation jet before *(A)* and after *(B)* an intravenous injection of a small dose (0.2 mL) of Albunex. The signal is much clearer after the injection of contrast material *(arrow).*

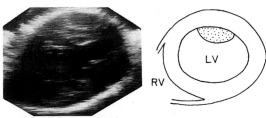

BEFORE IV MICROBUBBLES

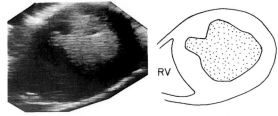

AFTER IV MICROBUBBLES

FIGURE 35–36. A papillary muscle short-axis view before *(upper panel)* and after *(lower panel)* the intravenous injection of Albunex. There is better endocardial definition after contrast material appears in the left ventricular cavity, and some posterior wall attenuation is also seen.

conditions such as a Cabrol procedure or Mustard operation could also be better visualized by color Doppler enhancement.

Regional and Global Left Ventricular Function

As already stated, the only U.S. Food and Drug Administration–approved use of Albunex is venous injection to better define the borders of the left ventricular cavity.[14] Other contrast agents are also currently undergoing clinical trials for the same purpose. The major areas in which this application is likely to be useful is in the definition of endocardial borders when they are not well seen during routinely obtained echocardiograms[14] and during stress (particularly dobutamine-induced) echocardiography.[115] Figure 35–36 is a papillary muscle short-axis view before (upper panel of figure) and after (lower panel of figure) the intravenous injection of Albunex. There is better endocardial definition after contrast material appears in the left ventricular cavity, and some posterior wall attenuation is also seen. This better definition of the endocardium with contrast agents can also potentially offer greater reliability for the estimation of the left ventricular ejection fraction. The endocardial borders are not well demonstrated during dobutamine echocardiography in about one fourth of all myocardial segments, and approximately three fourths of these segments are better visualized with the use of venous contrast agents[115]; this is particularly true for the lateral border.

Miscellaneous Uses

In a manner similar to that of cineangiography, the injection of contrast agents into the left ventricular cavity or the aortic root in the catheterization laboratory can be used to assess the severity of mitral and aortic regurgitation, respectively, during echocardiography. This is particularly useful in patients who are allergic to dyes or who have significant renal dysfunction. Preliminary experimental data suggest that this technique can be used to quantify the severity of mitral regurgitation by examining the relative washout rates of contrast material from the left atrial and left ventricular cavities.[116]

The pulmonary transit time of a tracer should be directly proportional to cardiac output. Contrast echocardiography, therefore, has the potential to assess cardiac output noninvasively by measuring the transit time of bubbles from the right to the left ventricle following a peripheral venous injection.[117] Since the transit time is proportional to both flow and volume, this technique can also be

used to assess pulmonary blood volume when cardiac output is known. Other applications of contrast echocardiography are also under development.

SUMMARY

Contrast echocardiography has experienced an exponential increase in applications over the past few years. The use of contrast material to study myocardial perfusion has afforded a new dimension to echocardiography that was not possible prior to the availability of this technique. Although the assessment of myocardial perfusion is possible today in the cardiac catheterization laboratory and the operating room, the routine use of this application in the noninvasive laboratory awaits the development of second- and third-generation contrast agents and better echocardiographic equipment. In the meanwhile, other nonmyocardial applications discussed in this chapter are likely to increase with the greater availability of commercially produced first-generation contrast agents. The field of contrast echocardiography is likely to evolve more rapidly within the next several years, as is its role in clinical cardiology.

References

1. Gramiak, R., and Shah, P.M.: Echocardiography of the aortic root. Invest. Radiol. 3:356, 1968.
2. Tei, C., Sakamaki, T., Shah, P.M., et al.: Myocardial contrast echocardiography: A reproducible technique of myocardial opacification for identifying regional perfusion defects. Circulation 67:585, 1983.
3. Kemper, A.J., O'Boyle, J.E., Sharma, S., et al.: Hydrogen peroxide contrast enhanced two-dimensional echocardiography: Real-time in-vivo delineation of regional myocardial perfusion. Circulation 68:603, 1983.
4. Feinstein, S.B., Ten Cate, F.J., Zwehl, W., et al.: Two-dimensional contrast echocardiography. I. In vitro development and quantitative analysis of echo contrast agents. J. Am. Coll. Cardiol. 3:14, 1984.
5. Gillam, L.D., Kaul, S., Fallon, J.T., et al.: Functional and pathologic effects of multiple echocardiographic contrast injections on the myocardium, brain and kidneys. J. Am. Coll. Cardiol. 6:825, 1985.
6. Moore, C.A., Smucker, M.L., and Kaul S.: Myocardial contrast echocardiography in humans. I. Safety: A comparison with routine coronary arteriography. J. Am. Coll. Cardiol. 8:1066, 1986.
7. Lang, R.M., Borow, K.M., Neumann, A., et al.: Effects of intracoronary injection of sonicated microbubbles on left ventricular contractility. Am. J. Cardiol. 60:166, 1987.
8. Keller, M.W., Glasheen, W., Teja, K., et al.: Myocardial contrast echocardiography without significant hemodynamic effects or reactive hyperemia: A major advantage in the imaging of myocardial perfusion. J. Am. Coll. Cardiol. 12:1039, 1987.
9. Reisner, S.A., Ong, L.S., Lichtenberg, G.S., et al.: Myocardial perfusion imaging by contrast echocardiography with use of intracoronary sonicated albumin in humans. J. Am. Coll. Cardiol. 14:660, 1989.
10. Christiansen, C., Kryvi, H., Sontum, P.C., et al.: Physical and biochemical characterization of Albunex, a new ultrasound contrast agent consisting of air-filled albumin microspheres suspended in a solution of human albumin. Biotechnol. Appl. Biochem. 19:307, 1994.
11. Hellebust, H., Christiansen, C., and Skotland, T.: Biochemical characterization of air-filled albumin microspheres. Biotechnol. Appl. Biochem. 18:227, 1993.
12. Walday, P., Tolleshaug, H., Gjoen, T., et al.: Biodistributions of air-filled albumin microspheres in rats and pigs. Biochem. J. 299:437, 1994.
13. Christiansen, C., Vebner, A.J., Muan, B., et al.: Lack of an immune response to Albunex, a new ultrasound contrast agent based on air-filled albumin microspheres. Int. Arch. Allergy Immunol. 104:372, 1994.
14. Feinstein, S.B., Cheirif, J., Ten Cate, F.J., et al.: Safety and efficacy of a new transpulmonary ultrasound contrast agent: Initial multicenter results. J. Am. Coll. Cardiol. 16:316, 1990.
15. Keller, M.W., Glasheen, W.P., and Kaul S.: Albunex: A safe and effective commercially produced agent for myocardial contrast echocardiography. J. Am. Soc. Echocardiogr. 2:48, 1989.
16. Ten Cate, F.J., Widimsky, P., Cornel, J.H., et al.: Intracoronary Albunex. Its effects on left ventricular hemodynamics, function, and coronary sinus flow in humans. Circulation 88(Part 1):2123, 1993.
17. Keller, M.W., Segal, S.S., Kaul, S., et al.: The behavior of sonicated albumin microbubbles in the microcirculation: A basis for their use during myocardial contrast echocardiography. Circ. Res. 65:458, 1989.
18. Jayaweera, A.R., Edwards, N., Glasheen, W.P., et al.: In vivo myocardial kinetics of air-filled albumin microbubbles during myocardial contrast echocardiography: Comparisons with radiolabeled red blood cells. Circ. Res. 74:1157, 1994.
19. Ismail, S., Jayaweera, A.R., Camarano, G., et al.: Albunex microbubbles mimic red blood cell transit through the human myocardium. Circulation 88(Suppl I):I-163, 1993.
20. Kemper, A.J., Force, T., Kloner, R., et al.: Contrast echocardiographic estimation

of regional myocardial blood flow after acute coronary occlusion. Circulation 72:1115, 1985.

21. Albers, V.M.: Underwater Acoustic Handbook. State College, Pennsylvania State University Press, 1960.

22. Hoff, L., Christiansen, C., and Skotland T.: Consideration about the contribution to acoustic backscatter from Albunex microspheres with different sizes. J. Ultrasound. Med. 13:181, 1994.

23. Iliceto, S., Caiati, C., Aragona, P., et al.: Improved Doppler signal intensity in coronary arteries after intravenous peripheral injection of a lung-crossing contrast agent (SHU 508A). J. Am. Coll. Cardiol. 23:184, 1994.

24. Porter, T., and Xie, F.: Visually detectable myocardial uptake with peripheral intravenous injections of sonicated dextrose albumin following incubation and inhalation with sulfur hexafluoride. J. Am. Soc. Echocardiogr. 7:S1, 1994.

25. Porter, T., and Xie, F.: Myocardial ultrasound contrast with intravenous perfluoropropane-enhanced sonicated dextrose albumin: Initial clinical experience in humans. J. Am. Coll. Cardiol. 25:39A, 1995.

26. Shapiro, J.R., Reisner, S.A., Lichtenberg, G.S., et al.: Intravenous contrast echocardiography with use of sonicated albumin in humans: Systolic disappearance of left ventricular contrast after transpulmonary transmission. J. Am. Coll. Cardiol. 16:1603, 1990.

27. Shandas, R., Sahn, D.J., Bales, G., et al.: Persistence of Albunex (ALB) ultrasound contrast agent: In vitro study of the effects of pressure and acoustic power on particle size, and the duration of contrast and Doppler effect. Circulation 82(Suppl. III):III-96, 1990.

28. Villanueva, F.S., Glasheen, W.P., Sklenar, J., et al.: Successful and reproducible myocardial opacification during two-dimensional echocardiography from right heart injection of contrast. Circulation 85:1557, 1992.

29. Skyba, D.M., Goodman, N.C., Jayaweera, A.R., et al.: Hemodynamic and safety characteristics of FS-069, a new contrast agent capable of producing myocardial opacification from a venous injection. J. Am. Soc. Echocardiogr. 7:S30, 1994.

30. Camarano, G.P., Jayaweera, A.R., Ismail, S., et al.: Detection of coronary stenoses and quantification of blood flow mismatch using myocardial contrast echocardiography during coronary hyperemia with FS-069, a new intravenous contrast agent. J. Am. Coll. Cardiol. 25:38A, 1995.

31. Camarano, G.P., Ismail, S., Goodman, N.C., et al.: Assessment of risk area during coronary occlusion and infarct size after reperfusion can be determined with myocardial contrast echocardiography using intravenous injections of FS-069, a new contrast agent. Circulation 90(Suppl I):I-68, 1994.

32. Grauer, S., Pantley, G.A., Xu, J., et al.: Aerosomes MRX115: Echocardiographic and hemodynamic characteristics of a new echo contrast agent that produces myocardial opacification after intravenous injection in pigs. Circulation 90(Suppl I):I-556, 1994.

33. Mulvagh, S.L., Foley, D.A., Klarich, K.K., et al.: Visualization of coronary arteries and measurement of coronary blood flow with transthoracic echocardiography after intravenous administration of a new echocardiographic contrast agent. J. Am. Coll. Cardiol. 25:228A; 1995.

34. Cotter, B., Kwan, O.L., Cha, Y.M., et al.: Dose-response characteristics, time-course, and hemodynamic responses to QW3600, an ultrasonic contrast agent capable of myocardial opacification by intravenous injection. J. Am. Coll. Cardiol. 23:393A, 1994.

35. Beppu, S., Matsuda, H., Shishido, T., et al.: Success of myocardial contrast echocardiography by peripheral venous injection: Visualization of area at risk. Circulation 88(Suppl I):I-401, 1993.

36. Gong, Z., Giraud, G., Pantley, G., et al.: Time course of chamber and myocardial contrast opacification with Echogen: A videodensitometric study in monkeys with microvascularization visualization studies in a cat mesentery model. Circulation 90(Part 2):I-556, 1994.

37. Grayburn, P.A., Erikson, J.M., and Velasco, C.E.: Assessment of myocardial risk area and infarct size by peripheral intravenous injection of a new phase shift echo contrast agent. Circulation 90(Part 2):I-555, 1994.

38. Jayaweera, A.R., Skyba, D.M., and Kaul, S.: Technical factors that influence the determination of microbubble transit rate during contrast echocardiography. J. Am. Soc. Echocardiogr. 8:198, 1995.

39. Skyba, D.M., Jayaweera, A.R., Goodman, N.C., et al.: Quantification of myocardial perfusion with myocardial contrast echocardiography during left atrial injection of contrast: Implication for venous injection. Circulation 90:1513, 1994.

40. Jayaweera, A.R., Sklenar, J., and Kaul, S.: Quantification of images obtained during myocardial contrast echocardiography. Echocardiography 11:385, 1994.

41. Schrope, B., Newhouse, V.L., and Uhlendorf, V.: Simulated capillary blood flow measurement using a nonlinear ultrasonic contrast agent. Ultrason. Imaging 14:134, 1992.

42. Monaghan, M.J., Metcalfe, J.M., Odunlami, S., et al.: Digital radiofrequency echocardiography in the detection of myocardial contrast following intravenous administration of Albunex. Eur. Heart J. 14:1200, 1993.

43. Reimer, K.A., and Jennings, R.B.: The "wavefront phenomenon" of myocardial ischemic cell death. II. Transmural progression of necrosis within the framework of ischemic bed size (myocardium at risk) and collateral flow. Lab. Invest. 40:633, 1979.

44. Schaper, W., Frenzel, H., and Hort, W.: Experimental coronary artery occlusion. I. Measurement of infarct size. Basic Res. Cardiol. 74:46, 1979.

45. Kaul, S., Glasheen, W.P., Oliner, J.D., et al.: Relation between anterograde blood flow through a coronary artery and the size of the perfusion bed it supplies: Experimental and clinical implications. J. Am. Coll. Cardiol. 17:1403, 1991.

46. Kaul, S., Pandian, N.G., Guererro, J.L., et al.: The effects of selectively altering the collateral driving pressure on regional perfusion and function in the occluded coronary bed in the dog. Circ. Res. 61:77, 1987.

47. Kaul, S., Kelly, P., Oliner, J.D., et al.: Assessment of regional myocardial blood

flow with myocardial contrast two-dimensional echocardiography. J. Am. Coll. Cardiol. 13:468, 1989.

48. Kaul, S., Pandian, N.G., Okada, R.D., et al.: Contrast echocardiography in acute myocardial ischemia. I. In vivo determination of total left ventricular "area at risk." J. Am. Coll. Cardiol. 4:1272, 1984.

49. Kaul, S., Glasheen, W., Ruddy, T.D., et al.: The importance of defining left ventricular area at risk in vivo during acute myocardial infarction: An experimental evaluation with myocardial contrast two-dimensional echocardiography. Circulation 75:1249, 1987.

50. Kaul, S., Pandian, N.G., Gillam, L.D., et al.: Contrast echocardiography in acute myocardial ischemia. III. An in vivo comparison of the extent of abnormal wall motion with the "area at risk" for necrosis. J. Am. Coll. Cardiol. 7:383, 1986.

51. Kaul, S., Gillam, L.D., and Weyman A.E.: Contrast echocardiography in acute myocardial ischemia. II. The effect of site of injection of contrast agent on the estimation of "area at risk" for necrosis after coronary occlusion. J. Am. Coll. Cardiol. 6:825, 1985.

52. Sabia, P.J., Powers, E.R., Jayaweera, A.R., et al.: Functional significance of collateral blood flow in patients with recent acute myocardial infarction. A study using myocardial contrast echocardiography. Circulation 85:2080, 1992.

53. Grill, H.P., Brinkner, J.A., Tanbe, J., et al.: Contrast echocardiographic mapping of collateralized myocardium in humans before and after coronary angioplasty. J. Am. Coll. Cardiol. 16:1594, 1990.

54. Lim, Y., Nanto, S., Lee, J., et al.: Coronary collaterals assessed with myocardial contrast echocardiography in healed myocardial infarction. Am. J. Cardiol. 66:556, 1990.

55. Okun, E.M., Factor, S.M., and Kirk E.S.: End-capillary loops in the heart: An explanation for discrete myocardial infarctions without border zones. Science 206:565, 1979.

56. Factor, S.M., Okun, E.M., and Kirk E.S.: The histological lateral border of acute canine myocardial infarction. A function of microcirculation. Circ. Res. 48:640, 1981.

57. Ito, H., Tomooka, T., Sakai, N., et al.: Lack of myocardial perfusion immediately after successful thrombolysis. A predictor of poor recovery of left ventricular function in anterior myocardial infarction. Circulation 85:1699, 1992.

58. Ragosta, M., Camarano, G.P., Kaul, S., et al.: Microvascular integrity indicates myocellular viability in patients with recent myocardial infarction: New insights using myocardial contrast echocardiography. Circulation 89:2562, 1994.

59. Lim, Y.-J., Nanto, S., Masuyama, T., et al.: Myocardial salvage: Its assessment and prediction by the analysis of serial myocardial contrast echocardiograms in patients with acute myocardial infarction. Am. Heart J. 128:649, 1994.

60. Agati, L., Voci, P., Bilotta, F., et al.: Influence of residual perfusion within the infarct zone on the natural history of left ventricular dysfunction after acute myocardial infarction: A myocardial contrast echocardiographic study. J. Am. Coll. Cardiol. 24:336, 1994.

61. Villanueva, F.S., Glasheen, W.D., Sklenar, J., et al.: Assessment of risk area during coronary occlusion and infarct size after reperfusion with myocardial contrast echocardiography using left and right atrial injections of contrast. Circulation 88:596, 1993.

62. Kloner, R.A., Ganote, C.E., and Jennings R.B.: The "no-reflow" phenomenon after temporary coronary occlusion in the dog. J. Clin. Invest. 54:1496, 1974.

63. White, F.C., Sanders, M., and Bloor C.M.: Regional redistribution of myocardial blood flow after coronary occlusion and reperfusion in the conscious dog. Am. J. Cardiol. 42:234, 1978.

64. West, P.N., Connors, J.P., Clark, R.E., et al.: Compromised microvascular integrity in ischemic myocardium. Lab. Invest. 38:677, 1978.

65. Villanueva, F.S., Glasheen, W.P., Sklenar, J., et al.: Characterization of spatial patterns of flow within the reperfused myocardium using myocardial contrast echocardiography: Implications for determining extent of myocardial salvage. Circulation 88:2596, 1993.

66. Johnson, W.B., Malone, S.A., Pantely, G., et al.: No reflow and extent of infarction during maximal vasodilation in the porcine heart. Circulation 78:462, 1988.

67. Vanhaecke, J., Flameng, W., Borgers, M., et al.: Evidence for decreased coronary flow reserve in viable postischemic myocardium. Circ. Res. 67:1201, 1990.

68. Sabia, P.J., Powers, E.R., Ragosta, M., et al.: An association between collateral blood flow and myocardial viability in patients with recent myocardial infarction. N. Engl. J. Med. 327:1825, 1992.

69. Gensini, G.G., and daCosta, B.C.B.: The coronary collateral circulation in living man. Am. J. Cardiol. 24:393, 1969.

70. Cohen, M.V.: Morphological considerations of the coronary collateral circulation in man. In Coronary Collaterals. New York, Futura Publishing, 1985, p. 1.

71. Jayaweera, A.R., and Kaul, S.: Quantification of myocardial blood flow with contrast echocardiography. Am. J. Card. Imaging 7:317, 1993.

72. Gould, K.L., and Lipscomb, K.: Effects of coronary stenoses on coronary flow reserve and resistance. Am. J. Cardiol. 34:48, 1974.

73. Jayaweera, A.R., Ismail, S., and Kaul, S.: Attenuation deforms time-intensity curves during contrast echocardiography: Implications for the assessment of transit rates. J. Am. Soc. Echocardiogr. 7:590, 1994.

74. Jayaweera, A.R., Matthew, T.L., Sklenar, J., et al.: Method for the quantitation of myocardial perfusion during myocardial contrast two-dimensional echocardiography. J. Am. Soc. Echocardiogr. 3:91, 1990.

75. Thompson, M.K., Starmer, C.F., Whorten, R.E., et al.: Indicator transit time considered as a gamma variate. Circ. Res. 14:502, 1964.

76. Marcus M.L.: Effects of coronary occlusion on myocardial perfusion. In The Coronary Circulation in Health and Disease. New York, McGraw-Hill, 1983, p. 221.

77. Lim, Y.J., Nanto, S., Masuyama, T., et al.: Visualization of subendocardial myocar-

dial ischemia with myocardial contrast echocardiography in humans. Circulation 79:233, 1989.

78. Cheirif, J., Zoghbi, W.A., Bolli, R., et al.: Assessment of regional myocardial perfusion by contrast echocardiography. II. Detection of changes in transmural and sub-endocardial perfusion during dipyridamole-induced hyperemia in a model of critical coronary stenosis. J. Am. Coll. Cardiol. 14:1555, 1989.

79. Kaul, S., Jayaweera, A.R., Glasheen, W.P., et al.: Myocardial contrast echocardiography and the transmural distribution of flow: A critical appraisal during myocardial ischemia not associated with infarction. J. Am. Coll. Cardiol. 20:1005, 1992.

80. White, C.W., Wright, C.B., Doty, D.B., et al.: Does the visual interpretation of the coronary angiogram predict the physiologic importance of a coronary stenosis? N. Engl. J. Med. 310:819, 1984.

81. Wilson, R.F., and White, C.W.: Intracoronary papavarine: An ideal coronary vasodilator for studies of the coronary circulation in conscious humans. Circulation 73:444, 1986.

82. Kern, M.J., Deligonal, U., Vandormael, M., et al.: Impaired coronary vasodilator reserve in the immediate postcoronary angioplasty period: Analysis of coronary artery flow velocity indexes and regional cardiac venous efflux. J. Am. Coll. Cardiol. 13:960, 1989.

83. Tillmanns, H., Leinberger, H., Neumann, F.J., et al.: Myocardial microcirculation in the beating heart: In vivo microscopic studies. *In* Spaan, J.A.E., Bruschke, A.V.G., and Gittenberger-de Groot, A.C. (eds.): Coronary Circulation. Dordrecht, The Netherlands, Martinus-Nijhoff, 1987, p. 88.

84. Kanatsuka, H., Sekiguchi, N., Aaki, K., et al.: Microvascular sites and mechanisms responsible for reactive hyperemia in the coronary circulation of the beating canine heart. Circ. Res. 71:912, 1992.

85. Fedor, J.M., McIntosh, D.M., Rembert, J.C., et al.: Coronary transmural myocardial blood flow responses in awake domestic pigs. Am. J. Physiol. 235:H435, 1978.

86. Rouleau, J., Boerboom, L.E., Surjadhana, A., et al.: The role of autoregulation and tissue diastolic pressures in the transmural distribution of left ventricular blood flow in anesthetized dogs. Circ. Res. 45:804, 1979.

87. Camarano, G., Jayaweera, A.R., Ismail, S., et al.: Measurement of myocardial blood volume is a preferable indicator of microvascular reserve than measurement of coronary blood flow: A study utilizing myocardial contrast echocardiography. J. Am. Soc. Echocardiogr. 7:S16, 1994.

88. Keller, M.W., Smucker, M.L., Burwell, L., et al.: Myocardial contrast echocardiography in humans. II. Assessment of coronary blood flow reserve. J. Am. Coll. Cardiol. 12:925, 1988.

89. Porter, T.R., D'Sa, A., Turner, C., et al.: Myocardial contrast echocardiography for the assessment of coronary blood flow reserve: Validation in humans. J. Am. Coll. Cardiol. 21:349, 1993.

90. Cheirif, J., Zoghbi, W.A., Raizner, A.E., et al.: Assessment of myocardial perfusion in humans by myocardial contrast echocardiography. I. Evaluation of regional coronary reserve by peak contrast intensity. J. Am. Coll. Cardiol. 11:735, 1988.

91. Perchet, H., Dupouy, P., Duval-Moulin, A., et al.: Improvement of subendocardial myocardial perfusion after percutaneous transluminal coronary angioplasty. A myocardial contrast echocardiography study with correlation between myocardial contrast reserve and Doppler coronary reserve. Circulation 91:1419, 1995.

92. Ismail, S., Jayaweera, A.R., Goodman, N.C., et al.: Detection of coronary artery stenoses and quantification of blood flow mismatch during coronary hyperemia with myocardial contrast echocardiography. Circulation 91:821, 1995.

93. Spotnitz, W.D., Keller, M.W., Watson, D.D., et al.: Success of internal mammary bypass grafting can be assessed intraoperatively using myocardial contrast two-dimensional echocardiography. J. Am. Coll. Cardiol. 12:196, 1988.

94. Goldman, M.E., and Mindich, B.P.: Intraoperative cardioplegia contrast echocardiography for assessing myocardial perfusion during open heart surgery. J. Am. Coll. Cardiol. 4:1029, 1984.

95. Keller, M.W., Spotnitz, W.D., Matthew, T.L., et al.: Intraoperative assessment of regional myocardial perfusion using quantitative myocardial contrast echocardiography: An experimental evaluation. J. Am. Coll. Cardiol. 16:1267, 1990.

96. Aronson, S., Lee, B.K., Liddicoat, J.R., et al.: Assessment of retrograde cardi-

oplegia distribution using contrast echocardiography. Ann. Thorac. Surg. 52:810, 1992..

97. Villanueva, F.S., Spotnitz, W.D., Jayaweera, A.R., et al.: Myocardial contrast echocardiography in humans: On-line intraoperative quantitation of regional myocardial perfusion during coronary artery bypass graft operations. J. Thorac. Cardiovasc. Surg. 104:1529, 1992.

98. Keller, M.W., Geddes, L., Spotnitz, W.D., et al.: Manifestations of reperfusion injury in the microcirculation following perfusion with hyperkalemic, hypothermic, cardioplegic solutions and blood perfusion: Effects of adenosine. Circulation 84:2485, 1991.

99. Villanueva, F.S., Kaul, S., Glasheen, W.P., et al.: Intraoperative assessment of the distribution of retrograde cardioplegia using myocardial contrast echocardiography. Surg. Forum 41:252, 1990.

100. Villanueva, F.S., Spotnitz, W.D., Glasheen, W.P., et al.: Physiology of retrograde cardioplegia delivery: Comparison with anterograde delivery with respect to myocardial cooling and nutrient blood flow. Am. J. Physiol. 268:H1555, 1995.

101. Ismail, S., Spotnitz, W.D., Jayaweera, A.R., et al.: Myocardial contrast echocardiography can be used to assess dynamic changes in microvascular function in vivo. J. Am. Coll. Cardiol. 25:246A, 1995.

102. Nath, S., Whayne, J.G., Kaul, S., et al.: Effects of radiofrequency catheter ablation on regional myocardial blood flow: Possible mechanism for late electrophysiologic outcome. Circulation 89:2667, 1994.

103. Fraker, T., Harris, P., Behar, V., et al.: Detection and exclusion of interatrial shunts by two-dimensional echocardiography and peripheral venous injection. Circulation 59:379, 1979.

104. Valdes-Cruz, L., Pieroni, D., Roland, J., et al.: Echocardiographic detection of intracardiac right-to-left shunts following peripheral venous injections. Circulation 54:558, 1976.

105. Weyman, A.E., Wann, L.S., Caldwell, R., et al.: Negative contrast echocardiography: A new method for detecting left-to-right shunts. Circulation 59:498, 1979.

106. Hopkins, W.E., Waggoner, A.D., and Barzilai, B.: Frequency and significance of intrapulmonary right-to-left shunting in end-stage hepatic disease. Am. J. Cardiol. 70:516, 1992.

107. Caldwell, S.H., Brantley, K., Dent, J., et al.: The hepatobiliary syndrome masquerading as pulmonary Langerhans-cell histocytosis. Ann. Intern. Med. 121:34, 1994.

108. Chen, D., Morganrath, J., Mardelli, T., et al.: Tricuspid regurgitation in tricuspid valve prolapse demonstrated with contrast cross-sectional echocardiography. Am. J. Cardiol. 46:983, 1980.

109. Meltzer, R.S., Van Hoogenhuyze, D.C.A., Serruys, P.W., et al.: The diagnosis of tricuspid regurgitation by contrast echocardiography. Circulation 63:1093, 1981.

110. Levine, R.A., Teicholz, L.E., Goldman, M.E., et al.: Microbubbles have intracardiac velocities similar to those of red blood cells. J. Am. Coll. Cardiol. 3:28, 1984.

111. Yock, P.G., and Popp, R.L.: Noninvasive estimation of right ventricular systolic pressure by Doppler ultrasound in patients with tricuspid regurgitation. Circulation 70:657, 1984.

112. Himelman, R.B., Stulbarg, M., Kircher, B., et al.: Noninvasive evaluation of pulmonary artery pressure during exercise by saline-enhanced Doppler echocardiography in chronic pulmonary disease. Circulation 79:863, 1989.

113. Nakatani, S., Imanishi, T., Terasawa, A., et al.: Clinical application of transpulmonary contrast-enhanced technique in the assessment of severity of aortic stenosis. J. Am. Coll. Cardiol. 20:973, 1992.

114. von Bibra, H., Becher, H., Firschke, C., et al.: Enhancement of mitral regurgitation and normal left atrial color Doppler flow signals with peripheral venous injection of a saccharide-based contrast agent. J. Am. Coll. Cardiol. 22:521, 1993.

115. Falcone, R.A., Markowitz, P.A., Perez, J.E., et al.: Intravenous Albunex during dobutamine stress echocardiography: Enhancement of left ventricular endocardial borders. Am. Heart J. 130:254, 1995.

116. Dent, J.D., Jayaweera, A.R., Glasheen, W.P., et al.: A mathematical model for the quantitation of mitral regurgitation: Experimental validation using contrast echocardiography. Circulation 86:553, 1992.

117. Galanti, G., Jayaweera, A.R., Villanueva, F.S., et al.: Transpulmonary transit of microbubbles during contrast echocardiography: Implications for estimating cardiac output and pulmonary blood volume. J. Am. Soc. Echocardiogr. 6:272, 1993.

CHAPTER

36 Stress Echocardiography

Thomas Ryan, M.D.

UNDERLYING PRINCIPLES ____ 504
METHODOLOGY ____ 504
Exercise Echocardiography ____ 504
Nonexercise Stress Echocardiography ____ 505
Imaging Techniques ____ 506
Digital-Imaging Techniques ____ 507

Interpretation of Stress Echocardiograms ____ 507
ACCURACY AND CLINICAL APPLICATIONS ____ 511
Detection of Coronary Artery Disease ____ 511
Localization of Coronary Artery Lesions ____ 512

Predicting the Extent and Severity of Disease ____ 512
Stress Echocardiography Versus Radionuclide Techniques ____ 514
Vasodilator Stress Echocardiography ____ 515
Atrial Pacing Stress Echocardiography ____ 516
Comparison of Various Stress Echocardiographic Techniques ____ 516
Stress Echocardiography After Coronary Revascularization ____ 517

Assessment of Myocardial Viability ____ 518
PROGNOSTIC VALUE OF STRESS ECHOCARDIOGRAPHY ____ 518
Predicting the Likelihood of Future Cardiac Events ____ 518
Postmyocardial Infarction Risk Stratification ____ 518
Preoperative Risk Assessment With Pharmacologic Stress Echocardiography ____ 519

During the past 15 years, stress echocardiography has evolved from an impractical research technique to a useful and ubiquitous clinical tool. The steady development of the field can be attributed to several factors, including improvements in image quality, growing clinical experience, and the application of digital imaging technology. Each of these factors has led to expanding use and, at the same time, contributed to improved accuracy. More recently, the increasing emphasis on cost containment in health care delivery has fostered continued growth of the field.

The basic premise underlying stress echocardiography is that myocardial ischemia leads to left ventricular dyssynergy that can be reliably detected with the use of two-dimensional echocardiography. Both endocardial motion and wall thickening are analyzed to determine the presence, extent, and location of wall motion abnormalities. When combined with a cardiovascular stress test, echocardiography can be used to distinguish *baseline* abnormalities from *transient* or *induced* wall motion changes. Global and regional left ventricular function are assessed at rest and during stress, providing both diagnostic and prognostic information.

This chapter focuses on the principles, methodology, and clinical applications of stress echocardiography. The various forms of stress echocardiographic techniques are presented, and the different approaches to wall motion analysis are discussed. Both the diagnostic and the prognostic applications of stress echocardiography are examined. The accuracy of each method is reviewed and compared with that of other stress testing modalities. Finally, guidelines for the proper use of stress echocardiography and its role in clinical decision-making are covered.

UNDERLYING PRINCIPLES

When cardiac function is assessed with echocardiography, the normal response to exercise is the development of hyperdynamic wall motion. This observation, first reported in tests using M-mode echocardiography in 1970,[1] provided new insight into the mechanical response of the normal left ventricle to stress and paved the way for the emergence of stress echocardiography. Dynamic exercise leads to an increase in endocardial excursion and wall thickening, especially in the upright posture. The hyperdynamic response is generally uniform and is associated with a reduction in end-systolic left ventricular cavity size but with little change in end-diastolic dimensions. With the patient in the supine posture, these changes may be less apparent because of the smaller rise in stroke volume.[2, 3] With termination of exercise, hypercontractility may transiently increase before returning to baseline within 2 to 4 minutes.[4]

The net effect of exercise on the left ventricle is a progressive increase in myocardial oxygen demand. When the delivery of oxygen is limited by the presence of a coronary artery lesion, supply is inadequate to meet the rising demand, and myocardial ischemia develops. This situation leads to a sequence of events referred to as the *ischemic cascade*. The classic work of Tennant and Wiggers in the 1930s demonstrated that regional dyssynergy was an early and predictable component of the ischemic process.[5] They were the first to describe, using an open-chest canine preparation, the dyskinetic left ventricular wall motion that occurs immediately after

coronary artery ligation. In the early 1970s, this same phenomenon was demonstrated with M-mode echocardiography.[6, 7]

Exercise-induced wall motion abnormalities develop relatively early in the course of ischemia, generally preceding angina and electrocardiographic changes. By comparing regional wall motion at baseline and during stress, it is possible to distinguish *resting* abnormalities, indicating prior infarction or hibernating myocardium, from *transient* dyssynergy, a specific marker of induced ischemia. The onset of an exercise-induced wall motion abnormality occurs soon after the development of a perfusion defect. With termination of exercise, the time course of resolution of regional dyssynergy is variable.[8, 9] Most wall motion abnormalities persist for several minutes, thereby allowing their detection with postexercise imaging. Although induced abnormalities may continue for as long as 30 minutes after cessation of exercise,[10] very rapid recovery of wall motion also occurs.[9, 11, 12]

METHODOLOGY

Exercise Echocardiography

Exercise echocardiography is generally performed using either a treadmill or a bicycle protocol (Table 36–1). In all cases, rest images are recorded to serve as a baseline for comparison. The parasternal long- and short-axis views and the apical four- and two-chamber views are commonly used in most protocols. Other views, such as the apical long-axis or subcostal-window, may also be included. Obtaining images *during* treadmill exercise is very difficult,[13] so most protocols rely on postexercise imaging.[14] Immediately after completion of exercise, the patient is moved from the treadmill to a table and placed in the left lateral decubitus position for imaging, which must be completed within 1 to 2 minutes. The advantages of this form of stress echocardiography are the widespread availability of treadmills and the wealth of clinical experience with this method of stress testing. The major disadvantage is the reliance on *postexercise imaging*. This approach assumes that wall motion abnormalities that develop during stress will persist long enough into recovery to be detected. Abnormalities that recover rapidly may be missed, causing false-negative results.[9, 11, 15]

TABLE 36–1. STRESS ECHOCARDIOGRAPHIC TECHNIQUES

Stress Methods	Imaging Modalities
Exercise	Two-dimensional echocardiography
Treadmill	Transesophageal echocardiography
Bicycle (upright, supine)	Doppler
Hand grip	Pulsed
Pharmacologic	Continuous-wave
Dobutamine	Color flow imaging
Arbutamine	
Dipyridamole	
Adenosine	
Atrial pacing	
Mental stress	

Bicycle exercise echocardiography can be performed using either upright or recumbent ergometry. The patient pedals at a constant cadence (usually 60 rpm) against an adjustable workload that is increased in a stepwise manner. Patient cooperation (to maintain the proper cadence) and coordination (to perform the pedaling motion) are mandatory for achieving adequate stress. The major advantage of bicycle exercise, compared with treadmill exercise, is the ability to obtain images both *during* and after exercise. Although imaging throughout exercise is technically possible, the interpretation is generally based on a comparison of rest images, peak images, and images obtained immediately after stress.

Obtaining a high-quality echocardiogram during exercise is challenging. With the patient supine, all the standard views generally can be recorded, even during vigorous exercise. The ability to obtain these images has been facilitated by the development of ergometers that allow left lateral decubitus positioning.[16] Proper patient support and stabilization, however, are critical to ensuring optimal performance. In the upright position, imaging is more technically difficult and is usually limited to apical and subcostal views.[17] Apical images are best recorded with the patient leaning forward over the handlebars, with the arms slightly extended. Subcostal views require a more lordotic posture and have the advantage of minimal lung interference. When one uses this method, special care must be taken to avoid apical foreshortening.

In addition to image acquisition, other fundamental differences exist between upright and supine exercise. Most patients are able to achieve a lower maximum level of exercise in the supine posture,[3] probably because of general inexperience with supine exercise and lack of proper muscle support, resulting in fatigue at an earlier stage. This limitation is partially offset by the development of ischemia at a lower workload during supine exercise. The explanation for this observation is based on hemodynamic differences between the two positions.[2, 3, 18] For a given level of stress, both end-diastolic volume and mean arterial blood pressure are greater in the supine position, owing in part to the enhanced venous return that results from leg elevation.[3] These alterations contribute to an elevation in wall stress that leads directly to an increase in myocardial oxygen demand and the potential for the earlier development of ischemia.[3, 18] In summary, no compelling superiority of either form of bicycle exercise has been demonstrated. Despite differences in hemodynamic response, both methods are capable of inducing ischemia. However, ease of image acquisition favors the supine posture. More practical issues, such as the cost of equipment and space requirements, favor upright bicycle ergometry.

Nonexercise Stress Echocardiography

Nonexercise stress echocardiography can be performed with either pharmacologic agents or cardiac pacing. Among the available pharmacologic agents, dobutamine, an adrenergic stimulant, and dipyridamole, a coronary vasodilator, have been used with the greatest frequency. These two drugs differ fundamentally in their mechanism of action and mode of inducing ischemia. Dobutamine increases heart rate and contractility by stimulating cardiac β-adrenergic receptors.[19] In addition, direct peripheral adrenergic effects combine with vascular reflex effects to produce an unpredictable vasoactive response. A gradual and modest increase in arterial blood pressure occurs most often. Occasionally, marked hypertension or varying degrees of hypotension may develop. The net effect of these phenomena is a dose-dependent increase in myocardial oxygen demand. In the normal heart, a significant augmentation of myocardial blood flow, and oxygen supply, occurs during dobutamine infusion.[20-22] However, when regional blood flow is limited by coronary disease, the increase in perfusion is inadequate to meet rising oxygen demand, and regional ischemia develops.

The predominant effect of dipyridamole is vasodilation. The action is mediated through inhibition of adenosine uptake, resulting in potentiation of the potent vasodilating effects of this endogenous chemical. *Normal coronary arteries* are especially responsive to dipyridamole's actions, creating a hyperemic effect in normal regions. Diseased coronary arteries, however, are relatively incapable of mounting a significant vasodilatory response. A "coronary steal" phenomenon develops, in which blood is diverted away from areas supplied by stenotic coronary arteries. Myocardial perfusion becomes increasingly heterogeneous, and oxygen supply to affected regions may decrease, resulting in hypoperfusion and the development of ischemia.[23-25]

The use of dobutamine as a stress echocardiographic method is predicated on the assumption that infusion of the drug in incremental doses will lead to myocardial ischemia and a resulting wall motion abnormality. The technique involves stepwise administration of the agent after a baseline echocardiogram has been recorded. A variety of protocols have evolved (Fig. 36–1). Typically, the infusion is begun at a dose of 5 μg/kg per minute and increased, in 3-minute stages, to a maximum of 30 to 40 μg/kg per minute. Images are obtained at low dose (usually 5 or 10 μg/kg per minute) and peak dose and may also be recorded at an intermediate dose level or after infusion (Fig. 36–2). Failure to develop a hyperdynamic wall motion response is considered abnormal and is most often indicative of ischemia.

In as many as 40 percent of patients, the heart rate response to dobutamine will be inadequate. To augment the chronotropic response, some investigators recommend the addition of atropine (administered intravenously in doses of 0.25 to 2.0 mg). Atropine is considered safe and is generally well tolerated.[26] In one study, the higher peak heart rate provided by the drug was associated with a significant increase in sensitivity for the detection of coronary artery disease.[27]

The major side effect of dobutamine infusion is the development of arrhythmias. Premature atrial and ventricular complexes are common. More clinically significant arrhythmias, such as ventricular tachycardia and atrial fibrillation, occur infrequently and generally respond to termination of the infusion. In one large series,[26] nonsustained ventricular tachycardia occurred in 3.8 percent of patients but was self-limited and rarely required specific therapy. Neither sustained ventricular tachycardia nor ventricular fibrillation occurred. Administration of an intravenous β-blocking agent has been used to treat the ischemia-related effects of the drug or to slow the ventricular response to atrial fibrillation. Death and myocardial infarction have occurred in association with dobutamine stress testing but are extremely rare. The acceptable safety profile

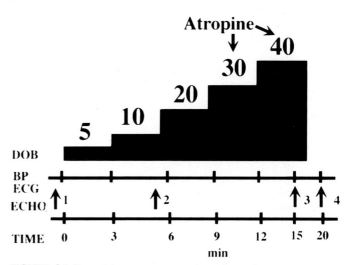

FIGURE 36–1. A dobutamine stress echocardiography (DSE) protocol. After baseline data are acquired, dobutamine (DOB) is infused, beginning at a dose of 5 μg/kg per minute and increasing, every 3 minutes, to a maximum dose of 40 μg/kg per minute. The blood pressure (BP) and ECG are recorded at each stage. Echocardiograms are recorded at baseline (no. 1), low dose (no. 2), peak dose (no. 3), and 5 minutes into recovery (no. 4). When necessary, atropine is given at the higher dose levels to augment the heart rate response. min = minutes.

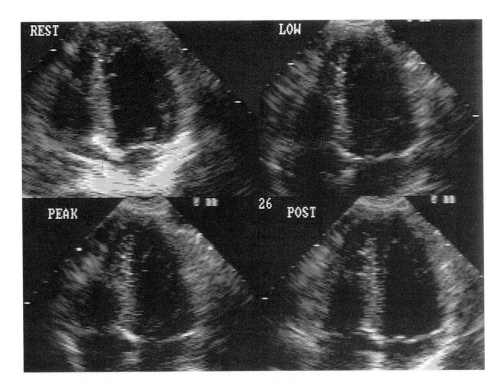

FIGURE 36–2. The quad-screen display of a dobutamine stress echocardiogram. Four-chamber views at baseline (REST), low dose (LOW), peak dose (PEAK), and recovery (POST) are simultaneously displayed with the use of digital imaging technology.

of the test is partly due to the ability to monitor wall motion throughout the infusion and, in doing so, to detect ischemia early in its course. By terminating the dobutamine infusion at a relatively early stage, the serious complications of ischemia can often be avoided.

Hypotension during dobutamine infusion has been reported in 10 to 20 percent of patients.[28] The significance of this development is quite different from that of exercise-induced hypotension. A decline in blood pressure is not a marker of severe ischemia,[28–30] nor is it associated with a poor prognosis.[28] Several mechanisms probably account for dobutamine-related hypotension. Some investigators have suggested a vasovagal reflex phenomenon.[29] In other cases, hyperdynamic wall motion may result in intracavitary obstruction.[30] In these patients, a dynamic left ventricular outflow-tract gradient can be demonstrated with Doppler imaging. Inadequate preload secondary to hypovolemia may be a risk factor.

Dipyridamole stress echocardiography is optimally performed with the use of the intravenous route of administration. The standard protocol uses a total dose of 0.56 mg/kg infused over 4 minutes, followed by 4 minutes of echocardiographic monitoring. If the test result remains negative, an additional 0.28 mg/kg is given over 2 minutes (for a total dose of 0.84 mg/kg). Echocardiographic monitoring is continued throughout the infusion and for at least 5 minutes afterward. Caffeine- and theophylline-containing products should be withheld for 12 hours prior to the test. The most common adverse effects of dipyridamole administration are headache, flushing, hypotension, and nausea. The use of dipyridamole is contraindicated in patients with bronchospastic lung disease. Aminophylline should be available during dipyridamole stress testing and can be used to readily reverse the hemodynamic and bronchospastic effects of the drug. Extensive experience with the test has confirmed its safety, and very few serious complications have been reported.[31]

In recent years, adenosine has also been used as a stress echocardiographic agent. The mechanism of action of this drug is very similar to that of dipyridamole, which acts by potentiating the effects of endogenous adenosine. It is a potent vasodilator and is characterized by a rapid onset and brief duration of action. Adenosine is administered intravenously at a dose of 0.14 mg/kg per minute infused over 6 minutes (cumulative dose, 0.84 mg/kg). Echocardiographic recording is performed during the final 1 to 2 minutes of the infusion. The short half-life of adenosine contributes to its safety and degree of patient tolerance. Significant bradyarrhythmias, including sinus bradycardia, sinus arrest, and impaired atrioventricular conduction, may occur during adenosine infusion but are usually very transient and well tolerated. The brief duration of action also has implications for echocardiographic imaging. The more transient the wall motion abnormality, the greater the likelihood that such abnormalities will be missed.

Another form of nonexercise stress echocardiography uses cardiac pacing.[32–35] In most cases, transesophageal atrial pacing is performed, often in conjunction with transesophageal imaging.[36, 37] A bipolar pacing device is positioned in the distal esophagus and is used to emit 10-msec impulses of sufficient output to capture the atria. Pacing is typically begun at 100 beats per minute and then increased every 2 minutes by 10 beats per minute. Echocardiographic monitoring may be transthoracic or transesophageal. The test provides a positive chronotropic stimulus but does not produce an inotropic stimulus. Therefore, hyperdynamic wall motion generally does not develop. Despite this limitation, feasibility and overall accuracy are acceptable, and the test appears to be a reasonable alternative when exercise is inadequate.[35] Potential problems include failure of atrial capture, atrioventricular block at higher heart rates, and patient intolerance.

Imaging Techniques

Transthoracic two-dimensional echocardiography is the primary imaging modality used for the assessment of ischemic heart disease. For stress testing, this technique is well suited to the detection and localization of wall motion abnormalities due to ischemia or prior infarction. The tomographic nature of ultrasound permits an unlimited number of imaging planes to be recorded, providing a complete assessment of the left ventricle. Regional and global systolic function, wall thickening, and endocardial excursion are evaluated with this technique. Its versatility is unsurpassed by any other imaging modality.

When transthoracic image quality is poor, transesophageal echocardiography may be used in conjunction with either pacing or pharmacologic stress.[37] In addition to being more "invasive," transesophageal stress echocardiography is somewhat limited with regard to the number of views that can be obtained. Reliance on single-plane transducer technology for stress echocardiography is not recommended. The use of biplane and multiplane transducers, however, permits a more complete evaluation of left ventricular wall motion. For most examinations, long-axis views from the esophagus and a series of transgastric short-axis planes provide an acceptable sampling of wall motion. Rapid repositioning of the endoscope to permit complete image acquisition within the allowable time frame requires experience and practice.

Doppler imaging plays a limited role in the field of stress echocardiography. In part this is due to the limited time frame during which imaging must be completed, making the acquisition of ancillary imaging data impractical. A unique feature provided by Doppler imaging is the ability to quantify global left ventricular systolic function. This is most often accomplished by recording the aortic or mitral flow-velocity integral, from which stroke volume and cardiac output can be derived.[38–40] By positioning a nonimaging probe in the suprasternal notch, one can measure aortic flow at rest and continuously during exercise. Because aortic cross-sectional area is constant, changes in the flow-velocity integral directly parallel changes in systolic function. In clinical studies, both stroke volume and flow acceleration have been measured during exercise testing to detect alterations in cardiac performance. Changes in aortic flow velocity correlate with severity of coronary artery disease and left ventricular dysfunction.[40] In one study,[39] the addition of Doppler imaging increased the sensitivity of wall motion analysis for the detection of disease. In addition to evaluating patients with ischemic heart disease, exercise Doppler echocardiography has also been used to assess the effects of drugs on cardiac function.[41] A more recent application of Doppler imaging analysis to stress testing has involved the detection of ischemic mitral regurgitation with color flow mapping.

Digital Imaging Techniques

The development and application of digital imaging techniques in the mid-1980s had a profound effect on the growth of stress echocardiography. Digital processing of ultrasound images converts analog data (recorded on videotape) into a digital format. Initially, digitization was performed "off-line" by manual processing of videotape recordings. Later, the process was automated and is now accomplished "on-line" by direct conversion of the video image into discrete bits of information recorded in binary code. With the use of a variety of storage media, the information is saved and then reassembled into a series of digital images.

The process of digitization, as applied to echocardiography, begins with identification of the R wave of the electrocardiogram. Using this as a starting point, the computer captures a series of frames of video images in real time. With the current generation of equipment, typically eight or more frames, each separated by 50 msec, are obtained. These images are digitized and displayed in a *cine loop*. The continuous loop may be as short as eight cells (approximately 350 msec and making up only a single systolic cycle) or as long as several minutes (analogous to a digital videotape). Once digitized, the images can be stored or displayed in a variety of ways. With stress echocardiography, side-by-side display of rest and stress views is the usual format.[42–44]

Digital imaging has several advantages when applied to stress echocardiography. Perhaps the most important of these is the versatility of display options available with digital recordings compared with analog recordings. A major limitation of videotape is the inability of displaying rest and stress images in a side-by-side format. When one uses videotape, the appreciation of stress-induced changes in wall motion requires *remembering* the resting study while viewing the stress study, and vice versa. Typically, the studies are reviewed repeatedly in an effort to confidently detect subtle changes. This is not only time-consuming but inherently inferior to side-by-side analysis of digital images, an approach that greatly increases the likelihood of identifying more subtle abnormalities. A second advantage of digital processing is the opportunity to edit the recording by selecting the cardiac cycles to

be used for the final cine loop. This allows elimination of images degraded by respiratory interference. Finally, because only a single cardiac cycle from each view is required to create the cine loop, postexercise imaging can be completed more quickly, thereby reducing the chance that an induced abnormality will resolve before it is detected.

Over the past decade, digital imaging technology has become an indispensable part of stress echocardiography and is now being applied to other areas of echocardiography.[45] Several issues, however, remain unresolved. There is still disagreement about how much of the ultrasound examination should be digitized and stored as the final study. Expanding the digital study to more than one cardiac cycle per view, for example, may prove desirable. With continued improvements in computer speed and storage capacity, the ability to record and save a more complete examination will be possible. As more information is stored, compromises in speed and ease of accessibility are inevitable. To accommodate larger data sets, *compression* of digital information will be used increasingly. How much compression can be tolerated without significantly compromising image quality remains unknown. Finally, standardization of the various aspects of digital imaging is desirable.[46] These include digital file formats, imaging parameters, compression algorithms, network standards, and storage media.

Interpretation of Stress Echocardiograms

Ischemia is manifested echocardiographically as a deterioration in regional systolic function. To make this determination, both wall thickening and endocardial excursion should be analyzed. Of the two parameters, a reduction in wall thickening may be the more specific marker of ischemia, because of the many factors that affect endocardial excursion, such as cardiac translation, left bundle branch block, and the postoperative state. Unfortunately, subjective interpretation of wall thickening is often difficult, so most analyses rely more heavily on wall motion changes.

With the use of multiple views, the entire left ventricle can be systematically interrogated. Regional wall motion is graded as normal, hypokinetic, akinetic, or dyskinetic (Fig. 36–3). Although a variety of schemes are available, use of the 16-segment model endorsed by the American Society of Echocardiography should be encouraged[47, 48] (Fig. 36–4). In the normal heart, stress causes both regional and global ventricular function to increase and wall motion to become hyperdynamic. Failure of the heart to respond in this manner is generally considered an abnormal response and is most often the result of ischemia (Fig. 36–5). It must be recognized, however, that the lack of a hyperdynamic response (i.e., *unchanged* wall motion) may be normal in certain situations. A low level of stress, severe hypertension, and drug therapy (especially β-adrenergic blockers) often preclude the development of hyperkinesis. In addition, *postexercise* wall motion may not appear hyperdynamic, especially if imaging is delayed for more than 1 or 2 minutes. Stress echocardiograms should be analyzed systematically, segment by segment, comparing rest and stress wall motion in each region. Global function, including ejection fraction, can also be evaluated to provide additional diagnostic data. For example, stress-induced dilation of the left ventricle is always abnormal and suggests the presence of multivessel coronary artery disease.

In stress echocardiography, a major goal of wall motion analysis is distinguishing ischemia from prior infarction. Regional wall motion abnormalities present at baseline are usually the result of previous myocardial infarction. More recently, it has been recognized that such abnormalities may be reversible, suggesting the presence of stunned or hibernating myocardium. Dobutamine echocardiography is being used increasingly to distinguish between these two possibilities (see later). The *resting* echocardiogram itself can also provide useful information. For example, if the myocardial segments are thin, echogenic (i.e., scarred), or dyskinetic, the likelihood of viability is low. On the other hand, if the segments are of full thickness and only hypokinetic, viability is much more likely.

Differentiating between ischemia and infarction requires com-

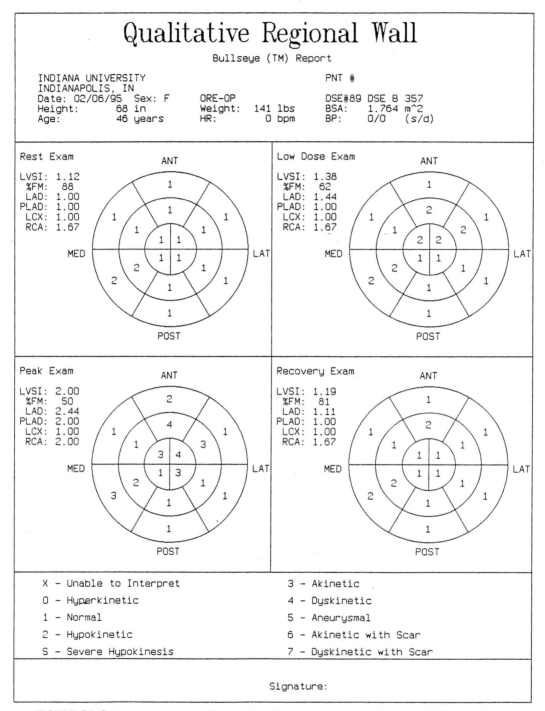

FIGURE 36–3. A computer-generated regional wall motion score report that uses a bull's-eye scheme. The left ventricle is divided into 16 segments, including 6 segments at the base, 6 segments at the midventricular level, and 4 segments at the apex. Wall motion is subjectively graded in each segment with the use of the scheme shown on the diagram. The grades are displayed for each of the different stages of the stress test. Global and regional wall motion score indices are automatically generated by the computer as shown.

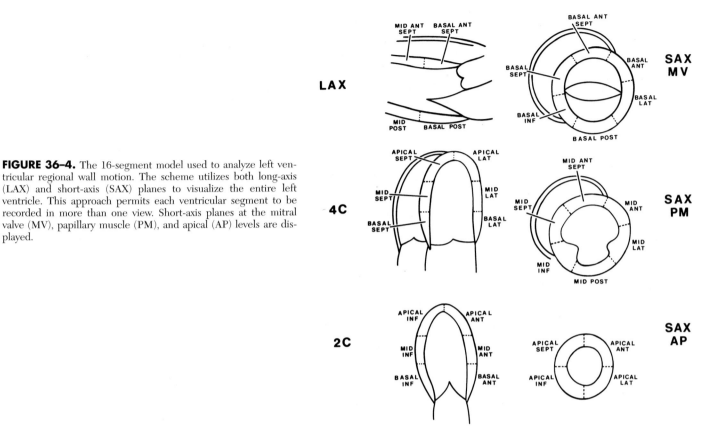

FIGURE 36–4. The 16-segment model used to analyze left ventricular regional wall motion. The scheme utilizes both long-axis (LAX) and short-axis (SAX) planes to visualize the entire left ventricle. This approach permits each ventricular segment to be recorded in more than one view. Short-axis planes at the mitral valve (MV), papillary muscle (PM), and apical (AP) levels are displayed.

parison of rest and stress images. A region that is normal at rest and deteriorates with stress is most likely ischemic. A region that is akinetic at rest and remains unchanged with stress is indicative of prior infarction. The significance of a resting wall motion abnormality that worsens with stress is less clear, which may be the result of ischemia developing in an area of *partial prior infarction* (analogous to a mixed-thallium defect).[49] However, other explanations, such as a change in regional loading conditions, are also plausible, and stress echocardiography may not permit distinction among these possibilities. Improvement during stress of a resting wall motion abnormality is uncommon. Normalization of mild resting hypokinesis is most likely a normal finding.[50] Stress-induced improvement of akinetic or dyskinetic regions may result from a tethering effect of adjacent normal segments that become hyperdynamic. A summary of the various wall motion responses encountered during stress echocardiography is provided in Table 36–2.

The location and extent of wall motion abnormalities can be correlated with the location of coronary artery lesions. However, individual variability in coronary distribution, especially of the pos-

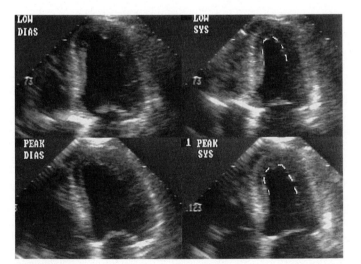

FIGURE 36–5. An abnormal dobutamine stress echocardiogram. On the left, end-diastolic (DIAS) images of the four-chamber view are presented. In the upper right quad, the low-dose systolic (LOW SYS) image shows normal endocardial excursion and wall thickening of the apex. In the lower right quad, at peak dose (PEAK SYS), the end-systolic image shows a decrease in both endocardial motion and wall thickening. This change is suggestive of ischemia involving the left anterior descending coronary artery.

TABLE 36–2. CLINICAL SIGNIFICANCE OF WALL MOTION RESPONSES TO STRESS

Wall Motion		
Rest	**Stress**	**Interpretation**
Normal	Increases	Normal
Normal	Unchanged	Normal vs. ischemia?
Normal	Decreases	Ischemia
Hypokinetic	Increases	Normal (stunned or hibernating°)
Hypokinetic	Unchanged	Infarction
Hypokinetic	Decreases	Infarction ± ischemia
Akinetic/dyskinetic	Increases	Stunned or hibernating°
Akinetic/dyskinetic	Unchanged	Infarction
Akinetic/dyskinetic	Decreases	Infarction

°With dobutamine only.

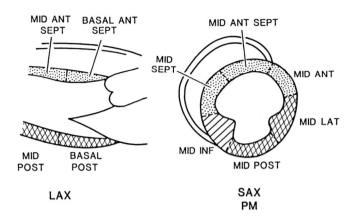

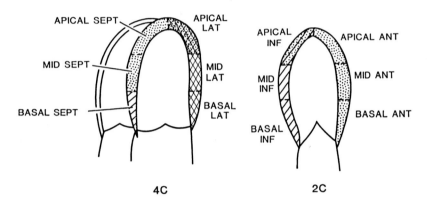

FIGURE 36–6. This diagram demonstrates how the 16 segments of the left ventricle can be recorded with the use of four views, including the parasternal long-axis (LAX) and short-axis (SAX) at the papillary muscle (PM) level, and the apical four-chamber (4C) and two-chamber (2C) views. The relationship between coronary artery distribution and each of the 16 segments is demonstrated. See text for details.

▨ LEFT ANTERIOR DESCENDING DISTRIBUTION
▨ RIGHT CORONARY ARTERY DISTRIBUTION
▨ CIRCUMFLEX DISTRIBUTION
▨ LEFT ANTERIOR DESCENDING/CIRCUMFLEX OVERLAP
▨ LEFT ANTERIOR DESCENDING/RIGHT CORONARY ARTERY OVERLAP

terior circulation, reduces the precision of these predictions. The scheme used at Indiana University for predicting coronary anatomy based on wall motion is shown in Figure 36–6. This approach uses two parasternal and two apical views and divides the left ventricle into 16 segments, as recommended by the American Society of Echocardiography. Note that some segments are designated "overlap" regions. Abnormalities in these segments should be interpreted on the basis of the presence or absence of dyssynergy in adjoining segments. For example, an abnormality in the apical-inferior segment is most likely due to disease in the left anterior descending artery if the anterior wall is also involved, or to disease in the right coronary artery if the inferoposterior wall is abnormal. Most studies have reported excellent results for identifying lesions in the left anterior descending and right coronary arteries,[51, 52] but with quite variable and sometimes very poor accuracy for detecting left circumflex artery lesions.[16] Several factors have been proposed to account for these findings. The left circumflex artery often supplies less myocardium than the other arteries, making detection of wall motion abnormalities more difficult. Optimal recording of lateral-wall endocardium is not always possible, which may contribute to false-negative results. Finally, in some cases, lateral-wall motion abnormalities are detected but are incorrectly ascribed to another vessel.

Subjective wall motion analysis is often challenging, and the existence of a learning curve must be acknowledged. Optimal results require training and experience on the part of the interpreter. There is, unfortunately, little information that addresses these issues to help guide the physician who seeks training in this field. The importance of training and experience as a determinant of competency has been addressed by Picano and colleagues in a study that compared diagnostic accuracy in two groups of interpreters.[12] A series of 50 stress echocardiograms were analyzed by inexperienced cardiologists (beginners) and experienced cardiologists (experts) in the field of stress echocardiography. Diagnostic accuracy, using an angiographic reference standard, was 62 ± 6 percent for beginners and 85 ± 3 percent for the experts, a highly significant difference. The study was repeated after the beginners had gained additional experience. Following a period of training that consisted of supervised interpretation of 100 studies, the accuracy of interpretation for the two groups was similar (83 ± 3 percent for beginners versus 86 ± 2 percent for experts). This study confirms the presence of a learning curve for stress echocardiography and provides some guidelines for defining minimal competency in the field.

In summary, interpretation of stress echocardiograms relies heavily on subjective analysis of wall motion and careful comparison of rest and stress images. A more objective and standardized approach to analysis is desirable, but currently it does not exist. Quantitative methods, such as ejection fraction, minor-dimension chord shortening, or center line, are often limited by image quality. Newer approaches, such as acoustic quantification, color-encoded wall motion, or Doppler tissue imaging, are still undergoing validation studies to determine their potential role in stress echocardiography.

TABLE 36–3. ACCURACY OF EXERCISE ECHOCARDIOGRAPHY: COMPARISON WITH CORONARY ANGIOGRAPHY

Author(s)	Reference	Method	n	Angio (%)	Sensitivity (%) Overall	SVD	MVD	No MI	Specificity (%)
Armstrong et al.	131	TME	95	≥50	88			80	87
Armstrong et al.	71	TME	123	≥50	87	81	93	78	86
Crouse et al.	54	TME	228	≥50	97	93	100		64
Quiñones et al.	53	TME	289	≥50	74	58	89		88
Marwick et al.	57	TME	150	≥50	84	79	96	87	86
Ryan et al.	66	TME	64	≥50	78	76	80	78	100
Galanti et al.	130	Upright bicycle	53	≥70	93	93	92		96
Pozzoli et al.	129	Upright bicycle	75	≥50	71	60	94		96
Sawada et al.	132	TME or upright bicycle	57	≥50	86	88	82		86
Hecht et al.	16	Supine bicycle	180	≥50	93	78	90	91	86
Hecht et al.	15	Supine bicycle	136	≥50	94	84	100	92	88
Ryan et al.	11	Upright bicycle	309	≥50	93	84	100	91	78

Angio = angiographic criteria for significant disease; MI = myocardial infarction; MVD = multivessel coronary artery disease; n = number of patients; SVD = single-vessel coronary artery disease; TME = treadmill.

ACCURACY AND CLINICAL APPLICATIONS

Detection of Coronary Artery Disease

In clinical studies published since 1984, the overall sensitivity of exercise echocardiography for the detection of angiographic coronary artery disease has ranged from 71[129] to 97 percent[54] (Table 36–3). With the use of dobutamine stress echocardiography, sensitivity has been reported as between 70[27] and 96 percent[56] (Table 36–4). A variety of factors affect accuracy and help account for these differences. Sensitivity is greatest in the presence of multivessel coronary artery disease, severe coronary stenoses, and an adequate exercise workload. Sensitivity is reduced in patients with single-vessel disease, in those with moderate severity of stenosis, and in those who fail to achieve 85 percent of their target heart rate. It is noteworthy that in at least one study,[57] image quality did not significantly affect overall accuracy. In some studies, sensitivity has also been correlated with coronary lesion location, being higher for the left anterior descending artery and lower for the left circumflex artery.[11]

Patient selection criteria have a profound effect on accuracy. For example, for the detection of coronary artery disease, sensitivity is higher when a large percentage of patients with prior myocardial infarction are included. Such patients contribute to a high sensitivity on the basis of resting wall motion abnormalities and may or may not develop induced ischemia. Among patients with *normal* resting wall motion, detection of disease depends on the ability to identify *induced* wall motion abnormalities. Sensitivity in this setting has ranged from 66[57] to 91 percent[16] for exercise echocardiography and 68[58] to 89 percent[59] for dobutamine stress. In general, stress echocardiography has a lower sensitivity but a higher specificity in patients with normal resting wall motion.

Accuracy in patients with prior myocardial infarction (and, hence, resting wall motion abnormalities) should be defined differently. In these patients, the diagnosis of coronary artery disease is rarely in doubt, and the stress test is usually performed to detect ischemia, the presence of multivessel disease, or both. Several studies using exercise[11, 57] and dobutamine[59] have demonstrated the ability of stress echocardiography to provide additional diagnostic information in patients with abnormal wall motion at rest. Between 70[11] and 80 percent[59] of patients with resting wall motion abnormalities *and* multivessel disease were identified.

Angiographic criteria for the presence or absence of disease also influence reported accuracy. In most published series, a 50 percent reduction in coronary artery diameter is used as the definition of *significant disease*. Stenoses of intermediate severity may or may not cause exercise-induced ischemia, leading some investigators to suggest that stress echocardiography may be used in such cases to assess the *functional significance* of these moderate lesions.[60] If, instead, a 70 percent diameter reduction is used as the criterion

TABLE 36–4. ACCURACY OF PHARMACOLOGIC STRESS ECHOCARDIOGRAPHY: COMPARISON WITH CORONARY ANGIOGRAPHY

Author(s)	Reference	Method	n	Angio (%)	Sensitivity (%) Overall	SVD	MVD	No MI	Specificity (%)
Sawada et al.	59	Dob	103	≥50	89	81	100	89	85
Cohen et al.	67	Dob	70	≥70	86	69	94		95
Mazeika et al.	73	Dob	50	≥70	78	50	75		93
McNeill et al.	27	Dob	80	≥50	70				88
Segar et al.	51	Dob	85	≥50	95			90	82
Marcovitz and Armstrong	56	Dob	141	≥50	96	95	97	87	66
Marwick et al.	80	Dob	217	≥50	72	66	77		83
Hoffman et al.	52	Dob	66	≥70	79	78	81	79	81
Martin et al.	55	Dob	40	≥50	76				60
Martin et al.	55	Aden	40	≥50	40				93
Martin et al.	55	Dip	40	≥50	56				67
Picano et al.	133	Dip	103	≥70	74	50	90		100
Picano et al.	134	Dip	75	≥70	56	37	86		100
Severi et al.	83	Dip	429	≥75	75	67	86		90
Zoghbi et al.	84	Aden	73	≥75	85	80	91	60	92
Marwick et al.	82	Aden	97	≥50	58	52	64		87

Aden = adenosine; Dip = dipyridamole; Dob = dobutamine; other abbreviations as in Table 36–3.

for positivity, the sensitivity of stress echocardiography would be expected to be higher.

The direct relationship between stenosis severity and the likelihood of a positive test result is well established. Hecht and associates[16] found a significantly higher sensitivity for vessels with 90 to 100 percent diameter narrowing compared with vessels with 50 to 70 percent stenosis (91 versus 81 percent, $P < .05$). Salustri and co-workers[61] compared echocardiography and single-photon emission computed tomography (SPECT) in 44 consecutive patients with single-vessel disease using a postbicycle exercise protocol. Coronary lesions were stratified as >70 percent, 50 to 70 percent, and <50 percent. The prevalence of an ischemic response with both imaging tests was directly related to lesion severity ($P < .001$). The percent diameter stenosis was moderately correlated with the ischemic wall motion score index (r = 0.62).

There is some evidence, though not conclusive, that sensitivity may be different among the various exercise modalities, specifically, treadmill and bicycle ergometry. The potential for "rapid recovery" of induced wall motion abnormalities could adversely affect the sensitivity of methods that rely on postexercise imaging, such as treadmill testing. It is well established that most induced wall motion abnormalities persist long enough into recovery to be readily detected.[10] The time course of recovery and the factors that affect the rate of resolution of ischemia are not completely clear.[8, 62, 63] The duration of ischemia, the extent and severity of hypoperfusion, and the presence or absence of coronary collateral flow are factors that likely play a role in this process.[64, 65]

The phenomenon of rapid recovery of wall motion and its effect on accuracy has been examined by several investigators. Presti and colleagues[9] were the first to describe the prompt resolution of wall motion abnormalities after bicycle exercise (Fig. 36–7). In their series of 104 consecutive patients, rapid recovery occurred in 10 of 29 patients with inducible dyssynergy at peak exercise. In 6 patients with an abnormal echocardiogram at peak exercise, postexercise wall motion was completely normal, resulting in a decrease in sensitivity from 100 percent at peak to 70 percent after exercise. Ryan and associates[11] studied 309 patients with upright bicycle exercise. In 39 patients (13 percent), a wall motion abnormality was present at peak but was not present after exercise. The sensitivity of peak and postexercise imaging were 91 and 83 percent, respectively. Using supine bicycle exercise, Hecht and co-workers[15] reported similar findings in a series of 136 patients. Postexercise

imaging had a sensitivity of 83 percent, compared with 94 percent at peak. The percent diameter stenosis of arteries supplying regions with rapid recovery was slightly less, compared with those in areas with persistent wall motion abnormalities (80.6 ± 16 percent versus 85.9 ± 14 percent, $P = .07$).

The specificity of exercise echocardiography ranges from 64[54] to 100 percent.[66] Reported values for dobutamine stress echocardiography are between 66[56] and 95 percent.[67] Much of this variation is explained on the basis of patient selection. For example, when only patients with normal resting wall motion are included, specificity is higher because ischemia is by far the most likely cause of an induced wall motion abnormality in this setting.[66] Conversely, left ventricular dysfunction at baseline may be due to other conditions, such as nonischemic cardiomyopathy. These patients may have abnormal stress echocardiograms in the absence of coronary artery disease. Exercise-induced wall motion abnormalities may occasionally occur in patients who do not have coronary artery disease.[68, 69]

As expected, lower specificity has generally been reported in studies in which sensitivity was quite high, which occurs primarily because of the subjective criteria used to define a positive and negative test result. Furthermore, the spectrum of wall motion response to stress is a continuum, with some overlap expected between normal and abnormal results.[50] For example, if one insists on hyperdynamic wall motion to interpret a test as normal, some patients who do not have coronary disease (who fail to manifest this hyperdynamic response) will be classified as abnormal, resulting in lower specificity. With the use of this same approach, however, relatively few false-negative results will occur, and sensitivity will be high. If the interpreter, instead, considers mild hypokinesis to be normal, sensitivity would decline, but specificity would improve. This inverse relationship between sensitivity and specificity has important implications for applying published data to clinical practice.

In many reported series, addressing the issue of specificity is difficult because of the inclusion of a relatively small number of patients without coronary disease. Such distribution may be expected to bias the interpreter, making it more likely that a test will be read as abnormal. An alternative approach is the determination of the *normalcy rate*. Normalcy refers to the probability of a normal test result in a population of patients with a very low pretest likelihood of disease. Most published series report normalcy rates of 93 to 100 percent.[16, 57, 70]

Localization of Coronary Artery Lesions

The ability of stress echocardiography to localize coronary artery lesions has been evaluated in several clinical studies. It may be particularly important in patients with known coronary anatomy or to demonstrate the functional significance of a given lesion or to determine which lesion is the most probable cause of ischemia. To predict coronary anatomy, left ventricular wall segments are correlated with a specific artery or its branch. A variety of factors affect the accuracy with which individual lesions can be identified (Table 36–5). For example, in patients with multivessel coronary artery disease, the induction of ischemia in the region supplied by the most severely diseased vessel may lead to termination of the test before abnormalities develop in more moderately diseased areas. Because of the relatively small amount of myocardium involved, lesions in distal arteries or smaller branches may be missed. The expected individual variability of coronary distribution must also be taken into account, especially with regard to the posterior circulation. In some series,[71] considerable overlap between the right and the left circumflex coronary arteries has been reported.

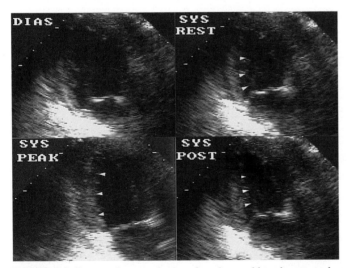

FIGURE 36–7. A quad-screen display of an abnormal bicycle stress echocardiogram. This study demonstrates the phenomenon of "rapid recovery." The end-diastolic (DIAS) two-chamber view is shown in the upper left quad. Systolic wall motion at baseline is normal (upper right, SYS REST). In the lower left quad at peak dose, there is akinesis of the inferobasal wall. In the lower right quad, during immediate recovery (SYS POST), there is recovery of endocardial excursion and wall thickening.

Predicting the Extent and Severity of Disease

Severity of disease can be defined in several ways, and exercise echocardiography is useful for making this determination. As would be expected, stress echocardiography is more sensitive in patients

TABLE 36–5. LOCALIZATION OF CORONARY ARTERY LESIONS

			Sensitivity (%)		
Author(s)	*Reference*	*Method*	*LAD*	*LCX*	*RCA*
Armstrong et al.	71	TME	71°	13°	85°
Pozzoli et al.	129	Upright bicycle	69	45	65
Hoffman et al.	52	Supine bicycle	85°	60°	82°
		Dob	83°	50°	82°
Marwick et al.	57	TME	77	67	70
Hecht et al.	16	Supine bicycle	95	78	81
Ryan et al.	11	Upright bicycle	79	36	79
			80°	17°	83°
Segar et al.	51	Dob	79	70	77

° = patients with single-vessel disease only.

LAD = left anterior descending coronary artery; LCX = left circumflex coronary artery; RCA = right coronary artery; other abbreviations as in Tables 36–3 and 36–4.

with multivessel disease compared with single-vessel disease. However, the *specific identification* of multivessel disease hinges on the demonstration of wall motion abnormalities in *more than one* vascular territory. Armstrong and colleagues[71] reported a sensitivity of treadmill exercise echocardiography of 97 percent for detection of coronary disease among patients with multivessel disease. For the specific identification of multivessel involvement, however, sensitivity was only 54 percent. Bicycle exercise echocardiography, using peak exercise imaging, may be superior for this purpose. Hecht and associates[15] correctly detected the presence of multivessel disease in 93 percent of patients. Predicting the exact number of diseased arteries was accomplished in 76, 68, and 68 percent of patients with one-, two-, and three-vessel disease, respectively. Also using bicycle exercise, Ryan and co-workers[11] reported a sensitivity of 95 percent in patients with multivessel disease. The number of diseased arteries was correctly determined in 186 of 309 patients (60 percent). Underestimation of the extent of disease occurred in 26 percent, and overestimation in 14 percent. Roger and col-

leagues[72] examined the incremental value of wall motion analysis, combined with clinical and other exercise variables, for the identification of multivessel coronary artery disease in 150 patients. The sensitivity and specificity for the determination of multivessel involvement was 73 and 70 percent, respectively (Fig. 36–8).

The ability to identify multivessel disease with dobutamine stress echocardiography is partly dependent on the stress protocol. If wall motion is carefully monitored and used as an end point for test termination, the likelihood of detecting disease in more than one coronary artery is relatively low—the study is stopped when the most severely diseased vessel produces ischemia. If the test is continued, however, the ability to induce multiple wall motion abnormalities has been demonstrated.[51, 67]

The relationship between exercise echocardiography and the stress electrocardiogram (ECG) has been examined by several investigators (Fig. 36–9). In every instance, wall motion analysis has been shown to be more sensitive and specific for the detection of coronary artery disease. Marwick and associates[57] reported a higher sensitivity of echocardiography, compared with the exercise ECG, even when patients with a nondiagnostic stress ECG were excluded (87 versus 63 percent, respectively, $P = .01$). Much of this improved sensitivity occurs in patients with false-negative results on exercise ECG. When the exercise ECG result is negative, the sensitivity of echocardiography has been reported as between 67[52] and 90 percent.[11] Specificity is also higher for exercise echocardiography, whether or not patients with a nondiagnostic ECG are included.[57] The superiority of the exercise echocardiogram, compared with the ECG, for detecting coronary artery disease is greatest in patients with single-vessel disease.[52, 66] The value of the ECG in dobutamine stress testing is quite low, and investigators have uniformly demonstrated the superiority of wall motion analysis for the detection of coronary artery disease.[55, 56, 67, 73]

Wall motion analysis is also very valuable in patients with a nondiagnostic ECG. Of 309 patients studied by Ryan and co-workers,[11] 104 had a nondiagnostic ECG. The most common cause of this result was an abnormal baseline ST segment, T wave, or both. The negative and positive predictive values of echocardiography in these patients were 82 and 93 percent, respectively. Even when patients with resting wall motion abnormalities were ex-

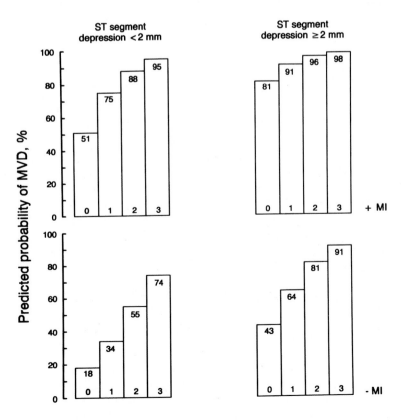

FIGURE 36–8. The predictive probability of multivessel coronary artery disease (MVD) is displayed as a function of history of myocardial infarction (MI), the presence or absence of significant ST-segment depression, and the number of abnormal left ventricular regions present on the postexercise echocardiogram (0 to 3). (From Roger, V.L., Pellikka, P.A., Oh, J.K., et al.: Identification of multivessel coronary artery disease by exercise echocardiography. J. Am. Coll. Cardiol. 24:109, 1994. Reprinted with permission from the American College of Cardiology.)

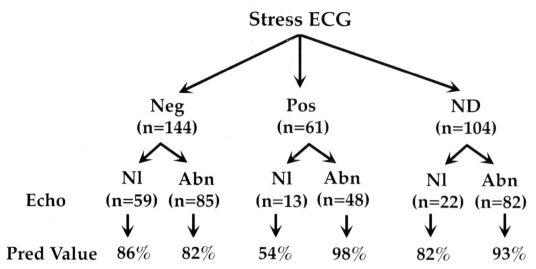

FIGURE 36–9. The diagnostic accuracy of bicycle exercise echocardiography when combined with the stress ECG. Predictive value (Pred Value) of the echocardiogram within each subgroup is shown on the bottom line. Accuracy of echocardiography in predicting angiographic coronary artery disease is high in each group, except for those with a positive stress ECG and a normal exercise echocardiogram. In these patients, echocardiography has a negative predictive valve of only 54 percent. Neg = negative stress ECG; Pos = positive stress ECG; ND = nondiagnostic stress ECG. (From Ryan, T., Segar, D.S., et al.: Detection of coronary artery disease with upright bicycle exercise echocardiography. J. Am. Soc. Echocardiogr. 6:186, 1993, with permission.)

cluded, echocardiography had a sensitivity of 83 percent and a specificity of 82 percent. The incremental value of echocardiography is less well studied in patients with a *positive* stress ECG. In most of these patients, a wall motion abnormality will develop, confirming the presence of ischemia. When the echocardiographic results are discordant, however, the positive stress ECG cannot be ignored. Ryan and colleagues[11] identified only 13 such patients (4 percent of their total) with a *normal* exercise echocardiogram in association with an *ischemic* stress ECG. Six of these patients had coronary disease, including two with three-vessel involvement. Thus, the negative predictive value of echocardiography in this setting was only 54 percent (see Fig. 36–9).

The ability of exercise echocardiography to assess the extent of myocardial involvement in the ischemic process provides an opportunity to use the test to examine the relationships among angina, the ECG, and the ischemic burden. In most studies, angina appears to be unrelated to the extent and severity of induced ischemia, as defined echocardiographically.[74–76] Hecht and associates[75] studied the relationship between the size of the induced wall motion abnormality and the presence or absence of angina and ST-segment changes. They identified three groups: (1) those with both chest pain and ST-segment depression (symptomatic ischemia), (2) those with ST-segment depression but no chest pain (asymptomatic ischemia), and (3) those with neither angina nor ST-segment depression (truly silent ischemia). The investigators found that regional dyssynergy without either chest pain or ECG changes was common and that ST-segment depression was the variable that correlated best with the extent of the wall motion abnormality. Wall motion abnormalities in patients with truly silent ischemia were smaller than in those with associated ST-segment depression.

Stress Echocardiography Versus Radionuclide Techniques

Several clinical studies have been performed that compared the various stress echocardiographic methods with radionuclide techniques. Any comparison between these imaging modalities must recognize that the two techniques record fundamentally different aspects of ischemia. Because hypoperfusion must occur before regional dyssynergy, it is generally assumed that a perfusion defect will precede the development of a wall motion abnormality. This suggests that perfusion scintigraphy will be more sensitive than stress echocardiography, particularly when exercise is terminated *after* the occurrence of hypoperfusion but *before* wall motion deteriorates. Conversely, echocardiography should be more specific, since it requires the development of a wall motion abnormality as the manifestation of ischemia.

Despite these theoretical differences, it is reasonable to expect stress echocardiography and radionuclide scintigraphy to provide similar and concordant information with respect to the presence, location, extent, and severity of coronary disease. These issues have been addressed in several clinical studies, the results of which are summarized in Table 36–6. In most series, the overall sensitivity and specificity of the two tests are quite similar. Hecht and co-workers[77] compared supine bicycle exercise echocardiography and treadmill tomographic thallium-201 imaging in 71 patients. There were no differences in overall sensitivity (90 versus 92 percent), specificity (80 versus 65 percent), or accuracy in individual vessels (88 versus 82 percent). Quinones and colleagues[53] examined the accuracy of treadmill exercise echocardiography and tomographic thallium-201 scintigraphy in 112 patients who also underwent coronary angiography. Sensitivity values for the two tests were nearly identical, whether the patient had one-, two-, or three-vessel disease. The specificities for echocardiography and thallium were 88 and 81 percent, respectively.

Concordance has also been evaluated in several studies. In the series of 289 patients reported by Quinones and associates,[53] both echocardiography and SPECT were normal in 137 patients and abnormal in 118, yielding an overall agreement of 88 percent. To distinguish between resting (i.e., fixed) and induced (i.e., reversible) abnormalities, the results from two methods agreed in 82 percent of regions. Within the abnormal regions, SPECT detected more reversible defects, whereas echocardiography detected more resting abnormalities. The most common source of discordant results involved areas exhibiting partial reversibility with SPECT but a fixed (or resting) wall motion abnormality with echocardiography. To account for this finding, the authors speculated that SPECT may be superior for the detection of ischemia within a zone of previous infarction.

Echocardiography and nuclear imaging techniques have also been compared with the use of pharmacologic stress. A variety of

TABLE 36–6. STUDIES COMPARING THE ACCURACY OF STRESS ECHOCARDIOGRAPHY AND RADIONUCLIDE IMAGING

			Echocardiography			Nuclear Imaging			
Author(s)	*Reference*	*n*	*Method*	*Sensitivity (%)*	*Specificity (%)*	*Method*	*Sensitivity (%)*	*Specificity (%)*	*Agreement (%)*
Pozzoli et al.	129	75	Bicycle	71	96	MIBI	84	88	88
Hecht et al.	77	71	Bicycle	90	80	SPECT	92	65	79
Quiñones et al.	53	289	TME	74	88	SPECT	76	81	88
Hoffman et al.	52	66	Bicycle	80	87	TME-SPECT	89	71	
Galanti et al.	130	53	Bicycle	93	96	Planar thal	100	92	
Marwick et al.	80	217	Dob	72	83	MIBI	76	67	
Marwick et al.	82	97	Dob	85	82	Aden-MIBI	86	71	
Forster et al.	78	105	Dob	75	89	MIBI	83	89	74
Takeuchi et al.	81	120	Dob	85	93	SPECT	89	85	81

MIBI = ^{99m}Tc-methoxyisobutyl isonitrile; planar thal = planar thallium-201; SPECT = single-photon emission computed tomography (using thallium-201); other abbreviations as in Tables 36–3 and 36–4.

different protocols, stress agents, and imaging modalities have been studied. For most techniques, the studies have demonstrated a similar degree of accuracy.[78–81] Marwick and co-workers[82] performed dobutamine and adenosine stress testing in conjunction with both echocardiography and SPECT imaging (with methoxyisobutyl isonitrile) in 97 consecutive patients. The results of the four different stress test combinations were compared with those of coronary angiography (Fig. 36–10). Sensitivity and overall accuracy were similar for dobutamine echocardiography, dobutamine methoxyisobutyl isonitrile, and adenosine methoxyisobutyl isonitrile. For adenosine echocardiography, however, both sensitivity (58 percent) and accuracy (69 percent) were significantly lower compared with the other three modalities.

It is clear from the data presented above that stress echocardiography and radionuclide imaging are capable of providing similar diagnostic information in most clinical situations. When one chooses among these tests, several issues must be considered. For example, to detect ischemia within an area of prior infarction, radionuclide imaging may be preferable. Exercise echocardiography is limited in its ability to detect ischemia in areas of abnormal resting wall motion. However, recent data suggest that dobutamine stress echocardiography may be able to provide this assessment.[49] The higher specificity of echocardiography reported in most series may be particularly important in certain patient subsets, such as those with left ventricular hypertrophy. Echocardiography also has the advantages of lower cost and lack of radiation exposure. The diagnostic information is available immediately, and patients are not required to return for delayed imaging. The additional information provided by echocardiography, such as data on valvular disease, may also be desirable. Conversely, nuclear techniques are more amenable to quantitative analysis and are clearly preferred when echocardiographic image quality is unacceptable. Finally, it is essential to consider local experience and expertise. Both forms of stress testing are technically challenging and operator-dependent. Extrapolation of the published data to local laboratories assumes an equivalent level of quality and has important implications for comparing the various methods.

Vasodilator Stress Echocardiography

Vasodilator stress echocardiography, using either dipyridamole or adenosine, is being utilized extensively, especially in Europe. To induce ischemia with dipyridamole, it appears necessary to use a higher dose (0.84 mg/kg) than is routinely employed for nuclear imaging protocols. This approach is safe[31] and acceptable sensitivity and specificity have been reported in most series (see Table 36–4). Severi and colleagues[83] studied 429 consecutive hospitalized patients with a history of chest pain but no prior myocardial infarction. Coronary disease was defined as a ≥75 percent reduction in luminal diameter of at least one major artery. Overall sensitivity and specificity were 75 and 90 percent, respectively. With the use of adenosine, which has a shorter duration of action, similar findings have been reported.[84] Other investigators, however, have achieved less success. For example, Mazeika and associates[85] examined 58 patients, 40 of whom had coronary artery disease. Dipyridamole-induced wall motion abnormalities developed in only 16 of these 40 patients (40 percent sensitivity), all of whom had multivessel disease.

An advantage of dipyridamole echocardiography is the opportunity to stratify a positive test result with respect to regional extent *and* time of onset of the wall motion abnormality. Picano and co-workers[86] compared coronary flow reserve (assessed with the use of positron emission tomography) and time duration from the beginning of infusion to the onset of the dyssynergy in a series of 11 patients with single-vessel disease. A significant correlation was found (r = 0.87) between the dipyridamole time and the functional severity of the lesion, as defined by the regional flow reserve (Fig. 36–11).

From the earlier discussion, it is evident that dipyridamole echocardiography is a reasonable alternative to other forms of nonexercise stress echocardiography. Feasibility and safety have been estab-

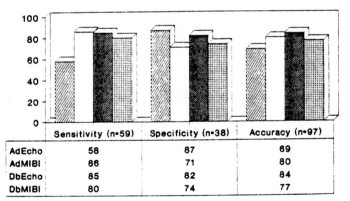

	Sensitivity (n=59)	Specificity (n=38)	Accuracy (n=97)
AdEcho	58	87	69
AdMIBI	86	71	80
DbEcho	85	82	84
DbMIBI	80	74	77

FIGURE 36–10. A bar graph demonstrating the sensitivity, specificity, and accuracy of dobutamine (Db) and adenosine (Ad) stress, when combined with echocardiography (Echo) and methoxyisobutyl isonitrile (MIBI) single-photon emission computed tomography (SPECT). The sensitivity of adenosine echo was significantly less than adenosine MIBI SPECT (*P* = .001), dobutamine echo (*P* = .001), and dobutamine MIBI SPECT (*P* = .01). The accuracy of adenosine echo was significantly less than that of adenosine MIBI SPECT (*P* < .0005), dobutamine echo (*P* = .001), and dobutamine MIBI SPECT (*P* = .005). The three latter tests did not differ from each other in sensitivity or accuracy, and none of the specificities differed significantly. (From Marwick, T., Willemart, B., D'Hondt, A. et al.: Selection of the optimal nonexercise stress for the evaluation of ischemic regional myocardial dysfunction and malperfusion. Circulation 87:345, 1993, with permission.)

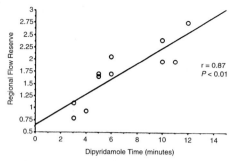

FIGURE 36–11. The relationship between regional coronary blood flow reserve and dipyridamole time in 11 patients with coronary artery disease and a positive dipyridamole echocardiography test. Please see text for details. (Adapted from Picano, E., Parodi, O., Lattanzi, F., et al.: Assessment of anatomic and physiologic severity of single-vessel coronary artery lesions by dipyridamole echocardiography: Comparison with positron emission tomography, and quantitative angiography. Circulation 89:753, 1994, with permission.)

lished. For most operators, it is probably less sensitive but more specific than competing modalities. An advantage of this technique is its demonstrated ability to assess the functional significance of a coronary artery lesion and to stratify the ischemic wall motion response accordingly.

Atrial Pacing Stress Echocardiography

Atrial pacing has also been used as an exercise-independent form of stress echocardiography. Imaging can be performed from either the transthoracic or, more commonly, the transesophageal window. Overall sensitivity and specificity for the detection of coronary disease are quite high (83 to 93 percent and 76 to 100 percent, respectively).[33-36] Accuracy is preserved in patients with single-vessel disease,[33, 34, 36] in those with a nondiagnostic stress ECG,[35] and in those with normal resting wall motion.[33, 34] Iliceto and colleagues[33] compared postexercise echocardiography and transesophageal atrial pacing in 78 consecutive patients. Echocardiography during atrial pacing was more sensitive (90 versus 82 percent) and less specific (84 versus 95 percent) compared with postexercise

testing. Among patients with normal resting wall motion, the improved sensitivity provided by atrial pacing was even greater (75 versus 56 percent). More recent data from this same laboratory suggest similar accuracy of posttreadmill exercise and atrial pacing echocardiography.[35] The test, however, is somewhat more invasive than other forms of stress echocardiography, and patient tolerance is understandably less. With the transesophageal approach, image quality is generally excellent. In some cases, however, an inability to maintain contact between the transducer and the esophagus occurs at higher heart rates.

Comparison of Various Stress Echocardiographic Techniques

Choosing among these different stress echocardiographic modalities is dependent on patient selection, the goal of testing, and the relative accuracy of each method. Several investigators have compared the accuracy of the different forms of pharmacologic stress echocardiography. In almost all cases, dobutamine echocardiography was more sensitive and less specific than either dipyridamole[58, 87] or adenosine[55, 82] echocardiography. Vasodilator drugs are quite capable of causing redistribution of coronary blood flow and are therefore ideally suited for use in conjunction with perfusion imaging agents, such as thallium-201. It is possible, however, that regional perfusion can be altered without a resultant wall motion abnormality.[88-90] This suggests that dipyridamole stress testing with echocardiography may be less sensitive than that with perfusion scintigraphy.[91] Furthermore, in an animal study comparing the severity of regional dysfunction induced by dobutamine and dipyridamole, dobutamine was associated with a consistently greater reduction in ischemic zone segment shortening compared with dipyridamole[92] (Fig. 36–12).

Comparisons between exercise and pharmacologic stress echocardiographic protocols have also been performed (Table 36–7). In such studies, patient selection criteria must be carefully considered when the results are evaluated. For example, if patients with poor exercise capacity are examined, it would be relatively easy to demonstrate the superiority of pharmacologic stress testing in that cohort. Thus, any comparison between the different stress techniques should separately address two issues: (1) the *feasibility* of the tests in an unselected patient population, and (2) the *accuracy*

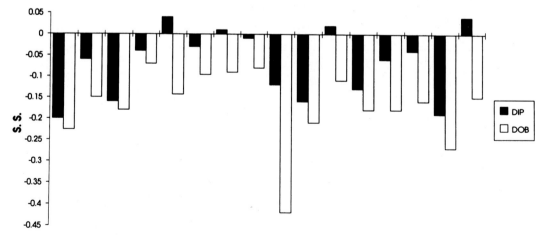

FIGURE 36–12. Magnitude of the ischemic wall motion response to dobutamine (DOB) and dipyridamole (DIP) stress in a series of 16 individual animals. Segment shortening (S.S.) was measured with sonomicrometry, and the data are displayed as changes from baseline values. In each animal, the magnitude of the change in segment shortening induced by pharmacologic stress is greater with dobutamine, compared with dipyridamole. (From Segar, D.S., Ryan, T., Sawada, S.G., et al.: Pharmacologically induced myocardial ischemia: A comparison of dobutamine and dipyridamole. J. Am. Soc. Echocardiogr. 8:9, 1995, with permission.)

TABLE 36–7. COMPARISON OF THE ACCURACY OF VARIOUS STRESS ECHOCARDIOGRAPHIC METHODS

Author(s)	Reference	n	Method	Sensitivity (%)	Specificity (%)	Accuracy (%)
Marwick et al.	82	97	Dob	85	82	84
			Aden	58	87	69
Hoffman et al.	52	66	Bicycle	80	87	82
			Dob	79	81	80
Cohen et al.	93	52	Bicycle	78	87	81
			Dob	86	87	87
Marangelli et al.	35	104	TME	89	88	88
			TAP	83	76	80
			Dip	43	92	63
Beleslin et al.	87	136	TME	88	82	87
			Dob	82	77	82
			Dip	74	94	77
Iliceto et al.	33	58	Bicycle	82	95	—
			TAP	90	84	—

TAP = transesophageal atrial pacing; other abbreviations as in Tables 36–3 and 36–4.

of the tests in a cohort of patients able to successfully complete each protocol.

The feasibility of the various stress echocardiographic modalities was examined by Marangelli and colleagues[35] in 104 consecutive patients with suspected coronary artery disease but no evidence of prior myocardial infarction. Treadmill exercise, transesophageal atrial pacing, and dipyridamole stress echocardiography were compared. Successful exercise testing was not possible in 24 of 104 (23 percent) patients because of an inability to exercise, poor image quality, or technical problems. Of the 82 patients referred for nonexercise stress testing, dipyridamole echocardiography was successfully completed in 80 (96 percent feasibility), and the pacing protocol in 63 (77 percent feasibility). However, because of the significantly higher accuracy of the exercise echocardiogram, as well as the additional functional information available, the authors concluded that exercise testing was the test of choice among patients able to adequately perform the test. Among patients unable to exercise, nonexercise stress echocardiography should be utilized.

The diagnostic accuracy of exercise compared with that of dobutamine stress echocardiography has been evaluated by several investigators. In all cases, the two tests have yielded similar results in patients able to successfully complete both protocols.[52, 87, 93] Cohen and associates[93] examined 52 patients, using supine bicycle exercise and dobutamine stress echocardiography. Sensitivity, specificity, and the ability to specifically identify one-, two-, and three-vessel disease were not statistically different between the two tests. However, the ischemic threshold consistently occurred at a lower heart rate and blood pressure during dobutamine compared with exercise stress. The authors concluded that the two tests demonstrate comparable diagnostic accuracy but produce ischemia by means of different physiologic mechanisms, thereby accounting for the lower ischemic threshold of the dobutamine test.

Stress Echocardiography After Coronary Revascularization

The goals of stress testing after coronary revascularization include the assessment of functional capacity, documentation of successful revascularization, and detection and localization of recurrent or persistent ischemia. Several factors combine to make this a challenging but important undertaking.[94] After coronary artery bypass surgery, exercise echocardiography can be utilized to identify nonrevascularized regions and to localize ischemia. Sawada and associates[95] examined 42 patients with upright bicycle exercise echocardiography at a mean of 6.3 years after coronary artery bypass surgery. Successful imaging was possible in 90 percent. For the detection of nonrevascularized vessels, echocardiography had a sensitivity of 94 percent and a specificity of 87 percent. With the use of a simplified scheme that divided the left ventricle into

anterior and posterolateral regions, accurate localization was possible in approximately 90 percent of patients. Crouse and co-workers reported similar results, using treadmill exercise.[96] These investigators demonstrated that exercise echocardiography was feasible and accurate for identifying recurrent ischemia after successful surgical revascularization. The application of pharmacologic stress echocardiography to this patient population has not been extensively studied.[97]

Stress echocardiography has also been used in patients undergoing coronary angioplasty. Both exercise[60, 98–102] and pharmacologic stress[103, 104] have been applied to this patient population. Most studies have demonstrated that stress echocardiography can be used to detect normalization of baseline wall motion[99] and to confirm improvement or resolution of ischemic wall motion abnormalities following angioplasty.[98] Localization of ischemia and detection of nondilated coronary stenoses can also be accomplished.[99, 102] The improvement in wall motion response usually occurs early, often within 24 hours after the intervention.[103, 104] Because of the limitations of angiography for gauging the severity of a coronary lesion after angioplasty, some investigators have proposed using stress echocardiography to assess the functional significance of disease.[60, 98]

A limitation of many of these studies is the selection bias that occurs when only patients who return for re-evaluation are studied. For example, if only patients who return for repeat angiography are included (presumably because of recurrent or persistent symptoms), the likelihood of restenosis is increased, and the interpretation of test results may be influenced accordingly. To avoid this situation, some investigators have studied a more nonselected population.[100, 101] Mertes and colleagues[100] applied bicycle exercise echocardiography to 86 patients following nonsurgical coronary revascularization. All subjects routinely underwent both the stress test and angiography, regardless of symptoms. For the detection of significant coronary disease, stress echocardiography had a sensitivity and specificity of 83 and 85 percent, respectively. Because of the high frequency of prior infarction within the cohort, the investigators also measured left ventricular end-systolic volume index. They postulated that an increase in end-systolic volume would be an additional marker of ischemia. The combination of wall motion and end-systolic volume analysis increased the sensitivity of the test to 90 percent.

The studies discussed above underscore the utility and limitations of stress echocardiography for the assessment of patients after revascularization procedures. By virtue of its ability to document inducible ischemia, the test has obvious utility in the postrevascularization patient, primarily to provide objective evidence on the presence or absence of ischemia and to correlate symptoms with an independent marker of disease. Thus, when a problem is suspected on clinical grounds, a stress echocardiogram can be used to confirm the diagnosis. An unresolved question is the *timing* of stress echocardiography after revascularization procedures, especially angioplasty. There are no data to support the application of stress echocardiography as a screening study to be routinely applied in asymptomatic patients. How wall motion analysis should be used for clinical decision-making after angioplasty, particularly in the absence of other indicators of ischemia, remains to be defined. Additional clinical studies are needed to clarify the proper role of stress echocardiography in this setting.

Assessment of Myocardial Viability

A more recent and rather novel application of stress echocardiography is the potential use of dobutamine for the detection of viable myocardium. It is now well established that regional akinesis is not always an irreversible state. Abnormally contracting segments may demonstrate functional improvement under two circumstances: (1) transient ischemia followed by reperfusion, which is often associated with temporary dyssynergy that improves spontaneously over time, that is, *stunned myocardium;* and (2) chronically ischemic but metabolically intact regions with the capacity to regain function when successful revascularization is undertaken, that is, *hibernating myocardium.*

The role of dobutamine echocardiography in assessing these two conditions and thereby distinguishing reversible from irreversible injury has been explored in several studies. The concept is based on experimental evidence that stunned but viable myocardium retains the ability to respond to β-adrenergic stimulation, resulting in augmented contractility.[105] Infarcted (irreversibly injured) myocardium does not respond in this manner. Piérard and colleagues were the first to apply this concept clinically.[106] They studied 17 patients who received thrombolytic therapy after anterior myocardial infarction. Dobutamine echocardiography (at 10 μg/kg per minute) and positron emission tomography were then performed within 7 ± 4 and 9 ± 5 days, respectively. Functional improvement in the infarct zone was predicted equally well by both tests, and concordant results occurred in 79 percent of segments. These results were extended by subsequent investigators, who studied larger and more heterogeneous patient groups.[49, 107, 108] The sensitivity and specificity of low-dose dobutamine echocardiography for predicting functional recovery is approximately 80 and 85 percent, respectively. The results correlate well with rest thallium-201 uptake,[109] and the test is superior to most other markers of viability, such as postextrasystolic potentiation, a small rise in creatine kinase enzyme, and absence of Q waves.[107]

Among patients with hibernating myocardium, dobutamine echocardiography is able to identify patients likely to demonstrate functional improvement in abnormal segments after revascularization. The accuracy of the test in this setting is similar to that of the results obtained in stunned myocardium.[110, 111]

Although these results are encouraging, some caution must be exercised when one applies them to clinical practice. The optimal protocol, particularly with respect to dobutamine dose, has not been agreed on universally. The changes in regional function used to define a positive or negative result are often subtle, thereby making the results difficult to replicate in routine clinical practice. To date, the number of patients studied has been relatively small, and long-term follow-up has not been reported. Furthermore, it is not clear *how much* left ventricular myocardium has to improve, and to what degree, for the findings to be clinically important. It is possible that a test to detect viable myocardium could be *too* sensitive and that a threshold must exist below which recovery of function is irrelevant. For example, if viability is correctly predicted in 1 of 16 left ventricular segments, how should this information alter patient management? It seems likely that dobutamine echocardiography will become a valuable method of assessing myocardial viability. However, the answers to these questions must be obtained before the test can be used routinely for this application.

PROGNOSTIC VALUE OF STRESS ECHOCARDIOGRAPHY

Predicting the Likelihood of Future Cardiac Events

The prognostic value of stress echocardiography depends on the ability of the test to induce and detect myocardial ischemia *and* the significance of that finding for determining the likelihood of future events. The association between ischemia and prognosis is well established,[112] so it is not surprising that stress echocardiography can be used for this purpose. In addition to the detection of ischemia, the *resting echocardiogram* also provides data on global left ventricular function and prior myocardial infarction, both of which have prognostic implications.

The prognostic role of exercise echocardiography has now been evaluated in several patient populations. Among patients with a normal stress echocardiogram, prognosis is generally quite favorable.[113] Krivokapich and co-workers[114] examined the ability of treadmill exercise echocardiography to predict cardiac events in 360 patients followed for at least 1 year. A positive stress echocardiogram, defined as a new or worsening wall motion abnormality, occurred in 18 percent of patients. The cardiac event rate was 34 percent in patients with a positive stress echocardiogram and 9 percent in those with a negative stress echocardiogram. The most powerful predictors of an event were poor exercise tolerance (6 minutes or less on the Bruce protocol) and an inducible wall motion abnormality. The investigators further demonstrated the complementary value of the echocardiogram and ECG during stress testing for risk assessment. When both were positive, the event rate was 50 percent, and when both were negative, the event rate was 6 percent. Similar findings have been reported with dobutamine stress echocardiography for risk stratification.[115]

The prognostic value of dipyridamole stress echocardiography has been well studied. Severi and colleagues[83] reported long-term follow-up (38 ± 14 months) in 429 patients who were hospitalized for evaluation of chest pain but had no evidence of prior myocardial infarction. With the use of multivariate analysis, the dipyridamole time (the duration from onset of infusion to positivity) was found to be the most powerful independent predictor of myocardial infarction and cardiac death. A unique feature of this study was that the stress echocardiographic results were stratified beyond a designation of normal or abnormal. The use of the dipyridamole time incorporates both the presence *and* the severity of ischemia and demonstrates the powerful predictive value of this approach.

The studies discussed above underscore the value of wall motion analysis in risk assessment. The type of stress echocardiography used does not appear to be an important factor. The absence of an inducible wall motion abnormality identifies a patient with an excellent prognosis and a low likelihood of a cardiac event over the ensuing year. On the other hand, inducible ischemia, as defined echocardiographically, is associated with a significantly increased risk. Risk assessment can be further refined by taking into account the stress ECG and, perhaps, other parameters of the stress echocardiogram, such as dipyridamole time or the number and extent of the wall motion abnormalities.

Postmyocardial Infarction Risk Stratification

One of the earliest applications of exercise echocardiography was for the purpose of postmyocardial infarction risk stratification. Once the accuracy of the technique for detecting ischemia in patients with prior myocardial infarction was established,[71] attention turned toward the *early* postinfarction period, in an effort to identify patients at increased risk for recurrent cardiac events.[71, 116, 117] These initial studies involved patients recovering from uncomplicated myocardial infarction who underwent stress testing 7 to 35 days after the event. Results of the test were correlated with angiography and clinical outcome. The mean follow-up period ranged from 12 weeks[116] to approximately 1 year.[117] Because most subjects had a resting wall motion abnormality, the echocardiogram was classified as negative in the absence of a *new* or an induced abnormality. A positive test was generally defined as regional dyssynergy *remote* from the infarct location. Worsening of wall motion within the infarct zone was also considered a positive result in one of these studies.[117]

Despite the relatively small population size of each study, the results were quite similar. During the convalescent period after uncomplicated myocardial infarction, an exercise-induced wall motion abnormality was predictive of an increased risk of subsequent cardiac events, identifying 63[117] to 80 percent[118] of these patients. The absence of inducible ischemia conferred a favorable prognosis, identifying 79[116] to 95 percent[118] of patients with a good outcome.

More recently, dipyridamole echocardiography has been well studied as a means of postinfarction risk stratification. Bolognese and colleagues were the first to explore this application.[76, 119, 120] They demonstrated the accuracy of dipyridamole echocardiography for detecting multivessel disease[119] and for assessing long-term prognosis. In a series of 151 patients followed for more than 18 months after myocardial infarction, dipyridamole echocardiography was an accurate means of risk stratification.[120] Event-free survival was 76 percent when the test was negative and 51 percent in patients with a positive test result (*P* < .01). The test had a sensitivity and specificity for detecting multivessel disease of 74 and 97 percent, respectively. These investigators further demonstrated the limited role of signs and symptoms for assessing risk. Among patients with an abnormal dipyridamole echocardiogram, the presence or absence of angina during the test did not correlate with extent of disease nor with event rate.[76]

The Echo Persantine Italian Cooperative (EPIC) Study Group recently reported the results of their multicenter study examining postinfarction risk stratification in elderly patients.[121] This ongoing trial included 190 patients older than 65 years of age who underwent dipyridamole echocardiography after uncomplicated myocardial infarction and were then followed for a mean of 14 months. The overall event rate was 36 percent in patients with a positive stress-echocardiogram and 10 percent in patients with a negative stress echocardiogram (*P* < .001). The death rate was also significantly higher among patients with a positive result, compared with a negative result (13 versus 3 percent, respectively, *P* < .01). Thus, the positive and negative predictive value of dipyridamole echocardiography for determining the likelihood of subsequent events was 52 and 83 percent, respectively.

Dobutamine has been less well studied for this purpose. Takeuchi and associates[49] examined 40 consecutive patients 1 month after myocardial infarction. They specifically addressed the issue of wall motion response within the infarct zone and correlated these results with tomographic thallium imaging and quantitative angiography. Worsening of infarct zone wall motion was associated with

residual ischemia and more severe stenosis of the infarct-related artery. Improvement in wall motion correlated with a lower likelihood of ischemia and less severe coronary narrowing. Other investigators have used dobutamine echocardiography for risk stratification, focusing on the detection of remote ischemia or other signs of multivessel disease. As discussed earlier, dobutamine has also been utilized for the identification of patients with stunned or hibernating myocardium after myocardial infarction.

Preoperative Risk Assessment With Pharmacologic Stress Echocardiography

Risk stratification is also performed in patients with known or suspected coronary artery disease prior to major surgical procedures. A variety of approaches to this problem are currently being used, including the detection of induced myocardial ischemia. When used in conjunction with clinical risk factors, the presence or absence of ischemia has been shown to be a powerful indicator of the likelihood of perioperative cardiac events. Dobutamine stress echocardiography is a useful technique for this purpose, especially in patients unable to adequately perform exercise testing, such as those with peripheral vascular disease. These patients have a high prevalence of coronary disease and, as a group, are at greatest risk for perioperative cardiovascular complications.

Six clinical trials have now been published, examining the role of dobutamine stress echocardiography for preoperative risk assessment.[122–127] The studies differ with respect to the definition of a positive and negative echocardiogram, and in only two[125, 127] were the echocardiographic results withheld from the managing physicians. A summary of the results of these studies is presented in Table 36–8. Both "hard" and "soft" end points are included. Despite the inherent differences in study design, striking similarities in the findings are noteworthy. Positive results occurred in 25 to 50 percent of patients. A normal stress echocardiogram was highly predictive of a favorable outcome (negative predictive value 93 to 100 percent). The predictive value of a positive result ranged from 17 to 78 percent for *all* events and from 7 to 44 percent for *hard* events, which included myocardial infarction and death. When multivariate analysis was performed,[127] an induced wall motion abnormality was the single most powerful predictor of an event.

The use of dobutamine stress echocardiography for preoperative risk stratification is rapidly gaining acceptance. Its sensitivity for identifying high-risk status is acceptable, with few false-negative results. Although these findings compare favorably with other forms of nonexercise stress testing, some issues remain unresolved. Perhaps most important are the questions of who should be tested and what should be done with a positive finding. The predictive value of a positive result is rather low, so most patients with a

TABLE 36–8. PREOPERATIVE RISK ASSESSMENT USING PHARMACOLOGIC STRESS ECHOCARDIOGRAPHY PRIOR TO MAJOR NONCARDIAC SURGERY

Author(s)	Reference	n°	Method	% Patients With Ischemia	Positive Predictive Value (%) "Hard" Events†	Positive Predictive Value (%) All Events	Negative Predictive Value (%)
Lane et al.	122	38	Dob	50	16	21	100
Tischler et al.	128	109	Dip	8	44	78	99
Lalka et al.	123	60	Dob	50	23	33	93
Eichelberger et al.	125	75	Dob	36	7	19	100
Langan et al.	126	74	Dob	24	17	17	100
Poldermans et al.	127	131	Dob	27	14	43	100
Dávila-Román et al.	124	88	Dob	23	10	20	100

°Number of patients who underwent elective vascular surgery.
†Myocardial infarction or death.
Abbreviations as in Table 36–4.

dobutamine-induced wall motion abnormality can undergo elective surgery without experiencing serious complications. Distinguishing these intermediate-risk patients from those who require further evaluation and treatment remains an important challenge. Perhaps a more detailed assessment of the extent and severity of the wall motion abnormality will prove useful for this purpose.

References

1. Kraunz, K., and Kennedy, J.: Ultrasonic determination of left ventricular wall motion in normal man: Studies at rest and after exercise. Am. Heart J. 79:36, 1970.
2. Steingart, R.M., Wexler, J., Slagle, S., et al.: Radionuclide ventriculographic responses to graded supine and upright exercise: Critical role of the Frank-Starling mechanism at submaximal exercise. Am. J. Cardiol. 53:1671, 1984.
3. Thadani, U., West, R.O., Mathew, T.M., et al.: Hemodynamics at rest and during supine and sitting bicycle exercise in patients with coronary artery disease. Am. J. Cardiol. 39:776, 1977.
4. Koike, A., Itoh, H., Doi, M., et al.: Beat-to-beat evaluation of cardiac function during recovery from upright bicycle exercise in patients with coronary artery disease. Am. Heart J. 120:316, 1990.
5. Tennant, R., and Wiggers, C.J.: The effect of coronary artery occlusion on myocardial contraction. Am. J. Physiol. 112:351, 1935.
6. Kerber, R.E., and Abboud, F.M.: Echocardiographic detection of regional myocardial infarction. Circulation 47:997, 1973.
7. Kerber, R.E., Marcus, M.L., Wilson, R., et al.: Effects of acute coronary occlusion on the motion and perfusion of the normal and ischemic interventricular septum. An experimental echocardiographic study. Circulation 54:928, 1976.
8. Athanasopoulos, G., Marsonis, A., Joshi, J., et al.: Significance of delayed recovery after digital exercise echocardiography. Br. Heart J. 66:104, 1991.
9. Presti, C.F., Armstrong, W.F., and Feigenbaum, H.: Comparison of echocardiography at peak exercise and after bicycle exercise in the evaluation of patients with known or suspected coronary artery disease. J. Am. Soc. Echocardiogr. 1:119, 1988.
10. Robertson, W.S., Feigenbaum, H., Armstrong, W.F., et al.: Exercise echocardiography: A clinically practical addition in the evaluation of coronary artery disease. J. Am. Coll. Cardiol. 2:1085, 1983.
11. Ryan, T., Segar, D.S., Sawada, S.G., et al.: Detection of coronary artery disease using upright bicycle exercise echocardiography. J. Am. Soc. Echocardiogr. 6:186, 1993.
12. Picano, E., Lattanzi, F., Orlandini, A., et al.: Stress echocardiography and the human factor: The importance of being expert. J. Am. Coll. Cardiol. 17:666, 1991.
13. Heng, M.K., Simard, M., Lake, R., et al.: Exercise two-dimensional echocardiography for diagnosis of coronary artery disease. Am. J. Cardiol. 54:502, 1984.
14. Berberich, S.N., Zager, J.R.S., Plotnick, G.D., et al.: A practical approach to exercise echocardiography: Immediate post exercise echocardiography. J. Am. Coll. Cardiol. 3:284, 1984.
15. Hecht, H.S., DeBord, L., Sotomayor, N., et al.: Supine bicycle stress echocardiography: Peak exercise imaging is superior to postexercise imaging. J. Am. Soc. Echocardiogr. 6:265, 1993.
16. Hecht, H.S., DeBord, L., Shaw, R., et al.: Digital supine bicycle stress echocardiography: A new technique for evaluating coronary artery disease. J. Am. Coll. Cardiol. 21:950, 1993.
17. Ginzton, L.E., Conant, R., Brizendine, M., et al.: Exercise subcostal two-dimensional echocardiography: A new method of segmental wall motion analysis. Am. J. Cardiol. 53:805, 1984.
18. Currie, P.J., Kelly, M.J., and Pitt, A.: Comparison of supine and erect bicycle exercise electrocardiography in coronary heart disease: Accentuation of exercise-induced ischemic ST depression by supine posture. Am. J. Cardiol. 52:1167, 1983.
19. Tuttle, R.R., and Mills, J.: Dobutamine: Development of a new catecholamine to selectively increase cardiac contractility. Circ. Res. 36:185, 1975.
20. Tuttle, R.R., Pollock, G.D., Todd, G., et al.: The effect of dobutamine on cardiac oxygen balance, regional blood flow, and infarction severity after coronary artery narrowing in dogs. Circ. Res. 41:357, 1977.
21. Leier, C.V., Heban, P.T., Huss, P., et al.: Comparative systemic and regional hemodynamic effects of dopamine and dobutamine in patients with cardiomyopathic heart failure. Circulation 58:466, 1978.
22. Kates, R.E., and Leier, C.V.: Dobutamine pharmacokinetics in severe heart failure. Clin. Pharmacol. Ther. 24:537, 1978.
23. Eagle, K.A., Singer, D.E., Brewster, D.C., et al.: Dipyridamole-thallium scanning in patients undergoing vascular surgery: Optimizing preoperative evaluation of cardiac risk. JAMA 257:2185, 1987.
24. Iskandrian, A.S., Heo, J., Askenase, A., et al.: Dipyridamole cardiac imaging. Am. Heart J. 115:432, 1988.
25. Picano, E., Simonetti, I., Masini, M., et al.: Transient myocardial dysfunction during pharmacologic vasodilation as an index of reduced coronary reserve: A coronary hemodynamic and echocardiographic study. J. Am. Coll. Cardiol. 8:84, 1986.
26. Mertes, H., Sawada, S.G., Ryan, T., et al.: Symptoms, adverse events, and complications associated with dobutamine stress echocardiography: Experience in 1118 patients. Circulation 88:15, 1993.
27. McNeill, A.J., Fioretti, P.M., El-Said, M.E., et al.: Enhanced sensitivity for detection of coronary artery disease by addition of atropine to dobutamine stress echocardiography. Am. J. Cardiol. 70:41, 1992.
28. Marcovitz, P.A., Bach, D.S., Mathias, W., et al.: Paradoxic hypotension during dobutamine stress echocardiography: Clinical and diagnostic implications. J. Am. Coll. Cardiol. 21:1080, 1993.
29. Mazeika, P.K., Nadazdin, A., and Oakley, C.M.: Clinical significance of abrupt vasodepression during dobutamine stress echocardiography. Am. J. Cardiol. 69:1484, 1992.
30. Pellikka, P.A., Oh, J.K., Bailey, K.R., et al.: Dynamic intraventricular obstruction during dobutamine stress echocardiography. A new observation. Circulation 86:1429–1432, 1992.
31. Picano, E., Marini, C., Pirelli, S., et al.: Safety of intravenous high-dose dipyridamole echocardiography. Am. J. Cardiol. 70:252, 1992.
32. Piérard, L.A., Serruys, P.W., Roelandt, J., et al.: Left ventricular function at similar heart rates during tachycardia induced by exercise and atrial pacing: An echocardiographic study. Br. Heart J. 57:154, 1987.
33. Iliceto, S., D'Ambrosio, G., Sorino, M., et al.: Comparison of postexercise and transesophageal atrial pacing two-dimensional echocardiography for detection of coronary artery disease. Am. J. Cardiol. 57:547, 1986.
34. Iliceto, S., Sorino, M., D'Ambrosio, G., et al.: Detection of coronary artery disease by two-dimensional echocardiography and transesophageal atrial pacing. J. Am. Coll. Cardiol. 5:1188, 1985.
35. Marangelli, V., Iliceto, S., Piccinni, G., et al.: Detection of coronary artery disease by digital stress echocardiography: Comparison of exercise, transesophageal atrial pacing and dipyridamole echocardiography. J. Am. Coll. Cardiol. 24:117, 1994.
36. Lambertz, H., Kreis, A., Trumper, H., et al.: Simultaneous transesophageal atrial pacing and transesophageal two-dimensional echocardiography: A new method of stress echocardiography. J. Am. Coll. Cardiol. 16:1143, 1990.
37. Zabalgoitia, M., Gandhi, D.K., Abi-Mansour, P., et al.: Feasibility and safety of transesophageal stress echocardiography. Am. J. Med. 303:90, 1992.
38. Mitchell, G.D., Brunken, R.C., Schwaiger, M., et al.: Assessment of mitral flow velocity with exercise by an index of stress-induced left ventricular ischemia in coronary artery disease. Am. J. Cardiol. 61:536, 1988.
39. Labovitz, A.J., Pearson, A.C., and Chaitman, B.R.: Doppler and two-dimensional echocardiographic assessment of left ventricular function before and after intravenous dipyridamole stress testing for detection of coronary artery disease. Am. J. Cardiol. 62:1180, 1988.
40. Bryg, R.J., Labovitz, A.J., Mehdirad, A.A., et al.: Effect of coronary artery disease on Doppler-derived parameters of aortic flow during upright exercise. Am. J. Cardiol. 58:14, 1986.
41. Harrison, M.R., Smith, M.D., Nissen, S.E., et al.: Use of Doppler echocardiography to evaluate cardiac drugs: Effects of propranolol and verapamil on aortic blood flow velocity and acceleration. J. Am. Coll. Cardiol., 11:1002, 1988.
42. Feigenbaum, H.: Exercise echocardiography. J. Am. Soc. Echocardiogr. 1:161, 1988.
43. Crawford, M.H.: Perspectives in exercise echocardiography: The role of digital acquisition and storage of images. Coronary Artery Dis. 2:531, 1991.
44. Feigenbaum, H.: Digital recording, display, and storage of echocardiograms. J. Am. Soc. Echocardiogr. 1:378, 1988.
45. Iliceto, S., D'Ambrosio, G., Scrutinio, D., et al.: A digital network for long-distance echocardiographic image and data transmission in clinical trials: The CEDIM study experience. J. Am. Soc. Echocardiogr. 6:583, 1993.
46. Thomas, J.D., and Khandheria, B.K.: Digital formatting standards in medical imaging: A primer for echocardiographers. J. Am. Soc. Echocardiogr., 7:67, 1994.
47. Ewy, G.A., Ronan, J.A., Jr., Appleton, C.P., et al.: ACC/AHA guidelines for the clinical application of echocardiography. A report of the American College of Cardiology/American Heart Association Task Force on Assessment of Diagnostic and Therapeutic Cardiovascular Procedures (Subcommittee to Develop Guidelines for the Clinical Application of Echocardiography). J. Am. Coll. Cardiol. 16:1505, 1990.
48. Schiller, N.B., Shah, P.M., and Crawford, M.: Recommendations for quantitation of the left ventricle by two dimensional echocardiography. J. Am. Soc. Echocardiogr. 2:358, 1989.
49. Takeuchi, M., Araki, M., Nakashima, Y., et al.: The detection of residual ischemia and stenosis in patients with acute myocardial infarction with dobutamine stress echocardiography. J. Am. Soc. Echo. 7:242, 1994.
50. Ginzton, L.E., Conant, R., Brizendine, M., et al.: Quantitative analysis of segmental wall motion during maximal upright exercise: Variability in normal adults. Circulation 73:268, 1986.
51. Segar, D.S., Brown, S.E., Sawada, S.G., et al.: Dobutamine stress echocardiography: Correlation with coronary lesion severity as determined by quantitative angiography. J. Am. Coll. Cardiol. 19:1197, 1992.
52. Hoffman, R., Lethen, H., Kleinhaus, E., et al.: Comparative evaluation of bicycle and dobutamine stress echocardiography with perfusion scintigraphy and bicycle electrocardiogram for identification coronary artery disease. Am. J. Cardiol. 72:555, 1993.
53. Quiñones, M.A., Verani, M.S., Haichin, R.M., et al.: Exercise echocardiography versus thallium-201 single-photon emission computed tomography in evaluation of coronary artery disease: Analysis of 292 patients. Circulation 85:1026, 1992.
54. Crouse, L.J., Harbrecht, J.J., Vacek, J.L., et al.: Exercise echocardiography as a screening test for coronary artery disease and correlation with coronary arteriography. Am. J. Cardiol. 67:1213, 1991.
55. Martin, T.W., Seaworth, J.F., Johns, J.P., et al.: Comparison of adenosine, dipyridamole, and dobutamine in stress echocardiography. Ann. Intern. Med. 116:190, 1992.
56. Marcovitz, P.A., and Armstrong, W.F.: Accuracy of dobutamine stress echocardiography in detecting coronary artery disease. Am. J. Cardiol. 69:1269, 1992.
57. Marwick, T.H., Nemec, J.J., Pahkow, F.J., et al.: Accuracy and limitations of

exercise echocardiography in a routine clinical setting. J. Am. Coll. Cardiol. 19:74, 1992.

58. Previtali, M., Lanzarini, L., Ferario, M., et al.: Dobutamine versus dipyridamole echocardiography in coronary artery disease. Circulation 83:27, 1991.

59. Sawada, S.G., Segar, D.S., Ryan, T., et al.: Echocardiographic detection of coronary artery disease during dobutamine infusion. Circulation 83:1605, 1991.

60. Sheikh, K.H., Bengtson, J.R., Helmy, S., et al.: Relation of quantitative coronary lesion measurements to the development of exercise-induced ischemia assessed by exercise echocardiography. J. Am. Coll. Cardiol. 15:1043, 1990.

61. Salustri, A., Pozzoli, M.M.A., Hermans, W., et al.: Relationship between exercise echocardiography and perfusion single-photon emission computed tomography in patients with single-vessel coronary artery disease. Am. Heart. J., 124:75, 1992.

62. Gavrielides, S., Kaski, J.C., Tousoulis, D., et al.: Duration of ST segment depression after exercise-induced myocardial ischemia is influenced by body position during recovery but not by type of exercise. Am. Heart J. 121:1665, 1991.

63. Homans, D.C., Sublett, E., Dai, X.Z., et al.: Persistence of regional left ventricular dysfunction after exercise-induced myocardial ischemia. J. Clin. Invest. 77:66, 1986.

64. Fujibayashi, Y., Yamazaki, S., Chang, B., et al.: Comparative echocardiographic study of recovery of diastolic versus systolic function after brief periods of coronary occlusion: Differential effects of intravenous nifedipine administered before and during occlusion. J. Am. Coll. Cardiol. 6:1289, 1985.

65. Freedman, S.B., Dunn, R.F., Bernstein, L., et al.: Influence of coronary collateral blood flow on the development of exertional ischemia and Q wave infarction in patients with severe single-vessel disease. Circulation, 71:681, 1985.

66. Ryan, T., Vasey, C.G., Presti, C.F., et al.: Exercise echocardiography: Detection of coronary artery disease in patients with normal left ventricular wall motion at rest. J. Am. Coll. Cardiol. 11:993, 1988.

67. Cohen, J.L., Greene, T.O., Ottenweller, J., et al.: Dobutamine digital echocardiography for detecting coronary artery disease. Am. J. Cardiol. 67:1311, 1991.

68. Douglas, P.S., O'Toole, M.L., and Woodlard, J.: Regional wall motion abnormalities after prolonged exercise in the normal left ventricle. Circulation 82:2108, 1990.

69. Fisman, E.Z., Pines, A., Ben-Ari, E., et al.: Left ventricular exercise echocardiographic abnormalities in apparently healthy men with exertional hypotension. Am. J. Cardiol. 63:81, 1989.

70. Bach, D.S., Hepner, A., Marcovitz, P.A., et al.: Dobutamine stress echocardiography: Prevalence of a nonischemic response in a low-risk population. Am. Heart J. 125:1257, 1993.

71. Armstrong, W.F., O'Donnell, J., Ryan, T., et al.: Effect of prior myocardial infarction and extent and location of coronary artery disease on accuracy of exercise echocardiography. J. Am. Coll. Cardiol. 10:531, 1987.

72. Roger, V.L., Pellikka, P.A., Oh, J.K., et al.: Identification of multivessel coronary artery disease by exercise echocardiography. J. Am. Coll. Cardiol. 24:109, 1994.

73. Mazeika, P.K., Nadazdin, A., and Oakley, C.M.: Dobutamine stress echocardiography for detection and assessment of coronary artery disease. J. Am. Coll. Cardiol. 19:1203, 1992.

74. Marwick, T.H., Nemec, J.J., Torelli, J., et al.: Extent and severity of abnormal left ventricular wall motion detected by exercise echocardiography during painful and silent ischemia. Am. J. Cardiol. 69:1483, 1992.

75. Hecht, H.S., DeBord, L., Sotomayor, N., et al.: Truly silent ischemia and the relationship of chest pain and ST-segment changes to the amount of ischemic myocardium: Evaluation by bicycle stress echocardiography. J. Am. Coll. Cardiol. 23:369, 1994.

76. Bolognese, L., Rossi, L., Sarasso, G., et al.: Silent versus symptomatic dipyridamole-induced ischemia after myocardial infarction: Clinical and prognostic significance. J. Am. Coll. Cardiol. 19:953, 1992.

77. Hecht, H.S., DeBord, L., Shaw, R., et al.: Supine bicycle stress echocardiography versus tomographic thallium-201 exercise imaging for the detection of coronary artery disease. J. Am. Soc. Echocardiogr. 6:177, 1993.

78. Forster, T., McNeill, A.J., Salustri, A., et al.: Simultaneous dobutamine stress echocardiography and technetium-99m isonitrile single-photon emission computed tomography in patients with suspected coronary artery disease. J. Am. Coll. Cardiol. 21:1591, 1993.

79. Hoffmann, R., Lethen, H., Kleinhans, E., et al.: Comparative evaluation of bicycle and dobutamine stress echocardiography with perfusion scintigraphy and bicycle electrocardiogram for identification of coronary artery disease. Am. J. Cardiol. 72:555, 1993.

80. Marwick, T., D'Hondt, A.M., Baudhuin, T., et al.: Optimal use of dobutamine stress for the detection and evaluation of coronary artery disease: Combination with echocardiography or scintigraphy, or both? J. Am. Coll. Cardiol. 22:159, 1993.

81. Takeuchi, M., Araki, M., Nakashima, Y., et al.: Comparison of dobutamine stress echocardiography and stress thallium-201 single-photon emission computed tomography for detecting coronary artery disease. J. Am. Soc. Echocardiogr. 6:593, 1993.

82. Marwick, T.H., Willemart, B., D'Hondt, A., et al.: Selection of the optimal nonexercise stress for the evaluation of ischemic regional myocardial dysfunction and malperfusion. Circulation 87:345, 1993.

83. Severi, S., Picano, E., Michelassi, C., et al.: Diagnostic and prognostic value of dipyridamole echocardiography in patients with suspected coronary artery disease: Comparison with exercise electrocardiography. Circulation 89:1160, 1994.

84. Zoghbi, W.A., Cheirif, J., Kleiman, N.S., et al.: Diagnosis of ischemic heart disease with adenosine echocardiography. J. Am. Coll. Cardiol. 18:1271, 1991.

85. Mazeika, P., Nihoyannopoulos, P., Joshi, J., et al.: Uses and limitations of high dose dipyridamole stress echocardiography for evaluation of coronary artery disease. Br. Heart J. 67:144, 1992.

86. Picano, E., Parodi, O., Lattanzi, F., et al.: Assessment of anatomic and physiologic severity of single-vessel coronary artery lesions by dipyridamole echocardiography: Comparison with positron emission tomography and quantitative angiography. Circulation 89:753, 1994.

87. Beleslin, B.D., Ostojic, M., Stepanovic, J., et al.: Stress echocardiography in the detection of myocardial ischemia: Head-to-head comparison of exercise, dobutamine, and dipyridamole tests. Circulation 90:1168, 1994.

88. Fung, A.Y., Gallagher, K.P., and Buda, A.J.: The physiologic basis of dobutamine as compared with dipyridamole stress interventions in the assessment of critical coronary stenosis. Circulation 76:943, 1987.

89. Jain, A., Suarez, J., Mahmarian, J.J., et al.: Functional significance of myocardial perfusion defects induced by dipyridamole using thallium-201 single-photon emission computed tomography and two-dimensional echocardiography. Am. J. Cardiol. 66:802, 1990.

90. Whitfield, S., Aurigemma, G., Pape, L., et al.: Two-dimensional Doppler echocardiographic correlation of dipyridamole-thallium stress testing with isometric handgrip. Am. Heart J. 121:1367, 1991.

91. Simonetti, I., Rezai, K., Rossen, J.D., et al.: Physiological assessment of sensitivity of noninvasive testing for coronary artery disease. Circulation 83 (Suppl III):43, 1991.

92. Segar, D.S., Ryan, T., Sawada, S.G., et al.: Pharmacologically induced myocardial ischemia: A comparison of dobutamine and dipyridamole. J. Am. Soc. Echocardiogr. 8:9, 1995.

93. Cohen, J.L., Ottenweller, J.E., George, A.K., et al.: Comparison of dobutamine and exercise echocardiography for detecting coronary artery disease. Am. J. Cardiol. 72:1226, 1993.

94. Lavie, C.J., Gibbons, R.J., Zinsmeister, A.R., et al.: Interpreting results of exercise studies after acute myocardial infarction altered by thrombolytic therapy, coronary angioplasty or bypass. Am. J. Cardiol. 67:116, 1991.

95. Sawada, S.G., Judson, W.E., Ryan, T., et al.: Upright bicycle exercise echocardiography after coronary artery bypass surgery. Am. J. Cardiol. 64:1123, 1989.

96. Crouse, L.J., Vacek, J.L., Beauchamp, G.D., et al.: Exercise echocardiography after coronary artery bypass grafting. Am. J. Cardiol. 70:572, 1992.

97. Bongo, A.S., Bolognese, L., Sarasso, G., et al.: Early assessment of coronary artery bypass graft patency by high-dose dipyridamole echocardiography. Am. J. Cardiol. 67:133, 1991.

98. Labovitz, A.J.: The effects of successful PTCA on left ventricular function: Assessment by exercise echocardiography. Am. Heart J. 117:1003, 1989.

99. Broderick, T., Sawada, S., Armstrong, W.F., et al.: Improvement in rest and exercise induced wall motion abnormalities following angioplasty: An exercise echocardiography study. J. Am. Coll. Cardiol. 15:591, 1990.

100. Mertes, H., Erbel, R., Nixdorff, U., et al.: Exercise echocardiography for the evaluation of patients after nonsurgical coronary artery revascularization. J. Am. Coll. Cardiol. 21:1087, 1993.

101. Heinle, S.K., Lieberman, E.B., Ancukiewicz, M., et al.: Usefulness of dobutamine echocardiography for detecting restenosis after percutaneous transluminal coronary angioplasty. Am. J. Cardiol. 72:1220, 1993.

102. Hecht, H.S., DeBord, L., Shaw, R., et al.: Usefulness of supine bicycle stress echocardiography for detection of restenosis after percutaneous transluminal coronary angioplasty. Am. J. Cardiol. 71:293, 1993.

103. Akosah, K.O., Porter, T.R., Simon, R., et al.: Ischemia-induced regional wall motion abnormality is improved after coronary angioplasty: Demonstration by dobutamine stress echocardiography. J. Am. Coll. Cardiol. 21:584, 1993.

104. McNeill, A.J., Fioretti, P.M., El-Said, E.M., et al.: Dobutamine stress echocardiography before and after coronary angioplasty. Am. J. Cardiol. 69:740, 1992.

105. Ellis, S.G., Wynne, J., Braunwald, E., et al.: Response of reperfusion-salvaged, stunned myocardium to inotropic stimulation. Am. Heart J. 107:13, 1984.

106. Piérard, L.A., DeLandsheere, C.M., Berthe, C., et al.: Identification of viable myocardium by echocardiography during dobutamine infusion in patients with myocardial infarction after thrombolytic therapy: Comparison with positron emission tomography. J. Am. Coll. Cardiol. 15:1021, 1990.

107. Smart, S.C., Sawada, S., Ryan, T., et al.: Low-dose dobutamine echocardiography detects reversible dysfunction after thrombolytic therapy of acute myocardial infarction. Circulation 88:405, 1993.

108. Watada, H., Ito, H., Oh, H., et al.: Dobutamine stress echocardiography predicts reversible dysfunction and quantitates the extent of irreversibly damaged myocardium after reperfusion of anterior myocardial infarction. J. Am. Coll. Cardiol. 24:624, 1994.

109. Marzullo, P., Parodi, O., Reisenhofer, B., et al.: Value of rest thallium-201/technetium-99m sestamibi scans and dobutamine echocardiography for detecting myocardial viability. Am. J. Cardiol. 71:166, 1993.

110. Cigarroa, C.G., DeFilippi, C.R., Brickner, M.E., et al.: Dobutamine stress echocardiography identifies hibernating myocardium and predicts recovery of left ventricular function after coronary revascularization. Circulation 88:430, 1993.

111. LaCanna, G., Alfieri, O., Giubbini, R., et al.: Echocardiography during infusion of dobutamine for identification of reversible dysfunction in patients with chronic coronary artery disease. J. Am. Coll. Cardiol. 23:617, 1994.

112. Pollock, S.G., Abbott, R.D., Boucher, C.A., et al.: Independent and incremental prognostic value of tests performed in hierarchical order to evaluate patients with suspected coronary artery disease. Circulation 85:237, 1992.

113. Sawada, S.G., Ryan, T., Conley, M., et al.: Prognostic value of a normal exercise echocardiogram. Am. Heart J. 120:49, 1990.

114. Krivokapich, J., Child, J.S., Gerber, R.S., et al.: Prognostic usefulness of positive or negative exercise stress echocardiography for predicting coronary events in ensuing twelve months. Am. J. Cardiol. 71:646, 1993.

115. Mazeika, P.K., Nadazdin, A., and Oakley, C.M.: Prognostic value of dobutamine

echocardiography in patients with high pretest likelihood of coronary artery disease. Am. J. Cardiol. 71:33, 1993.

116. Jaarsma, W., Visser, C., and Funke Kupper, A.: Usefulness of two-dimensional exercise echocardiography shortly after myocardial infarction. Am. J. Cardiol. 57:86, 1986.

117. Applegate, R.J., Dell'Italia, L.J., and Crawford, M.H.: Usefulness of two-dimensional echocardiography during low-level exercise testing early after uncomplicated myocardial infarction. Am. J. Cardiol. 60:10, 1987.

118. Ryan, T., Armstrong, W.F., O'Donnell, J.A., et al.: Risk stratification following acute myocardial infarction during exercise two-dimensional echocardiography. Am. Heart J. 114:1305, 1987.

119. Bolognese, L., Sarasso, G., Aralda, D., et al.: High dose dipyridamole echocardiography early after uncomplicated acute myocardial infarction: Correlation with exercise testing and coronary angiography. J. Am. Coll. Cardiol. 14:357, 1989.

120. Bolognese, L., Sarasso, G., Bongo, A.S., et al.: Stress testing in the period after infarction. Circulation 83:32, 1991.

121. Camerieri, A., Picano, E., Landi, P., et al.: Prognostic value of dipyridamole echocardiography early after myocardial infarction in elderly patients. J. Am. Coll. Cardiol. 22:1809, 1993.

122. Lane, R.T., Sawada, S.G., Segar, D.S., et al.: Dobutamine stress echocardiography for assessment of cardiac risk before noncardiac surgery. Am. J. Cardiol. 68:976, 1991.

123. Lalka, S.G., Sawada, S.G., Dalsing, M.C., et al.: Dobutamine stress echocardiography as a predictor of cardiac events associated with aortic surgery. J. Vasc. Surg. 15:831, 1992.

124. Dávila-Román, V.G., Waggoner, A.D., Sicard, G.A., et al.: Dobutamine stress echocardiography predicts surgical outcome in patients with an aortic aneurysm and peripheral vascular disease. J. Am. Coll. Cardiol. 21:957, 1993.

125. Eichelberger, J.P., Schwarz, K.Q., Black, E.R., et al.: Predictive value of dobutamine echocardiography just before noncardiac vascular surgery. Am. J. Cardiol. 72:602, 1993.

126. Langan, E.M., Youkey, J.R., Franklin, D.P., et al.: Dobutamine stress echocardiography for cardiac risk assessment before aortic surgery. J. Vasc. Surg. 18:905, 1993.

127. Poldermans, D., Fioretti, P.M., Forster, T., et al.: Dobutamine stress echocardiography for assessment of perioperative cardiac risk in patients undergoing major vascular surgery. Circulation 87:1506, 1993.

128. Tischler, M.D., Lee, T.H., Hirsch, A.T., et al.: Prediction of major cardiac events after peripheral vascular surgery using dipyridamole echocardiography. Am. J. Cardiol. 68:593, 1991.

129. Pozzoli, M.M.A., Fioretti, P.M., Salustri, A., et al.: Exercise echocardiography and technetium-99m MIBI single-photon emission computed tomography in the detection of coronary artery disease. Am. J. Cardiol. 67:350, 1991.

130. Galanti, G., Sciagrá, R., Comeglio, M., et al.: Diagnostic accuracy of peak exercise echocardiography in coronary artery disease: Comparison with thallium-201 myocardial scintigraphy. Am. Heart J. 122:1609, 1991.

131. Armstrong, W.F., O'Donnell, J., Dillon, J.C., et al.: Complementary value of two-dimensional exercise echocardiography to routine treadmill exercise testing. Ann. Intern. Med. 105:829, 1986.

132. Sawada, S.G., Ryan, T., Fineberg, N.S., et al.: Exercise echocardiographic detection of coronary artery disease in women. J. Am. Coll. Cardiol. 14:1440, 1989.

133. Picano, E., Lattanzi, F., Masini, M., et al.: High dose dipyridamole echocardiography test in effort angina pectoris. J. Am. Coll. Cardiol. 8:848, 1986.

134. Picano, E., Distante, A., Masini, M., et al.: Dipyridamole-echocardiography test in effort angina pectoris. Am. J. Cardiol. 56:452, 1985.

CHAPTER

37 Echocardiography in Coronary Artery Disease: Myocardial Ischemia and Infarction

Kirk T. Spencer, M.D.

Richard E. Kerber, M.D.

REGIONAL CONTRACTION ABNORMALITIES _____ 522
PROGNOSIS AFTER MYOCARDIAL INFARCTION _____ 525
COMPLICATIONS OF MYOCARDIAL INFARCTION _____ 526
Myocardial Stunning _____ 527
Infarct Expansion _____ 527
Direct Visualization of Coronary Arteries _____ 530

OTHER APPLICATIONS OF ECHOCARDIOGRAPHY IN CORONARY ARTERY DISEASE _____ 530
Ultrasonic Contrast Techniques _____ 530
Stress Echocardiography _____ 530
Intraoperative Transesophageal Echocardiography _____ 530
Intravascular Ultrasound _____ 530
Intracardiac Ultrasound _____ 530
Ultrasonic Tissue Characterization _____ 530
CONCLUSION _____ 530

Coronary atherosclerosis, the most common cause of cardiac disease in adults, characteristically declares itself by interrupting or reducing myocardial perfusion, causing ischemia or infarction. Echocardiography can be used in a variety of ways to detect ischemic heart disease:[1] it can demonstrate regional contraction abnormalities or can detect changes in wall motion or thickening, or it can display the complications of myocardial infarction, such as ventricular thrombi, ventricular aneurysms, and ventricular septal or papillary muscle rupture. These uses of echocardiography are emphasized in this chapter. Many other applications of echocardiography related to coronary artery disease—exercise ventricular function, coronary arterial imaging, myocardial perfusion by contrast techniques, and tissue characterization methods for detect-

ing myocardial fibrosis—are discussed in detail elsewhere in this book.

REGIONAL CONTRACTION ABNORMALITIES

Reductions in myocardial perfusion result in abnormalities of contraction, typically on a local or regional basis. Such reductions may be acute or chronic and yield hypokinesis (reduced systolic contraction), akinesis (absence of systolic contraction), or dyskinesis (systolic thinning or bulging) (Fig. 37–1). Such abnormalities are easy to detect with echocardiography and have been studied experi-

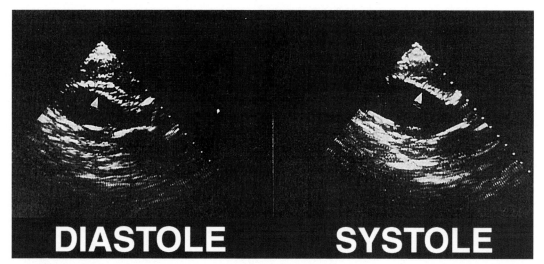

FIGURE 37–1. Two-dimensional echocardiogram, parasternal long-axis view. This view of a patient with an acute anteroseptal infarction shows systolic thinning and anterior bulging of the interventricular septum *(arrowhead)*. (From Pandian, N.P., Skorton, D.J., Kerber, R.E., et al.: Ischemic heart disease. *In* Talano, J.V., and Gardin, J.M. [eds.]: Textbook of Two-Dimensional Echocardiography. New York, Grune & Stratton, 1983, with permission.)

mentally and clinically for more than 20 years.[2] The relationship between coronary artery stenosis and regional wall motion is complex and determined by the balance of myocardial blood flow and myocardial demand. A stenosis that is not flow limiting at rest may become flow limiting with increased myocardial demand and produce a regional contraction abnormality. The echocardiographic location of the contraction abnormality suggests which coronary vessel is stenosed.

The presence of regional contraction abnormalities at rest strongly suggests the diagnosis of coronary disease. Not only can echocardiography demonstrate the presence of infarction, but also it may be used to quantify the extent of infarction. Several experimental and clinical studies[3–5] have shown a good correlation be-

tween the extent of wall motion abnormalities, as demonstrated by echocardiography, and the size or mass of an infarction (Fig. 37–2). All these studies have shown that the extent of regional dyskinesis overestimates the infarct size. This overestimation is probably due to the phenomenon of "adjacent nonischemic dyskinesis," that is, the observation that noninfarcted areas immediately adjacent to regions of ischemia or infarction develop contraction abnormalities. This condition may occur because myocardium adjacent to the infarct area may be "tethered" or placed under unfavorable regional loading conditions and appear dysfunctional. It is also clear that myocardium contiguous to infarcted areas may exhibit reversible ischemic dysfunction (stunning). In an experimental reperfusion model, the good correlation between dyskinesis and infarct

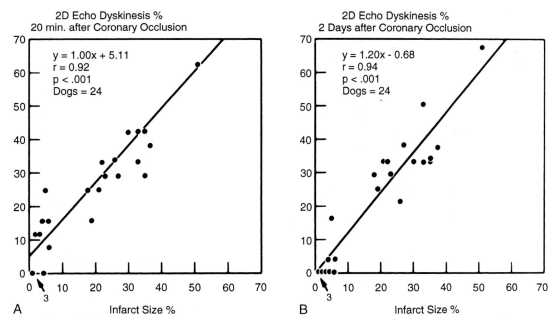

FIGURE 37–2. Relation between infarct size and the extent of dyskinesis by two-dimensional echocardiography at 20 minutes *(A)* and 2 days *(B)* after coronary occlusion. The percent dyskinesis was highly correlated with infarct size at both 20 minutes and 2 days, but echo-measured dyskinesis overestimated the size of infarction. (From Pandian, N.G., Koyanagi, S., Skorton, D.J., et al.: Relationships between two-dimensional echocardiographic wall thickening abnormalities, infarct size, and coronary risk area in normal and hypertrophied myocardium in dogs. Am. J. Cardiol. 52:1318, 1983, with permission.)

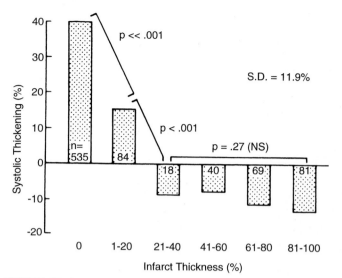

FIGURE 37–3. Relationship of percent wall thickening and transmural extent of necrosis. Systolic thinning did not appear until the extent of necrosis exceeded 20 percent of the wall thickness. (From Lieberman, A.N., Weiss, J.L., Jugdutt, B.I., et al.: Two-dimensional echocardiography and infarct size: Relationship of regional wall motion and thickening to the extent of myocardial infarct in the dog. Circulation 63:739, 1981, with permission of the American Heart Association, Inc.)

size in the setting of permanent coronary occlusion was lost once reperfusion was undertaken; the residual dyskinesis substantially overestimated the myocardium subsequently shown to be necrotic.[4]

The absence of regional contraction abnormalities does not exclude myocardial infarction. In experimental studies, Lieberman and associates showed that a "threshold" phenomenon exists: ab-

sence of dyskinesis did not exclude infarction involving less than 20 percent of the transmural myocardial thickness (Fig. 37–3).[6] Kerber and colleagues studied a closed-chest canine model of varying infarct size (Fig. 37–4) and showed that echocardiography was highly sensitive for the detection of large infarcts but often could not demonstrate dyskinesis in small nontransmural infarctions.[7] This finding is consistent with the clinical observation that between 20 and 40 percent of non-Q-wave myocardial infarctions are not associated with a regional wall motion abnormality.[8] Likewise, the lack of a contraction abnormality does not exclude severe coronary obstruction because of the chronic nature of coronary artery disease and collateralization.

Although the presence of a regional contraction abnormality may suggest coronary artery disease, it does not prove that acute myocardial infarction has occurred. A regional wall motion abnormality may represent one of many ischemic syndromes, including acute ischemia, acute infarction, prior infarction, silent ischemia, stunned myocardium, or hibernating myocardium. Stunned myocardium is noncontractile but viable with nearly normal coronary blood flow. Hibernating myocardium is noncontractile but viable with chronically low perfusion. Regional dyskinesis can also occur with coronary vasospasm, bundle branch blocks, and improper transducer alignment, as well as other noncoronary syndromes.[9–11]

The presence of a regional contraction abnormality in a patient with chest pain consistent with myocardial ischemia is useful. Current clinical and electrocardiographic criteria do not allow prompt identification of all patients with acute myocardial infarction. Conversely, approximately two thirds of patients admitted to hospital so that infarction may be ruled out do not have a myocardial infarction.[12, 13] Echocardiography may demonstrate a diagnostic regional contraction abnormality. Although a normal echocardiogram does not rule out ischemia, it does suggest that the area at risk is small. In a prospective analysis of patients suspected of having cardiac chest pain, echocardiography was sensitive for the detection of acute myocardial infarction (≥90 percent).[14–17] Patients with

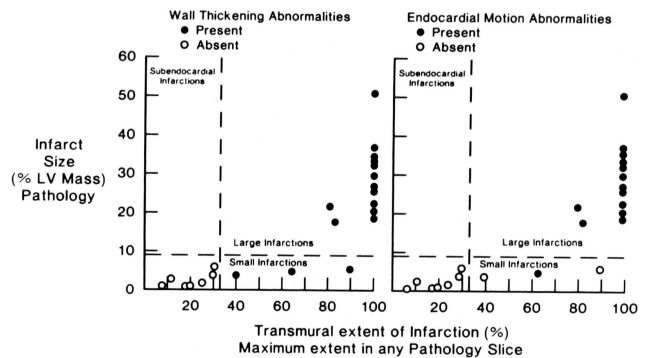

FIGURE 37–4. Relation between infarct size (% LV mass), maximal transmural extent of infarct, and two-dimensional echocardiographic abnormalities. Wall thickening and endocardial motion remained normal in slices with only small subendocardial infarcts but were invariably abnormal in larger infarcts that extended into the subepicardium. (From Pandian, N.G., Skorton, D.J., Collins, S.M., et al.: Myocardial infarct size threshold for two-dimensional echocardiographic detection. Sensitivity of systolic wall thickening and endocardial motion abnormalities in small vs. large infarctions. Am. J. Cardiol. 55:551, 1985, with permission.)

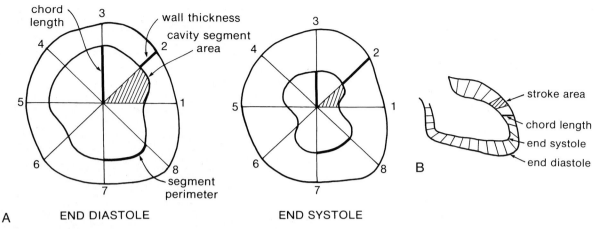

FIGURE 37–5. Indexes of regional left ventricular performance. *A,* Short-axis representation of LV at end-diastole and end-systole, showing change in chord length, wall thickness, cavity segment area, and segment perimeter during the cardiac cycle. *B,* Right anterior oblique representation of endocardial borders at end-diastole and end-systole, showing change of chord length and stroke area. (From Collins, S.M., et al.: Quantitative analysis of left ventricular function by imaging methods. *In* Miller, D.D. [ed.]: Clinical Cardiac Imaging. New York, McGraw-Hill, 1988, pp. 233–259, with permission.)

myocardial infarction not detected with echocardiography had small non-Q-wave myocardial infarctions with benign clinical courses. However, although most patients with regional wall motion abnormalities and chest pain are found to have coronary artery disease,[18] the positive predictive value of this finding for acute myocardial infarction is low. Most likely, this is so because these patients have other ischemic syndromes (e.g., unstable angina, prior infarction). Echocardiography may also reveal an alternative cardiac source of chest pain (mitral valve prolapse, pericarditis, aortic dissection).

The quantification of regional contraction abnormalities with echocardiography is of considerable importance. There are several indices of regional contraction. In general they are based on quantifying endocardial motion or myocardial wall thickening (Fig. 37–5).[19–21] Although these measurements have shown good reproducibility and accuracy compared with other techniques, they have in general proved too cumbersome or complex for routine clinical use. A detailed review of the quantitative echocardiographic assessment of regional left ventricular systolic function can be found in Chapter 27.

The clinical assessment of regional left ventricular function is generally done with a "semiquantitative" wall motion analysis. Multiple methods have been suggested, but all of them involve dividing the left ventricle into segments on several standard echocardiographic views. Each segment is then assigned a score based on the qualitative degree of abnormal wall motion and thickening. The American Society of Echocardiography has recommended a 16-segment model (Fig. 37–6) and a standardized scoring system (1 = normal; 2 = hypokinesis; 3 = akinesis; 4 = dyskinesis).[22] The overall left ventricular wall motion score is determined by totaling the individual segment scores.

PROGNOSIS AFTER MYOCARDIAL INFARCTION

The prognosis after myocardial infarction is determined by the extent of global dysfunction and residual functioning myocardium.[23] Several investigators have used echocardiographic techniques to derive prognostic information in postinfarct patients. The most common approach has been the development of a wall motion score index. Typically, the ventricle is divided into 9 to 16 segments, each of which is assigned a score based on severity of dysfunction (usually, endocardial motion abnormalities). In most systems, the higher the numerical score, the more severe or extensive the

dysfunction. Echocardiographic wall motion scores correlate well with infarct size as determined with electrocardiographic and pathologic studies.[24–28] As infarct size is one of the most potent predictors of prognosis after infarction, the echocardiographic wall motion score is a useful risk-stratification tool. Likewise, global left ventricular function (ejection fraction) is a potent predictor of mortality after infarction. Thus, echocardiographic techniques for estimating left ventricular ejection fraction are also prognostically useful. The clinical ability to measure ejection fraction has recently been enhanced with real-time endocardial edge detection systems.

A poor echocardiographic wall motion score identifies patients at risk for in-hospital mortality, as well as heart failure, malignant arrhythmias, and cardiogenic shock.[15, 29–31] Likewise, echocardio-

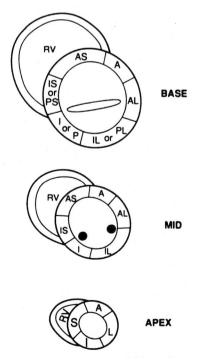

FIGURE 37–6. Suggested 16-segment model for evaluation of left ventricular regional wall motion abnormalities. (From Schiller, N.B., Shah, P.M., Crawford, M., et al.: Recommendations for quantitation of the left ventricle by two-dimensional echocardiography. J. Am. Soc. Echocardiogr. 22:358, 1989, with permission.)

graphic wall motion scores can prospectively identify patients who are at very low risk after infarction. The echocardiographic identification of high-risk patients for early aggressive intervention and low-risk patients for early hospital discharge has important patient management implications. Echocardiographic wall motion scores have been evaluated in multivariate analysis as predictors of mortality and morbidity and have been found to be stronger predictors than most clinical, laboratory, or hemodynamic parameters.[32–34]

Two-dimensional wall motion scores also predict long-term (posthospitalization) prognosis. Morbidity and mortality at 2 months and 1 year are correlated with left ventricular wall motion scores.[31, 32, 34, 35–38] Reinfarction and congestive heart failure are more common in patients with worse wall motion scores. Echocardiographic assessment of wall motion remote to infarction also has prognostic value with regard to severity of coronary artery disease and cardiac complications. Regional wall motion abnormalities remote to infarction are associated with multivessel coronary artery disease and increased morbidity.[18, 39–41]

COMPLICATIONS OF MYOCARDIAL INFARCTION

Echocardiography can be used to detect complications of myocardial infarction, including acute mechanical complications, such as ventricular septal defect, papillary muscle rupture, ventricular free wall rupture, and right ventricular infarction. In addition, echocardiography is invaluable in evaluating more chronic complications, such as myocardial stunning, infarct expansion, and ventricular thrombus formation.

Ventricular septal rupture typically occurs in a setting of single-vessel coronary disease, initial infarction, and absence of septal collateral vessels.[42] The rupture typically occurs in the muscular portion of the septum, often in the center of a septal aneurysm (Fig. 37–7). Prompt recognition is essential, as the mortality rate is

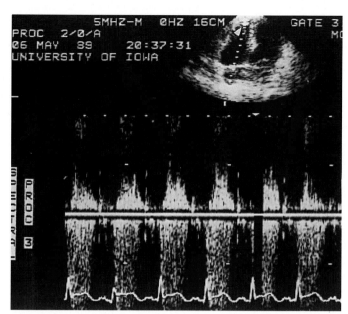

FIGURE 37–8. An example of a pulsed-wave Doppler recording in a patient with a postinfarction ventricular septal defect. *Upper panel,* The range gate *(arrow)* is in the right ventricle adjacent to the septum. *Lower panel,* There is an abnormal flow pattern in systole away from the transducer at the sampling point in the right ventricle, indicating left ventricular–to–right ventricular flow across a septal defect.

high. The actual defect may not always be visualized with two-dimensional echo. Doppler echocardiography is invaluable in demonstrating the high-velocity jet across the defect, either by pulsed-wave Doppler (Fig. 37–8) or by color Doppler techniques (Fig. 37–9). Left-to-right shunt volumes and right ventricle systolic pressures can also be estimated.[43] Recent data pooled from many studies suggest that the sensitivity of various transthoracic echocardiographic techniques for detection of ventricular septal rupture is as follows: two-dimensional echo, 58 percent; contrast echo, 86 percent; Doppler echo, 96 percent; and color flow Doppler, 100 percent.[44]

FIGURE 37–9. See Color Plate 10.

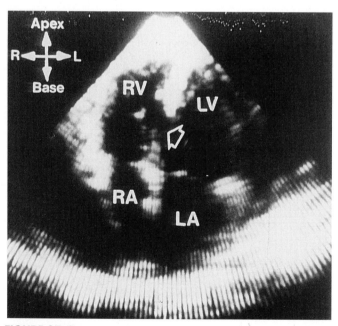

FIGURE 37–7. Apical four-chamber view in a patient with acute ventricular septal rupture secondary to myocardial infarction. The arrow shows the break in continuity between the junction of the proximal one third and distal two thirds of the septum. The right side of the septum actually was flail and moved in a chaotic manner. LA = left atrium; LV = left ventricle; RA = right atrium; RV = right ventricle. (From Mintz, G.S., et al.: Two-dimensional echocardiographic identification of surgically correctable complications of acute myocardial infarction. Circulation 64:91, 1981, with permission of the American Heart Association, Inc.)

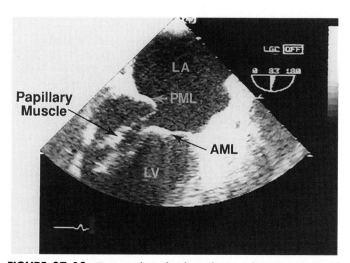

FIGURE 37–10. Transesophageal echocardiogram from a patient with recent acute myocardial infarction and mitral regurgitation. Partial disruption of the papillary muscle is evident with prolapse of the posterior mitral leaflet. AML = anterior mitral leaflet; PML = posterior mitral leaflet.

Papillary muscle rupture often presents in a manner that mimics that of ventricular septal rupture, that is, the appearance of a new systolic murmur in the setting of acute infarction, pulmonary edema, and/or shock. Echocardiography can establish the correct diagnosis, showing an abnormal papillary muscle appearance, often with a mobile mass attached to the mitral leaflet-chordae apparatus (Fig. 37–10). The leaflets may be flail. Doppler and color Doppler techniques show the mitral regurgitation well (Fig. 37–11); if there is rapid equilibration of left ventricular and atrial pressures, the instantaneous Doppler velocity decreases very rapidly from early to late systole (Fig. 37–12). Transesophageal echocardiography allows prompt diagnosis when transthoracic images are inadequate.[45–48] *Papillary muscle dysfunction* functionally yields mitral regurgitation, even when there is no anatomical rupture of the papillary muscle. Echocardiographically detected mitral regurgitation is common in patients after acute myocardial infarction and may be due to papillary muscle dysfunction or asynergy of the supporting myocardium.[49–51] Mitral regurgitation after myocardial infarction is most often mild but may be severe.

FIGURE 37–11. See Color Plate 10.

Myocardial rupture accounts for 10 to 15 percent of in-hospital deaths from acute infarction, which occur in anterior, inferior, and lateral infarcts, generally in older hypertensive patients with Q-wave infarctions. Echocardiographic recognition of free-wall rupture, although unusual because of rapid hemodynamic deterioration, has been demonstrated.[52]

Right ventricular infarction, which occurs in the setting of inferoposterior infarcts, can be diagnosed with echocardiography.[53–56] Echo features include akinesis or severe hypokinesis of the right ventricular free wall, usually with inferior or posterior septal hypokinesis. Other features include right ventricular dilation, interventricular septal flattening, tricuspid regurgitation, and reduced systolic excursion of tricuspid annulus.

Myocardial Stunning

All interventional studies of acute myocardial infarction that use serial echocardiography have demonstrated the phenomenon of postischemic dysfunction, or stunning.[57–62] Stunned myocardium is within the risk territory and has had flow restored (by percutaneous transluminal coronary angioplasty or thrombolysis, or spontaneously) yet remains dysfunctional. Thus, left ventricular function immediately after revascularization may not represent eventual left ventricular function. Serial echos after reperfusion show gradual improvement in regional left ventricular function from the early period after reperfusion up to days 10 to 14 but generally not beyond. Recovery of regional function after myocardial infarction seems related to the presence of a patent infarct artery[58, 59, 61, 62] and the interval between chest pain and reperfusion.[58, 59, 61] Future ischemic events seem to be more common in patients with significant stunning.[59] Two-dimensional echocardiography combined with low-dose dobutamine infusion has been used to distinguish stunned from nonviable myocardium after thrombolytic therapy.[63, 64] Stunned myocardium responds to low-dose inotropic stimulation. This technique correlates well with positron emission tomography scanning in the identification of stunned myocardium.[64]

Infarct Expansion

Infarct expansion occurs when a transmural infarct dilates and expands, so a greater proportion of the ventricular circumference is occupied by the infarct, even though the mass of the infarct does not increase (as distinct from extension of an existing infarct, i.e., new necrosis).[65] Infarct expansion may be a precursor to aneurysm

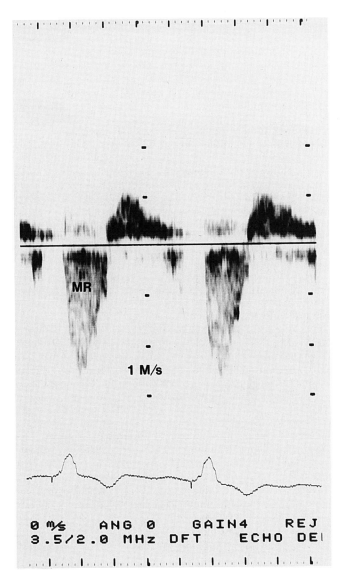

FIGURE 37–12. Continuous-wave Doppler in a patient with acute mitral regurgitation. The maximal velocity peaks early in systole and then decreases abruptly. This occurs presumably on the basis of a large "V" wave with rapid reduction of the pressure difference between the LA and the LV in middle-to-late systole. (From Kotler, M.N., Goldman, A.P., and Parry, W.R.: Acute consequences and chronic complications of acute myocardial infarction. *In* Kerber, R.E. [ed.]: Echocardiography in Coronary Artery Disease. Mt. Kisco, NY, Futura Publishing Co., 1988, p. 17, with permission.)

formation and myocardial wall rupture.[66, 67] Additionally, infarct expansion, along with left ventricular dilation, is part of the postinfarction process of cardiac remodeling. Left ventricular remodeling is important not only because it is a powerful predictor of left ventricular dysfunction and congestive heart failure[68] but also because there is ample evidence that it can be prevented or decreased with pharmacologic therapy.[69–71] Echocardiography is superbly suited to serially evaluating left ventricle size and shape and thus to detecting and quantifying ventricular remodeling. Echocardiographically, ventricular remodeling is marked by (1) an increase in infarct segment length, (2) myocardial thinning in the infarct zone, and (3) an increase in total size of the left ventricle.

Ventricular remodeling begins early after infarction and continues over a period of weeks to months. Infarct expansion is strongly correlated with the size and location of the infarct and is probably more common with a closed infarct-related artery.[68, 72–76] The extreme case of infarct expansion is the formation of a left ventricular aneurysm. *Left ventricular aneurysms* are generally defined as well-demarcated, bulging segments, present in diastole as well as systole but expanding even more in systole (Fig. 37–13). These aneurysms occur in as many as one third of acute infarction patients,[77] most often at the ventricular apex. Consequently, left ventricular aneurysms are best demonstrated by apical views; often oblique, nonstandard tomographic planes are required. In this respect, echocardiography has an advantage because multiple planes are available to the operator, as opposed to radiographic techniques that use standardized, fixed tomographic slices. Large aneurysms, or aneurysms that form early after a myocardial infarct, are associated with a poor prognosis.

Left ventricular pseudoaneurysms occur when an infarcted segment of myocardium ruptures but the hemopericardium is contained by adherent parietal pericardium; thus, in contrast with a true aneurysm, there is no myocardial tissue in the wall surrounding and containing the aneurysm. Most investigators have emphasized that by echocardiography the entrance or "neck" of the pseudoaneurysm is shown to be narrow in relation to the size of the pseudoaneurysm itself; this is in contrast with the wide opening into a true aneurysm.[77–79] A saccular or globular contour of the pseudoaneurysm is often present, as is thrombotic material in the pseudoaneurysm. Pseudoaneurysms are much less common than true aneurysms, and differentiation between an atypically appearing true aneurysm and a pseudoaneurysm may be difficult (Fig. 37–14).

Left ventricular thrombi are a common complication of myocardial infarction, usually in a dyskinetic left ventricular apex. In such patients, the incidence of thrombi is 30 percent.[80] Thrombi appear as echo-dense masses adjacent to but distinct from the underlying endocardium. Most investigators require visualization in at least two distinct planes to establish the diagnosis. Because the acoustic characteristics of thrombi and myocardium differ, ultrasonic tissue characterization techniques may afford another method of diagnosing thrombi.[81–83] Echocardiography has been found to be highly sensitive (77 to 95 percent) and specific (86 to 93 percent) in the detection of experimental and clinical left ventricular thrombi.[80, 84–86] Thrombi rarely occur in inferior infarctions. They occur 4 to 5 days after anterior infarction; more rapid development is associated with larger infarcts and higher mortality.[87–89]

The appearance of thrombi varies. They may be flat and layered,

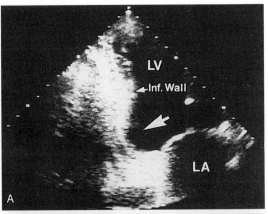
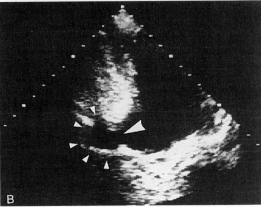

FIGURE 37–14. *A,* An apical two-chamber view in a patient with a large inferior wall infarction *(large arrow). B,* An off-axis view reveals a narrow communicating orifice *(large arrow).* The pseudoaneurysm is outlined by the *smaller arrows.* (From Kotler, M.N., Goldman, A.P., and Parry, W.R.: Acute consequences and chronic complications of acute myocardial infarction. *In* Kerber, R.E. [ed.]: Echocardiography in Coronary Artery Disease. Mt. Kisco, NY, Futura Publishing Co., 1988, p. 17, with permission.)

in part assuming the contour of the underlying infarcted myocardium, or they may protrude into the left ventricular cavity. The centers of established thrombi may liquefy, yielding a sonolucent appearance. Examples of these varying configurations are shown in Figures 37–15 to 37–17. Thrombi may be mobile, especially those that protrude into the ventricular cavity, or immobile. These varying morphologies have prognostic significance with regard to the risk of embolization. Thrombi that protrude into the left ventricular cavity, which are mobile and have sonolucent centers, have a substantially higher rate of embolization than do flat, layered, immobile thrombi.[83, 84, 90, 91] For example, Visser and associates reported 119 patients with left ventricular thrombi complicating acute myocardial infarction; 26 of these patients experienced embolic events.[83] A protruding thrombus was encountered in 23 (88 percent) of the 26 patients with embolism but in only 17 (18 percent) of 93 without emboli. Free mobility of the thrombus was seen in 15 (58 percent) of the 26 embolism patients, compared with 3 (3 percent) of 93 nonembolism patients. Similar results have been reported by other investigators.

When thrombi with a high embolic potential are detected, should the patient be given anticoagulant therapy? Prospective but nonrandomized studies have suggested a beneficial effect of such treatment; anticoagulated patients had a much lower rate of embolic events.[92, 93] However, Visser and associates found that of 12 patients with embolism complicating thrombus in acute infarction, 7 were already receiving oral anticoagulation therapy.[83] Large-scale prospective randomized studies of anticoagulation in echo-detected high-risk thrombi are needed; at present, however, there seems to be enough clinical evidence to recommend systemic anticoagulation (when there are no contraindications) for patients with acute

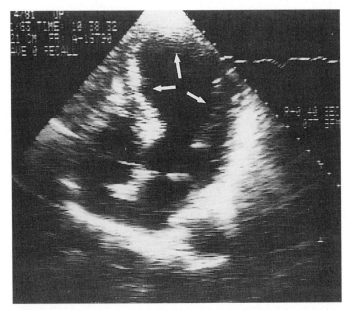

FIGURE 37–13. Apical four-chamber view. An apical left ventricular aneurysm is demonstrated by the arrows. (From McPherson, D.D., Taylor, A.L., Collins, S.M., et al.: Two-dimensional echocardiography in coronary artery disease: Present status and new directions. *In* Kotler, M.N., and Steiner, R.M. [eds.]: Cardiac Imaging: New Technologies and Clinical Applications. Philadelphia, F.A. Davis, 1986, with permission.)

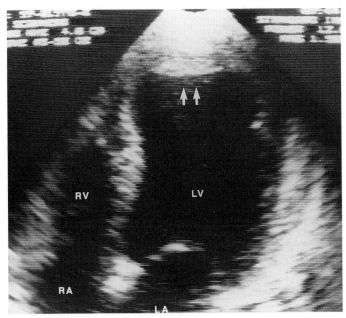

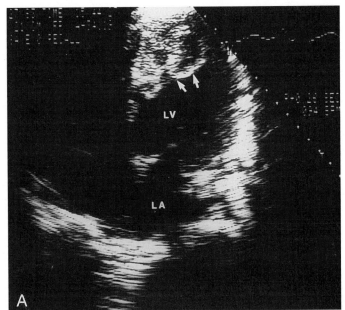

A

FIGURE 37-15. Apical four-chamber view illustrating a flat, layered ventricular thrombus located in the apex *(arrows)*. LA = left atrium; LV = left ventricle; RA = right atrium; RV = right ventricle. (From Vandenberg, B.F., Seabold, J.E., Schroder, E., et al.: Noninvasive imaging of left ventricular thrombi: Two-dimensional echocardiography and indium-111 platelet scintigraphy. Am. J. Card. Imaging 1:289, 1987, with permission.)

infarction and mobile, protruding, or sonolucent left ventricular thrombi. To search for these thrombi, Vandenberg and colleagues recommend an initial echocardiogram during the first week of admission after acute infarction; when the initial study shows no thrombus but apical dyskinesis is noted, the echocardiogram should be repeated prior to discharge.[94, 95]

Does anticoagulation of acute infarct patients prevent the forma-

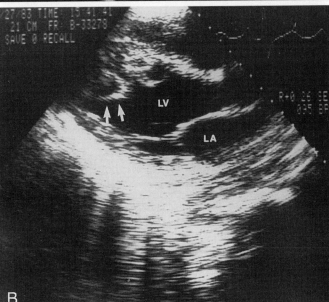

B

FIGURE 37-17. An apical left ventricular thrombus with areas of sonolucency *(arrows)*. *A,* Four-chamber apical view. *B,* Parasternal long-axis view. LV = left ventricle; LA = left atrium. (From Vandenberg, B.F., Seabold, J.E., Schroder, E., et al.: Noninvasive imaging of left ventricular thrombi: Two-dimensional echocardiography and indium-111 platelet scintigraphy. Am. J. Card. Imaging 1:289, 1987, with permission.)

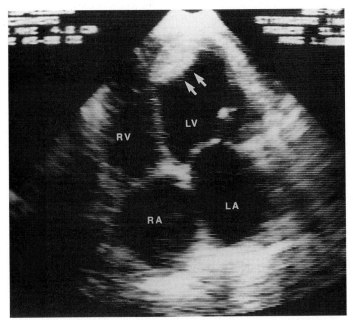

FIGURE 37-16. Four-chamber apical view illustrating an apical thrombus protruding into the left ventricular cavity *(arrows)*. LV = left ventricle; LA = left atrium; RV = right ventricle; RA = right atrium. (From Vandenberg, B.F., Seabold, J.E., Schroder, E., et al.: Noninvasive imaging of left ventricular thrombi: Two-dimensional echocardiography and indium-111 platelet scintigraphy. Am. J. Card. Imaging 1:289, 1987, with permission.)

tion of mural thrombi? Turpie and associates performed a randomized trial of low-dose versus high-dose subcutaneous heparin in 221 patients with acute anterior infarct.[96] The detection of left ventricular thrombus with echocardiography, rather than the occurrence of systemic embolism, was used as the primary outcome. Ventricular thrombi were observed by means of two-dimensional echocardiography on the 10th day after infarction in 10 of 95 patients (11 percent) in the high-dose heparin group (12,500 U every 12 hours) versus 28 of 88 patients (32 percent) in the low-dose group (5000 U every 12 hours) ($P = .0004$). There was no difference in the frequency of hemorrhagic complications. Thus, high-dose subcutaneous heparin therapy appears to be appropriate for anterior infarction patients.

Does anticoagulation affect *existing* thrombi? Kupper and co-workers found that in patients with established thrombi, 93 percent showed resolution or change in thrombus size and shape after treatment with oral anticoagulations.[88]

What is the effect of coronary artery thrombolytic therapy on the incidence of ventricular thrombus formation? Two prospective studies have provided different answers to this question: Eigler and associates showed a reduction in the rate of left ventricular mural thrombus formation after systemic thrombolysis.[97] More recently, however, Held and colleagues showed no difference in mural thrombus incidence in patients receiving systemic tissue plasminogen activator versus streptokinase versus no thrombolytic agent.[98] Patients with anterior infarctions in this series had a thrombus incidence of 33 percent, similar to the rate found in most other studies.

Direct Visualization of Coronary Arteries

Transthoracic echocardiography can visualize a portion of the left main and proximal left anterior descending coronary artery in 60 to 70 percent of patients.[99, 100] Calcifications and luminal abnormalities that represent atherosclerotic plaque can be identified.[101–103] Not only does transesophageal echocardiography allow the entire left main and proximal left anterior descending coronary artery to be viewed (50 to 100 percent of patients), but also the proximal circumflex and right coronary arteries can be seen, although less frequently.[104–108] Transesophageal echo is sensitive (80 to 90 percent) and specific (88 to 100 percent) for detection of significant left main coronary stenosis.[104, 105] Several investigators have used pulsed-wave Doppler echocardiography to measure proximal coronary artery blood flow velocity.[109, 110]

OTHER APPLICATIONS OF ECHOCARDIOGRAPHY IN CORONARY ARTERY DISEASE

Ultrasonic Contrast Techniques

Microbubbles contained in an injected solution are strong ultrasonic reflectors that can be easily detected with echocardiography. Extensive animal experimentation and initial human experience with these agents have shown that intra-aortic and intracoronary injections can be used to demonstrate myocardial perfusion and calculate myocardial risk area. Intravenous injection of these agents is used to opacify the left ventricle chamber after transpulmonary passage to improve endocardial definition. This technique is discussed in detail in Chapter 35.

Stress Echocardiography

Coronary arterial stenosis may have minimal effects at rest but may be profoundly flow limiting during exercise. Exploiting this phenomenon, researchers have long sought electrocardiographic changes during exercise as a marker of ischemic heart disease. Similarly, echocardiographically demonstrated exercise-induced dyskinesis is a marker for myocardial ischemia. In patients who are unable to exercise, pharmacologic stress echocardiography with dipyridamole or dobutamine has been extensively employed. This use of echocardiography is discussed in detail in Chapter 36.

Intraoperative Transesophageal Echocardiography

Echocardiography can be used to detect myocardial ischemia and infarction during cardiac surgery, via the transesophageal approach. Generally, the probe is inserted after the patient is anesthetized and manipulated into an appropriate esophageal position. Short-axis and four-chamber views can be obtained and monitored. Changes in ventricular size and regional contractility can be recognized, and appropriate adjustments made to correct hypovolemia

and improve coronary perfusion. Transient segmental wall abnormalities have been associated with transient ischemia, whereas persistent abnormalities have been associated with infarction. An extensive discussion of this approach is found in Chapter 39.

The cardiac structures can also be imaged during cardiac surgery with the use of transducers held directly on the epicardium. This technique is discussed in Chapter 39.

Intravascular Ultrasound

A new application of ultrasound uses very high frequency (20 to 40 MHz) miniaturized probes inserted into arteries and veins to image from an intraluminal position. Preliminary animal and human studies have shown excellent demonstration of normal and diseased arterial wall and atheromatous plaques. The expanding clinical utility of intravascular ultrasound is detailed in Chapter 40.

Intracardiac Ultrasound

This application uses 10- to 12.5-MHz probes inserted into the left ventricle and right ventricle to image the myocardium; it is a promising technique for evaluating ventricular function in the cardiac catheterization laboratory.[111]

There is good correlation between the extent of ischemic dyskinesis identified with intracardiac ultrasound and transthoracic echo.[112] The effect of catheter movement on the image has been found to be minimal.[113] In experimental investigations, this approach has been able to identify stunned but viable myocardium,[114] as well as right ventricular infarction.[115] Its potential uses include the on-line measurement of regional left ventricular wall thickening.[116]

Ultrasonic Tissue Characterization

As the ultrasonic pulse traverses tissue, the signal is attenuated by absorption and scattering. The degree of attenuation, absorption, and backscattering that occurs is specific for the tissue or medium traversed and is determined by the physical properties of the tissue itself. Changes in the tissue, such as those induced by ischemia or infarction, may result in characteristic alterations of these properties. The relationship of ultrasound-tissue interaction to tissue structure, known as ultrasound tissue characterization, is discussed in Chapter 41.

CONCLUSION

Echocardiography can be used to detect and characterize myocardial ischemia and infarction. This technique can be employed in the settings of acute infarction and chronic coronary disease, with or without angina. Because echocardiography is noninvasive, does not have side effects, and is portable, it is uniquely suitable for use in multiple settings—emergency departments, coronary care units, wards, clinics, and operating rooms. Echocardiography is accurate and well validated and, in most circumstances, should be the initial imaging technique used to evaluate the coronary patient.

References

1. Kerber, R.E. (ed.): Echocardiography in Coronary Artery Disease. Mt. Kisco, NY, Futura, 1988.
2. Kerber, R.E., and Abboud, F.M.: Echocardiographic detection of regional myocardial infarction. An experimental study. Circulation 47:997, 1973.
3. Pandian, N.G., Koyanagi, S., Skorton, D.J., et al.: Relationships between two-dimensional echocardiographic wall thickening abnormalities, infarct size and coronary risk area in normal and hypertrophied myocardium in dogs. Am. J. Cardiol. 52:1318, 1983.
4. Taylor, A.L., Kieso, R., Melton J., et al.: Echocardiographically detected dyskinesis, myocardial infarct size, and coronary risk region relationships in reperfused canine myocardium. Circulation 71:1292, 1985.
5. Weiss, J.L., Buckley, B.H., Hutchins, G.M., et al.: Two-dimensional echocardio-

graphic recognition of myocardial injury in man. Comparison with post-mortem studies. Circulation 63:401, 1981.
6. Lieberman, A.N., Weiss, J.L., Jugdutt, B.I., et al.: Two-dimensional echocardiographic and infarct size. Relationship of regional wall motion and thickening to the extent of myocardial infarct in the dog. Circulation 63:739, 1981.
7. Pandian, N.G., Skorton, D.J., Collins, S.M., et al.: Myocardial infarct size threshold for two-dimensional echocardiographic detection. Sensitivity of systolic wall thickening and endocardial motion abnormalities in small vs. large infarctions. Am. J. Cardiol. 55:551, 1985.
8. Armstrong, W.F.: Echocardiography in coronary artery disease. Prog. Cardiovasc. Dis. 30:267, 1988.
9. Pasquini, J.A., Gottdiener, J.S., Cutler, D.J., et al.: Myocarditis with transient left ventricular apical dyskinesis. Am. Heart J. 109:371, 1985.
10. Pollick, C., Cujec, B., Parker, S., et al.: Left ventricular wall motion abnormalities in subarachnoid hemorrhage. J. Am. Coll. Cardiol. 12:600, 1988.
11. Ellrodt, A.G., Riedinger, M.S., Kimchi, A., et al.: Left ventricular performance in septic shock. Reversible segmental and global abnormalities. Am. Heart J. 110:402, 1985.
12. Lee, T.H., Cook, E.F., Weisberg, M.G., et al.: Acute chest pain in the emergency room: Identification of low risk patients. Arch. Intern. Med. 145:65, 1985.
13. Schroeder, J.S., Lamb, I.K., and Harrison, D.C.: Patients admitted to the coronary care unit for chest pain: High-risk subgroup for subsequent cardiovascular death. Am. J. Cardiol. 39:829, 1977.
14. Sabia, P. Afrookteh, A., Touchstone, D.A., et al.: Value of regional wall motion abnormality in the emergency room diagnosis of acute myocardial infarction. Circulation 84:1–85, 1991.
15. Horowitz, R.S., and Morganroth, J.I.: Immediate detection of early high risk patients with acute myocardial infarction using two-dimensional echocardiographic evaluation of left ventricular regional wall motion abnormalities. Am. Heart J. 103:814, 1982.
16. Horowitz, R.S., Morganroth, J., Parrotoo, C., et al.: Immediate diagnosis of acute myocardial infarction by two-dimensional echocardiography. Circulation 65:323, 1982.
17. Oh, J.K., Shub, C., Miller, F.A., et al.: Role of two-dimensional echocardiography in the emergency room. Echocardiography 2:217, 1985.
18. Peels, C.H., Visser, C.A., Kupper, A.J., et al.: Usefulness of two-dimensional echocardiography for immediate detection of myocardial ischemia in the emergency room. Am. J. Cardiol. 65:687, 1990.
19. Borow, K.M.: Clinical assessment of contractility in the ischemic left ventricle. Mod. Concepts Cardiovasc. Dis. 57:35, 1988.
20. Collins, S.M., Kerber, R.E., and Skorton, D.J.: Quantitative analysis of left ventricular function by imaging methods. *In* Miller, D.D. (ed): Clinical Cardiac Imaging, New York, McGraw-Hill, 1988, pp. 233–259.
21. Force, T.L., and Parisi, A.F.: Quantitative methods for analyzing regional systolic function with two-dimensional echocardiography. *In* Kerber, R.E. (ed.): Echocardiography in Coronary Artery Disease. Mt. Kisco, NY, Futura, 1988.
22. Schiller, N.B., Shah, P.M., Crawford, M., et al.: Recommendations for quantitation of the left ventricle by two-dimensional echocardiography. J. Am. Soc. Echocardiogr. 22:358, 1989.
23. Vandenberg, B.F., and Kerber, R.E.: Regional wall-motion abnormalities and coronary artery disease: Prognostic implications. *In* Kerber, R.E. (ed.): Echocardiography in Coronary Artery Disease. Mt. Kisco, NY, Futura, 1988.
24. Nixon, J.V., Narahara, K.A., and Smitherman, T.C.: Estimation of myocardial involvement in patients with acute myocardial infarction by two-dimensional echocardiography. Circulation 62:1248, 1980.
25. Visser, C.A., Lie, K., Kan, G., et al.: Detection and quantification of acute isolated myocardial infarction by two-dimensional echocardiography. Am. J. Cardiol. 47:1020, 1981.
26. Shen, W.K., Khandheria, B.K., Edwards, W.D., et al.: Value and limitations of two-dimensional echocardiography in predicting myocardial infarct size. Am. J. Cardiol. 68:1143, 1991.
27. Heger, J.J., Weyman, A.E., Wann, L.S., et al.: Cross-sectional echocardiography in acute myocardial infarction, detection and localization of regional left ventricular asynergy. Circulation 60:531, 1979.
28. Wyatt, H.L., Meerbaum, S., Heng, M.K., et al.: Experimental evaluation of the extent of myocardial dyssynergy and infarct size by two-dimensional echocardiography. Circulation 63:607, 1981.
29. Nishimura, R.A., Tajik, A.J., Shub, C., et al.: Role of two-dimensional echocardiography in the prediction of in-hospital complications after acute myocardial infarction. J. Am. Coll. Cardiol. 4:1080, 1984.
30. Kan, G., Visser, C.A., Koolen, J.J., et al.: Short and long term predictive value of admission wall motion score in acute myocardial infarction: A cross-sectional echocardiographic study of 345 patients. Br. Heart J. 56:422, 1986.
31. Launbjerg, J., Berning, J., Fruergaard, P., et al.: Sensitivity and specificity of echocardiographic identification of patients eligible for safe early discharge after acute myocardial infarction. Am. Heart J. 124:846, 1992.
32. Berning, J., Steensgaard-Hanson, F.V., and Appleyard, M.: Prognostication in acute myocardial infarction by early echocardiographic estimation of left ventricular ejection fraction: Multivariate statistical comparison with a clinical prognostic index and its components. Dan. Med. Bull. 39:177, 1992.
33. Sahasakul, Y., Chaithiraphan, S., Panchavinnin, P., et al.: Multivariate analysis in the prediction of death in hospital after acute myocardial infarction. Br. Heart J. 64:2, 1990.
34. Pierard, L.A., Albert, A., Chapelle, J.P., et al.: Relative prognostic value of clinical, biochemical, echocardiographic, and haemodynamic variables in predicting in-hospital and one-year cardiac mortality after acute myocardial infarction. Eur. Heart J. 10:24, 1989.
35. Berning, J., Launberg, J., and Appleyard, M.: Echocardiographic algorithms for admission and predischarge prediction of mortality in acute myocardial infarction. Am. J. Cardiol. 69:1538, 1992.
36. Domingo, E., Alvarez, A., Garcia del Castillo, H., et al.: Prognostic value of segmental contractility assessed by cross-sectional echocardiography in first acute myocardial infarction. Eur. Heart J. 10:532, 1989.
37. Bhatnagar, S.K., Moussa, M.A.A., and Al-Yusuf, A.R.: The role of prehospital discharge two-dimensional echocardiography in determining the prognosis of survivors of first myocardial infarction. Am. Heart J. 109:472, 1985.
38. Nishimura, R.A., Reeder, G.S., Miller, F.A., et al.: Prognostic values of predischarge two-dimensional echocardiogram after acute myocardial infarction. Am. J. Cardiol. 53:429, 1984.
39. Stamm, R.B., Gibson, R.S., Bishop, H.L., et al.: Echocardiographic detection of infarct-localized asynergy and remote asynergy during acute myocardial infarction: Correlation with the extent of angiographic disease. Circulation 67:233, 1983.
40. Jaarsma, W., Visser, C.A., Van, M.J., et al.: Prognostic implications of regional hyperkinesia and remote asynergy of noninfarcted myocardium. Am. J. Cardiol. 58:394, 1986.
41. Shen, Z., Palma, A., Rajachandran, M., et al.: Prediction of single and multivessel coronary disease in patients after myocardial infarction according to quantitative ultrasound wall motion analysis. Am. Heart J. 125:949, 1993.
42. Kotler, M.N., Goldman, A.P., and Parry, W.R.: Acute consequences and chronic complications of acute myocardial infarction. *In* Kerber, R.E. (ed.): Echocardiography in Coronary Artery Disease. Mt. Kisco, NY, Futura, 1988, pp. 17–51.
43. Barron, J.V., Sahn, D.J., Valdes-Cruz, L.M., et al.: Clinical utility of two-dimensional Doppler echocardiographic techniques for estimating pulmonary to systemic blood flow ratios in children with left-to-right shunting, atrial septal defect, ventricular septal defect, or patent ductus arteriosus. J. Am. Coll. Cardiol. 3:169, 1984.
44. Buda, A.: The role of echocardiography in the evaluation of mechanical complications of acute myocardial infarction. Circulation 84:1–109, 1991.
45. Koenig, K., Wolfgang, K., Hofman, T., et al.: Transesophageal echocardiography for the diagnosis of rupture of the ventricular septum or left ventricular papillary muscle during acute myocardial infarction. Am. J. Cardiol. 59:362, 1987.
46. Chirillo, F., Totis, O., Caravzeani, A., et al.: Transesophageal echocardiographic findings in partial and complete papillary muscle rupture complicating acute myocardial infarction. Cardiology 81:54, 1992.
47. Stoddard, M.F., Keedy, D.L., and Kupersmith, J.: Transesophageal echocardiographic diagnosis of a papillary muscle rupture complicating acute myocardial infarction. Am. Heart J. 120:690, 1990.
48. Patel, A.M., Miller, F.A., Khandheria, B.K., et al.: Role of transesophageal echocardiography in the diagnosis of papillary muscle rupture secondary to myocardial infarction. Am. Heart J. 118:1330, 1989.
49. Barzilai, B., Gessler, C., Perez, J.E., et al.: Significance of Doppler-detected mitral regurgitation in acute myocardial infarction. Am. J. Cardiol. 61:220, 1988.
50. Alam, M., Thorstrand, C., and Rosenhamer, G.: Mitral regurgitation following first time acute myocardial infarction. Early and late findings by Doppler echocardiography. Clin. Cardiol. 16:30, 1993.
51. Loperfido, F., Biasucci, L.M., Pennesti, F., et al.: Pulsed Doppler echocardiography analysis of mitral regurgitation after myocardial infarction. Am. J. Cardiol. 58:692, 1986.
52. Desoutter, P., Halphen, C., and Haiat, R.: Two-dimensional echocardiographic visualization of free ventricular wall rupture in acute anterior myocardial infarction. Am. Heart J. 108:1360, 1984.
53. Goldberger, J.J., Himelman, R.B., Wolfe, C.L., et al.: Right ventricular infarction: Recognition and assessment of its hemodynamic significance by two-dimensional echocardiography. J. Am. Soc. Echocardiogr. 4:140, 1991.
54. Kaul, S., Tei, C., Hopkins, J.M., et al.: Assessment of right ventricular function using two-dimensional echocardiography. Am. Heart J. 107:526, 1984.
55. Jugdutt, B.I., Sussex, B.A., Sivaran, C.A., et al.: Right ventricular infarction: Two-dimensional echocardiographic evaluation. Am. Heart J. 107:505, 1984.
56. Cecchi, F., Zuppiroli, A., Favilli, S., et al.: Echocardiographic features of right ventricular infarction. Clin. Cardiol. 7:405, 1984.
57. Bourdilon, P., Broderick, T.M., Williams, E.S., et al.: Early recovery of regional left ventricular function after reperfusion in acute myocardial infarction assessed by serial two-dimensional echocardiography. Am. J. Cardiol. 63:641, 1989.
58. Ito, H., Tomooka, T., Sakai, N., et al.: Time course of functional improvement in stunned myocardium in risk area in patients with reperfused anterior infarction. Circulation 87:355, 1993.
59. Touchstone, D.A., Beller, G.A., Nygaard, T.W., et al.: Effects of successful intravenous reperfusion therapy on regional myocardial function and geometry in humans. J. Am. Coll. Cardiol. 13:1506, 1989.
60. Broderick, T.M., Bourdilon, P., Ryan, T., et al.: Comparison of regional and global left ventricular function by serial echocardiograms after reperfusion in acute myocardial infarction. J. Am. Soc. Echocardiogr. 2:315, 1989.
61. Otto, C.M., Stratton, J.R., Maynard, C., et al.: Echocardiographic evaluation of segmental wall motion early and late after thrombolytic therapy in acute myocardial infarction: The Western Washington Tissue Plasminogen activator emergency room trial. Am. J. Cardiol. 65:132, 1990.
62. Presti, C.F., Gentile, R., Armstrong, W.F., et al.: Improvement in regional wall motion after percutaneous transluminal coronary angioplasty during acute myocardial infarction: Utility of two-dimensional echocardiography. Am. Heart J. 115:1149, 1988.
63. Barilla, F., Gheorghiade, M., Alam, M., et al.: Low dose dobutamine in patients with acute myocardial infarction identifies viable but not contractile myocardium

and predicts the magnitude of improvement in wall motion abnormalities in response to coronary revascularization. Am. Heart J. 122:1522, 1991.

64. Pierard, L.A., DeLandsheere, C.M., Berthe, C., et al.: Identification of viable myocardium by echocardiography during dobutamine infusion in patients with myocardial infarction after thrombolytic therapy. Comparison with positron emission tomography. J. Am. Coll. Cardiol. 15:1021, 1990.

65. Meiztish, J.L., Berger, H.J., Plankey, M., et al.: Functional left ventricular aneurysm formation after acute transmural myocardial infarction. N. Engl. J. Med. 311:1001, 1984.

66. Jugdutt, B.I., and Michorowski, B.L.: Role of infarct expansion in rupture of the ventricular septum after acute myocardial infarction: A two-dimensional echocardiographic study. Clin. Cardiol. 10:641, 1987.

67. Hochman, J.S., and Bulkley, B.H.: The pathogenesis of left ventricular aneurysm: An experimental study in the rat model. Am. J. Cardiol. 50:83, 1982.

68. Jugdutt, B.I.: Identification of patients prone to infarct expansion by the degree of regional shape distortion on an early two-dimensional echocardiogram after myocardial infarction. Clin. Cardiol. 13:28, 1990.

69. Jugdutt, B.I., and Warnica, J.W.: Intravenous nitroglycerin therapy to limit myocardial infarct size, expansion and complications: Effect of timing, dosage, and infarct location. Circulation 78:906, 1988.

70. Pfeffer, M.A., Lamas, G.A., Vaughan, D.E., et al.: Effect of captopril on progressive ventricular dilatation after anterior myocardial infarction. N. Engl. J. Med. 319:80, 1988.

71. Pfeffer, M.A., Braunwald, E., Moye L.A., et al.: On behalf of the SAVE investigators. Effect of captopril on mortality and morbidity in patients with left ventricular dysfunction after myocardial infarction: Results of the Survival and Ventricular Enlargement Trial. N. Engl. J. Med. 327:669, 1992.

72. Picard, M.H., Wilkins, G.T., Ray, P.A., et al.: Natural history of left ventricular size and function after acute myocardial infarction: Assessment and prediction by echocardiographic endocardial surface mapping. Circulation 82:484, 1990.

73. Picard, M.H., Wilkins, G.T., Ray, P.A., et al.: Progressive changes in ventricular structure and function during the year after acute myocardial infarction. Am. Heart J. 124:24, 1992.

74. Siu, S.C., Nidorf, S.M., Galounbos, G.S., et al.: The effect of late patency of the infarct related coronary artery on left ventricular morphology and regional function after thrombolysis. Am. Heart J. 124:265, 1992.

75. Hirai, T., Fujita, M., Nakajima, H., et al.: Importance of collateral circulation for prevention of left ventricular aneurysm formation in acute myocardial infarction. Circulation 79:791, 1989.

76. Picard, M.H., Wilkins, G.T., Gillam, L.D., et al.: Immediate regional endocardial surface expansion following coronary occlusion in the canine left ventricle: Disproportionate effects of anterior versus inferior ischemia. Am. Heart J. 121:753, 1991.

77. Weyman, A.E., Peskoe, S.N., Williams, E.S., et al.: Detection of left ventricular aneurysms by cross-sectional echocardiography. Circulation 54:936, 1976.

78. Catherwood, E., Mintz, G.S., Kotler, M.N., et al.: Two-dimensional echocardiographic recognition of left ventricular pseudoaneurysm. Circulation 62:294, 1980.

79. Gatewood, R.P., and Nanda N.: Differentiation of left ventricular pseudoaneurysm from true aneurysm with two-dimensional echocardiography. Am. J. Cardiol. 46:869, 1980.

80. Visser, C.A., Kan, G., David, G.K., et al.: Two-dimensional echocardiography in the diagnosis of left ventricular thrombus: A prospective study of 67 patients with anatomic validation. Chest 83:228, 1983.

81. Asinger, R.W., Mikell, F.L., Sharma, B., et al.: Observations on detecting left ventricular thrombus with two-dimensional echocardiography. Emphasis on avoidance of false-positive diagnoses. Am. J. Cardiol. 47:145, 1981.

82. McPherson, D.D., Knosp, B.M., Kieso, R., et al.: Ultrasound characterization of acoustic properties of acute intracardiac thrombi: Studies in a new experimental model. J. Am. Soc. Echocardiogr. 1:264, 1988.

83. Visser, C.A., Kan,G., Meltzer, R.S., et al.: Embolic potential of left ventricular thrombus after myocardial infarction: A two-dimensional echocardiographic study of 119 patients. J. Am. Coll. Cardiol. 5:1276, 1985.

84. Ezekowitz, M.D., Wilson, D.A., Smith, E.O., et al.: Comparison of indium-111 platelet scintigraphy and two-dimensional echocardiography in the diagnosis of left ventricular thrombi. N. Engl. J. Med. 306:1509, 1983.

85. Stratton, J.R., Lighty, G.W., Pearlman, A.S., et al.: Detection of left ventricular thrombus by two-dimensional echocardiography: Sensitivity, specificity, and causes of uncertainty. Circulation 66:156, 1982.

86. Seabold, J.E., Schroder, E., Conrad, G.R., et al.: Indium-111 platelet scintigraphy and two-dimensional echocardiography for detection of left ventricular thrombus: Influence of clot size and age. J. Am. Coll. Cardiol. 9:1057, 1987.

87. Asinger, R.W., Mikell, F.L., Elsperger, J., et al.: Incidence of left ventricular thrombus after acute transmural myocardial infarction. N. Engl. J. Med. 305:297, 1981.

88. Kupper, A.J.F., Verheught, F.W.A., Peels, C.H., et al.: Left ventricular thrombus incidence and behavior studied by serial two-dimensional echocardiography in acute anterior myocardial infarction: Left ventricular wall motion systemic embolism and oral anticoagulation. J. Am. Coll. Cardiol. 13:1514, 1989.

89. Spirito, P., Bellotti, P., Chiarella, F., et al.: Prognostic significance and natural history of left ventricular thrombi in patients with acute anterior myocardial infarction—A two-dimensional echocardiographic study. Circulation 72:774, 1985.

90. Haughland, J.M., Asinger, R.W., Mikell, F.L., et al.: Embolic potential of left ventricular thrombi detected by two-dimensional echocardiography. Circulation 70:588, 1981.

91. Stratton, J.R., and Resuich, A.D.: Increased embolic risk in patients with left ventricular thrombi. Circulation 75:1004, 1987.

92. Keating, E.C., Gross, S.A., Schlamowitz, R.A., et al.: Mural thrombi in myocardial infarction. Am. J. Med. 74:989, 1983.

93. Weinrich, D.J., Burke, J.F., and Ferrel, J.P.: Left ventricular mural thrombi complicating acute myocardial infarction. Ann. Intern. Med. 100:789, 1984.

94. Vandenberg, B.F., Seabold, J.E., Schroder, E., et al.: Noninvasive imaging of left ventricular thrombi: Two-dimensional echocardiography and indium-111 platelet scintigraphy. Am. J. Cardiac. Imaging 1:289, 1987.

95. Vandenberg, B.F., and Kerber, R.E.: Left ventricular thrombi in acute and chronic coronary artery disease: The role of two-dimensional echocardiography. In Kerber, R.E. (ed.): Echocardiography in Coronary Artery Disease. Mt. Kisco, NY, Futura, 1988.

96. Turpie, A.G.G., Robinson, J.G., Doyle, D.J., et al.: Comparison of high-dose with low-dose subcutaneous heparin to prevent left ventricular mural thrombosis in patients with acute transmural anterior myocardial infarction. N. Engl. J. Med. 320:352, 1989.

97. Eigler, N., Maurer, G., and Shah, P.E.: Effect of early systemic thrombolytic therapy on left ventricular mural thrombus formation in acute myocardial infarction. Am. J. Cardiol. 54:261, 1984.

98. Held, A.C., Gore, J.M., Paraskos, J., et al.: Impact of thrombolytic therapy on left ventricular mural thrombi in acute myocardial infarction. Am. J. Cardiol. 62:310–311, 1988.

99. Douglas, P.S., Fiolkoski, J., Berko, B., et al.: Echocardiographic visualization of coronary artery anatomy in the adult. J. Am. Coll. Cardiol. 11:565, 1988.

100. Ryan, T., Armstrong, W.F., and Feigenbaum, H.: Prospective evaluation of left main coronary artery using digital two-dimensional echocardiography. J. Am. Coll. Cardiol. 7:807, 1986.

101. Rogers, E.W., Feigenbaum, H., Weyman, A.E., et al.: Possible detection of atherosclerotic coronary calcification by two-dimensional echocardiography. Circulation 62:1046, 1980.

102. Chandraratna, P.A.N., and Aronow, W.S.: Left main coronary artery patency assessed with cross-sectional echocardiography. Am. J. Cardiol. 46:91, 1980.

103. Rink, L.D., Feigenbaum, H., Godley, R.W., et al.: Echocardiographic detection of left main coronary artery obstruction. Circulation 65:719, 1982.

104. Yoshida, K., Yoshikawa, J., Hozumi, T., et al.: Detection of the left main coronary artery stenosis by transesophageal color Doppler and two-dimensional echocardiography. Circulation 81:1271, 1990.

105. Memmola, C., Iliceto, S., and Rizzon, P.: Detection of proximal stenosis of left coronary artery by digital transesophageal echocardiography: Feasibility, sensitivity and specificity. J. Am. Soc. Echocardiogr. 6:149, 1993.

106. Schrem, S.S., Tunick, P.A., Slater, J., et al.: Transesophageal echocardiography in the diagnosis of ostial left coronary artery stenosis. J. Am. Soc. Echo. 3:367, 1990.

107. Reichert, S.L., Visser, C.A., Koolen, J.J., et al.: Transesophageal examination of the left coronary artery with a 7.5 MHz annular array two-dimensional color flow Doppler transducer. J. Am. Soc. Echocardiogr. 3:118, 1990.

108. Erbel, R.: Transesophageal echocardiography. New window to coronary arteries and coronary blood flow. Circulation 83:339, 1991.

109. Yamagishi, M., Miyatake, K., Beppu, S., et al.: Assessment of coronary blood flow by transesophageal two-dimensional pulsed Doppler echocardiography. Am. J. Cardiol. 62:641, 1988.

110. Iliceto, S., Marangelli, V., Memmola, C., et al.: Transesophageal Doppler echocardiography evaluation of coronary blood flow velocity in baseline conditions and during dipyridamole-induced coronary vasodilation. Circulation 83:61, 1991.

111. Pandian, G., Kumar, R., Katz, S., et al.: Real-time intracardiac, two-dimensional echocardiography. Echocardiography 4:407, 1991.

112. McKay, C.R., Kieso, R., DeJong, S.C., et al.: Identification of myocardial risk areas by intracardiac ultrasound. Circulation 86: I-524, 1992.

113. Vandenberg, B.F., McKay, C.R., DeJong, S.C., et al.: Intracardiac ultrasound: Rotation and translation of left ventricular cavity area with a catheter stabilizing system. Circulation 88:I-70, 1993.

114. McKay, C.R., Spencer, K., Hanson, P., et al.: Intracardiac ultrasound and dobutamine can identify stunned myocardium in a canine model. J. Am. Coll. Cardiol. 21:75A, 1993.

115. Spencer, K.T., Smith, R.S., DeJong, S.C., et al.: Right ventricular and interventricular septal contraction in right ventricular infarction: Evaluation by intracardiac ultrasound. Circulation 88:I-69, 1993.

116. Spencer KT, DeJong SC, Smith RS, et al.: Intracardiac ultrasound on-line quantitative assessment of regional myocardial thickening: A new method. Circulation 88:I-220, 1993.

38 Transesophageal Echocardiography

Nelson B. Schiller, M.D.
Elyse Foster, M.D.

INDICATIONS FOR TRANSESOPHAGEAL
 ECHOCARDIOGRAPHY ____ 534
TECHNICAL CONSIDERATIONS ____ 534
Participating Personnel: Cardiologists,
 Anesthesiologists, Nurses, and
 Sonographers ____ 534
Physician Training Guidelines ____ 535
CONTRAINDICATIONS TO TRANSESOPHAGEAL
 ECHOCARDIOGRAPHY ____ 535
SAFETY OF TRANSESOPHAGEAL
 ECHOCARDIOGRAPHY ____ 536
TYPE AND LOCATION OF EQUIPMENT ____ 536
Echocardiographic Probes and Engines ____ 536
Other Equipment in the Transesophageal
 Echocardiography Laboratory ____ 537
TECHNICAL GUIDELINES ____ 537
The Procedure ____ 537
Sedation and Local Anesthesia ____ 537
Probe Passage and Manipulation ____ 537
STANDARD ANATOMY (VIEWS) OF
 TRANSESOPHAGEAL
 ECHOCARDIOGRAPHY ____ 537
Transverse-Plane Views (0 Degree) ____ 538
 Transverse Level 1 ____ 538
 Transverse Level 2 ____ 540
 Transverse Level 3 ____ 540
 Transverse Level 4 ____ 540
 Transverse Level 5 ____ 540
 Transverse Level 6 ____ 542
 Transverse Level 7 ____ 542
Longitudinal Planar Views (Biplane, Vertical, or
 Multiplanar 90 degrees) ____ 543
 Longitudinal Level 1 ____ 543
 Longitudinal Level 2 ____ 544
 Longitudinal Level 3 ____ 544
Multiplane Views ____ 544
EVALUATION OF THE LEFT VENTRICLE BY
 TRANSESOPHAGEAL
 ECHOCARDIOGRAPHY ____ 545
Systolic Function ____ 545

Diastolic Function by Transesophageal
 Echocardiography ____ 546
ISCHEMIC HEART DISEASE AND
 TRANSESOPHAGEAL
 ECHOCARDIOGRAPHY ____ 547
LEFT VENTRICULAR STRESS TESTING BY
 TRANSESOPHAGEAL
 ECHOCARDIOGRAPHY ____ 548
ENDOCARDITIS AND TRANSESOPHAGEAL
 ECHOCARDIOGRAPHY ____ 548
VALVE DISEASES ____ 550
Aortic Valve Disease ____ 550
 Aortic Stenosis ____ 550
 Aortic Insufficiency ____ 550
Mitral Valve Disease ____ 551
 Mitral Stenosis ____ 551
 Mitral Regurgitation ____ 552
Tricuspid and Pulmonary Valves ____ 555
Prosthetic Valve Evaluation ____ 555
PULMONARY ARTERIES ____ 556
INTRACARDIAC TUMORS, MASSES, SOURCE OF
 EMBOLISM, AND ROLE OF TRANSESOPHAGEAL
 ECHOCARDIOGRAPHY IN ATRIAL
 FIBRILLATION ____ 556
ATHEROSCLEROTIC PLAQUE IN THE DESCENDING
 AORTA AND CORONARY FLOW RESERVE IN
 CORONARY ARTERY DISEASE ____ 558
HEMODYNAMICS DERIVED FROM
 TRANSESOPHAGEAL ECHOCARDIOGRAPHY:
 APPLICATION IN CRITICAL CARE AND
 CARDIOPULMONARY RESUSCITATION ____ 559
AORTIC DISSECTION ____ 560
TRAUMA AND TRANSESOPHAGEAL
 ECHOCARDIOGRAPHY ____ 561
CONGENITAL HEART DISEASES AND
 TRANSESOPHAGEAL
 ECHOCARDIOGRAPHY ____ 561
FUTURE DEVELOPMENTS IN TRANSESOPHAGEAL
 ECHOCARDIOGRAPHY AND
 SUMMARY ____ 561

Transesophageal echocardiography (TEE) was first demonstrated by the pioneering experiments of Frazin and colleagues.[1] These initial efforts used an M-mode crystal on a modified steerable catheter ("lozenge on a string") and demonstrated that excellent images of the base of the heart could be obtained in patients in whom hyperinflated lungs had rendered surface imaging technically difficult. The technique failed to adequately image the left ventricle and languished until Hanrath and associates[2] demonstrated that a flexible gastroscope housing provided the ideal vehicle for delivering and manipulating an ultrasound transducer into an optimal retrocardiac esophageal position. These investigators first demonstrated that an M-mode crystal could reliably and reproducibly image the left ventricle, even during bicycle exercise.[2] In 1981, the authors' group at the University of California, San Francisco (UCSF), received one of Hanrath's gastroscope-mounted M-mode crystals and used it to demonstrate the value of intraoperative monitoring of left ventricular function. Based on these preliminary results, the Varian Corporation of Palo Alto produced two prototype gastroscope-mounted, phased-array, two-dimensional transducers, one of which went to Hanrath's group in Hamburg and the

TABLE 38–1. HISTORICAL DEVELOPMENT OF TRANSESOPHAGEAL ECHOCARDIOGRAPHY

1976	M-mode TEE (Frazin et al.[1])
1977	Two-dimensional *mechanical* probe (Hisanaga[°])
1981	Two-dimensional phased-array probe (Souquet et al.[3])
1982	Pulsed Doppler (Schluter et al.[4])
1986	Color flow imaging (de Bruijn[†])
1989	Biplane probe (Omoto et al.[9])
1989	Pediatric probe (Kyo et al.[10])
1992	Multiplane probe (Flachskampf[‡]; Roelandt[29])
1993	Dynamic three-dimensional imaging (Schneider et al.[11])

[°]Hisanaga, K., Hisanaga, A., Nagata, K., et al.: A new transesophageal real-time two-dimensional echocardiography system using flexible tubing and its clinical application. Proc. Jpn. Soc. Ultrasound Med. 32:43, 1977.

[†]deBruijn, N.P., Clements, F.M., and Kisslo, J.A.: Intraoperative transesophageal color flow mapping: Initial experience. Anesth. Analg. 66:386, 1987.

[‡]Flachskampf, F.A., Hoffman, R., Krebs, W., et al.: Initial clinical trial of a multiplane transesophageal echoscope. Z. Kardiol. 81:438, 1992.

other to the authors' group at UCSF.[3] In Hamburg several studies were performed in the outpatient arena[3–5] and included Doppler as well as two-dimensional imaging. At UCSF the authors' work centered on intraoperative imaging.[6–8] In both settings it was clear to those who saw these early images that they were superior in resolution and reliability to transthoracic echocardiography. By 1985, there were more than 30 centers worldwide that used this technique. However, its major growth period came after 1985, when Hewlett-Packard combined color flow Doppler imaging with a high-frequency 5-MHz phased-array probe. This refinement was followed by the development of probes capable of continuous-wave Doppler, a second or multiple imaging planes,[9] passage in small infants,[10] and registration of data sets suitable for three-dimensional reconstruction.[11] Based on these advances (Table 38–1) and on their enthusiastic acceptance by cardiologists, it is not surprising that between the time of publication of the last edition of this book and the time of writing of the second edition there have been more than 2000 new journal articles published on TEE. There is also ample evidence that TEE has become an indispensable tool in many clinical and intraoperative situations. The text that follows offers a comprehensive review of the clinical role of TEE, with particular emphasis on these indications that are now considered standard of practice.

INDICATIONS FOR TRANSESOPHAGEAL ECHOCARDIOGRAPHY

Transesophageal echocardiography is practiced in a variety of venues, each of which has its own group of indications. In the intraoperative venue, it is often an integral part of surgery involving heart valve disease, coronary artery disease, congenital conditions, and vascular disease. In the outpatient setting, its applications include judging the severity of valve disease, endocarditis and its complications, and ventricular, pericardial,[12, 13] and congenital diseases. In the disciplines dealing with critical care, it has been used in both the emergency room and the intensive care unit, particularly in evaluating patients with hypotension of unknown cause. Table 38–2 lists the indications for TEE.

For some of the indications listed in Table 38–2, transesophageal imaging is the first diagnostic modality used; for others, it supplements transthoracic echocardiography; and for still others it represents an emerging application whose benefit is as yet unestablished. Table 38–3 classifies the indications for TEE, listing each according to its place in the hierarchy of diagnostic procedures. Note that to provide many of these services, laboratories must be prepared to be available on a round-the-clock basis.

TECHNICAL CONSIDERATIONS

Participating Personnel: Cardiologists, Anesthesiologists, Nurses, and Sonographers

Elective TEE in outpatients or inpatients is usually performed by a cardiologist in a hospital setting, but there is growing interest in the use of this modality in office practice. Intraoperative echocardiography is performed primarily by anesthesiologists, but in many centers it is an interactive activity in which cardiologists routinely consult on problem findings that arise in the operating room and frequently read and report the results of the studies jointly. A high level of interaction and collaboration is certainly the case in the authors' institution and has resulted in the recent inauguration of a video connection between the adult and the pediatric echocardiography reading rooms and the cardiac operating rooms. This connection makes echocardiographic consultation continually available. All anesthesia residents rotate through the authors' laboratory while they are serving on the cardiovascular anesthesia rotation, and all operating room studies are interpreted at joint didactic reading sessions. In emergency nonelective studies in critical care units, cardiologists usually perform TEE. Again, close cooperation with anesthesiologists who attend critical care patients results in frequent interactions about these patients. Examples of this situation include the hypotensive patient who is awake and may require very careful sedation or even intubation so that TEE can be safely performed, or the patient with an endotracheal tube already in place in whom safe esophageal intubation is difficult and requires the use of a laryngoscope. The exact distribution of responsibilities among qualified practitioners of TEE varies from institution to institution, depending on the interest and availability of qualified physicians.

In addition to physician echocardiographers, nurses have become a part of many TEE laboratories. Nursing participation is especially important when use is made of conscious sedation. After the authors performed the first 100 elective studies without patient sedation, it became apparent that most patients felt quite uncomfort-

TABLE 38–2. INDICATIONS FOR TRANSESOPHAGEAL ECHOCARDIOGRAPHY

Intraoperative
Left and right ventricular function (global and segmental)
Interpretation of hemodynamic changes (especially hypotension)
Evaluation of the success of repairs to vessels, valves, and of congenital and acquired defects
Confirmation of preoperative diagnosis (especially in emergency situations)
Judging atherosclerotic burden (emergent evaluation of great vessels for plaque extent)
Trauma surgery (especially evaluation of the great vessels)

Ambulatory or Hospitalized (Noncritical Care) Patients
Endocarditis and its complications
Severity and etiology of native and prosthetic valve disorders
Diseases of the great vessels
Source of embolism
Cardiac tumors or masses
Pericardial and paracardiac disorders
Congenital heart disease
Coronary physiology and anatomy
Left and right ventricular function and anatomy (global and segmental)
Guidance of interventional and therapeutic procedures (valvular, electrophysiological, etc.)
Imaging during diagnostic stress testing
Left atrial and appendage function and contents prior to cardioversion

Critical Care
Differential diagnosis of acute hemodynamic compromise in myocardial infarction, post surgery, and general intensive care
Emergency room patients presenting with cardiopulmonary arrest, hypotension, chest pain, obtundation or severe chest injury.

TABLE 38–3. HIERARCHICAL INDICATIONS FOR TRANSESOPHAGEAL ECHOCARDIOGRAPHY

TEE First Modality Used (Transthoracic Echocardiography Supplemental)
Mechanism of mitral disruption
Abscess presence and location in endocarditis
Prosthetic mitral or tricuspid valve dysfunction (perivalvular leak, ring dehiscence, vegetation, pannus, or thrombus)
Cardiac source of embolus arising *directly* from a thrombus in the left atrium, plaque in the aortic arch, thrombus on a redundant interatrial septum, or *indirectly* from a paradoxical embolus crossing an atrial septal defect or patent foramen ovale
Dissection or intramural hematoma of the aorta
Intraoperative evaluation of left ventricular function, valve repair or replacement, and congenital heart disease palliation.

TEE Supplements Transthoracic Echocardiography
Native valve disease etiology and severity
Prosthetic valve obstruction and anterior periprosthetic aortic regurgitation
Initial detection of bulky vegetations in endocarditis
Left ventricular apical thrombus as source of embolus
Congenital heart disease
Left ventricular function evaluation
Hemodynamic abnormalities (high and low output, high and low filling pressures, etc.)

TEE Application Likely, Emerging or Under Study
Embolic risk estimation prior to atrial arrhythmia cardioversion
Embolic risk estimation prior to mitral stenosis balloon valvuloplasty
TEE imaging with atrial pacing or pharmacologic perturbation to detect provocable ischemia or abnormal coronary flow reserve
Guidance of therapeutic catheter-based procedures such as arrhythmia ablation or mitral stenosis valvuloplasty
Cause of cardiac arrest and effectiveness of CPR
Estimating likelihood of critical coronary disease from aortic arch plaque burden
Pulmonary embolism presence and severity

able during the procedure and that patient acceptance was poor. With the addition of conscious sedation, patient acceptance has vastly improved. The participation of a nurse with critical care experience is highly desirable in that it maximizes the safety of this procedure. If a nurse is not available, a second person such as a physician colleague should be in the examining room or close at hand to assist with unexpected problems.

The role of the sonographer in TEE is variable. In some laboratories,[14] the sonographer is responsible for optimizing the quality of the image during the study and, in a few cases, actually performs minor manipulations of the transducer once the physician has passed it. This latter role is controversial, but it is not without precedent. For example, in endoscopy laboratories, technicians sometimes perform supervised intubations.

Physician Training Guidelines

The American Society of Echocardiography (ASE) has published guidelines for physician training in TEE.[15] These guidelines represent the recommendations of a group of physicians who are highly experienced in the technique, and these recommendations are intended for the use of hospital practice committees, who alone have the authority to set standards of practice for staff members. The ASE training guidelines in general echocardiography, published in 1987,[16] form the basis for the 1992 transesophageal echocardiography recommendations, and they recognize three levels of training in echocardiography. Level I training is introductory exposure to echocardiography at a level likely to be encountered in the first year of fellowship. Level II physicians are those who, after fellowship, have accumulated an additional 6 months of extensive experience in interpreting echocardiograms but are not qualified to run a laboratory that supervises training and research. Level III physicians have had at least 1 full year of fellowship training devoted exclusively to echocardiography under the supervision of a Level III physician. As Table 38–4, a summary of the American Society of Echocardiography guidelines, shows, the ASE recommends at least Level II training before a physician is trained to perform TEE.

The ASE guidelines also describe the skills, cognitive and technical, required to perform TEE.[15] The cognitive skills listed include knowledge of appropriate indications, contraindications, and risks; understanding of the differential diagnostic considerations for each clinical situation; knowledge of the technical operation of ultrasound equipment and of the physics of echocardiography and Doppler ultrasound equipment and of the physics of echocardiography and Doppler ultrasound; knowledge of tomographic anatomy in the multiple planes presented in a transesophageal echocardiographic image; recognition of abnormal anatomy as imaged in a transesophageal echocardiographic format; knowledge of normal and morbid cardiovascular hemodynamics and how to derive such information from transesophageal echocardiographic information; knowledge of when to recognize inadequate data; knowledge of alternative technologies and their indications; and ability to communicate findings to the patient and the referring physician.

The technical skills cited by the ASE recommendations include proficiency in performing a standard transthoracic examination, proficiency in safely introducing the probe and adjusting it to obtain technically adequate images, and proficiency in the quantitation of the information.

CONTRAINDICATIONS TO TRANSESOPHAGEAL ECHOCARDIOGRAPHY

The absolute and relative contraindications for TEE,[17] independent of the setting, are listed in Table 38–5. They include recent (within 4 to 6 hours) oral intake, esophageal obstruction (mass or stricture) or diverticulum, prior esophageal surgery (esophagectomy, fundal-plication procedure), unevaluated active gastrointestinal bleeding, a perforated viscus, and an uncooperative patient. A history of dysphagia or previous mediastinal radiation may necessitate further investigation by means of barium swallow or esophagoscopy prior to blind intubation of the esophagus.

Relative contraindications include esophagitis, nonbleeding esophageal varices, severe cervical arthritis that limits neck flexion,

TABLE 38–4. RECOMMENDED TRAINING TO ACQUIRE AND MAINTAIN SKILLS IN TEE

Component	Objective	Duration	No. of Cases
Level II (general echo)	Competence in general echo	6 mo	300
Esophageal intubation	Skilled intubation	Variable	25
TEE examination	Skill in performance and interpretation	Variable	50
Continuing education	Retain competence	Annual	30–75

Adapted from Pearlman, A.S., Gardin, J.M., Martin, R.P., et al.: Guidelines for physician training in transesophageal echocardiography: Recommendations of the American Society of Echocardiography Committee for Physician Training in Echocardiography. J. Am. Soc. Echocardiogr. 5(2):187–194, 1992, with permission.

TABLE 38–5. CONTRAINDICATIONS TO
TRANSESOPHAGEAL ECHOCARDIOGRAPHY

Absolute
Recent (within 4–6 h) oral intake
Esophageal obstruction (mass or stricture) or diverticulum
Prior esophageal surgery (esophagectomy, fundal-plication procedure)
Undiagnosed active gastrointestinal bleeding
A perforated viscus
An uncooperative patient
Undiagnosed dysphagia

Relative
Previous mediastinal radiation
Esophagitis
Nonbleeding esophageal varices
Severe cervical arthritis limiting neck flexion
Compromised cardiac or respiratory status, increasing the risk of
    adequate sedation

and a compromised cardiac or respiratory status that increases the risk of adequate sedation. However, in the last case, if the information from TEE is critical to the care of unstable patients, endotracheal intubation for mechanical ventilation and airway protection should be considered.

SAFETY OF TRANSESOPHAGEAL ECHOCARDIOGRAPHY

Complications consequent to TEE are extremely uncommon. Daniel and co-workers[17] reporting on more than 10,000 studies from 15 European institutions, found that intubations succeeded 98.5 percent of the time. In 0.88 percent, the study was prematurely terminated because of patient intolerance, pulmonary complications, arrhythmias, angina, minor pharyngeal bleeding, and fatal hematemesis in one case of advanced esophageal carcinoma. Thus, with one death the mortality rate was 0.001 percent and the rate of significant morbidity 0.18 percent. Studies in the elderly[18] and in the critically ill[19–22] also confirm the universal impression that this procedure, when performed with appropriate precautions, is safe.

In any discussion of safety, some consideration must be given to the risk of endocarditis posed by the procedure itself. Most evidence points to TEE as carrying a very low burden of bacteremia and a low risk of endocarditis.[23–27] In the authors' own practice they continue to provide prophylaxis according to the guidelines of the American Heart Association when dealing with patients with

mitral regurgitation, prosthetic heart valves, or complex congenital heart disease. Part of this approach is colored by their experience with one patient with moderately severe mitral regurgitation, who developed endocarditis due to *Streptococcus sanguis* 1 week after TEE.[28] The authors' practice is to administer amoxicillin, 3 g orally, 1 hour before the procedure. In patients with penicillin allergy, the authors administer erythromycin or intravenous vancomycin, 1 g. Based on a lack of evidence favoring post-procedural prophylaxis, the authors have dropped the second antibiotic dose.

TYPE AND LOCATION OF EQUIPMENT

Echocardiographic Probes and Engines

The standard transesophageal echocardiographic probe is built around the housing of a standard upper gastrointestinal endoscope (Fig. 38–1A). This design consists of a flexible tube ranging from 8 mm (pediatrics) to 12 mm at its maximum diameter. Because of wires running longitudinally through the tube to the tip of the probe, where the transducer is mounted, it can be manipulated through a wide range of angles and positions at various levels. Because of the stiffness of the shaft, torque can be applied to the shaft of the probe, and the transducer can be rotated around the long axis of the shaft. These various manipulations allow the operator to obtain many views from a considerable variety of tomographic planes.

The first practical mass-produced probes had a single-plane, phased-array transducer whose 32 elements were aligned transversely to the long axis of its shaft. In 1989, biplane echocardiography was introduced[9] and was quickly adopted worldwide as the preferred method of imaging. Biplane probes are still commonly used and have replaced monoplane probes in most laboratories. These probes consist of two separate arrays of elements mounted sequentially at the tip of the probe. The distal element is oriented transversely (0 degree) and the proximal element longitudinally (90 degrees). To view a cardiac structure in both planes it is necessary to either advance or withdraw the probe slightly so that the target structure is centered relative to the transducer elements. In transverse imaging, the most important scanning maneuver is to advance and withdraw the probe, and in horizontal or longitudinal imaging, applying torque to the probe is most important.

By 1993, multiplane imaging was introduced[11, 29–31] and was judged to be a substantial improvement over biplane imaging. Multiplane probes rotate a single 64-element, phased array through 180 degrees by using a miniature clockwork mechanism located in the tip of the probe (See Fig. 38–1B). After our first year of experience, the authors have been able to successfully place this

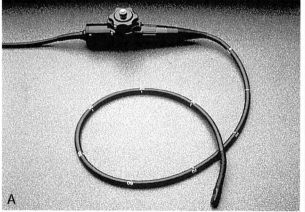
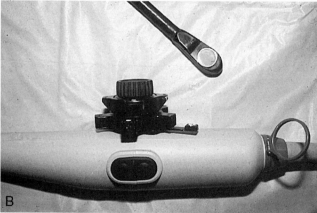

FIGURE 38–1. *A*, A commercially available, 64-element phased-array TEE probe, a gastroscope-like device. *B*, Close-up of a multiplane 64-element phased-array TEE probe. The circular disk-like transducer mounted in the probe tip can be controlled through 180 degrees with the switch mounted in the handle.

slightly larger probe with almost complete success. Another engineering approach in the development of multiplanar transesophageal echocardiographic imaging used a single-element mechanical transducer manipulated through a range of motion while oscillating along a single spatial plane. The authors' attempts to image with this modestly priced instrument were also satisfactory, but with lower color sensitivity. The multiplanar instrument has the advantage of allowing one to "dial in" a structure. For example, the aortic valve cannot usually be viewed en face unless the element is oriented at approximately 30 degrees from the transverse plane (see later text).

Based on almost 2 years of experience with multiplanar imaging, there is no question that it is now the "community standard" for TEE. Because a multiplanar device that rotates around a fixed point allows reconstruction of three-dimensionally rendered images, the importance of multiplanar capability will grow with the maturation of three-dimensional imaging.

Other Equipment in the Transesophageal Echocardiography Laboratory

A pulsed oximeter contributes substantially to the safety of TEE, especially when conscious sedation is used. Supplemental oxygen is mandatory for the same reason, and its use can be guided by pulsed oximetry. Blood pressure monitoring should be performed throughout the procedure, at the very least manually and, ideally, both manually and automatically. Suction equipment is also required to reduce the danger of airway compromise due to secretions and to ensure patient comfort. A "crash cart" for full resuscitation should be available in close proximity as a necessary adjunct to the safe performance of conscious sedation. Space and equipment for proper cleaning and storage of probes should be allotted. Note that the formalin-based material (Cydex) emits irritating fumes and should be properly vented. Bite guards, intravenous supplies, contrast agents, protective garments and goggles, and appropriate pharmacologic agents all are required.

TECHNICAL GUIDELINES

The Procedure

In all but dire emergencies, the patient's history, physical examination, and a recent surface echocardiogram should be reviewed prior to the study. A well-considered differential diagnosis and the views required to support each element in the differential should be carefully constructed *prior to* passing the probe. Written, informed consent is required in most institutions, except when emergent or extenuating conditions prohibit it. The patient should be in the fasting state for at least 4 hours and preferably for 6. If careful questioning fails to reveal gastrointestinal disease or drug allergy for protocol medications, antibiotic prophylaxis is given, if indicated. Electrocardiography, blood pressure, and oximetry are continually monitored throughout the procedure. Dentures should be removed and nasal oxygen begun if saturation falls below 95 percent. In the critical care setting, it may be necessary to remove the nasogastric tube to improve intraesophageal contact and to partially deflate the endotracheal tube to allow passage.

Sedation and Local Anesthesia

Some form of local lidocaine is used, with care taken to avoid overdosage. A useful end point is the suppression of the gag reflex, documented by stimulation of the posterior pharynx. In their patients, the authors use a combination of intravenous meperidine, 25 to 50 mg, and midazolam, 0.5 to 7 mg, to induce arousable sleep. Monitoring during this state should be performed with considerable care. In ventilated patients, the help of critical care nurses

and an anesthesiologist may be necessary. Such help is particularly important when paralytic agents, such as vecuronium, are required.

Probe Passage and Manipulation

After induction of adequate levels of sedation and ensurance of hemodynamic stability, the patient is turned into left recumbency, and the head is tilted forward so that the chin nearly rests on the chest. The examiner places the bite block in the proper direction over the probe (small end toward the tip) and lubricates the end of the probe with water-soluble gel. The authors have found that viscous lidocaine makes a good lubricant while it also serves to maintain upper pharyngeal analgesia. Wearing two sets of gloves (the outer pair can be removed if they become too slippery to manipulate the probe), the examiner places his or her left forefinger into the mouth and exerts forward traction on the base of the tongue while passing the probe toward the esophagus. The left forefinger can be used to keep the probe in the midline. Usually, the endoscopic controls are set so that the probe is slightly flexed and stiffened. As the probe passes the larynx, slight resistance is felt and the patient is asked to swallow while the probe is advanced. If the probe is passed by this point of narrowing with alacrity, gagging can be minimized. The probe is then advanced to about 35 cm from the incisors. At this point the probe is torqued, and the structures at the base of the heart are identified.

Because a study may be shortened by patient intolerance, it is best to seek the target structures in the order of their priority which will have been predetermined by the differential diagnosis. For example, in a patient with known mitral insufficiency who is suspected of having endocarditis, the mitral valve should be examined first, followed by the other valves. If there is time, other structures, such as the left ventricle and descending aorta, can and should be examined to produce a complete examination. Each structure should be examined in its longitudinal and transverse planes, as well as any intermediate planes that define its normality or pathology. Among the many factors that favor a successful examination are attention to optimizing the images by selection of appropriate depth settings and by limiting color flow interrogation to as small a sector as possible.

During the examination the operator needs to make sure that the study has been recorded properly and that all elements in the differential diagnosis have been addressed. After the probe has been withdrawn, the patient must be monitored until it is safe to ambulate. The authors insist that outpatients be accompanied for this examination and be instructed not to operate a motor vehicle or ride public transportation until the day after the examination.

STANDARD ANATOMY (VIEWS) OF TRANSESOPHAGEAL ECHOCARDIOGRAPHY

There is some disagreement as to what constitutes "standard" transesophageal echocardiographic views. For example, one school of thought[31] proposes that image orientation should conform to that adopted for surface imaging. However, to accomplish this consistency it is necessary to electronically invert some images during the course of the examination. In this chapter, all views are displayed with the apex of the fan at the top of the screen, so the top of the screen always identifies the position of the transducer.[11] This approach avoids the need to flip the image at an arbitrary point in the examination, and it keeps the most highly focused and resolved part of the image in one position on the video display. Its disadvantages include the need for visualizing the patient lying prone.

In the next discussion, the views and their anatomy are presented in terms of the distance of the transducer from the incisors. This value is given in centimeters, and the operator can easily determine it from the markings on the shaft of the transesophageal echocardiographic probe. Transverse plane views (0 degree) are presented first, followed by longitudinal views (90 degrees), and, finally, the multiplane, "in-between" views.

Transverse Plane Views (0 Degree)

Transverse Level 1

Transverse level 1 is 25 to 30 cm from incisors. At this level there are two technical problems. The first is interference with the image by air in the bronchus, and the second is gagging from upper esophageal stimulation by the widest portion of the probe. At this level, in the transverse plane the great vessels are seen—the ascending aorta and superior vena cava in short-axis, and the main pulmonary artery and its branches in long axis (Figs. 38–2A and 38–3A). The right pulmonary artery is seen best as it crosses

posterior to the aorta, whereas the left is often obscured by the air-filled left main bronchus. If the probe is rotated posteriorly, the descending aorta can be imaged (Fig. 38–4, *upper left*). At this level this structure appears circular, but with slight withdrawal the transverse arch can be seen and recognized by its tubular shape. Acquiring skill in imaging the main pulmonary artery branches and the descending aorta and arch is of great importance in treating critically ill patients suspected of having aortic dissection or pulmonary embolism. It is important here, and in all other views, to improve contact with gentle pressure on the wheel that allows the transducer to be anteriorly flexed. Similarly, if the probe is equipped with multiplanar capability, it is important to improve the image of the target structure by making slight changes in the angle of the transducer.

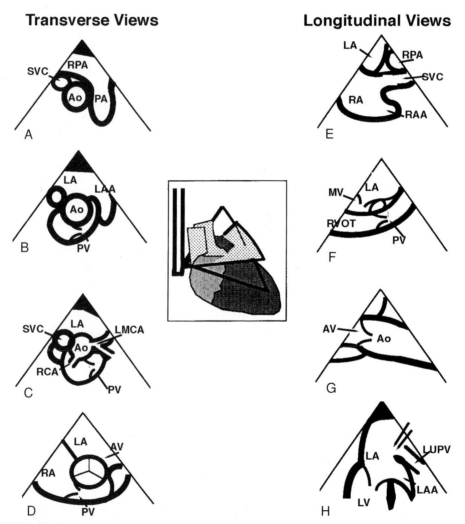

FIGURE 38–2. Transverse and longitudinal views from the base of the heart are shown diagrammatically. *A,* Transverse view of the relationship between the pulmonary artery bifurcation and the ascending aorta and superior vena cava. *B,* Transverse view of the aorta, superior vena cava, left atrium, and left atrial appendage with the pulmonary valve anteriorly. *C,* Transverse view of the upper portion of the aortic root and the origin of the left main and right coronary arteries. *D,* Transverse view, showing the short axis of the aortic valve with three-leaflet appearance. *E,* Longitudinal "bicaval" view centered on the superior vena cava and right atrial appendage. *F,* Longitudinal view of the right ventricular outflow tract, pulmonary valve, and main pulmonary artery. *G,* Longitudinal view of the aortic root and ascending aorta with the profile of the aortic valve and its relationship to the left ventricular outflow tract. *H,* Longitudinal view of the left atrial appendage and left upper pulmonary veins. Note that they are separated by a prominent fold that is a normal structure *(arrows).* PA = pulmonary artery; RPA = right pulmonary artery; SVC = superior vena cava; Ao = aorta; LA = left atrium; LAA = left atrial appendage; PV = pulmonary valve; LMCA = left main coronary artery; RCA = right coronary artery; AV = aortic valve; RA = right atrium; RAA = right atrial appendage; MV = mitral valve; RVOT = right ventricular outflow tract; LUPV = left upper pulmonary vein. (From Schneider, A.T., Hsu, T.-L., Schwartz, S.L., et al.: Single, biplane, multiplane, and three-dimensional echocardiography: Echocardiographic-anatomic correlations. Cardiol. Clin. 11:361, 1993, with permission.)

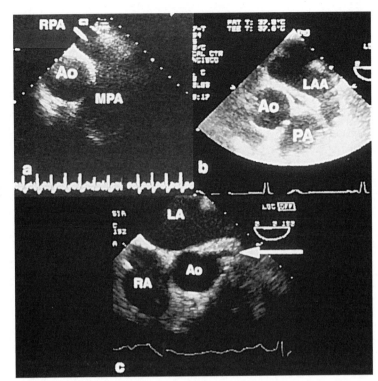

FIGURE 38–3. *A,* Transverse view of pulmonary artery bifurcation. *B,* Transverse view of left atrial appendage and ascending aorta. *C,* Transverse view showing origin of left main coronary artery *(solid arrow).* Abbreviations as in Figure 38–2.

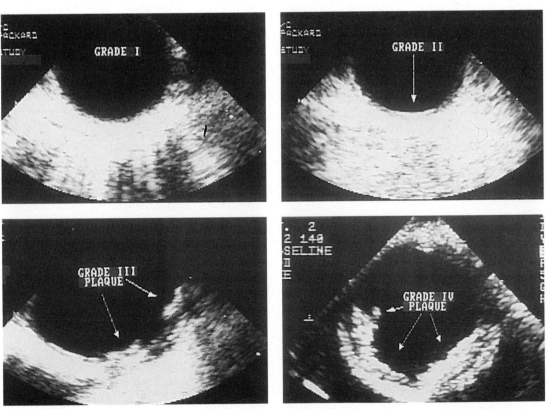

FIGURE 38–4. Transverse images of the descending aorta. *Upper Left,* Normal transverse aorta. *Upper Right,* Transverse aorta with intimal thickening (grade 2). *Lower Left,* Transverse aorta with minimally protruding plaque (grade 3). *Lower Right,* Transverse aorta with plaque with significant luminal incursion (grade 4). (From Fazio, G.P., Redberg, R.F., Winslow, T., et al.: Transesophageal echocardiographically detected atherosclerotic aortic plaque is a marker for coronary artery disease. J. Am. Coll. Cardiol. 21:144–150, 1993. Reprinted with permission from the American College of Cardiology.)

Transverse Level 2

Transverse level 2 is 28 to 35 cm. The structure at the top of the image fan (and, therefore, the one most posterior) is the left atrium. In the center of the image and immediately anterior to it is the proximal aorta. In the lower left part of the image is the right atrium, with the interatrial septum separating it from the left atrium. In the lower right part of the screen is part of the right ventricular outflow tract (see Fig. 38–2D). The proximal portion of the aorta has a variable appearance, depending on the relationship of the heart to the esophagus. In some, the aorta appears nearly in short axis, and in others it is off axis. With slight withdrawal, the coronary arteries come into view (see Figs. 38–2C and 38–3C). The left main coronary artery is easiest to image, and the right main coronary artery is more difficult. With multiplanar imaging or, in some patients, with careful manipulation of the probe, the left anterior descending coronary artery may be seen. At the level of the left main coronary artery, just above the aortic valve leaflets, the atrial appendage can be seen as a narrow-based triangular structure on the left side of the atrium. Careful manipulation of gains reveals the linear trabeculation (trabeculum carnae, so-called pectinate muscles) (see Figs. 38–2B and 38–3B). Further to the left of the appendage is the left upper pulmonary vein, running nearly parallel to the appendage. Separating the left atrial appendage from the left upper pulmonary vein is a prominent infolded portion of the atrial wall (see Figs. 38–2B and 38–3B). To the uninitiated viewer this fold has the appearance of a tumor, and in a few instances, patients have gone to surgery based on this misinterpretation. Because of the resemblance to a thrombus, this fold has been named facetiously the "warfarin ridge." The left upper pulmonary vein is seen simultaneously with and at the same level as the left atrial appendage; the right upper pulmonary vein is seen with the right atrial appendage. Also, lower pulmonary veins run toward the left atrium at right angles to the upper vein and appendage. The appendage can be explored with pulsed Doppler imaging to obtain flow patterns.[32] The pulmonary vein can also be studied with Doppler imaging[33] (Figs. 38–5 and 38–6). Torquing or rotating the probe along its long axis so that it is directed posteriorly results in a short-axis image of the descending aorta (see Fig. 38–4).

FIGURE 38–5. See Color Plate 10.

Transverse Level 3

This transverse level is 33 to 35 cm. Advancing the probe a few centimeters further reveals the left ventricular outflow tract and the basal part of the left ventricle (Figs. 38–7A and 38–8A). The proximal aorta and its relationship to the outflow tract is seen, as is the mitral valve dividing the left atrium from the left ventricle. In this view part of the right ventricle can be seen and, at times, a portion of the tricuspid valve. The view is mainly of value as a window on aortic insufficiency severity and, to a lesser extent, mitral regurgitation severity.

Transverse Level 4

Transverse level 4 is 35 to 37 cm. Further advancement reveals a four-chamber view (see Figs. 38–7B and 38–8B) with the atria side by side at the top of the image (see Fig. 38–13A) and the ventricles and their atrioventricular valves below. This view is an excellent starting point for both left ventricular diastolic inflow and mitral regurgitation studies. The anatomy of the mitral valve is well seen, as is that of the interatrial septum—particularly the thin *fossa ovalis* and, if present, associated patency. It is also possible to explore the atrium from this view and the other views mentioned

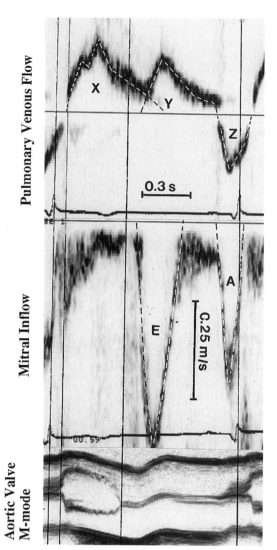

FIGURE 38–6. *Upper,* Pulsed-wave Doppler signal from within the left upper pulmonary vein showing the systolic (X) and diastolic (Y) components of atrial filling and the retrograde flow at the time of atrial contraction (Z). *Middle,* Mitral Doppler inflow signal taken from the tips of the mitral valve leaflets. *Lower,* Aortic valve M-mode pattern. These are displayed for timing purposes. E = early diastolic mitral filling wave; A = diastolic filling wave because of atrial contraction. (From Kuecherer, H.F., Kusumoto, F., Muhiudeen, I.A., et al.: Pulmonary venous flow patterns by transesophageal pulsed Doppler echocardiography: Relation to parameters of left ventricular systolic and diastolic function. Am. Heart J. 122:1683–1693, 1991, with permission.)

previously by rotating and flexing the probe. Although it appears as if the left ventricle is well seen, the apex is rarely visualized in this view, and critical information about global or segmental function is thus not provided. It is important to avoid being misled about ventricular function during the viewing of this foreshortened anatomic slice. It is best to confirm impressions from the gastric short axis (see later) or with surface imaging from the apex impulse.

Transverse Level 5

Transverse level 5 is 37 to 39 cm. Just beyond the four-chamber view, just proximal to the gastroesophageal junction, an improved image of the right ventricle and tricuspid valve and right atrium appears (see Figs. 38–7C and 38–8C). The most noteworthy feature

Transverse Views

Longitudinal Views

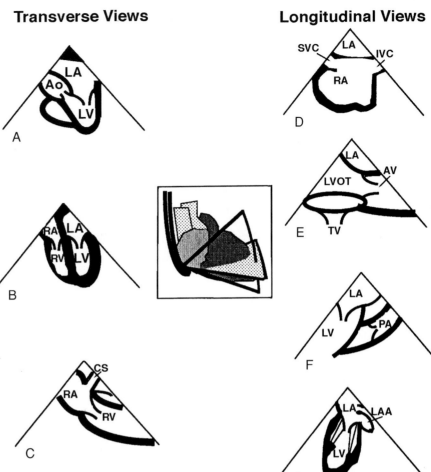

FIGURE 38–7. *A,* Transverse view at the level of the left ventricular outflow tract. *B,* Transverse four-chamber view. *C,* Transverse view of right ventricular inflow tract, showing the entrance of the coronary sinus into the right atrium. *D,* Longitudinal bicaval view showing the relationship of the venae cavae to the right atrium. *E,* Longitudinal view of the aortic root, aortic valve, and left ventricular outflow tract. *F,* Longitudinal view of left ventricular inflow tract. *G,* Longitudinal view of left ventricular inflow tract in relationship to left atrial appendage (two-chamber view). (From Schneider, A.T., Hsu, T.-L., Schwartz, S.L., et al.: Single, biplane, multiplane, and three-dimensional echocardiography: Echocardiographic-anatomic correlations. Cardiol. Clin. 11:361–387, 1993, with permission.)

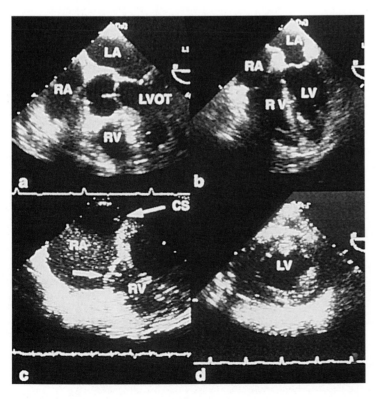

FIGURE 38–8. *A,* Transverse view of left ventricular outflow tract. *B,* Transverse four-chamber view. *C,* Transverse view of right ventricular inflow view with coronary sinus entering right atrium. *D,* Gastric transverse short-axis view.

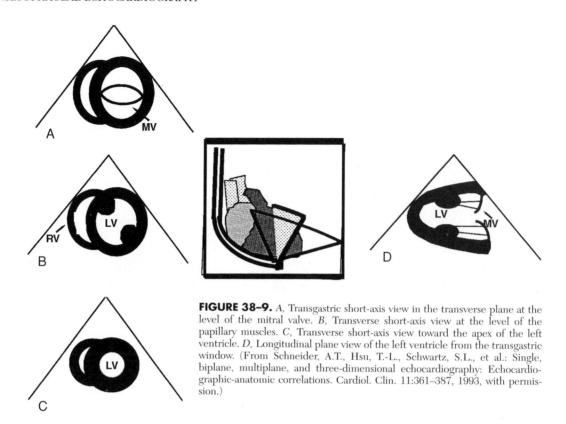

FIGURE 38-9. *A,* Transgastric short-axis view in the transverse plane at the level of the mitral valve. *B,* Transverse short-axis view at the level of the papillary muscles. *C,* Transverse short-axis view toward the apex of the left ventricle. *D,* Longitudinal plane view of the left ventricle from the transgastric window. (From Schneider, A.T., Hsu, T.-L., Schwartz, S.L., et al.: Single, biplane, multiplane, and three-dimensional echocardiography: Echocardiographic-anatomic correlations. Cardiol. Clin. 11:361–387, 1993, with permission.)

of this view is that the coronary sinus entering the right atrium is seen at the apex of the image. If preliminary research is confirmed, indicating that coronary sinus flow by Doppler imaging is an indicator of coronary arterial flow, then this view will increase in importance. Note that this view is quite similar to a posteriorly directed transthoracic apical four-chamber view.

Transverse Level 6

Transverse level 6 is 40 cm. When the probe is advanced further, slight resistance and patient discomfort are encountered, as the tip of the probe crosses the gastroesophageal junction. From this position it is usually necessary to anteflex the probe to ensure mucosal contact. It is also necessary to increase the depth of the field as the target, the short axis of the left ventricle, lies on the far field of the fan. With further slight manipulation, the mitral and papillary muscle levels of the left ventricular short axis can be imaged in turn (Figs. 38–9A to C and 38–10A to C; see Fig. 38–13C). The posteromedial papillary muscle is in the near field, the anterolateral in the far field. Both have an unusually bright appearance that is perfectly normal from this vantage point; this

hysteresis should serve as a cautionary observation to the difficulties that surround tissue characterization by ultrasound. Long experience with the use of this view in the operating room suggests that it is the most reliable for evaluating segmental and global left ventricular function.[34]

Transverse Level 7

Transverse level 7 is 40 to 45 cm. Early versions of TEE probes were limited in the degree of flexion that could be applied because of fear of injury to the patient. However, the extraordinary safety record of this procedure has resulted in slight increases in the range of motion of probes and the discovery that informative longitudinal views of the heart can be obtained from transgastric imaging (Fig. 38–11). The technique of obtaining these images involves advancing the probe to the fundus of the stomach and fully anteflexing it. These views are longitudinal views that include the apex of the left ventricle and are aligned with the great vessels. As such, they promise to allow left ventricular quantitation and to permit more reliable Doppler stroke volume and gradient determinations.

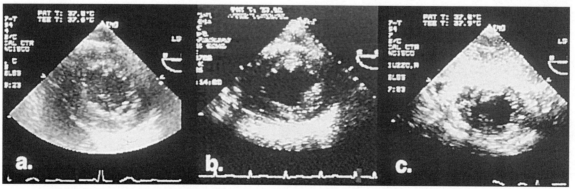

FIGURE 38-10. *A,* Transverse short-axis view at the mitral valve leaflet tips. *B,* Transverse short-axis view at the level of the papillary muscles. *C,* Transverse short-axis view near the apex of the left ventricle.

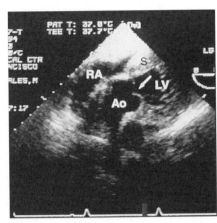

FIGURE 38–11. Deep gastric view of the left ventricular outflow tract and aortic root.

Longitudinal Planar Views (Biplane, Vertical, or Multiplanar 90 Degrees)

Historically, a second plane of imaging, the vertical or longitudinal, was added to the transverse by incorporating a second set of crystals into the probe (Fig. 38–12; see Figs. 38–2E to H, 38–7D to G, and 38–9D). In this way TEE evolved from monoplanar to biplane imaging. As stated, the disadvantage of separate crystal arrays for biplane imaging is that they impose the need to advance or withdraw the probe into position behind objects of interest, so that structures can be studied from orthogonal planes. Despite this disadvantage, the addition of biplane views was an immediate success in that it considerably expanded the comprehensiveness of the examination. Importantly, new views of the left ventricle, venae cavae, and aorta provided completely new information. Based on this universal experience, these authors consider biplane capability to be a minimum acceptable standard for laboratories. As will be seen, further experience with multiplane "any-angle" probes suggest that they may soon supplant biplane probes as a minimal requirement for the TEE laboratory.

As a general statement, imaging in the longitudinal view is accomplished successfully by maneuvers that differ considerably from the transverse view. Most importantly, the essence of this set of views and the largest gain in information are obtained from exerting torque, either clockwise or counterclockwise, on the probe. Although advancing the probe from one level to another is important, the bulk of information is gained through rotation. This strategy stands in contrast with that used in imaging in the transverse plane and is easy to understand when one considers that the long axis of the heart runs parallel to the long axis of both the body and the esophagus.

The longitudinal images described here are oriented with the cranial structures to the right of the viewer and the caudal structures to the left. As stated earlier, this particular system of image orientation is probably the most widely used; other experts have recommended inverting the images to conform to the orientation used in transthoracic imaging.[31]

Longitudinal Level 1

Starting at the level of the aortic valve and rotating the probe toward the right (clockwise) generates a view that demonstrates both venae cavae entering the right atrium (Figs. 38–2E, 38–7D, and 38–12, *upper left*). Features of the right atrium in this view are the atrial appendage (broad-based, with trabeculations extending beyond its ill-defined rim); the chaotically moving valve of the inferior vena cava (so-called Chiari's network or eustacian valve) demarcating the entrance of the inferior vena cava; the atrial septum; and a portion of the left atrium. From this view it is possible to follow the inferior vena cava to the entrance of the hepatic veins and the superior vena cava to its relationship to the right pulmonary artery. Rotating the transducer toward the center of the heart reveals the aortic root in long axis with a profile view of the aortic leaflets (see Figs. 38–2G, 38–7E, and 38–12, *lower left*). Anterior to the aortic valve is the best view of the right ventricular outflow tract (see Figs. 38–2F, 38–7F, and 38–12, *upper right*). This structure is seen at the bottom of the screen and can be followed to the pulmonary valve and main pulmonary artery. Rotating the probe counterclockwise and to the patient's left reveals a long axis view of the left ventricle, mitral valve, left atrium and

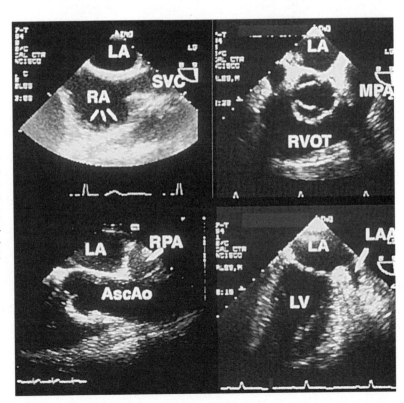

FIGURE 38–12. Longitudinal views: *Upper Left,* Bicaval view with right atrial appendage trabeculations extending beyond the rim of the broad-based appendage *(arrows).* The SVC is to the viewer's right. *Lower Left,* Long-axis view of the ascending aorta showing its relationship to the right pulmonary artery. *Upper Right,* Long-axis view of the right ventricular outflow tract and its relationship to the main pulmonary artery and aortic valve. *Lower Right,* Two-chamber view of the left ventricle showing the anterior wall and anteriorly placed left atrial appendage. The inferior wall is to the viewer's left.

atrial appendage (Fig. 38–13*B*; see Figs. 38–2*H*, 38–7*G*, and 38–12, *lower right*). This view of the left ventricle places the inferior wall to the left of the viewer and is similar to the apical two-chamber view seen on transthoracic echocardiography. Note that the posterior leaflet of the mitral valve is seen to the viewer's left.

Longitudinal Level 2

Passing the probe across the gastroesophageal junction in the transverse view allows viewing the left ventricle in the short axis (see Fig. 38–13*C*). From this level, switching into the longitudinal plane reveals a long-axis view of the ventricle, which is one of the most important views in that it reliably images the critically important inferobasal segment of the chamber (see Figs. 38–9*D* and 38–13*D*). It also demonstrates the papillary muscles and chordae tendineae in their most detailed presentation. Rotation toward the patient's right reveals a longitudinal view of the right ventricle, especially when that chamber is enlarged.

Longitudinal Level 3

Advancement of the probe into the deep gastric position shows the right ventricular outflow tract and pulmonary artery.

Multiplane Views

Probes equipped with multiplane capability[29] allow rotation of a single array of crystals through 180 degrees. This configuration allows structures and views to be fine-tuned for optimal imaging. For example, viewing the aortic valve in a "perfect" short axis is usually difficult or impossible with fixed single or biplane probes. In most patients, 30- to 45-degree imaging plane is required (Fig. 38–14). It has been shown, for example, that the stenotic aortic orifice can be accurately measured by planimeter and that the severity of obstruction can be measured from this plane.[36–39] It is evident that vegetations, valve abnormalities, and congenital abnormalities all can be studied more effectively with a multiplane probe. It is also evident that three-dimensional imaging is a natural outgrowth of this technology.[40]

Although it would be impossible to discuss all possible views available with multiplanar probes, a comment about how the authors conduct a multiplane examination is in order. With a jet of mitral regurgitation as an example, the examination begins with the transverse view of the mitral valve at the level of the left ventricle outflow tract and proceeds in 10-degree increments until about 120 degrees of rotation is reached. At each increment, the jet is optimized and its course traced by rotating the probe. In this way eccentric jets or perivalvular jets (in the case of a malfunctioning prosthesis) are most likely to be fully explored and demonstrated. In contrast with important pathologic conditions, normal structures need only be examined in the transverse or longitudinal planes, with slight adjustments in the plane of interrogation as needed for optimal visualization. In other words, it is best to anchor the examination to the standard biplane views, with the use of multiplane capability to refine objects of interest and relevance.

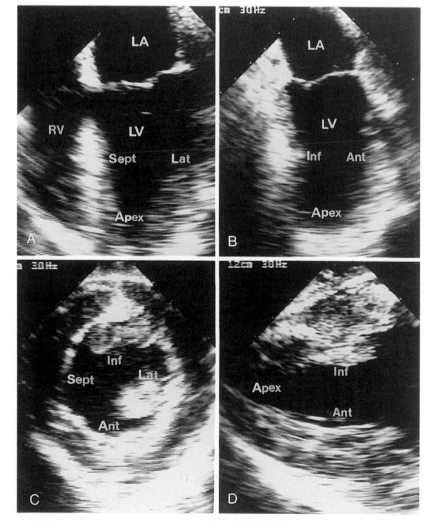

FIGURE 38–13. *A*, Transverse four-chamber view of the left ventricle. *B*, Longitudinal two-chamber view of the left ventricle. *C*, Gastric short-axis view at the level of the papillary muscles. *D*, Longitudinal view from the same level, showing the inferior and anterior papillary muscles.

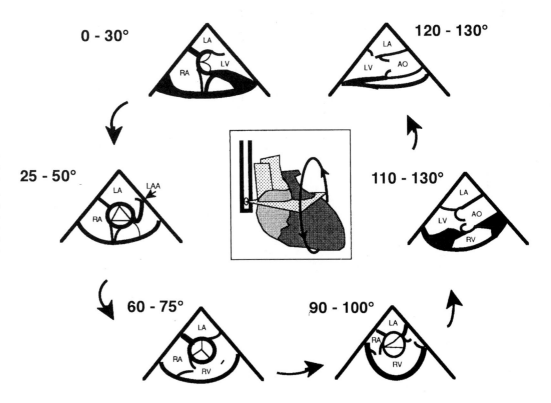

FIGURE 38–14. Diagram of impact on the images of serially changing the transducer through 150 degrees (see text). (From Schneider, A.T., Hsu, T.-L., Schwartz, S.L., et al.: Single, biplane, multiplane, and three-dimensional echocardiography: Echocardiographic-anatomic correlations. Cardiol. Clin. 11:361–387, 1993, with permission.)

EVALUATION OF THE LEFT VENTRICLE BY TRANSESOPHAGEAL ECHOCARDIOGRAPHY

Systolic Function

Transesophageal echocardiography displays most of the left ventricle with definition superior to that of transthoracic echocardiography. In particular, the full thickness of the myocardium, including the endocardium with its complex endoarchitecture, is seen with clarity. Unfortunately, most TEE views do not display the apical portion of the ventricle but rather a truncated or foreshortened version. This failing has the consequences of lowered sensitivity for ischemia and infarction limited to the apex, underrepresentation of chamber of volume, and misrepresentation of global function. For these reasons and because it usually can be obtained, most estimates of ventricular function (global and segmental) are made from a transgastric short-axis view (Fig. 38–15). Excluding as it does the long-axis behavior of the heart, this view must always be used with

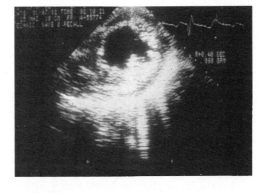
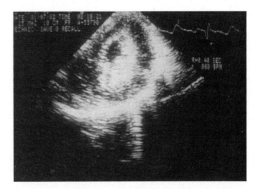
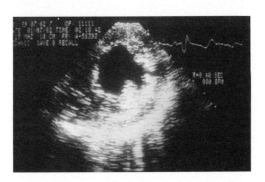
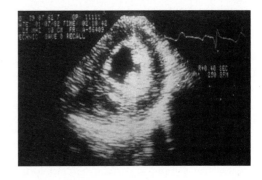

FIGURE 38–15. Short-axis gastric views in diastole *(left panels)* and systole *(right panels).* Upper panels show normal to hyperdynamic function, as judged by the small end-systolic area, which can be readily appreciated visually. At a later time, contractility has fallen, as shown by a slight increase in end-diastolic dimension *(lower left panel)* and a more obvious increase in end-systolic area *(lower right panel).*

some degree of caution. These caveats having been stated, the short axis remains a robust and reliable approach for judging left ventricular function. A competent TEE laboratory must be adept in its use. With the advent of biplane and multiplanar imaging this view can be supplemented with long-axis gastric views that approach the apex in some patients and image the base of the inferior wall reliably (see Figs. 38–9D and 38–13D).

Much of what the authors have learned about measuring systolic function comes from observations made by anesthesiologists using TEE in the operating theater.[34] In the authors' 15 years of experience with this technique, they feel strongly that what has been learned in the operating room is almost always directly applicable to the outpatient or critical care arenas. Therefore, in discussing systolic function or other aspects of left ventricular performance they will not make distinctions between knowledge acquired intraoperatively and that acquired outside that venue.

Most practitioners evaluate the left ventricle qualitatively. Studies have documented the validity of this approach for recognizing hypovolemia,[8, 41] the adverse effects of proximal cross-clamping of the aorta[6] and the influence of various anesthetic regimens on left ventricular function.[42–44]

Quantitation of the short-axis image of the left ventricle has been used mainly for research purposes. The validity of utilizing fractional area change or area ejection fraction as an analog of volume ejection fraction was tested by Urbanowicz and colleagues[45] who compared radionuclide blood pool imaging with TEE area ejection fraction in a group of patients in the postsurgical intensive care unit. They found that at lower ejection fractions (below 45 percent), the correlation between the reference standard blood pool image and the short axis measured by planimeter was linear, strongly confirming the usefulness of this measurement. At higher ejection fractions (normal and hypernormal), the correlation was poorer. Because discriminating among high ejection fractions is, at best, of minor clinical importance, the use of fractional short-axis area change can be considered to be rational. If one considers that the descent of the cardiac base represents longitudinal muscle function and is among the first properties to be altered in systolic dysfunction, it is to be expected that an index that is blind to longitudinal changes in cardiac dimensions would be effective once that vector of motion had been suppressed.

Moreover, the reproducibilty of measuring the area and fractional change of the short axis has been studied[34, 46] and found to be acceptable for clinical and investigational use.

The concept of using the short-axis area change for monitoring systolic function has become more attractive with the development and improvement of automatic border-detection technology. This computer-driven method requires a highly resolved image of the endocardium, which it is able to track on a frame-by-frame and beat-to-beat basis. Cahalan and associates[46] studied this technique and showed that it was reliable only for the most highly resolved images. This work and that of others[47–49] has led to recent improvements in this technique, which may soon enable the echocardiographer to continually measure systolic left ventricular function. Certainly in the outpatient setting, where it is impractical to interrupt the procedure to manually trace the outline of the ventricle, this development should be of considerable importance.

In transthoracic echocardiography (and, for that matter, in angiography and in the physiology laboratory), end-systolic volume is a parameter of cardiac function of considerable importance. This information has been derived from TEE by Gorcsan and co-workers,[50] who used automatic border detection to continuously compute end-systolic area measurements. These areas were digitized and integrated with femoral artery pressure to create real-time pressure volume loops.

Doppler evaluation of systolic performance is also feasible. Cardiac output has been measured from the pulmonary artery[51, 52] and left ventricular outflow tract[53] with the use of velocity-time integrals obtained by pulsed-wave Doppler and continuous-wave Doppler.[54] There is reason to believe that other flow signals, such as mitral inflow, may also provide cardiac output information.

Diastolic Function by Transesophageal Echocardiography

Mitral inflow, both singly and in combination with pulmonary venous flow, is the major source of clinically relevant information about diastolic left ventricular behavior. As with TEE, mitral inflow is recorded with the Doppler sample volume at the tips of the mitral leaflets in the transverse four-chamber (horizontal plane esophageal) view.[55, 56] Important diagnostic parameters derived from the mitral inflow signals include the ratio of peak early filling velocity to atrial filling velocity (E:A ratio), the deceleration time of early filling curve (DT), and the isovolumic relaxation time (IVRT) (see Fig. 38–6). Although there is considerable variability, two predominant patterns of flow have been recognized, reflecting the two major categories of diastolic dysfunction. An impairment in left ventricular relaxation is characterized by a decrease in the E:A ratio, which arises through a combination of prolongation of the deceleration time and an increase in the contribution of atrial contraction, the so-called A-wave dominant pattern (Fig. 38–16 left). This form of diastolic dysfunction occurs in hypertension and as the result of normal aging and, when seen, usually implies a normal mean filling pressure. Diminished left ventricular compliance is characterized by a "restrictive flow" pattern with an increased E:A ratio and a shortened isovolumic relaxation time and deceleration time (see Fig. 38–16 right). This pattern, which usually is accompanied by raised mean filling pressure, occurs not only in patients with restrictive cardiomyopathies such as amyloid heart disease but also in patients with acute and chronic cardiac decompensation associated with a variety of myopathic and pericardial conditions. As a patient decompensates, a pattern change from delayed relaxation to restriction occurs. At one point, as filling pressure rises to pathologic levels, the filling pattern will "pseudonormalize."

In applying these principles one must be aware that diastolic filling patterns cannot always be analyzed from a single observation, because they are influenced by a variety of factors, including loading conditions, heart rate, pericardial restraint, left atrial pressure and compliance, right and left ventricular interaction, coronary turgor, and intrinsic properties of left atrial and left ventricular muscle. For example, changes in loading conditions during cardiac surgery have been shown to influence filling patterns.[55] The interpretation of the mitral inflow pattern is greatly enhanced by exami-

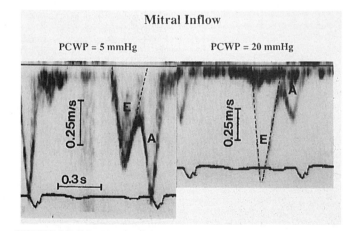

FIGURE 38–16. Mitral inflow, pulsed-wave Doppler: Effect of increased mean left atrial pressure on mitral inflow patterns. *Left,* Predominant late diastolic filling (A) of mitral flow in a patient with a wedge pressure of 5 mm Hg. *Right,* Decreased late diastolic filling (A) and increased early diastolic filling (E) in the same patient in response to an increase in mean wedge pressure to 20 mm Hg. (From Kuecherer, H.F., Muhiudeen, I.A., Kusumoto, F.M., et al.: Estimation of mean left atrial pressure from transesophageal pulsed Doppler echocardiography of pulmonary venous flow. Circulation 82:1127–1139, 1990, with permission. Copyright 1990, American Heart Association.)

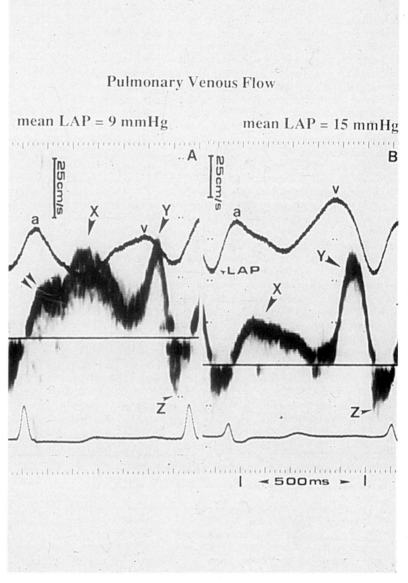

FIGURE 38–17. Effect of increased mean left atrial pressure (mean LAP) on pulmonary venous flow patterns. *Left,* Predominant systolic pulmonary venous flow velocities in patient with normal left LAP of 9 mm Hg. *Right,* Pulmonary venous flow velocity shifted toward early diastole (Y) in response to an increase in left atrial pressure to a mean of 15 mm Hg. Note that direct left atrial pressure measurement is displayed simultaneously with a pulmonary venous inflow tracing. The double arrowheads in the left panel and the single arrowhead in the left and right panels point to two separate systolic waves, which, when visible, indicate low filling pressures. (From Kuecherer, H.F., Muhiudeen, I.A., Kusumoto, F.M., et al.: Estimation of mean left atrial pressure from transesophageal pulsed Doppler echocardiography of pulmonary venous flow. Circulation 82:1127–1139, 1990, with permission. Copyright 1990, American Heart Association.)

nation of the pattern of pulmonary venous Doppler signal (Fig. 38–17). Transesophageal echocardiography has contributed substantially to our understanding of this hemodynamic parameter. The evaluation of pulmonary venous flow is interpreted in the section on hemodynamics and critical care.

ISCHEMIC HEART DISEASE AND TRANSESOPHAGEAL ECHOCARDIOGRAPHY

The use of echocardiography in ischemic disease is based on the rapid change in wall motion of a segment after interruption or critical decrease in its blood supply. This phenomenon occurs within a few seconds of the onset of ischemia, just after the onset of diastolic abnormalities and many seconds before angina and electrocardiographic changes. The continuous high-quality imaging of the left ventricle afforded by TEE during surgical procedures makes it ideally suited for the early detection of ischemia. This use of TEE was first reported by Beaupre and colleagues.[7] Shortly thereafter, Smith and associates[57] compared the prevalence of electrocardiographic changes to wall motion changes after coronary bypass and found TEE changes more predictive of postoperative myocardial infarction and of much greater yield. Using Holter

monitoring techniques, Leung and co-workers[58] also found TEE to be superior to electrocardiographic changes as a sign of ischemia. Leung and colleagues also found that hemodynamic changes were not predictive of ischemia and that ischemia was more common in the postbypass intensive care unit period than either before or during the procedure. Furthermore, postbypass ischemia on TEE was highly predictive of adverse outcome, whereas electrocardiographic changes were not. Others[59, 60] have also found changes in flow-directed catheter wedge pressures to be insensitive to ischemia.

The shortcomings of TEE in detection of intraoperative ischemia need to be considered. For example, Eisenberg and associates[61] found that *both* electrocardiographic changes and TEE lacked concordance and were thus of unproven value in monitoring ischemia intraoperatively. However, there were only 11 patients with events or adverse outcomes out of 174 ischemic instances. With improvements in surgical and anesthetic technique (possibly due in part to TEE itself), a much larger population of patients may be required to generate a large enough cohort with adverse outcomes. The reader is referred to Sutton and Cahalan[34] for a more thorough discussion of Eisenberg's study. Other limitations of the technique occur when conduction abnormalities, such as left bundle branch block or ventricular pacing, are encountered. In these circumstances, it can be difficult to distinguish the incoordinate contractions from delayed activation from those of an ischemic wall motion abnormality. Also, heterogeneity of contraction is not exclusive to ischemia. Cardiomyopathies frequently show regional wall motion abnormalities. Moreover, myocardial stunning may explain a wall motion abnormality in an adequately revascularized region. Differentiating this finding from ischemia due to an inadequate revascularization may be difficult. Perhaps in the future, newly developed ultrasound reflecting myocardial contrast agents will be used to document the adequacy of revascularization. Other possible influences that confound recognition of acute ischemia by means of TEE include volume changes and alterations in transducer position and/or angulation, creating *de novo* unmasking pre-existing wall motion abnormalities.

Finally, we should question whether TEE can be shown to influence the outcome of surgical procedures. Although it would be difficult to convince most cardiovascular anesthesiologists and recently trained surgeons to eliminate this modality, we are now in an era where third-party payers demand evidence of the cost effectiveness of diagnostic procedures. In one of the few studies available on this subject, Deutsch and co-workers[62] reported that among 100 cases of cardiovascular surgery, the technique was valuable in 10 percent of cases and essential in 2 percent. In contrast with this relatively low level of influence, Kato and colleagues[63] found that 30 percent of a group of 50 patients had an alteration in management that could be attributed to TEE. An important but unanswered question regarding the use of TEE in the operating room is whether it is more cost-effective and safe than traditional methods of monitoring. In the authors' institution, it has been calculated that if TEE *replaces* flow-directed pulmonary artery catheters, substantial savings accrue. Based on the authors' confidence in hemodynamic and functional information obtained from TEE, they frequently perform open heart surgery without the use of central catheters.

LEFT VENTRICULAR STRESS TESTING BY TRANSESOPHAGEAL ECHOCARDIOGRAPHY

Transesophageal echocardiography can be effectively combined with stress testing, because it provides stable and highly resolved images of the left ventricle. Practically speaking, the two modes of intervention that can be effectively performed with TEE are atrial pacing (esophageal and transvenous) and pharmacologic stress. Dynamic exercise or respiratory maneuvers would be likely to encounter low patient tolerance.

Lambertz and colleagues modified a probe so that pacing leads were embedded into the shaft at intervals from the tip to around 25 cm.[64–66] With this device, they studied 50 patients, using inducible wall motion abnormalities as an end point. They reported sensitivities of 85 percent for single-vessel disease and 100 percent for two- and three-vessel disease. They also studied 20 patients prior to vascular surgery and found that the location of a subsequently occurring intraoperative wall motion abnormality had been predicted by the induced wall motion abnormality in 6 subjects. In 60 patients after coronary angioplasty, they were able to detect

restenosis with a sensitivity and specificity very similar to those of perfusion scintigraphy. In the authors' own experience, the protective effects of anesthesia, antianginal medications, and confounding influences of altered preload make postinduction intraoperative pacing too insensitive for routine clinical application (M. Cahalan, personal communication). In some community hospital settings, the use of TEE and imaging has been shown to be a rapid and effective emergency room screening strategy (T. DonMichael, personal communication). Kamp and colleagues[67] have reported the inducement or increase in mitral regurgitation during pacing observed via TEE when the pacing induced a posterior wall motion abnormality. In a study of early post–myocardial infarction stress for risk stratification, Iliceto and associates[68] found that of the group with new transesophageal echocardiographic wall motion abnormalities after pacing, 65 percent had complications during follow-up, as opposed to 8 percent in a negative study. This form of imaging with pacing was twice as sensitive for predicting events as treadmill testing was in these same patients.

Pharmacologic agents used for stress testing during imaging with TEE include dobutamine, dipyridamole, and phenylephrine. Prince and co-workers[69] have reported a sensitivity of 90 percent and a specificity of 94 percent for the detection of coronary artery disease, using a standard dobutamine protocol. Dipyridamole was used in conjunction with TEE to evaluate the response of segmental wall motion to this agent before, immediately after, and several days after coronary artery surgery.[70] Among the few patients who remained positive, all had major events during the 1-year follow-up.

ENDOCARDITIS AND TRANSESOPHAGEAL ECHOCARDIOGRAPHY

The demonstration that M-mode echocardiography could visualize the vegetative masses that typify bacterial endocarditis gave cardiologists access to information that had been seen only on the operating or autopsy tables.[71, 72] Those of us who used this technique in the early 1970s soon saw both its strengths and its weaknesses. For example, localization of vegetations to the precise cusp of attachment was possible.[73] However, it was also apparent that for a mass to be detected by M-mode it had to exceed 5 mm in diameter.[73] Even when two-dimensional imaging supplanted M-mode as the imaging mode choice, evidence arose suggesting suboptimal sensitivity.[74] These suspicions were shown to be well founded when TEE was applied to the study of endocarditis.[75] However, it was not until almost a decade later when a number of studies addressed the sharp difference in sensitivity between transthoracic and TEE.

The role of TEE in endocarditis is a direct result of its high sensitivity in detecting the defining manifestation of the disease, valve vegetations. The comparison of the sensitivity of transthoracic echocardiography to that of TEE is an important issue, because if the two methods are similar in this regard, the less invasive and cheaper modality will be used.

There are at least five studies that address the differences in sensitivity between transthoracic echocardiography and TEE,[76–80] and these are presented in Table 38–6. Generally, these studies

TABLE 38–6. REPORTED SENSITIVITY AND SPECIFICITY OF TRANSTHORACIC AND TRANSESOPHAGEAL ECHOCARDIOGRAPHY FOR NATIVE VALVE ENDOCARDITIS

		TTE Sensitivity/Specificity	TEE Sensitivity/Specificity
Shively et al.[78] (1991) (n = 66)		44/98	94/100
Pedersen et al.[77] (1991) (n = 24)		50/–	100/–
Birmingham et al.[76] (1992) (n = 61)	Aortic	25/–	88/–
	Mitral	50/–	100/–
Sochowski and Chan[79] (1993) (n = 105)		–/–	91/–
Shapiro et al.[80] (1994) (n = 64)		60/91	87/91
Total (n = 256)		46/95	93/96

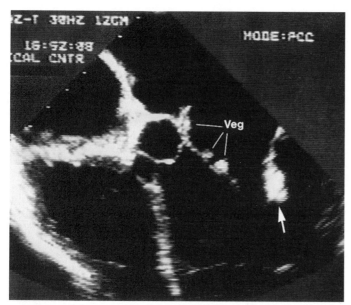

FIGURE 38–18. Transverse transesophageal echocardiographic four-chamber view in a patient with infectious endocarditis. Multiple small vegetations are seen studding the anterior mitral leaflet (Veg.). The large vegetation toward the base of the valve was the only one of the three seen on precordial imaging.

are considered positive when a valve abnormality (mass) has the characteristics that allow the process to be identified as a vegetation with a *high degree of certainty.* These characteristics include the texture of the mass, its location, characteristic motion, shape, and accompanying abnormalities. In general, experienced readers recognize a vegetation as having a gray scale and a low level of reflectance similar to that of the liver or middle myocardium (Fig. 38–18). Vegetations are usually positioned on the upstream side of the valve (e.g., on the atrial side of the mitral and ventricular side of the aortic valve in patients with mitral and aortic regurgitation, respectively), concentrated at the point at which a regurgitant or stenotic jet impinges on the valve or wall. The mass is usually amorphous and mobile. The mobility may be chaotic, appear to orbit around the valve, or have fine vibrations imparted by the jet. Abnormalities that accompany vegetations include periannular abscesses (solid or cystic) (Fig. 38–19), fistulas, and severe regurgitation. In prosthetic endocarditis, paravalvular leaks, valve dehiscence, and occasional obstruction are seen. Vegetations also characteristically prolapse into the upstream chamber, mitral vegetations into the atrium in systole, and aortic vegetations into the left ventricular outflow tract during diastole. As stated, they tend to flank the regurgitant jet. Characteristics that identify an abnormal mass as being unlikely to be a vegetation include high reflectivity, bistable appearance (white, not gray), fibrillar appearance with narrow base of attachment, and lack of associated regurgitation. These characteristics are used by experienced readers regardless of whether a transthoracic or transesophageal window is used (see Table 38–6).

FIGURE 38–19. See Color Plate 11.

The superior sensitivity of TEE is clearly and consistently documented by the studies listed in Table 38–6, in which the differences between modalities were strongly significant statistically. From these findings and from the study of Lowry and colleagues[81] it can be concluded that a negative transesophageal echocardiogram makes the probability of endocarditis very low. It does not, how-

ever, eliminate the possibility, and the echocardiographer should always temper interpretations with sound clinical judgment.

Prosthetic valve endocarditis is a special case. The materials used to construct these devices usually do not allow passage of ultrasound, and as a result, these valves shadow or obscure structures lying deep to the valve. For example, it is usually impossible to image the atrial side of the mitral prosthesis or the aortic side of the aortic prosthesis from a transthoracic approach. Transesophageal echocardiography solves this problem in mitral prostheses and improves it in aortic prostheses. When both mitral and aortic devices are present, the aortic device tends to obscure the mitral. Multiplanar devices have improved imaging in this situation. Tricuspid and pulmonic devices pose similar problems but can be effectively evaluated with TEE. Daniel and associates[82] reported on 33 cases of prosthetic endocarditis studied with both TEE and transthoracic echocardiography and found sensitivities of 82 and 36 percent, respectively. Alton and co-workers[83] reported similar findings, but with smaller numbers. In a study of TEE in 44 bioprosthetic valve patients going to surgery, Zabalgoitia and co-workers[84] found that transthoracic echocardiography had a sensitivity of 43 percent, whereas TEE sensitivity was 86 percent. In abscess identification, TEE was 100 percent sensitive, whereas transthoracic echocardiography was only 25 percent sensitive.

Once a native valve vegetation is identified, the attending physician is obligated to estimate the risk that the process poses to the patient's recovery or survival and to decide on an appropriate therapeutic plan. Most of these estimations and decisions can be made by a careful analysis of the clinical and transesophageal echocardiographic presentation. There are a few interesting and provocative studies that the clinician can use in making these decisions.[85–88] Using transthoracic echocardiography, researchers at Duke[88] looked at the site, size, mobility, shape, and attachment of vegetations. They found high interobserver agreement on the presence and location of vegetations but less agreement on the size, mobility, and shape. A vegetation size of more than 10 mm was associated with an embolic rate of more than 50 percent, whereas a vegetation size of less than 10 mm was associated with a rate of 42 percent. In general, they found that characteristics of vegetations from transthoracic echocardiography were not helpful in predicting complications. In applying transesophageal imaging to the same question, Mugge and colleagues[86] concurred with the lack of correlation between vegetation characteristics (except size) and prediction of embolic events. However, perhaps owing to the increased sensitivity of transesophageal imaging, they found a stronger association between vegetation size and embolic events than that in the Duke study, particularly when the vegetation was found on the mitral valve. A vegetation size of more than 10 mm was associated with an embolic rate of 46 percent, whereas one of less than 10 mm was associated with only a 20 percent risk ($P < .001$).

Perhaps the most useful study was that of Rohmann and colleagues,[85] who performed serial TEE in 83 patients and found that when a vegetation enlarged or remained static during 4 to 8 weeks of therapy, prognosis was much worse than for the group in whom the vegetation shrank with therapy. These differences were striking and included incidence of valve replacement (45 versus 2 percent), embolic events (45 versus 17 percent), abscess formation (13 versus 2 percent), and mortality (10 percent versus 0 percent) (for all $P < .05$). These data have allowed the authors to temporize in patients who present with large vegetations that tempt early surgical intervention before the appearance of complications. The authors frequently repeat the TEE after 7 days of antibiotic therapy and compare the size of the vegetations or vegetations. Although the authors' time scale is considerably shorter than the 4 to 6 weeks in Rohmann's study, the authors have frequently seen dramatic decreases in vegetation size after only 1 week of treatment.

Transesophageal echocardiography is also superior to transthoracic echocardiography in detecting the intracardiac complications of endocarditis. Valvular incompetence is a complication that arises directly from destruction of valve tissue or chordae. Rarely, a bulky vegetation may impede the coaptation of a substantial portion of the valve. Stenosis of an orifice is less common but can occur when a vegetation reaches sufficient size to intrude on a critical portion of the annulus area. Both regurgitation and stenosis caused by direct mechanical intrusion can be inferred from transesophageal findings and can be expected to improve with regression of the mass. In the presence of mechanical prostheses, vegetations can obstruct the valve orifice and interfere with leaflet closure; suture dehiscence and even liberation of the devices can occur. In prosthetic regurgitation or stenosis, when the annulus of the prosthesis is stable and when there is no paravalvular leak, it can be inferred that bulky vegetation is impeding leaflet motion.

Among the destructive complications of endocarditis, the severe morbidity associated with pyogenic complications, including abscess, fistula, and pseudoaneurysm, makes their recognition of paramount importance. All these processes occur in and around the valve annuli, affecting the fibrous and muscular soft tissue. These lesions may begin as cellulitis, probably spreading by local extension from the valve leaflet. The authors believe that it is often possible to recognize their early stage by noting an unusual thickening of the periannular region during vegetative endocarditis. The area of cellulitis can become necrotic and cavitary (abscess), develop into a blind pouch ("pseudoaneurysm"),[89] or invade a contiguous chamber to establish a communication (fistula). Examples of fistulous communications include aorta to left atrium (associated with a new continuous murmur) and left ventricle to right atrium. If the abscess extends into the septum, the conduction system may be interrupted or slowed, and a right bundle branch block with first degree atrioventricular block may ensue. In a landmark study of the effectiveness of TEE in detecting abscesses in endocarditis, Daniel and co-workers[90] studied 118 cases and found evidence of abscess formation in 37 percent. The mortality rate among those with abscess was 23 versus 14 percent for those without abscess. The sensitivity and specificity of transthoracic imaging were 28 percent and 99 percent, whereas those of transesophageal imaging were 87 and 95 percent. From these data it is evident that abscess-related lesions are relatively common in endocarditis (especially when the infecting organism is *Staphylococcus aureus*) and represent a subgroup that is at high risk for death. Transthoracic echocardiography is inadequate for detection of abscesses, because its sensitivity is far too low, and the extent of the lesion is unlikely to be appreciated.

In summary, TEE has an unassailable place in the diagnostic evaluation and management of endocarditis. It is far superior to surface imaging by dint of its greater sensitivity in detecting native valve vegetations, prosthetic valve vegetations, paravalvular abscess, and other pyogenic complications. A negative transesophageal study makes endocarditis unlikely, and a large vegetation that fails to shrink during therapy connotes a poor prognosis. Based on these considerations and clinical experience, it is the firm opinion of many experts that every patient with a strong possibility of endocarditis should undergo at least one transesophageal echocardiogram.

VALVE DISEASES

Aortic Valve Disease

Aortic Stenosis

Transthoracic Doppler echocardiography is an established method for determining the severity of aortic stenosis. However, unlike mitral stenosis, transthoracic echocardiography does not permit direct planimetry of a stenotic aortic valve. Stoddard and colleagues[36] demonstrated that TEE can image the stenotic orifice and that planimetry of that orifice produces a valve area determination with an excellent correlation with that determined by transthoracic echocardiography Doppler imaging (continuity equation). The correlation coefficient for this comparison was r = .93, the percent differences between the two methods was small (10 ± 9 percent),

and the TEE method correlated even more closely with the catheterization-determined valve area than did the transthoracic echocardiographic value (r = .91 versus 0.84). Two years after Stoddard's study, the availability of multiplane TEE probe technology enabled Hoffman and colleagues[39] to study 41 patients with calcific aortic stenosis. They were successful in obtaining a measurable orifice in 38 of 41. In the three patients with whom they were unsuccessful, the stenosis was obviously very severe ("pinhole stenosis"). The correlation coefficient with valve area by catheterization (Gorlin formula) was .95, and the prediction of severe stenosis (area < 0.75 cm^2) had a sensitivity of 96 percent. Based on the authors' own experience, imaging the aorta in a precise short axis is a requirement of this technique. With older monoplane or biplane probe technology, tedious manipulation are required for such imaging to be successful. With multiplane probes, almost all aortic valves can be seen in the short axis in a plane that is 30 to 45 degrees from the transverse (0 degree) (Fig. 38–20).

In conclusion, TEE allows the visualization of the true short axis of the aortic valve. In stenotic valves this view permits direct planimetry of the stenotic systolic orifice and has been shown to be accurate to a level that equals and may exceed that of the standard continuity equation as applied to Doppler transthoracic echocardiography.

Aortic Insufficiency

Transthoracic Doppler echocardiography grades the severity of aortic insufficiency by use of continuous-wave Doppler imaging of the regurgitant jet,[91] pulsed-wave Doppler imaging of reverse flow in the descending aorta,[92] and color flow Doppler imaging of the height of the regurgitant jet in the left ventricular outflow tract[93]; these methods are reliable and complementary. Planimetry of the maximal area that a color flow signal achieves in a receiving chamber (i.e., mitral regurgitation into the left atrium and aortic regurgitation into the left ventricle) also has been advanced as a reliable means of judging the severity of a regurgitant lesion.[94] Recent studies[95] have cast considerable doubt on the validity of this method.

There are relatively few studies of the incremental value of TEE in measuring the severity of aortic insufficiency; according to universal clinical experience, it is exquisitely sensitive to the most trivial amount of insufficiency. Smith and colleagues[96] compared the maximum area of the aortic regurgitation jet in the left ventricle by surface imaging to transesophageal imaging in the four-chamber view. Not surprisingly, the jet areas measured from TEE were consistently larger. Sutton and co-workers[97] evaluated flow reversal in the descending aorta intraoperatively and found that only patients with "severe" aortic insufficiency had flow reversal; the abnormality disappeared after valve replacement. It is noteworthy that Sutton used the ratio of the height of the regurgitant jet in the outflow tract to the outflow tract diameter as the reference standard for aortic insufficiency severity because this reliable transthoracic index had not been validated for transesophageal imaging (see Fig. 38–20). The authors' clinical experience strongly suggests that this method is transferable to TEE and that the longitudinal plane views of the aorta and left ventricular outflow tract (see Figs. 38–2 and 38–12*B*) are usually optimal for judging the severity of aortic insufficiency.

In the authors' experience, aortic insufficiency severity is best judged by combining data from transthoracic echocardiography and TEE. In performing the latter, the operator should obtain a short-axis view at the level of the leaflets. With omniplane capability this view is obtained at about 30 degrees and allows determination of the valve morphology (tricuspid or congenitally abnormal), the size of the limiting systolic orifice, and the size and location of the regurgitant jet. The ratio of the jet, as seen in short axis to the area subtended by the aortic ring, is a helpful means of judging the severity of the regurgitation.[98] In the transverse plane, advancing the probe to the level of the left ventricular outflow tract to the jet diameter. It is important to avoid exaggerating the diameter of eccentric jets that parallel the plane of the aortic cusps. In the

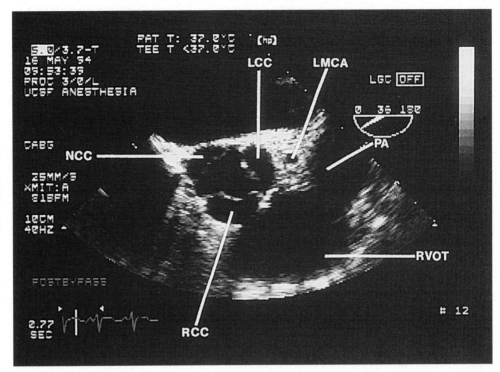

FIGURE 38–20. Short-axis view of the aortic valve obtained in early systole with the cusp partially opened. In this case, the transducer has been angled to 30 degrees from the transverse. LCC = left coronary cusp; RCC = right coronary cusp; NCC = noncoronary cusp; RVOT = right ventricular outflow tract; LMCA = left main coronary artery; PA = pulmonary artery.

longitudinal axis, the ascending aorta from the valve to the right pulmonary artery should be viewed in long axis (Fig. 38–21 *left*; see Fig. 38–12 *lower left*). Pathology of the aortic root and ascending aorta (e.g., aortoannular ectasia, type I aortic dissection and Marfan syndrome) should be excluded as the etiology of aortic valve insufficiency (Fig. 38–22). The leaflets should be inspected for evidence of malcoaptation and aortic valve prolapse. Moreover, directing the image to the plane that clearly demonstrates the coaptation of the aortic valve affords researchers another view of the regurgitant jet. It is important to obtain mitral inflow and regurgitant signals to seek evidence of restricted inflow from torrential regurgitation and diastolic mitral regurgitation from elevated filling pressures. In the authors' experience, the angles of interrogation imposed by the transesophageal window are usually suboptimal for measuring continuous-wave Doppler time intervals of the aortic insufficiency jet and pulsed-wave Doppler of reversed flow in the descending aorta. These variables are better determined from the transthoracic image.

FIGURES 38–21 AND 38–22. See Color Plate 11.

Mitral Valve Disease

Mitral Stenosis

Transthoracic echocardiography is the established method of detecting, quantitating, and judging the severity of mitral stenosis.[99] Transesophageal echocardiography has a growing role in mitral stenosis, which has paralleled the growth in catheter-based palliative interventions. These interventions require a transseptal puncture to deliver a dilating balloon along the path of blood flow and across the obstructed mitral orifice. When successful, these techniques offer dramatic relief of symptoms and may help a patient avoid the need for thoracotomy. Transesophageal echocardiography has been used in mitral stenosis *prior to the procedure* to identify atrial spontaneous contrast, atrial appendage thrombus (a contraindication to valvuloplasty felt to increase risk of stroke from catheter dislodgment of thrombus), and poor atrial appendage function[100] (Fig. 38–23) as well as to prejudge the likelihood of

success by evaluating the morphology of the mitral valve and its supporting apparatus. Transesophageal echocardiography has been used *during the procedure* to guide transseptal puncture and balloon placement and *after the procedure* to detect undesirable degrees of mitral regurgitation, to study the resolution of spontaneous contrast in response to relief of obstruction and the hemodynamic impact of the residual atrial septal defect resulting from the transseptal puncture, and to document the disappearance of atrial thrombi.

Spontaneous contrast in the left atrium is a dramatic finding on TEE. In its obvious form it appears as smoke-like, slowly swirling patterns in the left atrium (see Fig. 38–23 *left*). It is difficult to quantitate because it depends on transducer frequency and gain settings of the instrument. When frequencies higher than 5 MHz are used, low-intensity contrast can be seen in normal subjects without mitral regurgitation who have normal or slightly reduced cardiac output. When gain settings are too low or when there is bright light in the examination setting (such as in the operating room), higher grades of spontaneous contrast can be missed. In the authors' experience, this phenomenon should be sought with 5-MHz frequency, with the gains high enough to create uniform low-level background noise throughout the atrium. In its more intense forms, this finding has been shown to have important implications in mitral stenosis and in chronic atrial fibrillation of nonvalvular origin. In a study of 400 patients, Black and colleagues[101] found it in 19 percent, 95 percent of whom had either atrial fibrillation or mitral stenosis. In mitral stenosis and in nonvalvular atrial fibrillation, spontaneous contrast was the only independent predictor of embolism, stroke, or both. In another study, its presence was found to carry a relative risk ratio of 10.6 for mitral stenosis in sinus rhythm. Bernstein and co-workers[103] found that it did not predict anything but more severe degrees of stenosis, that is, it was a marker of stasis. Fatkin and colleagues[104] studied the hematologic correlates and found that spontaneous contrast was related to the presence of anticardiolipin antibody, a high sedimentation rate, and increased fibrinogen levels. Mugge and colleagues[100] pointed out the complementary nature of left atrial appendage function in assessing embolic risk. Those at highest risk had maximum contractile velocities in atrial fibrillation below 0.25 m per second. These patients also tended to have appendage thrombi.

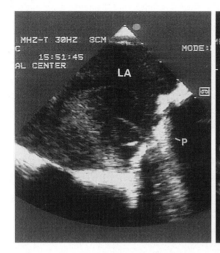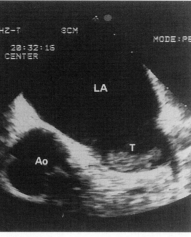

FIGURE 38–23. *Left,* Transesophageal echocardiographic demonstration of left atrial spontaneous contrast in a patient with a normally functioning mitral prosthesis (P). *Right,* A left atrial appendage thrombus (T) is illustrated in a patient with a recent peripheral thrombolic event. Ao = aortic root; LA = left atrium.

Levin and co-workers[105] reported using TEE criteria for judging the suitability of the valve for percutaneous balloon mitral valvuloplasty. Most authors, however, recommend relying on transthoracic echocardiography to judge the degree of mobility, calcification, subvalvular disease, and mitral regurgitation.

A number of reports have emphasized the importance of residual atrial septal defects after the transseptal procedure.[106–109] Although they concluded that these defects were small and usually insignificant, the left-to-right jet provides a convenient means of obtaining a Doppler gradient between the atria. Using the inferior vena cava response to respiration as a guide to right atrial pressure,[110] researchers found that the sum of the transseptal pressure difference and right atrial pressure provides a measure of left atrial pressure.

In summary, TEE is an integral part of modern diagnosis and treatment of mitral stenosis.

Mitral Regurgitation

Mitral regurgitation has been mentioned several times in this chapter, because its detection and evaluation pervades the practice of TEE. The success of TEE in the evaluation of mitral regurgitation is due to the proximity of the intraesophageal transducer to the left atrium; from this vantage point, the mitral regurgitation jet is generally in the direction of (i.e., axial or parallel to) the ultrasound beam. In situations that frustrate transthoracic echocardiography (e.g., acoustic shadowing from calcium or prosthesis), TEE provides an unimpeded view.

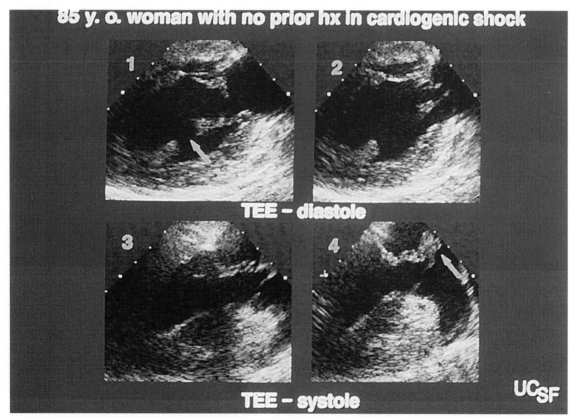

FIGURE 38–24. Ruptured papillary muscle: *Panel 1,* Longitudinal transgastric view showing discontinuity of anterolateral papillary muscle (PM) *(arrow). Panel 2,* Late diastolic frame showing free muscle head migrating toward the atrium. In early *(panel 3),* and middle *(panel 4)* systole, the PM head and its chordae prolapse deeply into the left atrium.

Transthoracic echocardiography is still the first line of evaluation in mitral regurgitation.[111–113] In most cases it is possible to accurately estimate the clinical severity and the etiology of a lesion with the use of this modality. However, there are many instances in which this estimation cannot be made with confidence, and TEE is indicated. The following discussion recommends and describes a diagnostic approach to mitral regurgitation that uses TEE to determine the etiology, to define its severity, and to guide its use in the operating room.

In nearly 90 percent of normal individuals, minor grades of mitral regurgitation are detected. These tiny jets arise from the center of the valve coaptation point and penetrate into the receiving chamber (i.e., the left atrium) for a short distance; their spectral Doppler envelopes are incomplete and of low density. Functional mitral insufficiency can be inferred when the valve is morphologically normal, but the left ventricle is either globally or segmentally abnormal. The color flow jet is usually central, occurring at a coaptation point that is marked by decreased contact area and displacement toward the left ventricle apex (the opposite of prolapse). Ischemic syndromes cause intermittent severe mitral regurgitation in association with segmental wall motion abnormalities. Dyskinesis of the muscle supporting one of the papillary muscles undermines the mitral apparatus and mitral regurgitation results. Papillary muscle rupture occurs most commonly in conjunction with myocardial infarction[114] and rarely in endocarditis[115] (Fig. 38–24).

Degenerative changes in the mitral valve are most commonly manifested by myxomatous change that thickens and elongates the leaflets and chordae and enlarges the annulus. Mitral prolapse of one or more of the three scallops of the posterior leaflet or of both leaflets is the hallmark of this condition, but its precise features have not been well studied by means of TEE beyond the original descriptions by Schluter and co-workers.[116] The most common complications of mitral prolapse are ruptured chordae tendineae which are the leading cause of severe nonrheumatic mitral regurgitation (Fig. 38–25). On transthoracic echocardiography the condition can usually be diagnosed by observing a flail portion of the mitral valve protruding into the left atrium in systole. Often, a remnant of the severed chord can be seen as a filamentous structure, moving with the flail portion of the leaflet. When the sickle-shaped scallop can be recognized the diagnosis is ensured but if,

as is often true, the mass is poorly defined, the differential between a liberated scallop and a vegetation can be impossible. Transesophageal echocardiography makes this differentiation with increased but by no means absolute certainty. Transesophageal echocardiography also is more precise in determining which of the three scallops of the posterior leaflet are involved. Such information is of importance in planning mitral valve repair. In the relatively common association between prolapse and vegetation it can be impossible by echocardiography to distinguish among the components of the prolapsing mass.

FIGURE 38–25. See Color Plate 11.

Postinflammatory (i.e., rheumatic) changes in the mitral valve are recognized by TEE by the same features used in transthoracic echocardiography. Valve thickening, immobility, doming into the ventricle, chordal foreshortening, and calcification support this diagnosis (Fig. 38–26). Mitral regurgitation in this condition is characterized by malcoaptation. Valve lesions related to systemic lupus erythematosus have been related to antiphospholipid antibodies, but this association is controversial, and antiphospholipid antibodies may occur in association with a unique syndrome apart from lupus.[117] These lesions cause focal areas of thickening, which concentrate on the atrial aspect of the valve toward the tips of the leaflets (Fig. 38–27), creating a club-like appearance. Occasionally, severe mitral regurgitation is associated with these lesions.

FIGURE 38–26. See Color Plate 12.

In judging the severity of mitral regurgitation, more than 20 variables can be examined.[118] With the use of this approach, severe lesions are readily recognized, but distinguishing between mild and moderate or moderate and severe mitral regurgitation can be difficult. In recent years it has been the authors' practice to use

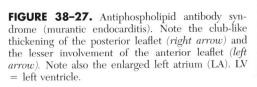

FIGURE 38–27. Antiphospholipid antibody syndrome (murantic endocarditis). Note the club-like thickening of the posterior leaflet *(right arrow)* and the lesser involvement of the anterior leaflet *(left arrow)*. Note also the enlarged left atrium (LA). LV = left ventricle.

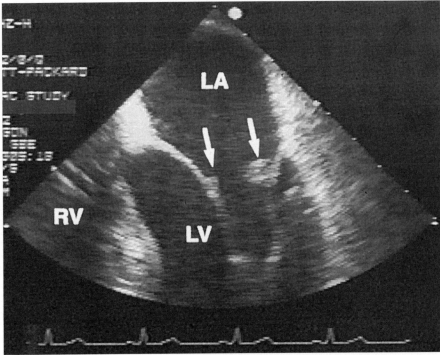

exercise-induced changes in pulmonary pressure to make this differentiation.[119]

The features of severe mitral regurgitation by color flow Doppler imaging arise from the high-energy transfer of a large volume of blood into the left atrium. On the ventricular side of the valve, proximal flow acceleration is seen as a concentric series of hemispheric rings of alternating colors, with each ring denoting an isovelocity of aliasing. The diameter of the ring closest to the regurgitant orifice is measured and in severe mitral regurgitation usually approaches 1 cm (see Fig. 38–25, *right panel*). As the color jet crosses the defect in the valve, the width of the jet exceeds 5 mm.[120, 121] As the jet enters the left atrium, the jet becomes eccentric and hugs the wall of the chamber. Once entrained on the wall (Coanda effect), the wall jet may completely circle the chamber. The jet also tends to penetrate the atrial appendage and one or more of the pulmonary veins. The color flow pattern in the receiving chamber is agitated and multidirectional; spontaneous contrast is absent.[122, 123] During most of its passage around the atrium the jet is broad and aliased. It must be emphasized that any aliased (mosaic) wall-hugging jet, however small in apparent area, should be considered as representing hemodynamically significant mitral regurgitation until proven otherwise. Some researchers have found the jet area in the left atrium on TEE to be an excellent guide to mitral regurgitation severity.[124] Because the entire left atrium cannot be seen at one time, the measurement of total jet size is problematic. Furthermore, careful study of most jets with appropriate frame rates and Nyquist limits reveal that they are not central jets but are entrained wall jets that do not lend themselves to "jet area measurement." On a technical note, the authors have observed that failure to carefully limit the area of color flow mapping results in low frame rates, low resolution, and excessive errors. The color flow examination should be directed only at the region of interest and cover as small a portion of the image fan as possible.

The spectral Doppler pattern of severe mitral regurgitation also has many features. The early diastolic mitral inflow pulsed-wave Doppler signal (E wave) obtained at the tips of the mitral leaflets is almost always increased to greater than 1.4 m per second. In a technically difficult transthoracic echocardiogram, this important clue may be the only finding that alerts a physician to the presence of severe mitral regurgitation. In addition to increased inflow velocity, the pattern is strongly E wave dominant, with a small A wave (E:A ratio >2). This pattern is identical to the restrictive inflow pattern and, in fact, has a similar origin in that filling pressures may be elevated in both situations. Whereas the velocity time integral of the mitral inflow signal is increased, the velocity time integral of the left ventricular outflow tract or pulmonary artery pulsed-wave Doppler systolic signal is normal or decreased. This discrepancy is analogous to the difference in pulmonic and aortic flow signals encountered in left-to-right shunts.

Evaluation of the pulmonary veins by TEE has provided insight into hemodynamics. In mitral regurgitation, this evaluation is a standard part of the examination and usually includes the left upper pulmonary vein, from which flow into the left atrium is usually axial to the beam of interrogation. In hemodynamically severe mitral regurgitation, the flow in one or more pulmonary veins, depending on jet direction, usually demonstrates systolic flow reversal[125–127] (Fig. 38–28). Normally, pulmonary venous flow into the left atrium is predominantly systolic; systolic reversal is paradoxical. It has been observed that mitral regurgitation jet flow may enter the pulmonary veins of only one lung and result in unilateral or unilobar pulmonary edema.[128] Once the authors became aware of this phenomenon, they observed a number of cases in their own practice; a few of these patients were initially misdiagnosed as having lobar pneumonia.

In studying the continuous wave Doppler systolic patterns of regurgitant mitral flow, several features should signal severe mitral regurgitation. If the flow signal can be aligned parallel to the beam, which is often difficult with severe eccentric jets, the jet will appear highly and uniformly dense throughout its duration, will have a well-defined envelope and may, in its late phases, show evidence of a "v-wave cutoff sign." This sign results from a rapid decrease in ventriculoatrial gradient as the large volume of regurgitant blood abruptly raises pressure in the left atrium. In severe decompensated mitral regurgitation, the tricuspid regurgitation peak velocity will be increased as the result of pulmonary hypertension.

Transesophageal echocardiographic two-dimensional imaging of the left ventricle and atrium contains numerous clues to severe mitral regurgitation. The left ventricle is spherically dilated and hyperdynamic. The left atrium is enlarged at peak systole and has an unusually pronounced change in volume that is visible during the cardiac cycle. The mitral valve itself may have one of the lesions consistent with severe mitral regurgitation, such as a flail

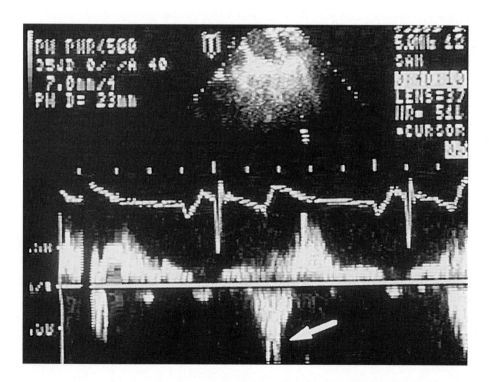

FIGURE 38–28. Spectral pulsed Doppler from the left upper pulmonary vein showing early to middle systolic flow reversal (*arrow*) in a patient with severe mitral regurgitation. Note that the normal pattern (shown in Figure 38–6) has been reversed in systole.

leaflet. In a situation analogous to the wall-hugging jet, the presence of evidence of valve disruption obligates the echocardiographer to seriously consider and exclude severe mitral regurgitation.

Intraoperative guidance of mitral valve repair in severe mitral regurgitation is an established indication for TEE; few, if any, centers performing this procedure undertake it without TEE.[129, 130] The environment in the cardiovascular surgical suite imposes unique demands on the cardiologist or the cardiovascular anesthesiologist-echocardiographer. The window of time in which an estimation of the importance of a lesion must be made is narrow, the working space crowded, and the ambient light excessive. No decision is more challenging than the one to put a patient back on cardiopulmonary bypass after an apparently unsuccessful mitral valve repair. In addition to methodically and efficiently evaluating the variables enumerated earlier, it is essential that the echocardiographer be aware of the hemodynamic state of the patient at the moment of imaging (Fig. 38–29). Postpump hypotension may lead to an erroneous conclusion about the presence of mitral regurgitation after repair, and blood pressure should be normalized before surgical decisions are made. On the one hand, important regurgitation may be missed because of low afterload in the presence of low systemic vascular resistance. However, one may note paradoxically significant mitral regurgitation that resolves once hypotension is corrected. In the latter case, the hypotension was usually on the basis of decreased left ventricular contractility and responds to inotropic agents. In the course of restoring blood pressure by volume and pharmacologic perturbations, heart size may decrease and contractility may improve. At this point, the enlarged mitral apparatus (particularly if it is myxomatous) is confined in the ventricle by the annuloplasty ring. During systole, this redundant tissue develops systolic anterior motion and creates a dynamic gradient in the left ventricular outflow tract. In the authors' experience this situation responds to decreasing catecholamines and increasing preload and rarely, if ever, requires further surgical intervention.[129]

FIGURE 38–29. See Color Plate 12.

Tricuspid and Pulmonary Valves

The tricuspid and pulmonary valves are the most difficult of the four valves to image with TEE. Both valves are thinner and deeper into the far field of the image, and the higher frequencies used in TEE tend to penetrate poorly. Multiplane capability is very helpful in imaging these valves, especially the pulmonary. Although the specific indications for TEE of these valves occur less frequently than the others, it is important to inspect them as a routine part of each examination.

Right-sided endocarditis affects the tricuspid valve far more commonly than the pulmonary valve. Although many experts recommend TEE when right-sided endocarditis is suspected, San Roman and colleagues[131] studied 48 intravenous drug users by means of both transthoracic echocardiography and TEE and concluded that sensitivities for detecting vegetations and grading and detecting tricuspid regurgitation were identical. In this series of younger and perhaps more easily imaged subjects, the two modalities detected the same vegetations. Transesophageal echocardiography did, however, give more detailed images of the vegetations. Publication of this paper occasioned a number of letters to the editor of the *Journal of the American College of Cardiology*,[132] citing cases in which TEE was absolutely essential to this diagnosis. For example, the authors and others have encountered immunologically challenged patients receiving chemotherapy or hyperalimentation who develop large vegetations on chronically placed central venous catheters in whom transthoracic echocardiography was nondiagnostic. Cohen and co-workers[133] collected 19 such patients and

found transthoracic echocardiography to have a sensitivity of only 26 percent. In nine of these patients, TEE led to a major change in management, such as surgery.

Tricuspid insufficiency can often be detected with TEE at an angle of interrogation that enables recording a complete continuous-wave Doppler signal, from which velocity measurements and right ventricular systolic pressure calculations can be made.[119] The characteristics of the jet, from which an estimation of severity can be made, may also be easier to appreciate with Doppler TEE than with transthoracic echocardiography. The etiology of tricuspid insufficiency may be evident only by means of TEE; for example, inclusion of the septal leaflet in forming a ventricular septal aneurysm to close a ventricular septal defect may be associated with severe tricuspid insufficiency and is, at times, difficult to visualize with surface imaging.[134] At other times, unusual manifestations of tricuspid regurgitant jets are encountered, such as the observation that these jets can contribute to the severity of right-to-left shunting in atrial septal defect by direct streaming through the defect.[135]

The pulmonary valve and right ventricular outflow tract are of interest primarily in congenital heart diseases. However, although rare, pulmonary valve endocarditis can occur. Most of the TEE literature on this condition is limited to single-case reports.[136–138] However, the authors encountered three cases shortly after acquiring biplane imaging capability,[139] suggesting that the condition might be more common than originally thought. Shapiro and colleagues[140] reported an additional three cases and also attributed their detection of those cases to the improved pulmonary valve imaging afforded with biplane capability.

In recent years there has been renewed interest in the Ross procedure, in which a normal pulmonary valve is used as an autograft to replace a badly diseased or deformed aortic valve. The repositioned pulmonary valve is replaced with a homograft.[141, 142] In this way females of child-bearing age can avoid chronic anticoagulation and its teratogenic potential. The authors have also used this technique in patients who have previously had aortic valve mechanical prostheses, allowing them to discontinue anticoagulation. As the popularity of this procedure increases, TEE will play a growing role in the chronic follow-up of these patients.

Pulmonic insufficiency can be readily identified with surface imaging. Although usually trivial, it is an important lesion in repaired tetralogy of Fallot, where it behaves like chronic aortic insufficiency in that it often takes several decades for it to manifest clinically. Unfortunately, in the longitudinal view, the presence of the ventricular septal patch may produce acoustic shadowing that frustrates views of the right ventricular outflow tract and pulmonary valve in repaired tetralogy of Fallot. Transesophageal echocardiography may play an important confirmatory role in cases in which the short duration of the pulsed-wave Doppler signal of severe regurgitant lesions can make detection less certain.

Prosthetic Valve Evaluation

Delineation of normal prosthetic valve function is usually possible with transthoracic echocardiography. Despite the acoustic shadowing that accompanies these devices, a Doppler signal that demonstrates normal transprosthetic flow velocity and flow duration usually suffices to exclude a stenotic or incompetent valve. In cases in which borderline findings appear, in which strong clinical suspicion of malfunction exists, or in which the echocardiogram is technically inadequate, TEE is the imaging method of choice.[143] Because TEE images are taken from a position posterior to the heart, the atrial side of the mitral and tricuspid valves can be seen. Transthoracic echocardiography images anteriorly, and the atria are situated in the far field, where resolution is low, and they are shadowed by the prosthesis. On the other hand, transthoracic echocardiography demonstrates the ventricular side of the valve that lies in its near field, whereas TEE does not. Both methods have difficulty with aortic prostheses, and the presence of mitral and aortic devices in the same patient may make the task of the echocardiographer more difficult. In most cases, however, the methods are complementary.

The physician evaluating a prosthetic device with TEE should be aware of the range of abnormalities that are possible in these devices and should match those possibilities to the patient's presentation. The major abnormalities encountered are as follows:

1. *Paravalvular regurgitation.* This abnormality can arise from broken or dehisced sutures, from a poorly seated ring, or from endocarditis (dehiscence) (Fig. 38–30). In the authors' experience hemolysis is a common but generally underappreciated complication of these leaks, especially in the mitral position.[144–146] A transesophageal echocardiogram is required to detect paravalvular leakage and should be routinely done when a prosthetic valve patient presents with severe anemia. The authors have also seen severe hemolysis occur after mitral valve repair, when regurgitation developed around the annuloplasty ring. To recognize these leaks, one must search with a high color frame rate and middle range Nyquist limits (35–50 cm/sec) *outside* the sewing ring in several views from several angles; sometimes, these jets are seen inadvertently when one examines other structures, such as the interatrial septum. The most severe form of paravalvular regurgitation is seen when there is dehiscence of a substantial portion of the sewing ring.[147] In this case there is severe regurgitation, which may be so torrential that the regurgitant flow is almost laminar. As in angiography, the sewing ring is seen to rock with each cardiac cycle. Both the laminar flow and the rocking motion of the ring may elude the inexperienced echocardiographer, delaying recognition of this life-threatening condition.

FIGURE 38–30. See Color Plate 12.

---

2. *Endocarditis.* See previous discussion.

3. *Obstruction due to pannus, thrombus, or vegetation.* If an unexpected rise in transprosthetic gradient from a baseline determination or from established normal values for valves of that type and size is encountered in a newly symptomatic patient, the possibility of critical obstruction should be considered. Clinical clues to this possibility include the age of the valve and the adequacy of anticoagulation. In a heterograft, the leaflets themselves may become calcified and immobile. Once the threshold of suspicion has been crossed, TEE should be strongly considered. In the case of suspected aortic pannus, the distal end of the left ventricular outflow tract should be searched both with imaging and with color flow. Pannus tends to lie close to the valve ring and can be easily overlooked. There can be a prevalve jet that suggests pannus which, on further searching with a variety of frequencies, angles, and gain settings, will be detected. In the mitral position, the same procedure should be followed. Finding a high grade of spontaneous contrast in the left atrium (with or without thrombi) or finding thrombus around the sewing ring should heighten suspicion of pannus formation. Thin fibrillar strands are also encountered on the mitral annulus and the left ventricular outflow tract. These structures are brightly reflective and highly mobile and may or may not be associated with a pathologic process.

4. *Regurgitation due to bioprosthetic degeneration or mechanical valve pannus, thrombus, or vegetation.* Physiologic regurgitation (the so-called seating puff of angiography) is universally encountered and dependent in degree on the type of prosthesis used. Typically, normally functioning mechanical valves, such as the bi-leaflet St. Jude, have up to four central regurgitant jets, whose features include low intensity and only minimal penetration into the atrium (Fig. 38–31), whereas the monodisc Medtronic-Hall valve has two jets, one of which is prominent (Fig. 38–32). Normally functioning heterografts are less likely to have these small regurgitant signals. Pathologic jets tend to be central, intense,

broad, and highly aliased, and they tend to hug the wall of the atrium, penetrating to its roof, continuing around its perimeter, and terminating where they began. The bioprosthetic leaflets can usually be seen and are either thickened or partially flail (Fig. 38–33). In the case of the mechanical valves, the offending mass or tissue can usually be seen, but the actual locus of obstruction may not be visible.

FIGURES 38–31 to 38–33. See Color Plate 13.

When a thrombus is present in the vicinity of the sewing ring and when obstruction is plausible clinically and suggested by Doppler imaging, consideration should be given to the use of thrombolysis. The other option is surgery, which, if thrombolysis fails, may be contraindicated by the augmented risk of bleeding. Vitale and co-workers[148] described their experience with 28 patients, 20 of whom were treated surgically and 8 with recombinant tissue plasminogen activator. There was one operative death and complete success and no deaths with thrombolysis. Dzavik and co-workers[149] reported a very similar experience and noted that the surgical mortality for this condition had approached 50 percent, so thrombolysis, despite potential hemorrhagic complications, may be the treatment of choice.

5. *Regurgitation due to strut fracture and disk liberation.* There has been considerable concern about large Bjork-Shiley monodisc valves because of their low but significant incidence of strut fracture, leading to liberation of the disk and rapid hemodynamic compromise. Fortunately, the authors have had only one such patient in their institution. In this case, clinical deterioration was so rapid that diagnostic TEE could not be performed. The patient was taken from the emergency room to surgery, based on clinical suspicion, and survived.

PULMONARY ARTERIES

During examination of the pulmonary valve with TEE, it is important to inspect the central pulmonary artery and the proximal branches. Dilation can be appreciated by comparing the vessel to the aorta. The main pulmonary artery is usually only slightly larger than the aorta, whereas the branches are smaller. The right and left branches are normally smaller than the ascending aorta. These comparisons are easier to make with TEE than with transthoracic echocardiography and can point to clinically important conditions such as pulmonary hypertension and shunts. When proficiency is gained in imaging the pulmonary artery and its branches, TEE can be used in the urgent workup of suspected large *acute* pulmonary embolism[150–152] and in *chronic* pulmonary hypertension associated with recurrent pulmonary emboli.[153]

INTRACARDIAC TUMORS, MASSES, SOURCE OF EMBOLISM, AND ROLE OF TRANSESOPHAGEAL ECHOCARDIOGRAPHY IN ATRIAL FIBRILLATION

Cardiac tumors are rare, being reported in fewer than 0.1 percent of autopsies.[154] Nonetheless, in the filtering process through which patients are referred to cardiologists and echocardiography laboratories, they constitute a subgroup that not only appears with regularity but in which dramatic relief of symptoms and reduction of mortality is often accomplished. Also, when the physician performs or interprets TEE, it is important to avoid overdiagnosis of cardiac masses. Like any highly magnified imaging system, TEE tends to exaggerate previously obscure normal structures.[155] For the unwary and inexperienced echocardiographer, misinterpretations may occur. On the left side of heart, the muscular septum dividing the left upper pulmonary vein from the atrial appendage, the atrial appendage trabeculations, ectopic chordae, bands, and trabeculations are potentially confounding normal structures. On the right side, Chiari's network, the septomarginal trabeculation, and the right atrioventricular groove are often confused with pathologic growths.

Left atrial myxoma is the most common tumor encountered and is usually recognized by transthoracic echocardiography. However, TEE has the advantages of better localizing its stalk and more clearly defining its characteristic appearance (cysts and bone islands), its mobility and any damage to the mitral valve[156, 157] (Fig. 38–34). Highly mobile tumors with broad bases of attachment have much higher embolic potential than the well encapsulated ones. Myxomas also occur on valves, but most often valve tumors are fibroelastomas[158, 159] (Fig. 38–35). Myxomas have also been found in the right ventricular outflow tract.[160] Other tumors, such as fibrosarcomas and rhabdomyomas, are rarely encountered. Metastatic tumors are also seen on occasion, with melanoma being among the more common.

Right-sided tumors tend to grow larger than left-sided tumors; TEE has distinct advantages in their localization and characterization.[161] Of particular interest are tumors that arise in the abdomen and pelvis and extend up the inferior vena cava into the right heart.[162–165] In imaging these tumors it is important to use the bicaval view, so that their origin in the inferior vena cava can be confirmed. Although these tumors are usually very large when encountered, a multidisciplinary approach between abdominal and cardiovascular surgeons can result in protracted palliation.

The heart and great vessels are implicated as the source of systemic arterial emboli in 10 percent of annual strokes and transient ischemic attacks.[154] Tumors can be a source of embolism, but the most commonly implicated structures and masses are left atrial appendage thrombus[166] (see Fig. 38–23), atrial septal aneurysm with patent foramen ovale (Fig. 38–36), left atrial spontaneous contrast (see Fig. 38–23), patent foramen ovale, and protruding aortic atheroma (see Fig. 38–4).

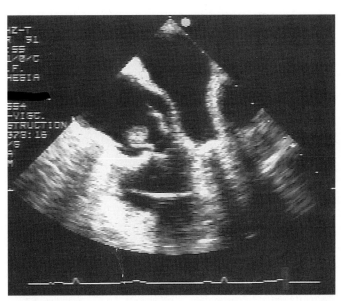

FIGURE 38–35. Aortic fibroelastoma. This transverse left ventricular outflow tract view during systole shows the open aortic valve leaflets with the right coronary cusp of the aortic valve, showing a round, almost tumor-like mass at its tip. This process is typical in appearance of a fibroelastoma.

All series that compare TEE with transthoracic echocardiography clearly show that the former is superior in yield in identifying potential sources for arterial emboli. For example, Pearson and colleagues,[166] in a study of 79 patients, found that the yield of potential sources of embolism rose from 15 to 57 percent when they compared transthoracic echocardiography with TEE in patients with pre-existing cardiac disease and from 19 to 39 percent in those without it.

As regards patent *foramen ovale,* some series report that almost 50 percent of individuals with cryptogenic stroke have this potential right-to-left shunt.[167] Because 25 percent of the normal population has this finding, others have suggested caution in interpretation of its presence.[168, 169] Also, the yield of TEE for detecting *patent foramen ovale* is only marginally better than that of transthoracic echocardiography, especially if right-sided contrast with Valsalva's maneuver is used.

Interatrial septal aneurysm (see Fig. 38–36) is closely related to patent foramen ovale in that most "aneurysms" are associated with a patent foramen. This finding can be recognized as a redundant, highly mobile membranous portion of the atrial septum. Schneider and colleagues first studied 23[170] and then 40 patients[171] with this entity. More than 83 percent had an associated patent foramen; in 52 percent there was a history of cerebrovascular accident, and in 27 percent transthoracic echocardiography did not reveal the redundant interatrial septum. The authors concluded that interatrial septal aneurysm should be sought by use of TEE in cases of unexplained stroke and, if found, treated with anticoagulation.

Lipomatous hypertrophy of the interatrial septum has been associated with arterial embolization, pulmonary emboli,[172] arrhythmias, and sudden death.[173] Most reports of this abnormality are single-case reports, and further study of the entity is being awaited. To the echocardiographer performing transthoracic echocardiography lipomatous hypertrophy of the interatrial septum is difficult to appreciate because the atrial septum sits in the far field of the image, where beam-spread artifact often obscures the details of the septum. With TEE the entity presents as a striking dumbbell-shaped interatrial septum that involves the septum *primum* and *venosus* portions but always spares the foramen ovale. In some cases this entity can be mistaken for a tumor, but its fatty nature is apparent from the intense shadowing it creates.

Thrombus in the atrial appendage can be detected only with TEE (see Fig. 38–23). The association between thrombus in this

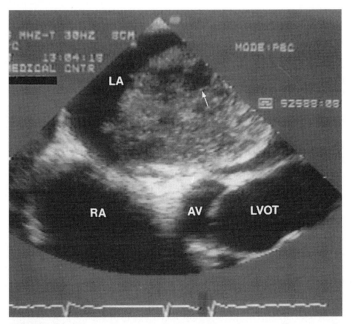

FIGURE 38–34. Transesophageal echocardiographic view, illustrating the characteristic cystic (*arrow*) acoustic findings that may be seen in benign myxomas. The brighter areas in the lower right portion of the tumor may represent calcification or bone formation, also typical of this lesion. Finally, on the edge of the mass toward the left atrial cavity, note that there are a few small protuberances or "daughter lesions." LA = left atrium; RA = right atrium; AV = aortic valve; LVOT = left ventricular outflow tract.

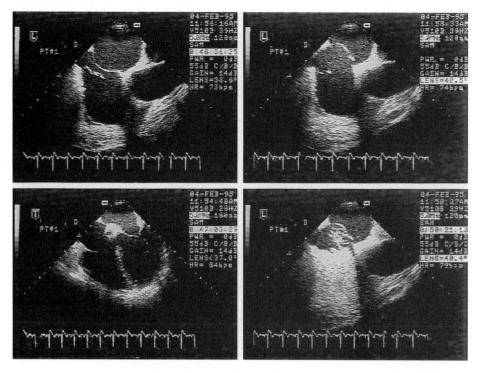

FIGURE 38–36. Atrial septal "aneurysm," Chiari network, and patent foramen ovale. *Upper Left Panel,* Longitudinal biatrial view with interatrial septum bulging from left to right. *Upper Right Panel,* Same view during a different phase of respiration with reversed curvature of the interatrial septum from right to left. The exact definition of an atrial septal aneurysm is not agreed on, so this prominent structure may merely represent an exaggeration of normal. *Lower Right Panel,* Postcontrast view with some contrast elements crossing the interatrial septum into the left atrium. *Lower Left Panel,* Normal four-chamber view in this patient points out the need for exact positioning over the middle portion of the foramen ovale so that both the Chiari remnant and the interatrial septal aneurysm can be appreciated.

structure and embolic stroke is established, as is the association between its dysfunction and the tendency to form thrombus.[100] In their study, Mugge and associates[100] demonstrated that when the appendage contractions fail to exceed 0.2 m per second, there is a strong association not only with atrial appendage thrombus and spontaneous contrast in the atrial cavity but also with embolic events.

Aortic arch and proximal descending aortic debris and plaque are gaining increasing attention as a previously unheralded source of cerebral emboli and infarction (see Fig. 38–4). Amarenco and colleagues[174] studied 250 patients with no known explanation for stroke with TEE and found 28 percent with plaque, as opposed to 8 percent in a control group of cerebrovascular accident patients with known causes for stroke. In a similar study Toyoda and co-workers[175] found aortic arch lesions in 42 percent but made the interesting original observation that those with complex or mobile plaque also tended to have calcification in the arch of the aorta on chest radiograph.

Few applications of TEE have "caught on" as quickly as its application to decision-making in atrial fibrillation. Because atrial fibrillation of more than a few days' duration is associated with embolic stroke, it has been standard practice to anticoagulate patients for 4 weeks prior to elective cardioversion. Based on the theory that an atrium demonstrated to be free from thrombus would allow immediate cardioversion, a number of studies that used TEE have been published. In perhaps the most quoted study, Manning and colleagues[176] performed TEE on 94 patients and found 12 with thrombi in the left atrium (most in the appendage). Of those free from thrombus, 78 successfully underwent cardioversion without embolic complications in the postcardioversion period. In a smaller study of 40 patients, Black and co-workers[177] did encounter one postcardioversion stroke in a patient with spontaneous contrast but no thrombus, as did Missault and co-workers[178] and Salka and associates.[179] Repeat TEE in Black's patient revealed the interim development of atrial appendage thrombus. This finding prompted the same group[180] to evaluate the impact of cardioversion on atrial function. Importantly, they found that atrial appendage function decreased in most patients after cardioversion and that new spontaneous contrast developed in 35 percent of patients in the immediate postcardioversion period. This study attributed these changes to postcardioversion stunning of the atrium and has provided a rationale for anticoagulating patients in the period immediately before and for at least 1 month after cardioversion.

ATHEROSCLEROTIC PLAQUE IN THE DESCENDING AORTA AND CORONARY FLOW RESERVE IN CORONARY ARTERY DISEASE

The descending aorta should be routinely imaged for a TEE examination to be considered complete. The authors have commonly observed varying degrees of intimal thickening and protruding or mobile masses that are variants of the atherosclerotic process. Because atherosclerosis is a generalized disease, the authors tested the hypothesis that this plaque is a marker for coronary artery disease.[181] In 61 patients who had TEE and angiography, the authors found 20 who were free from obstructive disease (but not of luminal irregularities) by means of angiography; only 2 of these 20 had aortic plaque. The presence of protruding plaque had a sensitivity and specificity for critical coronary stenosis of 90 percent and positive and negative predictive values of 95 and 82 percent. Another recent study has confirmed these observations.[182] A possible application for this information is in emergency situations, such as hemodynamic instability related to acute valve regurgitation, in which delaying surgery to perform coronary angiography is undesirable. In a such a situation the absence of aortic plaque might provide a rationale for proceeding directly to surgery.

Another approach to coronary artery disease that is in its formative stages uses the superior resolution of TEE to image the left anterior descending coronary artery and to sample its flow signal with pulsed-wave Doppler[183] (Fig. 38–37). During imaging, a coronary vasodilator such as dipyridamole[184, 185] or adenosine is infused, and the increase in flow is compared to the greater than twofold increase expected of a normal artery. This increase is an expression of coronary flow reserve. As a recent innovation, lung-crossing, left-sided ultrasound contrast agents have been given to augment the quality of coronary artery flow signals.[185, 186]

FIGURE 38–37. See Color Plate 13.

HEMODYNAMICS DERIVED FROM TRANSESOPHAGEAL ECHOCARDIOGRAPHY: APPLICATION IN CRITICAL CARE AND CARDIOPULMONARY RESUSCITATION

Transesophageal echocardiography can rapidly provide a comprehensive array of anatomic and hemodynamic variables. In critical care settings, where patients are often obtunded and mechanically ventilated, this modality can usually differentiate between the causes of hypotension, dyspnea, and chest pain. To reliably and safely apply TEE to critical care, skill, experience and multidisciplinary approach are essential. A working relationship among intensivists, anesthesiologists, and cardiologists is an integral part of every successful critical care TEE program.

Hemodynamic variables that are derived from TEE are comprehensive enough to provide accurate cross-sectional hemodynamic information; variables measured include cardiac output, left ventricular-atrial filling pressure, temporal distribution of filling, chamber preload, atrial interaction, and pulmonary pressure.

CARDIAC OUTPUT. The main pulmonary artery is the most convenient site from which to measure cardiac output. Its cross-sectional diameter can be measured and the velocity-time integral at that site obtained. The product of the cross-sectional area and the stroke distance (VTI) is stroke volume. The product of stroke volume and heart rate is cardiac output. This method was established in the operating room by comparing it to thermodilution cardiac output.[51] Although cardiac output by thermodilution is not an ideal reference standard, the pulsed-wave Doppler method was able to follow directional changes in that parameter. In our clinical experience with the method we have been encouraged by how consistently the pulsed-wave Doppler results match standard measurements and reflect the clinical situation. The deep gastric long-axis view has been reported to provide an additional window for sampling cardiac output by pulsed-wave Doppler interrogation of the left ventricular outflow tract.[187]

LEFT VENTRICULAR AND ATRIAL FILLING PRESSURES. Pulmonary venous flow patterns, mitral inflow signal configuration, and continuous-wave Doppler of mitral regurgitation contain information from which filling pressures can be estimated.

Transesophageal echocardiography at the base of the heart demonstrates the entrance of the four pulmonary veins into the left atrium. The left upper pulmonary vein flow is close to and parallel to the direction of the interrogating beam. Highly resolved color flow pulsed-wave Doppler images are readily obtained and help to guide positioning of the sample volume into the proximal 1 cm of the vein. Flow in the pulmonary veins is typical of central veins in that it is triphasic.[33, 108, 188, 189] The systolic phase is predominant, accounting for more than 55 percent of total flow integral (see Fig. 38–17, *left panel*). The second phase occurs in early diastole and is approximately 40 percent of the total. Both of these phases move in a central direction and occur as the result of atrial systolic filling and atrial diastolic emptying. The third phase is in late diastole and results from atrial contraction. In contrast to the first two phases, the atrial phase is retrograde and usually small. In conditions that alter left ventricular filling patterns, especially when filling pressures are elevated, systole becomes subordinate to diastole (see Fig. 38–17, *right panel*). Concurrently, retrograde atrial flow may increase and exceed in duration forward atrial flow across the mitral valve.[190] In severe mitral regurgitation, systolic flow reversal has been described as one of the signs of severity.[126]

Mitral inflow and pulmonary flow patterns are complementary.[54] For example, restrictive mitral inflow is characterized by a short isovolumic relaxation time, a normal or slightly elevated peak velocity, a short deceleration time, and a low A wave velocity. These features result in an increased E:A ratio and a pattern known as "pseudonormalization." A restrictive pattern on mitral inflow and decreased systolic fraction on pulmonary venous inflow are complementary, permitting confident recognition of elevated filling pressure. A prolonged retrograde pulmonary venous A wave and a shortened A wave on mitral inflow also connote elevated filling pressure (see Figs. 38–6, 38–16, and 38–17).

Mitral regurgitation continuous-wave Doppler signals are hemodynamically informative.[54] The Bernoulli equation, when applied to the peak systolic mitral regurgitation flow velocity, can be used to calculate the peak systolic gradient between the left atrium and the left ventricle. This value exceeds systemic arterial pressure by a value equal to left atrial pressure. In other words, the sum of the transmitral gradient and left atrial pressure equals systolic arterial pressure, and the difference of the arterial pressure and the left atrial pressure is the filling pressure. Other features of the mitral continuous-wave Doppler flow signal are the density of the signal (proportional to severity of regurgitation), the v-wave cutoff sign (see mitral regurgitation section), and the early systolic acceleration of the jet flow envelope (an expression of dP/dt).

THE LEFT VENTRICLE AND LEFT ATRIUM. Volume changes affect the size and shape of the left heart chambers. In acute hypovolemia, most normal hearts become hyperdynamic and develop very small end-systolic volumes. In preload sensitive hearts, contractility may decrease, but this situation is harder to recognize. In one example, a heart is rapidly atrially paced without any change in metabolic demands, and the contractility of the left ventricle visibly decreases while the chamber remains small. The left atrium in hypovolemia becomes tubular, and it may be possible to see the entire chamber and the pulmonary veins in one image. Similarly, the right atrium, venae cavae, and hepatic veins become small, and respiratory collapse might be appreciated. In congestive heart failure, especially if chronic, the left ventricle assumes a spherical state as it dilates. This appearance is strikingly different from the ellipsoid shape of the healthy heart. While one cannot determine the filling pressure from inspecting the ventricles and atria, observations of these features can reinforce the inferences drawn from Doppler data.

The behavior of the interatrial septum is a particularly important clue as to the left ventricular filling pressure.[191] Observations made on ventilated patients showed that in the euvolemic or hypovolemic state, the interatrial septum, normally curved to the right, will reverse curvature at end expiration at both end-systole and end-diastole. The cause of the rapid reversal in curvature has been documented with flow-directed catheters; it arises from a transient reversal in the pressure differential such that right atrial pressure transiently exceeds left atrial pressure during the expiratory phase of the ventilator cycle. This occurs only when pressures (pulmonary capillary wedge and central venous pressure) are low and nearly equal. If either atrium carries higher pressure, the atrial septum will remain bowed toward the lower pressure chamber. In mitral regurgitation, for example, the atrial septum bows from left to right, and this curvature is little affected by the respiratory cycle. In tricuspid regurgitation or pulmonary hypertension the curvature goes from right to left. It is worth emphasizing how useful this simple observation can be in "tying together" multiple variables and emerging with a clear picture of a patient's hemodynamics.

CRITICAL CARE. Indications for TEE in the critically ill are suspicion of significant valve disease, prosthetic dysfunction, hypotension, suspected right or left ventricular dysfunction, situations conducive to mediastinal or thoracic bleeding, suspicion of hypoxia arising from an intracardiac shunt, chest pain indicative of dissection of the aorta, severe chest trauma, myocardial infarction with shock and cardiopulmonary resuscitation.[22, 192] In reviewing our own experience with 83 transesophageal echocardiograms in the critical care setting[192] we noted the following indications for study: endocarditis (43 percent), suspected cardiac source of embolism (13 percent), hypotension (10 percent), mitral regurgitation (10 percent), left ventricular dysfunction (6 percent), and prosthetic dysfunction (4 percent). Unexpected findings in 21 of 83 led to a change in management in 17 percent or a referral for invasive examination in 22 percent. In 13 of 83, surgical intervention was performed based on TEE without further examination. In our own critical care experience, complications have been exceedingly rare.

The complications of myocardial infarction deserve special men-tion in the discussion of critical care. The cause of hemodynamic instability in the setting of acute myocardial infarction can often be elucidated noninvasively, using echocardiography, but technical limitations may limit transthoracic imaging. In mechanically ventilated patients, highly defined images of the endocardium, essential for accurate wall motion evaluation, may be impossible, and TEE may be required to define the extent of the wall motion abnormalities accurately. Other complications of myocardial infarction, such as the cause of acute mitral regurgitation, may not be recognized by transthoracic echocardiography. In particular, diagnosis of papillary muscle rupture[114] is much more difficult than might be intuitively imagined (see Fig. 38–24). Similarly, the diagnoses of ventricular septal defect (Fig. 38–38), pseudoaneurysm, and intramyocardial hematoma cannot be made with certainty with the use of transthoracic echocardiography.[122, 193, 194] These complications should be suspected when a postmyocardial infarction patient with low output is evaluated and is unexpectedly found to have hyperdynamic left ventricular function. This paradox should prompt use of TEE to search for papillary muscle rupture or acute ventricular septal defect.

FIGURE 38–38. See Color Plate 14.

CARDIOPULMONARY RESUSCITATION. Victims of cardiopulmonary arrest arrive in the same condition but with a wide variety of etiologies. Transesophageal echocardiography is ideally suited for rapid evaluation of the etiology of arrest and the effectiveness of cardiopulmonary resuscitation.[195] The authors performed TEE on 18 patients in cardiopulmonary arrest as they arrived in their emergency room. Blind esophageal intubation was rapidly accomplished and was possible in 14 and required laryngoscopy in the other 4. In 10 of 18, the diagnosis was established. In four patients with acute myocardial infarction the diagnosis was made before the electrocardiographic electrodes could be attached. In two patients, dilated cardiomyopathy was diagnosed; in two, hypertrophic cardiomyopathy; and in one, normal prosthetic valve function. Of the six successfully resuscitated in this group, two survived to leave the hospital.

Research using TEE has helped elucidate the mechanism of cardiopulmonary resuscitation. In 20 patients evaluated in the authors' institution, they found that during compressions the chambers decreased in size, the mitral valve closed, and the aortic valve opened. In addition, spontaneous contrast improved, and atrioventricular valve regurgitation appeared. These findings seem to confirm that the heart is acting like a pump, confirming the so-called cardiac pump theory.[196] In a few, however, the thoracic pump theory was supported by observation of open aortic and mitral valve during compression. In one patient, the right side appeared to be a passive conduit (thoracic pump), whereas the left side was an active pump. Thus, both theories are probably correct, with the cardiac pump probably playing a role in the majority of patients.

AORTIC DISSECTION

Acute dissection of the thoracic aorta almost always presents as an acute chest pain syndrome. It is a true medical emergency in which rapid diagnosis and treatment are crucial to optimal survival. An excellent review of the role of TEE in treating this condition has been written by Erbel,[197] to which the reader is referred for a comprehensive review.

Cardiac ultrasound, in general, and TEE, in particular, represent ideal methods for the evaluation of patients suspected of having dissection. Both rapid detection of the condition and the crucial distinction between proximal (type A or I, II) and distal (type B or III) can be made with confidence (Fig. 38–39). Furthermore, most

of the complications can be quickly detected. In particular, TEE can detect the epiphenomena of pericardial effusion, segmental wall motion abnormalities, aortic insufficiency, and pleural effusions, all of which impact heavily on the treatment plan and survival. The technique can also detect features of the dissection itself; these include the extent and location of the intimal flap, its sites of communication with the true lumen, thrombus within its lumen, and the important variant of dissection, the intramural hematoma. In the absence of suspicion of arch vessel involvement (a potential indication for angiography), it is now standard practice to refer patients directly to surgery without any further testing once dissection is identified.

FIGURE 38–39. See Color Plate 14.

Omoto's group at Saitama University, Japan, has performed a number of critical studies that have helped to establish the role of TEE in dissection.[198–201] For example, in their series, TEE has diagnostic accuracy of more than 95 percent, both in the preoperative diagnosis,[198] as the sole preoperative diagnostic tool[199] and as an intraoperative guide to surgery.[200] Reporting on the use of TEE in the emergency room and comparing its impact to aortography, Chan[202] found no impact on outcome that could be ascribed to aortography and thus advised its abandonment. Chirillo and colleagues[203] compared the speed of obtaining a TEE with angiography and found that the latter took a mean of 39 minutes longer. The only role that they found for angiography was in defining vascular complications. Lower sensitivity of angiography[204] also limits its usefulness.

Computed tomography (CT) and magnetic resonance imaging (MRI) compare more favorably to TEE than aortography. De Simone and co-workers[205] found that TEE had sensitivity, specificity, accuracy, and positive predictive accuracy of 97, 96, 98, and 97 percent, whereas the values for CT were 91, 89, 95, and 94 percent. MRI was used by Deutsch and co-workers[206] and compared to TEE in chronic dissection. In this setting TEE was deficient only in studying the arch vessels and details of the postsurgical anastomosis site. In a comparison of MRI to TEE, Nienaber and associates[207] reported that when these modalities were performed in random order, they differed only in a slightly lower specificity of TEE. They ascribed this difference to misinterpretation of findings in the portion of the aortic arch that is prone to artifact and often obscured by the air-filled bronchus. This "blind spot" has been reduced in size since the writing of this report by the addition of multiplanar imaging. However, it remains a potential pitfall for TEE, and physicians should have a low threshold for referring patients for MRI when interpretive difficulties are encountered with TEE in that area. It should be pointed out that even if the diagnostic capabilities of CT or MRI are similar to those of TEE, the latter can be performed at the bedside, can yield more comprehensive data about cardiac complications and function, can be completed more quickly, can be continued in the operating room, and is considerably cheaper. The dangers of transporting a patient to the imaging suite to receive a slower (but equivalent) study cannot be minimized.

In the European Cooperative Study,[208] the nature of the communication between the true lumen and the false lumen and its impact on outcome in acute and chronic patients was studied in 68 patients. Spontaneous healing occurred in only 8 percent. The identification of any effusion (pleural or pericardial) carried a 52 percent mortality rate. Interestingly, finding thrombus in the false lumen was associated with an 80 percent survival rate. Because TEE was used in the initial evaluation of these patients, the comparison of survival rates with those of controls led the investigators to conclude that preoperative mortality was reduced by TEE, because it allowed a rapid initiation of treatment.

Intramural hematoma is a variant of dissection that can pose considerable difficulties for the echocardiographer. By its nature, the dissection remains confined to the wall of the aorta and, in a patient presenting with classic chest pain, may appear as no more than a thickening of the wall. A lack of familiarity with this entity can lead to severe diagnostic error.[209, 210] Other artifacts, such as proximity of the great veins to the aorta, have occasionally been associated with diagnostic error[211, 212] as well as other artifacts and types of aneurysm.[213]

A final caveat: TEE was performed in the studies reported here by highly skilled and experienced physicians. The study of dissection requires considerable experience and a strong working relationship with surgical and anesthesia colleagues. The physician who lacks these essentials would do well to apply TEE data conservatively, if at all.

TRAUMA AND TRANSESOPHAGEAL ECHOCARDIOGRAPHY

There is a growing body of literature on the use of TEE in major trauma. Although this application of TEE is too new to have generated solid data on outcomes, the consensus in the literature is that the modality is extremely accurate and helpful in situations in which there is suspicion of aortic transection, cardiac contusion, mediastinal hematoma, valve damage, or pericardial tamponade.

Two earlier studies focused on the diagnosis of myocardial contusion, which is often difficult to confirm by noninvasive or invasive means. Shapiro and colleagues[214] evaluated 19 thoracic trauma patients with no prior cardiac history and radiographic mediastinal widening. In 12 patients (63 percent) there were abnormalities that included segmental left ventricular hypokinesis (contusion) in 5, tricuspid regurgitation in 3, aortic and mitral regurgitation in 1, aortic wall hematoma in 2, and pericardial effusion in 1. In another study, Brooks and associates reviewed 50 patients presenting with thoracic trauma[215] and found a higher yield for a wall motion abnormality typical of contusion by TEE (52 percent) than transthoracic echocardiography (12 percent). Moreover, in the 17 patients with mediastinal widening and angiographic confirmation, TEE correctly identified 3 aortic disruptions and 14 normal aortas. These authors independently concluded that the test was highly sensitive for contusion and was an excellent screening method for urgent evaluation of post-traumatic mediastinal widening.

In comparing thermal injury patients to multiple trauma subjects,[216] TEE was used to evaluate systolic and diastolic ventricular function. Systolic function was normal in both types of injury, but diastolic performance, as measured by Doppler mitral inflow, was abnormal in thermal injury but not traumatic injury.

There are several additional series that have more extensively addressed the issue of aortic injury. The descending thoracic aorta was the subject of a study of 11 patients with blunt chest trauma.[217] Of six positive aortograms three were shown to be false-positive, whereas TEE correctly identified all positives and negatives. In the largest study to date, Smith and colleagues[218] studied 101 patients, all of whom underwent aortography. The success rate of TEE was 93 percent with 12 percent demonstrating rupture either at surgery or autopsy. In all patients TEE made the correct diagnosis. Most importantly, it was tolerated in all without additional morbidity (despite high injury score), and it took only approximately 29 minutes to perform (as compared with approximately 76 minutes for aortography). Kearney and co-workers also addressed the issue of diagnostic efficiency in the trauma setting in a study of 69 patients suspected of aortic injury.[219] As in Smith's study, TEE was more rapidly performed than aortography (27 versus 76 minutes, $P < .05$) and more accurately predicted the presence or absence of aortic injury in each case (sensitivity and specificity = 100 percent) whereas aortography produced false-negative results in two. Although TEE appears to be safe, rapid, and accurate in the evaluation of multiple-injury patients suspected of having aortic injury, the diagnostic modality used must be determined not only by the efficacy of the technique but also by the experience of the available personnel in interpreting the potential findings. With the increasing deployment of TEE, it is likely that this technology will eventually become the standard of care for severe chest trauma. The roles of the cardiologist, cardiovascular anesthesiologist, emergency room physician, or trauma surgeon in performing these studies remain to be defined.

CONGENITAL HEART DISEASES AND TRANSESOPHAGEAL ECHOCARDIOGRAPHY

Transthoracic echocardiography provides most of the information needed to diagnose and treat congenital heart disease in children, because the chest wall provides a much lower impediment to the passage of ultrasound than it does in adults.

In centers specializing in congenital heart disease, TEE is growing in importance both in the guidance of intraoperative repair of both children and adults[220–223] and in the routine evaluation of clinically important questions in operated and unoperated children and adults.[224] Ritter[225] reported a 56 percent increment in information over transthoracic echocardiography in 127 patients as young as 1 day of age studied in both outpatient and intraoperative settings. Muhiudeen and colleagues[220] reported a much lower incremental value, but their studies were performed mostly in the pediatric cardiovascular surgical suite. Although multiplane imaging is usually desirable in complex congenital heart disease, it may not be possible in premature infants of low birth weight. Pediatric probes of small diameter are available for these newborns but are currently single plane.

One example of the important role of TEE in adult congenital heart disease is in the diagnosis of interatrial communications, where it has been found to be more accurate than transthoracic echocardiography in determining both size and location[226, 227] (Fig. 38–40). Saline contrast material should be used to confirm the presence of shunting, especially when the defect is equivocal according to two-dimensional and color flow imaging. Biplane and multiplane transesophageal views are particularly useful in identification of the sinus venosus type of atrial septal defect.

FIGURE 38–40. See Color Plate 15.

The diverse indications for use of TEE in treating congenital heart disease can be classified as intraoperative, interventional, and elective. Marelli and colleagues[224] list the following indications for TEE by these general uses (Table 38–7).

FUTURE DEVELOPMENTS IN TRANSESOPHAGEAL ECHOCARDIOGRAPHY AND SUMMARY

Transesophageal echocardiography is a technology-driven technique. Its rapid growth after 1986 occurred when high-resolution color flow mapping was incorporated into high-resolution, small, phased-array probes. Other expansions in its indications have occurred with the addition of biplane and multiplane capability, especially because neither of these advances required an appreciable increment in probe size. It can be expected that even smaller probe size with either unchanged or improved image quality will lead to the next rung in the evolution of TEE. Very small probes will allow neonatal or even fetal imaging and will merge inexorably into devices suitable for intravascular applications. In the adult patient, very small probes may increase tolerance and allow nasal intubation or long-term imaging. Central processing units that are

TABLE 38-7. INDICATIONS FOR TRANSESOPHAGEAL ECHOCARDIOGRAPHY IN CONGENITAL HEART DISEASE

Elective (Inpatient or Outpatient) Indications
Atrial septal defect—especially sinus venosus and anomalous pulmonary venous drainage
Pulmonary atrioventricular fistulae
Atrial baffle obstruction
Fontan obstruction
Outflow tract obstruction (right or left)
Coronary artery anomalies
Coarctation of the aorta
Late tetralogy repair complications
Atrioventricular valve insufficiency severity
Patch leaks—estimate severity
Exclude thrombus prior to electrophysiology study or cardioversion

Intraoperative Indications
Further define anomalies—unsuspected variations
Evaluate adequacy of surgical repair
Presence and degree of unrepaired residua

Interventional Indications
Aortic and pulmonic valvuloplasty guidance
Coarctoplasty guidance
Dilation of atrial baffle obstruction guidance
Guide device closure of intracardiac shunts

Adapted from Marelli, A.J., Child, J.S., and Perloff, J.K.: Transesophageal echocardiography in congenital heart disease in the adult. Cardiol. Clin. 11(3):505–520, 1993, with permission.

shared among several intensive care beds would make it possible to create an affordable system in which probes can be left in place for days at a time. Smaller probes will also facilitate interventional imaging. With a small intranasal probe, dynamic exercise should be possible. As images improve further, so will automatic edge-detection algorithms. Accurate automated border detection will generate reliable on-line information about systolic and diastolic function. This high-quality information will facilitate adjustment of cardioactive therapeutic agents. Other image-processing methods, such as Doppler tissue imaging, second harmonics, and videodensitometry, will mature and allow contrast-perfusion studies of segmental myocardial blood flow. Improved imaging will also lead to studies of Doppler flow in the coronary arteries for flow reserve quantitation and for detection of local obstruction. It will also be possible to sample coronary sinus flow for the same purpose.

Three-dimensional imaging may also be among the next wave of advances in technology.[11, 40, 228] In the authors' own experience with this method the images were generated quickly enough and were of sufficient quality to acquire and demonstrate them to a surgeon performing a cardiovascular procedure (Fig. 38–41). Even though the probe design was clumsy and the protocol required a second intubation at two points in the procedure, images were acquired that enabled the surgeon to visualize abnormalities, such as flail mitral posterior leaflets, in the same orientation and aspect as under direct visualization. Incorporation of this method into a multiplane probe should ensure its universal dissemination.

FIGURE 38–41. See Color Plate 15.

Whether or not TEE becomes the most common way of obtaining a cardiac ultrasound examination will depend on parallel developments in transthoracic echocardiography. If research in chest wall imaging leads to considerably augmented image quality, TEE will remain the ancillary imaging method. Currently, expertise in TEE is not widely available. It is not uncommon for studies submitted to medical centers for a "second opinion" to be incomplete or suboptimal. Developments in digital image acquisition,

storage, and transmission may allow less experienced practitioners to obtain expert guidance during an examination by consulting an on-line expert from a remote site.

In summary, TEE is an established method of cardiac diagnosis. Although TEE requires considerable expertise and is semi-invasive, its robust growth attests to the ascendant importance of high image quality. There is little question that the applications of this technique will continue to widen.

References

1. Frazin, L., Talano, J.V., Stephanides, L., et al.: Esophageal echocardiography. Circulation 54:102, 1976.
2. Hanrath, P., Kremer, P., Langenstein, B.A., et al.: Transesophageal echocardiography. A new method for dynamic ventricle function analysis. Dtsch. Med. Wochenschr. 106:523, 1981.
3. Souquet, J., Hanrath, P., Zitelli, L., et al.: Transesophageal phased array for imaging the heart. IEEE Trans. Biomed. Eng. 29:707, 1982.
4. Schluter, M., Langenstein, B.A., Hanrath, P., et al.: Assessment of transesophageal pulsed Doppler echocardiography in the detection of mitral regurgitation. Circulation 66:784, 1982.
5. Schluter, M., Kremer, P., and Hanrath, P.: Transesophageal 2-D echocardiographic feature of flail mitral leaflet due to ruptured chordae tendineae. Am. Heart J. 108(3, Part 1):609, 1984.
6. Roizen, M.F., Beaupre, P.N., Alpert, R.A., et al.: Monitoring with two-dimensional transesophageal echocardiography. Comparison of myocardial function in patients undergoing supraceliac, suprarenal-infraceliac, or infrarenal aortic occlusion. J. Vasc. Surg. 1:300, 1984.
7. Beaupre, P.N., Kremer, P.F., Cahalan, M.K., et al.: Intraoperative detection of changes in left ventricular segmental wall motion by transesophageal two-dimensional echocardiography. Am. Heart J. 107(5, Part 1):1021, 1984.
8. Beaupre, P.N., Roizen, M.F., Cahalan, M.K., et al.: Hemodynamic and two-dimensional transesophageal echocardiographic analysis of an anaphylactic reaction in a human. Anesthesiology 60:482, 1984.
9. Omoto, R., Kyo, S., Matsumura, M., et al.: Bi-plane color transesophageal Doppler echocardiography (color TEE): Its advantages and limitations. Int. J. Card. Imaging 4:57, 1989.
10. Kyo, S., Koike, K., Takanawa, E., et al.: Impact of transesophageal Doppler echocardiography on pediatric cardiac surgery. Int. J. Card. Imaging 4:41, 1989.
11. Schneider, A.T., Hsu, T.L., Schwartz, S.L., et al.: Single, biplane, multiplane, and three-dimensional transesophageal echocardiography. Echocardiographic-anatomic correlations. Cardiol. Clin. 11:361, 1993.
12. Schiavone, W.A., Calafiore, P.A., and Salcedo, E.E.: Transesophageal Doppler echocardiographic demonstration of pulmonary venous flow velocity in restrictive cardiomyopathy and constrictive pericarditis. Am. J. Cardiol. 63:1286, 1989.
13. Hutchison, S.J., Smalling, R.G., Albornoz, M., et al.: Comparison of transthoracic and transesophageal echocardiography in clinically overt or suspected pericardial heart disease. Am. J. Cardiol. 74:962, 1994.
14. Mays, J.M., Nichols, B.A., Rubish, R.C., et al.: Transesophageal echocardiography: A sonographer's perspective. J. Am. Soc. Echocardiogr. 4:513, 1991.
15. Pearlman A.S.,Gardin, J.M., Martin, R.P., et al.: Guidelines for physician training in transesophageal echocardiography: Recommendations of the American Society of Echocardiography Committee for Physician Training in Echocardiography. J. Am. Soc. Echocardogr. 5:187, 1992.
16. Pearlman, A.S., Gardin, J.M., Martin, R.P., et al.: Guidelines for optimal physician training in echocardiography. Recommendations of the American Society of Echocardiography Committee for Physician Training in Echocardiography. Am. J. Cardiol. 60:158, 1987.
17. Daniel, W.G., Erbel, R., Kasper, W., et al.: Safety of transesophageal echocardiography. A multicenter survey of 10,419 examinations. Circulation 83:817, 1991.
18. Ofili, E.O., and Rich, S.W.: Safety and usefulness of transesophageal echocardiography in persons aged greater or equal to 70 years. Am. J. Cardiol. 66:1279, 1990.
19. Oh, J.K., Seward, J.B., Khandheria, B.K., et al.: Transesophageal echocardiography in critically ill patients. Am. J. Cardiol. 66:1479, 1990.
20. Khoury, A.F., Afridi, I., Quinones, M.A., et al.: Transesophageal echocardiography in critically ill patients: Feasibility, safety, and impact on management. Am. Heart J. 127:1363, 1994.
21. Pearson, A.C., Castello, R., and Labovitz, A.J.: Safety and utility of transesophageal echocardiography in critically ill patient. Am. Heart J. 119:1083, 1990.
22. Foster, E., and Schiller, N.B.: Transesophageal echocardiography in the critical care patient. Cardiol. Clin. 11:489, 1993.
23. Steckelberg, J.M., Khandheria, B.K., Anhalt, J.P., et al.: Prospective evaluation of the risk of bacteremia associated with transesophageal echocardiography (see Comments). Circulation 84:177, 1991.
24. Voller, H., Spielberg, C., Schroder, K., et al.: Frequency of positive blood culture during transesophageal echocardiography. Am. J. Cardiol. 68:1538, 1991.
25. Gorge, G., Erbel, R., Henrichs, K.J., et al.: Positive blood culture during transesophageal echocardiography. Am. J. Cardiol. 65:1404, 1990.
26. Melendez, L.J., Chan, K.L., Cheung, P.K., et al.: Incidence of bacteremia in transesophageal echocardiography: A positive study of 140 consecutive patients. J. Am. Coll. Cardiol. 18:1650, 1991.
27. Nikutta, P., Mantey-Stiers, F., Becht, I., et al.: Risk of bacteremia induced by transesophageal echocardiography: Analysis of 100 consecutive procedures. J. Am. Soc. Echocardiogr. 5:168, 1992.
28. Foster, E., Kusumoto, F.M., Sobol, S.M., et al.: Streptococcal endocarditis tem-

porally related to transesophageal echocardiography. J. Am. Soc. Echocardiogr. 3:424, 1990.
29. Roelandt, J.R., Thompson, I.R., Vletter W.B., et al.: Multiplane transesophageal echocardiography: Latest evolution in an imaging revolution. J. Am. Soc. Echocardiogr. 5:361, 1992.
30. Sloth, J.R., Pedersen, E.M., Nygaard, H., et al.: Multiplane transesophageal Doppler echocardiography measurements of the velocity profile in the human pulmonary artery. J. Am. Soc. Echocardiogr. 7:132, 1994.
31. Seward, J.B., Khandheria, B.K., Freeman, W.K., et al.: Multiplane transesophageal echocardiography: Image orientation, examination technique, anatomic correlations, and clinical applications. Mayo Clin. Proc. 68:523, 1993.
32. Jue, J., Winslow, T., Fazio, G., et al.: Pulsed Doppler characterization of left atrial appendage flow. J. Am. Soc. Echocardiogr. 6(3, Part 1):237, 1993.
33. Kuecherer, H.F., Muhiudeen, I.A., Kusumoto, F.M., et al.: Estimation of mean left atrial pressure from transesophageal pulsed Doppler echocardiography of pulmonary venous flow. Circulation 82:1127, 1990.
34. Sutton, D.C., and Cahalan, M.K.: Intraoperative assessment of left ventricular function with transesophageal echocardiography. Cardiol. Clin. 11(3):389, 1993.
35. Hoffman, P., Stumpter, O., Rydelwska-Sadowska, W., et al.: Transgastric imaging: A valuable addition of the assessment of congenital heart disease by transverse plane transesophageal echocardiography. J. Am. Soc. Echocardiogr. 6:35, 1993.
36. Stoddard, M.F., Arce, J., Liddel, N.E., et al.: Two-dimensional transesophageal echocardiography determination of aortic valve area in adults with aortic stenosis. Am. Heart J. 122:1415, 1991.
37. Braksator, W., Kuch, M., Drexler, M., et al.: Multi-plane transesophageal echocardiography: The next step to 3 dimensional imaging of the heart. Kardiol. Pol. 39:454, (Discussion 460), 1993.
38. Gysan, D., Braun, P., Park, J.W., et al.: Planimetric quantification of aortic valve stenosis using multiplanar transesophageal echocardiography. Z. Kardiol. 82:794, 1993.
39. Hoffmann, R., Flachskampf, F.A., and Hanrath, O.: Planimetry of orifice area in aortic stenosis using multiplane transesophageal echocardiography. J. Am. Coll. Cardiol. 22:529, 1993.
40. Roelandt, J.R., ten Cate, F.J., Vletter, W.B., et al.: Ultrasonic dynamic three-dimensional visualization of the heart with a multiplane transesophageal imaging transducer. J. Am. Soc. Echocardiogr. 7(3, Part 1):217, 1994.
41. Leung, J.M., and Levine, E.H.: Left ventricular end-systolic obliteration as an estimate of inoperative hypovolemia. Anesthesiology 81:1102, 1994.
42. Kikura, M., and Ikeda, K.: Comparison of effects of sevoflurane/nitrous oxide and enflurane/nitrous oxide on myocardial contractility in humans. Load-independent and noninvasive assessment with transesophageal echocardiography. Anesthesiology 79:235, 1993.
43. Houltz, E., Gustavsson, T., Caidahl, K., et al.: Effects of surgical stress and volatile anesthetics on left ventricular global and regional function in patients with coronary artery disease. Evaluation by computer-assisted two-dimensional quantitative transesophageal echocardiography. Aneth. Analg. 75:679, 1992.
44. Mitchell, M.M., Prakash, O., Rulf, E.N., et al.: Nitrous oxide does not induce myocardial ischemia in patients with ischemic heart disease and poor ventricular function. Anesthesiology 71:526, 1989.
45. Urbanowicz, J.H., Shaaban, M.J., Cohen, N.H., et al.: Comparison of transesophageal echocardiography and scintigraphic estimates of left ventricular end-diastolic volume index and ejection fraction in patients following coronary artery bypass grafting (see Comments). Anesthesiology 72:607, 1990.
46. Cahalan, M.K., Ionescu, P., Melton, H., Jr., et al.: Automated real-time analysis of intraoperative transesophageal echocardiograms. Anesthesiology 78:477, 1993.
47. Gorcsan, J., III., Gasior, T.A., Mandarino, W.A., et al.: On-line estimation of changes in left ventricular stroke volume by transesophageal echocardiographic automated border detection in patients undergoing coronary artery bypass grafting. Am. J. Cardiol. 72:721, 1993.
48. Marangelli, V., Pellegrini, C., Piccinni, G., et al.: On-line assessment of left ventricular function by automatic border detection echocardiography during rest and stress conditions. Cardiologia 38:701, 1993.
49. Lancee, C.T., Rijsterborgh, H., and Bom, N.: Monitoring aspects of an ultrasonic esophageal transducer. Initial experience. Med. Prog. Technol. 13:131, 1988.
50. Gorcsan, J., III., Denault, A., Gasior, T.A., et al.: Rapid estimation of left ventricular contractility from end-systolic relations by echocardiographic automated border detection and femoral arterial pressure. Anesthesiology 81:553, 1994.
51. Muhiudeen, L.A., Kuecherer, H.F., Lee, D., et al.: Intraoperative estimation of cardiac output by transesophageal pulsed Doppler echocardiography. Anesthesiology 74:9, 1991.
52. Izzat, M., Regragui, I.A., Wilde, P., et al.: Transesophageal echocardiographic measurements of cardiac output in cardiac surgical patients. Ann. Thorac. Surg. 58:1486, 1994.
53. Stoddard, M.F., Prince, C.R., Ammash, N., et al.: Pulsed Doppler transesophageal echocardiographic determination of cardiac output in human beings: Comparison with thermodilution technique. Am. Heart J. 126:956, 1993.
54. Kuecherer, H.F., and Foster, E.: Hemodynamics by transesophageal echocardiography. Cardiol. Clin. 11:475, 1993.
55. Gorcsan, J., III., Diana, P., Lee, J., et al.: Reversible diastolic dysfunction after successful coronary artery bypass surgery. Assessment by transesophageal Doppler echocardiography. Chest 106:1364, 1994.
56. Hoit, B.D., Shao, Y., Gabel, M., et al.: Influence of loading conditions and contractile state on pulmonary venous flow. Validation of Doppler velocimetry. Circulation 86:651, 1992.
57. Smith, J.S., Cahalan, M.K., Benefiel, D.J., et al.: Intraoperative detection of myocardial ischemia in high-risk patients: Electrocardiography versus two-dimensional transesophageal echocardiography. Circulation 72:1015, 1985.
58. Leung, J.M., O'Kelly, B., Browner, W.S., et al.: Prognostic importance of postbypass regional wall-motion abnormalities in patients undergoing coronary artery bypass graft surgery. SPI Research Group. Anesthesiology 71:16, 1989.
59. van Daele, M.E., Sutherland, G.R., Mitchell, M.M., et al.: Do changes in pulmonary capillary wedge pressure adequately reflect myocardial ischemia during anesthesia? A correlative preoperative hemodynamic, electrocardiographic, and transesophageal echocardiographic study. Circulation 81:865, 1990.
60. Atkov, O., Akchurin, R.S., Tkachuk, L.M., et al.: Intraoperative transesophageal echocardiography for detection of myocardial ischemia. Herz 18:372, 1993.
61. Eisenberg, M.J., London, M.J., and Leung, J.M.: Monitoring for myocardial ischemia during noncardiac surgery: A technology assessment of transesophageal echocardiography and 12-lead electrocardiography: The Study of the Perioperative Ischemia Research Group. JAMA 268:210, 1992.
62. Deutsch, H.J., Curtis, J.M., Leischik R., et al.: Diagnostic value of transesophageal echocardiography in cardiac surgery. Thorac. Cardiovasc. Surg. 39:199, 1991.
63. Kato, M., Nakashima, Y., Levine, J., et al.: Does transesophageal echocardiography improve postoperative outcome in patients undergoing coronary artery bypass surgery? J. Cardiothorac. Vasc. Anesth. 7:285, 1993.
64. Lambertz, H., Kreis, A., Trumper, H., et al.: Simultaneous transesophageal atrial pacing and transesophageal two-dimensional echocardiography: A new method of stress echocardiography (see Comments). J. Am. Coll. Cardiol. 16:1143, 1990.
65. Hoffmann, R., Lambertz, H., Kasmacher, H., et al.: Transoesophageal stress echocardiography for pre-operative detection of patients at risk of intraoperative myocardial ischemia. Eur. Heart J. 13:1482, 1992.
66. Hoffmann, R., Kleinhans, E., Lambertz, H., et al.: Transoesophageal pacing echocardiography for detection of restenosis after percutaneous transluminal coronary angioplasty. Eur. Heart J. 15:823, 1994.
67. Kamp, O., de Cock, C.C., van Eenige, M.J., et al.: Influence of pacing-induced myocardial ischemia on left atrial regurgitant jet: A transesophageal echocardiography study. J. Am. Coll. Cardiol. 23:1584, 1994.
68. Iliceto, S., Caiati, C., Ricci, A., et al.: Prediction of cardiac events after uncomplicated myocardial infarction by cross-sectional echocardiography during transesophageal atrial pacing. Int. J. Cardiol. 28:95, 1990.
69. Prince, C.R., Stoddard, M.F., Morris, G.T., et al.: Dobutamine two-dimensional transesophageal echocardiographic stress testing for detection of coronary artery disease. Am. Heart J. 128:36, 1994.
70. Biagini, A., Maffei, S., Baroni, M., et al.: Early assessment of coronary reserve after bypass surgery by dipyridamole transesophageal echocardiographic stress test. Am. Heart J. 120:1097, 1990.
71. Dillon, J.C., Feigenbaum, H., Konecke, L.L., et al.: Echocardiographic manifestation of valvular vegetations. Am. Heart J. 86:689, 1973.
72. Spangler, R.D., Johnson, M.L., Holmes, J.H., et al.: Echocardiographic demonstration of bacterial vegetations in active infective endocarditis. JCU J. Clin. Ultrasound 1:126, 1973.
73. Hirschfeld, D.S., and Schiller, N.: Localization of aortic valve vegetations by echocardiography. Circulation 53:280, 1976.
74. Peterson, S.P., Schiller, N., and Stricker, R.B.: Failure of two-dimensional echocardiography to detect aspergillus endocarditis. Chest 85:291, 1984.
75. Lichtlen, P.R., Gahl, K., and Daniel, W.G.: Infectious endocarditis: Clinical aspects and diagnosis. Schweiz. Med. Wochenschr. 114:1566, 1984.
76. Birmingham, G.D., Rahko, P.S., and Ballantyne, F., III: Improved detection of infective endocarditis with transesophageal echocardiography. Am. Heart J. 123:774, 1992.
77. Pedersen, W.R., Walker, M., Olson, J.D., et al.: Value of transesophageal echocardiography as an adjunct to transthoracic echocardiography in evaluation of native and prosthetic valve endocarditis. Chest 100:351, 1991.
78. Shively, B.K., Gurule, F.T., Roldan, C.A., et al.: Diagnostic value of transesophageal compared with transthoracic echocardiography in infective endocarditis. J. Am. Coll. Cardiol. 18:391, 1991.
79. Sochowski, R.A., and Chan, K.L.: Implication of negative results on a monoplane transesophageal echocardiographic study in patients with suspected infective endocarditis. (see Comments). J. Am. Coll. Cardiol. 21:216, 1993.
80. Shapiro, S.M., Young, E., De Guzman, S., et al.: Transesophageal echocardiography in the diagnosis of infective endocarditis (see Comments). Chest 105:377, 1994.
81. Lowry, R.W., Zoghbi, W.A., Baker, W.B., et al.: Clinical impact of transesophageal echocardiography in the diagnosis and management of infective endocarditis. Am. J. Cardiol. 73:1089, 1994.
82. Daniel, W.G., Mugge, A., Grote, J., et al.: Comparison of transthoracic and transesophageal echocardiography for detection of abnormalities of prosthetic and bioprosthetic valves in the mitral and aortic position. Am. J. Cardiol. 71:210, 1993.
83. Alton, M.E., Pasierski, T.J., Orsinelli, D.A., et al.: Comparison of transthoracic and transesophageal echocardiography in evaluation of 47 Starr-Edwards prosthetic valves. J. Am. Coll. Cardiol. 20:1503, 1992.
84. Zabalgoitia, M., Herrera, C.J., Chaudry, F.A., et al.: Improvement in the diagnosis of bioprosthetic valve dysfunction by transesophageal echocardiography. J. Heart Valve Dis. 2:595, 1993.
85. Rohmann, S., Erber, R., Darius, H., et al.: Prediction of rapid versus prolonged healing of infective endocarditis by monitoring vegetation size. J. Am. Soc. Echocardiogr. 4:465, 1991.
86. Mugge, A., Daniel, W.G., Frank, G., et al.: Echocardiography in infective endocarditis: Reassessment of prognostic implications of vegetation size determined by the transthoracic and the transesophageal approach. J. Am. Coll. Cardiol. 14:631, 1989.

87. Mugge, A.: Echocardiographic detection of cardiac valve vegetations and prognostic implications. Infect. Dis. Clin. North Am. 7:877, 1993.

88. Heinle, S., Wilderman, N., Harrison, J.K., et al.: Value of transthoracic echocardiography in predicting embolic events in active infective endocarditis. Duke Endocarditis Service. Am. J. Cardiol. 74:799, 1994.

89. Akins, E.W., Slone, R.M., Wiechmann, B.N., et al.: Perivalvular pseudoaneurysm complicating bacterial endocarditis: MR detection in five cases. A.T.R. 156:1155, 1991.

90. Daniel, W.G., Mugge, A., Martin, R.P., et al.: Improvement in the diagnosis of abscesses associated with endocarditis by transesophageal echocardiography (see Comments). N. Engl. J. Med. 324:795, 1991.

91. Teague, S.M., Heinsimer, J.A., Anderson, J.L., et al.: Quantification of aortic regurgitation utilizing continuous wave Doppler ultrasound. J. Am. Coll. Cardiol. 8:592, 1986.

92. Touche, T., Prasquier, R., Nitenberg, A., et al.: Assessment and follow-up of patients with aortic regurgitation by an updated Doppler echocardiographic measurement of the regurgitant fraction in the aortic arch. Circulation 72:819, 1985.

93. Perry, G.J., Helmcke, F., Nanda, N.C., et al.: Evaluation of aortic insufficiency by Doppler color flow mapping. J. Am. Coll. Cardiol. 9:952, 1987.

94. Helmcke, F., Nanda, N.C., Hsiung, M.C., et al.: Color Doppler assessment of mitral regurgitation with orthogonal planes. Circulation 75:175, 1987.

95. von Bibra, H., Becher, H., Frischke, et al.: Enhancement of mitral regurgitation and normal left atrial color Doppler flow signals with peripheral venous injection of a saccharide-based contrast agent. J. Am. Coll. Cardiol. 22:521, 1993.

96. Smith, M.D., Harrison, M.R., Pinton, R., et al.: Regurgitant jet size by transesophageal compared with transthoracic Doppler color flow imaging. Circulation 83:79, 1991.

97. Sutton, D.C., Kluger, R., Ahmed, S.U., et al.: Flow reversal in the descending aorta: A guide to intraoperative assessment of aortic regurgitation with transesophageal echocardiography. J. Thorac. Cardiovasc. Surg. 108:576, 1994.

98. Veyrat, C., Ameur, A., Gourtchiglouian, C., et al.: Calculation of pulsed Doppler left ventricular outflow tract regurgitant index for grading the severity of aortic regurgitation. Am. Heart J. 108(3, Part 1):507, 1984.

99. Hatle, L.: Doppler echocardiographic evaluation of mitral stenosis. Cardiol. Clin. 8:233, 1990.

100. Mugge, A., Kuhn, H., Nikutta, P., et al.: Assessment of left atrial appendage function by biplane transesophageal echocardiography in patients with nonrheumatic atrial fibrillation: Identification of a subgroup of patients at increased embolic risk. J. Am. Coll. Cardiol. 23:599, 1994.

101. Black, I.W., Hopkins, A.P., Lee, L.C., et al.: Left atrial spontaneous echo contrast: A clinical and echocardiographic analysis. J. Am. Coll. Cardiol. 18:398, 1991.

102. Chimowitz, M.I., DeGeorgia, M.A., Poole, R.M., et al.: Left atrial spontaneous echo contrast is highly associated with previous stroke in patients with atrial fibrillation or mitral stenosis. Stroke 24:1015, 1993.

103. Bernstein, N.E., Demopoulos, L.A., Tunick, P.A., et al.: Correlates of spontaneous echo contrast in patients with mitral stenosis and normal sinus rhythm. Am. Heart J. 128:287, 1994.

104. Fatkin, D., Herbert, E., and Feneley, M.P.: Hematologic correlates of spontaneous echo contrast in patients with atrial fibrillation and implications for thromboembolic risk. Am. J. Cardiol. 73:672, 1994.

105. Levin, T.N., Feldman, T., Bednarz, J., et al.: Transesophageal echocardiographic evaluation of mitral valve morphology to predict outcome after balloon mitral valvotomy. Am. J. Cardiol. 73:707, 1994.

106. Arora, R., Jolly, N., Kalra, G.S., et al.: Atrial septal defect after balloon mitral valvuloplasty: A transesophageal echocardiographic study. Angiology 44:217, 1993.

107. Kronzon, I., Tunick, P.A., Goldfarb, A., et al.: Echocardiographic and hemodynamic characteristics of atrial septal defects created by percutaneous valvuloplasty. J. Am. Soc. Echocardiogr. 3:64, 1990.

108. Lai, L.P., Shyu, K.G., Hsu, K.L., et al.: Bidirectional shunt through a residual atrial septal defect after percutaneous transvenous mitral commissurotomy. Cardiology 83:205, 1993.

109. Rittoo, D., Sutherland, G.R., and Shaw, T.R.: Quantification of left-to-right atrial shunting and defect size after balloon mitral commissurotomy using biplane transesophageal echocardiography, color flow Doppler mapping, and the principle of proximal flow convergence (see Comments). Circulation 87:1591, 1993.

110. Kircher, B.J., Himelman, R.B., and Schiller, N.B.: Noninvasive estimation of right atrial pressure from the inspiratory collapse of the inferior vena cava. Am. J. Cardiol. 66:493, 1990.

111. Perry, G.J., and Bouchard, A.: Doppler echocardiographic evaluation of mitral regurgitation. Cardiol. Clin. 8:265, 1990.

112. Blumlein, S., Bouchard, A., Schiller, N.B., et al.: Quantitation of mitral regurgitation by Doppler echocardiography. Circulation 74:306, 1986.

113. Himelman, R.B., Kusumoto, F., Oken, K., et al.: The flail mitral valve: Echocardiographic findings by precordial and transesophageal imaging and Doppler color flow mapping. J. Am. Coll. Cardiol. 17:272, 1991.

114. Kranidis, A., Koulouris, S., Filippatos, G., et al.: Mitral regurgitation from papillary muscle rupture: Role of transesophageal echocardiography (see Comments). J. Heart Valve Dis. 2:529, 1993.

115. Habib, G., Guidon, C., Tricoire, E., et al.: Papillary muscle rupture caused by bacterial endocarditis: Role of transesophageal echocardiography. J. Am. Soc. Echocardiogr. 7:79, 1994.

116. Schluter, M., Thier, W., Hinrichs, A., et al.: Clinical use of transesophageal echocardiography. Dtsch. Med. Wochenschr. 109:722, 1984.

117. Roldan, C.A., Shively, B.K., Lau, C.C., et al.: Systemic lupus erythematous valve disease by transesophageal echocardiography and the role of antiphospholipid antibodies. J. Am. Coll. Cardiol. 20:1127, 1992.

118. Schiller, N.B., Foster, E., and Redberg, R.F.: Transesophageal echocardiography in the evaluation of mitral regurgitation. The twenty-four signs of severe mitral regurgitation. Cardiol. Clin. 11:399, 1993.

119. Himelman, R.B., Stulbarg, M., Kircher, B., et al.: Noninvasive evaluation of pulmonary artery pressure during exercise by saline-enhanced Doppler echocardiography in chronic pulmonary disease. Circulation 79:863, 1989.

120. Grayburn, P.A., Fehske, W., Omran, H., et al.: Multiplane transesophageal echocardiographic assessment of mitral regurgitation by Doppler color flow mapping of the vena contracta. Am. J. Cardiol. 74:912, 1994.

121. Tribouilloy, C., Shen, W.F., Quere, J.P., et al.: Assessment of severity of mitral regurgitation by measuring regurgitant jet width at its origin with transesophageal Doppler color flow imaging. Circulation 85:1248, 1992.

122. Hwang, J.J., Shyu, K.G., Hsu, K.L., et al.: Significant mitral regurgitation is protective against left atrial spontaneous echo contrast formation, but not against systemic embolism. Chest 106:8, 1994.

123. Movsowitz, C., Movsowitz, H.D., Jacobs, L.E., et al.: Significant mitral regurgitation is protective against left atrial spontaneous echo contrast and thrombus as assessed by transesophageal echocardiography. J. Am. Soc. Echocardiogr. 6:107, 1993.

124. Castello, R., Lenzen, P., Aguirre, F., et al.: Quantitation of mitral regurgitation by transesophageal echocardiography with Doppler color flow mapping: Correlation with cardiac catheterization. J. Am. Coll. Cardiol. 19:1516, 1992.

125. Klein, A.L., Obarski, T.P., Stewart, W.J., et al.: Transesophageal Doppler echocardiography of pulmonary venous flow: A new marker of mitral regurgitation severity. J. Am. Coll. Cardiol. 18:518, 1991.

126. Klein, A.L., Stewart, W.J., Barlett, J., et al.: Effects of mitral regurgitation on pulmonary venous flow and left atrial pressure: An intraoperative transesophageal echocardiographic study. J. Am. Coll. Cardiol. 20:1345, 1992.

127. Klein, A.L., Bailey, A.S., Cohen, G.I., et al.: Importance of sampling both pulmonary veins in grading mitral regurgitation by transesophageal echocardiography. J. Am. Soc. Echocardiogr. 6:115, 1993.

128. Roach, J.M., Stajduhar, K.C., and Torrington, K.G.: Right upper lobe pulmonary edema caused by acute mitral regurgitation. Diagnosis by transesophageal echocardiography. Chest 103:1286, 1993.

129. Freeman, W.K., Schaff, H.V., Khandheria, B.K., et al.: Intraoperative evaluation of mitral valve regurgitation and repair by transesophageal echocardiography: Incidence and significance of systolic anterior motion. J. Am. Coll. Cardiol. 20:599, 1992.

130. Maurer, G., Siegel, R.J., and Czer, L.S: The use of color flow mapping for intraoperative assessment of value repair. Circulation 84(Suppl 3):1250, 1991.

131. San Roman, J.A., Vilacosta, I., Zamorano, J.L., et al.: Transesophageal echocardiography in right-sided endocarditis. J. Am. Coll. Cardiol. 21:1226, 1993.

132. Chappell, J.H.: Transesophageal echocardiography in right-sided endocarditis (letter). J. Am. Coll. Cardiol. 22:1751, 1993.

133. Cohen, G.I., Klein, A.L., Chan, K.L., et al.: Transesophageal echocardiographic diagnosis of right-sided cardiac masses in patients with central lines. Am. J. Cardiol. 70:925, 1992.

134. Winslow, T.M., Redberg, R.F., Foster, F., et al.: Transesophageal echocardiographic detection of abnormalities of the tricuspid valve in adults associated with spontaneous closure of perimembranous ventricular septal defect. Am. J. Cardiol. 79:967, 1992.

135. Kai, H., Koyanagi, S., Hirooka, Y., et al.: Right-to-left shunt across atrial septal defect related to tricuspid regurgitation: Assessment by transesophageal Doppler echocardiography. Am Heart J. 127:578, 1994.

136. Mehta, T., Achong, D.M., and Oates, E.: Septic pulmonary embolic from pulmonic valvular endocarditis demonstrated by serial ventilation-perfusion lung imaging. Clin. Nucl. Med. 18:11, 1994.

137. Soding, P.F., Klinck, J.R., Kong, A., et al.: Infective endocarditis of the pulmonary value following pulmonary artery catheterization. Intensive Care Med. 20:222, 1994.

138. Puleo, J.A., Shammas, N.W., Kelly, P., et al.: Lactobacillus isolated pulmonic valve endocarditis with ventricular septal defect by transesophageal echocardiography. Am. Heart J. 128(6, Part 1):1248, 1994.

139. Winslow, T., Foster, E., Adams, J.R., et al.: Pulmonary valve endocarditis: Improved diagnosis with biplane transesophageal echocardiography. J. Am. Soc. Echocardiogr. 5:206, 1992.

140. Shapiro, S.M., Young, E., Ginzton, L.E., et al.: Pulmonic valve endocarditis as an underdiagnosed disease: Role of transesophageal echocardiography. J. Am. Soc. Echocardiogr. 5:48, 1992.

141. Kumar, N., Gallo, R., Gometza, B., et al.: Pulmonary autograft for aortic valve replacement in rheumatic disease: An ideal solution? J. Heart Valve Dis. 3:384, 1994.

142. Kouchoukos, N.T., Davila-Roman, V.G., Spray, T.L., et al.: Replacement of the aortic root with a pulmonary autograft in children and young adults with aortic-valve disease (see Comments). N. Engl. J. Med. 330:1, 1994.

143. Khandheria, B.K.: Transesophageal echocardiography in the evaluation of prosthetic valves. Cardiol. Clin. 11:427, 1993.

144. Dilip, K.A., Vachaspathy, P., Clarke, B., et al.: Haemolysis following mitral valve repair. J. Cardiovasc. Surg. 33:568, 1992.

145. Smith, R.E., and Berg, D.: Occult paravalvular leak in a clinically normal St. Jude's mitral valve presenting with life-threatening microangiopathic hemolytic anemia. J. Cardiovasc. Surg. 32:56, 1991.

146. Enzenauer, R.J., Berenberg, J.L., and Cassell, P., Jr.: Microangiopathic hemolytic anemia as the initial manifestation of porcine valve failure. South Med. J. 83:912, 1990.

147. Akamatsu, S., Ueda, N., Terazawa, E., et al.: Mitral prosthetic dehiscence with laminar regurgitation flow signals assessed by transesophageal echocardiography. Chest 104:1911, 1993.

148. Vitale, N., Renzulli, A., Cerasuolo, F., et al.: Prosthetic valve obstruction: Thrombolysis versus operation. Ann. Thorac. Surg. 57:365, 1994.

149. Dzavik, V., Cohen, G., and Chan, K.L.: Role of transesophageal echocardiography in the diagnosis and management of prosthetic valve thrombosis. J. Am. Coll. Cardiol. 18:1829, 1991.

150. Barton, C.W., Eisenberg, M.J., and Schiller, N.: Transesophageal echocardiographic diagnosis of massive pulmonary embolism during cardiopulmonary resuscitation. Am. Heart J. 127:1639, 1994.

151. Klein, A.L., Stewart, W.C., Cosgrove, D., III., et al.: Visualization of acute pulmonary emboli by transesophageal echocardiography. J. Am. Soc. Echocardiogr. 3:412, 1990.

152. Hunter, J.J., Johnson, K.R., Karagianes, T.G., et al.: Detection of massive pulmonary embolus-in-transit by transesophageal echocardiography. Chest 100:1210, 1991.

153. Dittrich, H.C., McCann, H.A., and Blanchard, D.G.: Cardiac structure and function in chronic thromboembolic pulmonary hypertension. Am. J. Card. Imaging 8:18, 1994.

154. Dressler, F.A., and Labovitz, A.J.: Systemic arterial embolic and cardiac masses. Assessment with transesophageal echocardiography. Cardiol. Clin. 11:447, 1993.

155. Stoddard, M.F., Liddel, N.E., Longaker, R.A., et al.: Transesophageal echocardiography: Normal variants and mimickers. Am. Heart J. 124:1587, 1992.

156. Alam, M., and Sun, I.: Transesophageal echocardiographic evaluation of left atrial mass lesions. J. Am. Soc. Echocardiogr. 4:323, 1991.

157. Shyu, K.G., Chen, J.J., Cheng, J.J., et al.: Comparison of transthoracic and transesophageal echocardiography in the diagnosis of intracardiac tumors in adults. J. Clin. Ultrasound 22:381, 1994.

158. Narang, J., Neustein, S., and Israel, D.: The role of transesophageal echocardiography in the diagnosis and excision of a tumor of the aortic valve. J. Cardiothorac. Vasc. Anesth. 6;68, 1992.

159. Thomas, M.R., Jayakrishnan, A.G., Desai, J., et al.: Transesophageal echocardiography in the detection and surgical management of a papillary fibroelastoma of the mitral valve causing partial mitral valve obstruction. J. Am. Soc. Echocardiogr. 6:83, 1993.

160. Ports, T.A., Schiller, N.B., and Strunk, B.L.: Echocardiography of right ventricular tumors. Circulation 56:439, 1977.

161. Alam, M., Sun, I., and Smith, S.: Transesophageal echocardiographic evaluation of right atrial mass lesions. J. Am. Soc. Echocardiogr. 4:331, 1991.

162. Allen, G., Klingman, R., Ferraris, V.A., et al.: Transesophageal echocardiography in the surgical management of renal cell carcinoma with intracardiac extension. J. Cardiovasc. Surg. 32:833, 1991.

163. Hasnain, J.U., and Watson, R.J.: Transesophageal echocardiography during resection of renal cell carcinoma involving the inferior vena cava. South Med. J. 87:273, 1994.

164. Treiger, B.F., Humphrey, L.S., Peterson, C., Jr., et al.: Transesophageal echocardiography in renal cell carcinoma: An accurate diagnostic technique for intracaval neoplastic extension. J. Urol. 145:1138, 1991.

165. Van Camp, G., Abdulsater, J., Cosyns B., et al.: Transesophageal echocardiography of right atrial metastasis of a hepatocellular carcinoma. Chest 105:945, 1994.

166. Pearson, A.C., Labovitz, A.J., Tatineni, S., et al.: Superiority of transesophageal echocardiography in detecting cardiac source of embolism in patients with cerebral ischemia of uncertain etiology. J. Am. Coll. Cardiol. 17:66, 1991.

167. Klotzsch, C., Janssen, G., and Berlit, P.: Transesophageal echocardiography and contrast-TCD in the detection of a patent foramen ovale: Experiences with 111 patients. Neurology 44:1603, 1994.

168. Konstadt, S.N., and Louie, E.K.: Echocardiographic diagnosis of paradoxical embolism and the potential for right to left shunting. Am. J. Card. Imaging 8:28, 1994.

169. DeRook, F.A., Comess, K.A., Alber, G.W., et al.: Transesophageal echocardiography in the evaluation of stroke. Ann. Intern. Med. 117:922, 1992.

170. Schneider, B., Hanrath, P., Vogel, P., et al.: Improved morphologic characterization of atrial septal aneurysm by transesophageal echocardiography: Relation to cerebrovascular events. J. Am. Coll. Cardiol. 16:1000, 1990.

171. Schneider, B., Hofmann, T., Meinertz, T., et al.: Diagnostic value of transesophageal echocardiography in atrial aneurysm. Int. J. Card. Imaging 8:143, 1992.

172. Zarauza, M.J., Alonso, F., Hildalgo, M., et al.: Lipomatous hypertrophy of the interatrial septum simulating an atrial mass in a patient with a pulmonary embolism: Its diagnosis by transesophageal echocardiography and percutaneous biopsy. Rev. Esp. Cardial. 46:761, 1993.

173. Jornet, A., Batalla, J., Reig, J., et al.: Lipomatous hypertrophy of the interatrial septum. Report of 2 cases reported in vivo. Rev. Esp. Cardiol. 45:601, 1992.

174. Amerenco, P., Cohen, A., Tzourio, C., Bertrand, B., et al.: Atherosclerotic disease of the aortic arch and the risk of ischemic stroke [see comments]. N. Engl. J. Med. 331:147, 1994.

175. Toyoda, K., Yasaka, M., Nagata, S., et al.: Aortogenic embolic stroke: A transesophageal echocardiographic approach. Stroke 23:1056, 1992.

176. Manning, W.J., Silverman, D.I., Gordon, S.P., et al.: Cardioversion from the atrial fibrillation without prolonged anticoagulation with the use of transesophageal echocardiography to exclude the presence of atrial thrombi (see Comments). N. Engl. J. Med. 328:750, 1993.

177. Black, I.W., Hopkins, A.P., Lee, L.C., et al.: Evaluation of transesophageal echocardiography before cardioversion of atrial fibrillation in noncoagulated patients. Am. Heart J. 126:375, 1993.

178. Missault, L., Jordaens, L., Gheeraert, P., et al.: Embolic stroke after unanticoagu-

179. Salka, S., Saeian, K., Sagar, K.B., et al.: Cerebral thromboembolization after cardioversion of atrial fibrillation in patients without transesophageal echocardiographic findings of left atrial thrombus. Am. Heart J. 126(3 Part 1):722, 1993.

180. Grimm, R.A., Stewart, W.J., Maloney, J.D., et al.: Impact of electrical cardioversion for atrial fibrillation on left atrial appendage function and spontaneous echo contrast: Characterization by simultaneous transesophageal echocardiography. J. Am. Coll. Cardiol. 22:1359, 1993.

181. Fazio, G.P., Redberg, R.F., Winslow, T., et al.: Transesophageal echocardiography detected atherosclerotic aortic plaque is a marker for coronary artery disease. J. Am. Coll. Cardiol. 21:144, 1993.

182. Tribouilloy, C., Shen, W.F., Peltier, M., et al.: Noninvasive prediction of coronary artery disease by transesophageal echocardiographic detection of thoracic aortic plaque in valvular heart disease. Am. J. Cardiol. 74:258, 1994.

183. Redberg, R.F., and Schiller, N.B.: Use of transesophageal echocardiography in evaluating coronary arteries. Cardiol. Clin. 11:521, 1993.

184. Iliceto, S., Marangelli, V., Memmola, C., et al.: Transesophageal Doppler echocardiography evaluation of coronary blood flow velocity in baseline conditions and during dipyridamole-induced coronary vasodilation (see Comments). Circulation 83:61, 191.

185. Iliceto, S., Caiati, C., Aragona, P., et al.: Improved Doppler signal intensity in coronary arteries after intravenous peripheral injection of a lung-crossing contrast agent (SHU 508A) (see Comments). Am. Coll. Cardiol. 23:184, 1994.

186. Redberg, R.F.: Coronary flow by transesophageal Doppler echocardiography: Do saccharide-based contrast agents sweeten the pot? (Editorial; Comment). J. Am. Coll. Cardiol. 23:191, 1994.

187. Darmon P.L., Hillel, Z., Mogtader, A., et al.: Cardiac output by transesophageal echocardiography using continuous-wave Doppler across the aortic valve. Anesthesiology 80:796 (Discussion 25A), 1994.

188. Kuecherer, H.F., Kusumoto, F., Muhiudeen, I.A., et al.: Pulmonary venous flow patterns by transesophageal pulsed Doppler echocardiography: Relation to parameters of left ventricular systolic and diastolic function. Am. Heart J. 122:1683, 1991.

189. Nishimura, R.A., Abel, M.D., Hatle, L.K., et al.: Relation of pulmonary vein to mitral flow velocities by transesophageal Doppler echocardiography. Effect of different loading conditions. Circulation 81:1488, 1990.

190. Rossvoll, O., and Hatle, L.K.: Pulmonary venous flow velocities recorded by transthoracic Doppler ultrasound: Relation to left ventricular diastolic pressures (see Comments). J. Am. Coll. Cardiol. 21:1687, 1993.

191. Kusumoto, F.M., Muhiudeen, I.A., Kuecherer, H.F., et al.: Response of the interatrial septum to transatrial pressure gradients and its potential for predicting pulmonary capillary wedge pressure: An intraoperative study using transesophageal echocardiography in patients during mechanical ventilation. J. Am. Coll. Cardiol. 21:721, 1993.

192. Foster, E., and Schiller, N.B.: The role of transesophageal echocardiography in critical care: USCF experience. J. Am. Soc. Echocardiolgr. 5:368, 1992.

193. Goldman, A.P., Glover, M.U., Mick, W., et al.: Role of echocardiography/Doppler in cardiogenic shock: Silent mitral regurgitation. Ann. Thorac. Surg. 52:296, 1991.

194. Topaz, O., and Taylor, A.L.: Interventricular septal rupture complicating acute myocardial infarction: From pathophysiologic features to the role of invasive and noninvasive diagnostic modalities in current management. Am. J. Med. 93:683, 1992.

195. Redberg, R.F., Tucker, K., and Schiller, N.B.: Transesophageal echocardiography during cardiopulmonary resuscitation. Cardiol. Clin. 11:529, 1993.

196. Redberg, R.F., Tucker, K.J., Cohen, T.J., et al.: Physiology of blood flow during cardiopulmonary resuscitation. A transesophageal echocardiographic study. Circulation 88:534, 1993.

197. Erbel, R.: Role of transesophageal echocardiography in dissection of the aorta and evaluation of degenerative aortic disease. Cardiol. Clin. 11:461, 1993.

198. Adachi, H., Kyo, S., Takamoto, S., et al.: Early diagnosis and surgical intervention of acute aortic dissection by transesophageal color flow mapping. Circulation 82(Suppl. 5):IV19, 1990.

199. Adachi, H., Omoto, R., Kyo, S., et al.: Emergency surgical intervention of acute aortic dissection with the rapid diagnosis by transesophageal echocardiography. Circulation 84(Suppl. 5):III14, 1991.

200. Kyo, S., Takamoto, S., Omoto, R., et al.: Intraoperative echocardiography for diagnosis and treatment of aortic dissection. Utility of color flow mapping for surgical decision making in acute stage. Herz 17:377, 1992.

201. Omoto, R., Kyo, S., Matsumura, M., et al.: Evaluation of biplane color Doppler transesophageal echocardiography in 200 consecutive patients. Circulation 85:1237, 1992.

202. Chan, K.L.: Impact of transesophageal echocardiography on the treatment of patients with aortic dissection (see Comments). Chest 101:406, 1992.

203. Chirillo, F., Cavallini, C., Longhini, C., et al.: Comparative diagnostic value of transesophageal echocardiography and retrograde aortography in the evaluation of thoracic aortic dissection. Am. J. Cardiol. 74:590, 1994.

204. Erbel, R., Mohr-Kahaly, S., Rennollet, H., et al.: Diagnosis of aortic dissection: The value of transesophageal echocardiography. Thorac. Cardiovasc. Surg. 35(SI):126, 1987.

205. De Simone, R., Haberbosch, W., Iarussi, D., et al.: Transesophageal echocardiography for the diagnosis of thoracic aorta aneurysms and dissections. Cardiologia 35:387, 1990.

206. Deutsch, H.J., Sechtem, U., Meyer, H., et al.: Chronic aortic dissection: Comparison of MR imaging and transesophageal echocardiography. Radiology 192:645, 1994.

207. Nienader, C.A., Spielmann, R.P., von Kodolitsch, Y., et al.: Diagnosis of thoracic

aortic dissection. Magnetic resonance imaging versus transesophageal echocardiography. Circulation 85:434, 1992.

208. Erbel, R., Oelert, H., Meyer, J., et al.: Effect of medical and surgical therapy on aortic dissection evaluated by transesophageal echocardiography. Implications for prognosis and therapy. The European Cooperative Study Group on Echocardiography (see Comments). Circulation 87:1604, 1993.

209. Mohr-Kahaly, S., Erbel, R., Kearney, P., et al.: Aortic intramural hemorrhage visualized by transesophageal echocardiography: Findings and prognostic implications. J. Am. Coll. Cardiol. 23:658, 1994.

210. Robbins, R.C., McManus, R.P., Mitchell, R.S., et al.: Management of patients with intramural hematoma of the thoracic aorta. Circulation 88(5, Part 2):III, 1993.

211. Thoele, D.G.: Anomalous inferior vena cava mimicking aortic dissection on transesophageal echocardiography. (Letter). Clin. Cardiol. 16:A12, 1993.

212. Torbicki, A., Jakubowska-Najniger, M., Stanislawska, J., et al.: Anomalous inferior vena cava mimicking aortic dissection on transesophageal echocardiography. Clin. Cardiol. 16:571, 1993.

213. Kronzon, I., Demopoulos, L., Schrem, S.S., et al.: Pitfalls in the diagnosis of thoracic aortic aneurysm by transesophageal echocardiography. J. Am. Soc. Echocardiogr. 3:145, 1990.

214. Shapiro, M.J., Yanofsky, S.D., Trapp, J., et al.: Cardiovascular evaluation in blunt thoracic trauma using transesophageal echocardiography (TEE) (see Comments). J. Trauma 31:835 (Discussion 839), 1991.

215. Brooks, S.W., Young, J.C., Cmolik, B., et al.: The use of transesophageal echocardiography in the evaluation of chest trauma. J. Trauma 32:761 (Discussion 765), 1992.

216. Kuwagata, Y., Sugimoto, H., Yoshioka, T., et al.: Left ventricular performance in patients with thermal injury or multiple trauma: A clinical study with echocardiography. J. Trauma 32:158 (Discussion 164), 1992.

217. Sparks, M.B., Burchard, K.W., Marrin, C.A., et al.: Transesophageal echocardiography. Preliminary results in patients with traumatic aortic rupture. Arch. Surg. 12:711 (Discussion 713), 1991.

218. Smith, M.D., Cassidy, J.M., Souther, S., et al.: Transesophageal echocardiography in the diagnosis of traumatic rupture of the aorta. N. Engl. J. Med. 332:356, 1995.

219. Kearney, P.A., Smith, D.W., Johnson, S.B., et al.: Use of transesophageal echocardiography in the evaluation of traumatic aortic injury. J. Trauma 34:696 (Discussion 701), 1993.

220. Muhiudeen, I.A., Roberson, D.A., Silverman, N.H., et al.: Intraoperative echocardiography for evaluation of congenital heart defects in infants and children (see Comments). Anesthesiology 76:165, 1992.

221. Muhiudeen, I.A., Roberson, D.A., Silverman, N.H., et al.: Intraoperative echocardiography in infants and children with congenital cardiac shunt lesions: Transesophageal versus epicardial echocardiography. J. Am. Coll. Cardiol. 16:1687, 1990.

222. Stevenson, J.G., Sorensen, G.K., Gartman, D.M., et al.: Transesophageal echocardiography during repair of congenital cardiac defects: Identification of residual problems necessitating reoperation. J. Am. Soc. Echocardiogr. 6:356, 1993.

223. Stumper, O.F., Elzenga, N.J., Hess, J., et al.: Transesophageal echocardiography in children with congenital heart disease: An initial experience. J. Am. Coll. Cardiol. 16:433, 1990.

224. Marelli, A.J., Child, J.S., and Perloff, J.K.: Transesophageal echocardiography in congenital heart disease in the adult. Cardiol. Clin. 11:505, 1993.

225. Ritter, S.B.: Transesophageal real-time echocardiography in infants and children with congenital heart disease. J. Am. Coll. Cardiol. 18:569, 1991.

226. Mehta, R.H., Helmcke, F., Nanda, N.C., et al.: Transesophageal Doppler color flow mapping assessment of atrial septal defect. J. Am. Coll. Cardiol. 16:1010, 1990.

227. Mehta, R.H., Helmcke, F., Nanda, N.C., et al.: Uses and limitations of transthoracic echocardiography in the assessment of atrial septal defect in the adult. Am. J. Cardiol. 67:288, 1991.

228. Foster, E., Redberg, R.F., and Schiller, N.B.: "Unroofing" the heart and aorta using 3-dimensional echocardiography. Circulation 88:349A, 1993.

CHAPTER

39 Intraoperative Echocardiography

William J. Stewart, M.D.

UNIQUE APPLICABILITY OF ECHOCARDIOGRAPHY TO INTRAOPERATIVE USE _____ 567
INTRAOPERATIVE ECHOCARDIOGRAPHIC METHODS _____ 567
Ultrasound Technology Applicable to Intraoperative Use _____ 567
Transesophageal Imaging Systems and Image Orientation _____ 567
The Complete Transesophageal Echocardiography Study _____ 568
Epicardial Echocardiographic Techniques and Imaging Planes _____ 568
Direct Epivascular Imaging of the Ascending Aorta _____ 569
Record Keeping and Communication for Intraoperative Echocardiography _____ 569
TRAINING FOR INTRAOPERATIVE ECHOCARDIOGRAPHY _____ 569
CHARACTERIZING VALVULAR AND VENTRICULAR FUNCTION WITH INTRAOPERATIVE ECHOCARDIOGRAPHY _____ 569
Quantifying Valvular Stenosis _____ 569
Quantitating Valvular Regurgitation _____ 570
Assessing Ventricular Systolic and Diastolic Function With Intraoperative Echocardiography _____ 570
PREPUMP INTRAOPERATIVE ECHOCARDIOGRAPHY IN VALVULAR SURGERY _____ 570
Echocardiographic Definition of the Mechanism of Valve Dysfunction _____ 570

Dependence of Severity of Valve Dysfunction on Loading Conditions _____ 570
Frequency of Changes in Surgery Based on Prepump Intraoperative Echocardiography _____ 571
POSTPUMP INTRAOPERATIVE ECHOCARDIOGRAPHY IN VALVULAR SURGERY _____ 571
Criteria for a Second Pump Run _____ 571
Complications Definable With Intraoperative Echocardiography _____ 571
Impact of Transesophageal Echocardiography Results on Postoperative Outcome _____ 571
INTRAOPERATIVE TRANSESOPHAGEAL ECHOCARDIOGRAPHY IN SPECIFIC VALVE OPERATIONS _____ 572
Valve Repair for Mitral Regurgitation _____ 572
Valvuloplasty and Balloon Valvulotomy for Mitral Rheumatic Valve Disease _____ 572
Valve Repair for Tricuspid Regurgitation _____ 573
Valve Repair for Aortic Regurgitation _____ 573
Stentless Human and Bioprosthetic Valves _____ 573
Standard Valve Replacement Surgery _____ 573
MYECTOMY FOR HYPERTROPHIC OBSTRUCTIVE CARDIOMYOPATHY _____ 573
SURGERY FOR CONGENITAL HEART DISEASE _____ 574
The Latest Arena to Shift from Epicardial Echocardiography to Transesophageal Echocardiography _____ 574

Changes in Operative Approach to Congenital
    Heart Surgery Based on Prepump and
    Postpump Intraoperative
    Echocardiography _____ 575
CORONARY ARTERY SURGERY _____ 575
Diagnosis of Intraoperative Ischemia _____ 575
Intraoperative Contrast
    Echocardiography _____ 576
Epicardial Visualization of Coronary
    Arteries _____ 576
TRANSPLANTATION AND SURGERY FOR SEVERE
    MYOCARDIAL DYSFUNCTION _____ 576
SURGERY FOR CARDIAC TRAUMA _____ 576
SURGERY FOR THORACIC AORTIC ANEURYSM
    OR DISSECTION _____ 576

Preoperative Diagnosis of Aortic Aneurysm or
    Dissection _____ 576
Intraoperative Echocardiography in Thoracic
    Aortic Aneurysm Surgery _____ 577
INTRAOPERATIVE MANAGEMENT OF FISTULAS
    DUE TO ENDOCARDITIS _____ 577
INTRAOPERATIVE DETECTION OF AORTIC
    ATHEROMA _____ 577
LIMITATIONS OF INTRAOPERATIVE
    ECHOCARDIOGRAPHY _____ 577
NEW ULTRASOUND TECHNOLOGY FOR FUTURE
    INTRAOPERATIVE USE _____ 578
CONCLUSIONS _____ 578

UNIQUE APPLICABILITY OF ECHOCARDIOGRAPHY TO INTRAOPERATIVE USE

The use of cardiac ultrasound to image the heart and great vessels during cardiac surgery is a logical extension of its increasingly useful role outside the operating room. Intraoperative echocardiography (IOE) is exciting because of its dramatic potential to have an immediate impact on patient outcome, probably more so than any other type of cardiovascular imaging.

Echocardiography has several advantages over other imaging modalities that are potentially applicable intraoperatively. The small ultrasound transducer can easily be introduced via the transesophageal echocardiography (TEE) approach or applied directly to the epicardial surface without major disruption of the operative process. In addition, echocardiography provides instantaneous images not requiring processing time. Echocardiography creates understandable images of cardiac and vascular anatomy, characterizes valvular morphology, estimates the severity of valvular stenosis and regurgitation, and characterizes ventricular systolic and diastolic function.

Studies performed immediately prior to cardiopulmonary bypass (*prepump*) help formulate surgical plans on the basis of current, accurate information about anatomy and physiology[1, 2] and provide a baseline for comparison after the surgery is completed. The findings of echocardiography following pulmonary bypass (*postpump*) may mandate immediate changes in surgical therapy in a percentage of cases,[3–6] which may prevent the need for subsequent reoperation and are predictive of subsequent outcome.[2, 7, 8]

This chapter focuses on the ability of IOE to assist with decision-making in patients undergoing surgery for valve repair, valve replacement, and coronary, myocardial, or congenital abnormalities.

INTRAOPERATIVE ECHOCARDIOGRAPHIC METHODS

Ultrasound Technology Applicable to Intraoperative Use

Echocardiograpic images contain information about cardiac structure and function. Principles of cardiac ultrasound used in standard transthoracic imaging are equally applicable during cardiac surgery. One must be careful to address each question with the appropriate ultrasound tool.

The *structure* of the heart, including the thickness and motion of walls, valves, or vascular structures, is imaged using M-mode and two-dimensional echocardiography utilizing the *amplitude* of reflections assessed from each location within the imaging field. *Flow* within the heart is imaged with Doppler echocardiography by assessing the *frequency shifts* of ultrasound reflections. Continuous-wave Doppler ultrasound can be used to measure maximum velocity of flow and thereby estimate pressure gradients. This requires parallel or nearly parallel alignment between the ultrasound beam and the direction of high-velocity flow. Pulsed Doppler is useful for looking at the time-varying velocity at one site within a vessel or chamber. Doppler color flow imaging is useful for spatial mapping of flow for evaluation of intracardiac shunts and valvular regurgitation. M-mode and color M-mode echocardiography are useful for timing cardiac motion and flow, respectively.

Instrument controls such as gain, transducer frequency, pulse repetition frequency, image angle, pulses per line, and depth must be appropriately chosen and optimized. The frame rate and sampling rate have a great impact on image quality and diagnostic potential. Attention must be given to the potential for ultrasound artifacts and aliasing. When surveying three-dimensional flow disturbances or cardiac structures with a one- or two-dimensional technique, the importance of using multiple image planes cannot be overemphasized.[9, 10]

Transesophageal Imaging Systems and Image Orientation

Modern applications of IOE began with the availability of color flow Doppler imaging with epicardial echocardiography, which preceded the availability of color flow mapping from TEE. In recent years, however, TEE has grown to become the method of choice for more than 90 percent of routine intraoperative imaging at the Cleveland Clinic (Fig. 39–1). TEE has several advantages over epicardial imaging—of great practical importance, the transducer does not enter the sterile field, and the study interferes less with the surgeon's activities.

A transesophageal transducer is a flexible endoscope with a set of crystals mounted on the tip. I use 3.5- to 5-MHz transducers for adults and 5- to 7-MHz transducers for children. After induction of anesthesia and endotracheal intubation, I suction the stomach, remove the nasogastric tube, lubricate the oropharynx with water-soluble gel, and insert the transducer into the esophagus. Insertion is performed blindly or with laryngoscopic guidance and is much easier and safer to carry out before placement of the anesthetic curtain and sterile drapes.

TEE is a safe procedure that adds much value when compared with the tiny risk to the patient.[11] Examination of the esophageal mucosa with fiberoptic endoscopy or autopsy within 24 hours of TEE has demonstrated no significant esophageal abnormalities.[12] Because of the rare incidence of esophageal or oropharyngeal trauma, however, caution is advised so that excessive force is avoided when placing the transducer.

TEE systems include three varieties: monoplane, biplane (with two planes perpendicular to each other), and multiplane (with one plane that can be rotated around 180 degrees). The standard

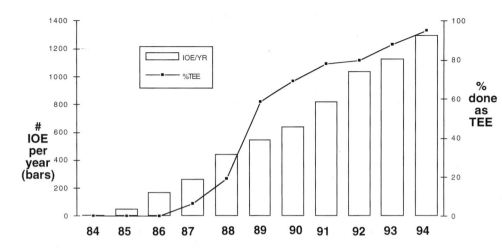

FIGURE 39-1. Growth in the number of intraoperative echocardiography (IOE) studies per year *(bars)* and in transesophageal echocardiography (TEE) as a percentage of intraoperative studies *(connected dots)* in 6340 patients studied from 1984 to 1994 at the Cleveland Clinic.

transverse transesophageal plane emanates from the scope with the image oriented perpendicular to the axis of the endoscope. The standard orientation is to have the near field at the top of the image. Therefore, the transverse orientation views the planes as if looking from a superior to an inferior direction. The view of the aortic valve is similar to the surgeon's view during an aortotomy, except that it is rotated about 180 degrees, with the posterior aspect of the image at the top and the left side of the patient to the right of the image. A set of transverse planes related to each other like a stack of coins can be obtained by pushing or pulling the probe to different levels of the esophagus, from the most inferior portion of the left ventricle (40 to 50 cm depth from the teeth) to the top of the aortic arch (18 to 22 cm depth). Variations in each plane may be obtained by slight rotations of the endoscope itself and minor flexion of the tip of the endoscope. Anterior flexion may be necessary for certain planes that are important for intraoperative diagnosis, such as the transgastric short-axis view of the mitral valve (Fig. 39–2). Flexion of the transverse plane to the patient's left is necessary to obtain a good short-axis view of the aortic valve.

Biplane transesophageal probes include the same crystal array for the transverse planes plus a second *longitudinal* set of crystals stacked proximal to the first set and oriented parallel to the long axis of the endoscope. Thus, the longitudinal image is oriented parallel to the axis of the endoscope. When the position of this plane is varied by rotation of the transducer, the image planes are related to each other like the positions of a door on a hinge.

Longitudinal views of the heart also show the near field at the top of the image, with more superior structures to the right of the image. The longitudinal image may require slight further adjustments; for example, flexion to the patient's left to obtain a long-axis view of the aortic valve.

Multiplane TEE transducers have a single linear array of crystals that can be moved with a tiny motor to rotate the plane around a line emanating at right angles from the axis of the scope. The transverse equivalent plane represents 0 degrees on the multiplane protractor. The longitudinal plane represents 90 degrees. The plane can be rotated from angles of 0 to 180 degrees, which is the transverse plane flipped right to left. To more fully understand in three dimensions the topography of a specific cardiac structure or flow pattern, it can be positioned in the middle of the image and observed during rotation of the multiplane image through all possible angles.

The Complete Transesophageal Echocardiography Study

For every patient, I begin the study by applying Willie Sutton's law, by "going for the money," answering first the most important clinical questions for that case. If the hemodynamics or the conditions for echocardiographic imaging deteriorate, at least the essential answers will be available. Thereafter, I advocate proceeding systematically through all four chambers, all four valves, and the great vessels, examining each in long- and short-axis views. Each portion is examined for its structural and flow characteristics.

Epicardial Echocardiographic Techniques and Imaging Planes

Epicardial echocardiography provides another intraoperative window to the heart and great vessels. In many respects, it is complementary to transesophageal imaging for intraoperative diagnosis. The complete IOE team should be capable of using either modality, as the situation demands. Although TEE has become the dominant modality, some disease states, including left ventricular outflow tract obstruction and ascending aortic atherosclerosis, are still best imaged with epicardial echocardiography. Epicardial echocardiography is also useful in situations in which TEE images cannot be obtained or are of inadequate quality.

For epicardial imaging of valvular, myocardial, and congenital abnormalities in adults, I use standard transthoracic transducers with frequencies of 2 to 5 MHz, mostly 3.5 MHz. Contamination of the sterile field is prevented by placing the transducer inside two sterile sleeves separated by sterile gel. The alternative, cold gas sterilization using ethylene oxide at a temperature of 100° F is awkward because it requires 48 hours of shelf time to allow gases to escape.

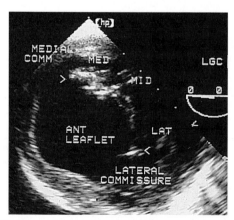

FIGURE 39-2. Transgastric short-axis view of the mitral valve recorded from a transesophageal transverse view (multiplane 0-degree angle), showing the position of the three scallops of the posterior leaflet medial (MED), middle (MID), and lateral (LAT), as well as the medial commissure (COMM) (>), and the lateral commissure (<). The anterior leaflet is seen on the lower left of the screen, and the posterior leaflet is toward the upper right.

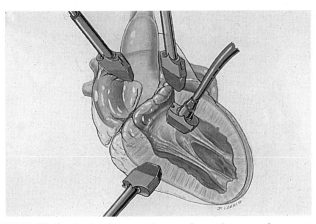

FIGURE 39–3. The four locations for transducer placement during epicardial intraoperative echocardiography. (From Cosgrove, D.M., and Stewart, W.J.: Mitral valvuloplasty. Curr. Probl. Cardiol. 14[7]:359, 1989.)

Because the heart is a moving target, intermittent transducer contact may occur, which causes loss of imaging continuity, yet inordinate transducer pressure can induce arrhythmias and disturb hemodynamics. My colleagues and I have developed a set of usable epicardial imaging planes (Fig. 39–3) that provide a complete intraoperative examination of the heart.[3, 4] The *parasternal equivalent* transducer position, with the transducer against the most anterior portion of the right ventricular outflow tract, obtains a set of images similar to those obtainable from the left parasternal window during transthoracic imaging. The *subcostal equivalent* transducer position is obtained by placing the transducer against the right ventricular free wall at the most inferior portion of the midsternal thoracotomy incision. Unfortunately, the apical window is unavailable during surgery, which makes it nearly impossible to orient a continuous-wave cursor parallel to mitral inflow with epicardial echocardiography.

Some of the best epicardial transducer windows I use do not have analogous counterparts in transthoracic imaging. The *aortopulmonary sulcus transducer position* is obtained by placing the longer side of the transducer against the right side of the main pulmonary artery, in the sulcus between it and the aorta, pointing the sector inferiorly and medially. The image resembles the parasternal equivalent long-axis image, but the aorta is angled more sharply to the top of the screen. The most difficult and most important epicardial image plane is the *aorta–superior vena cava transducer position*, obtained by placing the long side of the transducer against the right side of the ascending aorta and pointing inferiorly and to the left. This is the best view to evaluate left ventricular outflow tract velocity for estimating gradients in valvular and subvalvular stenosis, because the continuous-wave Doppler beam can be aligned parallel to flow.

Direct Epivascular Imaging of the Ascending Aorta

Five- to 7.5-MHz transducers are used for direct epivascular imaging of the ascending aorta. I prefer transducers that generate an image sector, but some centers use linear array transducers.[13] Long- and short-axis orientations are obtained by direct application of the transducer to the epiaortic surface. However, better images of the near wall of the aorta are obtained using a standoff device, such as a rubber glove partially filled with saline, to put the area of interest farther from the transducer and outside the near-field "bang" artifact.

Record Keeping and Communication for Intraoperative Echocardiography

A recording on videotape and a report should be made for each prepump and postpump study for interprofessional communica-

tions and medicolegal purposes. The results are also discussed immediately between members of the surgical and echocardiography teams.

TRAINING FOR INTRAOPERATIVE ECHOCARDIOGRAPHY

IOE is one of the most advanced forms of echocardiography in clinical practice. Judgments must be made "on the spot" that have a great impact on the outcome of surgery and the well-being of the patient. This immediacy requires the presence in the operating room of an expert in echocardiography. In teaching physicians to perform intraoperative TEE, the preceptor must be present in the operating room or connected to the operative team with a live connection of one-way video and two-way audio. Once clinical actions have been taken by the surgeon in response to the echocardiographic information, there is little use in second guessing on the basis of videotape review.

It has been recommended that training for TEE should follow completion of level II training in echocardiography, including mastery of all the basics of ultrasound diagnosis and at least 6 months or 300 studies of experience with transthoracic echocardiography.[14] This may not be practical for the practicing physician or the trainee in surgery or anesthesiology. I believe, however, that the equivalent of this training is necessary to provide the building blocks of complete understanding in the field.[15]

CHARACTERIZING VALVULAR AND VENTRICULAR FUNCTION WITH INTRAOPERATIVE ECHOCARDIOGRAPHY

Quantifying Valvular Stenosis

Continuous-wave Doppler echocardiography is used to record maximum velocity (V) to quantify the gradient (G) of valvular stenosis intraoperatively, using the simplified Bernoulli equation ($G = 4V^2$).[16] The cursor is directed parallel to flow, for example, mitral stenosis flow is recorded from the basilar TEE four-chamber or two-chamber views. Pressure half-time can also be used to estimate mitral valve area.[16] Aortic or subaortic gradients are best assessed with epicardial continuous-wave Doppler, as mentioned previously; they can also be estimated in some patients by continuous-wave Doppler imaging using the TEE transducer from deep transgastric views (Fig. 39–4).

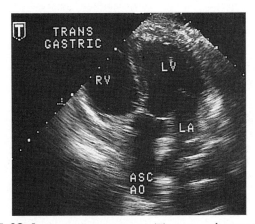

FIGURE 39–4. Transgastric transverse (T) view used to measure left ventricular outflow tract velocities with continuous wave Doppler imaging using a TEE probe. ASC AO = ascending aorta; LA = left atrium; LV = left ventricle; RV = right ventricle.

Quantitating Valvular Regurgitation

Regurgitation is assessed by measuring the size of the postjet flow disturbance[10] or the prejet flow acceleration,[17] or by looking at downstream or upstream effects on intravascular flow profiles. These methods are better than digital palpation of the heart for a thrill,[18] evaluation of the left atrial pressure V wave or the aortic pressure tracing, or filling the ventricle or aorta with saline with the left atrium open.[19] Doppler echocardiographiy has also supplanted contrast echocardiography for quantitation of valvular regurgitation.[6, 20–22]

Measuring the size of the left atrial mosaic color in systole correlates with the severity of mitral regurgitation by preoperative angiography,[10, 23] epicardial echocardiography,[24] and transthoracic echocardiography.[9] The amount of aortic regurgitation seen with preoperative angiography correlates with the width of the jet in the outflow tract seen with intraoperative TEE.[25] Color assessment of tricuspid regurgitation by IOE correlates with preoperative transthoracic echocardiography.[26] The amount of regurgitation on postpump IOE correlates with early postoperative transthoracic echocardiography for mitral regurgitation,[27] aortic regurgitation,[28] and tricuspid regurgitation.[29] Reversal of flow in the pulmonary vein velocity profile can also be used to determine the severity of mitral regurgitation, systolic reversal occurring in severe regurgitation.[30, 31]

Assessing Ventricular Systolic and Diastolic Function With Intraoperative Echocardiography

Assessing left ventricular size by TEE is reproducible[32] and is a useful gauge of the adequacy of intravascular volume replacement.[33–35] TEE can also assess the systolic function of the heart (which can be affected by many anesthetic agents), the adequacy of myocardial protection, and the effects of embolism of air or other material to the coronary bed.[36] Depiction of ventricular size by TEE provides indices of left ventricular preload that are as good or better than those provided by conventional invasive hemodynamic monitoring.[37] Intraoperative assessment by pulsed Doppler echocardiography of mitral and pulmonary vein flow profiles is also useful for determining ventricular diastolic function and optimizing filling dynamics.[38, 39]

PREPUMP INTRAOPERATIVE ECHOCARDIOGRAPHY IN VALVULAR SURGERY

IOE performed just prior to valvular surgery provides useful immediate information on valvular morphologic characteristics, the severity of regurgitation, stenotic gradients, and ventricular dysfunction, which adds to the accuracy of surgical planning.

Echocardiographic Definition of the Mechanism of Valve Dysfunction

A unique contribution of echocardiography in planning valvular surgery is its ability to characterize valvular morphologic features. The ability to repair a valve depends on the type of valve dysfunction and varies inversely with the extensiveness of the disease.[40] Valve repair is more technically demanding than valve replacement. To repair the mitral valve, the surgeon must understand the components of normal valvular function and address the specific dysfunction of that particular valve. Although the preoperative transthoracic echocardiogram usually provides sufficient information on the mechanism of dysfunction, IOE gives higher quality images, adding crucial additional understanding that facilitates optimal valve surgery.

Whether leaflet motion is normal, restricted, or excessive[41] on echocardiography[1] helps define the mechanism of mitral valve dysfunction. This aids the valve repair surgeon, whose open-heart appraisal is carried out in the absence of cardiac motion. Which leaflet is abnormal is determined from long-axis views. Short-axis views give a better appreciation of which portion of a leaflet is abnormal, such as distinguishing abnormalities of the medial, middle, or lateral scallop of the posterior mitral leaflet.

The jet direction is also helpful in defining the mechanism of dysfunction and the type of repair techniques needed.[1, 42] The color flow images of an aortic, tricuspid, or mitral leaflet that has excessive motion due to prolapse or flail demonstrate that the regurgitant jet is deflected to the opposite side of the receiving chamber (Fig. 39–5). In contrast, the jet tends to be directed toward a leaflet with restricted motion. A central jet direction is usually seen when the primary abnormality causing regurgitation consists of an equal amount of excessive or restricted motion of both leaflets, which is seen in patients with diffuse bileaflet prolapse or diffuse rheumatic valvular fibrosis and restriction, respectively.[1] A central jet also occurs commonly in patients with mitral regurgitation due to ventricular dilatation with normal mitral leaflets. The point of mitral coaptation is displaced toward the ventricular apex, with "relative mitral leaflet restriction" due to outward displacement of papillary muscles, a common result of ischemic heart disease.[43] In mitral regurgitation due to papillary muscle rupture or elongation, the jet emanates from the commissure on the side of the disruption.

FIGURE 39–5. See Color Plate 16.

Accurate prepump TEE information on the mechanism of dysfunction can predict the feasibility of repair[1, 40] and determine what other cardiac procedures are needed.[44] Assessing the degree of calcification can be helpful in planning the degree of debridement required.[45] Imaging vegetations helps determine that a valve is infected,[46, 47] which may influence the surgical approach. Finding a fistula[48] or abscess[49] may identify the need for an operation that is more extensive than simple valve surgery.[50]

Dependence of Severity of Valve Dysfunction on Loading Conditions

Some valve lesions are volatile and vary widely with fluctuations in loading conditions.[51] When differences are found between the results of prepump echocardiography and the preoperative transthoracic echocardiogram or catheterization information, however, careful consideration should be given to weighing the clinical relevance of each. Intravascular volume, preload, and afterload may be aberrant during intraoperative studies. Therefore, the true severity of ventricular and valvular dysfunction is more accurately depicted by preoperative transthoracic studies, which are usually performed with the patient in "street condition."

In some circumstances, the intraoperative echocardiographic study is tantamount to a focused in-depth consultation and should be handled with the same level of expertise and professionalism. It may be appropriate to use IOE for a last-minute assessment of the severity and mechanism of valve dysfunction,[7, 52] especially for lesions such as ischemic mitral regurgitation or an infected valve. However, *most* decisions on which surgical procedure should be performed should be made *prior to the patient entering the operating room*. Reduction in the amount of tricuspid regurgitation on the prepump study may result from sympatholysis or volume loss and should not dissuade the surgeon from carrying out the preoperative plan when tricuspid surgery seemed indicated on the basis of clinical and ambulatory assessments. Only in rare situations of dire emergency should IOE be the *only* mode of cardiac diagnosis.[53]

For example, tricuspid repair is indicated in patients who have clinical right-sided cardiac failure and structural tricuspid leaflet abnormalities causing severe tricuspid insufficiency. In patients undergoing surgery for left-sided valvular or myocardial problems, "functional" regurgitation with a structurally normal tricuspid valve is common. When severe and symptomatic, it should be repaired. However, predicting whether moderately severe regurgitation will improve merely with correction of the left-sided cardiac abnormality is difficult. Annuloplasty of a structurally normal regurgitant valve is probably needed when there is also annular dilatation[54] or right ventricular dysfunction that is out of proportion to the pulmonary hypertension.[55] Some patients who need tricuspid surgery on clinical examination do not show severe tricuspid regurgitation on color flow Doppler imaging in the operating room.[26]

Frequency of Changes in Surgery Based on Prepump Intraoperative Echocardiography

Of 426 consecutive patients undergoing IOE at Cleveland Clinic, changes in the operative mission based on the prepump echocardiogram were made in 40 patients (9 percent) (unpublished data). Most of these cases represented new lesions of other valves not noted at the time of preoperative studies. Most of the remainder represented significant new information about the mechanism of dysfunction that changed the directions of the surgical approach to the intended valve procedure. Other groups have reported that changes in the surgical plan based on the prepump echocardiogram were made in 11,[7] 16,[56] and 19 percent[2] of patients undergoing valvular surgery. Not all of these patients had the benefit of preoperative transthoracic echocardiography.

POSTPUMP INTRAOPERATIVE ECHOCARDIOGRAPHY IN VALVULAR SURGERY

IOE provides a "safety net" for checking the results of valve surgery prior to closing the chest. Through prevention of reoperations, IOE improves outcome in many nonprosthetic valve procedures. I believe that valve repair, homograft valve replacement, pulmonary autografts, stentless bioprosthetic valve replacement, and closure of periprosthetic fistulas *should not be performed without IOE.*

The postpump echocardiogram should be obtained after the patient has been weaned from cardiopulmonary bypass and intravascular volume, rhythm, and loading conditions have been normalized. The intraoperative study should investigate residual or new valvular regurgitation of all four valves, new complications of surgery, and ventricular size and performance.[57] When operating on patients with a mixture of valve lesions, one group found problems requiring changes in surgical management in 16 percent of patients.[56]

Criteria for a Second Pump Run

The policy at Cleveland Clinic is to put patients back on cardiopulmonary bypass for further surgery when they have postpump regurgitation that is moderate (2+) or greater in severity or when other complications are present. When there is a borderline amount of residual regurgitation, careful observation before administering protamine or decannulating the patient may show trends toward improvement or deterioration. In some cases, the systemic afterload should be increased with phenylephrine to bring out latent regurgitation that is likely to worsen later.

Of 6186 IOE studies that my colleagues and I have performed in the past 8 years, 5.8 percent have required further surgery during a return to cardiopulmonary bypass, prompted at least in part by IOE. Figure 39–6 shows that the frequency of second pump runs varies with the surgical mission.

When significant regurgitation is found on the postpump study after an initial attempt at valve repair, determination of the mechanism of valvular dysfunction by echocardiography is of even more importance. Immediate failure of valve repair is most commonly due to either poor understanding of the nature of the original problem or a surgical mishap.[58] Because the surgeon has already done his or her best to alleviate the problem, revised information regarding the current mechanism of dysfunction is helpful in guiding further repair, replacment, or other options.

Complications Definable With Intraoperative Echocardiography

Several other complications of cardiac surgery have been found in the early period after cessation of cardiopulmonary bypass. New ventricular dysfunction is the most common and is associated with an increase in postoperative complications and mortality.[2] Some other postpump TEE findings may warrant a second pump run. Iatrogenic aortic dissection or pseudoaneurysm can result from aortic cannulation.[59] New regurgitation may be found on an unoperated and previously normal valve.[60] Unsuspected mediastinal hematoma, tamponade (Fig. 39–7),[61] iatrogenic fistulas,[62] new myocardial infarction,[63] and iatrogenic atrial septal defect have also occasionally been seen and can often be corrected with further surgery during the same thoracotomy.

Impact of Transesophageal Echocardiography Results on Postoperative Outcome of Valvular Surgery

Because there is no valid control group for comparison of outcome in patients who undergo further surgery during a second run of cardiopulmonary bypass, it is impossible to determine the precise clinical impact of IOE. However, Sheikh and associates[2] reported 154 patients who had postpump TEE after valve surgery, a

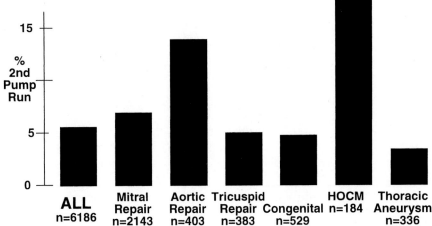

FIGURE 39–6. Frequency of second pump runs by valve lesion, from 1987 to 1994 at the Cleveland Clinic. HOCM = hypertrophic obstructive cardiomyopathy.

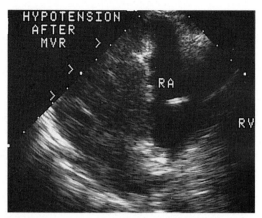

FIGURE 39–7. Transverse (T) image recorded after mitral valve replacement (MVR), showing a large hematoma (>) adjacent to the right atrium (RA) and right ventricle (RV), causing tamponade in a patient in whom hypotension occurred suddenly as the chest was closed.

subset of whom were found to have significant residual valvular dysfunction that was not immediately fixed. In this subset, there was a substantial excess in the morbidity (86 percent versus 15 percent) and mortality (43 percent versus 5 percent) rates over those patients in whom operation was performed concurrently but whose postpump echocardiographic results showed no significant valvular dysfunction.[2] In another study, patients with ischemic mitral regurgitation who had significant residual valvular dysfunction after repair had a markedly worse survival rate than did those whose postpump TEE showed good repair results.[7]

My colleagues and I have reported that a group of 73 patients whose postpump TEE showed mild or moderate regurgitation after mitral repair had a 10 percent reoperation rate in the following 3 years, compared with 4 percent in a group of matched patients in whom the postpump intraoperative echocardiogram showed an "echo-perfect" result with no regurgitation.[8] In a few reported patients, whose postpump severe regurgitation was ignored by the surgeon, early reoperation was required within a few months.[3, 23]

INTRAOPERATIVE TRANSESOPHAGEAL ECHOCARDIOGRAPHY IN SPECIFIC VALVE OPERATIONS

Valve Repair for Mitral Regurgitation

The most common indication for postpump IOE at many institutions is valve repair for mitral regurgitation. Prepump TEE is used

to refine the understanding of the mechanism of regurgitation, as detailed earlier. Using a scheme based on assessing the leaflet motion with echocardiography and the jet direction by color Doppler imaging (Table 39–1), IOE is accurate compared with the surgeon's assessment in more than 86 percent of cases.[1]

When moderate or more serious residual regurgitation is found by TEE after repair, reinstitution of cardiopulmonary bypass for further repair or valve replacement is appropriate. This has been reported in various frequencies ranging from 1 percent (1 of 62),[64] to 2 percent (5 of 246),[7] to 6 percent (5 of 88),[65] to 8 percent (11 of 143,[27] 8 of 100,[3] and 54 of 611),[66] to 10 percent (3 of 30).[20] In our experience with 2143 mitral repairs over the past 8 years, 154 patients (7.2 percent) had a postpump echocardiogram with residual regurgitation or other complications and underwent immediate further mitral surgery (see Fig. 39–6).

Dynamic outflow tract obstruction due to systolic anterior motion (SAM) of the mitral valve (Fig. 39–8) is one of the important complications that can occur in the setting of mitral valve repair,[27, 67] aortic valve replacement,[68] and other cardiac procedures.[69, 70] In milder cases, postpump dynamic outflow tract obstruction usually resolves with volume replacement and cessation of catecholamine administration.[71, 72] In some cases, however, the obstruction is severe and requires a second pump run for revision of the annuloplasty or valve replacement.[66, 67]

FIGURE 39–8. See Color Plate 16.

Valvuloplasty and Balloon Valvulotomy for Mitral Rheumatic Valve Disease

Another group of patients who benefit from IOE are those with rheumatic valve disease who are undergoing valve conservation procedures, ranging from mitral commissurotomy to extensive debridement, chordal stripping, and annuloplasty. Valve repair in these patients is more difficult than in myxomatous degeneration or ischemic mitral regurgitation. Relief of obstruction and no significant postrepair regurgitation are the important objectives.

Rather than surgery, many patients with pure rheumatic mitral stenosis now undergo balloon valvulotomy, for which transthoracic echocardiography[73] and TEE[74] are important adjuncts to patient selection. TEE is helpful during the performance of balloon valvulotomy for exclusion of thrombi, safe perforation of the atrial septum, accurate placement of the balloon, serial assessment of mitral regurgitation, and exclusion of tamponade.[75]

TABLE 39–1. UTILITY OF COLOR FLOW JET DIRECTION IN DETERMINING THE MECHANISM OF MITRAL REGURGITATION

Jet Direction	Mechanism	Most Common Causes
Anterior	Posterior leaflet flail	Myxomatous or endocarditis
	Posterior leaflet prolapse	Myxomatous
Posterior	Anterior leaflet flail	Myxomatous or endocarditis
	Anterior leaflet prolapse	Myxomatous
	Posterior leaflet restriction	Rheumatic or ischemic
Central	Balanced restriction	Rheumatic or ischemic
	Left ventricle dilatation	cardiomyopathy
Commissural	Papillary muscle elongation or disruption	Ischemic
	Commissural chordal rupture	Myxomatous or endocarditis
Eccentric origin	Leaflet perforation	Endocarditis
	Cleft	Congenital

Adapted from Stewart, W. J., Currier, P. J., Salcedo, E. E., et al.: Evaluation of mitral leaflet motion by echocardiography and jet direction by Doppler color flow mapping to determine the mechanism of mitral regurgitation. J. Am. Coll. Cardiol. 20:1353, 1992. With permission from the American College of Cardiology.

Valve Repair for Tricuspid Regurgitation

For the majority of patients undergoing surgery for tricuspid regurgitation, valve repair is the preferred procedure[41] and therefore IOE is useful. The prepump study defines the morphologic characteristics of the tricuspid valve, the presence of leaflet thickening, the degree to which leaflet support is abnormal, and right ventricular function. Intraoperative TEE can document the amount of regurgitation prior to cardiopulmonary bypass (Fig. 39–9) and, hopefully, resolution of the regurgitation afterward.[76]

FIGURE 39–9. See Color Plate 16.

After tricuspid repair, when the postpump intraoperative echocardiogram shows persistent tricuspid regurgitation that is moderate or severe (3+ or 4+), strong consideration should be given to a second cardiopulmonary bypass run for further repair or tricuspid valve replacement. This alternative is far better than discovering that the patient's left-sided valvular problem is improved but the tricuspid regurgitation warrants another operation at a future date. Suboptimal results on the postpump echocardiogram requiring a second pump run after tricuspid repair have been found in 20 of 383 patients (5.2 percent) over the past 8 years (see Fig. 39–6). Another study reported residual amounts of tricuspid regurgitation following repair, necessitating a second pump run in 5 to 10 percent of patients.[77]

One group has reported an innovative use of intraoperative TEE in performing DeVega tricuspid annuloplasty. By externalizing the annuloplasty sutures, the amount of annuloplasty can be adjusted after coming off cardiopulmonary bypass, based on the size of the tricuspid regurgitation jet shown on TEE.[29]

Valve Repair for Aortic Regurgitation

In patients undergoing aortic valve repair, IOE is useful in prepump refinement of the understanding of the mechanism of aortic regurgitation. For this purpose, I also separate aortic regurgitation into that associated with excessive, restricted, or normal leaflet motion. Aortic repair is feasible in a smaller and more selected group, mostly noncalcified valves that have aortic valve prolapse and either a bileaflet (Fig. 39–10) or trileaflet anatomy. Severe aortic regurgitation in the setting of normal valve morphology, with outward displacement of the sinotubular junction from an aneurysm of the ascending aorta, can also be repaired at the time of conduit placement.

Figure 39–10. See Color Plate 17.

Because aortic repair is technically more difficult than mitral repair, the incidence of second pump runs (Fig. 39–11) is higher. Moderate or more severe residual regurgitation requiring a return to cardiopulmonary bypass for further repair or replacement occurs in 10 to 12 percent of patients.[28, 78–81] In 403 patients who have undergone repair over the past 8 years, 58 (14.4 percent) have required further repair or replacement during the same thoracotomy procedure (see Fig. 39–6).

FIGURE 39–11. See Color Plate 17.

Stentless Human and Bioprosthetic Valves

For selected patients needing aortic valve replacment, some relatively new alternatives include the aortic homograft, the pulmonary autograft,[82] and the stentless bioprosthesis.[83] These options are particularly good in young patients and in those with active or recent endocarditis. IOE is also useful in these surgeries, in part because of the greater difficulty in suspending the valve appropriately.

Prepump TEE allows selection of an appropriate allograft size before aortic cross-clamping, which minimizes the delay for thawing the cryopreserved valve. Prior to the anticipated pulmonary autograft—the "Ross procedure"—IOE gives information about aortic root and pulmonary annular size and coronary ostial anatomy.

Immediately after implantation of a homograft or stentless valve, echocardiography is useful for checking for new or residual problems.[84] In our series of 80 patients undergoing homograft implantation, a second pump run was necessary in 12 percent of patients (unpublished data).

Standard Valve Replacement Surgery

In patients undergoing valve replacement with standard biologic or mechanical prostheses, TEE is an important tool in the preoperative work-up.[85, 86] However, intraoperative TEE makes a major contribution less often in this situation than in nonprosthetic surgery. Postpump TEE is sometimes useful for excluding prosthetic dysfunction and myocardial dysfunction[87] in patients who have unfavorable hemodynamics. After routine valve replacement, new periprosthetic leaks are suprisingly common, although they are usually small.[88] In occasional cases, I have detected new, larger perivalvular leaks early after surgery, which have been repaired on a second cardiopulmonary bypass run. Almost all transesophageal studies of normally functioning prosthetic valves show one or more small regurgitant jets, considered to be physiologic regurgitation. These are of no significance but must be distinguished from pathologic regurgitation.

In patients with severe periprosthetic regurgitation by prepump TEE, localization of the site aids in surgical management.[89] Postpump echocardiography after suture closure of the leak is useful in verifying its resolution or pointing out the need for further surgery.

MYECTOMY FOR HYPERTROPHIC OBSTRUCTIVE CARDIOMYOPATHY

For patients with hypertrophic cardiomyopathy with severe resting or latent obstruction and persistent symptoms despite maximal medical therapy, myectomy is an effective way to reduce symptoms and improve the prognosis. Baseline studies in the operating room prior to cardiopulmonary bypass are essential to characterize the location of hypertrophy,[90–93] determine the mechanism and extent of mitral regurgitation, and estimate the outflow gradient based on the maximal velocity recorded from epicardial continuous-wave Doppler imaging (Fig. 39–12) from the aorta–superior vena cava transducer position.[94]

On the postpump studies, the important parameters for echocardiographic study are the outflow tract gradient, the amount of mitral regurgitation, and the absence of an induced ventricular septal defect. If the postpump uninduced gradient is low, I routinely infuse isoproterenol to bring out latent obstruction, titrated from 2 to 10 μg per minute according to heart rate and outflow tract response. A postpump gradient greater than 50 mm Hg, either at rest or with provocation, warrants a second pump run; further myectomy of the site of persistent SAM-septal contact almost always eliminates the obstruction.[91] My colleagues and I studied 184 patients in the setting of myectomy and found that 34 patients (18.5 percent) had a suboptimal result on the postpump echocardiogram requiring further surgery. Most problems entailed

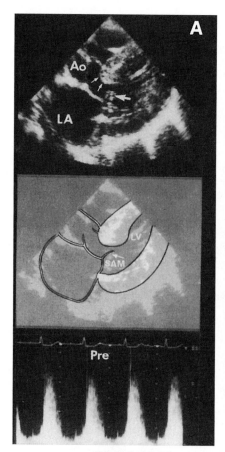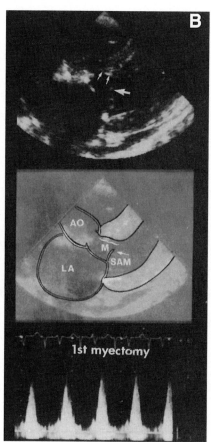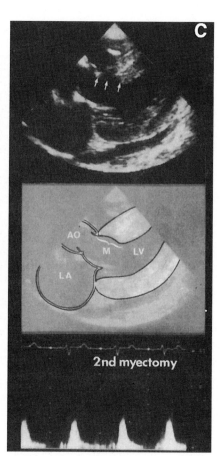

FIGURE 39–12. Initially unsuccessful myectomy for hypertrophic cardiomyopathy. *A, B,* and *C* show epicardial subcostal four-chamber equivalent images *(top)* and diagrams *(middle)* in systole and continuous wave Doppler spectra *(bottom,* with all calibrations at 1 m per second) recorded from the aorta–superior vena cava transducer position on the ascending aorta. *A,* Marked septal hypertrophy *(small arrows, top)* and systolic anterior motion (SAM) of the anterior mitral leaflet *(large arrow, top)* are present with the Doppler-derived outflow gradient of 80 mm Hg before operation. *B,* After initial myectomy *(M, middle),* with reduction in the septal bulge, SAM and an outflow gradient of 61 mm Hg persist. *C,* After the second pump run, the site of further myectomy *(M, middle)* extends longer and deeper, the SAM is eliminated, and the gradient is reduced to 19 mm Hg. AO = aorta; LA = left atrium; LV = left ventricle. (From Marwick, T.H., Stewart, W.J., Lever, H.M., et al.: Benefits of intraoperative echocardiography in the surgical management of hypertrophic cardiomyopathy. J. Am. Coll. Cardiol. 20:1066, 1992. With permission from the American College of Cardiology.)

persistent obstruction, but a quarter of the patients had intrinsic mitral valve dysfunction that before surgery could not be distinguished from that due to outflow tract obstruction. This is the highest percentage of second pump runs for any of the problems I have studied with IOE (see Fig. 39–6). An additional problem to watch for after myectomy is aortic regurgitation, which is reported in increased frequency postoperatively, presumably because of damage to the valve from the high velocity jet.[95]

SURGERY FOR CONGENITAL HEART DISEASE

IOE is an essential element of the intraoperative management of patients with selected types of congenital heart disease. It is useful to guide the assessment of anatomy and physiology before and after repair.

The Latest Arena to Shift from Epicardial Echocardiography to Transesophageal Echocardiography

Until the past few years, a larger percentage of intraoperative studies in patients with congenital heart disease were performed using the epicardial approach, merely because the available TEE devices were too large and could cause bronchial or aortic obstruction in small babies.[96, 97] More recently, tiny pediatric biplane transducers have been developed and have become the dominant mode of IOE in congenital heart disease, even in infants weighing as little as 3 to 5 kg.[101] In the pediatric age group, the transesophageal approach is used almost exclusively during the anesthetized state in the operating room or the intensive care unit rather than in the outpatient echocardiographic laboratory.

Even today the epicardial approach using a 5- to 7-MHz transducer is still better than TEE for intraoperative evaluation of right and left ventricular outflow tract morphologic features,[98] with alignment of a continuous-wave Doppler image parallel to the highest velocity flow. Epicardial echocardiography is also better than TEE in diagnosing a doubly committed subarterial ventricular septal defect.[99] Contrast echocardiographic injections from a peripheral vein (Fig. 39–13) or a pulmonary artery catheter should be combined with color flow imaging to identify shunts.[100]

FIGURE 39–13. See Color Plate 18.

IOE is particularly helpful for evaluating tetralogy of Fallot, transposition of the great arteries, abnormal pulmonary venous return, sinus venosus atrial septal defect, cor triatriatum,[102] complete atrioventricular valve repair, and correction of complex congenital heart disease.[103, 104] In pulmonary atresia, prepump TEE helps determine the size of the pulmonary artery confluence, which affects the surgical plan. Definition of anomalous pulmonary or systemic venous drainage (Fig. 39–14) may influence the preferred mode of cannulation and the feasibility of using retrograde cardioplegia.

Changes in Operative Approach to Congenital Heart Surgery Based on Prepump and Postpump Intraoperative Echocardiography

Prepump IOE improves on the preoperative transthoracic echocardiographic information, finding unsuspected additional defects and new morphologic information affecting the surgical approach in 3 percent (3 of 90)[105] to 13 percent (22 of 168) of patients.[106]

IOE after cardiopulmonary bypass is also extremely useful in complex congenital heart disease (Fig. 39–15) to look for persistent or new valvular regurgitation or outflow tract obstruction.[107] After atrial or ventricular septal defect repairs, tiny residual shunts are common[108] and subsequently close spontaneously in 80 percent of cases.[109] With larger persistent shunts seen by color or contrast imaging on the postpump echocardiogram, immediate revision should be considered because they are likely to become clinically significant and require surgery subsequently.[110]

FIGURE 39–15. See Color Plate 18.

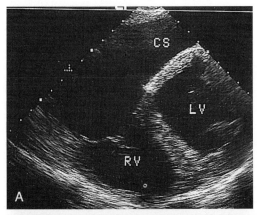

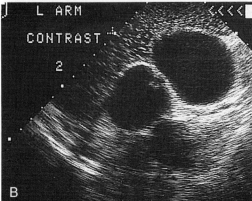

FIGURE 39–14. *A,* Transverse TEE image showing a massive coronary sinus (CS) posterior to the left ventricle (LV) with right ventricular (RV) enlargement. *B,* Transverse (T) image during contrast injection from the left (L) arm, showing contrast enhancement of the coronary sinus (*arrows*).

In a large series of postpump IOE, Ungerleider and colleagues found residua in 7 percent (22 of 328) of patients; the presence of persistent abnormalities on echocardiography was associated with adverse outcome.[111] One group found that the need for reoperation was correlated with the severity of left atrioventricular valve regurgitation as estimated by IOE following repair.[12]

IOE is also useful after the modified Fontan operation in diagnosing obstruction of atriopulmonary and cavopulmonary anastomoses, unsatisfactory atrial fenestration, residual cavoatrial shunting, and thrombi that cannot be identified by transthoracic echocardiography.[112] Residua after a Fontan operation leading to surgical revision were found in 18 percent (3 of 16)[113] to 47 percent (8 of 19) of patients.[114]

Of 529 patients that my colleagues and I studied with epicardial echocardiography or TEE during surgery for congenital heart disease over the past 8 years, 26 (4.9 percent) have required a second pump run for further surgery, at least in part because of the echocardiographic findings (see Fig. 39–6).

CORONARY ARTERY SURGERY

I do not routinely use IOE in all coronary artery operations. However, it is particularly useful in the presence of significant ventricular dysfunction to help manage inotropic agents and adjustments of intravascular volume status. It can also diagnose intraoperative ischemia on the basis of ventricular wall motion, determine perfusion territories using contrast echocardiography, and define coronary and graft anatomy using high-frequency epicardial echocardiography.

IOE can monitor patients for postpump improvement in contractile function of chronically ischemic segments.[35, 115–118] IOE is also useful in complications of infarction, such as acquired ventricular septal defect (Fig. 39–16), papillary muscle rupture,[53] ventricular free wall rupture,[119] and coronary bypass when combined with other missions such as valve operations.

FIGURE 39–16. See Color Plate 18.

Diagnosis of Intraoperative Ischemia

Intraoperative TEE is an accurate method of diagnosing ischemia during cardiac surgery.[120–122] Because wall motion abnormalities develop relatively early in the ischemic cascade, their identification is sensitive for determining new perfusion problems.

Accurate evaluation of ischemia is facilitated by comparison of side-by-side video loops, matched judiciously for the tomographic section of the left ventricle before and after development or resolution of the process. One must also be careful to take into account the loading conditions, pharmacologic effects, heart rate, and other factors influencing the inotropic state.

Although superficially it seems to be one of the elementary skills of an echocardiographer, the judgment required to diagnose ischemia and segmental contractile dysfunction accurately is one of the most difficult tasks in the field.[123] If sufficient training and echocardiographic expertise or sufficient numbers of imaging planes are not applied, detection of ischemia may not be accurate or add to other available clinical measures.[124]

New segmental abnormalities are occasionally found after seemingly successful coronary bypass operations.[63] A significant new wall motion abnormality can show that there has been immediate vein graft occlusion,[87] that the wrong vessel has been grafted, or that other arteries have unsuspected lesions. Clinically relevant ischemia must also be distinguished from global myocardial dysfunction resulting from transient metabolic factors or inadequate myocardial protection. Air embolism usually causes segmental dysfunction in the distribution of the right coronary artery because of the anterior position of its ostium[36]; this usually improves merely with resting on cardiopulmonary bypass.

Intraoperative Contrast Echocardiography

Numerous authors have documented the potential utility of IOE in quantitating regional myocardial perfusion using myocardial contrast echocardiography. The most common, available method is direct injection of 2 mL of sonicated 5 percent human albumin into the aortic root after application of the aortic cross-clamp or into the saphenous vein graft before the proximal anastomosis is made. Commercially produced albumin microspheres are now available for clinical use. Other agents are in development, including perfluorocarbons that generate bubbles by changing state at body temperature.[125]

Quantitative methods have been developed for intraoperative measurement of contrast myocardial enhancement from time-intensity curves.[126, 127] For example, the peak intensity of contrast enhancement within areas subtended by stenotic arteries with collaterals is significantly higher than that of areas with previous infarction. There is also a correlation between myocardial enhancement and increases in segmental wall thickening following revascularization.[128]

The sensitivity of contrast echocardiography for definition of the perfusion territory of each coronary artery is reasonable, although it appears to be lower for the right coronary artery. If the myocardium supplied by each graft can be clearly and consistently delineated, the tomographic views of a perfusion bed can provide a useful intraoperative tool.[129] Contrast studies also can guide the sequence of graft placement and thereby improve myocardial preservation.[130] Comparing the perfusion patterns of IOE contrast imaging delineates the myocardial regions predicted from coronary angiography the majority of the time.[131] The process of monitoring myocardial perfusion before and after coronary bypass operations has been reported.[132]

However, a good portion of the quantitative aspects of this technique have yet to be definitively validated. The time-intensity curves have been studied, but it is still not clear which parameters provide the most relevant information.[133] Variability in injection, imaging, and analysis techniques causes variability in data from time-intensity curves, which often precludes accurate quantification.[134] Therefore, the clinical role of this application is still uncertain, and it has not achieved widespread use.

Epicardial Visualization of Coronary Arteries

With high-frequency epicardial imaging, it is feasible to visualize the coronary vessels,[135, 136] localize stenoses and occlusions,[137] and evaluate the anastomoses of coronary grafts (Fig. 39–17). This technique can also be useful for finding the native arteries and localizing the site of maximal coronary stenosis.[138] Epicardial echocardiography can be particularly helpful while dissecting the heart free of scarring in reoperations. By direct visualization of graft anastomoses, epicardial echocardiography can diagnose errors in technique that can lead to unsatisfactory results.[139] The technique can also be useful in guiding surgical relief of a myocardial bridge over a coronary artery.[140]

FIGURE 39–17. See Color Plate 19.

In theory, epicardial visualization of coronary arteries should be popular because it permits the surgeon to evaluate the results of revascularization immediately. In practice, however, only the proximal right and left anterior descending arteries can be visualized,

and the transducer is large and cumbersome. Most surgeons rarely find a clinical need for this type of imaging.

TRANSPLANTATION AND SURGERY FOR SEVERE MYOCARDIAL DYSFUNCTION

IOE has also been used in patients with severe myocardial dysfunction who are undergoing heart transplantation, cardiomyoplasty, and placement of an aortic balloon pump or ventricular assist device. In patients undergoing orthotopic heart transplantation, IOE has been used to document ventricular and valvular function. In transplant recipients, tricuspid regurgitation may result from a mismatch in the size of the donor heart and the recipient pericardial cavity, resulting in distortion of the tricuspid valve ring. When the degree of tricuspid regurgitation assessed by IOE is moderate or more severe, one group advocates a reduction annuloplasty.[141]

TEE is of ready assistance when difficulty is encountered in "blind" passage of an intra-aortic balloon pump[142] and can diagnose and help to avoid trauma such as intimal dissection caused by suboptimal placement of the device.[143]

In latissimus dorsi cardiomyoplasty, epicardial echocardiography can document ventricular performance.[144] It is also useful for assessing filling dynamics during wrapping of the heart with the skeletal muscle. Most of the augmentation of myocardial performance cannot be seen until months later when the skeletal muscle has been trained with the pacing device.

IOE is useful in patients with cardiogenic shock who are receiving a left ventricular assist device either as a temporary external system or as an implantable device. Identification of apical thrombi and ascending aortic atheromas is important prior to placing the cannulas in those locations. In addition, one must exclude aortic insufficiency, which allows a flow loop to develop, and shunts like a patent foramen ovale, which cause hypoxia when the left ventricular assist device reduces left ventricular filling pressure.

SURGERY FOR CARDIAC TRAUMA

TEE is useful in identifying the presence and extent of trauma to the heart and great vessels. In penetrating missile wounds of the heart, IOE can localize the fragment and diagnose any resulting valvular dysfunction or shunt.[145] Traumatic aortic rupture can be diagnosed by TEE[146] and occurs most commonly at the site of suspension by the ligamentum arteriosum.

SURGERY FOR THORACIC AORTIC ANEURYSM OR DISSECTION

Preoperative Diagnosis of Aortic Aneurysm or Dissection

TEE is accurate and effective in characterizing thoracic aneurysms and has emerged as the first-line diagnostic method. The criteria for diagnosing dissection include imaging an intimal flap causing flow separation, defined by a differential in velocity by color Doppler imaging at the location of the flap (Fig. 39–18). Care must taken to avoid interpreting ultrasound artifacts as intimal flaps.[147, 148] Because of the rapidity of progression of aortic dissection, speed in diagnosis is important, which often makes TEE a better choice than magnetic resonance imaging, computerized tomography, or angiography for critically ill patients.

FIGURE 39–18. See Color Plate 19.

Intraoperative Echocardiography in Thoracic Aortic Aneurysm Surgery

Because an aortic dissection can progress overnight, prepump IOE is useful in updating the understanding of anatomy and physiology to include events that have transpired since preoperative studies. The prepump study finds new information that affects operative management in 18[149] to 20 percent of patients.[150] Identification of the proximal origin of the dissection and determination of concomitant aortic valve involvement significantly facilitate surgical repair. IOE aids in optimizing perfusion of distal organs by visualizing the location of entry and exit sites.[151]

The postpump study may also be useful in surgery on the thoracic aorta. After surgery for aortic dissection, TEE can verify sufficient flow in the major aortic branches and check for leakage at the suture lines.[149] As mentioned previously, aortic valve resuspension may also be checked by the postpump study.[151] Problems that needed further surgery before closure of the chest were found in 7 percent of patients in one series.[150] Of 336 patients studied at our institution with echocardiography during surgery for thoracic aortic aneurysms or dissections, or both, over the past 8 years, 12 patients (3.6 percent) had problems with the aortic valve, myocardial perfusion, or graft integrity sufficient to warrant a return to cardiopulmonary bypass for further surgery (see Fig. 39–6).

INTRAOPERATIVE MANAGEMENT OF PATIENTS WITH FISTULAS DUE TO ENDOCARDITIS

Echocardiography has greatly added to the accuracy of diagnosis in patients with endocarditis.[46] TEE is helpful in the intraoperative management of patients with deep tissue infections of the heart or multivalvular infections resulting from endocarditis.[49] Abscesses and fistulas occur most commonly in the area adjacent to a prosthesis or in patients with aortic valve endocarditis in which the regurgitant jet hits the anterior mitral leaflet and causes an endocardial abrasion with subsequent perforation or abscess formation.

The goals of the prepump TEE study are to determine the location of infection and to define the extent of the fistula. From a periaortic location, a fistula may form connecting the left ventricular outflow tract to the right ventricle (ventricular septal defect), the right atrium (like a "Gerbodi" ventricular septal defect), the left atrium (perforated anterior mitral leaflet), the atrial septum (into the left atrium, Fig. 39–19), or the aorta (periprosthetic leak). From a perimitral location, fistulas have been seen from the left ventricle to the left atrium (periprosthetic leak), the coronary sinus (with a shunt to the right atrium), or the pericardial space (pseudoaneurysm).

FIGURE 39–19. See Color Plate 20.

The first goal of surgery is to extirpate the infection by debriding all infected tissue, which sometimes requires excision of important structures of the heart such as portions of the aortic-mitral annulus. In such cases, reconstruction of those structures is important. It is best to avoid implanting prosthetic material, which creates a "foreign body phenomenon" and is likely to cause recurrence of infection. Homograft aortic valve replacement and valve repair are nonprosthetic options that may be superior in terms of avoiding subsequent recurrence of infections. Postpump TEE is again helpful after this type of challenging surgery to confirm resolution of the fistula flow or valve dysfunction and optimal reconstruction of the heart.

INTRAOPERATIVE DETECTION OF AORTIC ATHEROMA

Complications after cardiac surgery frequently result from embolization of atherosclerotic debris in the thoracic aorta that is dislodged by surgical manipulation. Although routine screening of all patients undergoing cardiac surgery is not feasible, IOE may be useful to optimize operative strategy in those who are older and have peripheral vascular atherosclerosis, diabetes, or aortic knob calcification seen on chest x-ray film. The frequency and severity of atheroma increase distally in the aorta, so transesophageal echocardiographic visualization of the descending aorta is most sensitive. Epivascular echocardiography has a greater impact on surgical management, however, because it is better at visualizing abnormalities of the ascending aorta, the usual site of cannulation, aortic cross-clamping, and the proximal anastomosis of coronary vein grafts.

IOE can identify a high-risk group—those with protruding (greater than 5-mm thickness) atheromas, particularly those that are mobile (Fig. 39–20). TEE data are predictive of stroke, which occurred in 25 percent of patients with mobile thoracic aortic atheroma versus 2 percent of those without.[152] In another series, patients with severe atherosclerotic changes seen by epicardial echocardiography had a 23 percent incidence of perioperative cerebrovascular complications and 15 percent mortality, compared with no strokes or deaths in patients with less than moderate atherosclerotic changes.[153]

Some authors have advocated changes in operative technique based on the echocardiographic findings of the severity and distribution of atheroma.[13] Cannulation of the femoral artery is an option, but this may cause worse problems if descending aortic atheromas are dislodged and embolized to the cerebral vessels by the reversal of flow. We have occasionally used brachiocephalic artery cannulation when the ascending aorta is full of atheroma. Hypothermic circulatory arrest and aortic arch debridement may be used in severe cases to reduce the incidence of stroke in patients carefully selected by IOE.[154]

LIMITATIONS OF INTRAOPERATIVE ECHOCARDIOGRAPHY

Simultaneous electrocautery or major surgical manipulation of the heart results in image degradation or distortion. If echocardiography is to be used in the operating room as a diagnostic procedure to answer important clinical questions, the operating room lights should be dimmed and other activities such as electrocautery suspended. The essential portions of intraoperative echocardiographic imaging can usually be completed in 5 minutes or less.

Because of their effects on valvular and ventricular function, loading conditions should be adjusted during intraoperative TEE

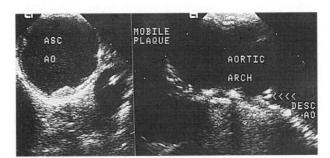

FIGURE 39–20. Epiaortic images of aortic atherosclerosis recorded with a 7-MHz transducer. *Left,* Short-axis epicardial image of the ascending aorta (ASC AO), showing sessile plaque especially on the lower portion of the image. *Right,* Long-axis epicardial image of the aortic arch and descending aorta (DESC AO), showing a mobile plaque (*arrows*).

to match ambulatory values.[51] The amplitude of reflected images and the amount of color flow on the instrument display vary greatly with instrument settings, such as gain and pulse repetition frequency, and with the adequacy of penetration and insonification of the area of interest. Obtaining diagnostic images requires good coupling between the transducer and the esophagus, an adequate signal-to-noise ratio, and orientation of image planes in understandable, standardized planes. The image is a two-dimensional plane cutting through the heart, which is obviously three-dimensional, so multiple orthogonal planes are needed to represent the overall cardiac performance and valvular function.[9]

It is important not to distract individuals from key responsibilities at times crucial for surgical or anesthetic observations and judgments, especially immediately following cessation of cardiopulmonary bypass. In a manner analogous to the pilot and copilot avoiding distractions during the takeoff and landing of an airplane, the surgeon and anesthesiologist must be attentive to the patient at the times crucial to intraoperative imaging. In this respect, it may be best to use a third individual, possibly a cardiologist or anesthesiologist trained in echocardiography, who can concentrate on the postpump imaging information.

NEW ULTRASOUND TECHNOLOGY FOR FUTURE INTRAOPERATIVE USE

Numerous applications of computer-based ultrasound processing technology have recently emerged into the realm of feasibility, with great potential for intraoperative use. Automated boundary detection is a way of automatically tracking the area of low amplitude (blood density) pixels within a region of interest.[155, 156] This technique is being investigated for potential intraoperative use in assessing ventricular function. Digital methods of assessing contrast intensity[126] and integrated backscatter may have a future role in optimizing the benefit of revascularization.[157] Doppler tissue imaging is a new method of tracking motion of the tissue of the heart that may have important applications.[158] Three-dimensional echocardiography has now passed the phase of feasibility testing and achieved the phase of clinical development for intraoperative use.[159] These new technologic developments may enhance our diagnostic acumen for intraoperative diagnosis with echocardiography in the future.

CONCLUSIONS

IOE is an extremely useful imaging modality for the care of patients undergoing selected types of cardiac surgery. The prepump echocardiogram provides a "road map" for valvular repair and other complex cardiac operations in the same way that the coronary arteriogram does for bypass surgery. The postpump intraoperative echocardiogram documents the success of the surgical mission or identifies the nature of problems requiring further surgery during the same procedure. IOE must be integrated with a good understanding of the clinical problems of the individual patient, the operative process, and the workings of the echocardiographic instrument. The rapid expansion of ultrasound technology promises to make IOE a most interesting field in the future.

References

1. Stewart, W.J., Currie P.J., Salcedo E.E., et al.: Evaluation of mitral leaflet motion by echocardiography and jet direction by Doppler color flow mapping to determine the mechanism of mitral regurgitation. J. Am. Coll. Cardiol. 20:1353, 1992.
2. Sheikh, K.H., de Bruijn, N.P., Rankin, J.S., et al.: The utility of transesophageal echocardiography and Doppler color flow imaging in patients undergoing cardiac valve surgery. J. Am. Coll. Cardiol. 15:363, 1990.
3. Stewart, W.J., Currie, P.J., Salcedo, E.E., et al.: Intraoperative Doppler color flow mapping for decision-making in valve repair for mitral regurgitation: Technique and results in 100 patients. Circulation 81:556, 1990.
4. Stewart, W.J., Currie, P.J., Agler, D.A., et al.: Intraoperative epicardial echocardiography: Technique, imaging planes, and use in valve repair for mitral regurgitation. Dynamic Cardiovasc. Imaging 1:179, 1987.
5. Mindich, B.P., Goldman, M.E., Fuster, V., et al.: Improved intraoperative evaluation of mitral valve operations utilizing two-dimensional contrast echocardiography. J. Thorac. Cardiovasc. Surg. 90:112, 1985.
6. Goldman, M.E., Mindich, B.P., Teichholz, L.E., et al.: Intraoperative contrast echocardiography to evaluate mitral valve operations. J. Am. Coll. Cardiol. 4:1035, 1984.
7. Sheikh, K.H., Bengtson, J.R., Rankin, J.S., et al.: Intraoperative transesophageal Doppler color flow imaging used to guide patient selection and operative treatment of ischemic mitral regurgitation. Circulation 84:594, 1991.
8. Fix, J., Isada, L., Cosgrove, D., et al.: Do patients with less than "echo-perfect" results from mitral valve repair by intraoperative echocardiography have different outcome? Circulation 88(Part 2):38, 1993.
9. Yoshida, K., Yoshikawa, J., Yamaura, Y., et al.: Assessment of mitral regurgitation by biplane transesophageal color Doppler flow mapping. Circulation 82:1121, 1990.
10. Helmcke, F., Nanda, N.C., and Hsiung, M.C.: Color Doppler assessment of mitral regurgitation with orthogonal planes. Circulation 75:175, 1987.
11. Daniel, W.G., Erbel, R., Kasper, W., et al.: Safety of transesophageal echocardiography: A multicenter survey of 10,419 examinations. Circulation 83:817, 1991.
12. Canter, C.E., Sekarski, D.C., Martin, T.C., et al.: Intraoperative evaluation of atrioventricular septal defect repair by color flow mapping echocardiography. Ann. Thorac. Surg. 48:544, 1989.
13. Wareing, T.H., Davila-Roman, V.G., Daily, B.B., et al.: Strategy for the reduction of stroke incidence in cardiac surgical patients. Ann. Thorac. Surg. 55:1400, 1993.
14. Pearlman, A.S., Gardin, J.M., Martin, R.P., et al.: Guidelines for physician training in transesophageal echocardiography: Recommendations of the American Society of Echocardiography Committee for Physician Training in Echocardiography. J. Am. Soc. Echocardiogr. 5:187, 1992.
15. Savage, R.M., Licina, M., Koch, C., et al.: Educational program for intraoperative transesophageal echocardiography. Anesth. Analg. 81:217, 1995.
16. Hatle, L., and Angelson, B.: Doppler Ultrasound in Cardiology: Physical Principles and Clinical Applications. Philadelphia, Lea & Febiger, 1985.
17. Vandervoort, P.M., Thoreau, D.H., Rivera, J.M., et al.: Automated flow rate calculations based on digital analysis of flow convergence proximal to regurgitant orifices. J. Am. Coll. Cardiol. 22:535, 1993.
18. Maurer, G., Czer, L.S., Chaux, A., et al.: Intraoperative Doppler color flow mapping for assessment of valve repair for mitral regurgitation. Am. J. Cardiol. 60:333, 1987.
19. Moulijn, A.C., Smulders, Y.M., Koolen, J.J., et al.: Intraoperative assessment of the mitral valve: Transesophageal Doppler echocardiography vs. left ventricular filling of the flaccid heart. Eur. J. Cardiothorac. Surg. 6:122, 1992.
20. Dahm, M., Iversen, S., Schmid, F.X., et al.: Intraoperative evaluation of reconstruction of the atrioventricular valves by transesophageal echocardiography. Thorac. Cardiovasc. Surg. 35:140, 1987.
21. Drexler, M., Erbel, R., Dahm, M., et al.: Assessment of successful valve reconstruction by intraoperative transesophageal echocardiography (TEE). Int. J. Card. Imaging 2:21, 1986.
22. Rafferty, T., Durkin, M., Elefteriades, J., et al.: Transesophageal echocardiographic evaluation of aortic valve integrity with antegrade crystalloid cardioplegic solution used as an imaging agent. J. Thorac. Cardiovasc. Surg. 104:637, 1992.
23. Reichert, S.L., Visser, C.A., Moulijn, A.C., et al.: Intraoperative transesophageal color-coded Doppler echocardiography for evaluation of residual regurgitation after mitral valve repair. J. Thorac. Cardiovasc. Surg. 100:756, 1990.
24. Kleinman, J.P., Czer, L.S., DeRobertis, M., et al.: A quantitative comparison of transesophageal and epicardial color Doppler echocardiography in the intraoperative assessment of mitral regurgitation. Am. J. Cardiol. 64:1168, 1989.
25. Rafferty, T., Durkin, M.A., Sittig, D., et al.: Transesophageal color flow Doppler imaging for aortic insufficiency in patients having cardiac operations. J. Thorac. Cardiovasc. Surg. 104:521, 1992.
26. Tanaka, M., Abe, T., and Hibi, N.: Intraoperative epicardial two-dimensional and pulsed Doppler echocardiography for assessing functional tricuspid regurgitation. J. Cardiol. 20:349, 1990.
27. Freeman, W.K., Schaff, H.V., Khandheria, B.K., et al.: Intraoperative evaluation of mitral valve regurgitation and repair by transesophageal echocardiography: Incidence and significance of systolic anterior motion. J. Am. Coll. Cardiol. 20:599, 1992.
28. Cosgrove, D.M., Rosenkranz, E.R., Hendren, W.G., et al.: Valvuloplasty for aortic insufficiency. J. Thorac. Cardiovasc. Surg. 102:571, 1991.
29. De Simone, R., Lange, R., Tanzeem, A., et al.: Adjustable tricuspid valve annuloplasty assisted by intraoperative transesophageal color Doppler echocardiography. Am. J. Cardiol. 71:926, 1993.
30. Klein, A.L., Stewart, W.J., Bartlett, J., et al.: Effects of mitral regurgitation on pulmonary venous flow and left atrial pressure: An intraoperative transesophageal echocardiographic study. J. Am. Coll. Cardiol. 20:1345, 1992.
31. Klein, A.L., Obarski, T.P., Stewart, W.J., et al.: Transesophageal Doppler echocardiography of pulmonary venous flow: A new marker of mitral regurgitation severity. J. Am. Coll. Cardiol. 18:518, 1991.
32. Deutsch, H.J., Curtius, J.M., Leischik, R., et al.: Reproducibility of assessment of left-ventricular function using intraoperative transesophageal echocardiography. Thorac. Cardiovasc. Surg. 41:54, 1993.
33. Roizen, M.F., Beaupre, P.N., Alpert, R.A., et al.: Monitoring with two-dimensional transesophageal echocardiography: Comparison of myocardial function in patients undergoing supraceliac, suprarenal-infraceliac, or infrarenal aortic occlusion. J. Vasc. Surg. 1:300, 1984.

34. Shintani, H., Nakano, S., Matsuda, H., et al.: Efficacy of transesophageal echocardiography as a perioperative monitor in patients undergoing cardiovascular surgery: Analysis of 149 consecutive studies. J. Cardiovasc. Surg. 31:564, 1990.

35. Voci, P., Bilotta, F., Scibilia, G., et al.: Reversal of left ventricular dysfunction early after coronary artery bypass grafting. Cardiologia 37:105, 1992.

36. Obarski, T.P., Loop, F.D., Cosgrove, D.M., et al.: Frequency of acute myocardial infarction in valve repairs versus valve replacement for pure mitral regurgitation. Am. J. Cardiol. 65:887, 1990.

37. Thys, D.M., Hillel, Z., Goldman, M.E., et al.: A comparison of hemodynamic indices derived by invasive monitoring and two-dimensional echocardiography. Anesthesiology 67:630, 1987.

38. Nishimura, R.A., Abel, M.D., Housmans, P.R., et al.: Mitral flow velocity curves as a function of different loading conditions: Evaluation by intraoperative transesophageal Doppler echocardiography. J. Am. Soc. Echocardiogr. 2:79, 1989.

39. Kuecherer, H.F., Muhiudeen, I.A., Kusumoto, F.M., et al.: Estimation of mean left atrial pressure from transesophageal pulsed Doppler echocardiography of pulmonary venous flow. Circulation 82:1127, 1990.

40. Cosgrove, D.M., and Stewart, W.J.: Mitral valvuloplasty. Curr. Probl. Cardiol. 14:359, 1989.

41. Carpentier, A., Deloche, A., Dauptain, J., et al.: A new reconstructive operation for correction of mitral and tricuspid insufficiency. J. Thorac. Cardiovasc. Surg. 61:1, 1971.

42. Himelman, R.B., Kusumoto, F., Oken, K., et al.: The flail mitral valve: Echocardiographic findings by precordial and transesophageal imaging and Doppler color flow mapping. J. Am. Coll. Cardiol. 17:272, 1991.

43. Stewart, W.J., Sun, J.P., Mayer, E., et al.: Mitral regurgitation with normal leaflets results from apical displacement of coaptation, not annular dilation. (Abstract.) Circulation 90:I-311, 1994.

44. Zhu, W.X., Oh, J.K., Kopecky, S.L., et al.: Mitral regurgitation due to ruptured chordae tendineae in patients with hypertrophic obstructive cardiomyopathy. J. Am. Coll. Cardiol. 20:242, 1992.

45. Marwick, T.H., Torelli, J., Obarski, T., et al.: Assessment of the mitral valve splitability score by transthoracic and transesophageal echocardiography. Am. J. Cardiol. 68:1106, 1991.

46. Mugge, E., Daniel, W.G., Frank, G., et al.: Echocardiography in infective endocarditis: Reassessment of prognostic implications of vegetation size determined by the transthoracic and the transesophageal approach. J. Am. Coll. Cardiol. 14:631, 1989.

47. van Herwerden, L.A., Gussenhoven, E.J., Roelandt, J.R., et al.: Intraoperative two-dimensional echocardiography in complicated infective endocarditis of the aortic valve. J. Thorac. Cardiovasc. Surg. 93:587, 1987.

48. Ballal, R.S., Mahan, E.F., III, Nanda, N.C., et al.: Aortic and mitral valve perforation: Diagnosis by transesophageal echocardiography and Doppler color flow imaging. Am. Heart J. 121(1 Pt. 1):214, 1991.

49. Daniel, W.G.: Improvement in the diagnosis of abscesses associated with endocarditis by transesophageal echocardiography. N. Engl. J. Med. 324:795, 1991.

50. Tingleff, J., Arendrup, H., and Pettersson, G.: Surgical repair of a postendocarditis abscess cavity in the heart guided by intraoperative transoesophageal echocardiography. Eur. J. Cardiothorac. Surg. 6:106, 1992.

51. Akamatsu, S., Terazawa, E., Kagawa, K., et al.: Evaluation of intraoperative transesophageal echocardiography. (Japanese.) J. Cardiol. 26:103, 1991.

52. Rankin, J.S., Livesey, S.A., Smith, L.R., et al.: Trends in the surgical treatment of ischemic mitral regurgitation: Effects of mitral valve repair on hospital mortality. Semin. Thorac. Cardiovasc. Surg. 1:149, 1989.

53. Goldman, A.P., Glover, M.U., Mick, W., et al.: Role of echocardiography/Doppler in cardiogenic shock: Silent mitral regurgitation. Ann. Thorac. Surg. 52:296, 1991.

54. Chopra, H.K., Nanda, N.C., Fan, P., et al.: Can two-dimensional echocardiography and Doppler color flow mapping identify the need for tricuspid valve repair? J. Am. Coll. Cardiol. 14:1266, 1989.

55. Farid, L., Dayem, M.K., Guindy, R., et al.: The importance of tricuspid valve structure and function in the surgical treatment of rheumatic mitral and aortic disease. Eur. Heart J. 13:366, 1992.

56. van Herwerden, L.A., Gussenhoven, W.J., Roelandt, J., et al.: Intraoperative epicardial two-dimensional echocardiography. Eur. Heart J. 7:386, 1986.

57. Kyo, S., Takamoto, S., Matsumura, M., et al.: Immediate and early postoperative evaluation of results of cardiac surgery by transesophageal two-dimensional Doppler echocardiography. Circulation 76:V113, 1987.

58. Marwick, T.H., Stewart, W.J., Currie, P.J., et al.: Mechanisms of failure of mitral valve repair: An echocardiographic study. Am. Heart J. 122:149, 1991.

59. Mohan, J.C., Reddy, K.N., Khanna, S.K., et al.: Pseudoaneurysm of the ascending aorta complicating cardiac surgery: Role of echocardiography in the diagnosis. Int. J. Cardiol. 31:33, 1991.

60. Johnston, S.R., Freeman, W.K., Schaff, H.V., et al.: Severe tricuspid regurgitation after mitral valve repair: Diagnosis by intraoperative transesophageal echocardiography. J. Am. Soc. Echocardiogr. 3:416, 1990.

61. D'Cruz, I.A., Overton, D.H., and Pai, G.M.: Pericardial complications of cardiac surgery: Emphasis on the diagnostic role of echocardiography. J. Card. Surg. 7:257, 1992.

62. Rosenzweig, B.P., Donahue, T., Attubato, M., et al.: Left ventricle-to-ascending aorta communication complicating composite graft repair undetected by aortography: Diagnosis by transesophageal echocardiography. J. Am. Soc. Echocardiogr. 4:639, 1991.

63. Smith, J.S., Cahalan, M.K., Benefiel, D.J., et al.: Intraoperative detection of myocardial ischemia in high-risk patients: Electrocardiography versus two-dimensional transesophageal echocardiography. Circulation 72:1015, 1985.

64. Mihaileanu, S., el Asmar, A.B., Acar, C., et al.: Intra-operative transoesophageal

65. Guyton, S.W., Paull, D.L., and Anderson, R.P.: Mitral valve reconstruction. Am. J. Surg. 163:497, 1992.

66. Stewart, W.J., Salcedo, E.E., and Cosgrove, D.M.: The value of echocardiography in mitral valve repair. Cleve. Clin. J. Med. 58:177, 1991.

67. Lee, K.S., Stewart, W.J., Lever, H.M., et al.: Mechanism of outflow tract obstruction causing failed mitral valve repair: Anterior displacement of leaflet coaptation. Circulation 88(Part 2):24, 1993.

68. Cutrone, F., Coyle, J.P., Novoa, R., et al.: Severe dynamic left ventricular outflow tract obstruction following aortic valve replacement diagnosed by intraoperative echocardiography. Anesthesiology 72:563, 1990.

69. Krenz, H.K., Mindich, B.P., Guarino, T., et al.: Sudden development of intraoperative left ventricular outflow obstruction: Differential and mechanism. An intraoperative two-dimensional echocardiographic study. J. Card. Surg. 5:93, 1990.

70. Goode, J.G., Baldeck, A.M., Berger, B.C., et al.: Intraoperative echocardiography for diagnosis of unsuspected hypertrophic cardiomyopathy. J. Cardiothorac. Vasc. Anesth. 6:449, 1992.

71. Webster, P.J., Raper, R.F., Ross, D.E., et al.: Pharmacologic abolition of severe mitral regurgitation associated with dynamic left ventricular outflow tract obstruction after mitral valve repair: Confirmation by transesophageal echocardiography. Am. Heart J. 126:480, 1993.

72. van Herwerden, L., Fraser, A.G., and Bos, E.: Left ventricular outflow tract obstruction after mitral valve repair assessed with intraoperative echocardiography: Noninterventional treatment. (Letter.) J. Thorac. Cardiovasc. Surg. 102:461, 1991.

73. Wilkins, G.T., Weyman, A.E., Abascal, V.M., et al.: Percutaneous balloon dilation of the mitral valve: An analysis of echocardiographic variables releted to outcome and the mechanism of dilatation. Br. Heart J. 60:299, 1988.

74. Casale, P.N., Whitlow, P., Currie, P.J., et al.: Transesophageal echocardiography in percutaneous balloon valvuloplasty for mitral stenosis. Cleve. Clin. J. Med. 56:597, 1989.

75. Goldstein, S.A., Campbell, A., Mintz, G.S., et al.: Feasibility of on-line transesophageal echocardiography during balloon mitral valvulotomy: Experience with 93 patients. J. Heart Valve Dis. 3:136, 1994.

76. Tanaka, M., Abe, T., Takashina, Y., et al.: Evaluation of secondary tricuspid regurgitation by intraoperative epicardial pulsed Doppler echocardiography. (Japanese.) J. Cardiol. 18:1083, 1988.

77. De Simone, R., Lange, R., Saggau, W., et al.: Intraoperative transesophageal echocardiography for the evaluation of mitral, aortic and tricuspid valve repair: A tool to optimize surgical outcome. Eur. J. Cardiothorac. Surg. 6:665, 1992.

78. Pretre, R., Faidutti, B., and Lerch, R.: Intraoperative TEE in aortic valve repair. Am. Heart J. 125:1822, 1993.

79. Stewart, W.J., Currie, P.J., Salcedo, E.E., et al.: Intraoperative echo in aortic valve repair. (Abstract.) Circulation 78:II-435, 1988.

80. Maurer, I., Regensburger, D., and Bernhard, A.: Aortic valve reconstruction in Rubinstein-Taybi syndrome: The valuable aid of transesophageal echocardiography. J. Cardiovasc. Surg. 32:327, 1991.

81. Baeza, O.R., Majid, N.K., Conroy, D.P., et al.: Combined conventional mechanical and ultrasonic debridement for aortic valvular stenosis. Ann. Thorac. Surg. 54:62, 1992.

82. Kumar, N., Prabhakar, G., Gometza, B., et al.: The Ross procedure in a young rheumatic population: Early clinical and echocardiographic profile. J. Heart Valve Dis. 2:376 1993.

83. McKay, R., and Ross, D.N.: Primary repair and autotransplantation of cardiac valves. Annu. Rev. Med. 44:181, 1993.

84. Bartzokis, T., St. Goar, F., DiBiase, A., et al.: Freehand allograft aortic valve replacement and aortic root replacement: Utility of intraoperative echocardiography and Doppler color flow mapping. J. Thorac. Cardiovasc. Surg. 101:545, 1991.

85. Alam, M., Serwin, J.B., Rosman, H.S., et al.: Transesophageal echocardiographic features of normal and dysfunctioning bioprosthetic valves. Am. Heart J. 121(4 Pt. 1):1149, 1991.

86. Karalis, D.G., Chandrasekaran, K., Ross, J.J., et al.: Single-plane transesophageal echocardiography for assessing function of mechanical or bioprosthetic valves in the aortic valve position. Am. J. Cardiol. 69:1310, 1992.

87. Deutsch, H.J., Curtius, J.M., Leischik, R., et al.: Diagnostic value of transesophageal echocardiography in cardiac surgery. Thorac. Cardiovasc. Surg. 39:199, 1991.

88. Abbruzzese, P.A., Meloni, L., Cardu, G., et al.: Intraoperative transesophageal echocardiography and periprosthetic leaks. (Letter.) J. Thorac. Cardiovasc. Surg. 101:556, 1991.

89. Meloni, L., Aru, G.M., Abbruzzese, P.A., et al.: Localization of mitral periprosthetic leaks by transesophageal echocardiography. Am. J. Cardiol. 69:276, 1992.

90. Syracuse, D.C., Gaudiani, V.A., Kastl, D.G., et al.: Intraoperative, intracardiac echocardiography during left ventriculomyotomy and myectomy for hypertrophic subaortic stenosis. Circulation 58(Suppl. I):I-24, 1978.

91. Marwick, T.H., Stewart, W.J., Lever, H.M., et al.: Benefits of intraoperative echocardiography in the surgical management of hypertrophic cardiomyopathy. J. Am. Coll. Cardiol. 20:1066, 1992.

92. Grigg, L.E., Wigle, E.D., Williams, W.G., et al.: Transesophageal Doppler echocardiography in obstructive hypertrophic cardiomyopathy: Clarification of pathophysiology and importance in intraoperative decision making. J. Am. Coll. Cardiol. 20:42, 1992.

93. Ius, P., Salandin, V., Zussa, C., et al.: Surgical treatment of left-ventricular outflow-tract obstruction guided by intraoperative transesophageal echocardiography. Thorac. Cardiovasc. Surg. 39:205, 1991.

94. Stewart, W.J., Schiavone, W.A., Salcedo, E.E., et al.: Intraoperative Doppler

echocardiography in hypertrophic cardiomyopathy: Correlations with the obstructive gradient. J. Am. Coll. Cardiol. 10:327, 1987.

95. Sasson, Z., Prieur, T., Skrobik, Y., et al.: Aortic regurgitation: A common complication after surgery for hypertrophic obstructive cardiomyopathy. J. Am. Coll. Cardiol. 13:63, 1989.

96. Gilbert, T.B., Panico, F.G., McGill, W.A., et al.: Bronchial obstruction by transesophageal echocardiography probe in a pediatric cardiac patient. Anesth. Analg. 74:156, 1992.

97. Lunn, R.J., Oliver, W.J., Hagler, D.J., et al.: Aortic compression by transesophageal echocardiographic probe in infants and children undergoing cardiac surgery. Anesthesiology 77:587, 1992.

98. Sreeram, N., Sutherland, G.R., Bogers, J.J., et al.: Subaortic obstruction: Intraoperative echocardiography as an adjunct to operation. Ann. Thorac. Surg. 50:579, 1990.

99. Muhiudeen, I.A., Roberson, D.A., Silverman, N.H., et al.: Intraoperative echocardiography in infants and children with congenital cardiac shunt lesions: Transesophageal versus epicardial echocardiography. J. Am. Coll. Cardiol. 16:1687, 1990.

100. Gussenhoven, E.J., van Herwerden, L.A., van Suylen, R.J., et al.: Recognition of residual ventricular septal defect by intraoperative contrast echocardiography. Eur. Heart J. 10:801, 1989.

101. Shah, P.M., Stewart, S., III, Calalang, C.C., et al.: Transesophageal echocardiography and the intraoperative management of pediatric congenital heart disease: Initial experience with a pediatric esophageal 2D color flow echocardiographic probe. J. Cardiothorac. Vasc. Anesth. 6:8, 1992.

102. Hogue, C.J., Barzilai, B., Forstot, R., et al.: Intraoperative echocardiographic diagnosis of previously unrecognized cor triatriatum. Ann. Thorac. Surg. 54:562 1992.

103. Ricou, F., Ludomirsky, A., Weintraub, R.G., et al.: Applications of intravascular scanning and transesophageal echocardiography in congenital heart disease: Tradeoffs and the merging of technologies. Int. J. Card. Imaging 6:221, 1991.

104. Cyran, S.E., Myers, J.L., Gleason, M.M., Weber, H.S., et al.: Application of intraoperative transesophageal echocardiography in infants and small children. J. Cardiovasc. Surg. 32:318, 1991.

105. Muhiudeen, I.A., Roberson, D.A., Silverman, N.H., et al.: Intraoperative echocardiography for evaluation of congenital heart defects in infants and children. Anesthesiology 76:165, 1992.

106. Gussenhoven, E.J., van Herwerden, L.A., Roelandt, J., et al.: Intraoperative two-dimensional echocardiography in congenital heart disease. J. Am. Coll. Cardiol. 9:565, 1987.

107. Hagler, D.J., Tajik, A.J., Seward, J.B., et al.: Intraoperative two-dimensional Doppler echocardiography: A preliminary study for congenital heart disease. J. Thorac. Cardiovasc. Surg. 95:516, 1988.

108. Wienecke, M., Fyfe, D.A., Kline, C.H., et al.: Comparison of intraoperative transesophageal echocardiography to epicardial imaging in children undergoing ventricular septal defect repair. J. Am. Soc. Echocardiogr. 4:607, 1991.

109. Hsu, Y.H., Santulli, T.J., Wong, A.L., et al.: Impact of intraoperative echocardiography on surgical management of congenital heart disease. Am. J. Cardiol. 67:1279, 1991.

110. Stumper, O., Fraser, A.G., Elzenga, N., et al.: Assessment of ventricular septal defect closure by intraoperative epicardial ultrasound. J. Am. Coll. Cardiol. 16:1672, 1990.

111. Ungerleider, R.M., Greeley, W.J., Sheikh, K.H., et al.: Routine use of intraoperative epicardial echocardiography and Doppler color flow imaging to guide and evaluate repair of congenital heart lesions: A prospective study. J. Thorac. Cardiovasc. Surg. 100:297, 1990.

112. Fyfe, D.A., Kline, C.H., Sade, R.M., et al.: Transesophageal echocardiography detects thrombus formation not identified by transthoracic echocardiography after the Fontan operation. J. Am. Coll. Cardiol. 18:1733, 1991.

113. Stumper, O., Sutherland, G.R., Sreeram, N., et al.: Role of intraoperative ultrasound examination in patients undergoing a Fontan-type procedure. Br. Heart J. 65:204, 1991.

114. Fyfe, D.A., Kline, C.H., Sade, R.M., et al.: The utility of transesophageal echocardiography during and after Fontan operations in small children. Am. Heart J. 122:1403, 1991.

115. Topol, E.J., Weiss, J.L., Guzman, P.A., et al.: Immediate improvement of dysfunctional myocardial segments after coronary revascularization: Detection by intraoperative transesophageal echocardiography. J. Am. Coll. Cardiol. 4:1123, 1984.

116. Ferrari, R., La Canna, G., Giubbini, R., et al.: Hibernating myocardium in patients with coronary artery disease: Identification and clinical importance. Cardiovasc. Drugs Ther. 6:287, 1992.

117. Simon, P., Mohl, W., Neumann, F., et al.: Effects of coronary artery bypass grafting on global and regional myocardial function: An intraoperative echocardiographic assessment. J. Thorac. Cardiovasc. Surg. 104:40, 1992.

118. Simon, P., Owen, A., Neumann, F., et al.: Immediate effects of mammary artery revascularization versus saphenous vein on global and regional myocardial function: An intraoperative echocardiographic assessment. Thorac. Cardiovasc. Surg. 3:228, 1991.

119. Maeta, H., Imawaki, S., Shiraishi, Y., et al.: Repair of both papillary and free wall rupture following acute myocardial infarction. J. Cardiovasc. Surg. 32:828, 1991.

120. Shah, P.M., Kyo, S., Matsumura, M., et al.: Utility of biplane transesophageal echocardiography in left ventricular wall motion analysis. J. Cardiothorac. Vasc. Anesth. 5:316, 1991.

121. Cahalan, M.K.: Pro: Transesophageal echocardiography is the "gold standard" for detection of myocardial ischemia. J. Cardiothorac. Anesth. 3:369, 1989.

122. Ellis, J.E., Shah, M.N., Briller, J.E., et al.: A comparison of methods for the detection of myocardial ischemia during noncardiac surgery: Automated ST-

123. Picano, E., Lattanzi, F., Orlandini, A., et al.: Stress echocardiography and the human factor: The importance of being expert. Am. J. Cardiol. 17:666 1991.

124. Eisenberg, M.J., London, M.J., Leung, J.M., et al.: Monitoring for myocardial ischemia during noncardiac surgery: A technology assessment of transesophageal echocardiography and 12-lead electrocardiography. The Study of Perioperative Ischemia Research Group. J.A.M.A. 268:210, 1992.

125. Matsuda, M., Kuwako, K., Sugishita, Y., et al.: Contrast echocardiography of the left heart by intravenous injection of perfluorochemical emulsion. (Jpn.) J. Cardiogr. 13(4):1021, 1983.

126. Villanueva, F.S., Glasheen, W.P., Sklenar, J., et al.: Characterization of spatial patterns of flow within the reperfused myocardium by myocardial contrast echocardiography. Circulation 88:2596, 1993.

127. Villaneuva, F.S., Spotnitz, W.D., Jayaweera, A.R., et al.: On-line intraoperative quantitation of regional myocardial perfusion during coronary artery bypass graft operations using myocardial contrast two-dimensional echocardiography. J. Thorac. Cardiovasc. Surg. 104:1524, 1992.

128. Hirata, N., Nakano, S., Taniguchi, K., et al.: Assessment of regional and transmural myocardial perfusion by means of intraoperative myocardial contrast echocardiography during coronary artery bypass grafting. J. Thorac. Cardiovasc. Surg. 104:1158, 1992.

129. Kabas, J.S., Kisslo, J., Flick, C.L., et al.: Intraoperative perfusion contrast echocardiography: Initial experience during coronary artery bypass grafting. J. Thorac. Cardiovasc. Surg. 99:536, 1990.

130. Keller, M.W., Spotnitz, W.D., Matthew, T.L., et al.: Intraoperative assessment of regional myocardial perfusion using quantitative myocardial contrast echocardiography: An experimental evaluation. J. Am. Coll. Cardiol. 16:1267, 1990.

131. Aronson, S., Lee, B.K., Wiencek, J.G., et al.: Assessment of myocardial perfusion during CABG surgery with two-dimensional transesophageal contrast echocardiography. Anesthesiology 75:433, 1991.

132. Spotnitz, W.D., Keller, M.W., Watson, D.D., et al.: Success of internal mammary bypass grafting can be assessed intraoperatively using myocardial contrast echocardiography. J. Am. Coll. Cardiol. 12:196, 1988.

133. Rovai, D., Nissen, S.E., Elion, J., et al.: Contrast echo washout curves from the left ventricle: Application of basic principles of indicator-dilution theory and calculation of ejection fraction. J. Am. Coll. Cardiol. 10:125, 1987.

134. Ten, C.F., Silverman, P.R., Sassen, L.M., et al.: Can myocardial contrast echo determine coronary flow reserve? Cardiovasc. Res. 26:32, 1992.

135. Sahn, D.J., Copeland, J.G., Temkin, L.P., et al.: Anatomic-ultrasound correlations for intraoperative open chest imaging of coronary artery atherosclerotic lesions in human beings. J. Am. Coll. Cardiol. 3:1169, 1984.

136. Kerber, R.E.: Echocardiographic assessment of atherosclerotic coronary lesions. Circulation 84(Suppl. 3):I322, 1991.

137. Isringhaus, H.: Intraoperative evaluation of coronary anatomy. Int. J. Card. Imaging 4:59, 1989.

138. McPherson, D.D., Hiratzka, L.F., Lamberth, W.C., et al.: Delineation of the extent of coronary atherosclerosis by high-frequency epicardial echocardiography. N. Engl. J. Med. 316:304, 1987.

139. Hiratzka, L.F., McPherson, D.D., Lamberth, W.C., et al.: Intraoperative evaluation of coronary artery bypass graft anastomoses using high-frequency epicardial echocardiography: Experimental validation and initial patient studies. Circulation 73:1199, 1986.

140. Watanabe, G., Ohhira, M., Takemura, H., et al.: Surgical treatment for myocardial bridge using intraoperative echocardiography: A report of two cases. J. Cardiovasc. Surg. 30:1009, 1989.

141. Haverich, A., Albes, J.M., Fahrenkamp, G., et al.: Intraoperative echocardiography to detect and prevent tricuspid valve regurgitation after heart transplantation. Eur. J. Cardiothorac. Surg. 5:41, 1991.

142. Koyanagi, T., Endo, M., Hashimoto, A., et al.: Intraoperative introduction of intra-aortic balloon catheter guided by transesophageal echocardiography. (Japanese.) Kyobu Geka 45:305, 1992.

143. Orihashi, K., and Oka, Y.: Intraluminal projection of descending thoracic aorta and intraaortic balloon pump catheter examined by transesophageal echocardiography in patients undergoing coronary artery bypass surgery. Hiroshima J. Med. Sci. 40:119, 1991.

144. Lange, R., Sack, F.U., Saggau, W., et al.: Performance of dynamic cardiomyoplasty related to the functional state of the heart. J. Card. Surg. 6:225, 1991.

145. Hassett, A., Moran, J., Sabiston, D.C., et al.: Utility of echocardiography in the management of patients with penetrating missile wounds of the heart. J. Am. Coll. Cardiol. 7:1151, 1986.

146. Ellis, J.E., and Bender, E.M.: Intraoperative transesophageal echocardiography in blunt thoracic trauma. J. Cardiothorac. Vasc. Anesth. 5:373, 1991.

147. Laurie, J.K., Appelbe, A., and Martin, R.P.: Detection of intimal flaps in aortic dissection by transesophageal echocardiography. Am. J. Cardiol. 69:1361, 1992.

148. Nienaber, C.A., Spielmann, R.P., von Kodolitsch, Y., et al.: Diagnosis of thoracic aortic dissection. Magnetic resonance imaging versus transesophageal echocardiography. Circulation 85:434, 1992.

149. Takamoto, S., Kyo, S., Adachi, H., et al.: Intraoperative color flow mapping by real-time two-dimensional Doppler echocardiography for evaluation of valvular and congenital heart disease and vascular disease. J. Thorac. Cardiovasc. Surg. 90:802, 1985.

150. Schippers, O.A., Gussenhoven, W.J., van Herwerden, L.A., et al.: The role of intraoperative two-dimensional echocardiography in the assessment of thoracic aorta pathology. Thorac. Cardiovasc. Surg. 36:208, 1988.

151. Goldman, M.E., Guarino, T., and Mindich, B.P.: Localization of aortic dissection

intimal flap by intraoperative two-dimensional echocardiography. J. Am. Coll. Cardiol. 6:1155, 1985.

152. Katz, E.S., Tunick, P.A., Rusinek, H., et al.: Protruding aortic atheromas predict stroke in elderly patients undergoing cardiopulmonary bypass: Experience with intraoperative transesophageal echocardiography. J. Am. Coll. Cardiol. 20:70, 1992.

153. Hosoda, Y., Watanabe, M., Hirooka, Y., et al.: Significance of atherosclerotic changes of the ascending aorta during coronary bypass surgery with intraoperative detection by echography. J. Cardiovasc. Surg. 32:301, 1991.

154. Ribakove, G.H., Katz, E.S., Galloway, A.C., et al.: Surgical implications of transesophageal echocardiography to grade the atheromatous aortic arch. Ann. Thorac. Surg. 53:758, 1992.

155. Gorscan, J., Gasior, T.A., Mandarino, W.A., et al.: Assessment of the immediate effects of cardiopulmonary bypass on left ventricular performance by on-line pressure-area relations. Circulation 89:180, 1994.

156. Perrino, A.C., Luther, M.A., O'Connor, T.Z., et al.: Automated border detection: Off-line validation of serial intraoperative measurements. Anesthesiology 81:3A, 1994.

157. Eaton, M.H., Lappas, D., Waggoner, A.D., et al.: Ultrasonic myocardial tissue characterization in the operating room: Initial results using transesophageal echocardiography. J. Am. Soc. Echocardiogr. 4:541 1991.

158. Fleming, A.D., Xia, S., McDicken, W.N., et al.: Myocardial velocity gradients detected by Doppler imaging. Br. J. Radiol. 67:679, 1994.

159. Pandian, N.G., Ludomirski, A., Cao, Q.L., et al.: Clinical application of 3 different modes of data acquisition for the performance of three-dimensional echocardiography. J. Am. Soc. Echocardiogr. 7:S45, 1994.

CHAPTER

40 Intravascular Ultrasound

Jeffrey M. Isner, M.D.

IN VITRO VALIDATION OF IVUS ____ 581
IVUS DETECTION OF "SILENT" PLAQUE ____ 582
TISSUE-PLAQUE CHARACTERIZATION ____ 582
USEFULNESS OF IVUS FOR QUANTIFYING VESSEL DIMENSIONS ____ 583
USEFULNESS OF IVUS FOR DEFINING THE MECHANISM OF BALLOON ANGIOPLASTY ____ 586
VASCULAR REMODELING ____ 591

USEFULNESS OF IVUS FOR GUIDING INTERVENTIONS ____ 592
INSTRUMENTS FOR COMBINED ULTRASOUND IMAGING AND PERCUTANEOUS REVASCULARIZATION ____ 597
THREE-DIMENSIONAL RECONSTRUCTION ____ 598
CURRENT LIMITATIONS OF IVUS FOR CLINICAL USE ____ 603

Advances in interventional technology have intensified the need for improved vascular imaging capabilities. Conventional contrast angiography has been the time-honored approach for lesion characterization and assessment. Angiography, however, remains limited by several factors, which have been well described previously.[1–10] These limitations relate principally to the fact that contrast angiography depicts the vessel lumen only; plaque and vessel wall are viewed as a "negative imprint" on the contrast-filled lumen. Although this phenomenon allows for characterization of lumen topography, irregularities in the plaque-wall topography may only be inferred from the negative imprint. Thus, angiography does not allow visualization or characterization of tissue elements below the intimal surface, which becomes particularly problematic in a vessel with diffuse disease, because the vessel may appear angiographically normal due to ubiquitous distribution of atherosclerotic plaque. Furthermore, contrast angiography is limited to a single planar view per injection; thus, information regarding the circumferential nature of the vessel-lumen interface cannot be directly recorded. Visualization of the vessel from alternative angles is possible but only at the expense of additional injections of contrast material. As a consequence of uniplanar viewing, direct measurement of luminal cross-sectional area is not feasible; instead, estimates of cross-sectional area must be derived from algorithms based on diameter measurements obtained from a single, potentially nonrepresentative plane.

Intravascular ultrasound (IVUS) imaging offers a potential solution to many of the limitations inherent in conventional contrast angiography. IVUS is unequivocally superior to contrast angiography in its ability to demonstrate detailed characteristics at the lumen-vessel wall interface, as well as depiction of structures within the plaque and vessel wall. Several investigators[11–15] have demonstrated that IVUS is exquisitely sensitive in detecting plaque and other details that are angiographically "silent." IVUS now provides the opportunity, for the first time, to accurately assess qualitative and quantitative effects of interventional therapy in vivo.[16–29] This advancement permits the clearer elucidation of the mechanisms by which balloon angioplasty increases luminal patency, as well as the device-specific effects of directional and rotational atherectomy, laser angioplasty, and stent deployment.

Technological developments, as well as an expanding library of clinical experience with image interpretation, have facilitated the clinical applications of IVUS. In this chapter, we review some of the early studies that laid the foundation for the current and potential future applications of IVUS, describe clinical experience with IVUS, and review the results of both combination (imaging-therapeutic) devices and three-dimensional reconstruction of serial IVUS images.

IN VITRO VALIDATION OF IVUS

Images of vessels derived from IVUS typically demonstrate a layered appearance surrounding the probe, as illustrated by the appearance of the normal arterial wall in Figure 40–1. The presentation of distinct layers is a consequence of the differing acoustic reflectivity of different tissues. Dense hyperreflective tissues are represented by bright echoes, and less dense tissues produce hypoechoic signals. Although the acoustic property of each tissue is critical in determining the brightness of the signal produced, it appears that "acoustic discrepancy" or "mismatch" (e.g., change in sonoreflectivity between adjacent structures) is the most important factor in defining the border between structures.[30] Accordingly, even a minor difference in tissue echogenicity can enable delineation of a border.

IVUS enables high-resolution imaging of vessel wall and lumen. Because of the intraluminal location of the probe and the ability of ultrasound energy to penetrate tissues, IVUS provides information regarding the arterial wall that was previously unavailable from in

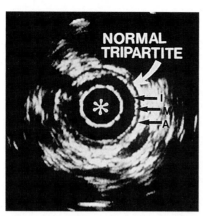

FIGURE 40–1. Architecture of the normal arterial wall as seen with IVUS. Asterisk indicates tranducer, positioned within arterial lumen. Three-layered appearance of normal arterial wall includes echogenic intima (I), echolucent media (M), and surrounding adventitia (A), again echogenic.

vivo examinations. Indeed, the experimental and clinical experience to date indicates that IVUS images correlate remarkably well with histologic examination, qualitatively as well as quantitatively. Numerous in vitro comparison studies have established the relationship between echos seen on IVUS images and structures seen histologically.[27, 30–36] Each layer of the arterial wall can be recognized from a typical ultrasound "signature": in normal muscular arteries, intima yields a hyperechoic signal; media a hypoechoic one; and adventitia a hyperechoic signal. Siegel and colleagues further confirmed the pathoanatomical correlates of the three layers by peeling away sequential layers of the vessel, using microdissection techniques.[37, 38] IVUS images were obtained at each stage of dissection and, despite the limitation of vessels being formalin-fixed, the results supported previous assignments of the three layers to intima, media, and adventitia. Pathologic or abnormal elements also have their own characteristic ultrasound appearance: for example, calcium consistently produces bright-echo reflections with acoustic shadowing or dropout of the subjacent ultrasound signal.

In addition to the qualitative similarity between IVUS and histology, quantitative measurements of the thickness of the arterial wall correlate remarkably well. Mallery and co-workers found correlation coefficients for total wall thickness and media alone of 0.85 and 0.83, respectively.[39] Potkin and associates found a similar correlation of 0.92 for linear wall thickness, including plaque and media combined.[33] Despite these results, because the correlation between IVUS and histologic measurements for intima alone is less than intima and media combined, there remains some controversy regarding the accuracy of IVUS in determining the thickness of the intimal layer. Several investigators have demonstrated that the inner echogenic layer shown in IVUS is often thicker than the intimal layer measured histologically.[40, 41] The presumed cause of this phenomenon is radial spreading, or "blooming," of the ultrasound reflections; that is, the signal created by the interface between blood and intima is sufficiently bright, relative to the subjacent echolucent media, that it "overlaps" into the medial area on the display screen.

Normal elastic arteries, in contrast with muscular arteries, do not demonstrate a distinct border between intima and media.[16, 31, 34, 42] Consequently, the vessel wall is more homogeneous and lacks the three-layered appearance. This situation is probably due to the presence of highly sonoreflective elastic and fibrous tissue in the medial layer. The absence of this tissue in muscular arteries renders the media more sonolucent and, therefore, creates the three-layered appearance.

Nishimura and associates observed in vitro that even muscular arteries may not exhibit the typical tripartite appearance when the intima is truly normal (e.g., only a few cell layers thick).[34] This finding was confirmed in vivo by Yeung and co-workers.[43] Whereas this phenomenon was originally presumed to be due to the relative lack of resolution of the 20-MHz device used in their study, work by Fitzgerald and colleagues confirmed the absence of an intimal signal in histologically normal vessels, even using a higher resolution 30-MHz instrument.[30] Explanted muscular coronary arteries from young patients (mean age = 27 years) had a homogeneous nonlayered IVUS appearance; in contrast, older (mean age = 42 years) vessels demonstrated the typical tripartite layering. Histologic analysis demonstrated that an intimal thickness of at least 178 μm was required to generate sufficient sonoreflectivity to be apparent on IVUS examination; in young normal patients, intimal thickness was typically less than 178 μm and, therefore, was sonographically silent. The implication of these findings is that intimal thickening advances with advancing age. Previous descriptions[27] of the three-layered appearance as the norm were based on studies from "relatively normal" vessels in patients with high-grade stenoses elsewhere; not unexpectedly, even so-called "normal" sites in these patients had evident intimal thickening. A second factor, which may account for the increased echogenicity of the intima with advancing age, is a gradual change in the composition of the intima, such that it is composed of more echogenic material; such an age-related change would be consistent with gradual loss in compliance and elasticity. Whether because of subtle intimal thickening or age-related changes in composition of the intimal layer, differences demonstrated by means of IVUS between "young" and "old" intima underscore the ability of IVUS to identify subtle abnormalities of the vascular wall.

IVUS DETECTION OF "SILENT" PLAQUE

Studies in the author's own laboratory,[27] as well as those of Tobis and associates,[44] Nissen and co-workers,[45] and Davidson and colleagues,[11] have shown that IVUS frequently demonstrates plaque not detected angiographically. Davidson and associates observed that among 46 percent of patients in whom plaque was identified by means of IVUS, the sites examined were normal, as shown with angiography. In reports[14, 46] comparing IVUS examinations with angiography in cardiac transplant recipients, St. Goar and co-workers demonstrated that among patients studied 1 year after cardiac transplantation, all exhibited intimal thickening in IVUS. Despite this finding, corresponding angiograms were normal in 42 of the 60 patients studied; in 21 of these 42, the thickening was severe or moderate. Likewise, angiography was found to be less sensitive than IVUS for assessment of progressive intimal thickening in transplant recipients.[47] The fact that diffuse, uniform intimal thickening would not be detected angiographically has been documented in multiple previous angiographic-histologic correlative studies.[6, 9] Interestingly, of the 20 patients studied by St. Goar and colleagues within 1 month after transplant, the intima was visualized in only 7 (35 percent); this finding is consistent with those described earlier regarding the "invisible"[48] nature of the intima on IVUS examination in young normal muscular arteries and suggests that the thickness of the intimal layer was less than 178 μm in these vessels (i.e., below the resolution level of the IVUS instrument).

In the author's own experience in imaging patients during interventional procedures, the finding of angiographically "silent" plaque has been the rule, rather than the exception. Angiographically normal sites, which are adjacent to lesions and which would typically be identified as "normal reference vessels," are almost always significantly diseased, as shown through IVUS. Again, this problem highlights one of the major liabilities of angiography: the degree of disease at one site is typically (and for lack of any other available standard) evaluated in relationship to a *normal-appearing* adjacent site.[5, 27]

TISSUE-PLAQUE CHARACTERIZATION

Previous studies have attempted to use IVUS to visualize plaque composition.[22, 31, 33, 34, 39] Fibrous plaque appears as bright, homoge-

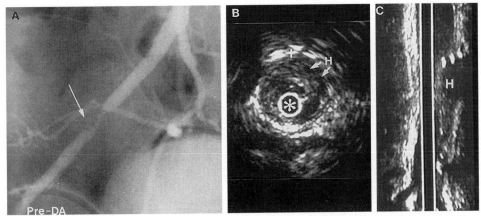

FIGURE 40–2. Angiographic and IVUS findings in a patient with crescendo claudication. *A,* Diagnostic arteriogram showing irregular, high-grade stenosis *(arrow)* in right external iliac artery. *B,* Two-dimensional intravascular ultrasound *(asterisk* indicates the ultrasound transducer) obtained before atherectomy shows heterogeneous plaque with hypoechoic foci that are consistent with plaque hemorrhage (H, *arrows*), suggesting plaque rupture as possible mechanism of patient's recent onset of symptoms. *C,* Three-dimensional reconstruction of serial IVUS images, showing right external iliac artery, narrowed by segmental stenosis that abuts ultrasound catheter, encroaching on lumen (hypoechoic foci of plaque hemorrhage, H, now seen in longitudinal disposition).

neous echos. Calcific deposits clearly and consistently generate intensely echogenic bright signals, which create an "acoustic shadow" that shields subjacent structures. In the author's experience, reproducible characterization of plaque as fibrous versus "fatty" is not as consistently possible when done by means of IVUS; this is almost certainly because, in part, few plaques are ever purely "fatty," and the lipid component of most plaques is, in fact, minor. In occasional cases, identification of thrombus by means of IVUS has been well documented.[20] Although some investigators have suggested that thrombus may be regularly distinguished from low-density plaque,[49] the author has not found any reliable characteristics to differentiate these two entities. Indeed, the appearance of thrombus may be variable even in the same patient. Seigel and associates likewise found IVUS to be insensitive for the identification of thrombus.[35] Detection of thrombus and associated unstable plaque appears to be one area in which angioscopy is superior to both IVUS and angiography.[50, 51]

In occasional cases, IVUS may be uniquely informative with regard to details of plaque-wall pathology. For example, the images shown in Figure 40–2 were recorded from a patient with onset of disabling claudication; hypoechoic foci that suggested plaque rupture and hemorrhage were responsible for the patient's accelerated symptoms.[52] Tissue obtained by directional atherectomy documented findings of plaque fissure and hemorrhage (Fig. 40–3), confirming plaque rupture as the mechanism for the patient's acute onset of symptoms.

FIGURE 40–3. See Color Plate 20.

Preliminary investigation using analysis of backscatter and "ice-pick" imaging may better define the acoustic properties of given tissues and allow more reproducible and accurate tissue characterization in vivo.[53]

USEFULNESS OF IVUS FOR QUANTIFYING VESSEL DIMENSIONS

The most critical advantage of IVUS for clinical work derives from its unequivocally superior capacity to define luminal dimensions, particularly cross-sectional area. Early in vitro studies by

Nishimura and co-workers demonstrated the accuracy (correlation coefficient = .98) of IVUS lumen measurements compared with those from histology.[34] Using live animals, Nissen and colleagues found a correlation for diameter between quantitative angiography and IVUS of .98 for normal sites and .89 for experimentally induced concentric stenoses.[45] Subsequent studies in humans found similarly close correlations (.80 to .95) between cross-sectional area in normal or nearly normal vessels, as measured with IVUS, versus those derived from quantitative angiography.[11, 15, 54] Diseased, non-dilated vessels demonstrated a lesser, but still respectable, correlation (r = .86).[15] Although these data demonstrate a good *correlation* between cross-sectional areas measured by IVUS and those derived from quantitative angiographic algorithms, the *absolute* values for area may differ substantially. Furthermore, because algorithms developed for quantitative angiography fail to address the problems posed by diffusely diseased vessels,[7] the *relative degree* of compromise of a given site may be better determined by use of IVUS.

To the extent that IVUS may directly demonstrate luminal cross-sectional area in cases in which angiography is complicated by certain anatomical factors, IVUS may be useful as a *diagnostic tool.* For example, angiographic assessment of the left main coronary artery has been a well-documented[5] source of angiographic ambiguity. IVUS imaging has been useful in such cases for elucidating the extent of luminal compromise (Fig. 40–4).[55] IVUS may also resolve lesion severity in instances in which the presence of bends, vessel overlap, or branch points obscures the border of contrast during angiography (Fig. 40–5). IVUS can also be particularly helpful in circumstances in which it is necessary to define components of the arterial wall. Although difficulty in assessing pathology is not uncommon in the tortuous coronary tree, IVUS may be specifically useful for defining the severity of aorto-ostial lesions in renal and mesenteric vessels (Figs. 40–6 and 40–7)[56]; stenoses at these sites are often difficult to visualize angiographically, because of their proximity to the aorta, the brisk flow of contrast, and the abundance of calcium.

After intervention, there is significantly more discrepancy between vessel dimensions determined with IVUS and angiography.[57] This phenomenon was graphically demonstrated in the assessment of 13 consecutive patients in whom the results of balloon (10) or laser (3) angioplasty were quantified with both quantitative angiographic analysis and intravascular ultrasound.[23] The minimal luminal diameter and cross-sectional area were calculated for interventional sites and nearby reference sites. The corresponding ultra-

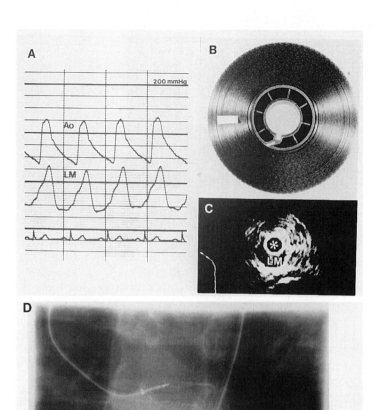

FIGURE 40–4. IVUS obviates need for multiple orthogonal views. *A,* In this patient, recurrent damping of coronary arterial pressure was observed on engaging left main (LM) coronary artery. *B,* Ambiguous angiographic appearance of LM required multiple angulated projections, resulting in protracted cine recording. *C,* IVUS inspection of LM promptly excluded significant LM stenosis. *D,* Cine frame of IVUS catheter in LM coronary artery. Ao = aorta; ° = IVUS catheter.

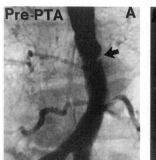
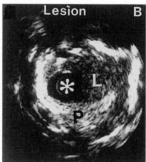
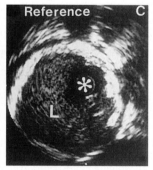

FIGURE 40–5. Superior imaging of eccentric aortic lesion with IVUS compared with that of angiography. This 63-year-old woman presented with accelerated bilateral buttocks claudication, occurring at 1 to 2 blocks. *A,* Conventional anteroposterior angiography failed to disclose any significant stenosis; mild irregularity *(arrow)* was seen within the distal aorta. After discovering a large pressure gradient, IVUS examination was performed. *B,* IVUS image depicts focal, eccentric plaque (P) narrowing the lumen (L) in distal aorta. *C,* IVUS from reference site distal to stenosis depicts normal lumen dimensions. After angioplasty-stent, gradient and symptoms resolved. ° = IVUS catheter.

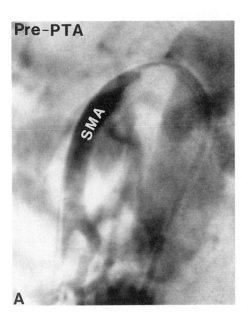
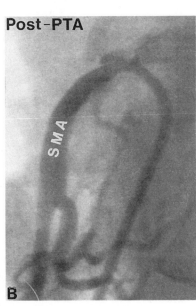

FIGURE 40–6. Balloon angioplasty (PTA) of superior mesenteric artery (SMA) in elderly woman with severe intestinal angina. *A,* Selective angiography before PTA demonstrates critical ostial stenosis. Angiogram depicted was obtained only after test injections in multiple other, less-optimal angles. *B,* Post-PTA plaque fracture is evident. Presence and distribution of calcium is difficult to discern with angiography and fluoroscopy.

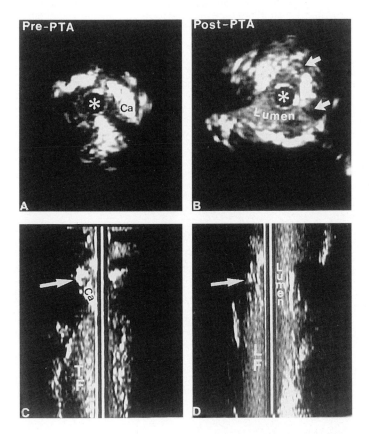

FIGURE 40–7. IVUS and sagittal three-dimensional reconstruction during balloon angioplasty (PTA) of superior mesenteric artery from Figure 40–6. *A,* IVUS before PTA demonstrates heavily calcified (Ca) plaque surrounding probe *(asterisk),* not appreciated by angiography (Fig. 40–6). *B,* IVUS after PTA shows enlargement of lumen because of increased separation-fracture *(arrows)* between calcific deposits. *C,* Sagittal image from serial IVUS frames reconstructs vessel longitudinally, in orientation similar to that of angiogram, and shows calcific plaque *(arrow)* encroaching on lumen, which has normal dimensions more distally. Coarse echoes in distal lumen indicate turbulent flow (TF) through stenosis. *D,* Sagittal view after PTA. Proximal lumen is partially enlarged at lesion site *(arrow)* and echo signals corresponding to blood flow are now more uniform, indicating more laminar flow (LF).

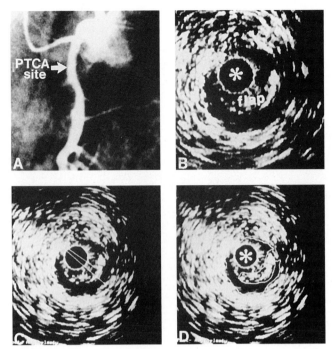

FIGURE 40–8. Angiographic versus IVUS assessment of postinterventional cross-sectional area. *A,* After balloon angioplasty (PTCA), morphology of PTCA site in proximal right coronary artery appears widely patent. *B,* IVUS image of PTCA site discloses tissue flap resulting from crescentic plaque fracture. *C,* Determination of post-PTCA luminal diameter, angiographically or even by IVUS using cross-sectional view is problematic: peninsular "flap" creates ambiguity regarding minimum versus maximum diameter. *D,* Determination of luminal cross-sectional area of even the complicated lumen resulting from PTCA is straightforward with the use of planimeter-measured area from IVUS cross-sectional image.

sound frames from both interventional and reference sites were digitized, and the minimal luminal diameter was measured directly; cross-sectional area was obtained by tracing the perimeter of the lumen. The luminal diameter for reference sites was measured as 3.9 mm with IVUS, versus 3.3 mm with quantitative angiography ($P < .05$). Regression analysis disclosed a correlation coefficient of 0.87. For cross-sectional area of *reference sites,* the absolute difference between ultrasound and angiography, 12.6 versus 9.6 mm², was also statistically significant ($P < .05$). Regression analysis disclosed a correlation coefficient of .92, similar to that calculated for analysis of luminal diameter. Luminal diameter for *interventional sites* was measured as 2.8 mm with IVUS, versus 1.8 mm with angiography ($P < .01$). Regression analysis disclosed a poorer correlation (.62) than that calculated for reference sites. Similarly, for cross-sectional area of interventional sites, there was a highly statistically significant difference between absolute measurements made by means of ultrasound (6.9) versus those made by means of quantitative angiography (2.8; $P < .01$).

There is good reason to believe that cross-sectional area measurements are more accurate when measured with IVUS than with quantitative angiography, especially after intervention. Figure 40–8 illustrates certain of the advantages inherent in IVUS imaging. First, IVUS provides accurate delineation of luminal borders and obviates the need for multiple orthogonal angiographic views. Second, IVUS provides the ability to directly planimeter cross-sectional area eliminating the dependence on algorithms that derive area from diameter measurements, algorithms that make potentially incorrect assumptions about luminal geometry. Third, in contrast with quantitative angiography, in which the catheter used for calibration may be located at a distance from the segment being measured, with IVUS the calibration instrument is, by definition, within the plane of measurement. Fourth, with IVUS, the area

being measured occupies nearly the entire field of view on the screen; in contrast, for angiographic analysis, the vascular region of interest involves only a small fraction of the cine frame from which it is measured.

USEFULNESS OF IVUS FOR DEFINING THE MECHANISM OF BALLOON ANGIOPLASTY

The most extensive clinical experience with IVUS to date, and the application in which IVUS appears to offer the greatest practical clinical use, has been in the assessment of the intravascular effects of percutaneous therapy in coronary and peripheral vessels. Contrast angiography, although routinely performed before and after instrumentation, provides only a profile of luminal diameter, rather than depiction of cross-sectional area; this fact, along with the other methodologic limitations described previously,[1, 2, 4–6] has compromised its usefulness for the study of angioplasty mechanisms. In vitro studies have demonstrated that IVUS consistently provides exquisite detail of morphologic alterations in the arterial wall and subjacent plaque that result from the barotrauma of balloon inflation.[33, 36, 58–60]

Experience with in vivo imaging after dilation has confirmed the in vitro data. In the few patients studied at necropsy after percutaneal transluminal angioplasty (post-PTA) in whom IVUS had also been performed, IVUS images displayed morphologic abnormalities identical to those seen by light microscopy (Fig. 40–9).[60, 61] The fact that IVUS routinely depicts tomographic full-thickness images of the arterial wall allows one to gain, in vivo, a perspective similar to that obtained from histologic examination. Furthermore, the performance of serial examinations in vivo provides documentation of pathologic alterations attributable to the specific instrumentation used. These unique features of IVUS have been used to good advantage in the study of the mechanisms by which balloon angioplasty improves lumina patency (Figs. 40–10 through 40–12). Observations derived from IVUS at the author's institution[27] and others[62] suggest that plaque fracture or dissection, or both, are associated with balloon dilation in the overwhelming majority of angiographically and hemodynamically successful procedures. Indeed, other data[63, 64] suggest that at least some degree of plaque fracture must be seen with IVUS to achieve a successful long-term result; vessels that display no tearing may be much more prone to recoil or to restenosis.

The relative contribution of plaque fractures, as opposed to other

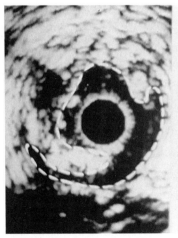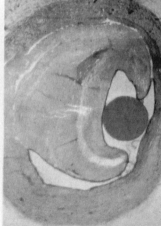

FIGURE 40–9. Correlation between IVUS and histology. *A,* IVUS image obtained from angioplasty (PTA) site in iliac artery, demonstrating extensive plaque fracture. Patient died 24 hours later from unrelated cause. *B,* Histologic section corresponding to PTA site in *A,* depicting morphologic features nearly identical to those seen with IVUS.

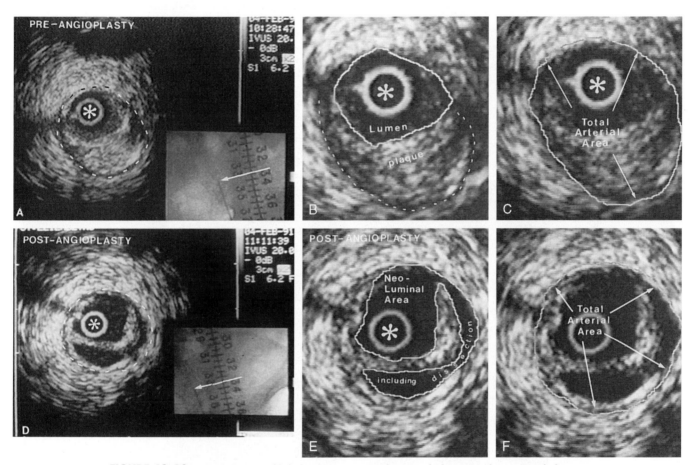

FIGURE 40–10. *A,* IVUS image of left iliac artery at site of stenosis before angioplasty. Asterisk denotes IVUS catheter. Echolucent band *(dashed line)* represents media of arterial wall. Split screen shows simultaneous fluoroscopic recording of catheter position during IVUS imaging; arrow marks position of IVUS transducer at time of image acquisition. *B,* Digitized IVUS image of stenosis site before angioplasty. Luminal area, confirmed by injection of agitated saline, is traced. Large eccentric plaque occupies area between lumen and media *(dashed line)* of vessel wall. *C,* Digitized IVUS image of stenosis site showing computerized tracing of medial border for assessment of total arterial area before angioplasty. *D,* IVUS image of same site in iliac artery after angioplasty. Dashed line traces medial border. Arrow confirms transducer location identical to preangioplasty site. *E,* Digitized postangioplasty image with computerized measurement of neoluminal area. Large, crescent-shaped dissection contributes significant portion of the neoluminal area. Injection of agitated saline confirmed that this dissection was functional part of postangioplasty lumen. *F,* Digitized IVUS image of postangioplasty artery with computerized measurement of total arterial area.

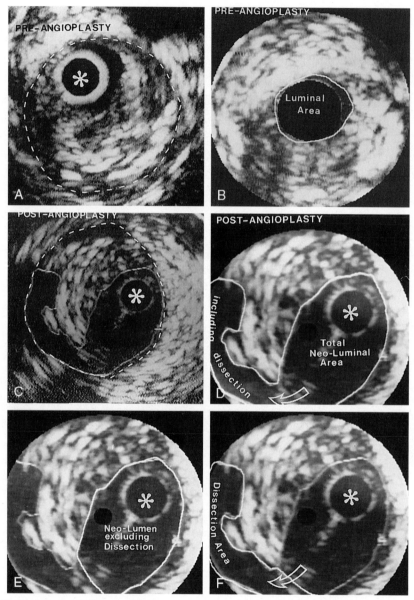

FIGURE 40–11. *A,* IVUS image of iliac artery at site of stenosis before angioplasty. Asterisk denotes IVUS catheter. Lumen of vessel, black and crescent-shaped, surrounds IVUS catheter. Dashed line marks outer border of the media of vessel wall. Area between lumen and media is filled with heterogeneous-appearing plaque. *B,* Digitized IVUS image at site of stenosis before angioplasty. Central black area represents computerized removal of IVUS catheter during digitizing process. Measurement of lumen area is demonstrated. *C,* IVUS image of same stenotic site, now after angioplasty. Dotted line along outer medial border denotes outer wall of the artery. Line tracing denotes neolumen, confirmed by injection of agitated saline during IVUS imaging. *D,* Digitized image of postangioplasty treatment site. Neoluminal area has now been measured and includes a large dissection. *E,* Tracing of the neolumen, excluding the area contributed by the dissection. *F,* Tracing of area contributed to neolumen by dissection area.

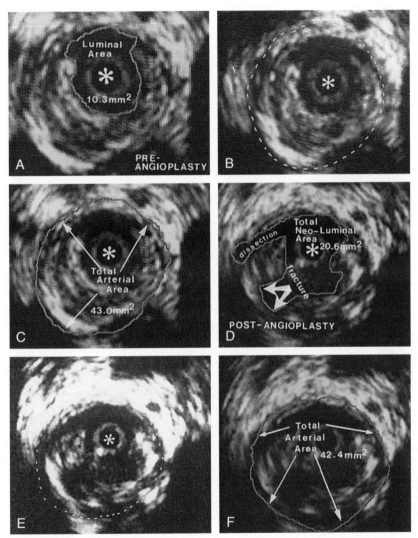

FIGURE 40–12. *A*, Digitized IVUS image of iliac artery before angioplasty, demonstrating measurement of luminal area. Asterisk marks IVUS catheter. *B*, primary unprocessed IVUS image from which digitized images were obtained. Dashed line traces media of vessel wall. *C*, Digitized image demonstrating measurement of total arterial area. *D*, Postangioplasty measurement of neoluminal area. Comparison with preangioplasty image (immediately to left) reveals that a significant part of the increase in luminal area is supplied by accessory lumen resulting from plaque fracture. *E*, Primary unprocessed IVUS image after angioplasty, from which digitized images for quantification were obtained. Dashed line traces outer border of media of arterial wall. *F*, Measurement of total arterial area after angioplasty from digitized IVUS image.

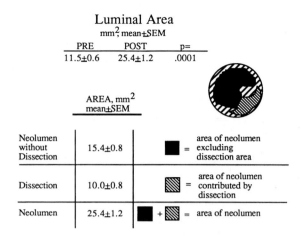

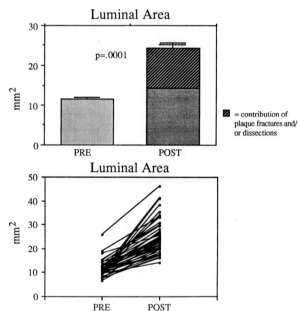

FIGURE 40–13. Luminal cross-sectional area measured with IVUS before and after angioplasty. *Top, Diagram,* Luminal area, excluding the contribution of plaque fractures and dissections, is represented in black; area contributed by fractures and dissections is represented by narrow diagonal stripes. Wide diagonal stripes denote atherosclerotic plaque. *Middle,* Bar graph showing luminal area (mean ± SEM) measured with IVUS before and after angioplasty for entire cohort. Area contributed by IVUS-defined plaque fractures and dissections is denoted by narrow diagonal stripes. *Bottom,* Graph showing luminal area before and after angioplasty measured with IVUS for 40 individual arteries.

factors, to the overall increase in luminal area seen after balloon angioplasty has been elucidated with IVUS (Figs. 40–13 and 40–14). Tobis and associates[36] demonstrated in vitro that diseased vessels subjected to balloon dilation tended to tear longitudinally at the thinnest region of the plaque; they suggested that these tears account for the enlargement of luminal cross-sectional area. Losordo and co-workers[65] evaluated IVUS images obtained before and after PTA performed in 40 patients and quantified the relative contributions of plaque fracture, plaque compression, and arterial stretch to the enhanced overall luminal area. Luminal cross-sectional area more than doubled, from 11.5 mm² before PTA to 25.4 mm² after PTA. The neolumen created by plaque fractures accounted for the majority (72 percent) of the total increase in luminal area. Compression of plaque was seen in all treated vessels and made an important but quantitatively less significant contribution to the postangioplasty increase in luminal area. Arterial stretching was demonstrated in only 25 percent of patients, and even in this group, its contribution to increased area was minimal. These

data confirm previous observations that suggest that plaque fracture constitutes the principal mechanism responsible for increased luminal patency after balloon angioplasty. These results consequently contradict conclusions based on earlier in vitro studies[66, 67] and a smaller in vivo study,[68] which implicated stretching of the vessel wall as a major factor contributing to increased lumen size.

In an attempt to categorize the degree of plaque fracture observed with IVUS after balloon angioplasty, Honye and colleagues[64] have identified six characteristic morphologic patterns of vessel disruption (Table 40–1). In their proposed scheme (Fig. 40–15), patterns A through D represent increasing degrees of plaque tearing and separation from subjacent structures, whereas pattern E represents stretching without obvious tearing. Of 66 coronary lesions subjected to balloon dilation, Honye and associates observed fairly equal distribution of the different morphologic subtypes, with a slight predominance in types B, C, and especially E. Interestingly, in their preliminary analysis, type E1 lesions displayed a greater tendency toward restenosis at 6-month follow-up.

Calcified plaque (Fig. 40–16) is detected with IVUS in most vessels undergoing angioplasty, a feature that is underappreciated in angiography and which may be important in understanding the mechanism of PTA. For example, Honye and co-workers identified

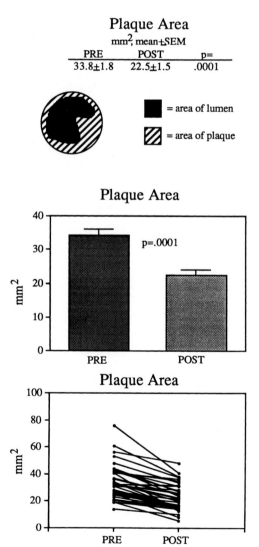

FIGURE 40–14. Plaque area before and after angioplasty. *Top, Diagram,* Lumen is indicated schematically in black; plaque is indicated by wide diagonal stripes. *Middle,* Bar graph showing plaque area (mean ± SEM) before and after angioplasty for entire cohort. *Bottom,* Graph showing plaque area before and after angioplasty measured with IVUS for 40 individual arteries.

TABLE 40–1. MORPHOLOGIC PATTERNS OF VESSEL DISRUPTION FOLLOWING PTCA

Type A: Partial-thickness tear in plaque, not extending to subjacent tissue
Type B: Full-thickness tear in plaque, extending to media, with separation of two edges of torn plaque
Type C: Full-thickness tear, with separation (dissection) of plaque from underlying media for arc of up to 180 degrees
Type D: Full-thickness tear, with separation of plaque extending circumferentially >180 degrees. Plaque largely or entirely pulled away from subjacent tissues
Type E: Stretching of concentric (E1) or eccentric (E2) plaque, without obvious separation or plaque fracture

Adapted from Honye, J., Mahon, D.J., Jain, A., et al. Morphological effects of coronary balloon angioplasty in vivo assessed by intravascular ultrasound. Circulation 85:1012, 1992. Copyright 1992, American Heart Association.

calcific deposits in 14 versus 83 percent of patients studied by means of angiography and ultrasound, respectively.[69] The author's experience has been similar.[22, 27] Waller and colleagues have previously suggested that tears and fractures typically occur along the border between calcific plaque and softer tissue[70]; assuming that such is the case, then the increased sensitivity of IVUS in detecting calcific deposits may be clinically relevant. Indeed, observations[71, 72] lend further support to the notion that the presence of calcium may predict the location and extent of plaque fracture. For example, Fitzgerald and associates[71] imaged 41 patients after angioplasty; they found that in 87 percent of patients with focal deposits of calcium who also demonstrated dissections, the fracture site was located adjacent to the calcified plaque. Furthermore, the extent of dissection was greater in the patients with calcified vessels than in those with noncalcified ones. To the extent that large dissections may portend a poor angioplasty outcome, including specifically a higher risk of abrupt closure, the detection and localization of calcium may become important practical applications of IVUS. Further studies are necessary, however, to discriminate the characteristic features or patterns of calcific deposition, which may be a harbinger of a poor percutaneous transluminal coronary angioplasty result.

FIGURE 40–16. See Color Plate 21.

Preliminary evidence from in vivo IVUS studies has also pro-

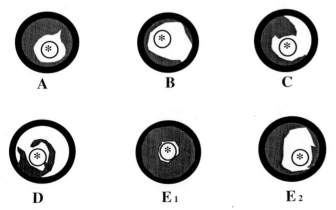

FIGURE 40–15. Classification of morphologic patterns of vessel disruption after percutaneous transluminal angioplasty. (After Honye, J., Mahon, D.J., Jain, A., et al.: Morphological effects of coronary balloon angioplasty in vivo assessed by intravascular ultrasound imaging. Circulation 85:1012, 1992, with permission. Copyright 1992, American Heart Association.)

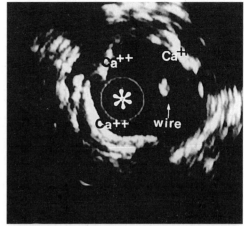

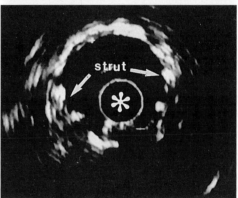

FIGURE 40–17. *Top,* Heavily calcified (Ca^{2+}) lesion with multiple plaque fractures after angioplasty. *Bottom,* Arterial wall trauma is effaced by deployed endovascular stent.

vided insight into the mechanisms by which directional atherectomy, stent deployment, and laser angioplasty enhance luminal area. In contrast with vessels undergoing balloon angioplasty, vessels in which directional atherectomy is performed demonstrate less prominent plaque–arterial wall disruption; instead, the perimeter of the neolumen is typically smooth and uninterrupted. In the author's initial series of patients,[27] no plaque cracks were observed on postatherectomy IVUS examination. Rather, discrete "bites" corresponding to individual passes of the cutting blade were often observed, consistent with tissue removal. Similar findings have been reported by Yock and co-workers,[73] Smucker and colleagues,[74] and Tenaglia and associates,[17] all of whom reported a relatively low incidence of plaque fracture. Controversy persists regarding the extent to which inflation of the eccentric balloon of the Simpson Atherocath contributes to increased luminal area; indeed, angiographic studies have suggested that the amount of tissue retrieved is not enough to account for the resultant increase in luminal diameter,[75, 76] and in certain cases it has been documented that the Dotter effect of the catheter and the effects of balloon inflation have produced the majority of luminal patency.

Signs of arterial wall trauma are most completely effaced on IVUS images recorded after delivery of an endovascular stent (Fig. 40–17): the extensive trauma observed at these same sites after balloon angioplasty (present implantation) suggests that stent implantation acutely ameliorates arterial wall pathology.[27, 77, 78]

VASCULAR REMODELING

The term vascular remodeling[79] has been clinically regarded as a naturally occurring adaptation to atherosclerosis[80] but, more recently, has been used to define a response of the vascular wall to percutaneous revascularization.[81] The former implies segmental arterial enlargement, whereas the latter involves segmental arterial constriction. The application of IVUS to both aspects of remodeling illustrates the utility of this imaging modality for studying pathogenetic mechanisms involving the intact arterial circulation of live patients. Glagov and co-workers[80] described the enlargement of atherosclerotic left main coronary arteries in a population of human hearts obtained post mortem. The conclusion that arterial enlargement occurred in response to the accumulation of atherosclerotic plaque was based on a regression analysis that correlated the size of the left main coronary arteries with the degree of atherosclerotic plaque accumulation. Subsequent, similarly performed pathologic studies[82] reproduced these findings. Epicardial echocardiography[83] was also used to compare coronary arterial dimensions in normal and atherosclerotic arteries, yielding similar results.

In vivo analysis of human arteries with the use of IVUS of paired adjacent normal and atherosclerotic arterial segments disclosed progressive focal dilation of the outer arterial wall in response to the incremental accumulation of atherosclerotic plaque (Fig. 40–18).[84] Quantitative analysis of arterial morphometry showed that as the cross-sectional area of plaque increased within a diseased vessel segment, the outer wall of the artery expanded in an attempt to compensate for this accumulation of plaque. Two points regarding the enlargement of arteries in response to plaque accumulation are worth emphasizing. First, the increase in total arterial area was proportional to the amount of plaque at the diseased site, as

demonstrated by the positive correlation between these variables. Second, the enlargement of the artery was a focal response that did not affect the adjacent normal segments of the artery.

Two important advantages of using IVUS provided a unique opportunity to demonstrate that arterial enlargement occurs as a local response of the artery wall to the development of atherosclerotic plaque. First, the collection of morphologic data was performed without the perturbation of tissue architecture, a prerequisite for standard pathologic examination.[85, 86] Second, because adjacent normal or nearly normal and diseased arterial segments were examined within the same artery, patients could serve as their own internal controls, avoiding the potential hazards of comparisons made between normal and abnormal individuals.

More recently, Post and colleagues[81] used the term remodeling to describe arterial constriction that develops after angioplasty and appears to constitute the pathogenetic mechanism that explains those cases of restenosis that lack a significant proliferative component. This concept was investigated in vivo by Mintz and co-workers,[87–89] who used IVUS to serially evaluate the acute and chronic responses to percutaneous revascularization in human patients. Because their approach permitted direct measurement of the areas of both wall and lumen, the authors' findings support the contention that late lumen loss is not limited to encroachment by atherosclerotic plaque but rather is related, in part, to a demonstrable reduction in total arterial cross-sectional area. These in vivo studies were extended to the lower extremity vasculature by Pasterkamp and associates. Using serial IVUS analyses of human patients undergoing percutaneous lower extremity revascularization,[90] they confirmed the interpretation that they had initially developed on the basis of live animal studies. Shown in Figure 40–19 is an extreme form of constrictive vascular remodeling due to stent collapse. IVUS clarified the basis for "restenosis" in this case and altered the proposed treatment strategy: whereas directional atherectomy had been planned, based on angiographic findings, recognition of stent collapse by IVUS dictated that balloon inflation alone be used to re-expand the collapsed stent.

USEFULNESS OF IVUS FOR GUIDING INTERVENTIONS

Although the ultimate role of IVUS vis-à-vis contrast angiography remains to be determined, the author has previously used IVUS as the primary (sole) imaging modality to guide interventional procedures.[91] In a series of 46 patients undergoing iliac or femoropopliteal revascularization, serial IVUS imaging was performed to assess the results of balloon dilation, directional atherectomy, and/or physiologic low-stress angioplasty. Decisions regarding whether the procedure result was satisfactory and whether to deliver further treatment were made on the basis of IVUS examinations alone, without any angiographic information. Repeat intervention was shown to be necessary with IVUS in approximately one third of patients; the specific adjunctive treatment modality, including repeat balloon inflation, adjunctive atherectomy, or stent deployment, was determined based on interpretation of the quantitative and qualitative findings on IVUS examination. Angiograms were performed after completion of the recanalization procedure, both to confirm the adequacy of the result by the traditional standard and to determine whether IVUS had failed to define a significant residual narrowing. In only 2 of 46 patients did information obtained on completion angiography indicate the need for repeat intervention.

A number of reports support the notion that IVUS enhances definition of residual luminal narrowing and morphometry after intervention and that this information may influence subsequent therapeutic management.[26, 92–95] Several of these studies have explored the lesion- and device-specific uses of IVUS[96–98] and, in addition to supporting its use to determine procedural outcome, suggest a potential role for IVUS in identifying the optimal inter-

FIGURE 40–18. Two-dimensional images and three-dimensional reconstruction of IVUS recording illustrating compensatory dilation. *Top Left,* Two-dimensional image shows minimal plaque. *Bottom Left,* Two-dimensional image shows moderate luminal narrowing. Corresponding sites on three-dimensional sagittal image (*top right*), indicated by arrows, show increased arterial diameter (media stripe to media stripe) at site of moderate atherosclerotic narrowing. As the three-dimensional cast image at bottom right shows, the effect of such focal dilation is to preserve similar luminal dimensions over entire length of diseased as well as normal artery.

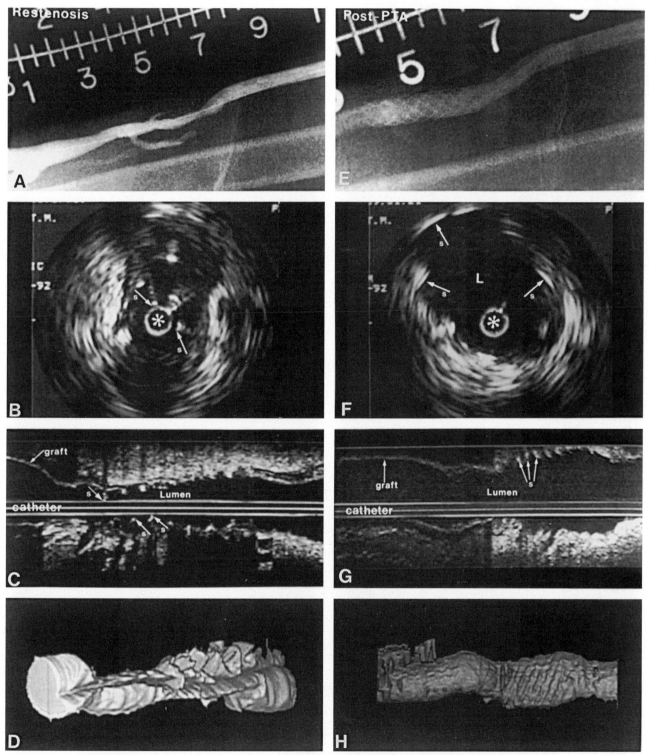

FIGURE 40–19. *A*, Restenosis of dialysis fistula appears by angiography to be due to neointimal thickening *(left)*. *B*, In fact, IVUS shows stent struts (s, *arrows*) abutting IVUS catheter. *C*, Sagittal three-dimensional reconstruction shows same finding in longitudinal format. *D*, Consequent luminal narrowing is illustrated by cast three-dimensional reconstruction. *E*, After angioplasty, angiographic luminal diameter is restored. IVUS (two-dimensional in *F*, three-dimensional sagittal in *G*) shows stent struts no longer abutting IVUS catheter. Luminal cast *(H)* shows augmented luminal patency.

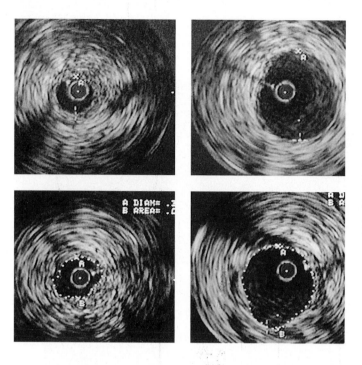

FIGURE 40–20. Use of IVUS to size interventional device. *Top Left,* Minimum luminal diameter of dialysis fistula measures 2.64 mm. Therefore, a burr measuring 3.0 mm in diameter is selected to perform rotational atherectomy. *Bottom Left,* Rotational atherectomy results in minimum lumen diameter of 3.0 mm. *Top Right,* Reference diameter of upstream segment of fistula measures 6.4 mm in minimum lumen diameter. An angioplasty (PTA) balloon (Blue Max, Boston Scientific) measuring 6 mm in diameter is selected for dilation. *Bottom Right,* Final cross-sectional area after PTA measures 6.0 mm in diameter.

ventional therapy. Examples of this phenomenon include determination of appropriate device-balloon size, based on accurate measurement of vessel dimensions (Fig. 40–20); selection of a directional, rather than a concentric atherectomy device, based on the finding of eccentric plaque; and choice of a device that is better suited for debulking of calcium, in the case of a heavily calcified lesion.

IVUS is uniquely suited for guidance in the deployment of endovascular stents (Fig. 40–21).[27, 77, 99–103] Whereas evaluation of the interface between stent struts and endoluminal surface is diffi-

cult with fluoroscopy (where one sees the stent but not the vessel wall) and angiography (where one sees the vessel but the contrast column may obscure the stent), such evaluation is straightforward when done with IVUS. IVUS is specifically useful during stent deployment in several respects. First, IVUS may assist in determining the need to stent a vessel after PTA, by identifying an inadequate luminal area (Fig. 40–22), severe plaque disruption, or the presence of a flow-limiting flap or dissection not apparent with angiography. Second, the target vessel may be measured with IVUS to ensure appropriate stent sizing (Fig. 40–23). Because balloon-

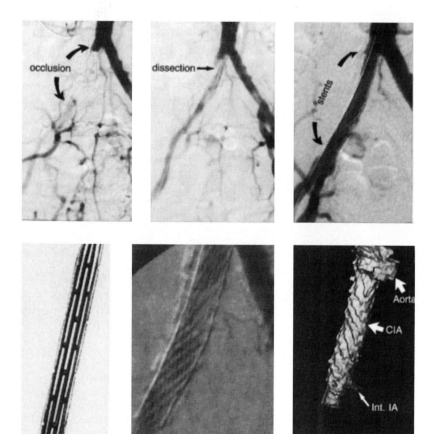

FIGURE 40–21. Amelioration of post-PTA dissection of iliac artery with the use of stents. *Top Left,* Baseline angiogram of occluded iliac artery. *Top Middle,* After angioplasty. *Top Right,* Following deployment of two Palmaz stents, an excellent angiographic result is obtained. *Bottom Left,* Unexpanded Palmaz stent. *Bottom Middle,* Digital radiographic image of deployed stents. *Bottom Right,* Three-dimensional reconstruction of serial IVUS images creates a "cast" of the vascular lumen of stented common iliac artery (CIA). Int. IA = internal iliac artery.

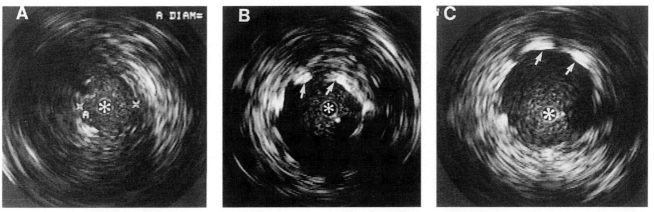

FIGURE 40–22. IVUS during subclavian PTA-stenting. *A,* IVUS after 7-mm balloon dilation. Maximum diameter measures 4.8 mm, indicating significant recoil. *B,* After stent deployment with 8-mm balloon, struts *(arrows)* still protrude slightly into lumen. *C,* Post-PTA 9-mm struts *(arrows)* now well apposed to arterial wall. ° = IVUS catheter.

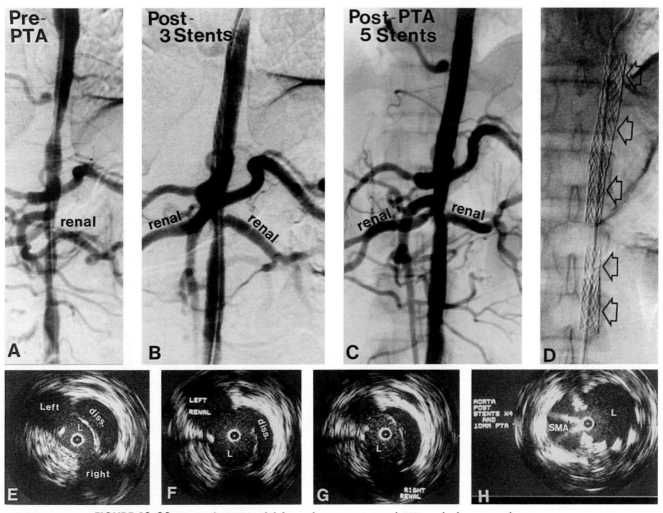

FIGURE 40–23. Revascularization of abdominal aortic stenosis with PTA–multiple stents under intravascular ultrasound (IVUS) guidance. This 30-year-old woman presented with malignant hypertension and nonpalpable femoral pulses due to abdominal aortic coarctation, thought to be secondary to Takayasu disease, now apparently quiescent. *A,* Angiogram before PTA demonstrates extensive disease in the aorta, both above and below the renal arteries. *B,* After PTA above and below the renal arteries and placement of three stents, result appears reasonable on angiography, although moderate stenosis remains below or at level of renal arteries. IVUS image *(E)* at takeoff of renals ("left" and "right") demonstrates large dissection (diss.), extending from proximal PTA site, encroaching on renal artery ostia and narrowing aortic lumen (L). *C,* Redilated aorta, with two additional stents, shows no encroachment at level of renal arteries; IVUS frames *(F)* and *(G)* confirm persistence of dissection (diss.), but concurrent enlargement of aortic lumen (L) and elimination of obstruction leading into renal arteries ("left renal," "right renal"). *D,* Stents *(arrows)* in aorta. *H,* IVUS of stent in middle aorta depicts struts overlying origin of superior mesenteric artery (SMA); struts cast "shadows" into SMA but do not compromise blood flow *(C).* Patient is asymptomatic and normotensive at 1-year follow-up.

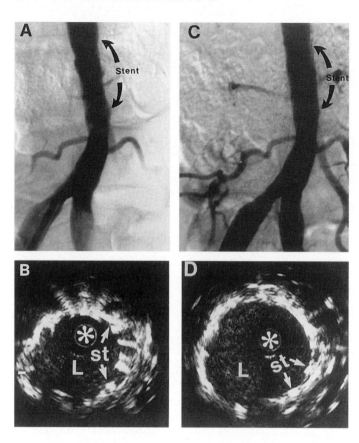

FIGURE 40–24. Stent underexpansion detected by IVUS. PTA and stent deployment in eccentric aortic lesion. *A,* Angiogram after deployment of Palmaz stent with 9-mm balloon depicts ostensibly good result, without obvious compromise in lumen or stent. *B,* Although lumen (L) is now enlarged compared with pre-PTA image, IVUS after 9-mm PTA-stent demonstrates stent underexpansion, with all struts (st) between 2 and 5 o'clock not in apposition to arterial wall. *C,* Angiogram following 12-mm PTA shows slight decrease in luminal irregularity where stent has been redilated *(arrows).* *D,* IVUS after 12-mm PTA demonstrates complete expansion of stent, with all struts (st) now completely apposed to arterial wall and overall lumen (L) area further increased.

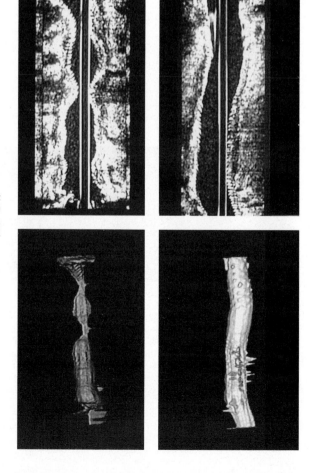

FIGURE 40–25. Suboptimal expansion of Wallstent (Schneider) "self-expanding" stent deployed in iliac artery is illustrated in sagittal *(top left)* and lumen cast *(bottom left)* three-dimensional reconstructions of IVUS recordings. Following supplementary balloon dilation, sagittal *(top right)* and cast *(bottom right)* images show satisfactory luminal dimensions.

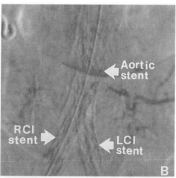

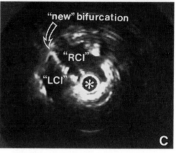

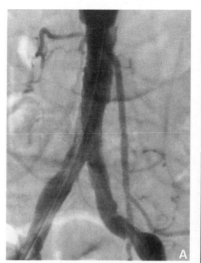

FIGURE 40–26. Percutaneous reconstruction of aortic bifurcation with balloon angioplasty and stent deployment. *A,* Final angiogram. *B,* Digital radiographic image of deployed aortic stent and common iliac stents. The latter were deployed with the "kissing balloon" technique. *C,* Cross-sectional IVUS image. Catheter in right common iliac (RCI) demonstrates interface of RCI and left common iliac (LCI) stents, that is, the "new bifurcation."

stent undersizing may predispose to abrupt closure and oversizing is associated with a hyperproliferative response leading to increased restenosis, exact sizing may directly affect clinical outcome. Third, IVUS permits identification of the origin, as well as end sites of a dissection, and thus easily identifies the longitudinal extent of the vessel that requires stenting. Fourth, IVUS may identify sites of inadequate stent expansion (Figs. 40–24 and 40–25) and, specifically, nonapposition of struts to the underlying arterial wall. This situation has been specifically implicated as a basis for stent thrombosis, and optimal stent expansion guided by IVUS has led some investigators to reduce the need for associated anticoagulation.[101, 102] Fifth, for complex deployment, as in the case of stenting the bifurcation of the distal aorta (Fig. 40–26), IVUS may facilitate stent positioning and, subsequently, can confirm the adequacy of the reconstructed bifurcation. Finally, IVUS is invaluable and perhaps uniquely capable of clarifying the basis for restenosis after stent deployment (Figs. 40–27 and 40–28).

INSTRUMENTS FOR COMBINED ULTRASOUND IMAGING AND PERCUTANEOUS REVASCULARIZATION

Initial attempts by Mallery and colleagues to combine intravascular ultrasound imaging with balloon angioplasty and/or mechanical atherectomy used a no. 4.5 Fr. balloon dilation catheter fitted with an array of eight 20-MHz transducers mounted radially around the catheter.[104] The transducers were positioned within and midway between the two ends of a 3.0-cm polyethylene balloon; images were recorded perpendicular to the long axis of the catheter, through the balloon.

Hodgson and associates,[105] performed in vivo imaging in normal canine coronary arteries, using an alternative design in which a ring of modified phased-array transducers were positioned *proximal* to the balloon. The design of this device was intended to permit

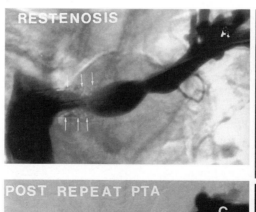

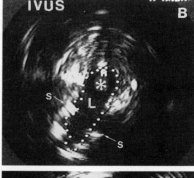

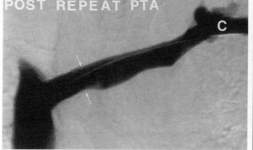

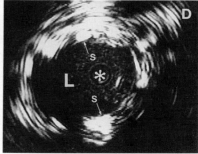

FIGURE 40–27. Restenosis due to eccentric stent collapse. *A,* Angiogram of subclavian vein proximal to a dialysis graft 4 months after angioplasty and Palmaz stent deployment. Narrowed contrast column within stent, whose edges *(arrows)* show full expansion, suggests classic restenosis due to neointimal proliferation. *B,* IVUS image from restenotic site depicts absence of neointimal growth within stent, but instead confirms eccentric collapse of the stent. Approximation of opposing struts *(arrows)* confers a narrowed, slit-like configuration to the stented lumen. *C,* Angiogram after repeat PTA depicts restoration of lumen. Contrast column now approaches stent borders *(arrows).* *D,* IVUS demonstrates re-expansion of stent to circular configuration, and enlargement of lumen (L) area.

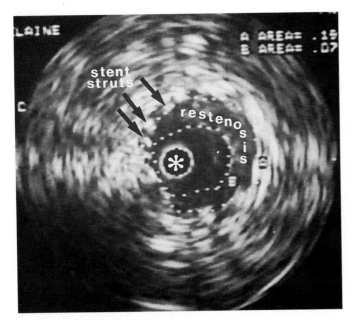

FIGURE 40–28. IVUS of restenosis within stent in renal artery. Stent configuration remains circular and fully expanded, but crescent of neointimal tissue growth ("restenosis") narrows the lumen cross-sectional area by approximately 50 percent. ° = IVUS catheter.

pre- and postdilation imaging without the requirement for multiple catheter exchanges. In vivo studies that used this so-called Oracle (Endosonics Inc., Pleasanton, CA) in humans during percutaneous transluminal coronary angioplasty[92, 106] suggest that images obtained immediately before and after balloon dilation using this device may influence procedural strategy.

Clinical investigation in the author's laboratory has confirmed that it is feasible to perform on-line IVUS imaging during percutaneous revascularization, monitoring the effects of angioplasty on the arterial wall *during* balloon inflation, as opposed to evaluating effects *post hoc,* as described earlier. The so-called balloon ultrasound imaging catheter (BUIC, Boston Scientific, Boston), which the author has used, is a hybrid device that incorporates both diagnostic and therapeutic functions, imaging through polyethylene balloon material, the thickness of which is standard for peripheral angioplasty balloons.[63] In 8 of 10 patients before PTA and 9 of 10 patients after PTA, images recorded from the BUIC permitted rapid quantitative analysis of minimum luminal diameter and luminal cross-sectional area. The measurements obtained were nearly indistinguishable from those recorded with a nonballoon ultrasound catheter.

Quantitative findings provided by the BUIC were specifically useful for defining the contribution of elastic recoil, long inferred as constituting a mechanical reason for loss of gain achieved during balloon inflation.[61, 107, 108] Previous investigators employed quantitative angiographic techniques to analyze the extent to which recoil complicates standard PTCA. For example, Nobuyoshi[108] observed that "restenosis" (>50 percent loss of gain in absolute diameter assessed by cinevideodensitometry) was already present in 27 (14.6 percent) of 185 patients or in 27 (11.4 percent) of 237 lesions by 1 day after PTCA and was, therefore, interpreted to represent evidence of elastic recoil.

Measurements recorded with the BUIC confirm the observations made with angiographic techniques and establish that the phenomenon of recoil is common to peripheral as well as coronary angioplasty and that such recoil is instantaneous. Interestingly, the single patient in the author's series in whom clinical evidence of restenosis has thus far been observed was the patient in whom recoil was most severe.

Finally, on-line ultrasound monitoring of balloon inflation also facilitates identification of the initiation of plaque fracture. Images recorded from the BUIC disclosed that plaque fractures were initiated by dilation at low (<2 atm) inflation pressures, which is consistent with previous clinical observations. For example, Hjemdahl-Monsen and associates found that most improvement in

luminal size occurred at inflation pressures <2 atm.[109] As suggested by Kleiman and co-workers,[110] any technique that permits immediate, on-line recognition of plaque fracture may theoretically be employed to modify the remainder of the dilation procedure in an attempt to prevent the development of a flow-limiting dissection.

Yock and colleagues have investigated a prototype catheter that combined a 30-MHz transducer with a modified version of the Simpson directional atherectomy catheter.[111] Preliminary experiments performed in vitro and in vivo demonstrated that this device could be used to monitor the depth to which plaque was mechanically excised. Furthermore, the availability of on-line imaging from within the cutting window of the device permits the operator to assign directionality to the subsequent cuts. The ability to selectively debulk plaque has obvious positive implications: by facilitating more complete and selective plaque removal and avoidance of normal elements in the arterial wall, the potential beneficial therapeutic effect of the Simpson device may be maximized.

The theoretical advantages of a combined laser–IVUS device are similar to those described earlier, including the enhanced ability to "aim" and thereby achieve precise tissue ablation and controlled plaque removal. Preliminary attempts to combine IVUS with laser ablation by Aretz and associates[112] and Linker and co-workers[113] suggested that the development of microcavitations during laser activation may preclude effective IVUS imaging. The author used a combination IVUS-laser catheter in vivo to guide and assess the results of laser-induced ablation of plaque.[114] The catheter consists of a conventional multifiber laser catheter, the wire-lumen of which has been used to accommodate a mechanical ultrasound transducer. Images recorded with IVUS simultaneously with excimer (308 nm) laser irradiation disclosed abrupt formation of cavitations, as previously described, that transiently attenuated the ultrasound image. On cessation of laser irradiation, normal blood flow cleared the excimer-generated gas, restoring the ultrasound image and documenting the extent of reduced plaque volume.

THREE-DIMENSIONAL RECONSTRUCTION

The introduction of three-dimensional reconstruction[21, 56, 62, 99, 115–126] has solved certain limitations inherent in the spatial display formats of current IVUS imaging systems. Conventional two-dimensional IVUS displays tomographic sections of the lumen and arterial wall in sequential fashion as a videotape recording. Comparison of individual segments examined by IVUS to adjacent or more distant segments requires repeated review of serially recorded images to reconstruct, in the mind's eye, the spatial relationship of the segments of interest. For example, while one tomographic image obtained during IVUS examination may offer high-resolution definition of a plaque fracture resulting from balloon angioplasty, details regarding the longitudinal distribution of the same plaque fracture at one site relative to proximal and distal sites cannot be displayed in a single image. In contrast, conventional angiography preserves the advantage of displaying each segment in longitudinal relationship to adjacent and more distant segments; once contrast media has opacified the artery of interest, any individual segment may be compared with adjacent and distant segments, limited only by the field of view.

For IVUS to provide the same capability, for example, to compare adjacent segments within the vessel, simultaneous viewing of the data from multiple sequential cross-sectional slices is necessary. The liability of IVUS that provides for only one tomographic view at a time, without a longitudinal perspective, may be resolved by "stacking" (Fig. 40–29) sequential IVUS frames recorded during a catheter pullback through a given vascular segment. Computer-based reconstruction of these serially acquired IVUS frames creates a longitudinal, three-dimensional format for IVUS data, thus preserving the benefits of detailed tomographic imaging while providing an efficient method of reviewing the cumulative IVUS data.

Original attempts to perform three-dimensional reconstructions in the author's laboratory involved the use of software (SigmaScan, Jandel Scientific, Corte Madera, CA) that required manual morphometric tracing of each serial tomographic image, followed by computer-aided reconstruction.[119] The more detail intended, the more images were required, and, consequently, the more labor-intensive was the reconstruction. The principal liability of this approach, however, is related to the fact that the modeling technique was based exclusively on boundary depiction and therefore allowed three-dimensional reconstruction of the lumen, but not the arterial wall. Such an approach would clearly squander one of the chief assets of intravascular ultrasound, namely, the capacity to image the vessel wall and thereby evaluate characteristics of the native wall, as well as pathologic alterations resulting from interventional therapies.

Automated three-dimensional reconstruction of intravascular ultrasound images was investigated in a preliminary fashion by Kitney and associates[127] with the use of voxel modeling. This approach considers each voxel, or volume element, as an extension of three-dimensional space of the digital image element, or pixel (picture element). Voxel modeling is a particularly attractive option for three-dimensional reconstruction of the vasculature because it preserves detailed ultrasound data and thereby allows representation of the arterial wall, rather than simply surface features that would limit the reconstruction to the arterial lumen.

To preserve information regarding the arterial wall and plaque in the reconstructed image, ImageComm Systems (Santa Clara, CA) developed for the author's institution a PC-based system that uses algorithms[128, 129] designed specifically for analysis of images recorded during IVUS examination (Omniview, Pura Labs, Brea, CA). This software employs a surface-rendering process predicated on segmented boundary formation but includes interpolative algorithms designed to link boundary elements and thereby preserve the capability of viewing the arterial wall as well as lumen. Three distinct display formats are currently available for reconstructed IVUS data: the so-called *sagittal, cylindrical,* and *lumen cast* modes. In the sagittal mode, a planar view of the IVUS data is displayed in longitudinal relief and can be revolved around the long axis of the IVUS catheter. The use of the sagittal format, in particular, not only facilitates comparative analysis of adjacent tomographic images but also offers the additional advantage of displaying the ultrasound data in a longitudinal profile-type format more familiar to the angiographer.

Although similar in orientation to an angiogram, sagittal reconstruction substantially augments the information available from conventional angiography in two important ways. First, limitless orthogonal views can be rendered by incremental rotation of the imaging plane about the reference catheter. Given the documented importance of orthogonal views in the assessment of luminal narrowing,[130] on the one hand, and the logistical factors that frequently obviate the possibility of obtaining orthogonal views, on the other, this feature may ultimately prove to be the principal advantage of three-dimensional reconstruction. Second, information regarding pathologic alteration of the arterial wall is provided simultaneously with the conventional assessment of luminal diameter narrowing. Experience with patients undergoing percutaneous revasculariza-

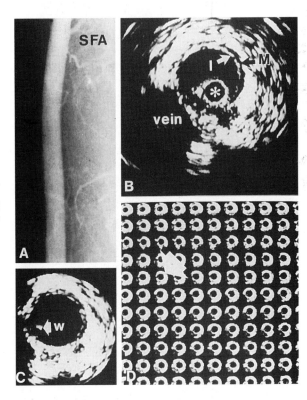

FIGURE 40–29. *A,* Angiogram of normal superficial femoral artery (SFA). *B,* Representative two-dimensional cross-sectional IVUS image of SFA (I = intima; asterisk = IVUS catheter) and adjacent vein. *C,* Digitized version of *B. D,* "Stack" of digitized two-dimensional IVUS images used to create three-dimensional reconstruction. (*Arrow* indicates image shown in *B* and *C.*)

tion indicates that certain features of arterial wall pathology are particularly well defined in such a longitudinal format. For example, three-dimensional reconstruction in the sagittal mode graphically demonstrated that recanalization of a lengthy total occlusion was achieved by tunneling a false lumen through calcified plaque (Figs. 40–30 and 40–31). Such a mechanism of recanalization has been previously described in vitro[131, 132] and is frequently inferred to occur in vivo.[133] Although the individual tomographic ultrasound images indicated creation of a "double-barrel" lumen, the full extent of pathologic disruption was more immediately apparent from inspection of the sagittal reconstructions. Similarly, sagittal reconstructions of balloon-dilated nonoccluded vessels demonstrates the longitudinal distribution of barotraumatic injury, otherwise evident as only local, isolated plaque fractures on the tomographic two-dimensional IVUS images. The use of the three-dimensional

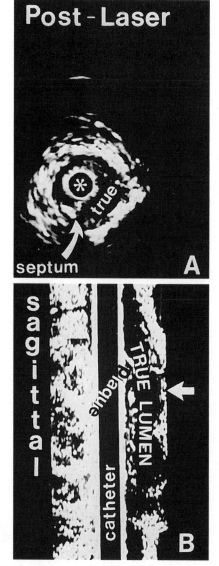

FIGURE 40–30. Subintimal channel created during recanalization of 8-cm occlusion in superficial femoral artery with guide wire (Terumo), followed by excimer laser angioplasty. *A,* Inspection by means of conventional two-dimensional reconstruction intravascular ultrasound demonstrates "double-barrel" lumen. IVUS probe *(asterisk)* in subintimal channel separated by "septum" from second ("true") lumen. *B,* Sagittal image rendered by on-line three-dimensional reconstruction depicts subintimal pathway of ultrasound catheter as it enters atherosclerotic plaque, which separates catheter from true lumen at right. Arrow depicts level of ultrasound frame shown in *A.*

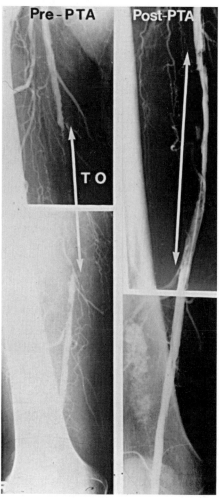

FIGURE 40–31. Angiograms before and after revascularization from patient illustrated in Figure 40–30. "Double-barrel" lumen is less well defined by angiography than with IVUS.

formats facilitates delineation of the extent of a dissection as well as selection and deployment of endovascular stents.

The cylindrical three-dimensional mode preserves the wall and lumen as an intact cylinder and thus provides true three-dimensional—as opposed to planar—views. Experience with the cylindrical format suggests that this mode of three-dimensional reconstruction, particularly when the reconstructed vascular segment is hemisected, is optimally suited for cases in which direct inspection of luminal topography is of special interest, such as analysis of implanted endovascular prostheses (Fig. 40–32). Details of the "cobblestone" neointima lining the stent cannot be appreciated angiographically, or even by intravascular ultrasound, when viewed in standard video format[77]; the algorithms developed to accomplish the cylindrical reconstruction serve the dual functions of both joining together the series of adjacent elements representing the neointima and then rotating the reconstructed image 90 degrees to permit viewing of the endoluminal surface en face. The sagittal reconstruction supplements the cylindrical format by facilitating analysis of arterial contour proximal and distal to the stent; such analysis is otherwise not feasible with the use of the unassembled tomographic images.

Although sagittal and cylindrical three-dimensional formats facilitate qualitative assessment of pathologic alterations involving arterial wall, neither format allows quantitative analysis of residual luminal cross-sectional area narrowing. Therefore, to take advantage of the unique ability to planimeter cross-sectional area from tomographic IVUS images, the lumen cast format was developed,[115, 116, 120, 123] reconstructing a cast of the lumen by isolating it from the underlying arterial wall. Each sequential stored IVUS frame is analyzed by projecting rays radially outward from the center of the transducer. Based on a preselected threshold value, these rays automatically detect the luminal border; the borders detected by the rays are integrated to create a disc-like cross-sectional area "map" for each IVUS frame. Maps from sequential frames are then stacked to create a three-dimensional cast of the lumen. The area of each map, or disc, is determined by precalibration with the known size of the IVUS probe, and the resulting series of cross-sectional area determinations is plotted linearly, allowing nearly instantaneous quantitative analysis of cross-sectional area along the entire length of the vascular segment examined. Inspection of the plot permits rapid identification of sites of residual cross-sectional narrowing.

Preliminary in vitro[134] and in vivo[120] investigations have provided evidence validating the algorithm employed for quantitative analysis in the lumen cast format. Although the lumen cast display forfeits information regarding qualitative alterations in the plaque and underlying wall, this format greatly facilitates on-line interpretation of the extent to which satisfactory luminal dimensions have been achieved. The cast graphically depicts residual sites of luminal narrowing and, as a cursor is directed to any suspicious site, provides automated quantitative assessment of luminal cross-sectional area and percent narrowing at that site. Moreover, because movement of the cursor to a specific level of the luminal cast simultaneously brings up the corresponding two-dimensional tomographic image on the upper left quadrant of the ImageComm workstation screen, the operator retains the option of inspecting the two-dimensional image to confirm the quantitative readout derived from analysis of the luminal cast. The author's experience with

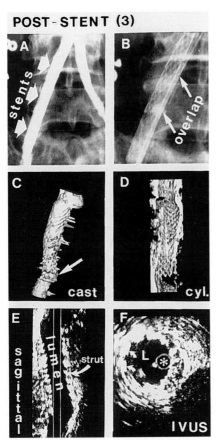

FIGURE 40–32. Angiogram (A) and plain film (B) show three stents in right common iliac artery. Final lumen is illustrated in three-dimensional reconstructions of IVUS images, shown here in lumen cast (C), cylindrical (cyl.) (D), and sagittal (E). Note cobblestone appearance of luminal surface of stent in cylindrical three-dimensional reconstruction (D). Representative two-dimensional IVUS image of stent is shown in F.

the lumen cast algorithm on-line during interventional procedures suggests that it is useful in accurately and rapidly identifying sites of residual narrowing, including sites that may otherwise be overlooked during routine two-dimensional IVUS examination because of their focal nature.

Certain limitations of current attempts to perform three-dimensional reconstruction must be acknowledged. First, it is apparent that the quality of the three-dimensional reconstructions can be only as good as the original two-dimensional images. Details that are absent from the original recordings will likewise be absent from the reconstructed images. For example, in instances in which calcific deposits are observed on the two-dimensional images to attenuate echoes from the subjacent plaque and/or wall, these portions of the plaque and/or wall will not be incorporated into the reconstructed image.

Second, "ring-down artifact," resulting from dead space in the acoustic transmission path and manifested on the two-dimensional image as a white halo immediately peripheral to the transducer, may obscure near-field structure in smaller, particularly stenotic vessels. In the author's preliminary work, such artifact was routinely masked out of the three-dimensional reconstructions; in cases in which reconstruction is applied to two-dimensional images with little or no lumen peripheral to the transducer, such masking can overestimate the three-dimensional depiction of luminal patency. Hopefully, current attempts by the manufacturers of mechanical transducer systems to eliminate such artifact will resolve this issue.

Third, whereas major branch points, such as the aortic bifurcation, are accurately depicted in the three-dimensional reconstruction, the two-dimensional images are otherwise reassembled as a straight tube. Sharp bends in the artery are not faithfully reconstructed on either the two- or the three-dimensional images. Although this is typically not a severe liability in evaluation of the peripheral and renal circulations, it may become more significant in the assessment of the more tortuous coronary circulation.

Fourth, three-dimensional reconstruction shares with conventional intravascular ultrasound imaging the difficulty of matching the rotational orientation of the ultrasound transducer to that of the imaged vessel. Furthermore, if the ultrasound probe is inadvertently twisted during the pullback recording, the three-dimensional reconstruction will reflect this rotational event.

Fifth, in most studies performed to date, the two-dimensional images have been acquired during a slow, timed catheter pullback; this strategy is intended to optimize the number of acquired images over a given segment length and provide equal representation for each portion of the artery in the reconstructed image. Such catheter pullback, however, is entirely operator dependent, and small variations in the rate of pullback may ultimately influence the three-dimensional representation. For example, if the catheter withdrawal rate is slowed during pullback through an abnormal segment of vessel and is subsequently accelerated through a more normal segment, the abnormal segment will occupy proportionally more than its true length of the resulting reconstruction. This phenomenon is particularly likely to occur when there is a tendency for the operator to slow catheter movement through abnormal segments to achieve closer inspection of morphologic disruptions. Modifications in acquisition technique include automated image registration using motorized pullback devices, rendering the technique less operator-dependent.[135]

Sixth, current software does not gate image acquisition to phases of the cardiac cycle. Although this is not a significant liability in three-dimensional reconstruction of peripheral vessels, it remains a major source of artifact in reconstruction of coronary and renal vessels.

Beyond these limitations, many of which are currently being addressed, the extent to which three-dimensional reconstruction will be used clinically is principally dependent on two factors: the time required for reconstruction and the prognostic implications of the resulting images. With regard to the former, image-processing time has been reduced considerably through a combination of modifications in software and memory expansion. Whereas early

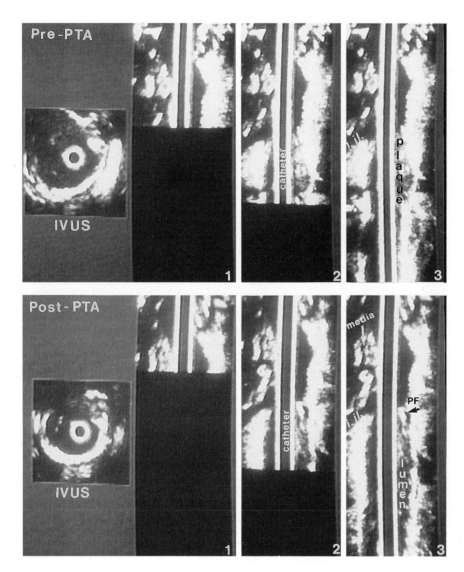

FIGURE 40–33. Real-time three-dimensional reconstruction of sagittal images during IVUS catheter pullback. *Upper Panel,* Pre-PTA, representative two-dimensional (2D) IVUS image stored from the beginning of the pullback is seen at left. This is one of the 220 individual images incorporated into sagittal three-dimensional reconstruction image, shown expanding in frames 1 to 3. IVUS catheter, located within vascular lumen, is abutted by atherosclerotic plaque (frame 3). Origin of internal iliac artery (i.il.) is demonstrated branching off to left one third of the way down reconstructed vessel. *Lower Panel,* Post-PTA, representative two-dimensional IVUS image is shown at left. Frames 1 to 3 depict expanding three-dimensional sagittal image, reconstructed concurrent with post-PTA IVUS pullback (e.g., real-time). In sagittal view shown in frame 3, lumen diameter is increased from that in pre-PTA image; plaque fracture (PF) in dilated site is demonstrated in longitudinal relief on reconstructed image. Reconstructed view facilitates assessment of longitudinal extent of plaque fracture resulting from balloon angioplasty.

FIGURE 40–34. In young children or transplant donors with pristine coronary arteries, the absence of any intimal thickening precludes demonstration with IVUS of a three-layered appearance. As intimal thickening first begins to develop, the three-layered appearance becomes visible. Subsequently, however, as atherosclerotic narrowing begins to encroach on the lumen, the plaque appears to also encroach on the intima-media border. As a result, the three-layered appearance is gradually eroded. With the development of a high-grade lesion, there is frequently little remaining of the three-layered appearance, making unambiguous demarcation of the internal and external elastic membranes (and, by inference, the media and the adventitia) less feasible.

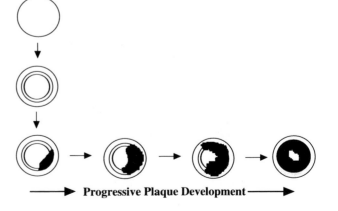

Progressive Plaque Development

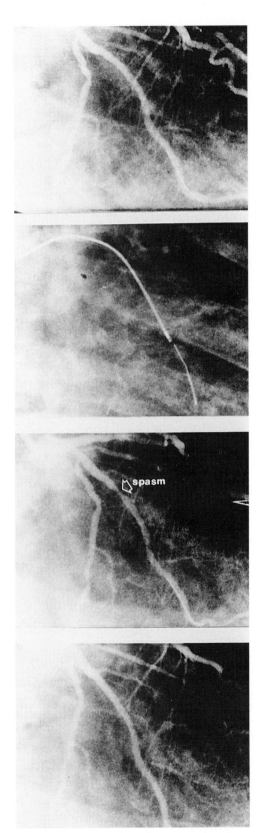

FIGURE 40–35. Coronary artery spasm induced by IVUS.

reconstructions typically required 20 to 40 minutes to assemble, current sagittal reconstructions are performed and visualized in real-time, concurrent with catheter pullback (Fig. 40–33).[117] Cylindrical and lumen cast reconstructions are routinely available within 30 seconds of completing the pullback recording.[122] Thus, the time required to reconstruct and review the reconstructed images is comparable to that required to review the video playback of a contrast angiogram.

CURRENT LIMITATIONS OF IVUS FOR CLINICAL USE

Initial clinical applications of IVUS have also revealed certain limitations of this technology. Perhaps the most decisive limitation concerns the inability of currently available IVUS devices to consistently discriminate boundaries between the three layers of the arterial wall at sites of severe narrowing by atherosclerotic plaque. With advanced degrees of atherosclerosis, the characteristic ultrasound patterns become blurred (Fig. 40–34). This is due principally to two factors: first, emaciation of the media typically accompanies progression of the atherosclerotic process.[136] Second, extensive calcific deposits, because they are often blanketed across the intimal-medial boundary and because they attenuate or "shadow" the ultrasound reflections from the deeper layers of the wall, further obscure the normal ultrasound depiction of the arterial wall. Ambiguity regarding the boundary between intimal thickening and media reduces the precision with which any given measurement of wall thickness can be determined to represent atherosclerotic plaque versus normal wall.[39]

A second limitation of all currently available IVUS devices is that the design of these devices allows only for side viewing. Because forward-viewing devices[137] are not yet available for routine clinical applications, IVUS cannot be currently employed to determine the composition (e.g., thrombus versus plaque) of a total occlusion prior to recanalization; nor can IVUS direct the advancement of a wire into an occluded segment. For that particular aspect of percutaneous interventional therapy, angioscopy may be superior. However, once through the occlusion, IVUS may identify whether the neolumen is intravascular or subintimal.[94]

Finally, it should be pointed out that the application of IVUS imaging is not without risk, especially in the coronary circulation.[138] Because of the relatively large size of catheters currently available, imaging must be performed more expeditiously than is usually the case in peripheral circulation. In addition, introduction of the IVUS catheter may occasionally precipitate spasm (Fig. 40–35)[139, 140]; accordingly, it is recommended that a final angiogram be recorded after IVUS examination of the coronary circulation.

References

1. Vlodaver, Z., Frech R., Van Tassel, R.A., et al.: Correlations of the ante-mortem arteriogram and the post-mortem specimen. Circulation 47:162, 1973.
2. Grondin, C.M., Dyrda, I., Pasternac, A., et al.: Discrepancies between cineangiographic and post-mortem findings in patients with coronary artery disease and recent myocardial revascularization. Circulation 49:703, 1974.
3. Pepine, C.J., Feldman, R.L., and Nichols, W.W.: Coronary arteriography: Potentially serious sources of error in interpretation. Cardiovasc. Med. 2:747, 1977.
4. Arnett, E.N., Isner, J.M., Redwood, C.R., et al.: Coronary artery narrowing in coronary heart disease: Comparison of cineangiographic and necropsy findings. Ann. Intern. Med. 91:350, 1979.
5. Isner, J.M., Kishel, J., Kent, K.M., et al.: Accuracy of angiographic determination of left main coronary arterial narrowing: Angiographic-histologic correlative analysis in 28 patients. Circulation 63:1056, 1981.
6. Isner, J.M., and Donaldson, R.F.: Coronary angiographic and morphologic correlation. Cardiol. Clin. 2:571, 1984.
7. de Feyter, P.J., Serruys, P.W., Davies, M.J., et al.: Quantitative coronary angiography to measure progression and regression of coronary atherosclerosis. Circulation 84:412, 1991.
8. Marcus, M.L., Skorton, D.J., Johnson, M.R., et al.: Visual estimates of percent diameter coronary stenosis: "A battered gold standard." J. Am. Coll. Cardiol. 11:882, 1988.
9. Dietz, W.A., Tobis, J.M., and Isner, J.M.: Failure of angiography to accurately depict the extent of coronary artery narrowing in three fatal cases of percutaneous transluminal coronary angioplasty. J. Am. Coll. Cardiol. 19:1261, 1992.
10. White, C.W., Wright, C.B., Doty, D.B., et al.: Does visual interpretation of the coronary arteriogram predict the physiologic importance of a coronary stenosis? N. Engl. J. Med. 310:819, 1984.
11. Davidson, C.J., Sheikh, K.H., Harrison, J.K., et al.: Intravascular ultrasonography versus digital subtraction angiography: A human in vivo comparison of vessel size and morphology. J. Am. Coll. Cardiol. 16:633, 1990.
12. Gussenhoven, W.J., Essed, C.E., Frietman, P., et al.: Intravascular echographic

assessment of vessel wall characteristics: A correlation with histology. Int. J. Card. Imaging 4:105, 1989.

13. Hodgson, J.McB., Graham, S.P., and Savakus, A.D.: Clinical percutaneous imaging of coronary anatomy using an over-the-wire ultrasound catheter system. Int. J. Card. Imaging 4:187, 1989.

14. St. Goar, F.G., Pinto, F.J., Alderman, E.L., et al.: Detection of coronary atherosclerosis in young adult heart using intravascular ultrasound. Circulation 86:756, 1992.

15. Nissen, S.E., Gurley, J.C., Grines, C.L., et al.: Intravascular ultrasound assessment of lumen size and wall morphology in normal subjects and patients with coronary artery disease. Circulation 84:1087, 1991.

16. Isner, J.M., Kaufman, J., Rosenfield, K., et al.: Combined physiologic and anatomic assessment of percutaneous revascularization using a Doppler guidewire and ultrasound catheter. Am. J. Cardiol. 71:70D, 1993.

17. Tenaglia, A.N., Buller, C.E., Kisslo, K.B., et al.: Mechanisms of balloon angioplasty and directional coronary atherectomy as assessed by intracoronary ultrasound. Am. J. Cardiol. 20:685, 1992.

18. Tenaglia, A.N., Tcheng, J.E., Kisslo, K.B., et al.: Intracoronary ultrasound evaluation of excimer laser angioplasty. (Abstract.) Circulation 86:I–516, 1992.

19. Yock, P.G., Fitzgerald, P.J., Linker, D.T., et al.: Intravascular ultrasound guidance for catheter-based coronary interventions. J. Am. Coll. Cardiol. 17:39B, 1992.

20. Comess, K., Fitzgerald, P.J., and Yock, P.G.: Intracoronary ultrasound imaging of graft thrombosis. N. Engl. J. Med. 327:1691, 1992.

21. Rosenfield, K., Kaufman, J., Pieczek, A., et al.: On-line three-dimensional reconstruction from 2D IVUS: Utility for guiding interventional procedures. (Abstract.) J. Am. Coll. Cardiol. 19:224A, 1992.

22. Rosenfield, K., Losordo, D.W., Ramaswamy, K., et al.: Qualitative assessment of peripheral vessels by intravascular ultrasound before and after interventions. (Abstract.) J. Am. Coll. Cardiol. 15:107A, 1990.

23. Rosenfield, K., Voelker, W., Losordo, D.W., et al.: Assessment of coronary arterial stenoses post-intervention by quantitative angiography versus intracoronary ultrasound in 13 patients undergoing balloon and/or laser coronary angioplasty. (Abstract.) J. Am. Coll. Cardiol. 17:46A, 1991.

24. The GUIDE Trial Investigators: Lumen enlargement following angioplasty is related to plaque characteristics. A report from the GUIDE trial. (Abstract.) Circulation 86:I–531, 1992.

25. Tobis, J.M., Mahon, D.J., Lehmann, K.G., et al.: Intracoronary ultrasound imaging after balloon angioplasty. (Abstract.) Circulation 82:III–676, 1990.

26. Mintz, G.S., Leon, M.B., Satler, L.F., et al.: Pre-intervention intravascular ultrasound imaging influences transcatheter coronary treatment strategies. (Abstract.) Circulation 86:I–323, 1992.

27. Isner, J.M., Rosenfield, K., Kelly, K., et al.: Percutaneous intravascular ultrasound examination as an adjunct to catheter-based interventions: Preliminary experience in patients with peripheral vascular disease. Radiology 175:61, 1990.

28. Gussenhoven, E.J., The, S.H.K., Serruys, P.W., et al.: Intravascular ultrasound and vascular intervention. J. Interven. Cardiol. 4:41, 1991.

29. Gurley, J.C., Nissen, S.E., Grines, C.L., et al.: Comparison of intravascular ultrasound and angiography following percutaneous transluminal coronary angioplasty. (Abstract.) Circulation 82:III–72, 1990.

30. Fitzgerald, P.J., St. Goar, F.G., Connolly, A.J., et al.: Intravascular ultrasound imaging of coronary arteries. Is three layers the norm? Circulation 86:154, 1992.

31. Gussenhoven, E.J., Essed, C.E., Lancee, C.T., et al.: Arterial wall characteristics determined by intravascular ultrasound imaging: An in vitro study. J. Am. Coll. Cardiol. 14:947, 1989.

32. Gussenhoven, E.J., Essed, C.E., Frietman, P., et al.: Intravascular ultrasonic imaging: Histologic and echographic correlation. Eur. J. Vasc. Surg. 3:571, 1989.

33. Potkin, B.N., Bartorelli, A.L., Gessert, J.M., et al.: Coronary artery imaging with intravascular high-frequency ultrasound. Circulation 81:1575, 1990.

34. Nishimura, R.A., Edwards, W.D., Warness, C.A., et al.: Intravascular ultrasound imaging: In vitro validation and pathologic correlation. J. Am. Coll. Cardiol. 16:145, 1990.

35. Siegel, R.J., Ariani, M., Fishbein, M.C., et al.: Histopathologic validation of angioscopy and intravascular ultrasound. Circulation 84:109, 1991.

36. Tobis, J.M., Mallery, J.A., Gessert, J.M., et al.: Intravascular ultrasound cross-sectional arterial imaging before and after balloon angioplasty in vitro. Circulation 80:873, 1989.

37. Coy, K.M., Maurer, G., and Siegel, R.J.: Intravascular ultrasound imaging: A current perspective. J. Am. Coll. Cardiol. 18:1811, 1991.

38. Siegel, R.J., Fishbein, M.C., Chae, J.S., et al.: Origin of the three-ringed appearance of human arteries by ultrasound: Microdissection with ultrasonic and histologic correlation. (Abstract.) J. Am. Coll. Cardiol. 15:17A, 1990.

39. Mallery, J.A., Tobis, J.M., Griffith, J.M., et al.: Assessment of normal and atherosclerotic arterial wall thickness with an intravascular ultrasound imaging catheter. Am. Heart J. 119:1392, 1990.

40. Yock, P.G., and Linker, D.T.: Intravascular ultrasound. Looking below the surface of vascular disease. Circulation 81:1715, 1990.

41. Webb, J.G., Yock, P.G., and Slepian, M.J.: Intravascular ultrasound: Significance of the three-layered appearance of normal muscular arteries. (Abstract.) J. Am. Coll. Cardiol. 15:17A, 1990.

42. Lockwood, G.R., Ryan, L.K., Gotlieb, A.I., et al.: In vitro high resolution intravascular imaging in muscular and elastic arteries. J. Am. Coll. Cardiol. 20:153, 1992.

43. Yeung, A.C., Ryan, T.J., Isner, J.M., et al.: Correlation of intravascular ultrasound characteristics with endothelium-dependent vasodilator function in the coronary arteries of cardiac transplant patients. Circulation 84:II–703, 1991.

44. Tobis, J.M., Mallery, J.A., Mahon, D.J., et al.: Intravascular ultrasound imaging of human coronary arteries in vivo. Circulation 83:913, 1991.

45. Nissen, S.E., Grines, C.L., Gurley, J.C., et al.: Application of a new phased-array

ultrasound imaging catheter in the assessment of vascular dimensions. In vivo comparison to cineangiography. Circulation 81:660, 1990.

46. St. Goar, F.G., Pinto, F.J., Alderman, E.L., et al.: Intracoronary ultrasound in cardiac transplant recipients: In vivo evidence of "angiographically silent" intimal thickening. Circulation 85:979, 1992.

47. Pinto, F.J., Chenzbraun, A., Botas, J., et al.: Feasibility of serial intracoronary ultrasound imaging for assessment of progression of intimal proliferation in cardiac transplant recipients. Circulation 90:2348, 1994.

48. Tuzcu, E.M., Hobbs, R.E., Rincon, G., et al.: Occult and frequent transmission of atherosclerotic coronary disease with cardiac transplantation. Insights from intravascular ultrasound. Circulation 91:1706, 1995.

49. Pandian, N.G., Kreis, A., and Brockway, B.: Detection of intraarterial thrombus by intravascular high frequency two-dimensional ultrasound imaging: In vitro and in vivo studies. Am. J. Cardiol. 65:1280, 1990.

50. Siegel, R.J., Chae, J.S., Forrester, J.S., et al.: Angiography, angioscopy, and ultrasound imaging before and after percutaneous balloon angioplasty. Am. Heart J. 120:1086, 1990.

51. Johnson, C., Hansen, D.D., Vracko, R., et al.: Angioscopy: More sensitive for identifying thrombus, distal emboli, and subintimal dissection. (Abstract.) J. Am. Coll. Cardiol. 13:146A, 1989.

52. Mecley, M., Rosenfield, K., Kaufman, J., et al.: Atherosclerotic plaque hemorrhage and rupture associated with crescendo claudication. Ann. Intern. Med. 117:663, 1992.

53. Yock, P.G., and Linker, D.T. Catheter-based two-dimensional ultrasound imaging. In Topol, E.J. (ed.): Textbook of Interventional Cardiology. Philadelphia, W.B. Saunders, 1993, pp. 816–827.

54. Tabbara, M., White, R.A., Cavaye, D., et al.: In vivo human comparison of intravascular ultrasonography and angiography. J. Vasc. Surg. 14:496, 1991.

55. Isner, J.M., and Rosenfield, K.: Enough with the fantastic voyage: Will IVUS pay in Peoria? Cathet. Cardiovasc. Diagn. 26:192, 1992.

56. Rosenfield, K., Losordo, D.W., Harding, M., et al.: Intravascular ultrasound of renal arteries in patients undergoing percutaneous transluminal angioplasty: Feasibility, safety, and initial findings, including 3-dimensional reconstruction of renal arteries. (Abstract.) J. Am. Coll. Cardiol. 17:204A, 1992.

57. Nakamura, S., Mahon, D.J., Maheswaran, B., et al.: An explanation for discrepancy between angiographic and intravascular ultrasound measurements after percutaneous transluminal coronary angioplasty. J. Am. Coll. Cardiol. 25:633, 1995.

58. Graham, S.P., Brands, D., Savakus, A.D., et al.: Utility of an intravascular ultrasound imaging device for arterial wall definition and atherectomy guidance. (Abstract.) J. Am. Coll. Cardiol. 13:222A, 1989.

59. Waller, B.F., Pinkerton, C.A., and Slack, J.D.: Intravascular ultrasound: A histologic study of vessels during life. The new "gold standard" for vascular imaging. Circulation 85:2305, 1992.

60. Waller, B.F., Orr, C.M., Pinkerton, C.A., et al.: Coronary balloon angioplasty dissections: "The Good, the Bad, and the Ugly." J. Am. Coll. Cardiol. 20:701, 1992.

61. Waller, B.F.: Pathology of new interventions used in the treatment of coronary heart disease. Curr. Probl. Cardiol. 11:666, 1986.

62. Coy, K.M., Park, J.C., Fishbein, M.C., et al.: In vitro validation of three-dimensional intravascular ultrasound for the evaluation of arterial injury after balloon angioplasty. J. Am. Coll. Cardiol. 20:692, 1992.

63. Isner, J.M., Rosenfield, K., Losordo, D.W., et al.: Combination balloon-ultrasound imaging catheter for percutaneous transluminal angioplasty. Circulation 84:739, 1991.

64. Honye, J., Mahon, D.J., Jain, A., et al.: Morphological effects of coronary balloon angioplasty in vivo assessed by intravascular ultrasound imaging. Circulation 85:1012, 1992.

65. Losordo, D.W., Rosenfield, K., Pieczek, A., et al.: How does angioplasty work? Serial analysis of human iliac arteries using intravascular ultrasound. Circulation 86:1845, 1992.

66. Farb, A., Virmani, R., Atkinson, J.B., et al.: Plaque morphology and pathologic changes in arteries from patients dying after coronary balloon angioplasty. J. Am. Coll. Cardiol. 16:1421, 1990.

67. Castaneda-Zuniga, W.R., Formanek, A., and Tadavarthy, M.: The mechanism of balloon angioplasty. Radiology 135:565, 1980.

68. The, S.H.K., Gussenhoven, E.J., Zhong, Y., et al.: Effect of balloon angioplasty on femoral artery evaluated with intravascular ultrasound imaging. Circulation 86:483, 1992.

69. Honye, J., Mahon, D.J., Nakamura, S., et al.: Enhanced diagnostic ability of intravascular ultrasound imaging compared with angiography. (Abstract.) Circulation 86:I-324, 1992.

70. Waller, B.F., Miller, J., Morgan, R., et al.: Atherosclerotic plaque calcific deposits: An important factor in success or failure of transluminal coronary angioplasty. (Abstract.) Circulation 78:II–376, 1988.

71. Fitzgerald, P.J., Ports, T.A., and Yock, P.G.: Contribution of localized calcium deposits to dissection after angioplasty. An observational study using intravascular ultrasound. Circulation 86:64, 1992.

72. Mintz, G.S., Douek, P., Pichard, A.D., et al.: Target lesion calcification in coronary artery disease: An intravascular ultrasound study. J. Am. Coll. Cardiol. 20:1149, 1992.

73. Yock, P.G., Fitzgerald, P.J., Sykes, C., et al.: Morphologic features of successful coronary atherectomy determined by intravascular ultrasound imaging. (Abstract.) Circulation 82:III–676, 1990.

74. Smucker, M.L., Scherb, D.E., Howard, P.F., et al.: Intracoronary ultrasound: How much "angioplasty effect" in atherectomy. (Abstract.) Circulation 82:III–676, 1990.

75. Penny, W.F., Schmidt, D.A., Safian, R.D., et al.: Insights into the mechanism of luminal improvement after directional coronary atherectomy. Am. J. Cardiol. 67:435, 1991.
76. Safian, R.D., Gelbfish, J.S., Erny, R.E., et al.: Coronary atherectomy. Clinical, angiographic, and histological findings and observations regarding potential mechanisms. Circulation 82:69, 1990.
77. Chokshi, S.K., Hogan, J., Desai, V., et al.: Intravascular ultrasound assessment of implanted stents. (Abstract.) J. Am. Coll. Cardiol. 15:29A, 1990.
78. Rutherford, R.B., Flanigan, D.P., Guptka, S.K., et al.: Suggested standards for reports dealing with lower extremity ischemia. J. Vasc. Surg. 4:80, 1986.
79. Isner, J.M.: Vascular remodeling. Honey, I think I shrunk the artery. Circulation 89:2937, 1994.
80. Glagov, S., Weisenberg, E., Zarins, C.K., et al.: Compensatory enlargement of human atherosclerotic coronary arteries. N. Engl. J. Med. 316:1371, 1987.
81. Post, M.J., Borst, C., and Kuntz, R.E.: The relative importance of arterial remodeling compared with intimal hyperplasia in lumen renarrowing after balloon angioplasty: A study in the normal rabbit and the hypercholesterolemic Yucatan micropig. Circulation 89:2816, 1994.
82. Zarins, C.K., Weisenberg, E., Kolettis, G., et al.: Differential enlargement of artery segments in response to enlarging atherosclerotic plaques. J. Vasc. Surg. 7:386, 1988.
83. McPherson, D.D., Hiratzka, L.F., Lambert, W.C., et al.: Delineation of the extent of coronary atherosclerosis by high-frequency epicardial echocardiography. N. Engl. J. Med. 316:304, 1987.
84. Losordo, D.W., Rosenfield, K., Kaufman, J., et al.: Focal compensatory enlargement of human arteries in response to progressive atherosclerosis in vivo documentation using intravascular ultrasound. Circulation 89:2570, 1994.
85. Glagov, S., Grande, J., Vesselinovitch, D., et al.: Quantitation of cells and fibers in histologic sections of arterial walls: Advantages of contour tracing on a digitizing plate. *In* McDonald, T.E., and Chandler, A.B. (eds.): Connective Tissues in Arterial and Pulmonary Disease. New York, Springer-Verlag, 1981, pp. 57–93.
86. Siegel, R.J., Swan, K., Edwards, G., et al.: Limitations of post-mortem assessment of human coronary artery size and luminal narrowing: Differential effects of tissue fixation and processing on vessels with different degrees of atherosclerosis. J. Am. Coll. Cardiol. 5:342, 1985.
87. Mintz, G.S., Kovach, J.A., Javier, S.P., et al.: Geometric remodeling is the predominant mechanism of late lumen loss after coronary angioplasty. (Abstract.) Circulation 88:I–654, 1993.
88. Mintz, G.S., Kovach, J.A., Pichard, A.D., et al.: Geometric remodeling is the predominant mechanism of clinical restenosis after coronary angioplasty. (Abstract.) J. Am. Coll. Cardiol. 23:138A, 1994.
89. Kovach, J.A., Mintz, G.S., Kent, K.M., et al.: Serial intravascular ultrasound studies indicate that chronic recoil is an important mechanism of restenosis following transcatheter therapy. (Abstract.) J. Am. Coll. Cardiol. 21:484, 1993.
90. Pasterkamp, G., Wensing, P.J.W., Post, J.M.J., et al.: Paradoxical arterial wall shrinkage may contribute to luminal narrowing of human atherosclerotic femoral arteries. Circulation 91:1444, 1995.
91. Isner, J.M., Rosenfield, K., Mosseri, M., et al.: How reliable are images obtained by intravascular ultrasound for making decisions during percutaneous interventions? Experience with intravascular ultrasound employed in lieu of contrast angiography to guide peripheral balloon angioplasty in 16 patients. (Abstract.) Circulation 82:III–440, 1990.
92. Hodgson, J.McB., and Nair, R.: Efficacy and usefulness of a combined intracoronary ultrasound-angioplasty balloon catheter: Results of the multicenter Oracle trial. (Abstract.) Circulation 86:I–321, 1992.
93. Fitzgerald, P.J., Muhlberger, V.A., Moes, N.Y., et al.: Calcium location within plaque as a predictor of atherectomy tissue retrieval: An intravascular ultrasound study. (Abstract.) Circulation 86:I-516, 1992.
94. Rees, M.R., Sivananthan, M.U., and Verma, S.P.: The role of intravascular ultrasound and angioscopy in the placement and followup of coronary stents. (Abstract.) Circulation 86:I-364, 1992.
95. Sahn, S., Rothman, A., Shiota, T., et al.: Acute and follow-up intravascular ultrasound findings after balloon dilation of coarctation of the aorta. Circulation 90:340, 1994.
96. Kimura, B.J., Fitzgerald, P.J., Sudhir, K., et al.: Guidance of directed coronary atherectomy by intracoronary ultrasound imaging. Am. Heart J. 124:1365, 1992.
97. Matar, F.A., Mintz, G.S., Pinnow, E., et al.: Multivariate predictors of intravascular ultrasound end points after directional coronary atherectomy. J. Am. Coll. Cardiol. 25:318, 1995.
98. Mintz, G.S., Potkin, B.N., Keren, G., et al.: Intravascular ultrasound evaluation of the effect of rotational atherectomy in obstructive atherosclerotic coronary artery disease. Circulation 86:1383, 1992.
99. Rosenfield, K., Losordo, D.W., Ramaswamy, K., et al.: Three-dimensional reconstruction of human coronary and peripheral arteries from images recorded during two-dimensional intravascular ultrasound examination. Circulation 84:1938, 1991.
100. Tenaglia, A.N., Kisslo, K., Kelly, S., et al.: Ultrasound guide wire-directed stent deployment. Am. Heart J. 125:1213, 1993.
101. Colombo, A., Hall, P., Nakamura, S., et al.: Intracoronary stenting without anticoagulation accomplished with intravascular ultrasound guidance. Circulation 91:1676, 1995.
102. Goldberg, S.L., Colombo, A., Nakamura, S., et al.: Benefit of intracoronary ultrasound in the deployment of Palmaz-Schatz stents. J. Am. Coll. Cardiol. 24:996, 1994.
103. Rosenfield, K., Schainfeld, R.M., Khan, W., et al.: Restenosis of stented dialysis conduits caused by stent collapse, not neointimal proliferation. J. Am. Coll. Cardiol. 25:262A, 1995.
104. Mallery, J.A., Gregory, K., Morcos, N.C., et al.: Evaluation of ultrasound balloon dilatation imaging catheter. (Abstract.) Circulation 76:IV–371, 1987.
105. Hodgson, J.M.B, Cacchione, J.G., Berry, J., et al.: Combined intracoronary ultrasound imaging and angioplasty catheter: Initial in vivo studies. Circulation 82:III–676, 1990.
106. Mudra, H., Blasini, R., Klauss, V., et al.: Diagnostic intracoronary ultrasound facility within a therapeutic balloon catheter has impact on PTCA strategy. (Abstract.) Circulation 86:I–324, 1992.
107. Sanders, M.: Angiographic changes thirty minutes following percutaneous transluminal coronary angioplasty. Angiology 36:419, 1985.
108. Nobuyoshi, M., Kimura, T., Nasaka, H., et al.: Restenosis after successful percutaneous transluminal coronary angioplasty: Serial angiographic follow-up of 229 patients. J. Am. Coll. Cardiol. 12:616, 1988.
109. Hjemdahl-Monsen, C.E., Ambrose, J.A., Borrico, S., et al.: Angiographic patterns of balloon inflation during percutaneous transluminal coronary angioplasty: Role of pressure-diameter curves in studying distensibility and elasticity of the stenotic lesion and the mechanism of dilation. J. Am. Coll. Cardiol. 16:569, 1990.
110. Kleiman, N.S., Raizner, A.E., and Roberts, R.: Percutaneous transluminal coronary angioplasty: Is what we see what we get? J. Am. Coll. Cardiol. 16:576, 1990.
111. Yock, P.G., Fitzgerald, P.J., Jang, Y.-T., et al.: Initial trials of a combined ultrasound imaging/mechanical atherectomy catheter. (Abstract.) J. Am. Coll. Cardiol. 15:105A, 1990.
112. Aretz, H.T., Martinelli, M.A., and LeDet, E.F.: Intraluminal ultrasound guidance of transverse laser coronary atherectomy. Int. J. Card. Imaging 4:153, 1989.
113. Linker, D.R., Bylock, A., and Amin, A.B.: Catheter ultrasound imaging demonstrates the extent of tissue disruption of excimer laser irradiation of human aorta. (Abstract.) Circulation 80:II–581, 1989.
114. Kasprzyk, D.J., Crowley, R.J., and Isner, J.M.: Excimer laser angioplasty in conjunction with intravascular ultrasonic imaging. SPIE Proc. Diagn. Ther. Cardiovasc. Intervent. II 1642:147, 1992.
115. Rosenfield, K., and Isner, J.M.: Quantitative analysis by 3-dimensional intravascular ultrasound. J. Interven. Cardiol. 4:205, 1992.
116. Isner, J.M., Rosenfield, K., Kelly, S., et al.: Percutaneous intravascular ultrasound for assessment of interventional techniques: Initial findings in patients undergoing balloon angioplasty, atherectomy, and endovascular stent implants. (Abstract.) Circulation 11:579, 1989.
117. Rosenfield, K., Kaufman, J., Langevin, R.E., et al.: Real-time three-dimensional reconstruction of intravascular ultrasound images of iliac arteries. Am. J. Cardiol. 70:412, 1992.
118. Schryver, T.E., Popma, J.J., Kent, K.M., et al.: Use of intracoronary ultrasound to identify the "true" coronary lumen in chronic coronary dissection treated with intracoronary stenting. Am. J. Cardiol. 69:1107, 1992.
119. DeJesus, S.T., Rosenfield, K., Gal, D., et al.: 3-Dimensional reconstruction of vascular lumen from images recorded during percutaneous 2-D intravascular ultrasound. (Abstract.) Clin. Res. 37:838A, 1989.
120. Rosenfield, K., Losordo, D.W., Ramaswamy, K., et al.: Quantitative analysis of luminal cross-sectional area from 3-dimensional reconstructions of 2-dimensional intravascular ultrasound: Validation of a novel technique. (Abstract.) Circulation 84:II–542, 1991.
121. Rosenfield, K., Harding, M., Pieczek, A., et al.: 3-Dimensional reconstruction of balloon dilated coronary, renal, and femoropopliteal arteries from 2-D intravascular ultrasound images: Analysis of longitudinal sagittal versus cylindrical views. (Abstract.) J. Am. Coll. Cardiol. 17:234A, 1991.
122. Rosenfield, K., Kaufman, J., Pieczek, A., et al.: Human coronary and peripheral arteries: On-line three-dimensional reconstruction from two-dimensional intravascular ultrasound scans. Radiology 184:823, 1992.
123. Rosenfield, K., Kaufman, J., Pieczek, A., et al.: Lumen cast analysis: A quantitative format to expedite on-line analysis for 3-D intravascular ultrasound images. (Abstract.) J. Am. Coll. Cardiol. 19:115A, 1992.
124. Rosenfield, K., Losordo, D.W., Harding, M., et al.: Three-dimensional reconstruction of coronary and peripheral vessels from 2-D IVUS images: Determination of optimal image acquisition rate during timed pullback. (Abstract.) J. Am. Coll. Cardiol. 17:262A, 1991.
125. Rosenfield, K., Losordo, D.W., Palefsky, P., et al.: On-line 3-D reconstruction of 2-D intravascular ultrasound images during balloon angioplasty: Clinical application in patients undergoing percutaneous balloon angioplasty. (Abstract.) J. Am. Coll. Cardiol. 17:156A, 1991.
126. Rosenfield, K., Losordo, D.W., Ramaswamy, K., et al.: 3-Dimensional reconstruction of intravascular ultrasound images recorded in 68 consecutive patients following percutaneous revascularization of totally occluded arteries: In vivo evidence that the neolumen frequently includes a subintimal component. (Abstract.) Circulation 84:II–686, 1991.
127. Kitney, R.I., Moura, L., and Straughen, K.: 3-D visualization of arterial structures using ultrasound and Voxel modeling. Int. J. Card. Imaging 4:177, 1989.
128. Raya, S.O., Udupa, J.K., and Barrett, W.A.: A PC-based 3D imaging system: Algorithms, software, and hardware considerations. Comput. Med. Imaging Graph. 14:353, 1990.
129. Raya, S.P.: SOFTVU: A software package for multidimensional medical image analysis. SPIE Proc. Med. Imaging IV 96:152, 1990.
130. Spears, J.R., Sandor, T., Baim, D.S., et al.: The minimum error in estimating coronary luminal cross-sectional area from cineangiographic diameter measurements. Cathet. Cardiovasc. Diagn. 9:119, 1983.
131. Tobis, J.M., Smolin, M., Mallery, J.A., et al.: Laser-assisted angioplasty in human peripheral artery occlusions: Mechanism of recanalization. J. Am. Coll. Cardiol. 13:1547, 1989.
132. Isner, J.M., Donaldson, R.F., Funai, J.T., et al.: Factors contributing to perforations resulting from laser coronary angioplasty: Observations in an intact human

post-mortem model of intra-operative laser coronary angioplasty. Circulation 72:II–191, 1985.

133. Melchior, J.P., Meir, B., Urban, P., et al.: Percutaneous transluminal coronary angioplasty for chronic total arterial occlusion. Am. J. Cardiol. 59:535, 1987.

134. Zientek, D.M., Rodriguez, E.R., Liebson, P.R., et al.: Validation of computerized three-dimensional reconstruction of intravascular ultrasound: Measurements of absolute luminal diameter and cross-sectional area in ex vivo human coronary arteries. J. Interven. Cardiol. 4:179, 1992.

135. Mintz, G.S., Keller, M.B., and Fay, K.G.: Motorized IVUS transducer pullback permits accurate quantitative axial length measurements. (Abstract.) Circulation 86:I-323, 1992.

136. Isner, J.M., Donaldson, R.F., Fortin, A.H., et al.: Attenuation of the media in coronary arteries in advanced atherosclerosis. Am. J. Cardiol. 58:937, 1986.

137. Evans, J.L., Ng, K.-H., Vonesh, M.J., et al.: Arterial imaging with a new forward-viewing intravascular ultrasound catheter. I: Initial studies. Circulation 89:712, 1994.

138. Hausmann, D., Erbel, R., Alibelli-Chemarin, M.-J., et al.: The safety of intracoronary ultrasound. A multicenter survey of 2207 examinations. Circulation 91:623, 1995.

139. Isner, J.M., Rosenfield, K., Losordo, D.W., et al.: Clinical experience with intravascular ultrasound as an adjunct to percutaneous revascularization. In Tobis, J.M., and Yock, P. (eds.): Intravascular Ultrasound Imaging. New York, Churchill Livingstone, 1992, pp. 171–197.

140. Alfonso, F., Macaya, C., Goicolea, J., et al.: Angiographic changes induced by intracoronary ultrasound imaging before and after coronary angioplasty. Am. Heart J. 125:877, 1993.

CHAPTER

41 Ultrasonic Characterization of Cardiovascular Tissue

Julio E. Pérez, M.D.

Mark R. Holland, Ph.D.

Benico Barzilai, M.D.

Scott M. Handley, Ph.D.

Byron F. Vandenberg, M.D.

James G. Miller, Ph.D.

David J. Skorton, M.D.

BASIC CONCEPTS OF ULTRASONIC TISSUE CHARACTERIZATION ____ 607
Definition of Acoustic Terms ____ 607
Approaches to Tissue Characterization and Measurement Techniques ____ 608
   Methods Based on Radiofrequency Data Analysis, Including Integrated Backscatter Imaging ____ 608
   Real-Time Backscatter Imaging ____ 609
   Methods That Display Acoustically Abnormal Tissue ____ 610
   Methods That Quantitate Echocardiographic Gray Level (Image) Data ____ 610
BIOLOGIC DETERMINANTS OF MYOCARDIAL ACOUSTIC PROPERTIES ____ 611
Collagen ____ 611
Scatterer Geometry ____ 611
Fiber Orientation ____ 612
Blood Flow–Water Content ____ 613
Other Determinants ____ 613
Dynamic Aspects of Scattering ____ 613
SPECIFIC DISEASE PROCESSES STUDIED BY ULTRASONIC TISSUE CHARACTERIZATION ____ 614

Acute Ischemia–Infarction ____ 614
Reperfused Myocardium ____ 615
Subacute and Chronic Infarction ____ 616
Myocarditis ____ 618
   Dilated Cardiomyopathy ____ 619
   Infiltrative-Restrictive Cardiomyopathy ____ 619
   Hypertrophic Cardiomyopathy ____ 620
   Experimental Cardiomyopathy ____ 621
Myocardial Effects of Pressure Overload: Arterial Hypertension ____ 621
Intracardiac Thrombus ____ 622
Myxoma ____ 622
Vegetations ____ 622
Myocardial Contusion ____ 622
Atherosclerosis ____ 622
Valvular Tissue ____ 622
Myocardial Effects of Diabetes Mellitus ____ 623
Cardiac Allograft Rejection ____ 623
Myocardial Effects of Cyanotic Congenital Heart Disease ____ 623
Aging ____ 623
CONCLUSIONS ____ 623

One of the important but unmet goals of cardiac diagnosis is the direct, noninvasive identification of tissue composition of cardiac structures. Certainly, abundant indirect information can be used to identify abnormal regions of the myocardium. For example, alterations in left ventricular contraction appearing in the setting of chest discomfort and electrocardiographic abnormalities suggest acute myocardial ischemia. Unfortunately, regional wall motion abnormalities are somewhat nonspecific and may appear in acute ischemia,[1] infarction, scar, and even nonischemic cardiomyopathy.[2] Similarly, alterations in cardiac enzymes in the same setting establish the presence of myocardial necrosis but do not differentiate between relatively diffuse subendocardial damage and localized transmural infarction. Thus, identifying the precise site, extent, and chronicity of ischemic myocardial injury is one of many possible situations in which current diagnostic techniques leave an important gap in the identification and characterization of regional myocardial abnormalities. At present, only endomyocardial biopsy, with its inherent limitations, permits the clinician to identify myocardial composition in a direct fashion.

Toward the goal of direct, yet noninvasive, myocardial tissue characterization, there has been increasing interest in the use of quantitative analysis of transmitted or reflected diagnostic ultrasound.[3-5] In particular, much information from experimental animal studies and a growing clinical investigative literature suggest that ultrasound interacts differently with abnormal, compared with normal, tissue. Thus, there has been interest in the use of ultrasound to identify acute and chronic abnormalities of myocardial composition and physiologic state—a field of investigation termed ultrasonic tissue characterization.[3] Ultrasonic cardiac tissue characterization may be defined as the identification and characterization of abnormalities in the physical or physiologic state of myocardium, based on analyzing interactions between ultrasound and tissue. The rationale for this field of study is that sufficient information is available in the ultrasound signal passing through or returning from myocardial tissue to identify the tissue as normal or abnormal and to indicate the nature of the abnormality.

Is the field of ultrasonic tissue characterization a new one? In fact, observations suggesting that ultrasound analyses might be capable of identifying abnormal soft tissue date back to the 1950s.[6] In the early 1970s, studies of experimental myocardial ischemia suggested that some acoustic properties were altered within minutes after acute coronary occlusion.[7] Why, then, has ultrasound tissue characterization not yet risen to the clinical horizon? Among many other problems, to be discussed subsequently, there has, until recently, been relatively little clinical research using ultrasound tissue characterization techniques. However, recent progress by several groups suggests the potential for clinical application in the near future.

BASIC CONCEPTS OF ULTRASONIC TISSUE CHARACTERIZATION

Definition of Acoustic Terms

Ultrasound travels within myocardium with a propagation speed that is determined by its density and compressibility. Other tissues that are much less compressible than myocardium, such as bone, exhibit much higher ultrasound propagation speeds.[8] Even among soft tissues, there are small differences in the velocity of ultrasound. For example, ultrasound velocity values increase progressively as waves travel through fat, water, liver, and muscle. All values of propagation speed for soft tissue are, however, close to the conventionally accepted value of approximately 1540 m per second. Even though this property may potentially lend itself to tissue differentiation, commercially available echocardiographic scanners assume a fixed propagation speed and therefore negate any role for acoustic velocity variations in characterizing tissue. Thus far, there has been very little work on differentiation of myocardial physical state, based on differences in propagation speed. However, studies on excised tissue indicate that there is a significant dependence of ultrasonic velocity on myocardial fiber direction.[9, 10]

The ultrasonic wavelength is the length of one cycle of the ultrasonic wave. The wavelength is given by the ratio of the propagation speed to the ultrasonic frequency used. The frequency is typically reported as a nominal or center frequency, as all transducers have some useful bandwidth or range extending from below to above this center frequency. Although, theoretically, decreasing the wavelength will improve resolution, this effect is limited by the fact that higher transmitted frequencies achieve less penetration through the chest wall into the myocardial region of interest. The diminished penetration of ultrasound with increasing frequency is due to higher attenuation as a function of frequency. Attenuation reduces the amplitude of the waves as the sound travels into the tissue of interest (i.e., it is depth related). The losses from attenuation can be due to reflection, scattering, or absorption (conversion into heat). We shall return to these concepts.

The product of propagation speed times the density of tissue yields the acoustic impedance (when attenuation effects are negligible). This product is usually fixed for a given tissue, although physiologic and dynamic interactions within the tissue may in theory modify the impedance; thus, it should not be considered a constant factor. One of the cardinal features of ultrasound that makes it powerful as a diagnostic tool is its property of being reflected when the waves reach a boundary between tissues (or areas within the same tissue) with different acoustic impedance values (e.g., different density and/or propagation speed values, an acoustic-impedance mismatch). When the incident wavelength is smaller than the dimension of the boundary, the reflection occurring is termed specular. In echocardiography, for example, specular reflection occurs at the interface between endocardium and blood and defines the borders or edges of cardiac muscle with respect to the cavities.

On the other hand, when the boundary (between the different tissues or components of a given tissue) is smaller than the wavelength of the incident wave, the type of reflection that takes place is called scattering. As opposed to specular reflections, scattering is a multidirectional phenomenon, in particular for heterogeneous media or in suspensions with particles, such as the blood stream. Among the multidirectional waves that result from scattering, those that are redirected back to the transmitting transducer are defined as being backscattered. Both the extent of backscatter and the degree of attenuation of a given tissue can be expressed in quantitative terms and are useful parameters for tissue characterization, in particular of myocardium. Both attenuation and backscatter are frequency dependent, although not necessarily in a linear fashion. Backscatter can be expressed as a function of frequency over the useful bandwidth of frequencies for a particular transducer. By averaging data over a range of frequencies, the variability in backscatter measurement related to phase interference and cancellation effects is minimized.[4, 11-24] The backscattered waves interfere with each other (i.e., constructive or destructive interference).[25] The phenomenon of phase cancellation from piezoelectric elements (the only type used in clinical echocardiographic systems) further compromises measurements. The effects are caused by distortions of the ultrasonic wave front resulting from inhomogeneities in the tissue, and they lead to degradation of the signal as it is received at the transducer. The effects are responsible for the speckle that is apparent in echocardiographic images.

To put into perspective the ultrasonic backscatter measurements of myocardium, we shall define three additional related parameters[26, 27]: backscatter transfer function, backscatter coefficient, and integrated backscatter. The detailed measurement techniques for these parameters are described in the next section. Briefly, the transducer is excited with an electrical voltage, and the power spectrum corresponding to the backscattered signal received from tissue is referenced to the power spectrum, obtained from a reference-perfect reflector, such as a steel plate, to obtain the backscatter transfer function. In this context, power spectrum refers to the plot of the ultrasonic energy returned from the tissue or reflector, with power as the ordinate and frequency as the abscissa. Integrated backscatter is defined as the frequency average of the backscatter transfer function (over the bandwidth of the transducer).

Although backscatter transfer function and integrated backscatter are useful relative measurements of the scattering efficiency of a selected volume of tissue, they are influenced by the aperture and focusing properties of the transducer used and by the attenuation of tissue. The backscatter coefficient can be obtained by multiplying the backscatter transfer function by factors that compensate for attenuation and the inverse solid angle subtended by the scattering volume.[26] The backscatter coefficient is an absolute measurement of the scattering properties of the volume of tissue.

As mentioned earlier, estimates of backscatter of tissue can be compromised by both phase cancellation effects at piezoelectric receivers and interference effects in the ultrasonic field. These effects combine to produce a phenomenon known as speckle in two-dimensional ultrasonic imaging.[28, 29] The term speckle was initially described in laser imaging and is defined as the pattern of gray shades in the image resulting from interference among the scattered waves.[25] It occurs whenever sound scatters from a surface whose irregularities are approximately equal to the wavelength of the sound. The interference pattern generated by the complex interaction between the ultrasonic beam and the individual scatterers or targets in tissue causes an uneven amplitude of noise, which gives a grainy or granular appearance to the image scan. This grainy pattern is superimposed on the tissue structural information. Because the grainy pattern degrades the resolution of an image, it is considered to be noise, and for imaging purposes a number of attempts have been made to reduce speckle in the image.[30-38] Two of these approaches are spatial averaging (making multiple discrete measurements within a region of tissue to provide a more reliable estimate of the average scattering properties of that region) and expressing the measurements in terms of integrated backscatter (frequency averaging).[26]

Approaches to Tissue Characterization and Measurement Techniques

Methods Based on Radiofrequency Data Analysis, Including Integrated Backscatter Imaging

To date, progress in quantitative myocardial tissue characterization has been possible because of significant advances in electrical engineering and physics applied to improving and modifying ultrasonic measurement and imaging systems. This technical evolution has been coupled with the interest of noninvasive cardiologists in providing echocardiography with quantitative power to distinguish normal from abnormal myocardium on the basis of intrinsic acoustic properties rather than myocardial dimensions or motion. Different groups of investigators have approached the problem of ultrasonic myocardial characterization with different instrumentation techniques and analysis systems. The strong dependence of standard echocardiographic data on specific instrumentation and operator system adjustments adds considerable subjectivity and thus variability to information extracted from these scans.

One important direction of research has relied on the analysis of unprocessed radiofrequency signals returning from myocardium. This approach has been used to quantify the degree of ultrasonic attenuation in transmission studies (in which excised tissue is studied in vitro with a transmitting transducer on one side of the tissue and a receiver on the other). Radiofrequency data analysis has also been used to quantify the extent of ultrasonic backscatter in pulse-echo studies (i.e., using the same transducer as transmitter and receiver as in conventional echocardiography) (Fig. 41–1). Attenuation is quantified by measuring the loss of signal due to transmission through a given thickness of tissue (in vitro), normalized to the loss of signal due to transmission through the same thickness of saline. By a substitution technique, the attenuation coefficient

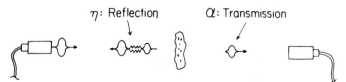

FIGURE 41–1. Attenuation (α) is most easily measured in transmission with separate transmitting and receiving transducers. Backscatter (η) is measured in reflection, with the same transducer serving as both transmitter and receiver.

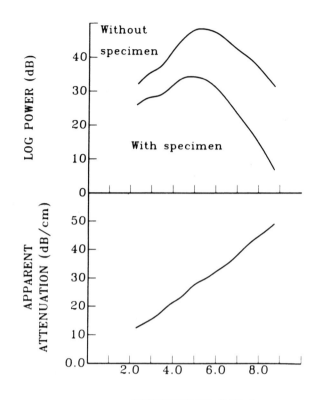

FIGURE 41–2. Plot of the ultrasonic energy transmitted with no specimen in the system and of that obtained with a specimen present (*top*). The attenuation versus frequency plot (*bottom*) is determined by subtracting the two curves shown at the top and correcting for the thickness of the specimen. (From Miller, J.G., Yuhas, D.E., Mimbs, J.W., et al.: Ultrasonic tissue characterization: Correlation between biochemical and ultrasonic indices of myocardial injury. Proc. I.E.E.E. Ultrasonics Symp. 76CH1120–5SU:33, 1976, © 1976 I.E.E.E.)

as a function of frequency is obtained (Fig. 41–2). The resulting slope (least-squares fit) is expressed in decibels per centimeter thickness of tissue per megahertz of useful frequency (dB/cm per MHz).

Although attenuation is an important quantitative descriptor of tissue architecture, it is difficult to measure in the heart in vivo. Thus, measurements of backscatter have been developed by detecting the signals reflected from a selected segment of myocardium. An electronic gate (typically, 3 μsec in duration) and the beam width define the volume of tissue of interest for measurements, avoiding specular reflections from endocardial and epicardial surfaces.[27] The backscatter transfer function (see earlier) is obtained by normalizing the backscattered signal power spectrum by the power spectrum corresponding to the reflection from a standard perfect-reflector surface. As mentioned earlier, integrated backscatter is the frequency average of the transfer function over the useful bandwidth of the transducer (Fig. 41–3) and is a measure of the total energy in the signal returned from the myocardium. These quantitative approaches offer the advantage of reducing the variability in measurements (i.e., due to interference and phase cancellation effects) and minimizing the effects of operator-dependent alteration of system controls that influence information derived from conventional echocardiographic data. Furthermore, integrated backscatter measurements have the potential to lend themselves to serial evaluation of the same segment of tissue. In addition, integrated backscatter can be estimated in the time domain, as well as in the more time-consuming approach of frequency-domain analysis with Fourier transforms alluded to previously. The estimate can be done by simply squaring and summing the time-domain signal to obtain an approximate value of integrated backscatter.[39]

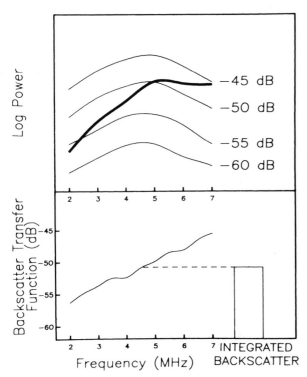

FIGURE 41–3. Backscatter transfer function and integrated backscatter obtained by interpolating the received power spectrum (*bold curve in top panel*), backscattered from myocardium with respect to the reference spectra from a stainless steel plate measured at 5-dB intervals. (From Miller, J.G., Perez, J.E., Mottley, J.G., et al.: Myocardial tissue characterization: An approach based on quantitative backscatter and attenuation. Proc. I.E.E.E. Ultrasonics Symp. 83CH1947–1:782, 1983, © 1983 IEEE.)

Real-Time Backscatter Imaging

To translate these quantitative measurements of acoustic properties of tissue into a clinically acceptable measurement or image format, a transitional step was taken to construct an M-mode–based system capable of measuring integrated backscatter in real time.[40] The next generation of this system was based on the adaptation of a commercial two-dimensional imaging device that uses conventional

phased-array transducers and computes in real time the integrated backscatter along each individual line of sight in the sector.[41–44] In the current implementation, once the summed intermediate-frequency signal has been formed from the output of the phased-array transducer, it can be sent to either the conventional video processing path or the integrated backscatter processor (Fig. 41–4). The processor incorporates digital hardware that produces a continuous signal that is proportional to the logarithm of integrated backscatter along each acoustic line in the image. The dynamic range of the integrated backscatter processor is more than 40 dB. The full dynamic range of the integrated backscatter data is mapped in 0.5-dB increments into the approximately 30-dB dynamic range available in the displayed video images. The output of the processor follows the remaining signal path through the scan converter as in the conventional image. Thus, the resulting image is created on the basis of integrated backscatter, and image resolution is reasonably well preserved (Fig. 41–5). The image is a quantitative, parametric image in which each picture element represents the value of relative integrated backscatter from data obtained in real time. The magnitude (in decibels) of the cyclic (diastolic-to-systolic) variation of integrated backscatter of a specific myocardial site is given by the logarithm of the ratio of backscattered energy in diastole to that in systole (see below for a more precise definition of the cyclic variation of myocardial backscatter). Over the range of transmit power used in the system, the magnitude of cyclic variation of integrated backscatter is essentially independent of transmit power. The current implementation of the system permits computation of the physiologic cardiac cycle—dependent variation in myocardial integrated backscatter, using an M-mode approach,[45] or directly from the two-dimensional image. Additional refinements in the future may permit quantitative comparison of absolute backscatter from patient to patient and among populations of patients with dissimilar myocardial pathology.

Recently, an approach that samples radiofrequency data corresponding to the entire sector during one cardiac cycle, without any data reduction technique or electrocardiographic triggering, has been developed.[46] Thus, all features of the signal can be studied, including integrated backscatter or signal spectral analysis. With this method, cyclic variation of myocardial integrated backscatter has been documented, and different regions of the myocardium can be compared in the same beat.

In addition, recent studies by investigators at Osaka University[47] have introduced an approach to obtain fully calibrated integrated

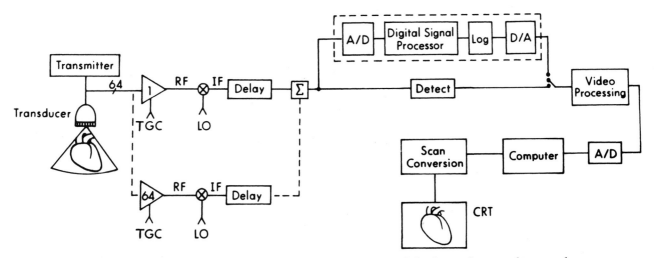

FIGURE 41–4. Diagram showing the modified signal processing path for the two-dimensional integrated backscatter imaging system. As in conventional imaging, the usual time-gain compensation (TGC) is used for attenuation. IF = intermediate-frequency signal; A/D = analog-to-digital conversion; D/A = digital-to-analog conversion; LO = low-pass filter; CRT = cathode ray tube; RF = radiofrequency. (From Vered, Z., Barzilai, B., Gessler, C.J., et al.: Ultrasonic integrated backscatter tissue characterization of remote myocardial infarction in human subjects. J. Am. Coll. Cardiol. 13:84, 1989. Reprinted with permission of the American College of Cardiology.)

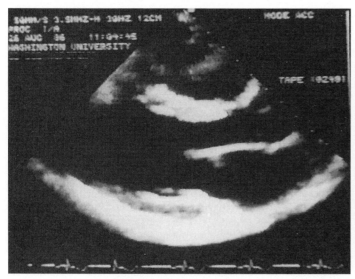 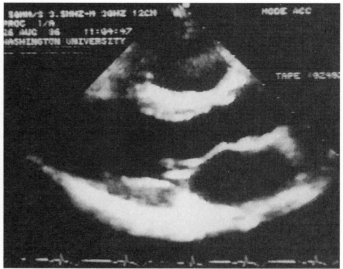

FIGURE 41–5. Diastolic *(left)* and systolic *(right)* still frames obtained with real-time integrated backscatter imaging in a normal subject. Diastolic-to-systolic decrease in myocardial integrated backscatter can be appreciated in the posterobasal and septal-basal segments. (From Perez, J.E., Miller, J.G., Barzilai, B., et al.: Progress in quantitative ultrasonic characterization of myocardium: From the laboratory to the bedside. J. Am. Soc. Echocardiogr. 1:294, 1988, with permission.)

backscatter images that should facilitate longitudinal clinical investigations in groups of patients or serial individual observations in a single patient. The measurement system developed consists of a commercially available echocardiograph interfaced with an analog-to-digital converter and a personal computer. Myocardial integrated backscatter is referenced to the backscatter power from the blood in the cavity in the vicinity of the myocardial tissue of interest. To correct for the attenuation or signal loss resulting from transmission through intervening tissue between the transducer and Doppler sample volume, the logarithmic power of Doppler signals scattering from the blood was subtracted from the logarithmic power of the myocardium at the region of interest. This approach renders measurements not only of the cyclic variation of myocardial backscatter but also of the myocardial backscatter itself, calibrated in decibels. This technique merits further studies for assessment of its stability and reproducibility in studies of populations.

Methods That Display Acoustically Abnormal Tissue

In addition to changes in overall myocardial echo amplitudes in the image (gray level), there are many recognizable changes in the spatial distribution or texture of these gray levels. Qualitative subjective descriptions of texture have used terms such as coarse or fine, uniform or nonuniform, and high-amplitude or low-amplitude echoes.[48] Obviously, these descriptions are strongly influenced by the experience and training of the operator and by equipment settings. Yet, this display-based approach has been used successfully by many investigators to describe the peculiar appearance of the ventricular septum in patients with hypertrophic cardiomyopathy[49] and the myocardium of patients with amyloid heart disease,[48] as well as the increased echogenicity of the ventricular septum (M-mode) in patients with remote myocardial infarction.[50]

Color encoding of conventional echocardiographic images with or without additional brightness modulation, as an alternative to gray scale displays, has been used to describe increased amplitude in segments of remote myocardial infarction[51] or eosinophilic myocardial disease.[52] These investigators, like Tanaka and associates,[53] have defined the pericardial reflection on two-dimensional views as exhibiting maximal intensity (or 100 percent). This pericardial reference has then been used to describe, in percentage values, the relative signal strength of normal-versus-abnormal regions. Because the human visual system is better able to distinguish among colors than among subtle changes in gray scale, this methodology has been used by other investigators as well. Other researchers

have described the evolution of scar maturation in dogs, followed serially with color-encoded images after experimental myocardial infarction.[54] Serial measurements were required, as opposed to a single set of observations of any one dog, to conclusively establish abnormal scar content.

The principal difficulty of these descriptive techniques is the subjective nature of the interpretation, which can be greatly altered by manipulation of the equipment settings. Other instrumentation-related considerations pertinent to this problem (and certainly to all other current approaches) involve changes in the time-gain compensation settings that may alter the acoustic signal, the use of nonlinear signal compression schemes, and reject and damping settings. Subjective setting of these controls in the system may mask or mimic pathologic processes. Others have proposed the use of "rational" (as opposed to conventional) time-gain compensation to better compensate for the attenuation suffered by round-trip travel of the signals into the tissue segment of interest. Conventional time-gain compensation may overcompensate, undercompensate, or both, leading to false differences in brightness (related to ultrasonic amplitude) that do not arise from true alterations in tissue structure.[55] In rational gain compensation, previously measured values for attenuation of blood and myocardium are assigned to define attenuation of a region along each line of sight in the image. This approach may improve detection of small scars in myocardium due to remote infarction[55] and has been implemented in the real-time integrated backscatter imaging[43] system to enable comparison of cyclic variation of myocardial integrated backscatter at different depths in the field (e.g., ventricular septum versus posterior wall values).

Methods That Quantitate Echocardiographic Gray Level (Image) Data

In addition to the use of data derived from radiofrequency signals (as used in the calculation of integrated backscatter) or visual inspection of images, in a third approach researchers have attempted to use quantitative analysis of video or image data. The motivations for choosing this approach include (1) the smaller data storage and processing requirements for video (as compared with radiofrequency) data and (2) the previously described abnormalities that may be seen by simple visual inspection of standard images, which suggests that information relevant to tissue ultrasonic properties may be extracted from images. The general approach consists of computer analysis of regional echo amplitude, including the spatial distribution (texture) of amplitudes in a quantitative, statistical fashion.[56] Assessment of regional echo amplitude first took the form of evaluating so-called first-order gray level attributes, such as average gray level (similar to image brightness), variance, skewness, and kurtosis of gray levels.[57] Quantitative analysis of first-order gray level data has proved useful for identification of infarction,[57] reperfusion,[58] and other abnormalities.

In contrast to the first-order gray level measurements, several groups have utilized quantitative analysis of spatial echo amplitudes in so-called texture analysis. Texture can be assessed by a number of measures[59–61] involving calculation of features of the two-dimensional spatial pattern of regional image gray levels (Fig. 41–6). These measures provide information concerning the heterogeneity of the gray levels and the relative size of the individual echo reflections and thus characterize the image texture. Quantitative texture measures have been used to demonstrate tissue changes due to myocardial contusion in closed-chest dogs[62] and cardiomyopathic changes in humans.[60] The methods can be applied in vivo to images from standard echocardiographic systems. Recent studies have employed two-dimensional autocorrelation function of the image sample as a mathematic measure, describing both the prominence and spacing between textural elements that make up an image.[63] This approach allowed differentiation between the myocardium of patients with hypertrophic cardiomyopathy and that of patients with pressure-overload hypertrophy in these studies. The main disadvantage of the aforementioned approaches lies in their dependence on instrumentation settings and probable lack of reproducibility among different laboratories.

BIOLOGIC DETERMINANTS OF MYOCARDIAL ACOUSTIC PROPERTIES

Diverse structural components of myocardium can influence its acoustic properties under physiologic and pathologic conditions.[26, 64] Ultrasonic tissue characterization for clinical application is directed primarily at delineation of the scattering properties of myocardial tissue.

Tissue elements responsible for scattering (i.e., scatterers) represent local regions of acoustic impedance mismatch.[65] The intensity

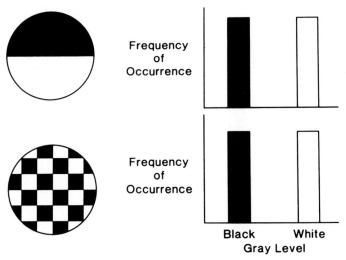

FIGURE 41–6. Concept of two-dimensional gray level texture. Two stylized digital regions of interest are shown (*left*). Because each region is half black and half white, the regions will display the same average gray level and identical gray level histograms (*right*). The obvious differences in the spatial distribution of black and white in the two regions, termed gray level texture, are not appreciated by simple inspection of average gray level or gray level histograms. (From Collins, S.M., and Skorton, D.J.: Cardiac Imaging and Image Processing. New York, McGraw-Hill, 1986, p. 199, with permission.)

of scattering depends on (1) the size, shape, and concentration of scatterers; (2) the difference in intrinsic acoustic impedance of the scatterers relative to the medium in which they reside; and (3) the spatial distribution of individual scatterers (e.g., random versus highly ordered). Myocardial elements responsible for scattering are much smaller than the wavelengths of ultrasound used for clinical imaging (wavelengths are 300 and 600 μm for 5-MHz and 2.5-MHz ultrasound, respectively). Various microstructural elements have been proposed as scatterers, including blood vessels, intact myocytes, and sarcomeres.[66]

Collagen

Collagen is a primary determinant of both scattering and attenuation of myocardial tissue. Studies have described the dependence of ultrasonic attenuation and scattering on myocardial collagen content and structure after experimental myocardial infarction.[67] Attenuation measurements were made in excised canine hearts and collagen content in regions of infarction was determined by assay of hydroxyproline. The attenuation coefficient increased and paralleled the hydroxyproline content in the infarct zone at each time interval.[68] The relationship between collagen content and ultrasonic attenuation and backscatter in dogs after myocardial infarction has been determined. Backscatter, attenuation, and hydroxyproline content progressively increased significantly in the infarct regions (Fig. 41–7).[69]

Further studies of isolated rabbit hearts excised 5 to 7 weeks after coronary artery occlusion and perfused with collagenase solutions were performed to determine the dependence of scattering and attenuation on the structural integrity of collagen in scar tissue after infarction.[68] Perfusion of infarct regions with collagenase markedly reduced ultrasonic backscatter. The concentration of hydroxyproline measured in the infarct regions remained unchanged after collagenase treatment. Thus, intact collagen, with its complex structural organization in regions of infarct scar tissue, appears to represent an important contributor to scattering.

Other studies have involved autopsied human hearts with fibrotic changes associated with remote infarction and have demonstrated a linear relationship between integrated backscatter and hydroxyproline content.[70] The magnitude of backscatter was greater in excised normal right ventricular segments than in normal left ventricular segments, corresponding to a higher collagen content in the right ventricle.[71] One study[72] extended these observations by detecting the highest backscatter values from canine right atrial wall tissue studied in vitro, followed by left atrial tissue, followed by the right ventricular myocardium, with the left ventricular myocardium exhibiting the lowest values. This pattern corresponds to the known regional concentration of collagen in different cardiac chamber walls. Some investigators have confirmed that the magnitude of backscatter is elevated in regions of myocardial infarction in both experimental animals and patients.[51, 54, 73–76]

Other investigators measured myocardial echo amplitude within 24 hours of endomyocardial biopsy in 25 patients after cardiac transplantation and found a modest but significant correlation between regional echo amplitude and tissue collagen content.[77] In these patients, the collagen content was judged to be within the physiologic normal range.

Scatterer Geometry

On the basis of measurements of the frequency dependence of scattering for normal myocardium, investigations have postulated that myocardial scatterers are comparable in size to cardiac myocytes.[78, 79] The relationship between the intensity of scattering and the frequency (f) of insonification can be described by a power law in which backscatter increases approximately as f^3 for normal myocardium.[26, 79] Theoretically, scatterers that are much smaller than a wavelength of sound are characterized by f^4 (Rayleigh scattering), and scatterers that are much larger than a wavelength

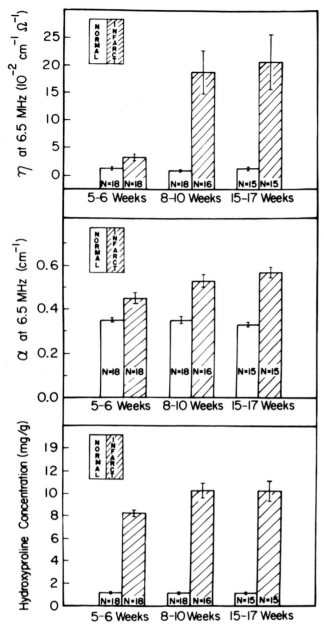

FIGURE 41-7. Comparison of the backscatter coefficient at 6.5 MHz (η, *top*), the attenuation coefficient at 6.5 MHz (α, *middle*), and the hydroxyproline concentration (*bottom*) in normal dog myocardium to values obtained from zones of infarction at three intervals after coronary artery occlusion. (From O'Donnell, M., Mimbs, J.W., and Miller, J.G.: The relationship between collagen and ultrasonic backscatter in myocardial tissue. J. Acoust. Soc. Am. 69:580, 1981, with permission.)

homogeneities increased significantly in cardiomyopathic hearts. Others have also reported that scattering intensity depends directly on cell size for a variety of tissues.[83] Thus, myocardial elements approximately the size of intact myocytes may be responsible in part for ultrasonic scattering under physiologic conditions. Electron microscopy studies have shown that cardiac myocytes are invested externally by a complex collagen matrix that provides structural support.[84] This microstructural arrangement (Fig. 41-8) of cells embedded in a collagen matrix may provide a sufficient local acoustic impedance mismatch to account for the scattering from normal myocardium.[65]

Further investigations directed to clarify the mechanisms for the cyclic variation of myocardial integrated backscatter suggest that changes in the effective size in the dominant scatterers may play an important role. Measurements of significant reductions in the frequency-dependence of myocardial backscatter from normal dogs from diastole to systole suggest that a cyclic enlargement of the dominant scatterers in tissue contributes to the cyclic variation measured.[85]

Other studies used a first-order model in which the scattering from myocardium was described in terms of Rayleigh scattering with the cardiac cycle variation in the scattering cross section. Absolute myocardial backscatter was described in these studies as a function of the frequency and phase of the cardiac cycle after their ultrasonic instrumentation was calibrated.[86]

Fiber Orientation

Myocardial acoustic properties also are influenced by the orientation of ventricular muscle fibers. Some studies have demonstrated that transmural ventricular muscle fiber bands spiral from endocardium to epicardium such that the predominant orientation of endocardial fiber bands is nearly perpendicular to the orientation of epicardial fibers.[87] The middle portion of the ventricular wall comprises mainly circumferentially oriented fiber bands. Some investigators have demonstrated that the magnitude of both ultrasonic attenuation and backscatter in excised heart tissue depends critically on the angle of insonification.[88-92] Attenuation is maximal when sound waves propagate parallel to or along the major fiber orientation and minimal in a direction perpendicular to the fiber orientation. Ultrasonic backscatter is maximal in a direction perpen-

of sound by f^o (specular scattering). The reduction of frequency dependence from approximately f^m to f^n, where $n < m$ after myocardial infarction, may indicate that the dominant myocardial scatterers are larger for infarcted than for normal myocardium and demonstrates the sensitivity of measurements of the frequency dependence of backscatter to pathologic replacement of normal myocytes by scar tissue after infarction.[80]

More detailed definition of the acoustic properties of biologic tissue has been attempted by the use of acoustic microscopy.[81] Insonification of thin histologic sections of autopsied normal and cardiomyopathic human myocardium with 200-MHz ultrasound have produced high-resolution, two-dimensional images of heart tissue.[82] These images reveal spatial variations of acoustic properties that are on the order of the size of cardiac myocytes for normal human myocardium. Furthermore, the dimensions of acoustic in-

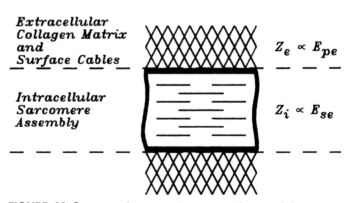

FIGURE 41-8. Proposed anatomical structure of myocardial scatterers. Myocardial scatterers are theorized to be approximately the size of myocytes. The Z_e (extracellular acoustic impedance) is proportional to the appropriate E_{pe} (extracellular parallel elastic modulus) and is identified with the extracellular collagen matrix and surface cables. The Z_i (intracellular acoustic impedance) is proportional to the appropriate E_{se} (series elastic element stiffness) and is identified with the intracellular sarcomere assembly and associated intracellular elastic fibers. If Z_e differs from Z_i at baseline, the juxtaposition of extracellular and intracellular elastic domain forms a scattering interface, composed of elastic elements with different baseline acoustic impedances. (From Wickline, S.A., Thomas, L.J., III, Miller, J.G., et al.: A relationship between ultrasonic integrated backscatter and myocardial contractile function. J. Clin. Invest. 76:2151, 1985, by copyright permission of the American Society for Clinical Investigation.)

dicular to the fibers and minimal in a direction parallel to or along the fiber axis. The same group has shown that integrated backscatter from canine myocardium measured in open-chest dogs is angle dependent but that the cardiac cycle-dependent variation of backscatter persists, regardless of the angle of insonification.[91]

Although skeletal and cardiac muscle are fundamentally different, some structural similarities have encouraged investigators to apply concepts about ultrasonic scattering properties studied in either type of laboratory tissue preparation. Recent studies have demonstrated that fiber orientation plays an important role in the alterations of skeletal muscle scattering induced by stretching.[93] In the orthogonal orientation, integrated backscatter was significantly increased with progressive stretching, but it changed very little (after minimal stretching) when the orientation was nearly parallel. The authors postulate that reorientation of the collagen surrounding the muscle fibers was most likely responsible for this observation.

Clinical studies in which the cyclic variation of myocardial integrated backscatter has been measured from parasternal and apical views have demonstrated the importance of fiber orientation on the measurements.[94] In 20 normal volunteers cyclic variation was demonstrable from parasternal but not from apical views, possibly because of angle-dependence of the predominant myocardial fiber orientation as seen from different views.

Blood Flow–Water Content

Tissue water content and hematocrit both influence myocardial scattering and attenuation. Studies in normal isolated rabbit hearts perfused with either Krebs-Henseleit buffer or whole blood showed that integrated backscatter increased by 200 percent after a brief washout with Krebs-Henseleit solution and returned to normal after perfusion with whole blood.[95] Perfusion with buffer of differing osmotic strengths to promote tissue edema resulted in increased tissue wet weight, accompanied by increased integrated backscatter that paralleled the extent of tissue edema. The accumulation of tissue edema early in the course of acute infarction results in decreased attenuation, in contrast to the increased attenuation observed in established infarct scars. Thus, both tissue water content and microvascular hematocrit may influence acoustic properties of myocardium. The presence or absence of blood flow itself may have a small impact on the absolute level of integrated backscatter. Additional studies reported minimal changes in integrated backscatter immediately following restoration of blood flow after 1 hour of coronary artery occlusion in dogs, associated with a lack of recovery of wall thickening after reperfusion.[96]

Further studies[97] have confirmed in open-chest dogs the negligible role of blood flow per se upon ultrasonic tissue parameters. Myocardial blood flow was varied from 0.8 to 12.9 mL/min/g, whereas the average myocardial ultrasonic gray level was measured off-line. Diastolic-to-systolic cyclic variation in intensity was noted but was not related to tissue blood flow, and neither was the segmental acoustic amplitude.

Nevertheless, reduction in coronary blood flow rate, perhaps resulting in very early manifestations of ischemia, can be detected by alterations in backscatter parameters. Some studies have documented marked blunting of integrated backscatter cyclic variation by reducing coronary flow rate by 50 percent in open-chest dogs,[98] in the absence of wall motion abnormalities in many of the animals. These results have been confirmed in clinical studies of transient ischemia,[99, 100] in which ultrasonic parameters were noted to be altered before mechanical dysfunction was evident.

Other Determinants

Myocardial acoustic properties may be influenced profoundly by disease entities that alter normal histologic architecture, such as the case of cardiac amyloidosis, which results in bright and speckled patterns manifested on conventional two-dimensional echocardiograms.[48] Other pathologic entities that entail infiltration or reorganization of myocardial tissue manifested by distinctive textural changes include hypertrophic cardiomyopathy, hemochromatosis, and eosinophilic endomyocardial disease.[101]

In addition, various intracardiac structures exhibit varying scattering as measured by radiofrequency analysis. Building on original observations[51, 53, 102] investigators have measured the pericardial interface as having the strongest reflection, with the septum exhibiting 22 percent of that of the pericardium, the posterior wall 17 percent, and the anterior mitral leaflet 5 percent.

Another source of variability in the measurements of myocardial acoustic properties may relate to inherent difficulties with the approach employed to obtain the measurement itself. Studies in which the cyclic variation of integrated backscatter was measured from septum or posterior wall shows small nonsignificant differences when measured repeatedly considering grouped data.[103] However, repeat measurements in individual subjects were not reliably reproduced because in this study, sampling of backscatter was limited to only two points in the cardiac cycle. Increased independent sampling and measurement from a backscatter waveform throughout the cardiac cycle,[104] is likely to improve reproducibility of the measurements. A method for incorporating this approach into a modified clinical echocardiographic scanner for determining the magnitude and time delay of the cyclic variation of integrated backscatter was recently described.[105]

Dynamic Aspects of Scattering

In addition to the determinants of backscatter in excised tissue or in vivo (averaged throughout the heart cycle), one study has shown that there is dynamic contribution of myocytes to the scattering process.[106] Investigators in that study demonstrated that backscatter intensity varies throughout the cardiac cycle, with maximal levels of scattering at end-diastole and minimal levels at end-systole (Fig. 41–9). The presence of cardiac cycle-dependent variation of backscatter intensity (or other measures of echo amplitude) has been widely confirmed in both experimental animals and human subjects.[106-111] The average magnitude of cyclic variation of backscatter is approximately 5 dB for normal myocardium. Cyclic variation of backscatter decreases substantially as a consequence of ischemic injury and recovers after reperfusion of injured but viable

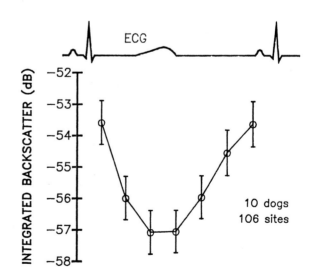

FIGURE 41–9. Cyclic variation of integrated backscatter in normal canine myocardium. (From Miller, J.G., Perez, J.E., Mottley, J.G., et al.: Myocardial tissue characterization: An approach based on quantitative backscatter and attenuation. Proc. I.E.E.E. Ultrasonics Symp. 83CH1947–1:782, 1983, © 1983 I.E.E.E.)

myocardial tissue in both experimental animals and human subjects.[96, 109, 111–114] Some studies have demonstrated that the magnitude and rate of change of physiologic cyclic variation of backscatter are related to intrinsic myocardial contractile performance[115] and are greater in subendocardial than in subepicardial regions. These results have been confirmed[111] and are consistent with the expectation of enhanced contractile performance in the subendocardium, as compared with that of the subepicardium.[65, 116] Isolated preparations of superfused canine myocardial papillary and frog skeletal gastrocnemius muscle also demonstrate a dependence of scattering intensity on muscle contractile state, independent of perfusion with blood.[117, 118] Other studies have described a quantitative relationship between the extent of cyclic variation of echo amplitude and the degree of segmental myocardial shortening as tested in normal humans, patients with cardiomyopathy, and patients with pulmonary hypertension.[119]

These observations indicate that acoustic properties of myocardium are related to contractile performance. Several hypotheses have been advanced to explain the cyclic alteration of myocardial acoustic properties and include cyclic alterations of myocardial elastic characteristics[65] and alterations of myocardial scatterer geometry.[118] However, no simple explanation as yet appears sufficient to account for the entire gamut of experimental observations.

SPECIFIC DISEASE PROCESSES STUDIED BY ULTRASONIC TISSUE CHARACTERIZATION

Acute Ischemia–Infarction

Among the qualitative observations from conventional echocardiograms, some studies detected early increases in regional echo amplitude as soon as 15 minutes after coronary occlusion.[120] The approximate size of the region exhibiting increased echo amplitude correlated with infarct size in experimental animals, as determined by histochemical techniques. Other studies identified a subset of patients with acute myocardial infarction, who exhibited a decrease in regional echo amplitude.[121] These patients had a higher risk of severe complications, including free wall rupture and death. Other investigators have attempted to improve the visual perception of differences in regional echo amplitude by using color encoding of the amplitude information, showing increases in echo amplitude during the evolution of myocardial infarction in experimental animals.[54]

In a series of studies using quantitative analysis of radiofrequency signals, various aspects of the acoustic characteristics of ischemia in experimental animals have been delineated. Initial studies reported decreases in acoustic impedance soon after coronary artery occlusion in dogs.[7, 122] In other early radiofrequency experiments, attenuation through excised myocardial specimens was measured in transmission studies. Significant decreases in attenuation in ischemic tissue were noted as soon as 15 minutes after coronary artery occlusion in dogs.[123] Decreased attenuation was noted for up to 24 hours after coronary artery occlusion and was thereafter replaced by an increase in attenuation. This study suggested that ischemic myocardial injury could be detected as early as 15 minutes after coronary occlusion, much sooner than light microscopic evidence of ischemic damage could be expected, and that the early decrease, followed by a later increase, in attenuation suggested that the stage of an acute injury could be estimated by using ultrasound methods.

With the use of reflected ultrasound, as opposed to attenuation measurements, integrated backscatter was shown to increase as soon as 1 hour after acute coronary artery occlusion in dogs.[95] Other studies used a fundamentally different calculation technique and identified an increase in the ratio of mean regional echo amplitude to the standard deviation of echo amplitudes within 30 minutes after coronary occlusion in dogs.[124]

Most of these results were based on the total amount of ultrasonic energy returning to the transducer, averaged throughout the cardiac cycle. The cyclic variation of ultrasound backscatter with cardiac contraction has been used as a variable to assess ischemic damage. Initial studies,[125] as subsequently confirmed,[108, 111] demonstrated that the normal cyclic variation of backscatter (decreasing with contraction) is blunted by ischemia (Fig. 41–10). This finding is now generally accepted to be an indication of the acute ischemic process. The physiologic basis of normal cardiac cycle-dependent backscatter variation has not been completely elucidated, but it may be related to cardiac contractile performance,[115] the elasticity of myocardial tissue,[65] and/or contraction-dependent variations in myocardial scatterer geometry.

Promising results have also been obtained in acute infarction by studying echocardiographic-image gray level characteristics. Investigators have used quantitative texture analysis to identify acute ischemia 2 hours after coronary occlusion in closed-chest dogs[126] (Fig. 41–11), as confirmed by others.[127] In addition, analysis of first-order gray level data demonstrated increased mean echo intensity on the septum 2 weeks after acute septal infarction in patients,[128] whereas analysis of skewness and kurtosis[57] was not contributory.

In additional animal experiments, investigators have postulated that the absolute myocardial wall thickness after myocardial ischemia made a major contribution in the measured integrated backscatter, suggesting that the elevation in backscatter after ischemia was primarily related to a decrease in wall thickness.[129] Others have demonstrated in experimental animals that the magnitude of cyclic variation of myocardial integrated backscatter exhibited a frequency-dependent increase[130] (i.e., higher magnitude when measured at 7 to 8 MHz, as opposed to 3 to 4 MHz). This pattern was useful in detecting the effects of acute ischemia and reperfusion, offering promise for implementation in humans (i.e., transesophageal or intracardiac imaging at higher frequencies).

Several clinical studies in the setting of acute myocardial ischemia have been added to the initial experience.[131] Recent studies using radiofrequency analysis of backscattered signals have demonstrated transient blunting (during stress testing) and subsequent recovery of the backscatter power in systole in patients with known anterior descending coronary artery disease.[132] In addition, the phase (delay of the nadir of cyclic backscatter variation) in the septum was increased transiently with subsequent normalization, whereas no appreciable changes occurred in the normally perfused posterior wall. These results in humans are concordant with those of previous studies in experimental animals.[96, 133] Other studies,[134] with the use of a system previously described,[86] demonstrated that

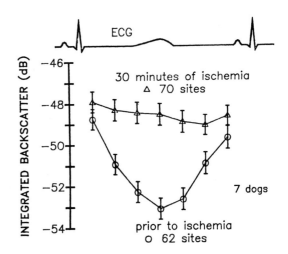

FIGURE 41–10. Blunting of the cyclic variation of backscatter and elevation of the time-averaged integrated backscatter after 30 minutes of myocardial ischemia in dogs. (From Miller, J.G., Perez, J.E., Mottley, J.G., et al.: Myocardial tissue characterization: An approach based on quantitative backscatter and attenuation. Proc. I.E.E.E. Ultrasonics Symp. 83CH1947–1:782, 1983, © 1983 I.E.E.E.)

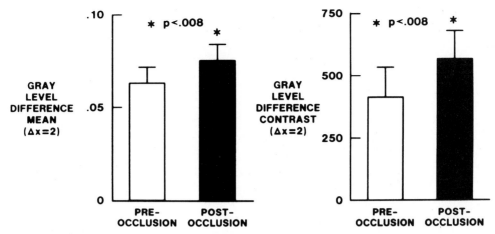

FIGURE 41–11. Efficacy of quantitative texture analysis in identifying acute ischemia. The data shown are for two quantitative texture parameters (gray level difference mean and contrast, both measured at a horizontal spacing [$\Delta \times$] of two pixels), measured before and after occlusion through the chest wall in nine dogs. Both texture parameters show significant alteration 2 hours after coronary occlusion. (From McPherson, D.D., Aylward, P.E., Knosp, B.M., et al.: Ultrasound characterization of acute myocardial ischemia by quantitative texture analysis. Ultrason. Imaging 8:227, 1986, with permission.)

patients with acute myocardial infarction studied within 36 hours of admission to a coronary care unit exhibit characteristic alterations in acoustic properties. Thus, the Fourier coefficient of amplitude (closely related to the magnitude of cyclic variation) was significantly lower in infarcted, as compared to normal myocardium, and the phase was significantly delayed. The sensitivity, specificity, and accuracy of the tissue characterization criteria were comparable to those of conventional echocardiographic detection of wall motion abnormalities.

In this regard, there have been three recent studies suggesting that alterations in myocardial acoustic properties resulting from acute ischemia actually precede, or are more sensitive than, the attendant mechanical dysfunction. Some studies[98] have been discussed previously under the section on blood flow-water content (see earlier). Marked reduction of the cyclic variation of integrated backscatter induced by reduction of coronary blood flow rate by 50 percent was associated with regional asynergy in only one third of the dogs. Similarly, other studies[135] suggest that ischemia induced by adenosine infusion in dogs with 75 percent reduction in coronary flow developed significant reductions in cyclic variation of integrated backscatter and increases in phase before any segmental dysfunction was evident. The same type of results is conveyed by two clinical studies.[99, 100] In one study[99] transient, short-lasting myocardial ischemia was detected in patients with vasospastic angina being exposed to ergonovine, as well as in patients with coronary artery disease subjected to dipyridamole stress and patients studied during coronary angioplasty. During transient ischemia, the myocardial region at risk exhibited increased mean gray amplitude, which was not related to the degree of dyssynergy induced. Furthermore, during angioplasty, elevation in myocardial gray levels (analogous to increased backscattering) was evident a mean of 10 seconds after occlusion at a time when no dyssynergy was detectable. In the second study myocardial gray levels were analyzed by transesophageal echocardiography in a given left ventricular wall segment of 15 patients in whom myocardial ischemia occurred intraoperatively, as detected by reversible akinesis or dyskinesis.[100] Patients were undergoing major abdominal or thoracic surgery, and ischemia occurred spontaneously and transiently. Ischemia was characterized by acute regional increases in echodensity and blunting of the normal pre-existing cyclic variation of gray levels. Furthermore, there was no correlation between the extent of dyssynergy and the degree of blunting of the cyclic variation, although there was a temporal association of the onset of dyssynergy with the onset of alterations in gray levels.

In summary, abnormal myocardial acoustic properties have been detected with induction of acute myocardial ischemia, but this relation is not solely mediated (either temporally or quantitatively) by the attendant alterations in mechanical function that accompany ischemia.

Reperfused Myocardium

The ability to identify successfully reperfused tissue (e.g., segments that remain viable despite temporary contractile abnormalities) and the ability to identify potentially viable myocardium to decide whether to attempt reperfusion are extremely important clinical issues in cardiovascular medicine at present. Echocardiographic tissue characterization data suggest that acoustic analysis techniques may aid in these determinations. To this end, initial studies demonstrated in an experimental canine preparation that alterations in ultrasound backscatter that occur after 20 minutes of coronary artery occlusion were reversed after 30 minutes of reperfusion.[136] In a study evaluating regional echo amplitude (gray level) data, researchers evaluated the effect of 3 hours of coronary occlusion, followed by 1 hour of reperfusion.[58] Viable myocardium demonstrated characteristic differences in mean echo amplitudes and skewness of gray level distributions, compared to those of regions that were infarcted (Fig. 41–12). Other studies[111, 113] have shown that the cardiac cycle-dependent variation in backscatter that is blunted by ischemia returns toward normal values after reperfusion. One group also[137] reported on the feasibility of distinguishing reversible from irreversible myocardial injury, measuring integrated backscatter Rayleigh 5 and the Fourier coefficient of amplitude modulation in two groups of dogs subjected to either 15 or 90 minutes of coronary artery occlusion. Brief ischemia increased integrated backscatter transiently with normalization after reperfusion, whereas the Fourier coefficient of amplitude modulation was transiently blunted with complete recovery. Prolonged occlusion rendered both parameters abnormal without correction after reperfusion. These results are concordant with previous studies[96] that demonstrated that the extent of alterations in the cyclic variation of backscatter resulting from ischemia (Fig. 41–13) and the magnitude of subsequent recovery after reperfusion are not merely related to the level of segmental wall thickening.[96] Similarly, studies have demonstrated in dogs[138] and patients[131] that cyclic variation of backscatter may recover after reperfusion at a time when wall motion and thickening abnormalities persist. Others have also demonstrated that persistently dysfunctional myocardium after 10 minutes of coronary artery occlusion, followed by reperfusion, exhibited normalization of the cyclic variation pattern but not the phase, despite restoration of myocardial blood flow.[133] In clinical studies similar to those previously discussed,[99, 100] investigators have

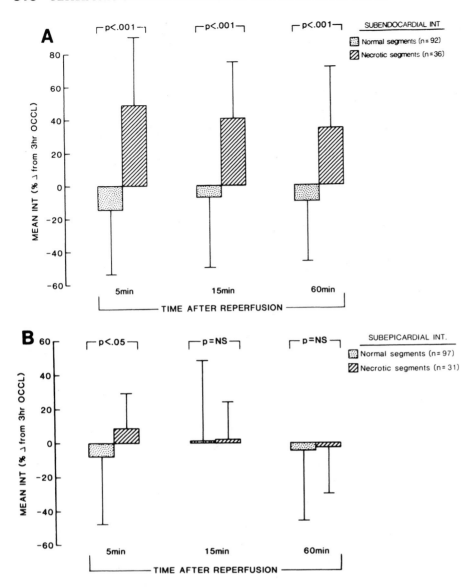

FIGURE 41–12. Alterations in mean echo intensities after coronary occlusion (OCCL) and reperfusion in dogs. *A* and *B* show data for subendocardial and subepicardial regions, respectively. The percent change in mean intensity in the subendocardial regions from 3 hours of coronary occlusion to 5, 15, and 60 minutes of reperfusion was significantly greater in necrotic tissue than in segments eventually shown to be salvaged. Results were somewhat similar only at 5 minutes of reperfusion in subepicardial regions. (From Haendchen, R.V., Ong, K., Fishbein, M.C., et al.: Early differentiation of infarcted and noninfarcted reperfused myocardium in dogs by quantitative analysis of regional myocardial echo amplitudes. Circ. Res. 57:718, 1985, with permission of the American Heart Association, Inc.)

described a causal relationship between occlusion of the supplying coronary artery and blunting of myocardial echo amplitude cyclic variation in patients undergoing coronary angioplasty.[139] The reduction in the variation was primarily due to an increase in end-systolic echo amplitude and was completely reversed following balloon deflation. In other studies,[140] closed-chest dogs with repeated 2-minute occlusions of the left anterior descending coronary artery, followed by coronary venous retroperfusion, were examined, measuring regional echo gray levels. When ischemia was treated by coronary venous retroperfusion, there was prevention of systolic increases in myocardial echo gray levels with preservation of the pattern of cyclic variation in backscatter observed at baseline. In concert these observations suggest that reperfused, viable, but "stunned" myocardium may be differentiated from necrotic tissue by ultrasound tissue characterization methods.

One inherent difficulty in the use of cyclic backscatter variation measurements in identifying acute infarction is the nonspecific nature of blunted cyclic variation. Decreases in cyclic variation of backscatter may occur in acute or chronic infarction. Studies have shown that analysis based on the frequency dependence of integrated backscatter can differentiate recently ischemic tissue from remotely infarcted myocardium in the same animal (Fig. 41–14), which suggests that future refinements in the assessment of parameters derived from radiofrequency data may be more specific for this differentiation.[80]

Subacute and Chronic Infarction

Myocardial infarction that has been present for a few days (but not long enough to result in significant deposition of collagen) also results in characteristic acoustic changes. Attenuation of infarcted myocardium was greater than that in normal tissue, beginning approximately 3 days after coronary occlusion.[123] In contrast, measurements made sooner (15 minutes to at least 24 hours) after occlusion demonstrated decreased attenuation as compared to normal attenuation. Therefore, very early changes in acoustic properties may be related to changes in myocardial perfusion, alterations in the formed elements of blood within the tissue region, and edema, whereas alterations in acoustic properties two or more days after coronary occlusion may be due to early cellular infiltration and other features of the necrotic process. Progressive increases in echo image amplitude, as displayed by a color-encoding technique, have been noted during evolving infarction.[54] Color encoding has been employed to detect regions of fibrosis in patients with remote myocardial infarction.[51, 75] Others have demonstrated in a closed-chest dog preparation of 48-hour-old myocardial infarction that the distribution of regional echo amplitudes differentiated infarcted from normal tissue.[57] Regions of myocardial infarction showed a decrease in the kurtosis (peakedness) of the echo amplitude distribution, as compared to that of normal myocardium (Fig. 41–15).

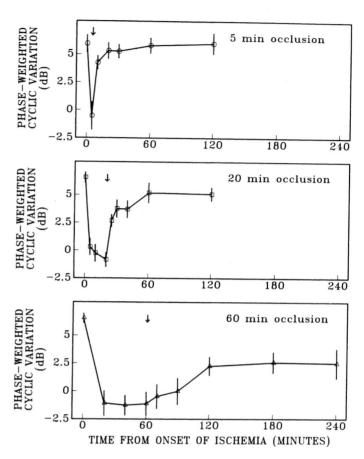

FIGURE 41-13. Changes in the phase-weighted amplitude of cyclic variation after coronary occlusion followed by reperfusion. The *top, middle,* and *bottom panels* represent responses of the phase-weighted amplitude for 5-, 20-, and 60-minute occlusions, respectively. The onset of reperfusion is denoted by an arrow. Each data point represents an average value for five dogs. Error bars represent standard error of the mean. (From Wickline, S.A., Thomas, L.J., III, Miller, J.G., et al.: Sensitive detection of the effects of reperfusion on myocardium by ultrasonic tissue characterization with integrated backscatter. Circulation 74:389, 1986, with permission of the American Heart Association, Inc.)

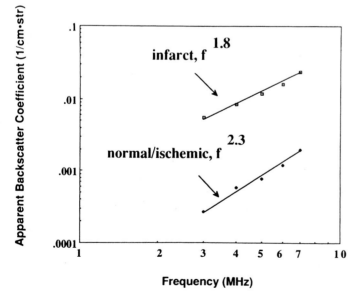

FIGURE 41-14. Backscatter coefficients for infarct and normal/ischemic myocardium. The backscatter coefficient for infarct is larger in magnitude and rises less rapidly with frequency (f) (not compensated for attenuation). (From Wear, K.A., Milunski, M.R., Wickline, S.A., et al.: Differentiation between acutely ischemic myocardium and zones of completed infarction on the basis of frequency dependent backscatter. J. Acoust. Soc. Am. 85:2634, 1989, with permission.)

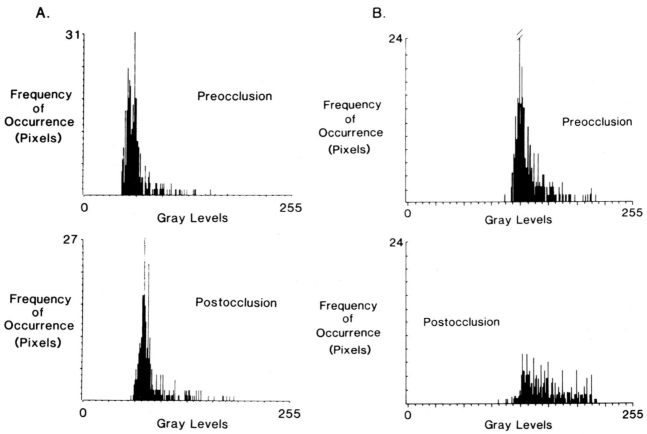

FIGURE 41–15. Gray level histograms (echo amplitude distributions) from infarcted and control myocardial regions before and 2 days after coronary occlusion in data acquired through the chest wall in dogs. *A,* Preocclusion and postocclusion gray level histograms from a control region; the shape of the histogram does not change between the two studies. *B,* Histograms from an infarcted region; the gray level distribution changes with a relatively higher frequency of higher gray levels postocclusion. (From Skorton, D.J., Melton, H.E., Jr., Pandian, N.G., et al.: Detection of acute myocardial infarction in closed-chest dogs by analysis of regional two-dimensional echocardiographic gray-level distributions. Circ. Res. 52:36, 1983, with permission of the American Heart Association, Inc.)

Using in vitro measurements of attenuation of excised myocardial specimens, researchers have shown marked increases in attenuation of the ultrasound signal that correlated well with increased collagen content at 2, 4, or 6 weeks after an acute myocardial infarction in dogs.[69] Studies of ultrasonic attenuation in excised tissue specimens had earlier established that the amount of change in attenuation in remote infarction correlated with the extent of injury assessed by creatine kinase levels.[141] Furthermore, integrated backscatter showed a substantial increase in remote experimental myocardial infarction.[79] Others studied specimens of fibrotic human myocardium and demonstrated a correlation between collagen content (assessed by hydroxyproline concentration) and integrated ultrasound backscatter (Fig. 41–16).[70] Other investigators have demonstrated[41] the applicability of integrated backscatter imaging for the precise localization of chronic experimental myocardial infarction correlated with gross pathology. Scarred myocardium lacked cyclic variation of integrated backscatter and exhibited higher values of relative backscatter. Using the same instrumentation, these observations were extended to humans with chronic myocardial infarction[44] (Fig. 41–17). Identification of scarred tissue was based on diminished cyclic variation of integrated backscatter and a prolonged time period from the R wave of the electrocardiogram to the nadir of the segmental integrated backscatter waveform. More recently, others have employed the same instrument to study 18 patients after a recent myocardial infarction, demonstrating that in regions of completed infarction in evolution the cyclic variation of integrated backscatter was significantly diminished, as compared to values from normal segments.[142]

In summary, these studies of chronic infarction suggest that the deposition of collagen as scar was responsible in part for the acoustic alterations manifested as increased attenuation and backscatter of abnormal tissue.

Myocarditis

The diagnosis of myocarditis frequently presents a clinical dilemma and eventually may require the performance of endomyocardial biopsy for confirmatory purposes. Conventional echocardiography typically discloses global systolic dysfunction without appreciable chamber dilation. Because this may be relatively nonspecific, additional diagnostic methods have been sought. Studies have reported on the quantitative analysis of echocardiographic regional image texture in 13 patients, of whom 8 had biopsy-proven myocarditis.[143] The parameter known as entropy (first-order analysis by texture) appeared to differentiate consistently patients with myocarditis from controls. Among second-order gray level statistical parameters, patients with myocarditis but also those with fibrosis had decreased entropy and higher angular second moment, as compared to controls. Therefore, although promising, the experience with tissue characterization in myocarditis is limited and there seems to be overlap in the groups of patients with inflammation and fibrosis with respect to texture analysis.

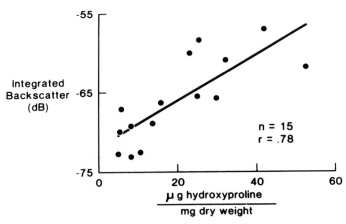

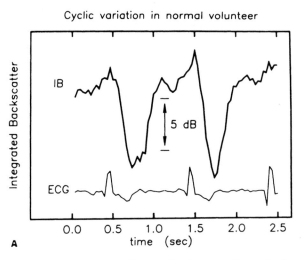

Cyclic variation in normal volunteer

A

FIGURE 41-16. Relationship between ultrasound integrated backscatter and collagen content in fibrotic myocardium. The data show a linear relationship between backscatter and hydroxyproline concentration in fibrotic human myocardium evaluated in vitro. (From Hoyt, R.H., Collins, S.M., Skorton, D.J., et al.: Assessment of fibrosis in infarcted human hearts by analysis of ultrasonic backscatter. Circulation 71:740, 1985, with permission of the American Heart Association, Inc.)

Dilated Cardiomyopathy

Based on previous tissue acoustic observations in animals and in patients with chronic myocardial infarction, one might expect the acoustic properties of dilated cardiomyopathies to include increased time-averaged ultrasound backscatter and a decrease in the cyclic variation of backscatter. Studies have noted that patients with dilated cardiomyopathy do exhibit a significant decrease in cyclic backscatter variation[43] (Fig. 41-18).

Other observations in dilated cardiomyopathy also support a role for ultrasound tissue characterization. The use of color encoding of echocardiographic data to enhance the perception of regional differences in backscatter increased echo brightness in patients with endomyocardial involvement due to hypereosinophilic cardiomyopathy.[52] Others have evaluated 16 patients with presumed dilated cardiomyopathy.[144] They measured the integrated value of the rectified radiofrequency signal emanating from the interventricular septum, taken as the backscatter index and expressed in percent normalized to the signal strength from the pericardium with the latter assumed to be 100 percent. All patients underwent endomyo-

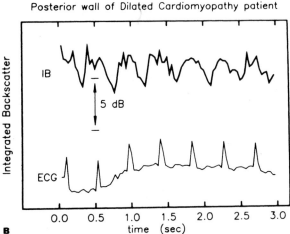

Posterior wall of Dilated Cardiomyopathy patient

B

FIGURE 41-18. Cyclic variation of integrated backscatter in the myocardium of a normal volunteer (*A*) and in the posterior wall of a patient with dilated cardiomyopathy (*B*). The patient with dilated cardiomyopathy exhibits significantly less cyclic variation of backscatter than does the normal volunteer. (From Vered, Z., Barzilai, B., Mohr, G.A., et al.: Quantitative ultrasonic tissue characterization with real-time integrated backscatter imaging in normal human subjects and in patients with dilated cardiomyopathy. Circulation 76:1067, 1987, with permission of the American Heart Association, Inc.)

cardial biopsies, which were stained with Masson's trichrome and studied for the extent of fibrosis. The percent integrated backscatter index was significantly higher in the presence of connective tissue area greater than 20 percent (eight patients) versus less than 20 percent. There was a significant correlation between percent integrated backscatter index and percent connective tissue area. In additional studies the frequency-dependence of backscatter was measured from biopsy specimens of explanted hearts of patients who underwent cardiac transplantation because of idiopathic cardiomyopathy.[145] The frequency dependence of backscatter increased progressively from epicardial to endocardial layer in conjunction with a progressive decrease in myofiber diameter. These results suggest that different types of cardiomyopathy exhibit distinct, heterogeneous transmural distributions of scattering structures.

In summary, the data on dilated cardiomyopathies indicate that regional echo intensity appears to be increased, cyclic variation in backscatter is blunted, and gray levels are altered.

Infiltrative-Restrictive Cardiomyopathy

Qualitative echocardiographic abnormalities in cardiac amyloidosis supplied some of the early motivation for ultrasound myo-

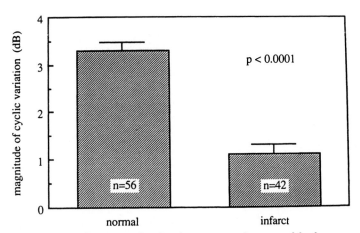

FIGURE 41-17. Magnitude of cyclic variation of integrated backscatter in normal versus remotely infarcted myocardium in clinical real-time backscatter imaging studies. Previously infarcted myocardium exhibited significantly less cardiac cycle-dependent variation in backscatter than did normal myocardium. (From Vered, Z., Barzilai, B., Gessler, C.J., et al.: Ultrasonic integrated backscatter tissue characterization of remote myocardial infarction in human subjects. J. Am. Coll. Cardiol. 13:84, 1989. Reprinted with permission of the American College of Cardiology.)

cardial tissue characterization, that is, the common clinical observation of abnormal tissue appearance in echocardiograms of patients with amyloidosis suggested that sufficient information was available in the ultrasound signal to differentiate these patients from normal persons. For example, an unusual "granular sparkling" appearance of the myocardium was noted in 90 percent of amyloid cases.[146] Others reported bright regional myocardial texture in a patient with amyloidosis.[147] In a systematic study of qualitative abnormalities in echocardiographic image texture, the histologic and clinical correlates of abnormal texture was evaluated as displayed on standard two-dimensional echocardiograms.[48] Of seven patients with amyloidosis in their study, three demonstrated "highly refractile echoes" (Fig. 41–19).

Quantitation of acoustic abnormalities in amyloidosis has been limited. The quantitative characteristics of echocardiographic image texture in patients with amyloid heart disease, hypertrophic cardiomyopathy, and hypertensive left ventricular hypertrophy and in normal persons was evaluated.[60] These investigators found that quantitative image texture analysis differentiated amyloidosis from hypertrophic cardiomyopathy and from normal myocardium. Others also used quantitative texture measures to differentiate amyloid-infiltrated myocardium from normal tissue in patients.[148]

Recently, studies have reported on their experience studying patients with β-thalassemia major and iron overload without overt signs of cardiac failure.[149] Integrated backscatter signals from the septum and the posterior wall were obtained and normalized to the signal strength of the pericardium (expressed in integrated backscatter percent). Twenty age- and sex-matched controls were also studied. The IB percent values were higher in patients with thalassemia major than in controls for both the septum and the posterior wall. Thus, myocardial reflectivity or backscatter is increased in these patients, probably because of iron deposits or secondary structural damage in the tissue, despite normal conventional echocardiographic indices of systolic function, indistinguishable from those of control subjects.

In summary, qualitative observations and preliminary quantitative analyses support a role for ultrasonic tissue characterization techniques in the diagnosis of infiltrative myopathy. This capability would be especially valuable in cases in which amyloid cardiomyopathy may mimic hypertrophic cardiomyopathy and in patients with thalassemia major.

Hypertrophic Cardiomyopathy

Early in the echocardiographic evaluation of hypertrophic cardiomyopathy, abnormalities in qualitative tissue appearance were noted. Initial reports noted an unusual "ground-glass" texture in the ventricular septum of some patients with hypertrophic cardiomyopathy.[49] Others noted that patients with hypertrophic cardiomyopathy exhibited bright echoes as well.[48] In the quantitative texture analytic study mentioned above[60] hypertrophic cardiomyopathy was

A

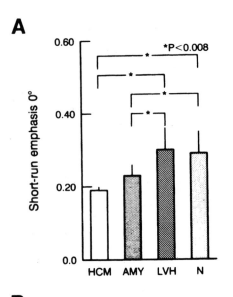

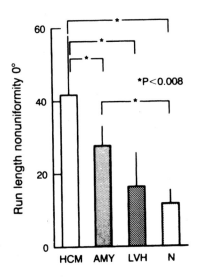

B

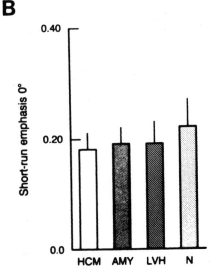

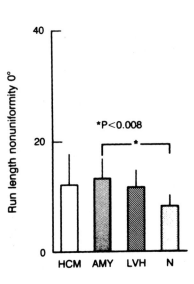

FIGURE 41-19. Differentiation of cardiomyopathies from normal myocardium in clinical echocardiograms, based on quantitative texture analysis. The graphs show selected gray level run length data obtained from end-diastolic long-axis clinical echocardiographic views of the ventricular septum (A) and posterior left ventricular wall (B) in patients with hypertrophic cardiomyopathy (HCM), amyloidosis (AMY), and left ventricular hypertrophy (LVH) and in normal persons (N). Quantitative parameters were able to differentiate both cardiomyopathies from those of normal persons and from each other. (From Chandrasekaran, K., Aylward, P.E., Fleagle, S.R., et al.: Feasibility of identifying amyloid and hypertrophic cardiomyopathy with the use of computerized quantitative texture analysis of clinical echocardiographic data. J. Am. Coll. Cardiol. 13:832, 1989. Reprinted with permission of the American College of Cardiology.)

differentiated from amyloidosis and from normal myocardium, based on quantitative features of echocardiographic image texture.

Recently, there have been several studies employing radiofrequency signal analysis involving this patient population. Twenty-five patients with classic echocardiographic findings of hypertrophic cardiomyopathy were studied with on-line radiofrequency analysis to obtain tissue reflectivity (analogous to integrated backscatter) of the septum and the posterior wall, both normalized to the signal of the pericardium and expressed as a percentage.[150] Results were compared to similar data in 25 normal age-matched control subjects. Patients with hypertrophic cardiomyopathy had values of backscatter significantly higher than those of normals in the septum and in the posterior wall. There was no correlation between the degree of reflectivity and left ventricular wall thickness. Thus, quantitative analysis of ultrasonic reflectivity can distinguish patients with hypertrophic cardiomyopathy independently from those with clinical features and conventional echocardiographic measurements. Others had already demonstrated that patients with hypertrophic cardiomyopathy had smaller values of cyclic variation of integrated backscatter in the septum, as compared to those of normal controls, whereas the posterior wall exhibited values not different from those of controls.[151] Additional recent work was carried out to differentiate hypertrophic cardiomyopathy from hypertensive cardiomyopathy, using a newly developed M-mode format-integrated backscatter imaging system capable of calibrating myocardial integrated backscatter with the power of Doppler signals from the blood[47] (see section on methods based on radiofrequency data analysis). With this new approach, cyclic variation of integrated backscatter and calibrated myocardial integrated backscatter were not different when researchers compared patients with hypertrophic cardiomyopathy to those with hypertensive hypertrophy. However, a transmural gradient in myocardial integrated backscatter (higher backscatter in the endocardial half than in the epicardial half of the wall) was present only in patients with hypertrophic cardiomyopathy. This finding suggests that differentiation among these patient groups is possible with this approach.

In summary, studies suggest that the altered architecture and fibrosis of hypertrophic cardiomyopathy may produce diagnostic abnormalities in myocardial acoustic properties.

Experimental Cardiomyopathy

Administration of doxorubicin to rabbits produced an anthracycline-induced experimental cardiomyopathy, in which increases in ultrasound-integrated backscatter were found in cardiomyopathic and fibrotic tissue.[152] Others reported the acoustic accompaniments of the spontaneous cardiomyopathy that occurs in the Syrian hamster[153]; these investigators noted increased regional ultrasound backscatter and increased heterogeneity of backscatter within regions of calcification and fibrosis.

In summary, ultrasound tissue characterization techniques show promise for identifying each of the major categories of cardiomyopathies. However, clinical data are preliminary, and standardization techniques have not yet been achieved.

Myocardial Effects of Pressure Overload: Arterial Hypertension

It has been demonstrated that myocardial hypertrophy alters the acoustic characteristics of myocardium.[154] Additional studies had documented increased echo intensities in the septum of patients with acquired valvular disease and essential hypertension with left ventricular hypertrophy and ST-T wave changes, as compared to data derived from normal controls.[155] Investigators postulated that these changes may be related to fibrosis in the tissue. In another study, two-dimensional echocardiograms were analyzed for regional echo intensity[156] to determine the relationship between STT wave changes, diastolic abnormalities, and echo intensity in patients with hypertrophy. They studied athletes, patients with hypertrophic cardiomyopathy, patients with secondary hypertrophy (who had

aortic stenosis, severe hypertension, coarctation, and subaortic stenosis) and controls. In patients with hypertrophy, regional echo amplitude was significantly increased in middle and basal septum and posterior wall. Patients with increased echo amplitude in any region had a higher incidence of ST-T changes and abnormalities of diastolic function than those with normal echo amplitude. In athletes, despite increases in left ventricular mass, there were no abnormalities in echo intensity or diastolic function. The increased echo intensity was attributed to myocardial fibrosis. Others have also demonstrated that the cyclic variation of myocardial integrated backscatter was reduced in the septum of patients with uncomplicated pressure-overload ventricular hypertrophy to a comparable extent, as was the case for patients with hypertrophic cardiomyopathy, as compared to that of normal controls.[151] The relation between wall thickness and tissue reflectivity has been further explored[157] in comparisons of wall thickness and integrated backscatter in open-chest pigs before and during coronary artery occlusion and after reperfusion. A distinct inverse relationship was found between the value of end-systolic integrated backscatter and myocardial wall thickness in an experimental preparation in which tissue collagen content would not play a role.

In contrast, a series of studies suggest that increased myocardial thickness per se does not alter the acoustic properties of the tissue, unless there are concomitant alterations in tissue composition or histology, which is presumed to be the case in patients with hypertrophic cardiomyopathy. Initially, integrated backscatter of myocardium (expressed as percent of pericardial reflection) was measured in athletes and in controls with a sedentary lifestyle.[158] Despite significantly greater wall thickness in the athletes, values for percent myocardial integrated backscatter were similar for both septum and posterior wall. When data from athletes and patients with hypertrophic cardiomyopathy with similar wall thickness were compared, the myocardial backscatter was significantly increased in the patients, as compared to the athletes. Thus, athletes and patients could be differentiated by backscatter analysis, despite comparable degrees of wall thickness. In other studies from this group, the same technique and acoustic measurements were used to study elite senior endurance athletes and normal age-matched controls with a sedentary lifestyle.[159] Despite greater left ventricular mass in the athletes, there were no significant differences among the two groups with respect to integrated backscatter measurements, suggesting that no significant pathologic structural changes had occurred in the older athletes' myocardium. Other studies from the same institution in patients with uncomplicated arterial hypertension lend further support to the notion that hypertrophy per se does not affect tissue acoustic parameters as indicators of myocardial structure.[160] These studies measured integrated backscatter of the myocardium in patients with hypertension and in age-matched control subjects. Hypertensive patients had higher values of mean blood pressure and left ventricular mass index than controls did but had similar values for backscatter. Therefore, these results suggest that in the absence of overt cardiac dysfunction, disproportionate connective tissue growth does not necessarily accompany the compensatory hypertrophic response to arterial hypertension in humans. These results are at variance with those of Naito and co-workers,[47] who reported that patients with hypertensive hypertrophy had values of cyclic variation and calibrated integrated backscatter similar to those of patients with hypertrophic cardiomyopathy. In this study they propose that the additional measurement of the transmural gradient in integrated backscatter is a differentiating feature among these groups. However, the hypertensive patients in the latter study[47] were older than those hypertensive patients in the former study,[160] which suggests that differences in collagen content related to aging may have played a role in accounting for the different results.

In summary, recent data suggest that in the absence of ischemia or other confounding events, myocardial wall thickness may influence tissue acoustic properties only when associated with alterations in collagen content or gross morphologic modifications, such as in hypertrophic cardiomyopathy or arterial hypertension associated with aging.

Intracardiac Thrombus

The acoustic properties of blood change substantially with the process of thrombus formation. After 24 hours of clot formation,[161] ultrasound backscatter from human blood increased by almost 19 dB. Some researchers have noted an unusual, speckled echocardiographic texture in thrombi (which was somewhat nonspecific and similar to that found in tumors).[162] In a more quantitative approach to assessment of the acoustic properties of ventricular thrombus, investigators[163] used stochastic analysis of radiofrequency ultrasound data to differentiate thrombus from artifact and intracardiac tumor. Others[164] evaluated the first-order gray level statistics of experimental ventricular thrombi in acutely infarcted dogs. Mean gray level, standard deviation, and skewness of regional gray levels all distinguished thrombus from intracavitary blood, and mean gray level and standard deviation distinguished thrombus from adjacent myocardium in views in which the regions of interest could be placed at similar depths of field (thus yielding data at approximately the same point along the time-gain compensation profile). Preliminary work with a real-time backscatter imaging system suggests that ventricular thrombi exhibit no significant cyclic variation of backscatter and have increased localized integrated backscatter, as compared to surrounding blood and adjacent myocardium.[165] In addition to the identification of a cardiac mass as a thrombus, ultrasound tissue characterization techniques may offer insight into the embolic potential of a thrombus. Other studies showed[166] that selected quantitative texture features of human intraventricular thrombi were of value in classifying thrombi as potentially embolic.

Myxoma

Studies carried out with the stochastic analysis method mentioned above were able to differentiate tumor from thrombus within the heart; the tumor was, however, not differentiated from artifact in those studies.[163] However, other studies, using neural network-based algorithms,[167] suggest that ultrasonic texture of tumors is different from that of thrombi.

Vegetations

Some studies have evaluated the echo amplitude characteristics of active versus healed valvular vegetations due to infective endocarditis.[168] Active (acute, culture-positive) vegetations exhibited relatively low echo amplitude, but the echo amplitude increased during healing. Presumably, these changes in echo amplitude were due to collagen deposition as vegetations healed.

Myocardial Contusion

Acute myocardial contusion causes a variety of pathologic sequelae, including intramyocardial hematomas and hemopericardium. Using an experimental model of myocardial contusion, investigators discovered that the quantitative features of echocardiographic image texture could be used to differentiate contused from normal myocardium.[62]

Atherosclerosis

There has been growing interest in characterization of the acoustic properties of the vascular wall to identify and define the composition of atherosclerotic plaque noninvasively. Early studies used a high-resolution scanner to image aortic and iliac vessels in vitro.[169] Fibrous, fibrofatty, and calcified lesions could be qualitatively differentiated by their characteristic ultrasonic image. Other studies

quantitatively assessed normal and atherosclerotic specimens of excised abdominal aorta[170]; they demonstrated increased integrated backscatter index in fibrofatty and calcified regions.

Some studies have shown that quantitative measurements of integrated backscatter differentiated calcified and fibrous regions from fibrofatty regions of human aorta (Fig. 41–20).[171] Others utilized high-frequency epicardial echocardiography intraoperatively to assess the acoustic characteristics of coronary arteries of patients at the time of cardiac surgery[172]; they demonstrated significant differences in the average gray level between atherosclerotic and normal coronary arterial wall. Early experience with intravascular ultrasound methods (i.e., catheter-mounted transducers) has also shown differences between qualitative and quantitative acoustic features of normal and atherosclerotic tissue.[173, 174] Thus, quantitative estimates of the energy reflected by the arterial wall give some insight into the composition of normal and atherosclerotic plaque in aorta, iliac, and coronary arteries.

Some investigators used the angle dependence of scattering to characterize arterial tissue; in their studies, they described a technique in which an oblique beam angle is used to limit the effect of the initial specular echo.[175] Others have measured the angle dependence of ultrasonic backscatter in arterial tissues.[176] A very directive pattern with a strongly angle-dependent backscatter was typical of calcified and fibrous plaques. Fatty samples were characterized by a nondirective pattern that was not significantly dependent on the angle of incidence of the ultrasonic beam.

Studies using acoustic microscopy (utilizing 27 or 50 Mhz) have been performed recently.[177, 178] The results of these investigations have further validated the important role of angle-dependence of backscatter power measurements and the significantly improved resolution conferred by the high interrogating frequency for detailed studies of vessel wall morphology. In contrast to these studies performed in vitro, clinical studies performed in vivo with images obtained by transesophageal echocardiography have detected a high incidence of unsuspected atherosclerotic plaques in the descending thoracic aorta in patients.[179] This approach may lend itself to future investigations of arterial tissue remodeling.

These observations suggest that definition of the composition of atherosclerotic plaque may be feasible, using quantitative ultrasonic techniques. In the future, these methods will be potentially applicable for the identification of peripheral vascular atherosclerosis and coronary atherosclerosis, when used intraoperatively or with intravascular ultrasonic catheters.

Valvular Tissue

Because conventional echocardiography has a relatively low specificity for evaluating calcific valve deposits, which has been shown

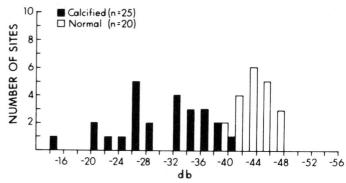

FIGURE 41–20. Distribution of echo amplitudes in normal and calcified aortic tissue. Calcified tissue exhibited significantly higher integrated backscatter values than normal aortic tissue. (From Barzilai, B., Saffitz, J.E., Miller, J.G., et al.: Quantitative ultrasonic characterization of the nature of atherosclerotic plaques in human aorta. Circ. Res. 60:459, 1987, with permission of the American Heart Association, Inc.)

to be an important factor in the outcome of interventional therapeutic procedures (surgery and balloon valvuloplasty), studies with tissue characterization have been carried out. After initial studies in vitro, preoperative studies in 33 patients who were scheduled to undergo mitral valve replacement via integrated backscatter measurements of the valves, using a 1-μsec acquisition gate in their system after obtaining images with a conventional 2.25 MHz transducer, were performed.[180] The valve tissue-integrated backscatter was expressed as a function of pericardial backscatter. The valves were subsequently excised and were submitted for histologic examination. The percent integrated backscatter was highest in patients with calcific valves, followed by that of patients with fibrotic valves, as compared to that from valves in older individuals without valvular disease who were age-matched for patients and young individuals with normal valves. This differentiation carried out in vivo holds promise for additional studies as valvuloplasty methods are more widely used.

Myocardial Effects of Diabetes Mellitus

Although patients with diabetes mellitus may be afflicted by cardiomyopathy, its prevalence and nature are controversial. Initial studies were performed to characterize myocardial acoustic properties in patients with insulin-dependent diabetes to determine whether ultrasound tissue characterization could detect changes potentially indicative of occult cardiomyopathy.[181] The magnitude of cyclic variation of myocardial ultrasound-integrated backscatter and its phase delay with respect to the onset of the cardiac cycle in the septum and posterior wall of the left ventricle were measured in patients with diabetes who had no overt cardiac disease. Despite normal ventricular systolic function by conventional echocardiography, cyclic variation of integrated backscatter was reduced in patients, as compared to that in controls. In addition, delay was significantly increased. Reduction of cyclic variation was greatest in patients with diabetes who also had neuropathy, as was the increase in delay vs. values in patients with diabetes but without neuropathy. Retinopathy and nephropathy were associated with abnormal myocardial acoustic properties as well. Furthermore, independent re-analysis of this data have confirmed the validity of these results.[182] Excellent receiver-operator curve values that approximate 0.9 were obtained when all four parameters (magnitude of cyclic variation of septum, magnitude of cyclic variation of posterior wall, delay of cyclic variation of the septum, and delay of cyclic variation of the posterior wall) were used for differentiation of patients with diabetes with noncardiac complications. Thus, abnormalities that may reflect fibrosis or other occult cardiomyopathic changes in patients with diabetes are readily detectable by means of myocardial tissue characterization, and they parallel the severity of noncardiac complications of diabetes.

Cardiac Allograft Rejection

The need for better noninvasive methods for surveillance of rejection in patients after cardiac transplantation has led to several studies using ultrasonic myocardial tissue characterization. Initial studies at Stanford included measurement of the cyclic variation of myocardial integrated backscatter in patients within 24 hours of endomyocardial biopsy.[183] Studies in 11 patients documented moderate acute rejection and disclosed reductions in the magnitude of cyclic variation in the septum and in the posterior wall, with subsequent normalization of the values after intensification of antirejection treatment and normalization of the biopsies. These studies attributed these results in the acoustic measurements to transient alterations in myocardial ultrastructure accompanying the rejection process. Similar results in detecting rejection have been obtained by several other investigators, who used digital image processing of conventional echocardiographic images,[184] and others who made use of a color-encoded gray scale method to quantitate myocardial echo amplitude.[185] Additional research documented in-

creases in myocardial echo amplitude by analysis of gray level histograms in an experimental animal preparation of heterotopic cardiac transplantation when antirejection medication was stopped.[186] In this study there was histologic confirmation of the acoustic measurements and, recently, these investigators have extended their experimental results to studies in humans with allograft rejection with comparable results.[187]

Myocardial Effects of Cyanotic Congenital Heart Disease

Because adults with nonrestrictive ventricular septal defects may have chronic hypoxemia that may lead to alterations in myocardial structure and function, investigators have recently used measurements of myocardial cyclic variation of integrated backscatter to define possible changes in tissue that may influence patients' clinical status.[188] As compared to age-matched controls, patients with a ventricular septal defect exhibited reduced values of cyclic variation in the septum and in the right ventricular free wall. As it was with results from other studies of patients with hypertrophy[158, 160] there was no correlation between backscatter and wall thickness or percent wall thickening in any of the myocardial walls studied. Histologic analysis obtained in three patients revealed interstitial and replacement fibrosis. These initial studies in this patient population suggest that the alterations in acoustic properties in tissue, despite preserved systolic function, may indicate subclinical manifestation of the adverse effects of chronic hypoxemia in myocardium, which could assist researchers in patient selection for cardiac transplantation in the future.

Aging

To define the effects of aging on myocardial structure by noninvasive means, studies have been carried out in subjects without cardiovascular disease (age, 22 to 71 years) by measuring the cyclic variation of myocardial integrated backscatter in the septum and posterior walls.[189] A significant correlation between the magnitude of cyclic variation of integrated backscatter and age of the subject for the posterior wall of the left ventricle was found but not for the septum. In the case of the septum, these investigators attributed the lack of significance to the inability to exclude specular septal echoes from the region of interest. Therefore, acoustic properties of myocardium appear to be influenced somewhat by aging, which stresses the need for age-matched controls in clinical studies.

CONCLUSIONS

Abundant experimental evidence supports the idea that ultrasound interacts differently with normal and abnormal cardiovascular tissue. Ultrasonic tissue characterization techniques have been demonstrated by means of a variety of methods and different investigative groups to be accurate in identifying acute myocardial ischemia, reperfusion, infarction, and scar deposition.[190] Cardiomyopathies, intracardiac masses, and atherosclerotic plaque also may be characterized by using ultrasonic analysis methods. Although these techniques are still considered investigational, very promising recent clinical results support their potential in the clinical setting. Further work remains to be accomplished before widespread clinical application can be strongly endorsed. In particular, the various stages of acute myocardial infarction cannot currently be differentiated solely on the basis of time-averaged backscatter or cyclic backscatter variation. Adding information on the frequency dependence of backscatter may help to make this clinically critical distinction. Techniques based on analysis of echocardiographic image (gray level) data are quite dependent on instrumentation variables, such as user adjustments of the imaging system. These instrumentation-related sources of variability will need to be minimized by standardization of the data acquisition method or by correction for variations in instrument settings.

Despite these remaining problems, the long history of successful experimental observations with ultrasonic tissue-characterization techniques and significant progress in clinical studies and observations support further development of this diagnostic approach to myocardial and vascular structural characteristics.

References

1. Falsetti, H.L., Marcus, M.L., Kerber, R.E., et al.: Quantification of myocardial ischemia and infarction by left ventricular imaging. (Editorial.) Circulation 63:747, 1981.
2. Wallis, D.E., O'Connell, J.B., Henkin, R.E., et al.: Segmental wall motion abnormalities in dilated cardiomyopathy: A common finding and good prognostic sign. J. Am. Coll. Cardiol. 4:674, 1984.
3. Linzer, M. (ed.): Ultrasonic tissue characterization. II. National Bureau of Standards Special Publication 525. Washington, D.C., U.S. Government Printing Office, 1979.
4. Miller, J.G., Perez, J.E., and Sobel, B.E.: Ultrasonic characterization of myocardium. Prog. Cardiovasc. Dis. 28:85, 1985.
5. Skorton, D.J., and Collins, S.M.: Characterization of myocardial structure with ultrasound. *In* Greenleaf, J. (ed.): Tissue Characterization With Ultrasound. Vol. II. Results and Applications. Boca Raton, Fla, CRC Press, 1986, p. 123.
6. Wild, J.J., Crafford, H.D., and Reid, J.M.: Visualization of the excised human heart by means of reflected ultrasound or echography. Am. Heart J. 54:903, 1957.
7. Namery, J., and Lele, P.P.: Ultrasonic detection of myocardial infarction in dog. Proc. IEEE Ultrasonics Symp. 72CH0708–8 SU:491, 1972.
8. Kremkau, F.W.: Ultrasound. *In* Kremkau, F.W. (ed.): Diagnostic Ultrasound: Physical Principles and Exercises. New York, Grune & Stratton, 1980, p. 5.
9. Hoffmeister, B.K., Verdonk, E.D., Wickline, S.A., et al.: Effect of collagen on the anisotropy of quasi-longitudinal mode ultrasonic velocity in fibrous soft tissues: A comparison of fixed tendon and fixed myocardium. J. Acoust. Soc. Am. 96:1957, 1994.
10. Verdonk, E.D., Wickline, S.A., and Miller, J.G.: Anistropy of ultrasonic velocity and elastic properties in normal human myocardium. J. Acoust. Soc. Am. 92:3039, 1992.
11. Marcus, P.W., and Carstensen, E.L.: Problems with absorbtion measurements of inhomogeneous solids. J. Acoust. Soc. Am. 58:1334, 1975.
12. Busse, L.J., Miller, J.G., Yuhas, D.E., et al.: Phase cancellation effects: A source of attenuation artifact eliminated by a CdS acoustoelectric receiver. Ultrasound Med. Biol. 3:1519, 1977.
13. Klepper, J.R., Brandenburger, G.H., Busse, L.J., et al.: Phase cancellation, reflection, and refraction effects in quantitative ultrasonic attenuation tomography. Proc. I.E.E.E. Ultrasonics Symp. 77:182, 1977.
14. Klepper, J.R., Brandenburger, G.H., Mimbs, J.W., et al.: Application of phase insensitive detection and frequency dependent measurements to computed ultrasonic attenuation tomography. I.E.E.E. Trans. Biomed. Eng. BME-28:186, 1981.
15. Kelly, M.P., and Liu, C.N.: Tomographic reconstruction of ultrasonic attenuation with correction for refractive errors. IBM J. Res. Dev. 25:71, 1981.
16. Shung, K.K., and Dzierzanowksi, J.M.: Effects of phase cancellation on scattering measurements. Ultrason. Imaging 4:56, 1982.
17. Busse, L.J., and Miller, J.G.: Detection of spatially nonuniform ultrasonic radiation with phase sensitive (piezoelectric) and phase insensitive (acoustoelectric) receivers. J. Acoust. Soc. Am. 70:1377, 1981.
18. Busse, L.J., and Miller, J.G.: A comparison of finite aperture phase sensitive and phase insensitive detection in the near field of inhomogeneous material. Proc. I.E.E.E. Ultrasonics Symp. 81:617, 1981.
19. Schmitt, R.M., Meyer, C.R., Carson, P.L., et al.: Error reduction in through transmission tomography using large receiving arrays with phase-insensitive signal processing. I.E.E.E. Trans. Sonics Ultrasonics SU-31-251, 1984.
20. Fitting, D.W., Carson, P.L., Giesey, J.J., et al.: A two-dimensional array receiver for reducing refraction artifacts in ultrasonic computed tomography of attenuation. I.E.E.E. Trans. Ultrason. Ferroelec. Freq. Contr. UFFC-34:346, 1987.
21. Johnson, P.H., and Miller, J.G.: Phase-insensitive detection for measurement of backscattered ultrasound. I.E.E.E. Trans. Ultrason. Ferroelec. Freq. Contr. UFFC-33:713, 1986.
22. Holland, M.R., and Miller, J.G.: Phase-insensitive and phase-sensitive quantitative imaging of scattered ultrasound using a two-dimensional pseudo-array. Proc. I.E.E.E. Ultrasonics Symp. 88:815, 1988.
23. Flax, S.W., and O'Donnell, M.: Phase aberration correction using signals from point reflectors and diffuse scatterers: Basic principles. IEEE Trans. Ultrason. Ferroelec. Freq. Contr. 35:758, 1988.
24. Trahey, G.E., Zhao, D., Miglin, J.A., et al.: Experimental results with a real-time adaptive ultrasonic imaging system for viewing through distorting media. I.E.E.E. Trans. Ultrason. Ferroelec. Freq. Contr. 37:418, 1990.
25. Shawker, T.H., Garra, B.S., and Insana, M.F.: Ultrasonic tissue characterization: Fundamental concepts and clinical applications. *In* Sanders, R.C., and Hill, M.C. (eds.): Ultrasound Annual 1985. New York, Raven Press, 1985, p. 93.
26. Miller, J.G., Perez, J.E., Mottley, J.G., et al.: Myocardial tissue characterization: An approach based on quantitative backscatter and attenuation. Proc. I.E.E.E. Ultrasonics Symp. 83CH1947–1:782, 1983.
27. O'Donnell, M., Bauwens, D., Mimbs, J.W., et al.: Broadband integrated backscatter: An approach to spatially localized tissue characterization in vivo. Proc. I.E.E.E. Ultrasonics Symp. 79CH1482–9:175, 1979.
28. Abbot, J.G., and Thurstone, F.L.: Acoustic speckle: Theory and experimental analysis. Ultrason. Imaging 1:303, 1979.
29. Burckhardt, C.B.: Speckle in ultrasound B-mode scans. I.E.E.E. Trans. Sonics Ultrasonics SU-25:1, 1978.
30. Smith, S.W., Trahey, G.E., and Von Ramm, O.T.: Two-dimensional arrays for medical ultrasound. Proc. I.E.E.E. Ultrasonics Symp. 91CH3079-1:625, 1991.
31. Trahey, G.E., and Freiburger, P.D.: An evaluation of transducer design and algorithm performance for two dimensional phase aberration correction. Proc. I.E.E.E. Ultrasonics Symp. 91CH3079-2:1181, 1991.
32. O'Donnell, M., and Pai-Chi, L.: Aberration correction on a two-dimensional anisotropic phased array. Proc. I.E.E.E. Ultrasonics Symp. 91CH3079-2:1189, 1991.
33. Wu, F., Fink, M., Mallart, R., et al.: Optimal focusing through aberrating media: A comparison between time reversal mirror and time delay correction techniques. Proc. I.E.E.E. Ultrasonics Symp. 91CH3079-2:1195, 1991.
34. Kanda, R., Sumino, Y., Takamizawa, K., et al.: An investigation of wavefront distortion correction: Correction using averaged phase information and the effect of correction in one and two dimensions. Proc. I.E.E.E. Ultrasonics Symp. 91CH3079-2:1201, 1991.
35. Karaman, M., Atalar, A., Koymen, H., et al.: Experimental analysis of a computationally efficient phase aberration correction technique. Proc. I.E.E.E. Ultrasonics Symp. 92CH3118-1:619, 1992.
36. Cassereau, D., Chakroun, N., Wu, F., et al.: Synthesis of a specific wavefront using 2D full and sparse arrays. Proc. I.E.E.E. Ultrasonics Symp. 92CH3118-N1:563, 1992.
37. Fitting, D.W., Norton, S.J., and Fortunko, C.M.: Adaptive array imaging in inhomogeneous media. Proc. I.E.E.E. Ultrasonics Symp. 92CH3118-1:653, 1992.
38. Dorme, C., Fink, M., and Prada, C.: Focusing in transmit-receive mode through inhomogeneous media: The matched filter approach. Proc. I.E.E.E. Ultrasonics Symp. 92CH311801:629, 1992.
39. Perez, J.E., Madaras, E.I., Sobel, B.E., et al.: Quantitative myocardial characterization with ultrasound. Automedica 5:201, 1984.
40. Thomas, L.J., III, Wickline, S.A., Perez, J.E., et al.: A real-time integrated backscatter measurement system for quantitative cardiac tissue characterization. I.E.E.E. Trans. Ultrason. Ferroelec. Freq. Contr. UFFC—33:27, 1986.
41. Barzilai, B., Thomas, L.J., III, Glueck, R.M., et al.: Detection of remote myocardial infarction with quantitative real-time ultrasonic tissue characterization. J. Am. Soc. Echocardiogr. 1:179, 1988.
42. Thomas, L.J., III, Barzilai, B., Perez, J.E., et al.: Quantitative real-time imaging of myocardium based on ultrasonic integrated backscatter. I.E.E.E. Trans. Ultrason. Ferroelec. Freq. Contr. 36: 466, 1989.
43. Vered, Z., Barzilai, B., Mohr, G.A., et al.: Quantitative ultrasonic tissue characterization with real-time integrated backscatter imaging in normal human subjects and in patients with dilated cardiomyopathy. Circulation 76:1067, 1987.
44. Vered, Z., Barzilai, B., Gessler, C.J., et al.: Ultrasonic integrated backscatter tissue characterization of remote myocardial infarction in human subjects. J. Am. Coll. Cardiol. 13:84, 1989.
45. Milunski, M., Canter, C.E., Wickline, S.A., et al.: Cardiac cycle-dependent variation of integrated backscatter is not distorted by abnormal myocardial wall motion in human subjects with paradoxical septal motion. Ultrasound Med. Biol. 15:311, 1989.
46. Bijnens, B., Herregods, M.C., Nuyts, J., et al.: Acquisition and processing of the radio-frequency signal in echocardiography: A new global approach. Ultrasound Med. Biol. 20:167, 1994.
47. Naito, J., Masuyama, T., Tanouchi, J., et al.: Analysis of transmural trend of myocardial integrated ultrasound backscatter for differentiation of hypertrophic cardiomyopathy and ventricular hypertrophy due to hypertension. J. Am. Coll. Cardiol. 24:517, 1994.
48. Bhandari, A.K., and Nanda, N.C.: Myocardial texture characterization by two-dimensional echocardiography. Am. J. Cardiol. 51:817, 1983.
49. Martin, R.D., Rakowski, H., French, J., et al.: Idiopathic hypertrophic subaortic stenosis viewed by wide-angle phased-array echocardiography. Circulation 59:1206, 1979.
50. Rasmussen, S., Corya, B.C., Feigenbaum, H., et al.: Detection of myocardial scar tissue by M-mode echocardiography. Circulation 57:230, 1978.
51. Logan-Sinclair, R.B., Wong, C.M., and Gibson, D.G.: Clinical applications of amplitude processing of echocardiographic images. Br. Heart J. 45:621, 1981.
52. Davies, J., Gibson, D.G., Foale, R., et al.: Echocardiographic features of eosinophilic endomyocardial disease. Br. Heart J. 48:434, 1982.
53. Tanaka, M., Teresawa, Y., and Hikichi, H.: Qualitative evaluation of the heart tissue by ultrasound. J. Cardiogr. 7:515, 1977.
54. Parisi, A.F., Nieminen, M., O'Boyle, J.E., et al.: Enhanced detection of the evolution of tissue changes after acute myocardial infarction using color-coded two-dimensional echocardiography. Circulation 66:764, 1982.
55. Melton, H.E., and Skorton, D.J.: Rational gain compensation for attenuation in cardiac ultrasonography. Ultrason. Imaging 5:214, 1983.
56. Aylward, P.E., McPherson, D.D., Kerber, R.E., et al.: Ultrasound tissue characterization in ischemic heart disease. Echocardiography 3:385, 1986.
57. Skorton, D.J., Melton, H.E., Jr., Pandian, N.G., et al.: Detection of acute myocardial infarction in closed-chest dogs by analysis of regional two-dimensional echocardiographic gray-level distributions. Circ. Res. 52:36, 1983.
58. Haendchen, R.V., Ong, K., Fishbein, M.C., et al.: Early differentiation of infarcted and noninfarcted reperfused myocardium in dogs by quantitative analysis of regional myocardial echo amplitudes. Circ. Res. 57:718, 1985.
59. Galloway, M.M.: Texture analysis using gray level run lengths. Comput. Graph. Image Process 4:172, 1975.
60. Chandrasekaran, K., Aylward, P.E., Fleagle, S.R., et al.: Feasibility of identifying

amyloid and hypertrophic cardiomyopathy with the use of computerized quantitative texture analysis of clinical echocardiographic data. J. Am. Coll. Cardiol. 13:832, 1989.

61. Weszka, J.S., Dyer, C.R., and Rosenfeld, A.: A comparative study of texture measures for terrain classification. I.E.E.E. Trans. Syst. Man. Cybernetics SMC-6-269, 1976.

62. Skorton, D.J., Collins, S.M., Nichols, J., et al.: Quantitative texture analysis in two-dimensional echocardiography: Application to the diagnosis of experimental myocardial contusion. Circulation 68:217, 1983.

63. Solomon, S.D., Kytomaa, H., Celi, A.C., et al.: Myocardial tissue characterization by autocorrelation of two-dimensional ultrasonic backscatter. J. Am. Soc. Echocardiogr. 7:631, 1994.

64. Perez, J.E., Miller, J.G., Barzilai, B., et al.: Progress in quantitative ultrasonic characterization of myocardium: From the laboratory to the bedside. J. Am. Soc. Echocardiogr. 1:294, 1988.

65. Wickline, S.A., Thomas, L.J., III, Miller, J.G., et al.: A relationship between ultrasonic integrated backscatter and myocardial contractile function. J. Clin. Invest. 76:2151, 1985.

66. Rose, J.H., Kaufmann, M.R., Wickline, S.A., et al.: A proposed microscopic elastic wave theory for ultrasonic backscatter from myocardial tissue. J. Acoust. Soc. Am. 97:1, 1995.

67. Miller, J.G., Yuhas, D.E., Mimbs, J.W., et al.: Ultrasonic tissue characterization: Correlation between biochemical and ultrasonic indices of myocardial injury. Proc. I.E.E.E. Ultrasonics Symp. 76(CH1120–5):33, 1976.

68. Mimbs, J.W., O'Donnell, M., Bauwens, D., et al.: The dependence of ultrasonic attenuation and backscatter on collagen content in dog and rabbit hearts. Circ. Res. 47:49, 1980.

69. O'Donnell, M., Mimbs, J.W., and Miller, J.G.: The relationship between collagen and ultrasonic attenuation in myocardial tissue. J. Acoust. Soc. Am. 65:512, 1979.

70. Hoyt, R.H., Collins, S.M., Skorton, D.J., et al.: Assessment of fibrosis in infarcted human hearts by analysis of ultrasonic backscatter. Circulation 71:740, 1985.

71. Hoyt, R.H., Skorton, D.J., Collins, S.M., et al.: Ultrasonic backscatter and collagen in normal ventricular myocardium. Circulation 69:775, 1984.

72. Baello, E.B., McPherson, D.D., Conyers, D.J., et al.: Ultrasound study of acoustic properties of the normal canine heart: Comparison of backscatter from all chambers. J. Am. Coll. Cardiol. 8:880, 1986.

73. Chandraratna, P.A.N., Ulene, R., Nimalasuriya, C., et al.: Differentiation between acute and healed myocardial infarction by signal averaging and color-encoding echocardiography. Am. J. Cardiol. 56:381, 1984.

74. Hikichi, H., and Tanaka, M.: Ultrasono-cardiotomographic evaluation of histologic changes in myocardial infarction. Jpn. Heart J. 22:287, 1981.

75. Shaw, T.R.D., Logan-Sinclair, R.B., Surin, C., et al.: Relation between regional echo intensity and myocardial connective tissue in chronic left ventricular disease. Br. Heart J. 51:46, 1984.

76. Shimazu, T., Nishioka, H., Fujiwara, M., et al.: Quantitative integrated backscatter characterization in canine myocardium. J. Cardiogr. 16:799, 1986.

77. Lythall, D.A., Bishop, J., Greenbaum, R.A., et al.: Relationship between myocardial collagen and echo amplitude in non-fibrotic hearts. Eur. Heart J. 14:344, 1993.

78. Shung, K.K., and Reid, J.M.: Ultrasonic scattering from tissue. Proc. IEEE Ultrasonics Symp. CH12364-ISU:230, 1977.

79. O'Donnell, M., Mimbs, J.W., and Miller, J.G.: The relationship between collagen and ultrasonic backscatter in myocardial tissue. J. Acoust. Soc. Am. 69:580, 1981.

80. Wear, K.A., Milunski, M.R., Wickline, S.A., et al.: Differentiation between acutely ischemic myocardium and zones of completed infarction on the basis of frequency dependent backscatter. J. Acoust. Soc. Am. 85:2634, 1989.

81. Kolosov, O.V., Levin, V.M., Mayev, R.G., et al.: The use of acoustic microscopy for biological tissue characterization. Ultrasound Med. Biol. 13:477, 1987.

82. Linker, D.T., Angelsen, B.A.J., and Popp, R.L.: Acoustic microscopy of normal and myopathic human myocardium: Implications for ultrasonic tissue characterization. (Abstract.) J. Am. Coll. Cardiol. 9:211A, 1987.

83. Fei, D.Y., and Shung, K.K.: Ultrasonic backscatter from mammalian tissues. J. Acoust. Soc. Am. 78:871, 1985.

84. Caulfield, J.B., and Borg, T.K.: The collagen network of the heart. Lab. Invest. 40:364, 1979.

85. Wear, K.A., Milunski, M.R., Wickline, S.A., et al.: Contraction-related variation in frequency dependence of acoustic properties of canine myocardium. (Abstract.) Ultrason. Imaging 11:143, 1989.

86. Rhyne, T.L., Sagar, K.B., Wann, S.L., et al.: The myocardial signature: Absolute backscatter, cyclical variation, frequency variation, and statistics. Ultrason. Imaging 8:107, 1986.

87. Streeter, D.D., Jr., and Hanna, W.T.: Engineering mechanics for successive states in canine left ventricular myocardium. II. Fiber angle and sarcomere length. Circ. Res. 33:656, 1973.

88. Mottley, J.G., and Miller, J.G.: Anisotropy of the ultrasonic backscatter of myocardial tissue. I. Theory and measurements in vitro. J. Acoust. Soc. Am. 83:755, 1988.

89. Klepper, J.R., Brandenburger, G.H., Mimbs, J.W., et al.: Application of phase insensitive detection and frequency dependent measurements to computed ultrasonic attenuation tomography. I.E.E.E. Trans. Biomed. Eng. 28:186, 1981.

90. Brandenburger, G.H., Klepper, J.R., Miller, J.G., et al.: Effects of anisotropy in the ultrasonic attenuation of tissue on computed tomography. Ultrason. Imaging 3:113, 1981.

91. Madaras, E.I., Perez, J.E., Sobel, B.E., et al.: Anistropy of the ultrasonic backscatter of myocardial tissue. II. Measurements in vivo. J. Acoust. Soc. Am. 83:762, 1988.

92. Mottley, J.G., and Miller, J.G.: Anistropy of the ultrasonic attenuation in soft tissues: Measurements in vitro. J. Acoust. Soc. Am. 88:1203, 1990.

93. Hete, B., and Shung, K.K.: Scattering of ultrasound from skeletal muscle tissue. I.E.E.E. Trans. Sonics Ultrasonics 40:4, 1993.

94. Vandenberg, B.F., Rath, L., Shoup, T.A., et al.: Cyclic variation of ultrasound backscatter in normal myocardium is view dependent: Clinical studies with a real-time backscatter imaging system. J. Am. Soc. Echocardiogr. 2:308, 1989.

95. Mimbs, J.W., Bauwens, D., Cohen, R.D., et al.: Effects of myocardial ischemia on quantitative ultrasonic backscatter and identification of responsible determinants. Circ. Res. 49:89, 1981.

96. Wickline, S.A., Thomas, L.J., III, Miller, J.G., et al.: Sensitive detection of the effects of reperfusion on myocardium by ultrasonic tissue characterization with integrated backscatter. Circulation 74:389, 1986.

97. Marini, C., Ghelardini, G., Picano, E., et al.: Effects of coronary blood flow on myocardial grey level amplitude in two dimensional echocardiography: An experimental study. Cardiovasc. Res. 27:279, 1993.

98. Reisner, S.A., Kumar, K.N., Ernst, A., et al.: Quantitative integrated backscatter during different coronary flow levels. (Abstract.) J. Am. Coll. Cardiol. 15:90A, 1990.

99. Picano, E., Faletra, F., Marini, C., et al.: Increased echo-density of transiently asynergic myocardium in humans: A novel echocardiographic sign of myocardial ischemia. J. Am. Coll. Cardiol. 21:199, 1993.

100. Pingitore, A., Kozakova, M., Picano, E., et al.: Acute myocardial gray level intensity changes detected by transesophageal echocardiography during intraoperative ischemia. Am. J. Cardiol. 72:465, 1993.

101. Skorton, D.J., and Collins, S.M.: Clinical potential of ultrasound tissue characterization in cardiomyopathies. J. Am. Soc. Echocardiogr. 1:69, 1988.

102. Lattanzi, F., Picano, E., Mazzarisi, A., et al.: In vivo radiofrequency ultrasound analysis of normal human heart structures. J. Clin. Ultrasound 15:371, 1987.

103. Stuhlmuller, J.E., Skorton, D.J., Burns, T.L., et al.: Reproducibility of quantitative backscatter echocardiographic imaging in normal subjects. Am. J. Cardiol. 69:542, 1992.

104. Mohr, G.A., Vered, Z., Barzilai, B., et al.: Automated determination of the magnitude and time delay ("phase") of the cardiac cycle dependent variation of myocardial ultrasonic integrated backscatter. Ultrason. Imaging 11:245, 1989.

105. Mobley, J., Feinberg, M.S., Gussak, H.M., et al.: On-line implementation of algorithm for determination of magnitude and time delay of cyclic variation of integrated backscatter in an echocardiographic imager. (Abstract.) 19th International Symposium on Ultrasonic Imaging and Tissue Characterization, Washington, D.C., June 1994. Ultrason. Imaging 16:49, 1994.

106. Madaras, E.I., Barzilai, B., Perez, J.E., et al.: Changes in myocardial backscatter throughout the cardiac cycle. Ultrason. Imaging 5:229, 1983.

107. Collins, S.M., Skorton, D.J., Prasad, N.V., et al.: Quantitative echocardiographic image texture: Normal contraction-related variability. IEEE Trans. Med. Imaging 4:185, 1985.

108. Fitzgerald, P.J., McDaniel, M.M., Rolett, E.L., et al.: Two-dimensional ultrasonic variation in myocardium throughout the cardiac cycle. Ultrason. Imaging 8:241, 1986.

109. Hajduczki, I., Jaffe, M., Areeda, J., et al.: Ultrasonic backscatter and 2D echocardiographic wall motion analysis during PTCA. (Abstract.) Circulation 778:II-442, 1988.

110. Olshansky, B., Collins, S.M., Skorton, D.J., et al.: Variation of left ventricular myocardial gray level in two-dimensional echocardiograms as a result of cardiac contraction. Circulation 70:972, 1984.

111. Sagar, K.B., Rhyne, T.L., Wartlier, D.C., et al.: Intramyocardial variability in integrated backscatter: Effects of coronary occlusion and reperfusion. Circulation 75:436, 1987.

112. Fitzgerald, P.J., McDaniel, M.D., Rolett, E.L., et al.: Two-dimensional ultrasonic tissue characterization: Backscatter power, endocardial wall motion and their phase relationship for normal, ischemic and infarcted myocardium. Circulation 76:850, 1987.

113. Glueck, R.M., Mottley, J.G., Miller, J.G., et al.: Effect of coronary artery occlusion and reperfusion on cardiac cycle-dependent variation of myocardial ultrasonic backscatter. Circ. Res. 56:683, 1985.

114. Wickline, S.A., Mohr, G.A., Shoup, T.A., et al.: Delineation of improved contractile performance after thrombolysis in acute myocardial infarction with real-time two-dimensional ultrasonic integrated backscatter. (Abstract.) J. Am. Coll. Cardiol. 11:99A, 1988.

115. Wickline, S.A., Thomas, L.J., III, Miller, J.G., et al.: The dependence of myocardial ultrasonic integrated backscatter on contractile performance. Circulation 72:183, 1985.

116. Sabbah, H.N., Marzilli, M., and Stein, P.D.: The relative role of subendocardium and subepicardium in left ventricular mechanics. Am. J. Physiol. 240:H920, 1981.

117. Glueck, R.M., Mottley, J.G., Sobel, B.E., et al.: Changes in ultrasonic attenuation and backscatter of muscle with state of contraction. Ultrasound Med. Biol. 11:605, 1985.

118. Wear, K.A., Shoup, T.A., and Popp, R.L.: Ultrasonic characterization of canine myocardial contraction. I.E.E.E. Trans. Ultrason. Ferroelect. Freq. Cont. 33:347, 1986.

119. Lythall, D.A., Logan-Sinclair, R.B., Ilsley, C.J.D., et al.: Relation between cyclic variation in echo amplitude and segmental contraction in normal and abnormal hearts. Br. Heart J. 66:268, 1991.

120. Fraker, T.D., Jr., Nelson, A.D., Arthur, J.A., et al.: Altered acoustic reflectance on two-dimensional echocardiography as an early predictor of myocardial infarct size. Am. J. Cardiol. 53:1699, 1984.

121. Werner, J.A., Speck, S.M., Greene, H.L., et al.: Discrete intramural sonolucency:

A new echocardiographic finding in acute myocardial infarction. (Abstract.) Am. J. Cardiol. 47:404, 1981.

122. Lele, P.P., and Namery, J.: A computer-based ultrasonic system for the detection and mapping of myocardial infarcts. Proc. San Diego Biomed. Symp. 13:121, 1974.

123. Mimbs, J.W., O'Donnell, M., Miller, J.G., et al.: Changes in ultrasonic attenuation indicative of early myocardial ischemic injury. Am. J. Physiol. 236:H340, 1979.

124. Schnittger, I.A., Vieli, A., Heiserman, J.E., et al.: Ultrasonic tissue characterization: Detection of acute myocardial ischemia in dogs. Circulation 72:193, 1985.

125. Barzilai, B., Madaras, E.I., Sobel, B.E., et al.: Effects of myocardial contraction on ultrasonic backscatter before and after ischemia. Am. J. Physiol. 247:H478, 1984.

126. McPherson, D.D., Aylward, P.E., Knosp, B.M., et al.: Ultrasound characterization of acute myocardial ischemia by quantitative texture analysis. Ultrason. Imaging 8:227, 1986.

127. Chandrasekaran, K., Chu, A., Greenleaf, J.F., et al.: 2D echo quantitative texture analysis of acutely ischemic myocardium. (Abstract.) Circulation 74:II-271, 1986.

128. Kawamura, K., Hishida, H., Sakabe, Y., et al.: Quantitative evaluation and color display of echo intensity two-dimensional echocardiography. J. Cardiogr. 15:1199, 1985.

129. Rijsterborgh, H., Mastik, F., Lancee, C.T., et al.: The relative contributions of myocardial wall thickness and ischemia to ultrasonic myocardial integrated backscatter during experimental ischemia. Ultrasound Med. Biol. 17:41, 1991.

130. Wear, K.A., Milunski, M.R., Wickline, S.A., et al.: The effect of frequency on the magnitude of cyclic variation of backscatter in dogs and implications for prompt detection of acute myocardial ischemia. I.E.E.E. Trans. Sonics Ultrasonics 38:5, 1991.

131. Milunski, M.R., Mohr, G.A., Perez, J.E., et al.: Ultrasonic tissue characterization with integrated backscatter: Acute myocardial ischemia, reperfusion, and stunned myocardium in patients. Circulation 80:491, 1989.

132. Vitale, D.F., Lauria, G., Pelaggi, N., et al.: Reproducibility of myocardial ultrasonic backscatter parameters in man. Comp. Cardiol. 293, 1992.

133. Barzilai, B., Vered, Z., Mohr, G.A., et al.: Myocardial ultrasonic backscatter for characterization of ischemia and reperfusion: Relationship to wall motion. Ultrasound Med. Biol. 16:391, 1990.

134. Saeian, K., Rhyne, T.L., and Sagar, K.B.: Ultrasonic tissue characterization for diagnosis of acute myocardial infarction in the coronary care unit. Am. J. Cardiol. 74:1211, 1994.

135. Shen, Z., Palma, A., Nanna, M., et al.: Ultrasonic tissue characterization of ischemic myocardium in response to pharmacologic stress test. (Abstract.) Circulation 84:II-705, 1991.

136. Rasmussen, S., Lovelace, E., Knoebel, S.B., et al.: Echocardiographic detection of ischemic and infarcted myocardium. J. Am. Coll. Cardiol. 3:733, 1984.

137. Sagar, K.B., Pelc, L.R., Rhyne, T.L., et al.: Role of ultrasonic tissue characterization to distinguish reversible from irreversible myocardial injury. J. Am. Soc. Echocardiogr. 3:471, 1990.

138. Milunski, M.R., Mohr, G.A., Wear, K.A., et al.: Early identification with ultrasonic integrated backscatter of viable but stunned myocardium in dogs. J. Am. Coll. Cardiol. 14:462, 1989.

139. Lythall, D.A., Gibson, D.G., Kushwaha, S.S., et al.: Changes in myocardial echo amplitude during reversible ischemia in humans. Br. Heart J. 67:368, 1992.

140. Hajduczki, I., Jaffe, M., Areeda, J., et al.: Preservation of regional myocardial ultrasonic backscatter and systolic function during brief periods of ischemia by synchronized coronary venous retroperfusion. Am. Heart J. 122:1300, 1991.

141. Mimbs, J.W., Yuhas, D.E., Miller, J.G., et al.: Detection of myocardial infarction in vitro based on altered attenuation of ultrasound. Circ. Res. 41:192, 1977.

142. Vandenberg, B.F., Stuhlmuller, J.E., Rath, L., et al.: Diagnosis of recent myocardial infarction with quantitative backscatter imaging: Preliminary results. J. Am. Soc. Echocardiogr. 4:10, 1991.

143. Ferdeghini, E.M., Pinamonti, B., Picano, E., et al.: Quantitative texture analysis in echocardiography: Application to the diagnosis of myocarditis. J. Clin. Ultrasound 19:263, 1991.

144. Picano, E., Pelosi, G., Marzilli, M., et al.: In vivo quantitative ultrasonic evaluation of myocardial fibrosis in humans. Circulation 81:58, 1990.

145. Wong, A.K., Verdonk, E.D., Hoffmeister, B.K., et al.: Detection of unique transmural architecture of human idiopathic cardiomyopathy by ultrasonic tissue characterization. Circulation 86:1108, 1992.

146. Siqueira-Filho, A.G., Cunha, C.L.P., Tajik, A.J., et al.: M-mode and two-dimensional echocardiographic features in cardiac amyloidosis. Circulation 63:188, 1981.

147. Chiaramida, S.A., Goldman, M.A., Zema, M.J., et al.: Real-time cross-sectional echocardiographic diagnosis of infiltrative cardiomyopathy due to amyloid. J. Clin. Ultrasound 8: 58, 1980.

148. Pinamonti, B., Picano, E., Ferdeghina, E.M., et al.: Quantitative texture analysis in two-dimensional echocardiography: Application to the diagnosis of myocardial amyloidosis. J. Am. Coll. Cardiol. 14:666, 1989.

149. Lattanzi, F., Bellsotti, P., Picano, E., et al.: Quantitative ultrasonic analysis of myocardium in patients with thalassemia major and iron overload. Circulation 87:748, 1993.

150. Lattanzi, F., Spirito, P., Picano, E., et al.: Quantitative assessment of ultrasonic myocardial reflectivity in hypertrophic cardiomyopathy. J. Am. Coll. Cardiol. 17:1085, 1991.

151. Masuyama, T., St. Goar, F.G., Tye, T.L., et al.: Ultrasonic tissue characterization of human hypertrophied hearts in vivo with cardiac cycle-dependent variation in integrated backscatter. Circulation 80:925, 1989.

152. Mimbs, J.W., O'Donnell, M., Miller, J.G., et al.: Detection of cardiomyopathic

changes induced by doxorubicin based on quantitative analysis of ultrasonic backscatter. Am. J. Cardiol. 47:1056, 1981.

153. Perez, J.E., Barzilai, B., Madaras, E.I., et al.: Applicability of ultrasonic tissue characterization for longitudinal assessment and differentiation of calcification and fibrosis in cardiomyopathy. J. Am. Coll. Cardiol. 4:88, 1984.

154. Tanaka, M., and Terasawa, Y.: Echocardiography evaluation of the tissue character in myocardium. Jpn. Circ. J. 43:367, 1979.

155. Sakabe, Y., Hishida, H., Kajiwara, K., et al.: Amplitude analysis of two-dimensional echocardiograms in patients with left ventricular hypertrophy. Jpn. Soc. Ultrasound Med. Proceedings. Sapporo, Japan, June 1984.

156. Shapiro, L.M., Moore, R.B., Logan-Sinclair, R.B., et al.: Relation of regional echo amplitude to left ventricular function and the electrocardiogram in left ventricular hypertrophy. Br. Heart J. 52:99, 1984.

157. Rijsterborgh, H., Mastik, F., Lancee, C.T., et al.: Ultrasonic myocardial integrated backscatter and myocardial wall thickness in animal experiments. Ultrasound Med. Biol. 16:29, 1990.

158. Lattanzi, F., DiBello, V., Picano, E., et al.: Normal ultrasonic myocardial reflectivity in athletes with increased left ventricular mass. A tissue characterization study. Circulation 85:1828, 1992.

159. DiBello, V., Lattanzi, F., Picano, E., et al.: Left ventricular performance and ultrasonic myocardial quantitative reflectivity in endurance senior athletes: An echocardiographic study. Eur. Heart. J. 14:358, 1993.

160. Gigli, G., Lattanzi, F., Lucarini, A.R., et al.: Normal ultrasonic myocardial reflectivity in hypertensive patients. Hypertension 21:329, 1993.

161. Shung, K.K., Fei, D.Y., Yuan, Y.W., et al.: Ultrasonic characterization of blood during coagulation. J. Clin. Ultrasound. 12:147, 1984.

162. Bhandari, A.K., Nanda, N.C., and Hicks, D.G.: Two-dimensional echocardiography of intracardiac masses: Echo pattern—histopathology correlation. Ultrasound Med. Biol. 8:673, 1982.

163. Green, S.E., Joynt, L.F., Fitzgerald, P.J., et al.: In vivo ultrasonic tissue characterization of human intracardiac masses. Am. J. Cardiol. 51:231, 1983.

164. McPherson, D.D., Knosp, B.M., Kieso, R.A., et al.: Ultrasound characterization of acoustic properties of acute intracardiac thrombi: Studies in a new experimental model. J. Am. Soc. Echocardiogr. 1:264, 1988.

165. Vandenberg, B.F., Kieso, R.A., Fox-Eastham, K., et al.: Characterization of acute experimental left ventricular thrombi with quantitative backscatter imaging. Circulation 81:1017, 1990.

166. Lloret, R.L., Cortada, X., Bradford, J., et al.: Classification of left ventricular thrombi by their history of systemic embolization using pattern recognition of two-dimensional echocardiograms. Am. Heart J. 110:761, 1985.

167. Gerber, T.C., Foley, D.A., Zheng, Y., et al.: Echocardiographic tissue characterization using a neural network: Differentiation between tumor and thrombus. (Abstract.) J. Am. Soc. Echocardiogr. 6:S30, 1993.

168. Tak, T., Rahimtoola, S.H., Kumar, A., et al.: Value of digital image processing of two-dimensional echocardiograms in differentiating active from chronic vegetations of infective endocarditis. Circulation 78:116, 1988.

169. Wolverson, M.K., Bashiti, H.M., and Peterson, G.J.: Ultrasonic tissue characterization of atheromatous plaques using a high resolution real-time scanner. Ultrasound Med. Biol. 9:599, 1983.

170. Picano, E., Landini, L., Distante, A., et al.: Different degrees of atherosclerosis detected by backscattered ultrasound: An in vitro study on fixed human aortic walls. J. Clin. Ultrasound 11:375, 1983.

171. Barzilai, B., Saffitz, J.E., Miller, J.G., et al.: Quantitative ultrasonic characterization of the nature of atherosclerotic plaques in human aorta. Circ. Res. 60:459, 1987.

172. McPherson, D.D., Sirna, S.J., Haugen, J.A., et al.: Acoustic properties of normal and atherosclerotic human coronary arteries: In vitro and in vivo observations. (Abstract.) Circulation 76:IV-43, 1987.

173. Gussenhoven, E.J., Essed, C.E., Lancee, C.T., et al.: Arterial wall characteristics determined by intravascular ultrasound imaging: An in vitro study. (Abstract.) J. Am. Coll. Cardiol. 14:947, 1989.

174. Linker, D.R., Yock, P.G., Thapliyal, H.V., et al.: In vitro analysis of backscattered amplitude from normal and diseased arteries using a new intraluminal ultrasonic catheter. (Abstract.) J. Am. Coll. Cardiol. 11:4A, 1988.

175. Shung, K.K., Hughes, D., Yujani, Y.W., et al.: C-mode imaging of arterial atherosclerotic lesion surfaces using oblique incidence. (Abstract.) Ultrason. Imaging 9:47, 1987.

176. Picano, E., Landini, L., Distante, A., et al.: Angle dependence of ultrasonic backscatter in arterial tissues: A study in vitro. Circulation 72:572, 1985.

177. De Kroon, M.G., Van der Wal, L.F., Gussenhoven, W.J., et al.: Backscatter directivity and integrated backscatter power of arterial tissue. Int. J. Card. Imaging 6:265, 1991.

178. Shepard, R.K., Miller, J.G., and Wickline, S.A.: Quantification of atherosclerotic plaque composition in cholesterol-fed rabbits with 50-MHz acoustic microscopy. Arterioscler. Thromb. 12:1227, 1992.

179. Lanza, G.M., Zabalgoitia-Reyes, M., Frazin, L., et al.: Plaque and structural characteristics of the descending thoracic aorta using transesophageal echocardiography. J. Am. Soc. Echocardiogr. 4:19, 1991.

180. Lattanzi, F., Picano, E., Landini, L., et al.: In vivo identification of mitral valve fibrosis and calcium by real-time quantitative ultrasonic analysis. Am. J. Cardiol. 65:355, 1990.

181. Perez, J.E., McGill, J.B., Santiago, J.V., et al.: Abnormal myocardial acoustic properties in diabetic patients and their correlation with the severity of disease. J. Am. Coll. Cardiol. 19:1154, 1992.

182. Wagner, R.F., Wear, K.A., Perez, J.E., et al.: Quantitative assessment of myocardial ultrasonic tissue characterization via ROC analysis of Bayesian classifiers. J. Am. Coll. Cardiol. 7:1706, 1995.

183. Masuyama, T., Valantine, H.A., Gibbons, R., et al.: Serial measurement of integrated ultrasonic backscatter in human cardiac allografts for the recognition of acute rejection. Circulation 81:829, 1990.

184. Lieback, E., Vilser, J., Bettman, M., et al.: Digital image processing of echocardiographic images by means of mathematical morphology and texture analysis—a new method to recognition of cardiac rejection. (Abstract.) Eur. Heart J. 13:358, 1992.

185. Lythall, D., Gibson, D., Swanson, K., et al.: Quantitative analysis of myocardial echo amplitude—A useful marker of cardiac rejection. (Abstract.) Circulation 80:II-676, 1989.

186. Stempfle, H.U., Angermann, C.E., Kraml, P., et al.: Serial changes during acute cardiac allograft rejection: Quantitative ultrasound tissue analysis versus myocardial histologic findings. J. Am. Coll. Cardiol. 22:310, 1993.

187. Angermann, C., Nassau, K., Drewell, R., et al.: Time averaged myocardial integrated backscatter measurements allow to identify and estimate severity of acute allograft rejection after heart transplantation in man. (Abstract.) Circulation 90:I-326, 1994.

188. Hopkins, W.E., Waggoner, A.D., and Gussak, H.: Quantitative ultrasonic tissue characterization of myocardium in cyanotic adults with an unrepaired congenital heart defect. Am. J. Cardiol. 74:930, 1994.

189. Masuyama, T., Nellessen, U., Schnittger, I., et al.: Ultrasonic tissue characterization with a real time integrated backscatter imaging system in normal and aging human hearts. J. Am. Coll. Cardiol. 14:1702, 1989.

190. Miller, J.G., Barzilai, B., Milunski, M.R., et al.: Myocardial tissue characterization: Clinical confirmation of laboratory results. Proc. I.E.E.E. Ultrasonics Symp. 89CH2791-2:1029, 1989.

Note: Page numbers in *italics* refer to illustrations. Page numbers followed by t indicate tables. Plate numbers refer to color sections; Plates 1 to 21 follow page 296, and Plates 22 to 35 follow page 892.

A wave, Doppler, in diastole, 342

Abdomen, computed tomography of, radiation dose in, 1206t

Abscesses, in endocarditis, magnetic resonance imaging of, 755, *756*
transesophageal echocardiography of, 549, 550, Plate 11

Absorption rate, specific, 1216

Acetate, carbon-11–labeled. See *Carbon-11 acetate.*

Acetoacetyl coenzyme A, in ketone metabolism, myocardial, 41, *42*

Acetrizoic acid, as contrast agent, *146*, 147

Acetyl coenzyme A, in myocardial metabolism, 34, *35*, 1172, *1173*
in tricarboxylic acid cycle, 41–42

Acetylcholine, in cardiac nervous system, 1052, 1053, *1053*
in neurotransmission, 1188

Acoustic impedance, in ultrasonography, in tissue characterization, 607

Acoustic noise, definition of, 1209

Acoustic quantitation, in ejection fraction measurement, 304–306, *305*, *306*

Acquisition matrix, definition of, 1209

Acquisition time, definition of, 1212

Acquisition window, definition of, 1209

Action potentials, in myocardial contraction, 23

Acyl coenzyme A, in myocardial metabolism, 39–41, *40*, *41*, 1173, *1173*
in positron emission tomography, 1069–1072, *1070*
in single-photon emission imaging, 1022, *1022*

Acyl coenzyme A dehydrogenase deficiency, and cardiomyopathy, positron emission tomography in, 1183, *1183*

Adenosine, and coronary blood flow changes, magnetic resonance imaging of, 737, *739*
contraindications to, with cardiac imaging, 79
for stress induction, 11
in echocardiography, 506
of coronary artery disease, 515
in positron emission tomography, 1094, *1094t*, 1096, 1097, *1097t*
in radionuclide imaging, 974, *974*, 975
in ultrafast computed tomography, 849

Adenosine monophosphate, cyclic, and ventricular function, 23

Adenosine triphosphate, in diastole, 336–337
in excitation-contraction coupling, 20–22, *22*
in magnetic resonance spectroscopy, 675, *676*, 784–790, *785*, *787t*, *788*, *789*
in myocardial metabolism, 42–43, *1173*, 1173–1174

Adenylyl cyclase, in cardiac neurotransmission, 1187
in desensitization, 1198

Adipose tissue. See *Fat.*

Adrenergic receptors, blockers of, in cardiac denervation, 1198
in ventricular function, 23, 29, 30
physiology of, 1186–1188
positron emission tomography of, 1189–1192, *1191*, *1193–1195*
in cardiac desensitization, 1198
in cardiomyopathy, hypertrophic, 1197–1198

Adrenergic receptors (*Continued*)
in heart failure, 1197
in myocardial ischemia, 1197

Adriamycin (doxorubicin), cardiotoxicity of, 958
nervous system dysfunction with, 1057

Aerosomes, in contrast echocardiography, 482

AF-DX 116, as cholinergic receptor antagonist, 1187–1188
in positron emission tomography, 1193

Afterload, atrial, and diastolic filling, 342
changes in, effect of, on left ventricular function, 27, 29
definition of, 8

Aging, and left ventricular function changes, Doppler echocardiography of, *347*, 347–349, *348*
cardiomyopathy in, echocardiography of, 396, 398–399
myocardium in, ultrasonic tissue characterization of, 623

AH23848, in prevention of thrombosis, indium-111–imaging of, 1046

ALARA principle, in radiation protection, 122

Albumin, in microbubbles, in contrast echocardiography, 481–485, *482–484*, Plate 8
in positron emission tomography, of myocardial blood flow, 1065, *1066*
indium-111–labeled, in myocardial perfusion imaging, 964, *965*

Albunex, in contrast echocardiography, 481, 483, *483*

Aldosterone, in cardiomyopathy, 1174

Aliasing, definition of, 1209

Allergy, to contrast agents, 157–158
in pulmonary angiography, 208

Alveolar edema, in congestive heart failure, 139, *139*

Amino acids, in myocardial metabolism, 45
radiolabeled, in positron emission tomography, 1075

Aminophylline, for dipyridamole-induced ischemia, 974

Amipaque, as contrast agent, *146*, 147

Ammonia, nitrogen-13–labeled. See *Nitrogen-13 ammonia.*

Amplatz technique, in coronary angiography, 228, 228–229

Amplification, in echocardiography, 284–285, *286*
in magnetic resonance imaging, 646, *647*

Amyloidosis, and cardiomyopathy, echocardiography in, 352, 354–355, 355–357, 361, 402, *402*, Plates 3 and 4
ultrasonic tissue characterization in, 613, 619–620, *620*

Analog optical disk, in cineangiography, 115

Analog-to-digital conversion, 60. See also *Digital.*

ANALYZE software, 812, 816, *816–818*

Anaphylactoid reaction, to contrast agents, 157–158

Anesthesia, for transesophageal echocardiography, 537

Aneurysms, and ventricular septal rupture, in myocardial infarction, 526, *526*
in contrast ventriculography, 167, *169*
of aorta, and thrombosis, indium-111 platelet imaging of, 1042, *1042*

Aneurysms (*Continued*)
angiography of, 202, *203*
imaging of, 99
magnetic resonance imaging of, 99, 705, *705–707*
radiography of, 134, *135*
surgery for, echocardiography in, 576–577
ultrafast computed tomography of, *855*, 855–856, *856*
of atrial septum, echocardiography of, 457–459, *459*
transesophageal, 557, *558*
of femoral artery, and thrombosis, indium-111 platelet imaging of, 1042
of left ventricle, after infarction, magnetic resonance imaging of, 726
calcification of, radiography of, *142*, 143
infarct expansion and, echocardiography of, 527–528, *528*
of pulmonary artery, angiography of, 215, *218*
with ventricular septal defect, surgery for, echocardiography in, Plate 18

Angina, diagnosis of, imaging in, 78
drugs for, continuation of, before angiography, 226
in coronary artery disease, angiography in, indications for, 221
myocardial perfusion in, radionuclide imaging of, 989t, 989–990
pacing-induced, glucose in, 1118
radionuclide angiography in, with severe stenosis, 949t, 949–951, *950*
radionuclide angiography in, in diagnosis, 947t, 947–949, *948*, 948t
in patient management, 954
in prognosis, *951–953*, 951–954

Angiography, and radiation exposure, 122, 122t
cerebral, radiation dose in, 1206t
contrast agents in, 144–162. See also *Contrast agents.*
definition of, 1209
digital, 251–268. See also *Digital angiography.*
fluoroscopic, 113–115
of aorta, 202, *202*
image contrast in, 107–110, *109*, *110*
image formation in, 105–110, *106–110*, 107t
in atrial volume measurement, 192–193
in left ventricular volume measurement, vs. echocardiography, 298, 298–300, *299*, 301t
of aorta, 199–207. See also *Aortography.*
of congenital heart disease, 90–92
magnetic resonance imaging in, 674
of coronary arteries, 220–248. See also *Coronary angiography.*
of left heart, in anatomic imaging, 1, 2
of mitral valve, 53, *54*
pulmonary, 208–218. See also *Pulmonary angiography.*
radionuclide, 923–958. See also *Radionuclide angiography.*
vs. intravascular ultrasonography, 581, *582*
x-ray production for, 104

Angioma, of pericardium, ultrafast computed tomography of, 870

Angioplasty, myocardial ischemia after, color Doppler imaging of, 360, Plate 3
percutaneous transluminal, and left ventricular function changes, Doppler echocardiography of, 329
peripheral, thrombosis after, indium-111 platelet imaging of, 1042
positron emission tomography after, of myocardial blood flow, 1107–1108, 1108
of myocardial metabolism, 1140
ultrasonography of, intravascular, 586–591, 586–591, 591t, Plate 21
in surgical guidance, 592–597, 594–598
combined instrumentation for, 597–598
in vessel measurement, 583, 585, 586, 586
three-dimensional reconstruction in, 598–603, 600–602
vascular remodeling in, 591–592, 593
Angiosarcoma, echocardiography of, 475, 475–476
Angiotensin, in cardiomyopathy, 1174
Angiotensin-converting enzyme inhibitors, effect of, on diastolic function, 28–29
Angiovist. See Diatrizoate.
Angular frequency, definition of, 1209
Angular momentum, definition of, 1209
Annexin V, in imaging of thrombosis, 1047
Annotation, definition of, 1209
Annuloaortic ectasia, and aneurysm, magnetic resonance imaging of, 705, 706
Annulus fibrosus, of aortic valve, 50, 51, 51
of mitral valve, 51, 51, 54
Anode, in x-ray production, 104
Anomalous pulmonary venous return, echocardiography of, 440–441, 441, 442, Plate 7
Antenna, definition of, 1209
Anthracycline, and cardiomyopathy, ultrasonic tissue characterization in, 621
Antibodies, antimyosin. See Antimyosin antibodies.
antiphospholipid, in lupus erythematosus and mitral regurgitation, transesophageal echocardiography of, 553, 553
in imaging of thrombosis, antifibrin, 1046, 1046–1047, Plate 30
anti-PADGEM, 1047
Anticoagulants, for myocardial infarction, assessment of, echocardiography in, 529–530
for thrombosis, assessment of, indium-111 platelet imaging of, 1038–1039, 1039
ultrafast computed tomography in, 867, 867
Antifibrin antibodies, in imaging of thrombosis, 1046, 1046–1047, Plate 30
Antihistamines, before coronary angiography, 226
Antimyosin antibodies, in imaging, of myocardial necrosis, 1013–1014, 1014
accuracy of, 1015, 1015–1016
in infarct sizing, 1017–1019, 1018, 1019
right ventricular, 1017
with positron emission tomography, 1124, 1125
with thallium-201 perfusion imaging, 1016–1017, 1017
of myocarditis, 87
Antiphospholipid antibodies, in lupus erythematosus, and mitral regurgitation, transesophageal echocardiography of, 553, 553
Aorta, aneurysms of. See Aneurysms, of aorta.
angioplasty of, stenting after, ultrasonic guidance of, 595–597

Aorta (Continued)
anomalies of, ultrafast computed tomography of, 879
atherosclerotic plaque of, echocardiography of, 99
blood flow in, measurement of, in congenital heart disease, magnetic resonance imaging in, 681, 681
with left-to-right shunting, Doppler echocardiography in, 430, 431
coarctation of, echocardiography of, 434–435, 435
imaging of, 91
magnetic resonance imaging of, 678, 698–700, 699
subclavian artery anomaly with, 696–697
congenital diseases of, imaging of, 99
magnetic resonance imaging of, 696–699, 696–700
descending, connection of, to pulmonary artery, echocardiography of, 424–427, 424–427, 431, Plate 7
echocardiography of, intraoperative, 569, 576–577, Plate 19
transesophageal, 538, 538, 539, 540
embryology of, 692, 692–693
enlargement of, radiography of, 131–134, 135, 136
in coronary artery anomalies, angiography of, 236t, 236–237, 237
inflammation of, magnetic resonance imaging of, 708, 709
magnetic resonance imaging of, techniques of, 693–696, 694, 695
radiography of, interpretation of, 127–128
transposition of, with pulmonary artery, echocardiography of, 439, 439–440, 440, 442, 445–448, 447
magnetic resonance imaging of, 678, 679
after surgery, 689, 689–690, 690
ultrafast computed tomography of, 876–877, 877–882
trauma to, angiography of, 204–207, 206
echocardiography of, transesophageal, 561
imaging of, 96–97
magnetic resonance imaging of, 708, 708
ultrafast computed tomography of, 852–859
contrast agents in, 854–855
radiation dose in, 855
scanners for, 853, 853–854, 854
ultrasonography of, intravascular, in vessel measurement, 583, 584
Aortic arch, anomalies of, magnetic resonance imaging of, 696–698, 696–698
embolism from, echocardiography of, transesophageal, 558
Aortic dissection, angiography of, 202–204, 203–205
echocardiography of, intraoperative, 576–577, Plate 19
transesophageal, 560–561, Plate 14
imaging of, 99
magnetic resonance imaging of, 700–705, 701–704
radiography of, 134, 136
ultrafast computed tomography of, 856–858, 856–859
Aortic regurgitation, contrast ventriculography in, 167, 169
echocardiography of, 372–376, 373–376, 501, Plates 4 and 5
intraoperative, 571, 573, Plate 17
imaging of, 85
left ventricular enlargement with, radiography of, 128, 129
magnetic resonance imaging of, 85, 710, 711
through prosthetic valve, echocardiography of, 388–389

Aortic regurgitation (Continued)
ultrafast computed tomography of, 825–826, 826, 827
Aortic root, angiography of, in coronary artery assessment, 256
after bypass surgery, 257, 257
dilatation of, echocardiography of, aortic regurgitation in, 372–373, 373
vs. mass lesion, 456, 457
in Marfan syndrome, magnetic resonance imaging of, 764
Aortic stenosis, calcification in, radiography of, 141, 141–142
congenital, balloon valvuloplasty for, 91
echocardiography of, 431–434, 432–434
echocardiography of, 366–372, 367, 368, 370–372
transesophageal, 550, 551
imaging of, 84–85
magnetic resonance imaging of, 85, 713–715, 713–717
Aortic valve, anatomy of, 50–51, 51, 52
balloon valvuloplasty of, echocardiography of, 389
disorders of, and left ventricular hypertrophy, magnetic resonance imaging in, 768
with coarctation, magnetic resonance imaging of, 700
function of, normal, 55, 55, 56
in ventriculography, with left ventricular hypertrophy, 52, 52
insufficiency of, radionuclide angiography of, 956–958, 956–958
transesophageal echocardiography of, 550–551, Plate 11
prosthetic, and distortion, in magnetic resonance imaging, quantitative, 764, 764
regurgitation through, Doppler echocardiography of, 388–389
transesophageal echocardiography of, 555–556, Plate 13
pseudomass of, echocardiography of, 454–457, 456
replacement of, Ross procedure for, transesophageal echocardiography after, 555
transesophageal echocardiography of, 538, 540, 541, 543, 543
with double-outlet right ventricle, echocardiography of, 437, 437
Aortitis, magnetic resonance imaging of, 708, 709
Aortography, 199–207
filming methods in, 200–202, 200–202
of aneurysms, 202, 203
of aortic dissection, 202–204, 203–205
of aortic trauma, 204–207, 206
risks of, 200
technique of, 199–200
Appearance time and density analysis, in digital angiography, of coronary circulation, 262, 262–264, 263, Plate 1
Archival storage, of digital images, 117–118
Array coil, definition of, 1209
Array processor, definition of, 1209
Arrhythmia, autonomic nervous system in, radionuclide imaging of, 1059
cardiac gating in, in magnetic resonance imaging, 647–648, 648, 649
coronary angiography and, 224–225, 225t
denervation and, positron emission tomography of, 1198
dobutamine and, in stress echocardiography, 505
in radionuclide angiography, equilibrium, 943
ventricular, and valvar dysfunction, 57
intractable, coronary angiography in, 222
Arteriography. See Angiography.
Arteriovenous fistula, pulmonary, angiography of, 214–215, 217

Arteriovenous fistula (Continued)
  ultrafast computed tomography in, 861
Arteriovenous malformations, pulmonary,
  contrast echocardiography of, 499
  imaging of, 100
Arteritis, Takayasu, magnetic resonance
  imaging of, 708, 709
  pulmonary artery in, angiography of, 215,
    217
Artifacts, definition of, 1209
Artificial intelligence, in interpretation of
  radionuclide images, 919–920
Aspartate, in myocardial metabolism, 38–39,
  39
Aspirin, and platelet uptake, after carotid
  endarterectomy, 1041–1042
  effect of, on thrombosis, indium-111 plate-
    let imaging of, left ventricular,
    1038, 1039
  prosthetic materials in, 1045, 1046
Asplenia, atrial situs inversus with,
  echocardiography of, 445, 446
  magnetic resonance imaging of, 676
Atherectomy, intravascular ultrasonic
  guidance of, 592, 594
  combined instrumentation for, 597–598
Atherosclerosis, angioplasty for. See
  Angioplasty.
  aortic, and aneurysm, magnetic resonance
    imaging of, 705, 705
  echocardiography of, complex plaque in,
    99
    intraoperative, 577, 577
    transesophageal, 558
  of carotid arteries, and thrombosis, indium-
    111 platelet imaging of, 1039t, 1039–
    1042, 1040t, 1041
  of coronary arteries. See Coronary arteries,
    disease of.
    angiography of, 220–248. See also Coro-
      nary angiography.
  peripheral, and thrombosis, indium-111
    platelet imaging of, 1042–1043
  ultrasonography of, intravascular, calcifica-
    tion in, 590–591, 591, Plate 21
    limitations of, 604, 605, 605
    vascular remodeling in, 591–592, 592
    without angiographic detection, 582
    tissue characterization in, 582–583, 583,
      622, 622, Plate 20
Athletes, myocardial tissue characterization in,
  ultrasonic, 621
Atoms, in x-ray absorption, 103
Atrial fibrillation, in Doppler
  echocardiography, of left ventricular
  function, 350, 351
  in radionuclide angiography, equilibrium,
    943
Atrial filling wave, in diastole, 342
Atrial pacing, with positron emission
  tomography, of myocardial fatty acid
  metabolism, in ischemia, 1115, 1116
Atrial septal defect, echocardiography of, 422,
  423, 423–424, Plate 7
  in blood flow measurement, 431
  transesophageal, 561, Plates 8 and 15
  magnetic resonance imaging of, 673, 678,
    678, 682–685, 684
  right ventricular enlargement with, radiogra-
    phy of, 132, 133
  surgery for, echocardiography in, 575, Plate
    18
  ultrafast computed tomography of, 876, 877
Atrial septum, aneurysm of, echocardiography
  of, 457–459, 459
  transesophageal, 557, 558
Atrial situs ambiguus, echocardiography of,
  442, 445, 446
  magnetic resonance imaging of, 676
Atrial situs inversus, echocardiography of,
  442, 445, 445

Atrial situs inversus (Continued)
  magnetic resonance imaging of, 676, 677,
    678
  with dextrocardia, radiography of, 143, 143
Atrioventricular groove, fat in,
  echocardiography of, vs. mass lesion, 457
Atrioventricular node, conduction through,
  changes in, contrast agents and, 154
Atrioventricular septal defects,
  echocardiography of, 427–430, 428–430,
  Plate 7
Atrioventricular valve, anomalies of, ultrafast
  computed tomography of, 877
  common, with atrioventricular septal de-
    fects, echocardiography of, 427–430,
    428–430, Plate 7
  with single ventricle, magnetic resonance
    imaging of, 677, 679
Atrium (atria), in diastolic function, after
  Mustard operation, magnetic resonance
  imaging of, 690
  left. See Left atrium.
  myxoma of, ultrafast computed tomography
    of, 864, 864–865, 865
  pressure in, and early filling wave, 338,
    340, 341
    valvar function and, 54–56, 55, 56
  right. See Right atrium.
  systolic function of, and diastolic filling, 342
  volume of, measurement of, angiography
    in, 192–193
Atropine, before coronary angiography, 226
  with dobutamine, in stress echocardiogra-
    phy, 505
Attenuation, in positron emission tomography,
  901, 903, 903–904
  in radionuclide imaging, of myocardial per-
    fusion, 983
  in single-photon emission computed tomog-
    raphy, 898–899, 899
  of x-rays, 103
Autonomic nervous system. See Nervous
  system.
Axillary artery, catheterization through, for
  aortography, 199–200
Axillary vein, valves in, as surrogates for
  cardiac valves, 57

Backprojection, in image reconstruction, in
  computed tomography, 797, 797–798
Backscatter, in ultrasonography, in tissue
  characterization, 607–610, 609, 610
Bacteremia, after endoscopy, in
  transesophageal echocardiography, 450
Bacterial infection, and endocarditis, mitral
  regurgitation with, 381, 381
Balloon angioplasty. See Angioplasty.
Balloon occlusion, in pulmonary angiography,
  210
Balloon pump, intra-aortic placement of,
  echocardiography in, 576
Balloon ultrasound imaging catheter, 598
Balloon valvuloplasty, for congenital heart
  disease, 90–92
  of aortic valve, echocardiography of, 389
Balloon valvulotomy, for mitral stenosis, in
  rheumatic disease, 572
Bandwidth, definition of, 1209
Barium enema, and radiation dose, 1206t,
  1207t
Basal viscous resistance, to coronary blood
  flow, 9
Baseline, definition of, 1209
Bay u3405, in prevention of thrombosis, with
  prosthetic materials, indium-111 platelet
  imaging of, 1046
Beam hardening, in computed tomography,
  794–795
  ultrafast, of myocardial perfusion, 846,
    846–847

Becquerel, in radiation dosimetry, 1205,
  1205t
Benadryl (diphenhydramine), for allergy, to
  contrast agents, 208, 226
Benzodiazepine receptors, in positron
  emission tomography, 1075, 1193–1194
Benzovesamicol, in positron emission
  tomography, of cholinergic receptors,
  1196
Bernoulli equation, in Doppler
  echocardiography, of aortic stenosis,
  366–367, 369
Beta-methyl-heptadecanoic acid, in
  myocardial metabolic imaging, 1025
Bicycle, in stress induction. See Exercise.
Biopsy, in myocarditis, 87
Biplane cineangiography, 114
Bismuth germanate, in positron emission
  tomography, 901
Bjork-Shiley prosthetic valve, dysfunction of,
  transesophageal echocardiography of, 556
Bladder, radiation dose to, in radionuclide
  imaging, 1207t
Bloch equations, definition of, 1209
Blood, changes in, contrast agents and, 159
  in magnetic resonance imaging, 635–637,
    636t
Blood cells, radiolabeled, in angiography, 942
  in imaging, and radiation dose, 1207t
Blood flow, coronary. See Coronary arteries,
  blood flow in.
  in myocardial perfusion. See Myocardial
    perfusion.
  in ultrasonic tissue characterization, of myo-
    cardium, 613
  magnetic resonance imaging of, in congeni-
    tal heart disease, 674, 674–675, 675
    quantitative, 774–779, 775–778
  shunting in. See Shunt(ing).
  ultrafast computed tomography of, in con-
    genital heart disease, 872–875, 873,
    875, 876
    indicator-dilution method in, 824–825,
      825
  velocity of, measurement of, Doppler ultra-
    sound in, 292–293, 292–294
Blood pressure, changes in, contrast agents
  and, 151, 151–155, 153–154
  elevated. See Hypertension.
  reduced, after pulmonary angiography, 211
    dobutamine and, in stress echocardiogra-
      phy, 506
Blood vessels. See also specific vessels, e.g.,
  Vena cava.
  dilation of, contrast agents and, 151, 151
  endothelial changes in, contrast agents and,
    159
  imaging of. See Angiography.
  ultrasonography of, intravascular, 581–603.
    See also Ultrasonography, intravascu-
    lar.
Blood volume, changes in, contrast agents
  and, 150t, 150–151, 151
Blue toe syndrome, microemboli and,
  indium-111 platelet imaging of, 1042
Blurring, of x-ray image, 106–107, 107t, 108
BMIPP. See Iodine-123 betamethyl
  iodophenyl pentadecanoic acid.
Boltzmann distribution, definition of,
  1209–1210
Boltzmann's constant, in magnetic resonance
  imaging, 630
Bone, disorders of, in chest radiography, 126,
  127
Bone marrow, radiation dose to, in diagnostic
  radiology, 1206t, 1207t
Border detection, in segmentation, in digital
  imaging, 69–70
Brachial artery, catheterization through, for
  coronary angiography, 227, 229
Bradycardia, contrast agents and, 154, 155

Brain, computed tomography of, radiation dose in, 1206t
lipids in, in magnetic resonance imaging, 635
radiation dose to, in radionuclide imaging, 1207t
Braking radiation, 103, *105*
Breast, carcinoma of, metastasis of, to heart, echocardiography of, 468, *469*
radiation dose to, in diagnostic radiology, 1206t
Bremsstrahlung, 103, *105*
Brightness linearity, in fluoroscopy, 113
Bromine-76 bromobenzylguanidine, in positron emission tomography, of presynaptic neurotransmission, 1196
Bronchoconstriction, with pulmonary embolism, and timing of angiography, 211
Bubbles, in contrast echocardiography, 481–485, *482–484*, Plate 8
in positron emission tomography, of myocardial blood flow, 1065, *1066*
Bulbis cordis, embryology of, 692–693
Bulboventricular loop, in congenital heart disease, echocardiography of, 442
Bulk magnetization, in magnetic resonance imaging, 630–632, *630–632*
Bundle branch block, as contraindication to pulmonary angiography, 208
Bypass grafts. See *Coronary arteries, bypass surgery of.*

Calcification, extracardiac, radiography of, 143, *143*
in aortic stenosis, *141*, 141–142, 366
in coronary artery disease, in ultrafast computed tomography, 829–833, *830–832*
in mitral regurgitation, 381
intracardiac, of thrombi, ultrafast computed tomography of, *866*, 866–867
radiography of, *141*, 141–143, *142*
of aortic transection, traumatic, magnetic resonance imaging of, 708, *708*
of atherosclerotic plaque, intravascular ultrasonography of, 590–591, *591*, Plate 21
of mitral annulus, echocardiography of, 459, *459*
of papillary muscles, echocardiography of, 459, *460*
of pulmonary emboli, ultrafast computed tomography of, 860, *860*
Calcium, binding of, by contrast agents, and reduced myocardial contractility, 153, *154*
in myocardial function, 20–24, *22*
Calcium-channel blockers, effect of, on diastolic function, 29
on ventricular function, 23
Cameras, in cineangiography, 114
in digital imaging, 60
in fluoroscopy, *112*, 112–113, *113*
in single-photon emission computed tomography, multihead, 895–896, *896*
scintillation, in radionuclide imaging, 889–891, *889–891*
angiographic, *925*, 925–926
Cancer, drugs for, and cardiotoxicity, radionuclide imaging of, angiographic, 958
nervous system in, 1059
metastatic, to heart, echocardiography of, 468, *469*
of esophagus, echocardiography of, vs. cardiac mass lesion, 457, *458*
of pericardium, echocardiography of, 408, *409*, 416, 468, *469*
metastatic, 468, *469*
ultrafast computed tomography of, 869, *870*

Cancer *(Continued)*
of pulmonary arteries, angiography of, 216, *218*
radiation exposure and, 122t, 122–123
Carbohydrates, in myocardial metabolism, 34–39, *36–39*. See also *Myocardial metabolism.*
Carbon dioxide, oxygen-15–labeled, in positron emission tomography, of myocardial blood flow, 1084
Carbon monoxide, radiolabeled, in positron emission tomography, in ventricular function assessment, 1078–1080
Carbon-11, in positron emission tomography, in ventricular function assessment, in carbon monoxide labeling, 1078
of cardiac nerves, 1188–1192, 1195–1196, 1198
of myocardial blood flow, in albumin microsphere labeling, 1065
of myocardial metabolism, in amino acid labeling, 1075
Carbon-11 acetate, in positron emission tomography, and radiation dose, 1207t
of myocardial metabolism, 1068t, *1073*, 1073–1075, *1074*, 1075t
after infarction, 1119–1120
coronary artery anatomy in, 1123–1124
thrombolysis in, 1124–1128, *1129*
in cardiomyopathy, dilated, 1175–1176
future of, 1183
in acyl coenzyme A dehydrogenase deficiency, 1183, *1183*
in coronary artery disease, 1132–1133
in ischemia, acute, 1115, 1118–1119
Carbon-11 benzovesamicol, in positron emission tomography, of cholinergic receptors, 1196
Carbon-11 hydroxyephedrine, in positron emission tomography, of cardiac nerves, 1075, 1198
Carbon-11 palmitate, in imaging, of myocardial metabolism, historical aspects of, 1021
tissue kinetics of, 1021, 1023–1025
in positron emission tomography, and radiation dose, 1207t
of myocardial metabolism, 1068t, 1068–1072, *1069–1071*, 1074–1075
after infarction, 1120, 1123
in cardiomyopathy, dilated, 1174–1178, *1175*, *1177*, *1180*, Plate 35
hypertrophic, 1180–1181
in acyl coenzyme A dehydrogenase deficiency, 1183, *1183*
in ischemia, acute, 1114–1115, *1116*, 1118–1119
study conditions in, standardization of, 1166–1167
Carbon-13, spectrum of, in magnetic resonance imaging, 784, *785*
Carbon-14 palmitate, in imaging, of myocardial metabolism, 1021, 1023, 1024
Carbonyl cyanide *m*-chlorophenylhydrazone, and cell injury, imaging of, single-photon emitting tracers for, 966
Carcinoid syndrome, and tricuspid regurgitation, echocardiography of, 385
and tricuspid stenosis, echocardiography of, 383, *384*, 385
Carcinoma. See *Cancer.*
Cardiac cycle, effect of, on ultrasonic tissue characterization, *613*, 613–614
mechanics of, *24*, 24–25, *25*
Cardiac gating, in computed tomography, limitations of, 800
in magnetic resonance imaging, 647–648, *647–649*
of aorta, 694
of cardiomyopathy, hypertrophic, 745

Cardiac gating *(Continued)*
of pericardium, 752, 753t
quantitative, 763
in myocardial perfusion imaging, in coronary artery disease, 983
in positron emission tomography, 1076, *1078*
in radionuclide angiography, first-pass, 930
in radionuclide imaging, 892–893, *893*, *894*
in myocardial viability assessment, 1007
Cardiac output, increased, contrast agents and, 152–153, *153*
measurement of, magnetic resonance imaging in, 769, *771*, 774, 776
ultrafast computed tomography in, in congenital heart disease, 873
Cardiac tamponade, echocardiography in, 354, *354*, 409–413, *410–413*
Cardiomegaly, radiography of, interpretation of, 76
Cardiomyopathy, classification of, 745, 1172, 1172t
dilated, echocardiography of, 87–88, 399–402, *400–402*
Doppler, 357
imaging of, 87–88
single-photon emitting tracers in, 1026t, 1031–1032
magnetic resonance imaging of, 747–751, *750*, *751*
spectroscopic, 1173–1174
nervous system dysfunction with, radionuclide imaging of, 1058
positron emission tomography in, in acyl coenzyme A dehydrogenase deficiency, 1183, *1183*
of myocardial blood flow, 1110
of myocardial metabolism, 1167, 1174–1178, *1175*, *1177–1180*, Plate 35
ultrasonic tissue characterization in, 619, *619*
doxorubicin-induced, 958
nervous system dysfunction with, 1057
experimental, ultrasonic tissue characterization in, 621
hypertrophic, contrast ventriculography of, 165, *166*, 168
echocardiography of, 395–399, *396–399*, Plate 6
Doppler, 355–357
imaging of, 88
single-photon emitting tracers in, 1026t, 1032, Plate 30
magnetic resonance imaging of, 745–747, *746–749*
myocardial mass measurement in, 769
nervous system dysfunction with, positron emission tomography of, 1197–1198
radionuclide imaging of, 1058
obstructive, myectomy for, echocardiography in, 573–574, *574*
positron emission tomography in, of myocardial blood flow, 1095t, 1110
of myocardial metabolism, 1178–1181, *1180*, *1181*
ultrasonic tissue characterization in, 620–621
in Duchenne muscular dystrophy, metabolism in, positron emission tomography of, 1181–1183, *1182*
infiltrative, ultrasonic tissue characterization in, 619–620, *620*
with hemochromatosis, left ventricular function in, Doppler echocardiography of, 329, *330*
magnetic resonance spectroscopy of, 789, *789*
metabolism in, systemic, abnormalities of, 1174

Cardiomyopathy (Continued)
myocardial metabolism in, positron emission tomography of, future of, 1183–1184
indications for, 1166
radionuclide angiography in, 956
restrictive, echocardiography of, 402, 402–403
imaging of, 88
magnetic resonance imaging of, 751, 751–752, 752
Cardiomyoplasty, echocardiography in, 576
Cardioplegia, in coronary bypass surgery, contrast echocardiography of, 495–498, 496–498
Cardiopulmonary resuscitation, transesophageal echocardiography with, 560
Cardiotoxicity, antitumor therapy and, radionuclide imaging of, angiographic, 958
nervous system in, 1059
Carnitine, in myocardial metabolism, 40, 40–41, 1172, 1173
Carotid artery, common, magnetic resonance imaging of, 699, 700
in aortic dissection, computed tomography of, 857, 857
thrombosis of, indium-111 platelet imaging of, 1039t, 1039–1042, 1040t, 1041
Carrier frequency, in Doppler ultrasound, 296
Cataracts, radiation exposure and, 123
Catecholamines, in myocardial metabolism, 44
in myocardial stimulation, for viability assessment, vs. positron emission tomography, 1159–1161
in ventricular function, 23, 30
Catheters, balloon ultrasound imaging, 598
echocardiography of, vs. cardiac mass lesions, 459, 461, 462
for aortography, 199–200
for pulmonary angiography, 209
in angiography, of congenital heart disease, 90–92
in aortic valve measurement, vs. Doppler echocardiography, 369, 372
in congenital heart disease, transesophageal echocardiographic guidance of, 449–450, Plate 8
in pericardial pressure measurement, 28
Cathode, in x-ray production, 104
Cedars-Sinai method, in myocardial perfusion assessment, with thallium imaging, 905–907, 905–907, 910
in radionuclide ventriculography, 914–917, 915–918
Cells, injury to, imaging of, single-photon emitting tracers for, 966, 966–967
Centerline method, in left ventricular wall motion assessment, 176, 179, 182, 186
echocardiographic, 314, 315
in magnetic resonance imaging, 727, 728
Cerebral blood vessels, angiography of, radiation dose in, 1206t
Cerebrovascular accident, carotid artery stenosis and, risk assessment for, indium-111 platelet imaging in, 1039t, 1039–1041, 1040t
Cerebrovascular disorders, coronary angiography and, 224, 225t
CGP 12177, carbon-11–labeled, in positron emission tomography, of cardiac nervous system, 1188, 1190, 1192
Chang's method, of attenuation correction, in single-photon emission computed tomography, 898
Chemical shift, definition of, 1210
in magnetic resonance spectroscopy, 785–786, 786, 787

Chemotherapy, toxicity of, to heart, radionuclide imaging of, angiographic, 958
nervous system in, 1059
Chest, pain in. See Angina.
Chest radiography, 126–143. See also Radiography.
Chiari network, echocardiography of, vs. mass lesions, 453, 453–454
Children, congenital heart disease in. See Congenital heart disease and specific disorders, e.g., Tetralogy of Fallot.
Chlorpromazine, before coronary angiography, 226
Cholesterol, elevated blood level of, myocardial blood flow in, 1095t
Cholinergic receptors, muscarinic, in cardiac innervation, 1187–1188
positron emission tomography of, 1189–1193, 1190, 1195
in presynaptic neurotransmission, 1196
Chordae tendineae, disorders of, and mitral regurgitation, 381
Chromium-51, in platelet labeling, in imaging of thrombosis, 1035
Chromosomal abnormalities, and cardiomyopathy, hypertrophic, 1178–1179
Chronic obstructive pulmonary disease, radionuclide angiography in, 939
right ventricular enlargement with, 131, 134
Cigarette smoking, and carbon-11 ketanserin concentration, in positron emission tomography, 1189
and myocardial ischemia, positron emission tomography of, 1106, 1106–1107
Cine acquisition, in angiography, of aorta, 113–115, 202, 202
in magnetic resonance imaging, 648–650, 649
myocardial tagging in, 668, 668, Plate 22
of aorta, 695, 695
of cardiomyopathy, hypertrophic, 746, 748
of coronary bypass grafts, 741, 741t
of myocardial function, 668, Plates 22 and 23
of myocardial infarction, 724–726, 725
of myocardial ischemia, inducible, 726–728, 727, 728
of valvular disease, 708, 710, 711
quantitative, 760–761, 761
of left ventricular function, myocardial tagging in, 771–774, 772, 773
in ultrafast computed tomography, 854, 864, 872
Cine film, in archival storage, of digital images, 117
Citrate synthetase, in tricarboxylic acid cycle regulation, 42
Citric acid cycle, in myocardial metabolism, 1172, 1173
Coagulation, impairment of, contrast agents and, 159
Coarctation, of aorta, angioplasty for, stenting after, 595
echocardiography of, 434–435, 435
imaging of, 91
magnetic resonance imaging of, 678, 698–700, 699
subclavian artery anomaly with, 696–697
Coherence, in magnetic resonance imaging, definition of, 1210
Coils, in magnetic field generation, definition of, 1210
Cold, in cardiac stress induction, in positron emission tomography, 1097
Collagen, in myocardium, in ultrasonic tissue characterization, 611, 612
in infarction, 611, 612, 618, 619

Collagen (Continued)
in ventricular compliance, in diastole, 337
Collateral circulation, coronary, angiography of, 238–239
positron emission tomography of, 1104–1106, 1105
Collimation, in computed tomography, 799
in positron emission tomography, 901, 902, 902, 903
in single-photon emission computed tomography, 898, 899
of gamma rays, in radionuclide imaging, 890
of x-rays, 105
Colon, radiation dose to, in radionuclide imaging, 1207t
Color flow Doppler imaging, 293–295, 294, 295t, Plate 1. See also Doppler echocardiography.
instrument settings for, 295–296
transducer configurations for, 296, 296
Compact disks, in digital image storage, 118
Compressive resistance, to coronary blood flow, 10
Compton scatter, in single-photon emission computed tomography, 897–898
of x-rays, 103
Computed tomography, after trauma, cardiovascular, 96–98
equipment for, in conventional scanning, 798, 798–799
in spiral scanning, 799–800
historical aspects of, 793–794
image reconstruction in, 795–798, 796, 797
in coronary blood flow measurement, 17, 17
of aortic aneurysm, 99
of aortic dissection, 99, 202–203
vs. echocardiography, transesophageal, 560
of aortic regurgitation, 85
of aortic stenosis, 85
of aortic trauma, 205–207, 206
of arteriovenous malformations, pulmonary, 100
of cardiomyopathy, 88
of congenital heart disease, 91, 92
of coronary artery disease, 82, 83
of heart anatomy, 2
of mitral regurgitation, 86
of mitral stenosis, 85
of myocardial perfusion, 4
of pericardial mass lesions, 94–95
of pericarditis, 93, 94
of pulmonary blood vessels, 218
of ventricular function, 2, 3
physics of, 794–795, 795
quantitation in, 58–60, 59, 59t
radiation dose in, 803–805, 804, 805, 805t, 1206t
scan times in, 800, 801
single-photon emission. See Single-photon emission computed tomography.
ultrafast, 793–886. See also Ultrafast computed tomography.
Computers, in digital image processing, 60, 63, 70. See also Digital images.
in interpretation of radionuclide images, artificial intelligence in, 919–920
in magnetic resonance imaging, 647
in radionuclide imaging, 890, 890
Conduction, atrioventricular, changes in, contrast agents and, 154
Congenital heart disease. See also specific structures, e.g., Aorta, and disorders, e.g., Ventricular septal defects.
cyanotic, myocardium in, ultrasonic tissue characterization of, 623
echocardiography of, 420–451. See also Echocardiography.
transesophageal, 561, 562t, Plate 15

Congenital heart disease (*Continued*)
  imaging of, 90–92
    interpretation of, 76
  magnetic resonance imaging of, 672–690.
      See also *Magnetic resonance imaging.*
  ultrafast computed tomography of, 871–
      886. See also *Ultrafast computed to-
      mography.*
Congestive heart failure, magnetic resonance
    spectroscopy of, 789
  radiography of, 134–139, *138, 139*
Conray (iothalamic acid), as contrast agent,
    146, 147, 149, 149t
Continuity equation, in Doppler
    echocardiography, of aortic stenosis, 369,
    371
Contraction, excitation coupled with, in
    myocardial function, 20–22, *22*
Contrast, definition of, 1210
  in angiographic image, 107–110, *109, 110*
  in image intensification, 111
  in ultrafast computed tomography, 805–
      808, 807t, *808*
  magnetization transfer, definition of, 1213
Contrast agents, 144–162
  anaphylactoid reaction to, 157–158
  and gastrointestinal disorders, 159
  and pulmonary dysfunction, 159
  and vasodilation, 151, *151*
  definition of, 1210
  effect of, on blood, 159
    on cardiac electrophysiology, 154–156,
        155, 156
    on intravascular volume, 150t, 150–151,
        151
    on kidneys, *158,* 158–159, 162
    on myocardial contractility, 153–154,
        153–155
    on systemic arterial pressure, 151, *152*
    on vascular endothelium, 159
    on ventricular filling pressure, 151–152,
        152
  historical aspects of, *145,* 145–148, *146*
  in aortography, 200
  in coronary angiography, 159–162, *160,*
      161t
    and complications, 225
  in echocardiography. See *Echocardiogra-
      phy.*
  in magnetic resonance imaging, 652–664
    cardiovascular response to, 655–656
    distribution of, in myocardium, 654–655
    effect of, on signal intensity, 654, *654,*
        655
    magnetic properties of, 653, *653*
    of coronary occlusion, acute, 656, *656,*
        657
    of myocardial infarction, 656–658, *658–*
        661, 722–724, *723–725*
    of myocardial perfusion, 659–664, *662–*
        664
    of myocardial viability, 658–659, *660, 661*
  in pulmonary angiography, 209
    allergy to, 208
  in ultrafast computed tomography, in exper-
      imental imaging, 813–814, *814, 815*
    of cardiac masses, 864
    of congenital heart disease, 872, 872t
    of coronary artery disease, 833
    of great vessels, 854–855
    of myocardial perfusion, in regional vas-
        cular volume measurement, 847–
        848, *847–849*
      intra-arterial, 843–845, *844,* 850
      intravenous, 840–843, *840–843,* 849–
          850
      kinetics of, 848–849, *849*
    of pericardium, 864, 868
  in ventriculography, 164–187. See also *Ven-
      triculography, contrast.*
  performance criteria for, 144–145

Contrast agents (*Continued*)
  toxicity of, acute, 149t, 149–150
Contrast washout analysis, in digital
    angiography, of coronary circulation, *259,*
    259–261, *260*
Contrast-to-noise ratio, definition of, 1210
Contusion, of myocardium, echocardiography
    of, transesophageal, 561
Copper-PTSM, in positron emission
    tomography, of myocardial blood flow,
    1066, 1067, 1085
Cor pulmonale, radiography of, 131, *134*
Cor triatriatum sinister, echocardiography of,
    459, *461*
Coronary angiography, 220–248
  after bypass surgery, 230, 256–257, *257,*
      267, *267*
  anatomy in, 233–235, *234*
  as outpatient procedure, 230–232, 232t
  common problems in, 247–248
  complications of, 223–226, 225t
  contraindications to, 223
  contrast agents in, effect of, on myocardial
      contractility, 153–154, *153–155*
  digital, 120–121
    in anatomic imaging, 255–256
  findings in, vs. postmortem examination,
      239–240
  historical aspects of, 220–221
  image enhancement in, histogram equaliza-
      tion in, 64, *66*
  indications for, 221–223, *223*
  interpretation of, 241–247, *242–246,* 247t
    variability in, 240, *240*
  magnetic resonance imaging in, 732–741
    echo planar technique in, 739, *740*
    in blood flow measurement, 777–779,
        778
    in blood flow velocity assessment, 736–
        737, *739*
    in patients with stents, 734–736, *739*
    in stenosis, 734, 737t, *737–739*
    of anomalous arteries, 737–739, *740*
    of bypass grafts, 739–741, *741,* 741t, *742*
    of stenosis, 734, 737t, *737–739*
    technical aspects of, 732–734, *732–737,*
        736t
  of bridging, 239
  of collateral vessels, 238–239
  of congenital anomalies, 235–238, *236,*
      236t, *237*
  patient management in, 226–227
  performance standards in, 248
  radiation dose in, 1206, 1206t
  radionuclide, of stenotic vessels, first-pass,
      935–939, 937t, *938,* 938t, *939,*
      Plates 27 and 28
    in diagnosis, 947t, 947–949, *948,* 948t
    in patient management, 954
    in prognosis, *951–953,* 951–954
    in severe disease, 949t, 949–951, *950*
  techniques of, 227–230, *228, 229, 231*
  view selection in, 232–233, *233, 234*
  vs. stress echocardiography, 511, 511t
Coronary arteries, anatomy of, 233–235, *234*
  and myocardial metabolism, in positron
      emission tomographic studies, after
      infarction, 1123–1124
  imaging of, 2
  angiography of, 220–248. See also *Coro-
      nary angiography.*
  blood flow in. See also *Myocardial ischemia*
      and *Myocardial perfusion.*
    and ventricular function, 30–31
    assessment of, digital angiography in,
        methods of, 257–264, *258–263,*
        Plate 1
    determinants of, 9, *9–11, 10*
    in ultrasonic tissue characterization, of
        myocardium, 613
    measurement of, imaging techniques for,
        17, *17–18, 18*

Coronary arteries (*Continued*)
  bypass surgery of, angiography of, 230
    digital, 256–257, *257,* 267, *267*
    echocardiography of, contrast, 495–498,
        496–498
      pericardial effusion in, 408, *408*
      stress testing in, 517–518
    magnetic resonance imaging of, 739–741,
        741, 741t, *742*
    radionuclide imaging before, in myocar-
        dial viability assessment, 996
    ultrafast computed tomography of, 833
  calcification of, radiography of, 143, *143*
  collateral, angiography of, 238–239
    positron emission tomography of, 1104–
        1106, *1105*
  digital imaging of, future of, 70
  disease of, and blood flow changes, 11–17,
      13–17
    and collateral circulation, 15–17
    and myocardial infarction, acute, 82–83
      prognosis after, echocardiography in,
          525–526
    and myocardial ischemia, with regional
        wall motion abnormalities, echocar-
        diography of, 522–525, *523–525*
    asymptomatic, angiography in, 222
    chronic, 83
    computed tomography of, ultrafast, 829–
        834, *830–832*
    contrast echocardiography of, 494–495,
        495, Plate 10
    detection of, 81–82
    diastolic function in, Doppler echocardi-
        ography of, 357–358
    digital angiography of, 264–267, *264–267*
    echocardiography of, intracardiac tech-
        nique in, 530
      intravascular technique in, 530
      stress, 511t, 511–514, *512–514*
        vasodilators in, 515–517, *516,* 517t
        vs. radionuclide imaging, 514–515,
            515, 515t
      tissue characterization in, 530
      transesophageal, 558, Plate 13
    epidemiology of, 220
    imaging of, interpretation of, 76
    indium-111 platelet imaging of, 1037,
        1037t
    magnetic resonance spectroscopy of,
        787–788, *788*
    morphology of, 244–247, *245, 246,* 247t
    myocardial blood flow in, positron emis-
        sion tomography of, 1094–1110. See
        also *Positron emission tomography.*
    myocardial metabolism in, imaging of,
        single-photon emission tracers in,
        1026t, 1029–1031, *1030, 1031*
    positron emission tomography of,
        1129–1135, 1130t, 1131t, 1139–
        1141, *1141, 1142,* 1142t, Plates 33
        and 34
      histopathology with, 1135–1139,
          1136–1138, Plate 35
      in prognosis, 1161–1165, *1162,*
          1162t, *1164,* 1165t
      indications for, 1165–1166
    myocardial perfusion in, 971–991. See
        Myocardial perfusion.
    nervous system dysfunction with, radionu-
        clide imaging of, 1057
    physiology of, 241, *242–244*
    prognosis of, 241–244, *245*
    radionuclide angiography of, first-pass,
        935–939, 937t, *938,* 938t, *939,*
        Plates 27 and 28
      in diagnosis, 947t, 947–949, *948,* 948t
      in patient management, 954
      in prognosis, *951–953,* 951–954
      in severe stenosis, 949t, 949–951, *950*

Coronary arteries (*Continued*)
    surgery for, echocardiography in, 575–
        576, Plate 19
    ultrafast computed tomography of, 826
    ventricular wall motion in, contrast ven-
        triculography of, 194–198, *197*
  echocardiography of, contrast, 530
    direct visualization in, 530
    stress, 530
    transesophageal, *538, 539, 540*
  magnetic resonance imaging of, 669–670,
    671
  occlusion of, and cardiomyopathy, dilated,
    magnetic resonance imaging of, 749,
    750
    and left ventricular wall motion abnor-
        malities, contrast ventriculography
        of, 176, 182, *186*
    and myocardial infarction. See *Myocar-
        dial infarction.*
    magnetic resonance imaging of, contrast
        agents in, *656, 656, 657*
  spasms of, intravascular ultrasonography
    and, *605, 605*
  trauma to, imaging of, 96, *97*
  ultrafast computed tomography of, 813–
    814, *815, 817, 818*
  ultrasonography of, intravascular, in vessel
    measurement, 583, *584, 586*
Coronary cusp, as aortic valve pseudomass,
    echocardiography of, 454–457, *456*
Coronary flow reserve, assessment of, contrast
    echocardiography of, 494
  definition of, 11
  in coronary artery disease, 14, *15, 16*
Coronary sinus, dilated, echocardiography of,
    454, *455*
Correlation time, in magnetic resonance
    imaging, 1210
Creatine kinase, in thallium-201 tomography,
    of myocardial perfusion, 911
Creatine phosphate, in myocardial
    metabolism, 43
Creatinine, in renal failure, contrast
    agent–induced, 159
Cryogens, with superconducting magnets, in
    magnetic resonance imaging, 643–645,
    646, 1210
Cryostats, definition of, 1210
Curie, in radiation dosimetry, 1205, 1205t
Cyanide, and cell injury, imaging of, single-
    photon emitting tracers for, 966
Cyanosis, in congenital heart disease,
    echocardiography in, 436–441,
    437–442, Plate 7
  imaging in, 92
  surgery for, magnetic resonance imaging
    after, 685–689, *688, 689*
  ultrafast computed tomography of, in
    myocardial tissue characterization,
    623
Cyclic adenosine monophosphate, and
    ventricular function, 23
Cysts, echinococcal, echocardiography of, 474,
    475
  pericardial, computed tomography of, ul-
    trafast, 869–870, *870*
  echocardiography of, *417, 418, 468, 470,*
    474–475
  imaging of, 94

Dacron, in arterial grafts, and thrombosis,
    indium-111 platelet imaging of, 1045,
    1046
Decibels, in ultrasound measurement,
    275–276, 276t
Decoupling, definition of, 1210
Demodulators, in magnetic resonance
    imaging, 646, *647*

Densitometry, x-ray, 121–122
Deoxyhemoglobin, in magnetic resonance
    imaging, 636, 636t
Dephasing gradient, definition of, 1210
Desensitization, cardiac, positron emission
    tomography of, 1198
Desipramine, in positron emission
    tomography, of presynaptic
    neurotransmission, 1195–1196
Detective quantum efficiency, in image
    intensification, 111
Dextrocardia, echocardiography of, 448, *449,
    450*
  radiography of, 143, *143*
Diabetes, and renal injury, contrast agents in,
    158
  myocardial effects of, ultrasonic tissue char-
    acterization of, 623
  myocardial metabolism in, 43–44, 47
  neuropathy with, cardiac, radionuclide im-
    aging of, 1058
Dialysis, fistula for, and vascular remodeling,
    ultrasonography of, 592, *593*
  atherectomy in, ultrasonic guidance of,
    592–594, *594*
Diamagnetic substances, definition of, 1210
Diaphragm, radiography of, interpretation of,
    127
Diastasis, valvar function in, 54, *55*
Diastole, early filling wave in, 338–342, *340,
    341*
  mitral valve in, 51, *52, 53*
  ventricular function in. See also *Left ventri-
    cle, function of.*
    determinants of, 25t, 25–29, *26, 28*
    echocardiography of, 306
      Doppler, 336–362. See also *Doppler
        echocardiography.*
    imaging of, 3
    in cardiomyopathy, dilated, 401, *401*
      hypertrophic, 397–398, *399*
      restrictive, 403
    physiology of, 336–338, *337–339*
Diatrizoate, as contrast agent, adverse effects
    of, clinical trials of, 160–161
  and heart rate changes, *155*
  and renal injury, 158, *158*
  and repolarization, 155, *156*
  and systemic arterial pressure, *152*
  and ventricular fibrillation, 156, *157*
  anticoagulant effect of, 159
  effect of, on cardiac output, *153*
    on intravascular volume, 150, *151*
    on myocardial contractility, 153, *154*
    on ventricular filling pressure, *152*
  historical aspects of, *146, 147*
  iodine concentration in, 148–149, 149t
  toxicity of, acute, 149t, 149–150
Diazepam, hydrogen-3–labeled, in positron
    emission tomography, of benzodiazepine
    receptors, 1194
  in sedation, for coronary angiography, 226
Dietary changes, for coronary artery disease,
    myocardial blood flow after, positron
    emission tomography of, 1108, Plate 32
Diffusion, definition of, 1210
Digital angiography, 251–268
  in ventricular function assessment, 252t,
    252–255, 253t, *254, 255*
  of aorta, 200–202
  of coronary arteries, after bypass grafts,
    256–257, *257, 267, 267*
    in anatomic assessment, 255–256
    in assessment of circulation, methods of,
        257–264, *258–263*, Plate 1
    stenotic, 264–267, *264–267*
  of pulmonary vessels, 209
  subtraction method in, 120
Digital images, characteristics of, 60–63,
    61–63
  data compression in, 120

Digital images (*Continued*)
  enhancement of, filtering in, 67–69, *68, 69,*
    118–119, *119*, 119t
  geometric operations in, 64–67
  point operations in, 63–64, *64–67*
  in aortography, 200–202, *201*
  in clinical diagnosis, 78–80
  in quantitation, 58–60, *59*, 59t
  in stress echocardiography, 507
  interpretation of, goals of, 1–6
    perception in, 72–77, *73, 75*
  processing of, 118–120, *119*, 119t
    future of, 70
  segmentation of, 69, 69–70
  storage of, 116–118, 117t
    viewers for, 118
    workstations for, 118
Digital scan conversion, in echocardiography,
    286–288, *287, 288*
Digital subtraction angiography, 120
  of aorta, 200–202
  of pulmonary vessels, 209
Digitalis (digoxin), and ventricular function,
    23, 30
Diodrast (iodopyracet), as contrast agent, *146,*
    147
Diphenhydramine (Benadryl), for allergy, to
    contrast agents, 208, 226
Dipole, magnetic, definition of, 1212
Dipole-dipole interaction, definition of, 1210
Dipyridamole, and platelet uptake, after
    carotid endarterectomy, 1041–1042
  for stress induction, 11, 15
    in echocardiography, 79, 505, 506
      after myocardial infarction, 488, 519,
        Plate 9
      of coronary artery disease, 515–517,
        516, 517t
      before revascularization, 519, 519t
      transesophageal, 548
  in magnetic resonance imaging, 727, 728
    of myocardial perfusion, 661–663, *662*
    of regional ventricular wall motion,
        770
  in positron emission tomography, of myo-
    cardial blood flow, 1094t, 1094–
    1097, *1095, 1096*, 1097t
  precautions with, 1166
  in radionuclide imaging, of myocardial
    perfusion, *974*, 974–975
    before noncardiac surgery, 990, 990t
  in ultrafast computed tomography, of
    myocardial perfusion, 849
  in prevention of thrombosis, with pros-
    thetic materials, indium-111 platelet
    imaging of, 1045, *1046*
Distortion, in image intensification, 111
  in magnetic resonance imaging, quantita-
    tive, 763t, 763–764, *764*
  pincushion, of digital images, 121
Diuretics, and diastolic function changes, 28
Diverticulum, aortic, magnetic resonance
    imaging of, 696, *696, 697, 698*
DMIPP, in imaging, of myocardial
    metabolism, 1025–1026
Dobutamine, and ventricular function,
    systolic, 30
  for stress induction, in echocardiography,
    505, *505–506, 506*
    after myocardial infarction, 519
    in myocardial viability assessment, 518
      vs. positron emission tomography,
        1159–1161
      vs. radionuclide imaging, 1008
    of coronary artery disease, 81–82
      before revascularization, 519t, 519–
        520
      vs. radionuclide imaging, *515*, 515t,
        515–517, *516*, 517t
    transesophageal, 548
  in magnetic resonance imaging, 668–669,
    727, *727–728*, Plate 23

Dobutamine (*Continued*)
in myocardial viability assessment, vs. positron emission tomography, 1160–1161
of regional ventricular wall motion, 770
in positron emission tomography, of myocardial blood flow, 1094, 1094t, 1097, 1097t
in radionuclide imaging, of myocardial perfusion, 974, *974, 975*
Dopamine, and ventricular function, systolic, 30
Doppler A wave, 342
Doppler E wave, 338–342, *340, 341*
Doppler echocardiography. See also *Echocardiography.*
in aortic surgery, 576, Plate 19
in evaluation, of diastolic function, 336, *546*, 546–547, *547*
A wave in, 342
after cardiac transplantation, 357
and prognosis, 358
clinical approach to, 345–346, 349
color M-mode recording in, 359–361, Plate 3
continuous-wave imaging in, 358–359, *360*
E wave in, 338–342, *340, 341*
in amyloidosis, cardiac, 352, 354–355, *355–357*
in cardiac tamponade, 354, *354*
in cardiomyopathy, dilated, 357 hypertrophic, 355–357
in congenital heart disease, 358
in coronary artery disease, 357–358
in hypertensive heart disease, 357
in pericarditis, constrictive, 350–354, *352, 353*
left ventricular filling pressure in, 358
measurements in, 346t, 346–349, *347, 348*, 348t
mitral deceleration in, 338, *339*
mitral velocity patterns in, 342–344, *343, 344*
pitfalls in, 349–350, 350t, *351*
pulmonary venous velocity patterns in, 344–345, *345*
of prosthetic valves, 388, *388–389*
of systolic function, 324–333, 546
left ventricular, 325t, 325–331, *326–330*
right ventricular, 331–333, *332*
vs. ultrasonic imaging, 325
of valvuloplasty, 389
in stress testing, 507
of aortic regurgitation, 374–376, *375, 376*, Plates 4 and 5
with prosthetic valve, 388–389
of aortic stenosis, 366–369, *368, 370–372*
congenital, 432–433, *433*
of atrial septal defects, 423, 423–424, Plate 7
of atrioventricular septal defects, 430, Plate 7
of cardiomyopathy, dilated, 401, *401* hypertrophic, 396–398, *398, 399*, Plate 6
of coarctation of aorta, 435, *435*
of mitral regurgitation, 381–383, 554, Plates 5 and 11
of mitral stenosis, *378*, 378–380, *379*
of myocardial infarction, with mitral regurgitation, 527, *527*, Plate 10
with papillary muscle rupture, 527, Plate 10
with ventricular septal rupture, 526, *526*, Plate 10
of patent ductus arteriosus, 424–427, *425–427*, Plate 7
of pericarditis, constrictive, 415, *416*
of pulmonary regurgitation, 387, Plate 6

Doppler echocardiography (*Continued*)
of pulmonary stenosis, 387
of pulmonary vein, 540, *540*, Plate 10
of shunting, left-to-right, in quantitation, 430–431
of total anomalous pulmonary venous return, 441, Plate 7
of tricuspid regurgitation, 385, *385–386, 386*, Plate 5
of tricuspid stenosis, 383–384, *385*
of valvular stenosis, intraoperative, 569, *569*
of ventricular septal defects, 422–423, Plate 6
signal enhancement in, contrast techniques in, 499–501, *500*
Doppler tissue imaging, 361, Plates 3 and 4
Doppler ultrasound, 291–296
in color flow imaging, 293–295, *294*, 295t, Plate 1
in measurement of blood flow velocity, 292–293, *292–294*
instrument settings for, 295–296
principles of, 292
transducer configurations for, 296, *296*
Double-outlet right ventricle, echocardiography of, 437, *437, 438*
Doxorubicin, cardiotoxicity of, 958
nervous system dysfunction with, 1057
Duchenne muscular dystrophy, cardiomyopathy in, positron emission tomography in, 1181–1183, *1182*
Ductus arteriosus, embryology of, 693
in aortic arch anomalies, 697
patent, echocardiography of, 424–427, *424–427*, 431, Plate 7
Dynamic range, definition of, 1210
Dynamic spatial reconstructor, Mayo, in ultrafast computed tomography, 811–814, *811–815*
ANALYZE software for, 812, 816, *816–818*
Dyspnea, diagnosis of, radionuclide angiography in, 958
Dysprosium, in magnetic resonance imaging, 653, 654
of myocardial viability, 658–659, *660, 661*

E₁ fragment, of fibrin, in imaging of thrombosis, 1047
E wave, Doppler, 338–342, *340, 341*
Ebstein anomaly, and tricuspid regurgitation, echocardiography of, 385
echocardiography of, 437–438, *438*
imaging of, 92
magnetic resonance imaging of, 712
repair of, echocardiography of, vs. mass lesion, *462, 463*
right atrial enlargement in, radiography of, 131, *131*
with transposition of great arteries, echocardiography of, 447
Echinococcal cyst, echocardiography of, 474, *475*
Echo offset, definition of, 1210
Echo planar imaging, 651, *651–652*
definition of, 1210
of cardiomyopathy, dilated, 750–751 hypertrophic, 746, *749*
of congenital heart disease, 674, *674*
of coronary arteries, 739, *740*
of myocardial function, 668
of myocardial ischemia, induced, 728, 731, *731*
of myocardial perfusion, 661
quantitative, 761, *761*
Echo time, definition of, 1217
Echocardiography, 273–291
after trauma, cardiovascular, 96–98
beam insertion in, 278

Echocardiography (*Continued*)
biologic effects of, 289–290
B-mode images in, 281–284, *282–286*
continuous loop display in, 288–289
contrast, in coronary bypass surgery, 495–498, *496–498*
in Doppler signal enhancement, 499–501, *500*
microbubble agents in, 481–485, *482–484*, Plate 8
of coronary arteries, 530 stenotic, 494–495, *495*, Plate 10
of left ventricular function, 501, *501*
of microvascular function, 498, *498–499, 499*
of myocardial perfusion, 485–499
in assessment of viability, after infarction, 486–489, *487–489*, Plate 9
in detection of infarction, *485*, 485–486, *486*, Plate 9
in quantification, 489–494, *490–493*
of shunts, 499, *500*
digital scan conversion in, 286–288, *287, 288*
Doppler. See *Doppler echocardiography.*
focusing in, 279–281, *279–281*
freeze-frame display in, 288–289
historical aspects of, 273–274
image formation in, 285–286, *286, 287*
in anatomic imaging, 1–2
in clinical diagnosis, 78, 80
in left ventricular mass estimation, 306–307, *307, 308*
in left ventricular volume measurement, 300, *300–301*
in myocardial viability assessment, vs. positron emission tomography, 1159–1161
intraoperative, 566–578
epicardial, 568–569, *569*
future technology in, 578
in aortic surgery, 576–577, *577*, Plate 19
in congenital defect repair, 574–575, *575*, Plate 18
in coronary artery repair, 575–576, Plate 19
in heart transplantation, 576
in myectomy, for hypertrophic cardiomyopathy, 573–574, *574*
in valvular surgery, 570–573, *571, 572*, 572t, Plates 16 and 17
limitations of, 577–578
of aortic atheroma, 577, *577*
of fistula repair, in endocarditis, 577, Plate 20
of left ventricular function, 570
of valvular regurgitation, 570
of valvular stenosis, 569, *569*
techniques of, 567–569, *568, 569*
training for, 569
vs. other imaging methods, 567
mechanical waves in, 275
of aneurysms, aortic, 99
of atrial septum, 457–459, *459*
of aortic coarctation, 434–435, *435*
of aortic dissection, 99
of aortic regurgitation, 85, 372–376, *373–376*, 501, Plates 4 and 5
of aortic stenosis, 84–85, 366–372, *367, 368, 370–372*
of atrial septal defects, *422, 423*, 423–424, Plate 7
of atrioventricular septal defects, 427–430, *428–430*, Plate 7
of cardiac tamponade, 354, *354*, 409–413, *410–413*
of cardiomyopathy, 395–403
dilated, 87–88, 399–402, *400–402*
hypertrophic, 395–399, *396–399*, Plate 6
restrictive, *402*, 402–403
of congenital heart disease, 90–92, 420–451

Echocardiography (*Continued*)
in segmental analysis, 441–445, *442–446*
transesophageal, 449–450, Plate 8
with cyanosis, 436–441, *437–442*, Plate 7
of coronary artery disease, 83
direct visualization in, 530
intracardiac technique in, 530
intravascular technique in, 530
tissue characterization in, 530
of dextrocardia, 448, *449, 450*
of epicardial fat, 459, *460*
of hypoplasia, of left heart, 435, *436*
of right heart, 438, *439*
of left atrial congenital membrane, 459, *461*
of left ventricular outflow obstruction, 431–435, *432–436*
of mass lesions, 452–476
extracardiac, 468, *470*
vs. intracardiac surgical devices, 459–463, *461, 462*
vs. normal structural variants, *453–456, 453–457*
of mitral annulus, calcified, 459, *459*
of mitral regurgitation, 85–86, 380, *380–383, 381*, Plate 5
of mitral stenosis, 85, 376–380, *377–379*
of myocardial infarction, right ventricular, 320, 527
with infarct expansion, 527–530, *528, 529*
with myocardial stunning, 527
with papillary muscle rupture, 526, 527, *527*, Plate 10
with ventricular septal rupture, 526, *526*, Plate 10
of myocardial ischemia, with regional contraction abnormalities, 522–525, *523–525*
of myocarditis, 87
of papillary muscles, calcified, 459, *460*
of patent ductus arteriosus, 424–427, *424–427*, Plate 7
of pericardial absence, 417
of pericardial cysts, 417, *418*, 468, *470, 474–475*
of pericardial effusion, 405–409, *406–409*
of pericardial hematoma, 417
of pericardial malignancy, 408, *409*, 416, 468, *469*
of pericardial tamponade, 94
of pericardial trauma, 416–417
of pericarditis, acute, 93, 416
chronic, 416
constrictive, 94, 413–416, *413–417*
of pericardium, normal, 404–405, *405*
of prosthetic valves, 387–389, *388*
of pulmonary regurgitation, 387, Plate 6
of pulmonary stenosis, 387
of right ventricular outflow obstruction, 435–436, *436*
of thrombi, in left atrium, 377–378, 465, *465–466, 466*
in left ventricle, 466–468, *467, 468*
in right atrium, 463, *463*
in right ventricle, *464, 465*
of transposition of great arteries, 439, *439–440, 440, 442, 445–448, 447*
of tricuspid regurgitation, 384–387, *385, 386*, Plate 5
of tricuspid stenosis, 383–384, *384, 385*
of tumors, metastatic, 468, *469*
primary, benign, 469–475, 471t, *471–475*
malignant, 475, *475–476, 476*
of univentricular heart, *448, 448–449*
of valvular function, 4
of valvular heart disease, 365–389
of valvuloplasty, 389
of ventricular function, 2, 3
systolic, 297–320
regional, 307–317, *309, 311–316*, Plate 2

Echocardiography (*Continued*)
right, 317–320, *318, 319*
volume measurements in, *298–300, 298–303*, 301t, *302*, Plates 1 and 2
vs. Doppler imaging, 325
of ventricular septal defects, 420–423, *421, 422*, Plate 6
postprocessing in, 288
preprocessing in, 288
pulse transmission in, 278, *278*
resolution in, 278–280, *278–280*
signal amplification in, 284–285, *286*
signal reception in, 284, *286*
single-beam systems in, display from, 281
stress, 503–520. See also *Stress testing, in echocardiography.*
transesophageal, 533–562. See also *Transesophageal echocardiography.*
ultrasound generation in, 275, *275*, 275t
ultrasound transmission in, 275–277, 276t, *277*
EchoGen, in contrast echocardiography, 482
Eddy currents, definition of, 1210–1211
Edema, in magnetic resonance imaging, 635–636
with contrast agents, 655
pulmonary, in congestive heart failure, 139, *139*
Editing, spectral, definition of, 1216
Eisenmenger syndrome, imaging of, 92
shunting in, contrast echocardiography of, 499, *500*
Ejection fraction, measurement of, echocardiography in, 301t, 303–306, *304–306*
radionuclide angiography in, after myocardial infarction, 954–955, *955*
equilibrium, 944, 944t, 946
in chest pain, in diagnosis, 948, *948*, 948t
in prognosis, *951–953*, 951–954
first-pass, in data interpretation, 932
in data processing, 928–930, 929t
of coronary artery disease, 936–937, 937t
in valvular disease, 956–958, *956–958*
ultrafast computed tomography in, 822, 824, *824*
ventriculography in, contrast, 175, *176*
radionuclide, 913–919, *915–920*, Plate 24
Ejection velocity, left ventricular, assessment of, Doppler echocardiography in, 325, *326, 327–330, 328–330*
magnetic resonance imaging in, 769
ultrafast computed tomography in, stress testing with, 834
right ventricular, assessment of, Doppler echocardiography in, 331
Elderly, cardiomyopathy in, echocardiography of, 396, 398–399
left ventricular function changes in, Doppler echocardiography of, *347, 347–349, 348*
myocardium in, ultrasonic tissue characterization of, 623
Electrocardiography, after myocardial infarction, with positron emission tomography, 1122–1124, *1125*
before positron emission tomography, of myocardial blood flow, with stress testing, 1098
during coronary angiography, 226–227
in cardiac gating, in magnetic resonance imaging, of aorta, 694
of cardiomyopathy, hypertrophic, 745
of pericardium, 752, 753t
in positron emission tomography, 1076, *1078*
in myocardial ischemia, vs. positron emission tomography, of myocardial metabolism, 1141–1146, *1143, 1144, 1146*

Electrocardiography (*Continued*)
of coronary artery disease, vs. stress echocardiography, 513–514, *514*
with radionuclide angiography, first-pass, 926
Electron-beam computed tomography, 793–886. See also *Ultrafast computed tomography.*
Electrons, transport of, in myocardial metabolism, 41–42
Embolism. See also *Thrombosis.*
echocardiography of, transesophageal, 557, *558*
left ventricular thrombosis and, after myocardial infarction, 468
risk assessment for, indium-111 platelet imaging in, 1038, *1038*
pulmonary, angiography of, 210–214, *211–216*
computed tomography of, 218
ultrafast, 859–861, *860*
imaging of, 100
indium-111 platelet imaging of, 1043
magnetic resonance imaging of, 218
with papillary fibroelastoma, echocardiography of, 473, *474*
Emory University method, in thallium tomography, of myocardial perfusion, 907–909, *908, 909*, Plate 23
Endarterectomy, carotid, indium-111 platelet imaging after, 1039t, *1041*, 1041–1042
End-diastolic volume, measurement of, by contrast ventriculography, 170–171, *172, 175*
by echocardiography, 301t
Endocardial tube, embryology of, 692–693
Endocarditis, abscess in, magnetic resonance imaging of, 755, *756*
as complication of transesophageal echocardiography, 536
echocardiography of, transesophageal, 548t, 548–550, *549*, Plate 11
prosthetic valve infection in, Plate 13
fistulas with, surgery for, echocardiography in, 577, Plate 20
infectious, and aortic aneurysm, magnetic resonance imaging of, 705, *706*
and aortic regurgitation, echocardiography of, 372
and mitral regurgitation, 381, *381*
and tricuspid regurgitation, echocardiography of, 385
Löffler's, Doppler echocardiography in, 354
valves in, ultrasonic tissue characterization of, 622
Endocardium, blood flow in, contrast echocardiography of, 493–494
fibroelastosis of, and cardiomyopathy, echocardiography of, 402–403
ischemia of, magnetic resonance imaging of, 669, *669*
motion of, in left ventricular systolic function, echocardiography of, 311, *311*
after myocardial infarction, 314–317, *316*, Plate 2
Endomyocardial fibrosis, and tricuspid stenosis, echocardiography of, 383
Doppler echocardiography in, 354
Endoscopy, in transesophageal echocardiography, and bacteremia, 450
Endothelium-derived relaxing factor, in coronary blood flow, 11, 13–14
End-systolic pressure-volume relations, measurement of, digital angiography in, 253–255
echocardiography in, 306
magnetic resonance imaging in, in congenital heart disease, 680–681, *680–682*
End-systolic volume, measurement of, contrast ventriculography in, 171

End-systolic volume (*Continued*)
echocardiography in, 301t
Enema, barium, and radiation dose, 1206t, 1207t
Energy, production of, in myocardial metabolism, 34, 35, 45, 1172–1174, *1173*
Energy level, in magnetic field, definition of, 1211
Epicardial blood flow, contrast echocardiography of, 493–494
Epicardial echocardiography, intraoperative, 568–569, *569*
in congenital defect repair, 574
in coronary artery surgery, 576, Plate 19
Epicardial fat pad, echocardiography of, 459, *460*
vs. pericardial effusion, 408–409
Epinephrine, radiolabeled, in positron emission tomography, of presynaptic neurotransmission, 1195–1196
Equilibrium, thermal, definition of, 1217
Erythrocytes, radiolabeled, and radiation dose, 1207t
in angiography, 942
Esophagus, carcinoma of, echocardiography of, vs. cardiac mass lesion, 457, *458*
echocardiography through. See *Transesophageal echocardiography.*
Eustachian valve, in congenital heart disease, echocardiography of, *442,* 442–443
persistent, echocardiography of, vs. mass lesions, 453, *453*
Excitation, in magnetic resonance imaging, definition of, 1211
selective, definition of, 1216
volume-selective, definition of, 1218
Excitation-contraction coupling, in myocardial function, 20–22, *22*
Excretory urography, radiation dose in, 1206t
Exercise, effect of, on myocardial metabolism, 44
in stress induction, with echocardiography, 504t, 504–505
rapid recovery after, and accuracy of results, 512, *512*
with radionuclide angiography, equilibrium, 942–943, *943*
first-pass, 926–927, *927*
with radionuclide imaging, in myocardial viability assessment, 998t, 998–1002, *999–1001*
of myocardial perfusion, in coronary artery disease, 973–974
with ultrafast computed tomography, 833–834
Eyes, movement of, in image search, 74
protection of, against radiation, 123

Fab fragments, in antifibrin antibodies, in imaging of thrombosis, 1046–1047
in antimyosin antibodies, in imaging of myocardial necrosis, 1014, 1015
FADH$_2$, in myocardial metabolism, 34, 41–43
Fallot's tetralogy. See *Tetralogy of Fallot.*
False tendons, of left ventricle, echocardiography of, vs. mass lesions, 454, *454*
Faraday shield, definition of, 1211
Fast computed tomography, 793–886. See also *Ultrafast computed tomography.*
Fasting, effect of, on myocardial metabolism, 43
Fat, epicardial, echocardiography of, 459, *460*
vs. pericardial effusion, 408–409
in atrioventricular groove, echocardiography of, vs. mass lesion, 457
in magnetic resonance imaging, 635
metabolism of, myocardial, 39–41, *40–42*
Fatty acids, in myocardial metabolism, 39–41, *40, 41, 43,* 1172–1173, *1173*

Fatty acids (*Continued*)
defects of, and cardiomyopathy, positron emission tomography in, 1183, *1183*
in iodine-123 imaging, in cardiomyopathy, vs. positron emission tomography, 1177–1178
in positron emission tomography, with carbon-11 palmitate, 1069, *1070*
in ischemia, 1114–1115, *1116,* 1118–1119
in single-photon emission imaging, after infarction, 1028–1029, *1029*
historical aspects of, 1021
in coronary artery disease, 1026t, 1029–1031, *1030, 1031*
technical aspects of, 1027, Plate 29
tissue kinetics of, 1021–1027, *1022–1025,* 1023t, 1026t
vs. positron emission tomography, 1161
Fatty tumors, echocardiography of, 473–474, *475*
pericardial, imaging of, 94–95
ultrafast computed tomography of, 870
Femoral artery, aneurysm of, and thrombosis, indium-111 platelet imaging of, 1042
catheterization through, for aortography, 199
for coronary angiography, 227, 229
ultrasonography of, intravascular, after angioplasty, 590–591, Plate 21
three-dimensional reconstruction in, *599, 600*
Femoral vein, catheterization through, for pulmonary angiography, 209
Ferritin, in magnetic resonance imaging, 636
Ferromagnetic crystals, in contrast agents, in magnetic resonance imaging, 653, *653*
Ferromagnetism, definition of, 1211
Fibrin, antibodies to, in imaging of thrombosis, *1046,* 1046–1047, Plate 30
Fibroelastoma, echocardiography of, transesophageal, 557, *557*
endomyocardial, and tricuspid stenosis, echocardiography of, 383
papillary, echocardiography of, 473, *474*
Fibroelastosis, endocardial, and cardiomyopathy, echocardiography of, 402–403
Fibroma, echocardiography of, 471–473, *474*
Fibrosa, of pericardium, anatomy of, 752
Fick method, in stroke volume determination, 169, *170*
Field echo, definition of, 1211
Field gradient, magnetic, definition of, 1212
Field lock, definition of, 1211
Filament current, in x-ray production, 104
Filling factor, definition of, 1211
Filling wave, atrial, 342
early, 338–342, *340, 341*
Filtered backprojection, in image reconstruction, in computed tomography, 797, 797–798
Filtering, in digital image enhancement, 67–69, *68, 69,* 118–119, *119,* 119t
in Doppler ultrasound, 295–296
in single-photon emission computed tomography, *896,* 896–897, *897*
of x-rays, 105, *105*
Filters, vena caval, for pulmonary embolism, 214, *216*
Fistula, for renal dialysis, and vascular remodeling, ultrasonography of, 592, *593*
atherectomy for, ultrasonic guidance of, 592–594, *594*
of coronary artery, angiography of, 235–236, *236*
of pulmonary artery, angiography of, 214–215, *217*
ultrafast computed tomography of, 861

Fistula (*Continued*)
with endocarditis, surgery for, echocardiography in, 577, Plate 20
Flavine-adenine dinucleotide, in myocardial metabolism, 34, 41–43
Flip angle, definition of, 1211
Flow compensation, definition of, 1211
in magnetic resonance imaging, 650, *650*
Flow effects, definition of, 1211
Flow velocity paradoxus, in cardiac tamponade, 411, *412*
Flow-related enhancement, definition of, 1211
Fluorine-18 benzovesamicol, in positron emission tomography, of cholinergic receptors, 1196
Fluorine-18 fluorobenzylguanidine, in positron emission tomography, of presynaptic neurotransmission, 1196
Fluorine-18 2-fluoro-2-deoxyglucose, in positron emission tomography, and radiation dose, 1207t
of myocardial metabolism, 1068t, *1072,* 1072–1075, 1076, *1077, 1086,* 1086–1088, *1087,* 1088t, Plate 31
after infarction, 1119–1122, *1121–1123*
coronary artery anatomy and, 1123–1124
thrombolysis and, 1124–1128, *1126, 1129*
in cardiomyopathy, dilated, 1176–1177, *1178, 1179*
hypertrophic, *1180,* 1180–1181, *1181*
in Duchenne muscular dystrophy, *1182,* 1182–1183
in clinical management, 1167
in coronary artery disease, 1129–1135, 1130t, 1139–1141, *1142,* Plates 33 and 34
histopathology with, 1135–1139, *1136,* Plate 35
in prognosis, 1161–1165, *1162, 1164*
in ischemia, 1115–1118, *1117, 1119,* Plate 33
ventricular wall thickening with, 1146–1147
vs. electrocardiography, *1143,* 1143–1145, *1144, 1146*
vs. perfusion defect imaging, 1154–1159, *1155*
vs. thallium-201 scintigraphy, 1148–1153, *1149–1151*
study conditions in, standardization of, 1166–1167
vs. single-photon emission computed tomography, with radioiodinated fatty acids, 1161
Fluorine-18 6-fluorodopamine, in positron emission tomography, of presynaptic neurotransmission, 1196
Fluorine-18 6-fluoronorepinephrine, in positron emission tomography, of presynaptic neurotransmission, 1196
Fluorine-18 metaraminol, in positron emission tomography, of cardiac nerves, 1075
in presynaptic neurotransmission, 1194–1195
Fluorine-18 misonidazole, in positron emission tomography, 1075–1076
Fluorobenzylguanidine, fluorine-18–labeled, in positron emission tomography, of presynaptic neurotransmission, 1196
2-Fluoro-2-deoxyglucose. See *Fluorine-18 2-fluoro-2-deoxyglucose.*
6-Fluorodopamine, fluorine-18–labeled, in positron emission tomography, of presynaptic neurotransmission, 1196
Fluorometaraminol, fluorine-18–labeled, in positron emission tomography, of presynaptic neurotransmission, 1194–1195

6-Fluoronorepinephrine, fluorine-18–labeled, in positron emission tomography, of presynaptic neurotransmission, 1196
Fluoroscopy, digital, of coronary arteries, in anatomic assessment, 255–256
in angiography, 113–115
of aorta, 202, *202*
progressive scan, 120
technical aspects of, 111–113, *112, 113*
Focal spot blur, of x-ray image, 106–107, *108*
Focal spot size, in x-ray production, 104, *105*
Focusing, in echocardiography, 279–281, *279–281*
Focusing cup, in x-ray production, 104
Fontan procedure, magnetic resonance imaging after, *682, 685–689, 688, 689*
Foramen ovale, patent, shunting in, contrast echocardiography of, 499
transesophageal echocardiography of, 557
Force-frequency response, in myocardial contraction, 23
Forward mapping, in digital image enhancement, 64, *67*
Fourier imaging, partial, definition of, 1214
Fourier transform, aliasing in, 1209
definition of, 1211
in digital image enhancement, 67, *68*
in magnetic resonance imaging, 641, *641*
two-dimensional, definition of, 1218
Fractionation principle, in positron emission tomography, of myocardial blood flow, 1082
Frame-mode acquisition, in radionuclide imaging, 893–894
in angiography, equilibrium, 942, *943*
Frank-Starling mechanism, in ventricular function, 29, *29*–30
Free induction decay, definition of, 1211
in magnetic resonance imaging, 631
Frequency, angular, definition of, 1209
definition of, 1211
resonance, definition of, 1215
Frequency domain filters, in digital image enhancement, 67–69, *69*
Frequency encoding, definition of, 1211
in magnetic resonance imaging, 640–643, *641, 642*
Fungal infection, in endocarditis, and abscess, magnetic resonance imaging of, 755, *756*
Furifosmin, in myocardial perfusion imaging, 963, 964t, 966–968
in coronary artery disease, 991

G proteins, in cardiac neurotransmission, 1187, *1188*
Gadolinium, as contrast agent, in magnetic resonance imaging, 653–655, *654, 655*
of coronary occlusion, *656, 657*
of myocardial infarction, 656–658, *658–661, 722–724, 722–725*
of myocardial ischemia, induced, 728–731, *729–731*
definition of, 1211
Gallium, in albumin microsphere labeling, in positron emission tomography, of myocardial blood flow, 1065
in imaging, of myocarditis, 87
Gamma cameras, in radionuclide imaging, 889–891, *889–891*
angiographic, 925, *925–926*
Gamma rays, in positron emission tomography, 901–903
in radionuclide imaging, detection of, *888, 888–889, 889*
Gastroepiploic artery, in coronary bypass, angiography of, 230
Gastrointestinal tract, disorders of, contrast agents and, 159
Gating, cardiac. See *Cardiac gating.*

Gating (*Continued*)
definition of, 1211
multiple, in single-photon emission computed tomography, 900, *901*
respiratory, in magnetic resonance imaging, 650–651
quantitative, 763
Gauss, definition of, 1211
Gender, and left ventricular function variations, in Doppler echocardiography, *347, 348,* 349
Genetic abnormalities, and cardiomyopathy, hypertrophic, 1178–1179
Ghost images, in magnetic resonance imaging, of aorta, 693–694
Glucose, myocardial metabolism of, 34–35, *36, 37,* 37–38
positron emission tomography of, *1086, 1086–1088, 1087,* 1088t
after infarction, 1119–1122, *1121–1123*
thrombolysis and, 1124–1128, *1126*
carbon-11 palmitate in, 1069, *1070*
fluorine-18 2-fluoro-2-deoxyglucose in, *1072,* 1072–1073
in clinical management, 1167
in coronary artery disease, 1129–1135, 1130t, 1139–1141, *1142,* Plates 33 and 34
histopathology with, 1135–1139, *1136,* Plate 35
in ischemia, acute, 1115–1118, *1117, 1119,* Plate 33
ventricular wall thickening with, 1146–1147
vs. electrocardiography, *1143,* 1143–1145, *1144, 1146*
vs. perfusion defect imaging, 1154–1159, *1155*
vs. thallium-201 scintigraphy, 1148–1153, *1149–1151*
Glycogen, myocardial metabolism of, 35–37, *36*
GMP-140, antibody to, in imaging of thrombosis, 1047
Gold-195m, in angiography, 924
Gorlin formula, in aortic valve measurement, 369
Gradient, definition of, 1211
of magnetic field, in magnetic resonance imaging, 640, *640*
rephasing, definition of, 1215
Gradient coils, definition of, 1211
Gradient echo, definition of, 1211
in magnetic resonance imaging, of congenital heart disease, *673,* 673–674
Gradient moment nulling, definition of, 1211
Gradient pulse, spoiler, definition of, 1217
Gradient systems, in magnetic resonance imaging, *645,* 645–647
Gray, in radiation dosimetry, 1205, 1205t
Gray level, in digital imaging, *62,* 62–63, *63*
in segmentation, 69, *69,* 70
modification of, in image enhancement, 63–64, *64–67*
in ultrasonic tissue characterization, 610–611, *611*
Gray-scale transformations, in digital image processing, 118
Guanethidine, in radionuclide imaging, of cardiac nervous system, 1054, *1054*
Guanosine triphosphate–binding proteins, in neurotransmission, 1187, *1188*
Gyromagnetic ratio, definition of, 1211

h wave, atrial, in valvar function, 55–56, *56*
Hancock prosthetic mitral valve, Doppler echocardiography of, 388, *388*
Hanning filter, in single-photon emission computed tomography, 897, *897*
Heart. See also specific structures, e.g., *Right atrium,* and disorders, e.g., *Cardiomyopathy.*

Heart (*Continued*)
imaging of. See specific techniques, e.g., *Magnetic resonance imaging.*
transplantation of. See *Transplantation, of heart.*
Heart block, complete, pulmonary angiography and, 208
Heart failure, congestive, magnetic resonance spectroscopy of, 789
radiography of, 134–139, *138, 139*
nervous system in, positron emission tomography of, 1196–1197
radionuclide imaging of, 1057–1058
Heart rate. See also specific abnormalities, e.g., *Tachycardia.*
and ventricular function, 30
changes in, effect of, on Doppler echocardiography, of left ventricular function, 350
reduced, contrast agents and, 154, *155*
Heat, in ultrasonography, biologic effects of, 289–290
Helical computed tomography, equipment for, 799–800
Hemangioma, of pericardium, ultrafast computed tomography of, 870
Hematocrit, in ultrasonic tissue characterization, of myocardium, 613
Hematoma, cardiac, magnetic resonance imaging of, 754, *754, 755, 756*
in aortic dissection, magnetic resonance imaging of, 700–705, *701–704*
transesophageal echocardiography of, 560–561
pericardial, after cardiac surgery, echocardiography of, 417
vs. cardiac tamponade, 410–411, *411*
Hemipericardium, left, absence of, radiography of, 140–141, *141*
Hemochromatosis, and cardiomyopathy, dilated, magnetic resonance imaging of, 751
infiltrative, left ventricular function in, Doppler echocardiography of, 329, *330*
restrictive, echocardiography of, 402
Hemoglobin, in magnetic resonance imaging, 636t, 636–637
Hemopericardium, with aortic aneurysm, magnetic resonance imaging of, 705, *707*
Hemorrhage, in lung, ultrasound and, 290
in magnetic resonance imaging, 635–637, 636t
intramyocardial, after infarction, 726, *726*
Hemosiderin, in magnetic resonance imaging, 636, 636t
Heparin, before coronary angiography, 224, 226
effect of, on left ventricular thrombosis, indium-111 platelet imaging of, 1038
for myocardial infarction, assessment of, echocardiography in, 529–530
for pulmonary embolism, assessment of, angiography in, 211–213
Hepatic vein, blood flow in, Doppler echocardiography of, 347
in tricuspid regurgitation, 385, *385*–386
Hepatopulmonary syndrome, arteriovenous shunting in, contrast echocardiography of, 499
Hernia, hiatal, echocardiography of, vs. cardiac mass lesion, 457, *458*
Hertz, definition of, 1211
Hexabrix. See *Ioxaglate.*
Hiatal hernia, echocardiography of, vs. cardiac mass lesion, 457, *458*
Hibernation, after myocardial ischemia, radionuclide imaging of, 997, *997*
Histamine, in anaphylactoid reaction, to contrast agents, 157

Homogeneity, in magnetic resonance imaging, definition of, 1211–1212
Hounsfield units, in image reconstruction, in computed tomography, 796–797
Hydatid cyst, echocardiography of, 474, 475
Hydrogen, nuclear magnetic resonance in, 629
  in water, in biologic tissue, 634, 634–635, 635
  spectrum of, in magnetic resonance imaging, 784, 785
Hydrogen-3, in positron emission tomography, of cardiac receptors, 1188–1193
  of presynaptic neurotransmission, 1195
Hydroxyapatite, pyrophosphate binding to, in technetium-99m imaging, of myocardial necrosis, 1012–1013
3-Hydroxybutyrate, in ketone metabolism, myocardial, 41, 42
6-Hydroxydopamine, in nerve degeneration, before radionuclide imaging, 1055
Hydroxyephedrine, carbon-11–labeled, in positron emission tomography, of cardiac nerves, 1075
  in denervation, 1198
Hydroxyproline, in ultrasonic tissue characterization, in myocardial infarction, 618, 619
Hypaque. See Diatrizoate.
Hypercholesterolemia, myocardial blood flow in, 1095t
Hyperemia, cardiac, induced. See Stress testing.
  reactive, after myocardial infarction, contrast echocardiography of, 487–488, 488, Plate 9
Hypertension, and heart disease, Doppler echocardiography in, 357
  and myocardial pressure overload, ultrasonic tissue characterization in, 621–622
  pulmonary, as contraindication to angiography, 208
  in congenital heart disease, assessment of, magnetic resonance imaging in, 689
  right ventricular enlargement with, radiography of, 131, 132–134
  ultrafast computed tomography in, 861
  with cardiomyopathy, hypertrophic, echocardiography of, 396, 398–399
  positron emission tomography in, of adrenergic receptors, 1197
Hyperthyroidism, maternal, and cardiomyopathy, hypertrophic, 1179
Hypoplastic left heart syndrome, echocardiography of, 435, 436
Hypoplastic right heart syndrome, echocardiography of, 438, 439
Hypotension, after pulmonary angiography, 211
  dobutamine and, in stress echocardiography, 506

IHDA, in imaging of myocardial metabolism, 1022–1024, 1024, 1025, 1026t, 1026–1027
  after infarction, 1028–1029, 1029
  in cardiomyopathy, 1031
  in coronary artery disease, 1029, 1030
IHPA, in imaging of myocardial metabolism, 1022–1024, 1023, 1026t, 1026–1027
  after infarction, 1028
  in cardiomyopathy, 1026t, 1031
Iliac artery, angioplasty of, intravascular ultrasonography of, 586–589
  stenting of, intravascular ultrasonography in, in surgical guidance, 594, 596
  three-dimensional reconstruction in, 601, 602

Image acquisition time, definition of, 1212
Image search, in cardiac image interpretation, 73–74
Imagent-US, in contrast echocardiography, 482
Immunoglobulin G, in antimyosin antibody, in imaging of myocardial necrosis, 1014
Impedance, acoustic, in ultrasonography, in tissue characterization, 607
  to coronary blood flow, measurement of, 9, 9–11, 10
Impedance matching layers, in echocardiography, 278
Impulse response analysis, in digital angiography, of coronary circulation, 261, 261
Indicator-dilution methods, historical aspects of, 836–837
  in computed tomography, 837–838, 838
  flow algorithms in, 838–840, 839
  ultrafast, in blood flow measurement, 824–825, 825
  in congenital heart disease, 872–874, 873
  in digital angiography, of coronary circulation, 258–259, 259
Indium-111, in antimyosin antibody imaging, of myocardial necrosis, 1014
  in infarct sizing, 1018, 1018
  with positron emission tomography, 1124, 1125
  with thallium-201 perfusion imaging, 1016, 1016–1017, 1017
  of myocarditis, 87
  in myocardial perfusion imaging, 964, 965
  platelets labeled with, in imaging of thrombosis, 1034–1047. See also Thrombosis.
Indobufin, effect of, on left ventricular thrombi, indium-111 platelet imaging of, 1039
Inductance, definition of, 1212
Infants, congenital heart disease in. See Congenital heart disease and specific disorders, e.g., Ventricular septal defects.
Infarction. See Myocardial infarction.
Inhomogeneity, in magnetic resonance imaging, definition of, 1212
Innominate artery, magnetic resonance imaging of, 699, 700
Inotropic stimulation, in myocardial viability assessment, vs. positron emission tomography, 1159–1161
Insulin, and myocardial metabolism, of glucose, 44
  of protein, 47
Intensification, of x-ray image, 110–111
Interatrial septum, aneurysm of, echocardiography of, 457–459, 459
  transesophageal, 557, 558
Interpulse times, definition of, 1212
Intestines, radiation dose to, in radionuclide imaging, 1207t
Intravenous urography, radiation dose in, 1206t
Inversion, in magnetic resonance imaging, definition of, 1212
Inversion time, definition of, 1217–1218
Inversion transfer, definition of, 1215–1216
Inversion-recovery, in magnetic resonance imaging, definition of, 1212
Iodine, as contrast agent, concentration of, 148, 148–149, 149t
  historical aspects of, 145, 145–148, 146
  toxicity of, acute, 149t, 149–150
  in antimyosin antibody imaging, of myocardial necrosis, 1014
Iodine-123, in fatty acid labeling, in imaging of myocardial metabolism, 1021–1027, 1022–1025, 1023t, 1026t
  in cardiomyopathy, vs. positron emission tomography, 1177–1178

Iodine-123 betamethyl iodophenyl pentadecanoic acid (BMIPP), in imaging, of cardiomyopathy, hypertrophic, 1032, Plate 30
  vs. positron emission tomography, 1181
  of myocardial metabolism, 1022, 1025–1026
  after infarction, 1028, 1029
  in coronary artery disease, chronic, 1031
Iodine-123 iodophenyl pentadecanoic acid (IPPA), in imaging, and radiation dose, 1207t
  of myocardial metabolism, 1022, 1023, 1024–1027, 1025, 1026t, Plate 29
  after infarction, 1028
  in cardiomyopathy, 1026t, 1031–1032
  in coronary artery disease, chronic, 1029–1031, 1030, 1031
  vs. positron emission tomography, 1161
  in single-photon emission computed tomography, in myocardial viability assessment, 1007
Iodine-123–iodoheptadecanoic acid (IHPA), in imaging of myocardial metabolism, 1022–1024, 1023, 1026t, 1026–1027
  after infarction, 1028
  in cardiomyopathy, 1026t, 1031
Iodine-123–iodohexadecanoic acid (IHDA), in imaging of myocardial metabolism, 1022–1024, 1024, 1025, 1026t, 1026–1027
  after infarction, 1028–1029, 1029
  in cardiomyopathy, 1031
  in coronary artery disease, 1029, 1030
Iodixanol, as contrast agent, 146, 148
  effect of, on ventricular filling pressure, 152
  iodine concentration in, 149, 149t
  toxicity of, acute, 149t, 149–150
Iodopyracet, as contrast agent, 146, 147
Iohexol, as contrast agent, adverse effects of, clinical trials of, 161
  and renal injury, 158, 158
  historical aspects of, 146, 147
  iodine concentration in, 149, 149t
  toxicity of, acute, 149t, 149–150
Iopamidol, as contrast agent, and heart rate changes, 155
  and systemic arterial pressure, 152
  and ventricular fibrillation, 156
  effect of, on cardiac output, 153
  on ventricular filling pressure, 152
  historical aspects of, 146, 147
  iodine concentration in, 149, 149t
Iothalamic acid, as contrast agent, 146, 147, 149, 149t
Ioversol, as contrast agent, and heart rate changes, 155
  and repolarization, 155, 156
  and systemic arterial pressure, 152
  and ventricular fibrillation, 157
  effect of, on cardiac output, 153
  on ventricular filling pressure, 152
  historical aspects of, 146, 147
  iodine concentration in, 149, 149t
Ioxaglate, as contrast agent, and pulmonary dysfunction, 159
  anticoagulant effect of, 159
  effect of, on intravascular volume, 150, 151
  on ventricular filling pressure, 152
  iodine concentration in, 149, 149t
IPPA. See Iodine-123 iodopheynl pentadecanoic acid.
Iridium-191m, in radionuclide angiography, 924
Iron, as contrast agent, in magnetic resonance imaging, 653

Iron (*Continued*)
  in thalassemia, and cardiomyopathy, ultra-
    sonic tissue characterization in, 620
Ischemia, cerebral, carotid artery stenosis
    and, indium-111 platelet imaging in,
    1039t, 1039–1042, 1040t, *1041*
  myocardial. See *Myocardial ischemia*.
  renal medullary, contrast agents and, 158
Isocitrate dehydrogenase, in tricarboxylic acid
    cycle regulation, 42
Isonitriles. See also specific compounds, e.g.,
    Technetium-99m sestamibi.
  in myocardial perfusion imaging, 963–968,
    964t, *966*
Isotropic motion, definition of, 1212
Isovue. See *Iopamidol*.

Jekyll-Hyde syndrome, 56, *56*
Judkins technique, in coronary angiography,
    227–228, *228*
Jugular vein, valves in, as surrogates for
    cardiac valves, 57

K shells, atomic, in x-ray absorption, 103
Kerley's B lines, in chest radiography, 126,
    127
  in congestive heart failure, 139, *139*
Ketanserin, carbon-11–labeled, in positron
    emission tomography, of cardiac nervous
    system, 1189
Ketones, myocardial metabolism of, 41, *42*,
    43
Kidneys, carcinoma of, metastatic, to heart,
    echocardiography of, 468, *469*
  disorders of, dialysis for, fistula for, and vas-
    cular remodeling, ultrasonography
    of, 592, *593*
    atherectomy in, ultrasonic guidance
      of, 592, *593*
  in renin-angiotensin system, abnormalities
    of, in cardiomyopathy, 1174
  infarction of, with aortic dissection, com-
    puted tomography of, 858
  injury to, contrast agents and, *158*, 158–
    159, 162
  radiation dose to, in radionuclide imaging,
    1207t
Kimray-Greenfield vena caval filter, for
    pulmonary embolism, angiography of,
    214, *216*
Kommerell diverticulum, magnetic resonance
    imaging of, 696, *696*
Krebs cycle, positron emission tomography of,
    in cardiomyopathy, dilated, 1175–1176
K-space, definition of, 1212
  in magnetic resonance imaging, in fre-
    quency encoding, 641–643, *642*

Lactate, in myocardial metabolism, 38
Lag, in fluoroscopy, 113
Lambert-Beer law, in computed tomography,
    794
Laplace relation, in ventricular mechanics, 24
Large intestine, radiation dose to, in
    radionuclide imaging, 1207t
Larmor equation, definition of, 1212
Larmor frequency, chemical shift in, 1210
  definition of, 1212
  in magnetic resonance imaging, in fre-
    quency encoding, 640, *641*
    in slice selection, 639–640, *640*
  in nuclear magnetic resonance, 629–632,
    632, *637*
  magnetic induction field in, 1209
Laser surgery, in atherectomy, instruments
    for, 598

Latissimus dorsi muscle, in cardiomyoplasty,
    ventricular performance with,
    echocardiography of, 576
Lattice, in magnetic resonance, definition of,
    1212
Lead, in radiation protection, 123
Leaflets, of aortic valve, 50–51, *51*
  of mitral valve, 51, *52–54*
Left atrial appendage, echocardiography of,
    vs. mass lesion, 457, *457*
Left atrium. See also *Atrium (atria)*.
  blood flow in, transesophageal echocardiog-
    raphy of, 559
  congenital membrane of, echocardiography
    of, 459, *461*
  echocardiography of, transesophageal, 538,
    540, Plate 10
  enlargement of, radiography of, 128, *130*
  in cardiac tamponade, echocardiography of,
    410, *410*
  junction of, with pulmonary vein, echocardi-
    ography of, vs. mass lesion, 457, *457*
  location of, in congenital heart disease,
    echocardiography in, 443, *443–446*,
    445
  pressure in, and left ventricular function,
    25, 27
  thrombosis in, echocardiography of, *465*,
    465–466, *466*
    indium-111 platelet imaging of, 1039
    with mitral stenosis, echocardiography of,
      377–378
  volume of, measurement of, magnetic reso-
    nance imaging in, 767
Left bundle branch block, as contraindication
    to pulmonary angiography, 208
Left hemipericardium, absence of,
    radiography of, 140–141, *141*
Left ventricle. See also *Ventricle(s)*.
  aneurysm of, after infarction, echocardiogra-
    phy of, 527–528, *528*
    magnetic resonance imaging of, 726
  calcification of, radiography of, *142*, 143
  blood flow in, measurement of, magnetic
    resonance imaging in, 777
    transesophageal echocardiography in,
      559
  Doppler tissue imaging of, 361, Plates 3
    and 4
  dysfunction of, coronary angiography in,
    222
  echocardiography of, transesophageal, 540–
    544, *541–544*
  ejection from, and valvar function, 55, *55*
  enlargement of, radiography of, 128, *129*
  false tendons of, echocardiography of, vs.
    mass lesions, 454, *454*
  filling pressure in, estimation of, Doppler
    echocardiography in, 358
  function of, assessment of, ambulatory mon-
    itoring in, 943–944
    contrast echocardiography in, 501, *501*
    contrast ventriculography in, *193*, 193–
      194, *194*
    digital angiography in, 252t, 252–255,
      253t, *254*, *255*
    magnetic resonance imaging in, 769–
      774, *771–773*
    nuclear stethoscope in, 891–892
    positron emission tomography in, after
      revascularization, 1130t, 1130–
      1135, 1131t, 1140–1141, 1142t
      image acquisition in, 1077–1078
    radionuclide angiography in, first-pass,
      932, 933, *933*, *934*, Plate 26
    ultrafast computed tomography in,
      822, 823–825, *825*
      in congenital heart disease, 875
    VEST in, 892
  determinants of, in diastole, 25t, 25–29,
    26, *28*

Left ventricle (*Continued*)
  diastolic, echocardiography of, trans-
    esophageal, *546*, 546–547, *547*
    in early filling wave, *340*, 341, *341*
  echocardiography of, intraoperative, 570
  ejection fraction in. See *Ejection frac-
    tion*.
  imaging of, 2–3
  in congenital heart disease, magnetic res-
    onance imaging of, 679–682, *680–
    683*
  in exercise stress testing, with ultrafast
    computed tomography, 834
  systolic, assessment of, Doppler echocar-
    diography in, 325t, 325–331, *326–
    330*
    echocardiography in, 297–317. See
      also *Echocardiography*.
    echocardiography of, transesophageal,
      545, 545–546
    in cardiomyopathy, dilated, echocardi-
      ography of, 399–402, *400–402*
    regional, echocardiography of, 307–
      317, *309*, *311–316*, Plate 2
  hypertrophy of, in cardiomyopathy, echocar-
    diography of, 395–396, *396*, *397*
  magnetic resonance spectroscopy of,
    789
  nervous system dysfunction with, radionu-
    clide imaging of, 1058
  subaortic cone in, 52, *52*
  in cardiac tamponade, echocardiography of,
    410, *411*
  in congenital heart disease, location of,
    echocardiographic, 443, *443–445*
  magnetic resonance imaging of, 676–677
  mass of, estimation of, echocardiography in,
    306–307, *307*, 308
    ultrafast computed tomography in,
      822, 823, *823*
  obstructed outflow from, congenital, echo-
    cardiography of, 431–435, *432–436*
    with transposition of great arteries, echo-
      cardiography of, 447–448
  output of, radionuclide angiography of, 946
  pseudoaneurysm of, after infarction, echo-
    cardiography of, 527–528, *528*
    magnetic resonance imaging of, 726,
      726
  stress in, measurement of, contrast ventricu-
    lography in, 175–176, *178*
    magnetic resonance imaging in, 773,
      773
  stress testing of, transesophageal echocardi-
    ography in, 548
  thrombosis in, echocardiography of, 466–
    468, *467*, *468*
    after infarction, 528–530, *529*
    indium-111 platelet imaging of, 1037t,
      1037–1039, *1038*, *1039*
  volume of, measurement of, contrast ven-
    triculography in, 167–176, *170–178*
    echocardiography in, 298–300, *298–
      303*, 301t, *302*, Plates 1 and 2
    magnetic resonance imaging in, 764t,
      764–766, *765–768*, 768t
    radionuclide angiography in, 929, *945*,
      945–946
    radionuclide ventriculography in, 915–
      916
  wall motion in, contrast ventriculography
    of, 176–182, *179–186*, 188, *189–191*
    in myocardial ischemia, echocardiogra-
      phy of, transesophageal, 547–548
    magnetic resonance imaging of, 726–
      728, *727*, *728*
    regional, contrast ventriculography of,
      194–198, *195–197*
    in myocardial ischemia, echocardiogra-
      phy of, 522–525, *523–525*
    with metabolic abnormalities, in pos-
      itron emission tomography,
      1146–1147

Left ventricle (*Continued*)
    radionuclide angiography of, 944–945, *945*
    segmental, magnetic resonance imaging of, 769
    radionuclide ventriculography in, 916, *916, 917*
    stress echocardiography of, 507–510, *508, 509,* 509t
    wall thickening in, in ischemia, magnetic resonance imaging of, 769–771
Leiomyoma, of pericardium, computed tomography of, ultrafast, 870
Ligamentum arteriosus, development of, 693
Ligands, in positron emission tomography, of cardiac receptors, 1189–1194, *1190, 1191, 1193–1195*
    of presynaptic neurotransmission, 1194–1196, *1196*
Line spread function, of image resolution, 106
Linear array transducers, in echocardiography, *282,* 282–283, *283*
Linearity, in fluoroscopy, 113
Lipids. See *Fat.*
Lipoma, echocardiography of, 473–474, *475*
    pericardial, imaging of, 94–95
    ultrafast computed tomography of, 870
List-mode acquisition, in radionuclide imaging, 894–895
    in angiography, equilibrium, 942
Liver, radiation dose to, in radionuclide imaging, 1207t
    with indium-111 platelet imaging, of thrombosis, 1035, 1036
    transplantation of, pulmonary assessment before, contrast echocardiography in, 499
Localization techniques, definition of, 1212
Löffler's endocarditis, Doppler echocardiography in, 354
Longitudinal magnetization, definition of, 1212
Longitudinal relaxation, definition of, 1212
    in magnetic resonance imaging, 631–633, *632, 633*
Lookup table, in digital image enhancement, 63–64, *64, 65*
Lungs. See also *Pulmonary* entries and *Respiration.*
    arteriovenous malformations in, imaging of, 100
    arteriovenous shunting in, contrast echocardiography of, 499
    atelectasis of, vs. aortic dissection, computed tomography of, *857, 858*
    congestion of, diuretics for, and diastolic function changes, 28
    dysfunction of, contrast agents and, 159
    dysplasia of, congenital, angiography in, 216–217
    effusion in, vs. pericardial effusion, echocardiography of, 409, *409*
    hemorrhage in, ultrasound and, 290
    obstructive disease of, chronic, radionuclide angiography in, 939
      right ventricular enlargement with, 131, *134*
    perfusion of, measurement of, ultrafast computed tomography in, in congenital heart disease, 874
    radiation dose to, in diagnostic radiology, 1206t
    radiography of, interpretation of, 127
    sequestration of, pulmonary angiography in, 216
    tumors of, echocardiography of, 468, *470*
    vascular diseases in, imaging of, 100
Lupus erythematosus, and mitral regurgitation, 553, *553*
Lymphoma, extension of, to heart, ultrafast computed tomography of, 865, *865*

Lymphoma (*Continued*)
  non-Hodgkin, echocardiography of, 468, *470*
Lymphosarcoma, cardiac, primary, echocardiography of, 476

Macromolecules, in proton exchange, with water, in magnetic resonance imaging, 634–635, *635*
Macroscopic magnetization vector, definition of, 1212
Magnetic dipole, definition of, 1212
Magnetic disks, in digital image storage, 117
Magnetic field, definition of, 1212
Magnetic field gradient, definition of, 1212
Magnetic induction, definition of, 1212
Magnetic moment, definition of, 1212–1213
Magnetic resonance, definition of, 1213
Magnetic resonance imaging, 629–790
    after Fontan procedure, *682,* 685–689, *688, 689*
    after Mustard operation, *689,* 689–690, *690*
    after Senning operation, *689,* 689–690, *690*
    after trauma, cardiovascular, 96–97
    cardiac gating in, 647–648, *647–649*
    cine acquisition in, 648–650, *649.* See also *Cine acquisition.*
    computers in, 647
    contrast agents in, 652–664
      cardiovascular response to, 655–656
      distribution of, in myocardium, 654–655
      effect of, on signal intensity, 654, *654, 655*
      magnetic properties of, 653, *653*
    definition of, 1213
    echo planar imaging in, *651,* 651–652. See also *Echo planar imaging.*
    flow compensation in, 650, *650*
    frequency encoding in, 640–643, *641, 642*
    future developments in, 670–671
    gradient systems in, *645,* 645–647
    image analysis protocols for, 670
    image enhancement in, lookup table in, 64, 65
    in coronary angiography, 732–741. See also *Coronary angiography, magnetic resonance imaging in.*
    integrated approach to, 667–671, *668–671,* Plates 22 and 23
    magnets for, 643–645, *646*
    multislice imaging in, 643, *645*
    of aorta, in congenital anomalies, *696–699,* 696–700
      techniques of, 693–696, *694, 695*
    of aortic aneurysm, 99, 705, *705–707*
    of aortic branch vessels, 699, *700*
    of aortic dissection, 99, 202–203, 700–705, *701–704*
      vs. echocardiography, transesophageal, 560
    of aortic regurgitation, 85, 710, *711*
    of aortic stenosis, 85, 713–715, *713–717*
    of aortic trauma, 708, *708*
    of atrial septal defect, *678,* 678, 682–685, *684*
    of cardiomyopathy, 88
      dilated, 747–751, *750, 751*
        vs. positron emission tomography, metabolic, 1177
      hypertrophic, 745–747, *746–749*
      restrictive, *751,* 751–752, *752*
    of congenital heart disease, 91, 92, 672–690
      anatomical segmental analysis in, 675–679, *677–679*
      technical options in, 673–675, *673–676*
      ventricular functional assessment in, 679–682, *680–683*
    of coronary artery disease, 82, 83
    of coronary occlusion, acute, 656, *656, 657*

Magnetic resonance imaging (*Continued*)
    of coronary vessels, 669–670, *671,* 739, *740*
    of endocardial ischemia, 669, *669*
    of heart anatomy, 2
    of heart disease, interpretation of, 76–77
    of mitral regurgitation, 86, 710, *711, 712,* 713
    of mitral stenosis, 85, 712–713
    of myocardial function, *668,* 668–669, Plates 22 and 23
    of myocardial infarction, 719–722, *719–726, 720,* 720t, *721*
      cine imaging in, 724–726, *725*
      contrast agents in, 656–658, *658–661,* 722–724, *723–725*
      in diagnosis of complications, 726, *726*
    of myocardial ischemia, 719–742
      inducible, 726–731, *727–731*
    of myocardial perfusion, 4, 5, 669, *670*
      contrast agents in, 659–664, *662–664*
    of myocardial tissue characteristics, 5–6
    of myocardial viability, 658–659, *660, 661*
      with inotropic stimulation, vs. positron emission tomography, 1160–1161
    of myocarditis, 87
    of pericardial mass lesions, 94–95
    of pericarditis, 93–94
    of pericardium, 752–754, *753,* 753t, *754*
    of pulmonary blood vessels, 218
    of pulmonary emboli, vs. ultrafast computed tomography, 861
    of pulmonary stenosis, 712
    in tetralogy of Fallot, *684,* 685
    of tricuspid valve disorders, 712, *712*
    of valvular disease, 708–710, *711*
    of ventricular function, 2, 3
    phase encoding in, 643, *644, 645*
      respiratory-ordered, 650–651
    physics of, 629–633, *630–633*
      in biologic tissue, 633–637, *634, 635,* 636t, 637t
    quantitative, 59, 60, 759–780
      automated analysis of, *779,* 779–780, *780*
      error sources in, 763t, 763–764, *764*
      of atrial volume, 767
      of blood flow, 774–779, *775–778*
      of left ventricular function, 769–774, *771–773*
      of myocardial mass, 768–769, *770*
      of ventricular volume, left, 764t, *764–766, 765–768,* 768t
        right, 766–767
      resolution in, 761–763, *762*
      techniques for, 760–761, *761*
    radiofrequency systems in, 645–646, *647*
    rapid-excitation, definition of, 1215
    relaxation times in, 637, 637t, 637–638
    respiratory gating in, 650–651
    slice selection in, 639–640, *640*
    spectroscopic, 784–790. See also *Magnetic resonance spectroscopy.*
    surface coils in, 651
    terminology in, 1209–1218
    workstations in, 647
Magnetic resonance spectroscopy, 784–790
    definition of, 1213
    future of, 790
    heart spectrum in, 784–785, *785*
    metabolite quantification in, 786–787
    of cardiomyopathy, 789, *789*
      dilated, 1173–1174
      hypertrophic, vs. positron emission tomography, metabolic, 1181
    of congenital heart disease, 675, *676*
    of congestive heart failure, 789
    of myocardial infarction, 788–789
    of myocardial ischemia, 787–788, *788*
    of transplanted heart, 789–790
    technique of, 785, *785–786, 786*
Magnetic shielding, definition of, 1213
Magnetic susceptibility, definition of, 1213

Magnetic tape, in digital image storage, 117–118

Magnetization, definition of, 1213
  longitudinal, definition of, 1212
  transverse, definition of, 1218

Magnetization transfer, definition of, 1213

Magnetization transfer contrast, definition of, 1213

Magnetization transfer rate, in water, in magnetic resonance imaging, 634

Magnetization vector, macroscopic, definition of, 1212

Magnets, for magnetic resonance imaging, 643–645, 646

Magnification, of digital images, 121
  of x-ray image, 110

Malate, in myocardial metabolism, 38–39, 39

Malonyl CoA, in lipid metabolism, myocardial, 41

Mammary artery, internal, angiography of, 230, 231
  in coronary bypass grafts. See Coronary arteries, bypass surgery of.

Manganese, as contrast agent, in magnetic resonance imaging, 653

Marfan syndrome, aortic aneurysm in, angiography of, 202, 203
  magnetic resonance imaging of, 705, 706
  aortic regurgitation in, echocardiography of, 373–374
  aortic root in, magnetic resonance imaging of, 764

Mass lesions. See also specific types, e.g., Thrombosis.
  echocardiography of, 452–476. See also Echocardiography.

Matrix size, in digital imaging, 60–62, 61
  in magnetic resonance imaging, quantitative, 762–763

Mayo dynamic spatial reconstructor, in ultrafast computed tomography, 811–814, 811–815
  ANALYZE software for, 812, 816, 816–818

MD-76. See Diatrizoate.

Mechanical waves, in ultrasound, in diagnostic imaging, 276t, 276–277, 277
  physics of, 274, 274–275

Mediastinum, tumors of, extension of, to heart, magnetic resonance imaging of, 755–757, 757

Medtronic-Hall prosthetic valve, dysfunction of, transesophageal echocardiography of, 556, Plate 13

Meglumine, as contrast agent, 147, 149, 149t

Mental stress, and myocardial ischemia, positron emission tomography of, 1106, 1106

Meperidine, in sedation, for coronary angiography, 226
  for transesophageal echocardiography, 537

Mesenteric artery, angioplasty of, intravascular ultrasonography of, 583, 585

Mesothelioma, of pericardium, ultrafast computed tomography of, 869, 870

Metabolism, myocardial, 34–48. See also Myocardial metabolism.

Metahydroxyephedrine, in positron emission tomography, of presynaptic neurotransmission, 1195–1196

Metaiodobenzylguanidine (MIBG), analogs of, in positron emission tomography, of presynaptic neurotransmission, 1196
  in radionuclide imaging, of cardiac nervous system, 1054, 1054–1059, 1055, 1055t, 1057
  iodine-123–labeled, in myocardial metabolic imaging, in cardiomyopathy, vs. positron emission tomography, 1177–1178, 1181

Metaraminol, fluorine-18–labeled, in positron emission tomography, of cardiac nerves, 1075
  in presynaptic neurotransmission, 1194–1195

Methemoglobin, in magnetic resonance imaging, 636, 636t

Methiodide-QNB, in positron emission tomography, of cardiac neurotransmission, 1189–1190, 1190, 1192–1193, 1195

Methylglucamine, as contrast agent, 147, 149, 149t

β-Methyl-heptadecanoic acid, in imaging, of myocardial metabolism, 1025

Methylprednisolone, before contrast radiography, in prevention of anaphylaxis, 158

Methysergide toxicity, and tricuspid stenosis, echocardiography of, 383

Metrizamide, as contrast agent, 146, 147

MIBG. See Metaiodobenzylguanidine.

Microbubbles, in contrast echocardiography, 481–485, 482–484, Plate 8
  in positron emission tomography, of myocardial blood flow, 1065, 1066

Microvasculature, myocardial, function of, contrast echocardiography of, 498, 498–499, 499

Midazolam, in transesophageal echocardiography, 537

Misonidazole, fluorine-18–labeled, in positron emission tomography, 1075–1076

Mitochondria, in lipid metabolism, myocardial, 40, 40–41

Mitral annulus, calcification of, echocardiography of, 459, 459
  Doppler tissue imaging of, 361, Plate 4

Mitral regurgitation, after myocardial infarction, echocardiography of, 527, 527, Plate 10
  contrast ventriculography in, 166, 167, 168
  echocardiography of, 380, 380–383, 381, Plate 5
    contrast, 501
    Doppler, continuous-wave, 358–359, 360
    in left ventricular function assessment, 350
    transesophageal, 552–554, 552–555, Plates 11 and 12
    multiplane views in, 544
  imaging of, 85–86
  in cardiomyopathy, dilated, echocardiography of, 401
    magnetic resonance imaging of, 749–750, 751
    hypertrophic, echocardiography of, 398
    magnetic resonance imaging of, 746–747
  left atrial enlargement with, radiography of, 128, 130
  magnetic resonance imaging of, 710, 711, 712, 713
    in blood flow quantitation, 777
  stroke volume in, measurement of, Doppler echocardiography in, 325, 327, 330–331
  ultrafast computed tomography of, 825–826

Mitral stenosis, echocardiography of, 376–380, 377–379
  transesophageal, 551–552, 552
  imaging of, 4, 85
  left atrial enlargement with, radiography of, 128, 130
  magnetic resonance imaging of, 712–713
  rheumatic disease and, echocardiography of, left atrial thrombosis in, 465, 465
  right ventricular enlargement with, radiography of, 131, 133

Mitral valve, anatomy of, 51–53, 51–54
  blood flow through, delayed relaxation in, 342, 343

Mitral valve (Continued)
  echocardiography of, transesophageal, 546, 546–547, 547
  functional importance of, 344, 344
  measurement of, magnetic resonance imaging in, 777
  nitroglycerin and, 345, 345
  normal, 342, 343
  physiology of, 337–338, 338, 339
  with restrictive filling, 342–344, 343, 344
  dysfunction of, without structural change, 56, 56–57
  echocardiography of, intraoperative, 568, 568, 570–572, 571, 572, 572t, Plate 16
    transesophageal, 538, 540, 540, 542, 542
  function of, normal, 54–56, 55, 56
  infection of, in endocarditis, transesophageal echocardiography of, 549, 549
  insufficiency of, radionuclide angiography of, 956
  prolapse of, contrast ventriculography in, 167, 169
  myxoma in, ultrafast computed tomography of, 864, 864
  prosthetic, echocardiography of, Doppler, 388, 388
    transesophageal, 555–556, Plates 12 and 13
  replacement of, hematoma after, magnetic resonance imaging of, 755, 756
  systolic anterior motion of, in hypertrophic cardiomyopathy, echocardiography of, 396, 398
  with double-outlet right ventricle, echocardiography of, 437, 437

M-mode echocardiography. See also Echocardiography.
  color Doppler, 359–361, Plate 3
  in left ventricular volume measurement, 300
  of pericarditis, constrictive, 413–415, 413–415
  of right ventricular function, systolic, 317

Mobin-Uddin vena caval filter, for pulmonary embolism, 214

Moderator band, of right ventricle, echocardiography of, vs. mass lesions, 454, 454

Modulation transfer function, of image resolution, 106

Modulators, in magnetic resonance imaging, 646, 647

Moiré pattern, in digital scan conversion, in echocardiography, 287, 287

Momentum, angular, definition of, 1209

Monitors, in fluoroscopy, 113

Monoamine oxidase, in cardiac nervous system, 1052, 1053

Monoclonal antibodies, antimyosin. See Antimyosin antibodies.

Motion, and artifacts, in single-photon emission computed tomography, 900
  and blurring, of x-ray image, 107
  and perception, in image interpretation, 73, 73
  correction for, in radionuclide angiography, 930–931, Plate 26

Movie-mode imaging. See Cine acquisition.

MQNB, in positron emission tomography, of cardiac neurotransmission, 1189–1190, 1190, 1192–1193, 1195

MRX-115, in contrast echocardiography, 482

Multiple echo imaging, definition of, 1213

Multiple gating, in single-photon emission computed tomography, 900, 901

Multislice imaging, definition of, 1213
  in magnetic resonance imaging, 643, 645
  quantitative, 760, 761
  in ultrafast computed tomography, 802

Muscarinic cholinergic receptors, in cardiac innervation, 1187–1188

Muscarinic cholinergic receptors (*Continued*)
positron emission tomography of, 1189–1193, *1190, 1195*
in presynaptic neurotransmission, 1196
Muscular dystrophy, Duchenne, cardiomyopathy in, positron emission tomography in, 1181–1183, *1182*
Mustard operation, magnetic resonance imaging after, *689,* 689–690, *690*
ultrafast computed tomography after, 876–877, *878–881*
Mycotic infection, in endocarditis, and abscess, magnetic resonance imaging of, 755, *756*
Myectomy, for cardiomyopathy, echocardiography in, 573–574, *574*
Myelography, spinal, endocarditis after, magnetic resonance imaging of, 755, *756*
Myocardial infarction, as complication of coronary angiography, 224, 225t
contrast ventriculography of, in assessment of thrombolysis, 188–192, *193*
ventricular wall motion in, 188, *189–191*
coronary angiography after, indications for, 221–222
coronary artery disease and, 82–83
echocardiography of, contrast, 485, 485–486, *486,* Plate 9
in prognosis, 525–526
infarct expansion in, 527–530, *528, 529*
left ventricular function in, regional, 307–310, 314–317, *316,* Plate 2
left ventricular thrombosis in, *467,* 467–468
myocardial stunning in, 527
myocardial viability in, 486–489, *487–489,* Plate 9
papillary muscle rupture in, *526,* 527, *527,* Plate 10
right ventricular, 320, 527
transesophageal, hemodynamic changes in, 559–560, Plate 14
ventricular septal rupture in, *526, 526,* Plate 10
with stress induction, in risk assessment, 518–520, 519t
magnetic resonance imaging of, 719–722, *720,* 720t, *721*
cine imaging in, 724–726, *725*
contrast agents in, 656–658, *658–661,* 722–724, *723–725*
in diagnosis of complications, 726, *726*
in myocardial mass estimation, 768–769
spectroscopic, 788–789
metabolism after, imaging of, single-photon emitting tracers in, 1028–1029, *1029*
positron emission tomography of, 1119–1122, *1121–1123*
after thrombolysis, 1124–1129, *1125, 1126, 1129*
coronary artery anatomy and, 1123–1124
electrocardiography with, 1122–1123
indications for, 1165–1166
vs. perfusion studies, 1156–1159
radionuclide imaging of, angiographic, 954–956, *955*
in assessment of necrosis, 1012–1019
accuracy of, 1014–1016, *1015*
antimyosin antibodies in, 1013–1014, *1014*
dual-isotope, *1016,* 1016–1017, *1017*
in infarct sizing, 1017–1019, *1018, 1019*
indications for, 1016
right ventricular, 1017
technetium-99m pyrophosphate in, 1012–1013, *1013*
in risk assessment, 988–989, 989t
nervous system dysfunction in, 1057, *1057*

Myocardial ischemia, after angioplasty, color Doppler imaging of, 360, Plate 3
and cardiomyopathy, dilated, 399
and hibernation, radionuclide imaging of, 997, *997*
and stunning, radionuclide imaging of, 996–997
and ventricular wall motion abnormalities, contrast ventriculography of, 176
and ventricular wall thickening, magnetic resonance imaging of, 769–771
effect of, on myocardial metabolism, 44–45
of protein, 47
on ventricular function, 31
regional, echocardiography of, 307, 310
electrocardiography in, vs. positron emission tomography, of myocardial metabolism, 1141–1146, *1143, 1144, 1146*
evaluation of, echocardiography in, transesophageal, 547–548
imaging of, single-photon emitting tracers for, 967–968, *968*
in coronary artery surgery, echocardiography of, 575–576
in stress echocardiography, 504
magnetic resonance imaging of, 652–653
in induced ischemia, 726–731, *727–731*
magnetic resonance spectroscopy of, 787–788, *788*
positron emission tomography in, metabolic, 1113–1168. See also *Positron emission tomography.*
of adrenergic receptors, 1197
of cardiomyopathy, dilated, 1176
ventricular wall motion in, regional abnormalities of, echocardiography of, 522–525, *523–525*
Myocardial metabolism, 34–48
after reperfusion, 44–45
and energy production, 34, *35,* 45
biochemistry of, 1172–1174, *1173*
imaging of, 5
with single-photon emitting tracers, 1020–1032
after infarction, 1028–1029, *1029*
historical aspects of, 1021
in cardiomyopathy, 1026t, 1031–1032, Plate 30
in coronary artery disease, 1026t, 1029–1031, *1030, 1031*
technical aspects of, 1027, Plate 29
tissue kinetics in, 1021–1027, *1022–1025,* 1023t, 1026t
magnetic resonance spectroscopy of, 786–787, 787t
of carbohydrates, 34–39, *36–39*
of lipids, 39–41, *40–42*
phosphate in, magnetic resonance spectroscopy of, 675, *676*
positron emission tomography of, 1113–1184. See also *Positron emission tomography.*
proteins in, 45–47, *46*
substrate interactions in, 43–45
tricarboxylic acid cycle in, 34, *35,* 41–43
Myocardial perfusion, 8–18
after infarction, thallium-201 imaging of, with antimyosin antibody imaging, of necrosis, *1016,* 1016–1017, *1017*
contrast echocardiography of, 485–499
in assessment of viability, after infarction, 486–489, *487–489,* Plate 9
in detection of infarction, 485, 485–486, *486,* Plate 9
in quantification, 489–494, *490–493*
imaging of, 4–5, *17,* 17–18
single-photon emitting tracers for, 963–968, 964t, *965–968*
vs. positron emission tomography, of myocardial metabolism, 1153–1159, *1155–1157*

Myocardial perfusion (*Continued*)
magnetic resonance imaging of, 4, 5, 669, *670*
contrast agents in, 659–664, *662–664*
radionuclide imaging of, 904–912
angiographic, 937–938, *938,* Plate 28
in coronary artery disease, 971–991
before noncardiac surgery, 990, 990t
diagnostic accuracy of, with technetium-99m, 982, *982–983*
with thallium-201, 979t–981t, *979–982*
image processing in, 975–979, *977–979,* Plate 28
in angina, 989t, 989–990
in asymptomatic patients, 983–984, *984*
in symptomatic patients, *984,* 984–985
individual artery assessment in, 985t, 985–986
planar techniques in, 975
risk assessment in, 986t, 986–988, *987, 988*
after myocardial infarction, 988–989, 989t
single-photon emission computed tomography in, 975
technetium-99m in, in investigational agents, 990–991
kinetics of, 973
thallium-201 in, *910,* 910–911, 972–973
planar methods in, 904–907, *905–907*
tomography in, with technetium-99m sestamibi, 911–912, *912*
with thallium-201, 907–911, *908–910,* Plate 23
restoration of, after ischemia, magnetic resonance imaging of, contrast agents in, 657–658, *660*
in animal studies, 720, 722, 723, *723*
metabolism after, 44–45
ultrasonic tissue characterization in, 615–616, *616, 617*
ultrafast computed tomography of, 835–850. See also *Ultrafast computed tomography.*
in congenital heart disease, 874–875
Myocardial tagging, in magnetic resonance imaging, 668, *668,* Plate 22
quantitative, automated analysis with, 779, *780*
of left ventricular function, 771–774, *772, 773*
Myocarditis, imaging of, 87
ultrasonic tissue characterization in, 618
Myocardium, blood flow to. See also *Myocardial ischemia* and *Myocardial perfusion.*
positron emission tomography of, 1094–1110. See also *Positron emission tomography.*
cardioplegia in, in coronary bypass surgery, contrast echocardiography of, 495–498, *496–498*
contractility of, assessment of, 8
effect of contrast agents on, 153–154, *153–155*
contraction of, abnormalities of, imaging of, 3
contrast agent distribution in, in magnetic resonance imaging, 654–655
contusion of, imaging of, 96, *97*
transesophageal echocardiography of, 561
in ventricular function, 20–24, *21, 22*
energetics of, 31–32, *32*
magnetic resonance imaging of, *668,* 668–669, Plates 22 and 23
mass of, measurement of, contrast ventriculography in, 175, *177*
magnetic resonance imaging in, 768–769, *770*

Myocardium (*Continued*)
    microvascular function in, contrast echocardiography of, *498*, 498–499, *499*
    oxygen consumption in, 8, 9, 31–32, *32*
    physiology of, in diastole, 336–337
    positron emission tomography of, in quantitative studies, 912–913, Plates 23 and 24
        tracer kinetics in, 1080–1081, *1081*
    restrictive diseases of, Doppler echocardiography in, 352, 354–355, *355–357*
    tissue characteristics of, imaging of, 5–6
    ultrasonography of. See *Ultrasonography.*
    viability of, assessment of, magnetic resonance imaging in, 658–659, *660, 661*
        positron emission tomography in, vs. inotropic stimulation, 1159–1161
        radionuclide imaging in, 996–1009
            in hibernation, 997, *997*
            in stunning, 996–997
            iodine-123 phenylpentadecanoic acid in, 1007
            technetium in, 1004–1007, *1005, 1006*, Plate 29
            thallium in, 997–1004, 998t, *998–1001, 1003, 1004*
        stress echocardiography in, 518
    wall of, thickening of, radionuclide imaging of, 912
Myocytes, injury to, imaging of, single-photon emitting tracers for, *966*, 966–967
    metabolism in, positron emission tomography of, 1113–1114
Myosin, antibodies to. See *Antimyosin antibodies.*
Myotonic dystrophy, cardiomyopathy in, metabolism in, positron emission tomography of, 1182–1183
Myxedema, and pericardial effusion, magnetic resonance imaging of, 753–754, *754*
Myxoma, atrial, ultrafast computed tomography of, *864*, 864–865, *865*
    cardiac, echocardiography of, 469–471, *471–473*
        transesophageal, 557, *557*
        magnetic resonance imaging of, 754–755, *755*
        ultrasonic tissue characterization in, 622

NAD, in myocardial metabolism, 34, 41–44
NADH, in myocardial metabolism, 34, 41–44
Nausea, contrast agents and, 159
Nembutal, in sedation, for magnetic resonance imaging, of aorta, 693
Neo-Iopax, as contrast agent, 147
Nephropathy, contrast agents and, *158*, 158–159, 162
Nervous system, cardiac, disorders of, in cardiomyopathy, 1174
    neurotransmitters in, 1052–1053, *1053*, 1186–1187
    physiology of, 1186–1188
    positron emission tomography of, cholinergic receptors in, 1189–1193, *1190, 1195*
        in cardiomyopathy, hypertrophic, 1197–1198
        in denervation, 1198
        in desensitization, 1198
        in heart failure, 1196–1197
        in myocardial ischemia, 1197
        presynaptic neurotransmission in, 1194–1196, *1196*
        technique of, 1188–1189
        tracers for, 1075
    radionuclide imaging of, 1052–1060
        future of, 1059–1060
        indications for, 1059
        scintigraphy in, 1053–1059, *1054, 1055, 1057*

Net magnetization, in magnetic resonance imaging, 630–632, *630–632*
Neurotransmitters. See *Nervous system.*
Nicotinamide-adenine dinucleotide, in myocardial metabolism, 34, 41–44
Nitric acid, in coronary blood flow, 11, 13–14
Nitrogen-13, in amino acid labeling, in positron emission tomography, 1075
Nitrogen-13 ammonia, in positron emission tomography, and radiation dose, 1207t
    of myocardial blood flow, 1065–1066, *1066*, 1068, 1076, *1077*, 1082–1086, *1083, 1084*, 1094, *1095, 1096*, 1098, Plates 31 and 32
        after post-infarction thrombolysis, 1124, *1126*, 1127, 1128
        with metabolic studies, after infarction, 1119–1122, *1121–1123*
            coronary artery anatomy in, 1123–1124
            in coronary artery disease, 1130, 1131, 1135, 1140, *1141*
            histopathology with, 1135, *1136*, 1137, Plate 35
            in prognosis, 1163, 1164, *1164*
            in ischemia, 1115–1118, *1119*, Plate 33
            vs. electrocardiography, *1143*, 1143–1145, *1144*
            vs. thallium scintigraphy, 1148, *1149–1151*, 1151
            in perfusion defect assessment, 1154–1157, *1157*
        of myocardial perfusion, with metabolic studies, in cardiomyopathy, dilated, 1176–1177, *1178, 1179*
            hypertrophic, *1180*, 1180–1181, *1181*
            in Duchenne muscular dystrophy, 1182, *1182*
Nitroglycerin, before coronary angiography, 226
    effect of, on blood velocity, 345, *345*
Nitroprusside, effect of, on diastolic function, 28, *28*
NOET, in myocardial perfusion imaging, 963, 964t, 966, 968
Noise, acoustic, definition of, 1209
    definition of, 1213
    in digital imaging, 116
        reduction of, 119–120
    in magnetic resonance imaging, quantitative, 763, 764
    in ultrafast computed tomography, 808, *808*, 809t
    in x-ray image formation, 110
    ratio of, to contrast, definition of, 1210
        to signal, definition of, 1216
Norepinephrine, in cardiac nervous system, 1052–1054, *1053, 1054*, 1186–1188
    in cardiomyopathy, hypertrophic, 1179–1180
    in positron emission tomography, in heart failure, 1196–1197
        of presynaptic neurotransmission, 1195, 1196
Nuclear magnetic resonance imaging, 629–790. See also *Magnetic resonance imaging.*
Nuclear Overhauser enhancement, in magnetic resonance spectroscopy, 785
Nuclear spin, definition of, 1213
Nuclear spin quantum number, definition of, 1213
Nuclear stethoscope, in radiation detection, 891–892
Nutation, definition of, 1213
Nyquist limit, definition of, 1213
    in Doppler measurement, of blood flow velocity, 293, *294*

Object size correction, in single-photon emission computed tomography, 899
Omnipaque. See *Iohexol.*
Optiray. See *Ioversol.*
Orientation, definition of, 1213
Osler-Weber-Rendu disease, pulmonary artery malformations in, 861
Osteosarcoma, cardiac, echocardiography of, 476
Ovaries, radiation dose to, in diagnostic radiology, 1206t, 1207t
    with indium-111 platelet imaging, of thrombosis, 1035
Overhauser enhancement, in magnetic resonance spectroscopy, 785
2-Oxoglutarate dehydrogenase, in tricarboxylic acid cycle regulation, 42
Oxygen, myocardial consumption of, 8, 9, 31–32, *32*
Oxygen-15, carbon monoxide labeled with, in positron emission tomography, in left ventricular function assessment, 1078–1080
    water labeled with, in imaging, and radiation dose, 1207t
        in positron emission tomography, of myocardial blood flow, *1066*, 1066–1068, 1083–1086, *1084*, 1094
            after infarction, 1124–1127
Oxyhemoglobin, in magnetic resonance imaging, 636t

P280, radiolabeled, in imaging of thrombosis, 1047
Pacemakers, and ischemia, ventricular function in, 31
    and tachycardia, with coronary vasodilation, 11, *12*
    in echocardiography, stress, 506, 516
        vs. cardiac mass lesions, 459–463, *461, 462*
    in magnetic resonance imaging, 1213
    with positron emission tomography, of myocardial metabolism, in ischemia, 1115, *1116*
PADGEM protein, antibody to, in imaging of thrombosis, 1047
Pain, in chest. See *Angina.*
Palmitate, carbon-11–labeled. See *Carbon-11 palmitate.*
Pannus, and prosthetic valve dysfunction, echocardiography of, 556
Papaverine, and hyperemia, in digital angiography, 262, Plate 1
    in coronary vasodilation, 11
Papillary fibroelastoma, echocardiography of, 473, *474*
Papillary muscles, calcification of, 459, *460*
    rupture of, in myocardial infarction, *526*, 527, *527*, Plate 10
15-Para-iodophenyl pentadecanoic acid (IPPA). See *Iodine-123 iodophenyl pentadecanoic acid.*
15-Para-iodophenyl-3,3-dimethyl pentadecanoic acid, in imaging, of myocardial metabolism, 1025–1026
15-Para-iodophenyl-3-R,S-methyl pentadecanoic acid. See *Iodine-123 betamethyl iodophenyl pentadecanoic acid.*
Paramagnetism, definition of, 1213–1214
    in contrast agents, in magnetic resonance imaging, 653, 654
Partial Fourier imaging, definition of, 1214
Partial saturation, definition of, 1214
Partial saturation spin echo, definition of, 1214
Partial volume effects, in magnetic resonance imaging, quantitative, 763

Partial volume effects (*Continued*)
 in positron emission tomography, 1078–1079, *1079*
Patent ductus arteriosus, echocardiography of, 424–427, *424–427*, 431, Plate 7
Patent foramen ovale, shunting in, contrast echocardiography of, 499
 transesophageal echocardiography of, 557
Penicillin, prophylactic use of, with transesophageal echocardiography, in congenital heart disease, 450
Peptides, in myocardial metabolism, 45–46, *46*
Perfluorpropane, in albumin microspheres, in contrast echocardiography, 482
Perfusion, myocardial, 8–18. See also *Myocardial perfusion.*
Pericardial effusion, computed tomography of, ultrafast, 869, *869*
 echocardiography of, 405–409, *406–409*
 magnetic resonance imaging of, 753–754, *754*
Pericardial tamponade, imaging of, 94
Pericardiocentesis, for cardiac tamponade, echocardiography during, 412–413, *413*
Pericarditis, acute, echocardiography of, 416
 imaging of, 93–94
 chronic, echocardiography of, 416
 constrictive, echocardiography of, 413–416, *413–417*
  Doppler, 350–354, *352, 353*
  imaging of, 94
  ultrafast computed tomography of, 825, *826*, 869, *870*
 magnetic resonance imaging of, 752, 753, *753*
Pericardium, absence of, echocardiography of, 417
 anatomy of, 752
 blood in, with aortic aneurysm, magnetic resonance imaging of, 705, *707*
 cancer of, echocardiography of, 408, *409*, 416, 468, *469*
 cysts of, echocardiography of, 417, *418*, 468, *470*, 474–475
  ultrafast computed tomography of, 869–870, *870*
 echocardiography of, normal, 404–405, *405*
 effect of, on ventricular function, in diastole, 27–28
 hematoma of, after cardiac surgery, echocardiography of, 417
  vs. cardiac tamponade, 410–411, *411*
 magnetic resonance imaging of, 752–754, *753*, 753t, *754*
 mass lesions of, imaging of, 94–95
 radiography of, 139–141, *139–141*
 trauma to, echocardiography of, 416–417
  imaging of, 96, *97*
 ultrafast computed tomography of, 867–870, *868–870*
  contrast agents in, 864, 868
  imaging sequences in, 863–864
  radiation dose in, 864, 868
Permeability, in magnetic resonance imaging, definition of, 1214
Persistent truncus arteriosus, echocardiography of, 440, *440, 441*
Phantom, definition of, 1214
Phase, definition of, 1214
Phase analysis, in radionuclide ventriculography, 917–919, *918, 919,* Plate 24
Phase correction, definition of, 1214
Phase cycling, definition of, 1214
Phase encoding, definition of, 1214
 in magnetic resonance imaging, 643, *644, 645*
  respiratory-ordered, 651
  quantitative, 761, *761*
Phase mapping, in magnetic resonance imaging, of aorta, 695, *695–696*

Phase-contrast technique, in magnetic resonance imaging, of blood flow, in coronary arteries, 736–737, 777–779, *778*
 quantitative, 774, 775
Phased array transducers, in echocardiography, 283–284, *284, 285*
Phenol, in nerve degeneration, before radionuclide imaging, 1055, 1056
Phenylephrine, radiolabeled, in positron emission tomography, of presynaptic neurotransmission, 1195
Phenylpropanolamine, and metaiodobenzylguanidine concentration, in imaging of nervous system, 1056
Phosphates, in myocardial metabolism, in magnetic resonance spectroscopy, 675, *676*
Phosphines. See also specific compounds, e.g., *Technetium-99m tetrofosmin.*
 in myocardial perfusion imaging, 963–968, 964t, *965*
Phosphocreatine, in magnetic resonance spectroscopy, 675, *676*, 784, 786–790, 787t, *787–789*
 in myocardial metabolism, 675, *676*, 1173–1174
Phosphofructokinase, in myocardial metabolism, 37, *37–38*, 43
Phosphorus, in magnetic resonance spectroscopy, 784, *785*
 in congenital heart disease, 675, *676*
Photoelectric effect, in x-ray absorption, 103
Photons. See also entries at *Single-photon.*
 detection of, in radionuclide imaging, 888, 888–889, *889*
 in x-rays, 102–103
 scatter of, in ultrafast computed tomography, of myocardial perfusion, *846, 846–847*
Piezoelectricity, in ultrasound, 275, *275*, 275t
Pincushion distortion, of digital images, 121
Pindolol, carbon-11–labeled, in positron emission tomography, of cardiac nervous system, 1190, *1192*
Pirenzepine, as cholinergic receptor antagonist, 1187–1188
Pixels, in digital imaging, 60–69, 1214
PK-11195, in positron emission tomography, 1075, 1194
Planar imaging, definition of, 1214
Plaque, arteriosclerotic. See *Atherosclerosis.*
Plasminogen activator, for pulmonary embolism, angiography after, 213–214
 in thrombolysis, for myocardial infection, positron emission tomography after, 1124–1125
 radiolabeled, in imaging of thrombosis, 1047
Platelets, indium-111–labeled. See *Indium-111.*
Pleural effusion, vs. pericardial effusion, echocardiography of, 409, *409*
Point spread function, of image resolution, 106
Polar mapping, of myocardium, in radionuclide imaging, 912–913, Plates 23 and 24
Polysplenia, atrial situs ambiguus with, echocardiography of, 445, *446*
 magnetic resonance imaging of, 676
Polytetrafluoroethylene, in prosthetic grafts, and thrombosis, indium-111 platelet imaging of, 1045, *1046*
Positron emission tomography, 1063–1199
 attenuation in, 901, *903*, 903–904
 future of, 1088
 image acquisition in, 1076–1080, *1077–1079*, Plate 31
 of cardiomyopathy, 88
 of coronary arteries, in blood flow measurement, 17, *17*

Positron emission tomography (*Continued*)
 stenotic, 81–83
 of myocardial blood flow, after heart transplantation, 1095t, 1109–1110
 image acquisition in, 1098, Plate 32
 image analysis in, *1098*, 1098–1099
 in cardiomyopathy, 1095t, 1110
 in coronary artery disease, *1099*, 1099–1100
  accuracy of, 1100t, 1100–1101
  after treatment, 1107–1108, *1108*, Plate 32
  collateral vessels in, 1104–1106, *1105*
  in asymptomatic patients, 1107
  limitations of, 1104
  localization in, 1101, *1101*
  preclinical, 1103, *1104*
  transient ischemia in, *1106*, 1106–1107, *1107*
  vasodilator capacity in, 1101–1103, *1102*
  vs. single-photon emission computed tomography, 1099, 1103–1104, *1104*, 1105t
 in syndrome X, 1095t, 1108–1109
 regional, 1081–1086, *1083, 1084*, 1094t, 1094–1096, *1095*, 1095t, *1096*
  stress testing in, 1094t, 1094–1096, *1095*, 1095t, *1096*
   electrocardiography with, 1098
   selection of agents for, 1096–1097, 1097t
 of myocardial infarction, vs. magnetic resonance imaging, 725–726
 of myocardial metabolism, 5
  after infarction, 1119–1122, *1121–1123*
   coronary artery anatomy and, 1123–1124
   electrocardiography with, 1122–1123
   thrombolysis in, 1124–1129, *1125, 1126, 1129*
  in cardiomyopathy, dilated, 1174–1178, *1175, 1177–1180*, Plate 35
   future of, 1183–1184
   hypertrophic, 1178–1181, *1180, 1181*
   in acyl coenzyme A dehydrogenase deficiency, 1183, *1183*
   in Duchenne muscular dystrophy, 1181–1183, *1182*
  in clinical management, 1167–1168
  in coronary artery disease, 1129–1135, 1130t, 1131t, 1139–1141, *1141, 1142*, 1142t, Plates 33 and 34
   histopathology with, 1135–1139, *1136–1138*, Plate 35
   in prognosis, 1161–1165, *1162*, 1162t, *1164*, 1165t
  in ischemia, 1113–1168
   acute, 1114–1119, *1116, 1117, 1119*, Plate 33
    ventricular wall motion abnormalities with, 1146–1147
   vs. electrocardiography, 1141–1146, *1143, 1144, 1146*
   vs. perfusion defect imaging, 1153–1159, *1155–1157*
   vs. thallium scintigraphy, 1147–1153, 1148t, *1149–1151*
  indications for, 1165–1166
  of glucose, *1086*, 1086–1088, *1087*, 1088t
  patient care during, 1166
  study conditions in, standardization of, 1166–1167
 of myocardial perfusion, 4–5
 of myocardium, in viability assessment, vs. inotropic stimulation, 1159–1161
  vs. single-photon emission computed tomography, 1008
   with technetium, 1006, Plate 29
  quantitative, 912–913, Plates 23 and 24
 of nervous system, cardiac, 1186–1199

Positron emission tomography (*Continued*)
in cardiomyopathy, hypertrophic, 1197–1198
in denervation, 1198
in desensitization, 1198
in heart failure, 1196–1197
in myocardial ischemia, 1197
in presynaptic neurotransmission studies, 1194–1196, *1196*
in receptor studies, 1189–1194, *1190, 1191, 1193–1195*
technique of, 1188–1189
quantitation in, 58, 60
scanners in, 900–903, *901–903*
tracers in, 1064, 1064t
in cardiac nerve imaging, 1075
kinetics of, 1080–1081, *1081*
of myocardial blood flow, 1064t, 1064–1068, *1065, 1066*
of myocardial metabolism, 1068t, 1068–1075, *1069–1074*, 1075t, Plate 31
Potassium, in myocardial contraction, 23
in myocardial perfusion imaging, 963, 964t
Practolol, carbon-11–labeled, in positron emission tomography, of cardiac nervous system, 1188–1190, 1192
Preamplifiers, in magnetic resonance imaging, 646, *647*
Precession, definition of, 1214
steady-state free, definition of, 1217
Prednisone, for allergy, to contrast agents, in pulmonary angiography, 208
Preload, atrial, and diastolic filling, 342
Premature ventricular contractions, in radionuclide angiography, equilibrium, 943
first-pass, 927–928, *928*
Pressure, and volume, end-systolic, 29, *29*–30
measurement of, in congenital heart disease, magnetic resonance imaging in, 680–681, *680–682*
in diastole, 26–27
in ventricular energetics, 32, *32*
in ventricular mechanics, *24*, 24–25, *25*
left ventricular, measurement of, contrast ventriculography in, 194, *194*
Pressure overload, and left ventricular hypertrophy, 31
Pressure waves, atrial, in normal function, 55–56, *56*
Probes, in magnetic resonance imaging, definition of, 1214
Progressive scan fluoroscopy, 112–113, 120
Promethazine, before coronary angiography, 226
Propagation speed, in ultrasonography, in tissue characterization, 607
Propranolol, and left ventricular function changes, Doppler echocardiography of, 329
carbon-11–labeled, in positron emission tomography, of cardiac nervous system, 1188–1190, 1192
Prostacyclin, in coronary blood flow, 11, 13
Prostaglandin I$_2$, in prevention of thrombosis, with prosthetic materials, indium-111 platelet imaging of, 1045–1046
Prosthetic materials, and thrombosis, indium-111 platelet imaging of, 1043t, 1043–1046, *1044–1046*
Prosthetic valves, and distortion, in magnetic resonance imaging, quantitative, 764, *764*
evaluation of, echocardiography in, 387–389, *388*
transesophageal, 555–556, Plates 12 and 13
Protein, in myocardial metabolism, 45–47, *46*
Protons, in nuclear magnetic resonance, 629–633, *630–633*
in biologic tissue, 633–635, 637t
Pseudoaneurysm, after myocardial infarction, echocardiography of, 527–528, *528*

Pseudoaneurysm (*Continued*)
magnetic resonance imaging of, 726, *726*
of aorta, angiography of, *201*, 204, *206*
thoracic, magnetic resonance imaging of, 705, *705, 706*
PTSM, in positron emission tomography, of myocardial blood flow, *1066, 1067*, 1085
Pulmonary. See also *Lungs.*
Pulmonary angiography, 208–218
contraindications to, 208
in congenital lung dysplasia, 216–217
indications for, 208
of aneurysm, 215, *218*
of arterial stenosis, 215, *217*
of arteriovenous fistula, 214–215, *217*
of embolism, 210–214, *211–216*
of sequestration, 216
of tumors, 216, *218*
of varices, 215
technique of, 208–210
Pulmonary arteries, anatomy of, 210
aneurysm of, angiography of, 215, *218*
angiography of, 208–218. See also *Pulmonary angiography.*
anomalies of, contrast echocardiography of, 499
imaging of, 100
ultrafast computed tomography of, 877, *877–879, 882–885*
blood flow in, in cardiac tamponade, echocardiography of, 411, *412*
in congenital heart disease, magnetic resonance measurement of, 681, *682*
after surgery, 685–689, *688, 689*
with left-to-right shunting, measurement of, Doppler echocardiography in, 430–431
compression of, by aortic aneurysm, computed tomography of, 855
connection of, to descending aorta, 424–427, *424–427*, 431, Plate 7
echocardiography of, transesophageal, 538, *538, 539*, 543, *543*, 556
embolism of, imaging of, 100, 210–214, *211–216*, 218
indium-111 in, 1043
enlargement of, radiography of, 134, *137, 138*
in identification of cardiac chambers, in echocardiography, of congenital heart disease, 443, *443*
in tetralogy of Fallot, echocardiography of, 437, *437*
left coronary artery origin from, angiography of, 236
pressure in, echocardiographic measurement of, in cardiomyopathy, 401
radiography of, 126, 127
stenosis of, angiography of, 215, *217*
thrombosis of, echocardiography of, *464*, 465
transposition of, with aorta, echocardiography of, *439*, 439–440, *440*, 442, 445–448, *447*
magnetic resonance imaging of, 678, *679*
after surgery, 689, *689–690, 690*
ultrafast computed tomography of, 876–877, *877–882*
tumors of, angiography of, 216, *218*
ultrafast computed tomography of, 813, *815*, 859–861, *860*
Pulmonary capillaries, albumin microbubbles in, in contrast echocardiography, 481
wedge pressure in, measurement of, radionuclide angiography of, 946
Pulmonary disease, chronic obstructive, radionuclide angiography in, first-pass, 939
right ventricular enlargement with, radiography of, 131, *134*
Pulmonary edema, in congestive heart failure, radiography of, 139, *139*

Pulmonary hypertension, as contraindication to angiography, 208
in congenital heart disease, assessment of, magnetic resonance imaging in, 689
right ventricular enlargement with, radiography of, 131, *132–134*
ultrafast computed tomography in, 861
Pulmonary regurgitation, echocardiography of, 387, Plate 6
in tetralogy of Fallot, magnetic resonance imaging of, *684, 685, 686, 687*
Pulmonary sequestration, angiography of, 216
Pulmonary stenosis, congenital, balloon valvuloplasty for, 91
echocardiography of, 435–436, *436*
echocardiography of, 387
magnetic resonance imaging of, 712
in tetralogy of Fallot, *684, 685*
Pulmonary transit time, assessment of, contrast echocardiography in, 501
Pulmonary valve, atresia of, echocardiography of, 438, *439*
blood flow through, echocardiography of, in pericarditis, 415, *415*
disorders of, imaging of, 86
transesophageal echocardiography of, 555
in tetralogy of Fallot, echocardiography of, 437, *437*
Pulmonary veins, abnormalities of, ultrafast computed tomography of, 875, *876*, 877–879, *884*
anatomy of, 210
anomalous connection of, angiography of, 217
echocardiography of, 440–441, *441, 442*, Plate 7
blood flow in, in mitral regurgitation, echocardiography of, Doppler, 382
transesophageal, 554, *554*
measurement of, Doppler echocardiography in, 347, *348*, 348t
in pericarditis, constrictive, 351, *353*
velocity patterns of, in diastole, 344–345, *345*
echocardiography of, in congenital heart disease, 443, *443*
transesophageal, 540, *540*, Plate 10
enlargement of, radiography of, 134
in cardiomyopathy, pressure measurement in, echocardiographic, 401
in congestive heart failure, radiography of, 139, *139*
in transposition of great arteries, surgery of, magnetic resonance imaging after, 689, 689–690, *690*
junction of, with left atrium, echocardiography of, vs. mass lesion, 457, *457*
radiography of, 126, 127
varices of, angiography of, 215
Pulse, radiofrequency, definition of, 1214
Pulse length, definition of, 1214
Pulse programmer, definition of, 1214
Pulse sequences, in magnetic resonance imaging, acronyms for, 1214–1215
definition of, 1214
in slice selection, 640, *640*
Pulse width, definition of, 1214
Pyrophosphate, technetium-99m, in imaging of myocardial necrosis, 1012–1013, *1013*
accuracy of, 1015
in infarct sizing, 1017–1019, *1019*
right ventricular, 1017
Pyruvaldehyde-bis-(thiosemicarbazone), in positron emission tomography, of myocardial blood flow, *1066, 1067*
Pyruvate, in myocardial metabolism, 37, 37–38, *38*

Q3, in myocardial perfusion imaging, 963
in coronary artery disease, 991

Q12, in myocardial perfusion imaging, 963, 964t, 966–968
  in coronary artery disease, 991
Q waves, in electrocardiography, in myocardial ischemia, vs. positron emission tomography, 1141–1146, *1143*, *1144*, *1146*
QNB, in positron emission tomography, of cardiac neurotransmission, 1188–1190, *1190*, 1192–1193, *1195*
Quantitation, acoustic, in ejection fraction measurement, 304–306, *305*, *306*
  in cardiac imaging, 58–60, *59*, 59t
  in digital imaging, 116
  errors in, 62, *62–63*
  in magnetic resonance imaging, 759–780. See also *Magnetic resonance imaging, quantitative.*
Quantitative analysis, of digital images, 121–122
Quantum detection efficiency, in image intensification, 111
Quantum noise, in x-ray image formation, 110
Quantum number, nuclear spin, definition of, 1213
  spin, definition of, 1217
Quenching, definition of, 1215
Quinuclidinyl benzilate (QNB), in positron emission tomography, of cardiac neurotransmission, 1188–1190, *1190*, 1192–1193, *1195*

Rad, in radiation dosimetry, 1205, 1205t
Radian, definition of, 1215
Radiation, detection of, nuclear stethoscope for, 891–892
  VEST for, 892
  dose of, in computed tomography, 803–805, *804*, *805*, 805t
    ultrafast, of great vessels, 855
    measurement of, 1205, 1205t
      in medical exposure, 1205–1208, 1206t, 1207t
      in natural exposure, 1206
      with indium-111 platelet imaging, of thrombosis, 1035
  protection against, 122t, 122–124
Radiofrequency, definition of, 1215
Radiofrequency data analysis, in ultrasonic tissue characterization, 608, *608*
Radiofrequency pulse, definition of, 1214
  in magnetic resonance imaging, 631, *631*
Radiofrequency systems, in magnetic resonance imaging, 645–646, *647*
Radiography. See also specific techniques, e.g., *Ultrafast computed tomography.*
  aortic enlargement in, 131–134, *135*, *136*
  calcifications in, 141–143, *141–143*
  contrast agents in, 144–162. See also *Contrast agents* and specific agents, e.g., *Iodine.*
  of aortic aneurysm, 99
  of aortic dissection, 99
  of aortic stenosis, 84
  of cardiac chamber enlargement, 128–131, *129–134*
  of cardiomyopathy, dilated, 87
  of chest, 126–143
    interpretation of, sequence of, 127–128
    normal, 128, *129*
    positional abnormalities in, 143, *143*
    purposes of, 126
    radiation dose in, 1206t, 1207t
    technical aspects of, 126–127
  of congestive heart failure, 134–139, *138*, *139*
  of heart anatomy, 1
  of left ventricular size, in aortic regurgitation, 85

Radiography (*Continued*)
  in mitral regurgitation, 85
  of mitral stenosis, 85
  of myocarditis, 87
  of pericarditis, 93, 94
  of pericardium, 139–141, *139–141*
  of pulmonary artery embolism, 100
  of pulmonary blood vessel enlargement, 134, *137*, *138*
  paracardiac densities in, 143
Radionuclide angiography, equilibrium, 941–958
  after myocardial infarction, 954–956, *955*
  in cardiotoxicity, after antitumor therapy, 958
  in chest pain, in diagnosis, 947t, 947–949, *948*, 948t
    in patient management, 954
  in dyspneic patient, 958
  of cardiomyopathy, 956
  of coronary artery disease, in prognosis, *951–953*, 951–954
    severe, 949t, 949–951, *950*
  of diastolic function, 946–947
  of ejection fraction, 944, 944t, 946
  of left ventricular output, 946
  of left ventricular volume, *945*, 945–946
  of left ventricular wall motion, regional, 944–945, *945*
  of regurgitant fraction, 946
  of valvular heart disease, 956–958, *956–958*
  technical aspects of, 942–944, *943*
  vs. first-pass, 939
  first-pass, 923–939
    data acquisition in, *924*, 924–927, *925*, *927*, Plate 24
    data interpretation in, *931*, 931–934, *933–936*, Plates 26 and 27
    data processing in, 927–931, *928*, 929t, *930*, Plates 25 and 26
    of coronary artery disease, 935–939, 937t, *938*, 938t, *939*, Plates 27 and 28
    vs. equilibrium method, 939
  of aortic regurgitation, 85
  of ejection fraction, vs. ultrafast computed tomography, 824, *824*
  of mitral regurgitation, 86
  of myocardial infarction, vs. magnetic resonance imaging, 725, *725*
Radionuclide imaging, 887–1060. See also specific agents, e.g., *Technetium.*
  future developments in, 919–920
  image acquisition in, 892–895, *893*, *894*
  in positron emission tomography, 900–904, *901–903*. See also *Positron emission tomography.*
  in single-photon emission computed tomography, 895–897, *895–900*, *899–901*, 900t. See also *Single-photon emission computed tomography.*
  in ventriculography, in myocardial quantitative studies, 913–919, *915–919*, Plate 24
  of cardiac anatomy, 1
  of coronary artery disease, vs. digital angiography, 266, *266*, *267*
  of coronary artery disease, vs. stress echocardiography, 514–515, *515*, 515t
  of myocardial necrosis, 1012–1019
    accuracy of, 1014–1016, *1015*
    antimyosin antibodies in, 1013–1014, *1014*
    dual-isotope, *1016*, 1016–1017, *1017*
    indications for, 1016
    right ventricular, 1017
    technetium-99m pyrophosphate in, 1012–1013, *1013*
  of myocardial perfusion, 904–912. See also *Myocardial perfusion.*

Radionuclide imaging (*Continued*)
  planar methods in, 904–907, *905–907*
  single-photon emitting tracers in, 963–968, 964t, *965*, *967*, *968*
  tomography in, with technetium-99m sestamibi, 911–912, *912*
    with thallium-201, 907–911, *908–910*, Plate 23
  vs. contrast echocardiography, 489
  of myocardium, in assessment of viability, 996–1009
    in hibernation, 997, *997*
    in stunning, 996–997
    iodine-123 phenylpentadecanoic acid in, 1007
    technetium in, 1004–1007, *1005*, *1006*, *1008*, Plate 29
    thallium in, 997–1004, 998t, *998–1001*, *1003*, *1004*
  of nervous system, cardiac, 1052–1060, *1054*, *1055*, *1057*
  of thrombosis. See *Thrombosis.*
  radiation detection in, principles of, *888*, 888–889, *889*
  scintillation cameras in, 889–891, *889–891*
  ventilation-perfusion, of pulmonary artery embolism, 100
Radon's equation, in image reconstruction, in computed tomography, 793–794
Ramp filter, in single-photon emission computed tomography, 896, *896–897*, *897*
Ramp time, definition of, 1215
Rapid-excitation magnetic resonance imaging, definition of, 1215
Rastelli's operation, magnetic resonance imaging after, 685
Receiver, in magnetic resonance imaging, definition of, 1215
Receiver dead time, in magnetic resonance imaging, definition of, 1215
Receiver operating characteristic analysis, in image interpretation, 75, *75–76*
Red blood cells, radiolabeled, in angiography, equilibrium, 942
  in imaging, and radiation dose, 1207t
Reference compound, definition of, 1215
Reflection, in ultrasound transmission, 276–277, *277*
Refraction, in ultrasound transmission, 276–277, *277*
Region growing, in segmentation, in digital imaging, 69
Region partitioning, in segmentation, in digital imaging, 69
Rejection, of transplanted heart, magnetic resonance imaging of, 751
  myocardial blood flow in, positron emission tomography of, 1095t, 1109
  ultrasonic tissue characterization in, 623
Relaxation, myocardial, in ventricular filling, 26
Relaxation rates, definition of, 1215
Relaxation time, definition of, 1215
  in magnetic resonance imaging, 631–633, *632*, *633*
  of heart, 637, 637t, 637–638
  spin-lattice, definition of, 1217
  spin-spin, definition of, 1217
Rem, in radiation dosimetry, 1205, 1205t
Renal. See *Kidneys.*
Renin-angiotensin-aldosterone system, abnormalities of, in cardiomyopathy, 1174
Renografin. See *Diatrizoate.*
Reperfusion, myocardial, magnetic resonance imaging of, after infarction, in animal studies, 720, *722*, *723*, *723*
  contrast agents in, 657–658, *660*

Reperfusion (Continued)
metabolism after, 44–45
ultrasonic tissue characterization in, 615–616, 616, 617
Repetition time, definition of, 1218
Rephasing gradient, definition of, 1215
Repolarization, prolonged, contrast agents and, 154–155, 156
Reserpine, and metaiodobenzylguanidine uptake, in imaging, of cardiac nervous system, 1055
radiolabeled, in positron emission tomography, of presynaptic neurotransmission, 1195
Resistance, to coronary blood flow, measurement of, 9, 9–11, 10
Resolution, in digital imaging, definition of, 60
in echocardiography, 278–280, 278–280
in image formation, in cardiac angiography, 106–107, 107, 107t, 108
in image intensification, 111
in magnetic resonance imaging, quantitative, 761–763, 762
in positron emission tomography, 902–903
in single-photon emission computed tomography, 895, 895
in ultrafast computed tomography, 805–808, 806–808, 807t
spatial, definition of, 1216
Resolution element, definition of, 1215
Resonance, definition of, 1215
nuclear. See also Magnetic resonance imaging.
physics of, 629–633, 630–633
Resonance frequency, definition of, 1215
Respiration, and hemodynamic changes, in cardiac tamponade, 411, 412
in pericarditis, constrictive, 416, 417
and motion artifacts, in magnetic resonance imaging, gating for, 650–651
of aorta, 693–694
phase encoding for, 650–651
quantitative, 761, 761, 763
Reverse mapping, in digital image enhancement, 64–67
Reversibility analysis, in myocardial perfusion assessment, 906
Rhabdomyoma, echocardiography of, 471, 473
Rhabdomyosarcoma, echocardiography of, 476, 476
Rheumatic disease, and aortic regurgitation, echocardiography of, 372
and mitral regurgitation, echocardiography of, 381
intraoperative, 572
transesophageal, 553, Plate 12
magnetic resonance imaging of, 712, 713
and mitral stenosis, echocardiography of, 377, 377
left atrial thrombosis in, 465, 465
magnetic resonance imaging of, 712–713
and tricuspid regurgitation, surgery for, echocardiography in, Plate 16
and tricuspid stenosis, echocardiography of, 383
Ribonucleic acid (RNA), in myocardial protein metabolism, 45, 46, 46
Right atrium. See also Atrium (atria).
angiosarcoma of, echocardiography of, 475, 475–476
Chiari network in, echocardiography of, vs. mass lesions, 453, 453–454
echocardiography of, transesophageal, 538, 540, 543, 543
enlargement of, radiography of, 128–131, 130, 131
in cardiac tamponade, echocardiography of, 409–411, 410, 411
junction of, with superior vena cava, echocardiography of, vs. mass lesion, 456, 457

Right atrium (Continued)
location of, in congenital heart disease, echocardiographic, 442–445, 443–446
magnetic resonance imaging in, 676, 677, 678
pulmonary venous drainage into, echocardiography of, 440–441, 441, 442, Plate 7
systolic function of, Doppler echocardiography of, 331, 332, 332
thrombi in, echocardiography of, 463, 463
volume of, measurement of, magnetic resonance imaging in, 767
Right ventricle. See also Ventricle(s).
blood flow into, measurement of, Doppler echocardiography in, 342, 343, 347
magnetic resonance imaging in, 777
double-outlet, echocardiography of, 437, 437, 438
ejection fraction of, radionuclide angiography of, 946
enlargement of, radiography of, 131, 132–134
function of, assessment of, digital angiography in, 255, 255
imaging of, 3
in radionuclide angiography, first-pass, 929–930, 930
systolic, echocardiography of, 317–320, 318, 319
Doppler, 331–333, 332
in cardiac tamponade, echocardiography of, 409–411, 410, 411
in congenital heart disease, location of, echocardiography in, 442, 443, 443–445
morphology of, magnetic resonance imaging of, 676–677, 679
infarction of, echocardiography of, 527
necrosis after, radionuclide imaging of, 1017
interaction of, with left ventricle, in diastolic function, 27–28
in systolic function, 30
moderator band of, echocardiography of, vs. mass lesions, 454, 454
obstructed outflow from, congenital, echocardiography of, 435–436, 436
systolic pressure in, in tricuspid regurgitation, Doppler measurement of, 386, 386
thrombi in, echocardiography of, 464, 465
transesophageal echocardiography of, 540, 541, 542
ventriculography of, 192
volume of, measurement of, magnetic resonance imaging in, 766–767
RNA, in myocardial protein metabolism, 45, 46, 46
RO 5-4864, in positron emission tomography, of benzodiazepine receptors, 1194
Roentgenography. See Radiography.
Ross procedure, in aortic valve replacement, transesophageal echocardiography after, 555
Rotating frame of reference, in magnetic resonance imaging, 1215
Rotating frame zeugmatography, in magnetic resonance spectroscopy, 785–786, 786
Rotating reference frame, in magnetic resonance imaging, 631–633, 632
Rubidium, in imaging, and radiation dose, 1207t
of myocardial perfusion, 963, 967, 968
in positron emission tomography, 1075
of myocardial blood flow, 1066, 1067, 1068, 1085, 1094, 1098
with metabolic studies, in coronary artery disease, 1139, 1162, 1163
in ischemia, 1117, 1117, 1118
in perfusion defect assessment, 1156, 1156

St. Jude prosthetic valve, transesophageal echocardiography of, 556, Plates 13 and 15
Sampling, in digital imaging, 60, 115–116
definition of, 1215
Saphenous vein, in coronary bypass grafts. See Coronary arteries, bypass surgery of.
Sarcoidosis, and cardiomyopathy, echocardiography of, 402
Doppler, 354
Sarcoma, of heart, echocardiography of, 475, 475–476, 476
of pulmonary arteries, angiography of, 216
Sarcomeres, myocardial, 20, 21
Saturation, in magnetic resonance imaging, definition of, 1214, 1215
Saturation recovery, definition of, 1215
Saturation transfer, definition of, 1215–1216
Scatter, acoustic, in ultrasonography, 277, 277
in tissue characterization, 607–608
in radionuclide imaging, of myocardial perfusion, in coronary artery disease, 983
in single-photon emission computed tomography, 897–898
of x-rays, 103
reduction of, in angiography, 109, 110
Scatter radiation, protection against, 123
Schoonmaker technique, in coronary angiography, 229, 229
Scimitar syndrome, pulmonary blood vessels in, angiography of, 217
ultrafast computed tomography of, 875, 876
Scintigraphy. See Radionuclide imaging and specific agents, e.g., Thallium-201.
Scintillation (gamma) cameras, in radionuclide imaging, 889–891, 889–891
angiographic, 925, 925–926
Scintillation counter, in radionuclide imaging, 888, 888–889, 889
Secobarbital, in sedation, for coronary angiography, 226
Secundum atrial septal defect, right ventricular enlargement with, radiography of, 132
Sedation, for coronary angiography, 226
for magnetic resonance imaging, 693
for transesophageal echocardiography, 537
Selectan, as contrast agent, 145, 146
Selective excitation, definition of, 1216
Senning operation, magnetic resonance imaging after, 689, 689–690, 690
ultrafast computed tomography after, 876
Sensitive plane, definition of, 1216
Sequestration, pulmonary, angiography of, 216
Serosa, of pericardium, anatomy of, 752
Sestamibi. See Technetium-99m sestamibi.
Shaded-surface displays, in image reconstruction, three-dimensional, 59, 59, 60
Shadow phenomenon, in ultrafast computed tomography, of myocardial perfusion, 487, 846, 846
Shielding, active, definition of, 1209
magnetic, definition of, 1213
Shift reagents, definition of, 1216
Shim coils, definition of, 1216
Shimming, definition of, 1216
Shunt(ing), contrast echocardiography of, 499, 500
in atrial septal defect, echocardiography of, 423, 423–424, Plate 7
magnetic resonance imaging of, 673, 682, 684, 685
in atrioventricular septal defect, echocardiography of, 427, 430, Plate 7
in congenital heart disease, in surgical management, magnetic resonance imaging of, 685
right-to-left, echocardiography of, 436–438, 437–439

Shunt(ing) (Continued)
    ultrafast computed tomography of, 873, 873–874, 875
    in patent ductus arteriosus, echocardiography of, Plate 7, 424–427, 424–427
    in ventricular septal defect, echocardiography of, 422, 422–423, Plate 6
    left-to-right, quantitation of, Doppler echocardiography in, 430–431
        magnetic resonance imaging in, 774, 776
        radiography of, interpretation of, 76
        radionuclide angiography of, 933–934, 935, 936, Plate 27
    pulmonary arteriovenous, contrast echocardiography of, 499
Sievert, in radiation dosimetry, 1205, 1205t
Signal averaging, definition of, 1216
Signal-to-noise ratio, definition of, 1216
    in digital imaging, 116
Simpson's rule, in myocardial mass measurement, 769
    in quantitation, for digital image processing, 59
    in volume measurement, atrial, 767
        left ventricular, 298, 299, 765, 765–766, 768
        right ventricular, 767
Single-photon emission computed tomography, image acquisition in, 895
    image interpretation in, 897–900, 899, 900, 900t
    image reconstruction in, 896, 896–897, 897
    in cardiomyopathy, hypertrophic, vs. positron emission tomography, 1181
    in coronary artery disease, 81–83
        chronic, myocardial metabolism in, 1026t, 1029–1031, 1031
        vs. stress echocardiography, 514–515, 515, 515t
        with positron emission tomography, 1099, 1103–1104, 1104, 1105t, 1132
    in myocardial viability assessment, vs. positron emission tomography, 1008
        metabolic, 1148t, 1148–1153, 1149–1151
        with iodine-123–phenylpentadecanoic acid, 1007
        with technetium, 1004–1007, 1008
        with thallium, 998–1004, 1000, 1001, 1003
    multihead cameras in, 895, 895–896, 896
    multiple-gated, 900, 901
    of cardiac nervous system, 1052, 1054, 1055t
    of myocardial infarction, vs. magnetic resonance imaging, 725
    of myocardial metabolism, 5, 1027
        after infarction, 1028, 1029
        vs. positron emission tomography, 1161
    of myocardial necrosis, 1013
    of myocardial perfusion, in coronary artery disease, 975
        diagnostic accuracy of, 981t, 981–982
        image processing in, 976–979, 977–979, Plate 28
        individual artery assessment in, 985t, 985–986
        vs. positron emission tomography, of myocardial metabolism, 1154–1156, 1155, 1159
        with thallium contrast, 907–911, 908–910, Plate 23
    of myocardial wall thickening, 912
    of thrombosis, with indium-111–labeled platelets, 1036, 1036
    resolution in, 895, 895
Single-photon emitting tracers. See also specific agents, e.g., Thallium-201.
    in imaging, of cellular injury, 966, 966–967
    of myocardial metabolism, 1020–1032

Single-photon emitting tracers (Continued)
    after infarction, 1028–1029, 1029
    historical aspects of, 1021
    in cardiomyopathy, 1026t, 1031–1032, Plate 30
    in coronary artery disease, 1026t, 1029–1031, 1030, 1031
    technical aspects of, 1027, Plate 29
    tissue kinetics in, 1021–1027, 1022–1025, 1023t, 1026t
    of myocardial perfusion, 963–968, 964t, 965, 967, 968
Single-photon imaging, multiwire gamma camera in, 891
Situs ambiguus, atrial, echocardiography of, 442, 445, 446
    magnetic resonance imaging of, 676
Situs inversus, atrial, echocardiography of, 442, 445, 445
    magnetic resonance imaging of, 676, 677, 678
    with dextrocardia, radiography of, 143, 143
Slice, in imaging, definition of, 1216
Slice selection, in magnetic resonance imaging, 639–640, 640
    quantitative, 762
Slice thickness, definition of, 1216
Small intestine, radiation dose to, in radionuclide imaging, 1207t
Smoking, and carbon-11 ketanserin concentration, in positron emission tomography, 1189
    and myocardial ischemia, positron emission tomography of, 1106, 1106–1107
Sodium, in myocardial contraction, 22, 23
Sodium iodide, in positron emission tomography, 901
Sodium iodide thallium detector, in radionuclide imaging, 888, 888–889
Solid state memory, in digital image storage, 117
Sones technique, in coronary angiography, 227, 228
Sorenson's method, of attenuation correction, in single-photon emission computed tomography, 898
Spatial filtering, in digital image enhancement, 67, 68, 118–119, 119
Spatial resolution, definition of, 1216
Spatially localized spectroscopy, definition of, 1216
Specific absorption rate, definition of, 1216
Speckle, in ultrasonography, in tissue characterization, 608
Spectral editing, definition of, 1216
Spectral line, definition of, 1216
Spectrometer, definition of, 1216
Spectroscopy, in magnetic resonance imaging, 784–790. See also Magnetic resonance spectroscopy.
    spatially localized, definition of, 1216
Spectrum, definition of, 1216
Spin, in magnetic resonance, definition of, 1216
    nuclear, definition of, 1213
Spin density, definition of, 1216
Spin echo, definition of, 1216
    partial saturation, definition of, 1214
Spin quantum number, definition of, 1217
Spin tagging, definition of, 1217
Spin-echo imaging, definition of, 1216–1217
Spin-lattice relaxation, 631–633, 632, 633, 1217
Spin-spin coupling, definition of, 1217
Spin-spin relaxation, 633, 633, 1217
Spin-warp imaging, definition of, 1217
Spinal cord, myelography of, endocarditis after, magnetic resonance imaging of, 755, 756
Spine, disorders of, in chest radiography, 126, 127

Spine (Continued)
    radiography of, radiation dose in, 1206t
Spiral computed tomography, equipment for, 799–800
Spleen, anomalies of, atrial situs inversus with, echocardiography of, 445, 446
    magnetic resonance imaging of, 676
    radiation dose to, in radionuclide imaging, 1207t
    with indium-111 platelet imaging, of thrombosis, 1035, 1036
Split-and-merge techniques, in segmentation, in digital imaging, 69
Spoiler gradient pulse, definition of, 1217
ST segment, in electrocardiography, in myocardial ischemia, vs. positron emission tomography, of metabolism, 1145–1146
Starvation, and myocardial protein metabolism, 47
Steady-state free precession, definition of, 1217
Stenting, after balloon angioplasty, ultrasonography of, 600, 601, 602
    arterial, ultrasonography of, in surgical guidance, 594–597, 594–598
        vascular remodeling in, 592, 593
    intracoronary, magnetic resonance angiography in, 734–736, 739
Stethoscope, nuclear, in radiation detection, 891–892
Stewart-Hamilton technique, in indicator-dilution imaging, 836, 838–839
Stimulated echo, definition of, 1217
Strain, in ventricular mechanics, 24
Streptokinase, in thrombolysis, for myocardial infarction, positron emission tomography after, 1124, 1125, 1126
Stress, in ventricular mechanics, 24
    mental, and myocardial ischemia, positron emission tomography of, 1106, 1106
Stress testing, in echocardiography, 503–520
    drug-induced ischemia in, 505, 505–506, 506
    exercise in, 504t, 504–505
    image interpretation in, 507–510, 508–510, 509t
    imaging techniques in, 506–507
    in myocardial viability assessment, vs. radionuclide imaging, 1008
    of coronary arteries, 530
        stenotic, 511t, 511–514, 512–514
        after revascularization, 517–518
        atrial pacing in, 516
        vasodilators in, 515–517, 516, 517t
        vs. radionuclide imaging, 514–515, 515, 515t
    of left ventricular function, regional, 309
    of myocardial viability, 518
    principles of, 504
    prognostic value of, 518–520, 519t
    transesophageal, 506–507
        of left ventricle, 548
    in magnetic resonance imaging, of left ventricle, 726–731, 727–731
    in positron emission tomography, of myocardial blood flow, 1094t, 1094–1096, 1095, 1095t, 1096
        electrocardiography with, 1098
        selection of agents for, 1096–1097, 1097t
    in radionuclide angiography, equilibrium, 942–943
        first-pass, 926–927, 927
    in radionuclide imaging, of myocardial perfusion, in coronary artery disease, 973–975, 974
    in single-photon emission computed tomography, of myocardial perfusion, in coronary artery disease, 981–982

Stress testing (*Continued*)
    in thallium-201 scintigraphy, in myocardial
        viability assessment, vs. positron emis-
        sion tomography, 1147–1152, 1148t,
        1149–1151
    in ultrafast computed tomography, 833–834
Stroke, carotid artery stenosis and, risk
        assessment for, indium-111–labeled
        platelet imaging in, 1039t, 1039–1041,
        1040t
Stroke volume, in mitral stenosis, in valve
        area estimation, 379
    measurement of, by contrast ventriculogra-
        phy, 169, *170*, 175
        Doppler echocardiography in, 325, 327,
            327–328, 330
            in mitral regurgitation, 325, 327, 330–
                331
        in congenital heart disease, magnetic res-
            onance imaging in, 681, *681*
        in mitral regurgitation, echocardiography
            in, 382
        magnetic resonance imaging in, 769, *771*
        ultrafast computed tomography in, 823,
            824
Structured noise, in x-ray image formation,
        110
Stunning, after myocardial ischemia,
        echocardiography of, 307, 310
    magnetic resonance imaging of, 668,
        Plate 23
    radionuclide imaging of, 996–997
Subaortic cone, in ventriculography, 52, *52*
Subclavian artery, aberrant, right, ultrafast
        computed tomography of, 862, *862*
    with aortic arch anomalies, magnetic reso-
        nance imaging of, 696, 696–697, *698*
    in aortic dissection, computed tomography
        of, 857, *857*
    magnetic resonance imaging of, 699, *700*
Subclavian vein, angioplasty of, stenting after,
        ultrasonic guidance of, 595, *597*
Succinyl CoA, in myocardial metabolism, 41,
        42, *42*
Sulfinpyrazone, for thrombosis, left
        ventricular, 1039
    preventive use of, with prosthetic materi-
        als, 1046
Suloctidil, for thrombosis, preventive use of,
        with prosthetic materials, 1046
Superconducting magnets, for magnetic
        resonance imaging, 643–645, *646*
Superconductor, definition of, 1217
Superparamagnetic compounds, as contrast
        agents, in magnetic resonance imaging,
        653, 653–655
Suppression, definition of, 1217
Surface coils, definition of, 1217
    in magnetic resonance imaging, 651
Susceptibility, magnetic, definition of, 1213
Sutures, in heart transplantation,
        echocardiography of, vs. mass lesions,
        457, *458*
Sympathetic nervous system. See *Nervous
        system.*
Syndrome X, myocardial blood flow in,
        positron emission tomography of, 1095t,
        1108–1109
Systemic lupus erythematosus, and mitral
        regurgitation, 553, *553*
Systole, atrial, valvar function in, 54, *55*
    mitral valve in, 51, *52*, *53*
    ventricular function in. See also *Left ventri-
        cle, function of.*
        imaging of, 2–3
        right, echocardiography of, 317–320, *318*,
            319

T1 relaxation, in magnetic resonance imaging,
        631–633, *632*, *633*, 1217

T1 relaxation (*Continued*)
    of heart, 637, *637*, 637t
$T1_\rho$ relaxation, in magnetic resonance
        imaging, 632–633
T2 relaxation, in magnetic resonance imaging,
        633, *633*, 1217
    of heart, 637, 637t
T2' relaxation, in magnetic resonance
        imaging, 633, 1217
Tachycardia, effect of, on Doppler
        echocardiography, of left ventricular
        function, 350
    pacing-induced, and coronary vasodilation,
        11, *12*
    ventricular, nervous system in, radionuclide
        imaging of, 1058
Tagging, myocardial, in magnetic resonance
        imaging, 668, *668*, Plate 22
    quantitative, automated analysis with,
        779, 780
        of left ventricular function, 771–774,
            772, *773*
Takayasu arteritis, magnetic resonance
        imaging of, 708, *709*
    pulmonary artery in, angiography of, 215,
        217
Tamponade, cardiac, echocardiography of,
        354, *354*, 409–413, *410–413*
    pericardial, imaging of, 94
Tantalum-178m, in radionuclide angiography,
        924
Teboroxime, technetium-99m, in myocardial
        perfusion imaging, 963–968, 964t,
        965, *966*
    in coronary artery disease, 973, 982–
        983
Technetium. See also *Radionuclide imaging.*
Technetium-94m, in positron emission
        tomography, of myocardial blood flow,
        1066, 1067–1068
Technetium-99m, energy spectrum of, in
        radionuclide imaging, 889
    in antimyosin antibody imaging, of myocar-
        dial necrosis, 1014
    in imaging, of coronary artery disease,
        81–83
        of myocardial perfusion, 963–968, 964t,
            965, *966*
    in radionuclide angiography, equilibrium, in
        red blood cell labeling, 942
        first-pass, 924
Technetium-99m furifosmin, in myocardial
        perfusion imaging, 963, 964t, 966–968
    in coronary artery disease, 991
Technetium-99m hexamethyl-
        propyleneamineoxime, in platelet
        labeling, in imaging of thrombosis, 1035
Technetium-99m pyrophosphate, in imaging
        of myocardial necrosis, 1012–1013,
        1013
    accuracy of, 1015
    in infarct sizing, 1017–1019, *1019*
        right ventricular, 1017
    vs. antimyosin antibodies, 1014
Technetium-99m Q3, in myocardial perfusion
        imaging, 963
    in coronary artery disease, 991
Technetium-99m sestamibi, in imaging, and
        radiation dose, 1207t
    in myocardial viability assessment, 1004–
        1007, *1005*, *1006*, *1008*, Plate 29
    of myocardial perfusion, 4, 963–967,
        964t, *966*
        in coronary artery disease, diagnostic
            accuracy of, 982, *982*
        image processing with, 976–979, *979*
        kinetics of, 973
        in ischemia, vs. positron emission to-
            mography, of myocardial metabo-
            lism, 1154–1155, *1155*
        tomographic, 911–912, *912*

Technetium-99m sestamibi (*Continued*)
    of myocardial tissue characteristics, 5
    in single-photon emission computed tomog-
        raphy, of coronary artery disease, with
        positron emission tomography, 1132
    vs. thallium-201, 900, *900*, 900t
Technetium-99m teboroxime, in myocardial
        perfusion imaging, 963–967, 964t, *965*,
        966
    in coronary artery disease, 973, 982–983
Technetium-99m tetrofosmin, in myocardial
        perfusion imaging, 963–968, 964t, *965*
    in coronary artery disease, 990–991
Teflon (polytetrafluoroethylene), in prosthetic
        grafts, and thrombosis, indium-111
        platelet imaging of, 1045, 1046
Teichholz model, in left ventricular volume
        measurement, by magnetic resonance
        imaging, 766, 768
Teratoma, of pericardium, ultrafast computed
        tomography of, 870
Tesla, definition of, 1217
Testes, radiation dose to, in diagnostic
        radiology, 1206t, 1207t
Tethering, of nonischemic myocardium, 310
Tetralogy of Fallot, echocardiography of, 437,
        437
    imaging of, 92
    repair of, magnetic resonance imaging
        after, *684*, 685, *686*, 687
        pulmonic insufficiency after, transesopha-
            geal echocardiography after, 555
    right ventricular enlargement in, radiogra-
        phy of, 131, *133*
Tetrofosmin, technetium-99m, in myocardial
        perfusion imaging, 963–968, 964t,
        965
    in coronary artery disease, 990–991
Thalassemia, and cardiomyopathy, ultrasonic
        tissue characterization in, 620
Thallium-201. See also *Radionuclide imaging.*
    in imaging, and radiation dose, 1207t
        of coronary artery disease, 81–83
            vs. digital angiography, 264, *266*, *267*
            vs. stress echocardiography, 514, 515t
        of myocardium, in nongated acquisition,
            892
    in viability assessment, 79, 997–1004,
        998t, *998–1001*, *1003*, *1004*
        vs. positron emission tomography, of
            metabolism, 1147–1153, 1148t,
            1149–1151
    tissue characteristics in, 5
    in myocardial perfusion imaging, 4, 963–
        968, 964t, *965–968*
        after infarction, with antimyosin antibody
            imaging, of necrosis, *1016*, 1016–
            1017, *1017*
        in cardiomyopathy, dilated, vs. positron
            emission tomography, 1174–1176
        in coronary artery disease, before noncar-
            diac surgery, 990, 990t
            diagnostic accuracy of, 979t–981t,
                979–982
            image processing with, 975–976, *977*,
                978, Plate 28
            in asymptomatic patients, 983–984,
                984, 984–985
            individual artery assessment in, 985t,
                985–986
            kinetics of, 972–973
            risk assessment in, 986t, 986–988
                after infarction, 988–989, 989t
        in ischemia, vs. positron emission tomog-
            raphy, of myocardial metabolism,
            1154, 1156
        in planar methods, 904–907, *905–907*
        in tomography, 907–911, *908–910*, Plate
            23
        vs. magnetic resonance imaging, contrast,
            663, *663*, *664*

Thallium-201 (Continued)
in single-photon emission computed tomography, vs. technetium-99m, 900, *900*, 900t
radiation from, detection of, instruments for, 888, 888–889
Thebesian veins, in cardioplegia, in coronary bypass surgery, contrast echocardiography of, 497, *497*
Thermal equilibrium, definition of, 1217
Thermal injury, in ultrasonography, 289–290
Three-dimensional reconstruction, in digital cardiac imaging, *59*, 59t, 59–60
future of, 70
in ultrafast computed tomography, of congenital heart disease, 879, 885
in ultrasonography, intravascular, 598–603, *599–602*
Thrombolysis, coronary angiography after, 222
for myocardial infarction, assessment of, echocardiography in, 530
contrast, 487, *487*, 488
positron emission tomography in, 1124–1129, *1125, 1126, 1129*
radionuclide angiography in, 955
ventriculography in, 188–192, *193*
for pulmonary embolism, assessment of, angiography in, 211–214, *215*
Thrombosis. See also *Embolism.*
and prosthetic valve dysfunction, transesophageal echocardiography of, 556
echocardiography of, left atrial, *465*, 465–466, *466*
with mitral stenosis, 377–378
left ventricular, 466–468, *467, 468*
after myocardial infarction, 528–530, *529*
pulmonary arterial, *464*, 465
right atrial, *463*, 463
right ventricular, *464*, 465
in aortic dissection, magnetic resonance imaging of, 700–705, *701–704*
indium-111 platelet imaging of, 1034–1047
in arteries, 1039t, 1039–1043, 1040t, *1041, 1042*
coronary, 1037, 1037t
in left atrium, 1039
in left ventricle, 1037t, 1037–1039, *1038, 1039*
in veins, 1043
technical aspects of, 1034–1037, *1036*
valvular, 1037, 1037t
with prosthetic materials, 1043t, 1043–1046, *1044–1046*
intracardiac, calcification of, radiography of, *142*, 142–143
ultrafast computed tomography of, 865–867, *866, 867*
ultrasonic tissue characterization in, 622
intracavitary, in cardiomyopathy, dilated, echocardiography of, 402, *402*
of atrial appendage, echocardiography of, transesophageal, 551, 552, 557–558
radionuclide imaging of, experimental agents in, *1046*, 1046–1047, Plate 30
with aortic aneurysm, ultrafast computed tomography of, 855, *856*
Thromboxane A$_2$, in coronary blood flow, 11
Thyroid, disorders of, and pericardial effusion, magnetic resonance imaging of, 753–754, *754*
ectopic tissue of, in heart, magnetic resonance imaging of, 755
hyperfunction of, maternal, and cardiomyopathy, hypertrophic, 1179
radiation dose to, and cancer risk, 122t, 123
in radionuclide imaging, 1207t
Ticlopidine, for thrombosis, indium-111 platelet imaging after, 1039, 1046
Tidal wave, in valvar function, 55

Time-density analysis, 122
Time-gain compensation, in echocardiography, 284–285, *286*
Time-of-flight technique, definition of, 1217
in magnetic resonance imaging, of blood flow, in coronary arteries, 737, 777
quantitative, 774, *775*
Tissue plasminogen activator, for pulmonary embolism, angiography after, 213–214
in thrombolysis, for myocardial infection, positron emission tomography after, 1124–1125
radiolabeled, in imaging of thrombosis, 1047
Tobacco smoking, and carbon-11 ketanserin concentration, in positron emission tomography, 1189
and myocardial ischemia, positron emission tomography of, *1106*, 1106–1107
Tomography. See specific types, e.g., *Positron emission tomography.*
Total anomalous pulmonary venous return, echocardiography of, 440–441, *441, 442*, Plate 7
t-PA, for pulmonary embolism, angiography after, 213–214
in thrombolysis, for myocardial infarction, positron emission tomography after, 1124–1125
radiolabeled, in imaging of thrombosis, 1047
Transducers, in Doppler ultrasound, 296, *296*
in echocardiography, 278–280, *279, 280*
linear array, 282, *282–283, 283*
phased array, 283–284, *284, 285*
Transesophageal echocardiography, 533–562
anesthesia for, 537
contraindications to, 535–536, 536t
development of, 533–534, 534t
equipment for, *536*, 536–537
future developments in, 561–562, Plate 15
hemodynamic measurements with, 559–560, Plate 14
in cardiac output assessment, 559
in diastolic function assessment, 346
in pericarditis, constrictive, 351, 353
in stress testing, 506–507, 548
indications for, 534, 534t, 535t
intraoperative, 567–568, *568*
in congenital defect repair, 574–575, *575*
longitudinal views in, 543–544, *543–545*
multiplane views in, 544, *545*
of aortic atherosclerosis, 558
of aortic dissection, 560–561, Plate 14
of aortic insufficiency, 550–551, Plate 11
of aortic regurgitation, 372
of aortic stenosis, 550, *551*
of atrial septal aneurysm, 459, *459*
of atrial septal defect, 561, Plate 15
of cardiomyopathy, hypertrophic, 397
of congenital heart disease, 449–450, 561, 562t, Plates 8 and 15
of coronary arteries, intraoperative, 530
stenotic, 558, Plate 13
of endocarditis, 548t, 548–550, *549*, Plate 11
of epicardial fat, 459, *460*
of esophageal carcinoma, 457, *458*
of fibroelastoma, papillary, 473, *474*
of intracardiac devices, 461, *462*
of ischemic heart disease, 547–548
of left atrial membrane, congenital, 459, *461*
of left ventricle, in functional evaluation, diastolic, 545, 546–547, *547*
systolic, *545*, 545–546
stress testing in, 548
of lymphoma, *470*
of mitral regurgitation, 381, 552–554, *552–555*, Plates 11 and 12
of mitral stenosis, 551–552, *552*

Transesophageal echocardiography (Continued)
of myxoma, 471
of papillary muscle disruption, after infarction, 526
of prosthetic valves, 555–556, Plates 12 and 13
of pseudomasses, cardiac, 453–457, *454–457*
of pulmonary arteries, 538, *538, 539, 543, 543, 556*
of pulmonary valve disorders, 555
of thrombi, in left atrium, 465, *466, 466*
in right atrium, 463, *463*
in right ventricle, *464*, 465
of trauma, cardiovascular, 561
of tricuspid valve disorders, 555
of tumors, cardiac, 556–557, *557*
of ventricular septal defect, 560, Plate 14
personnel in, 534–535, 535t
safety of, 536
technique of, 537
transverse views in, 537–542, *538–543*, Plate 10
Transfer function analysis, in digital angiography, of coronary circulation, 261, *261*
Transit time analysis, in digital angiography, of coronary circulation, 257–258, *258*
Transplantation, of heart, assessment for, positron emission tomography in, of myocardial metabolism, 1166
donor evaluation for, coronary angiography in, 222
echocardiography of, intraoperative, 576
evaluation after, coronary angiography in, 222, *223*
Doppler echocardiography in, 357
magnetic resonance imaging in, 751
spectroscopic, 789–790
positron emission tomography in, of myocardial blood flow, 1095t, 1109–1110
radionuclide imaging in, of nervous system, 1058–1059
rejection of, magnetic resonance imaging of, 751
ultrasonic tissue characterization in, 623
sutures in, echocardiography of, vs. mass lesions, 457, *458*
of liver, pulmonary assessment before, contrast echocardiography in, 499
Transposition of great arteries, echocardiography of, *439*, 439–440, *440, 442, 445–448, 447*
magnetic resonance imaging of, 678, *679*
after surgery, 689, *689–690, 690*
ultrafast computed tomography of, 876–877, *877–882*
Transverse magnetization, definition of, 1218
Transverse (spin-spin) relaxation, in magnetic resonance imaging, 633, *633*, 1217
Trauma, cardiovascular, imaging of, 95–98
transesophageal echocardiography of, 561
to aorta, angiography of, 204–207, *206*
magnetic resonance imaging of, 708, *708*
to heart, surgery for, echocardiography in, 576
to pericardium, echocardiography of, 416–417
Treadmill, in stress induction. See *Exercise.*
Tricarboxylic acid cycle, in myocardial metabolism, 34, *35*, 41–43
in positron emission tomography, with carbon-11 acetate, 1074
Tricuspid regurgitation, echocardiography of, 384–387, *385, 386*, Plate 5
Doppler, 331–332
color flow mapping in, Plate 1
contrast technique with, 499–500, *500*

Tricuspid regurgitation (*Continued*)
  intraoperative, 570–571, *571*, 573, Plate
    16
  imaging of, 86
  magnetic resonance imaging of, 712, *712*
  right atrial enlargement with, radiography
    of, 131, *131*
  with ventricular arrthythmia, 56–57
Tricuspid stenosis, echocardiography of,
    383–384, *384*, *385*
  imaging of, 86
  magnetic resonance imaging of, 712
Tricuspid valve, abnormalities of, with
    transposition of great arteries,
    echocardiography of, 447
  atresia of, echocardiography of, 437, *438*
  magnetic resonance imaging of, 712
  blood flow through, in cardiac tamponade,
    echocardiography of, 411, *412*
  magnetic resonance imaging of, after
    Mustard operation, 689–690, *690*
  after Senning operation, 689–690, *690*
  measurement of, in congenital heart dis-
    ease, magnetic resonance imaging
    in, 682, *683*
  Ebstein anomaly of, echocardiography of,
    437–438, *438*
  after surgical repair, vs. mass lesion,
    462, *463*
  magnetic resonance imaging of, 712
  echocardiography of, transesophageal, 540,
    541, 555
  in identification of cardiac chambers, in
    echocardiography, of congenital heart
    disease, 443, *443*
  myxoma of, computed tomography of, ul-
    trafast, 865, *865*
  surgery of, hematoma after, magnetic reso-
    nance imaging of, 755, *756*
Triggering, definition of, 1218
Triphenyltetrazolium chloride, in
    echocardiography, after myocardial
    infarction, 488, Plate 9
Tritium, in positron emission tomography, of
    cardiac receptors, 1188–1193
  of presynaptic neurotransmission, 1195
Triton-X, and cell injury, imaging of, single-
    photon emitting tracers for, 966
Truncus arteriosus, embryology of, 692–693
  persistent, echocardiography of, 440, *440*,
    441
Tuberous sclerosis, rhabdomyoma with,
    cardiac, echocardiography of, 471, *473*
Tumor(s), drugs for, and cardiotoxicity,
    radionuclide imaging of,
    angiographic, 958
  nervous system in, 1059
  echocardiography of, 452–476
    vs. normal structural variants, 453–456,
      453–457
  of heart, computed tomography of, *864*,
    864–865, *865*
    ultrafast, contrast agents in, 864
      imaging sequences in, 863–864
      radiation dose in, 864
    magnetic resonance imaging of, 754–757,
      754–757
  metastatic, echocardiography of, 468, *469*
  primary, benign, echocardiography of,
    469–475, 471t, *471–475*
    classification of, 468–469, 471t
    malignant, echocardiography of, 475,
      475–476, *476*
  transesophageal echocardiography of,
    556–557, *557*
  ultrasonic tissue characterization in, 622
  of lung, echocardiography of, 468, *470*
  of pericardium, echocardiography of, 408,
    409, 416, 468, *469*
    metastatic, 468, *469*
    ultrafast computed tomography of, 869,
      870, 871

Tumor(s) (*Continued*)
  of pulmonary arteries, angiography of, 216,
    218
Tuning, definition of, 1218
TurboFLASH technique, in magnetic
    resonance imaging, of myocardial
    ischemia, induced, 728–729, *729*, *730*

Ultrafast computed tomography, 793–886
  acquisition sequences in, 802–803, *803*
  advantages of, 827
  cost of, *826*, 827
  data handling in, 801–802
  disadvantages of, *826*, 827
  equipment for, 800–802, *801*
    evolution of, 811
    Mayo dynamic spatial reconstructor in,
      811–814, *811–815*
      ANALYZE software for, 812, 816,
        816–818
    technical strengths of, 810
    technical weaknesses of, 810–811
  geometrical accuracy of, 808–810, *810*
  image analysis in, 76, 814–816, *816–818*
  image display in, 802, 812, 814–816, *816–
    818*
  image processing in, 802, 812
  image reconstruction in, 802, 812
  multislice mode in, 802
  need for, in cardiac imaging, 800
  noise in, 808, *808*, 809t
  number linearity in, 808, 810t
  of aortic aneurysms, 855, 855–856, *856*
  of aortic dissection, 856–858, *856–859*
  of cardiac masses, contrast agents in, 864
    imaging sequences in, 863–864
    radiation dose in, 864
  of cardiac tumors, *864*, 864–865, *865*
  of cardiovascular structure, technical as-
    pects of, 820t, 820–823, *821*, *822*
  of congenital heart disease, 871–886
    atria in, 876, *877*
    blood flow analysis in, 872–875, *873*,
      875, *876*
    future of, 879–886
    imaging protocols in, 872, 872t
    pulmonary vessels in, 877, 877–879, *882–
      885*
    three-dimensional reconstruction in, 879,
      885
    transposition of great arteries in, 876–
      877, *877–882*
    vena cava in, 876, *877*
    ventricles in, 877, *877*
      function assessment of, 875
  of coronary artery disease, 826, 829–834,
    830–832
  of great vessels, 852–862
    advantages of, 858–859
    contrast agents in, 854–855
    disadvantages of, 859
    equipment for, 853, 853–854, *854*
    radiation dose in, 855
  of left ventricular function, 822, 823–825,
    825
  of left ventricular mass, 822, 823, *823*
  of myocardial perfusion, 835–850
    artifacts in, 845–847, *846*
    contrast agents in, intra-arterial, 843–
      845, *844*, 850
      intravenous, 840–843, *840–843*, 849–
        850
      kinetics of, 848–849, *849*
    flow algorithms in, 838–840, *839*
    indicator-dilution methods in, historical
      aspects of, 836–837
    recommended methods for, 849–850
    regional transfer function in, 850
    regional vascular volume in, 847–848,
      848, *849*

Ultrafast computed tomography (*Continued*)
  of pericarditis, constrictive, 825, *826*
  of pericardium, 867–870, *868–870*
    contrast agents in, 864
    imaging sequences in, 863–864
    radiation dose in, 864, 868
  of pulmonary arteries, 813, *815*, 859–861,
    860
  of subclavian artery, right, aberrant, 862,
    862
  of thoracic disorders, noncardiac, 826–827
  of thrombi, intracardiac, 865–867, *866*, *867*
  of valvular regurgitation, 825–826, *826*, *827*
  of vena caval lesions, *861*, 861–862
  performance characteristics in, 803
  radiation dose in, 803–805, *804*, *805*, 805t
  resolution in, 805–808, *806–808*, 807t
  single-slice mode in, 802
  uniformity in, 808, *809*, 809t
  x-ray detection in, 801
  x-ray production in, 801
Ultrafast magnetic resonance imaging, of
    myocardial ischemia, induced, 728–731,
    729–731
Ultrasonography, Doppler, 291–296. See also
    Doppler ultrasound.
  heat in, biologic effects of, 289–290
  in tissue characterization, 606–624
    goals of, 606–607
    methods of, 608–611, *608–611*
    myocardial acoustic properties in, 611–
      614, *612*, *613*
    of atherosclerosis, 622, *622*
    of myocardium, after reperfusion, 615–
      616, *616*, *617*
      in aging, 623
      in arterial hypertension, 621–622
      in cardiomyopathy, 618–621, *619*, *620*
      in congenital heart disease, cyanotic,
        623
      in contusion, 622
      in diabetes mellitus, 623
      in infarction, acute, 614
        subacute, 616–618, *618*, *619*
      in ischemia, 606–607
        acute, *614*, 614–615, *615*
      in myxoma, 622
      in transplant rejection, 623
      inflamed, 618
      with thrombosis, intracardiac, 622
    of valvular vegetations, in endocarditis,
      622
    terminology of, 607–608
  intravascular, 581–603
    in guidance of surgical interventions,
      592–597, *594–598*
      combined instrumentation for, 597–
        598
    in vessel measurement, 583–586, *584–
      586*
    limitations of, *604*, 605, *605*
    of angioplasty, 586–591, *586–591*, 591t,
      Plate 21
    of arteriosclerosis, angiographically unde-
      tected, 582
      in tissue-plaque characterization, 582–
        583, *583*, Plate 20
    of vascular remodeling, 591–592, *592*,
      593
    three-dimensional image reconstruction
      in, 598–603, *599–602*
    validation of, in vitro, 581–582, *582*
  mechanical waves in, 275
  of heart, 273–291. See also *Echocardiogra-
    phy.*
  piezoelectricity in, 275, *275*, 275t
  sound wave transmission in, 275–277, 276t,
    277
Undersampling, in digital imaging, 62, *62*
Uniformity correction, in single-photon
    emission computed tomography, 899

Univentricular heart, echocardiography of, *448*, 448–449
  magnetic resonance imaging of, 676–677, *679*
Urinary bladder, radiation dose to, in radionuclide imaging, 1207t
Urography, intravenous, radiation dose in, 1206t
Urokinase, for pulmonary embolism, assessment of, angiography in, 211–214
Urokon, as contrast agent, *146*, 147
Uroselectan, as contrast agent, 145, *146*, 147

v wave, atrial, 54–56, *56*
Valve(s). See also specific valves, e.g., *Aortic valve*.
  disease of, congenital, imaging of, 91
    echocardiography of, 365–389
    magnetic resonance imaging of, 708–710, *711*
    surgery for, coronary angiography before, 222
  dysfunction of, venous surrogate valvar function in, 57
    without structural change, *56*, 56–57
  function of, imaging of, 3–4
    normal, 53–56, *55*, *56*
  infection of. See *Endocarditis*.
  insufficiency of, radionuclide angiography of, *933*, 935
  of left heart, anatomy of, 50–53, *51–54*
  prosthetic, and distortion, in magnetic resonance imaging, quantitative, 764, *764*
    evaluation of, echocardiography in, 387–389, *388*
      transesophageal, 555–556, Plates 12 and 13
    imaging in, 86
    regurgitation through, contrast ventriculography of, 175, *176*
    echocardiography of, intraoperative, 570
    magnetic resonance imaging of, 774–777, *777*
    radionuclide angiography of, 946
    replacement of, hematoma after, magnetic resonance imaging of, 755, *756*
  stenosis of, blood flow measurement in, magnetic resonance imaging in, 777
    echocardiography of, intraoperative, 569, *569*
  surgery of, echocardiography in, 570–573, *571*, *572*, 572t, Plates 16 and 17
  thrombosis of, indium-111 platelet imaging of, 1037, 1037t
  trauma to, imaging of, 97
  ultrasonic tissue characterization of, 622–623
Valvuloplasty, evaluation of, Doppler echocardiography in, 389
  for congenital heart disease, 90–92
  for mitral disease, and aortic regurgitation, echocardiography of, *379*, *379*
    rheumatic, 572
Valvulotomy, balloon, for mitral rheumatic disease, 572
Varices, pulmonary, angiography of, 215
Vascoray, as contrast agent, *146*, 147, 149, 149t
Vascular ring, in aortic arch anomalies, magnetic resonance imaging of, 697, *698*
Vasoconstriction, and coronary blood flow, 11, *12*
  with pulmonary embolism, and timing of angiography, 211
Vasodilation, and coronary blood flow, 11, *12*
  contrast agents and, 151, *151*
Vasodilators, and left ventricular function changes, Doppler echocardiography of, 329

Vasodilators (*Continued*)
  in stress echocardiography, 505, 506
    of coronary artery disease, 515–517, *516*, 517t
Vector, definition of, 1218
Vena cava, blood flow in, measurement of, Doppler echocardiography in, 347, 348t
  catheterization through, in pulmonary angiography, 209
  congenital abnormalities of, ultrafast computed tomography of, 876, *877*
  echocardiography of, in congenital heart disease, 443, *443*
    transesophageal, 538, *538*, 543, *543*
  filters in, for pulmonary embolism, 214, *216*
  inferior, in cardiac tamponade, echocardiography of, 411
    lymphoma extension through, ultrafast computed tomography of, 865, *865*
    junction of, with right atrium, echocardiography of, vs. mass lesion, *456*, 457
    pulmonary vein drainage to, angiography of, 217
  superior, disorders of, ultrafast computed tomography in, *861*, 861–862
    engorgement of, in pericarditis, magnetic resonance imaging of, 752, *753*
    enlargement of, radiography of, 128
    left, persistent, echocardiography of, vs. mass lesions, 454, *455*
Ventilation-perfusion imaging, of pulmonary embolism, 100, 210–211
  vs. ultrafast computed tomography, 859, 861
Ventricle(s), filling pressure of, changes in, contrast agents and, 151–152, *152*
  function of, 19–32
    cardiac hypertrophy and, 31
    coronary blood flow and, 30–31
    determinants of, in diastole, 25t, 25–29, *26*, *28*
      in systole, 29, 29–30
    mechanics of, 24, 24–25, *25*
    myocardial energetics in, 31–32, *32*
    myocardium in, 20–24, *21*, *22*
  inversion of, after correction of great artery transposition, ultrafast computed tomography of, 877, *882*
  left. See *Left ventricle*.
  muscle fibers in, acoustic properties of, in ultrasonic tissue characterization, 612–613
  myopathy of. See *Cardiomyopathy*.
  premature contraction of, in radionuclide angiography, equilibrium, 943
    first-pass, 927–928, *928*
  right. See *Right ventricle*.
  single, echocardiography of, *448*, 448–449
    magnetic resonance imaging of, 676–677, *679*
  thallium-201 scintigraphy of, in testing of viability, 79
Ventricular arrhythmia, and valvar dysfunction, 57
  intractable, coronary angiography in, 222
Ventricular fibrillation, contrast agents and, 155–156, *156*
Ventricular septal defects, echocardiography of, 420–423, *421*, *422*, Plate 6
  in blood flow measurement, 431
  intraoperative, Plate 18
  transesophageal, 560, Plate 14
  with pulmonary stenosis, 435, *436*
  imaging of, 91
  magnetic resonance imaging of, 678–679
  ultrafast computed tomography of, 877, *877*
  with transposition of great arteries, echocardiography of, 447, *447*
Ventricular septum, rupture of, myocardial infarction and, 526, *526*, Plate 10

Ventricular tachycardia, nervous system in, radionuclide imaging of, 1058
Ventriculography, contrast, 164–187
  applications of, 187–198
  in coronary artery disease, 188–192, *189–191*, *193*
  in functional assessment, vs. digital angiography, 252t, 252–253, 253t
  in volume determination, 167–176, *170–178*, *193*, 193–194
    vs. magnetic resonance imaging, 766, *767*
  in wall motion assessment, regional, 194–198, *195–197*
  of right ventricle, 192
  qualitative assessment of, 165–167, *165–169*
  technique of, 164–165
  of myocardial infarction, vs. magnetic resonance imaging, 725, *725*
  radionuclide, in anatomic imaging, 1
    in myocardial quantitative studies, 913–919, *915–919*, Plate 24
    of coronary artery disease, vs. digital angiography, 266, *266*, *267*
  subaortic cone in, 52, *52*
Verapamil, and left ventricular function changes, Doppler echocardiography of, 329
  for hypertrophic cardiomyopathy, evaluation of, Doppler echocardiography in, 355–357
Vesamicol, in positron emission tomography, of cholinergic receptors, in presynaptic neurotransmission, 1196
VEST, in left ventricular function monitoring, ambulatory, 943
  in radiation detection, 892
Video camera. See also *Cine acquisition*.
  in cineangiography, 115
  in digital imaging, 60
  in fluoroscopy, *112*, 112–113, *113*
Videodensitometry, in digital angiography, of left ventricle, 253
Viral infection, and pericarditis, magnetic resonance imaging of, 753, *753*
Viscous resistance, basal, to coronary blood flow, 9
Vision, and perception, in image interpretation, 72–74, *73*
Visipaque. See *Iodixanol*.
Volume, and pressure, end-systolic, 29, 29–30
  in diastole, 26–27
  in ventricular energetics, 32, *32*
  in ventricular mechanics, 24, 24–25, *25*
Volume imaging, definition of, 1218
Volume overload, and left ventricular hypertrophy, 31
Volume-selective excitation, definition of, 1218
Vomiting, contrast agents and, 159
Voxels, definition of, 1218
  in digital imaging, 60
  in intravascular ultrasonography, in three-dimensional reconstruction, 599
  in magnetic resonance imaging, quantitative, 761–762, *762*

Warfarin, effect of, on left ventricular thrombi, indium-111 platelet imaging of, 1039, *1039*
Washout rate profiles, in myocardial perfusion assessment, by thallium scintigraphy, *906*, 906–907, *907*
Water, in biologic tissue, in magnetic resonance imaging, *634*, 634–635, *635*
  contrast agents in, 655
  in myocardial tissue, in ultrasonic tissue characterization, 613

Water (*Continued*)
  oxygen-15–labeled, in imaging, and radiation dose, 1207t
  in positron emission tomography, of myocardial blood flow, *1066*, 1066–1068, 1083–1086, *1084*, 1094
    after infarction, thrombolysis and, 1124–1127
Wavelengths, in ultrasonography, 275, 275t
  in tissue characterization, 607
Wire-frame displays, in image reconstruction, three-dimensional, *59*, 59–60
Workstations, in magnetic resonance imaging, 647

x descent, in valvar function, 55, 56
Xanthines, effect of, on pharmacologic stress testing, with radionuclide imaging, 974
Xenon-133, in myocardial perfusion imaging, 963
X-rays, collimation of, 105
  detection of, in radionuclide imaging, principles of, *888*, 888–889, *889*
  exposure to, control of, 105
  filtration of, 105, *105*
  image produced by, formation of, 105–110, *106–110*, 107t
  in cineangiography, 113–115

X-rays (*Continued*)
  in fluoroscopy, 111–113, *112*, *113*
  physics of, and use of contrast agents, 144
  production of, 103–104
  properties of, 102–103
  radiographic applications of. See specific techniques, e.g., *Angiography*.

y descent, in valvar function, 54, 55

Zeugmatography, rotating frame, in magnetic resonance spectroscopy, 785–786, *786*

ISBN 0-7216-7127-6